THE EXERCISE PROFESSIONAL'S GUIDE TO PERSONAL TRAINING

A Client-centered Approach to Inspire Active Lifestyles

AMERICAN COUNCIL ON EXERCISE®

EDITORS

SABRENA JO, MS

CEDRIC X. BRYANT, PHD, FACSM

LANCE C. DALLECK, PHD

CHRISTOPHER S. GAGLIARDI, MS

DANIEL J. GREEN

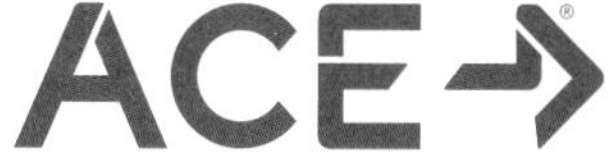

Library of Congress Control Number: 2020901979

ISBN 978-1-890720-76-6

Printed in the United States of America

A B C D

Distributed by:
American Council on Exercise
4851 Paramount Drive
San Diego, CA 92123
(858) 576-6500
(858) 576-6564 FAX
ACEfitness.org

Project Editor: Daniel J. Green
Technical Editors: Cedric X. Bryant, PhD, FACSM, Lance C. Dalleck, PhD, Chris Gagliardi, MS, Todd Galati, MA, Sabrena Jo, MS, and Jessica Matthews, DBH
Art Direction: Karen McGuire and Devon Browning
Creative Design and Cover Design: Rick Gray
Production: Nancy Garcia
Photography: Vertex Photography
Anatomical Illustrations: James Staunton
Stock images: Getty.com, AdobeStock.com
Index: Kathi Unger
Cover and exercise models: Rebekah Abrahim, Suzanne Austin, Courtney Brickner, Devon Browning, Jermaine Castaneda, Jacque Crockford, Chris Gagliardi, Sabrena Jo, Chris Kiepfer, Jeremiah Lafica, Nika Schiazza, Jessica Talbi, Tiffany Tate, Nicole Thompson, and Amanda Wigley
Production Services provided by Westchester Education Services of Dayton, Ohio — A U.S. Employee-owned Company

Acknowledgments:
Thanks to the entire American Council on Exercise staff for their support and guidance through the process of creating this textbook. Thank you to Hoist Fitness for hosting photo shoots for this publication.

NOTICE
The field of health and wellness is ever-changing. As new research and clinical experience broaden our knowledge, changes in programming and standards are required. The authors and the publisher of this work have checked with sources believed to be reliable in their efforts to provide information that is complete and generally in accord with the standards accepted at the time of publication. However, in view of the possibility of human error or changes in industry standards, neither the authors nor the publisher nor any other party who has been involved in the preparation or publication of this work warrants that the information contained herein is in every respect accurate or complete, and they are not responsible for any errors or omissions or the results obtained from the use of such information. Readers are encouraged to confirm the information contained herein with other sources.

ACE's Mission Is to Get People Moving.

P20-001

Table of Contents

Authors

Lance C. Dalleck, PhD, is a professor of Exercise and Sport Science and High Altitude Exercise Physiology at Western Colorado University in Gunnison, Colorado. His primary research interests include prevention of chronic diseases through evidence-based interventions (exercise and nutrition) and quantifying the energy expenditure of outdoor and non-traditional types of physical activity. Dr. Dalleck has published more than 100 peer-reviewed articles, delivered over 50 conference proceedings, and written 10 book chapters. He also serves on the Scientific Advisory Panel for the American Council on Exercise.

Todd Galati, MA, is the Senior Director of Standards and Practice Advancement for the American Council on Exercise. He holds a bachelor's degree in athletic training, a master's degree in kinesiology, and four ACE certifications (Certified Medical Exercise Specialist, Personal Trainer, Health Coach, and Group Fitness Instructor). Prior to joining ACE, Galati was a program director with the University of California, San Diego School of Medicine, where he researched the effectiveness of youth fitness programs in reducing risk for cardiovascular disease, obesity, and type 2 diabetes. Galati's experience includes teaching biomechanics, applied kinesiology, and anatomy classes at California State University, San Marcos and San Diego State University, working as a research physiologist with the U.S. Navy, personal training in medical fitness facilities, and coaching endurance athletes.

Sabrena Jo, MS, is the Director of Science and Research for the American Council on Exercise and ACE Liaison to the Scientific Advisory Panel. Jo has been actively involved in the fitness industry since 1987. As an ACE Certified Group Fitness Instructor, Personal Trainer, and Health Coach, she has taught group exercise and owned her own personal-training and health-coaching businesses and is a relentless pursuer of finding ways to help people start and stick with physical activity. Jo is a former full-time faculty member in the Kinesiology and Physical Education Department at California State University, Long Beach. She has a bachelor's degree in exercise science as well as a master's degree in physical education/biomechanics from the University of Kansas.

Natalie Digate Muth, MD, MPH, RDN, FAAP, FACSM, is a board-certified pediatrician, obesity medicine specialist, and registered dietitian. She directs a healthy weight clinic in Carlsbad, California, and is an Adjunct Assistant Professor at UCLA Fielding School of Public Health. She is a member of the Motivational Interviewing Network of Trainers. Dr. Muth has published over 100 articles, books, and book chapters, including *Coaching Behavior Change* (ACE, 2014), *ACE Fitness Nutrition Manual* (ACE, 2013), *Family Fit Plan: A 30-Day Wellness Transformation* (American Academy of Pediatrics, 2019), *The Picky Eater Project: 6 Weeks to Healthier, Happier Family Mealtimes* (American Academy of Pediatrics, 2016), *"Eat Your Vegetables!" and Other Mistakes Parents Make: Redefining How to Raise Healthy Eaters* (Healthy Learning, 2012), the textbook *Sports Nutrition for Allied Health Professionals* (F.A. Davis, 2014), and several chapters in the *ACE Diabetes Prevention Lifestyle Coaching Handbook* (ACE, 2019). She holds a Bachelor of Science degree in psychology and physiological science from UCLA, and a Master of Public Health and Medical Doctor degree from the University of North Carolina-Chapel Hill.

Mark S. Nagel, EdD, teaches in the Sport and Entertainment Management Department at the University of South Carolina. Dr. Nagel has published extensively in a variety of areas of sport management, including law, finance, and marketing. Prior to becoming a professor, Dr. Nagel worked in campus recreation and intercollegiate athletics.

Lauren Shroyer, MS, ATC, is the Senior Director of Product Development at the American Council on Exercise. Shroyer, who is a NATA-BOC Certified Athletic Trainer, started her career as an ATC at a Division I university for almost four years, where her primary role was the administration of post-injury and post-surgical rehabilitation programs for student-athletes across 20 sports. Since moving to a career in the fitness industry, her specialization has been working with clients, both athletes and non-athletes, who are struggling with chronic injuries and conditions, including professional athletes, Olympic athletes, and retired athletes, as well as weekend warriors and those who have never led an active lifestyle but strive for improved strength and movement capability in the face of chronic conditions. In addition to her practical experience, Shroyer has held several positions in fitness operations, from brick-and-mortar studios to online personal training. Shroyer has a bachelor's degree in psychology from the University of Illinois and a master's degree in athletic training from Illinois State University.

James S. Skinner, PhD, FACSM, specializes in exercise physiology, is a Professor Emeritus in the Department of Kinesiology at Indiana University, and has conducted over 55 years of research on the relationships among exercise, training, genetics, and health. He is the Senior Advisor on Exercise Science for ACE and a member of the ACE Scientific Advisory Panel. A former president of the American College of Sports Medicine (ACSM), he is one of five principal investigators of the HERITAGE Family Study on the role of genetics in the response of cardiovascular disease and diabetes risk factors after training. He has received the ACSM's Honor Award and over $50 million in grants from various resources. In 2011, he received the Doctor Honoris Causa from Semmelweis University in Budapest, Hungary. He has published over 300 articles, six books, and 21 educational DVDs and has lectured in 67 countries in English, French, German, and Spanish.

Foreword

I earned my American Council on Exercise (ACE) Personal Trainer certification in 1995. I remember how excited I was to "officially" be a trainer. Although I didn't know exactly where, who, when, or even how I was going to train, the excitement I had knowing that I could change people's lives for a living genuinely fired me up.

Twenty-five years later, I am extremely grateful for the life that "training" has allowed me to have: thousands of pounds lost by my clients and gym members, self-esteem and confidence boosted, kids and athletes recognizing their potential and attaining their goals, Super Bowls won, World Series won, MVPs earned, relationships saved, quality of lives sky-rocketed from kids to grandmas and grandpas in their 80s, bodies and minds transformed, and, most importantly, millions of lives changed across the globe.

I call that IMPACT. And that has driven me for the past 20+ years of my fitness career. I started my business, Fitness Quest 10, in 2000 to change lives. It was a small 2,000-square-foot training studio that combined one-on-one training with Pilates, yoga, and massage therapy. I was a one-man show with no clients, no money, and no business plan. Heck, looking back, I really didn't know exactly what I wanted to do "when I grew up." But I had a lot of passion to help people improve their lives.

Today, things are quite a bit different than yesteryear. I lead a team of 42 people at my gym. I lead a Mastermind group of several hundred fitness entrepreneurs yearning to be their best in training, business, leadership, and personal growth. I write books. And I travel the world speaking and presenting to ignite people's bodies, minds, and souls. That's what fires me up. I still train athletes. I still train kids. And I still train regular "Joes" and "Janes" yearning for the most in life.

One thing is consistent amidst all the changes since 1995. I've maintained my ACE Personal Trainer Certification. I take great pride in the fact that I'm ACE Certified and that ACE has provided me the foundation to create and live my purpose in life.

Just like I have evolved and changed in my 25-year career, ACE has continued to lead and forge ahead in this ever-changing, yet always incredible, industry. As a matter of fact, for the past 35 years, ACE has been the standard bearer for excellence in the health and fitness industry. More specifically, ACE's personal training textbooks have served not only as essential tools for those preparing to enter the industry, but also as go-to references for newcomers and veteran personal trainers alike. One of the keys to that continued excellence is ACE's ability to evolve by using feedback from established exercise professionals to help steer the direction of its textbooks and push the industry forward.

I have personally relied on ACE's textbooks and resources for years and have made them mandatory resources for my staff at Fitness Quest 10 and in my Mastermind program.

It is an absolute honor to write the foreword to *The Exercise Professional's Guide to Personal Training*. It's the perfect example of that evolution over time in our industry. This new textbook offers a comprehensive client-centered approach to personal training that focuses on behavior change, client empowerment, and evidence-based personalized programming. From the ACE Mover Method™ features that appear throughout the textbook offering sample client–personal trainer interactions and effective coaching techniques to the ACE IFT Model Exercise Programming Template offered in Chapter 11, ACE has provided the ultimate blueprint for success, not only for you as a personal trainer, but also for each of your clients.

Whether your career goals center on training competitive athletes, women during and after pregnancy, older adults working to improve their quality of life, or youth setting the groundwork for a lifetime of physical activity, the American Council on Exercise will be an invaluable partner every step of the way. Make good use of this textbook and all else that ACE has to offer and you will be well on your way to a promising and rewarding career in the fitness industry.

The world needs more life-transformers and personal trainers who are committed to radiating more positivity in the world. I believe that with the right certification, education, training, mindset, and commitment to excellence, you can be one of the select few who have the opportunity to call themselves, "personal trainer." That, my friend, is a badge of honor.

I believe that everyone has a life worth telling a story about. It's up to you to create "your story." Dive into this book, as I know it will significantly impact you.

Best of luck and I hope our paths cross soon. I can't wait to hear your story someday!

Much love... and tons of IMPACT!

Todd Durkin, MS, CSCS
Owner, Fitness Quest 10 & Todd Durkin Enterprises
Author, *The WOW Book* and *The IMPACT Body Plan*
2017 Jack LaLanne Award for Lifetime Achievement
2005 ACE Personal Trainer of the Year
2004 IDEA Personal Trainer of the Year
ACE Certified since 1995

Introduction

The American Council on Exercise is proud to introduce *The Exercise Professional's Guide to Personal Training*. This all-new textbook serves as the most current and comprehensive personal training resource to date, providing a practical guide for empowering clients to make lasting lifestyle changes through increased physical activity, improved fitness, and meaningful behavior change. Our goal when putting together this textbook was to meet the needs of personal trainers at every stage of their careers, from deciding whether to work as an employee or independent contractor to owning one's own fitness facility, from training people who strive for general fitness to specializing in a niche clientele that allows you to increase your income and become a recognized expert in your community.

Section I: Introduction consists of two chapters, the first of which explains the role and scope of personal trainers, including professional responsibilities and ethics, as well as the personal trainer's role as part of the healthcare continuum and in allied healthcare. The second chapter in this section introduces the ACE Integrated Fitness Training® (ACE IFT®) Model, which is explored in substantially more depth later in the textbook. This chapter also introduces the ACE Mover Method™, which encompasses the philosophy by which personal trainers can empower clients to make behavioral changes to improve their health, fitness, and overall health.

Section II: A Client-centered Approach to Personal Training includes four chapters. This section begins with a discussion of behavioral theory models and principles of behavior change; continues by exploring effective communication, goal setting, and teaching techniques within the framework of the client–personal trainer relationship; and includes an exploration of preparticipation health screening with a goal of removing any unnecessary barriers to clients becoming more physically active. Finally, this section concludes with a chapter on nutrition for health and fitness, including the ACE Position Statement on Nutrition Scope of Practice for Personal Trainers.

Section III: Assessments, Programming, and Progressions includes five chapters that form the heart of this textbook, beginning with a chapter on resting assessments and anthropometric measurements, which can be used as a baseline against which to measure future progress. These include heart rate, blood pressure, and circumference measurements. This is followed by a chapter on cardiorespiratory training, including coverage of the physiological adaptations to acute and chronic cardiorespiratory exercise, assessments of cardiorespiratory fitness, and the three phases of the Cardiorespiratory Training component of the ACE IFT Model.

This is followed by two chapters on muscular training, the second component of the ACE IFT Model. The first chapter covers the foundations and benefits of muscular training, as well as principles and variables of program design. The second muscular training chapter covers functional, movement, and load/speed assessments that correspond to the three phases of the Muscular Training component of the ACE IFT Model.

Finally, this section concludes with a chapter on integrated exercise programming that ties everything together to provide a greater understanding of the ACE IFT Model and the evidence base that supports it. The cornerstone of this chapter is the ACE IFT Model Exercise Programming Template, which personal trainers can use to develop and progress exercise programs, along with three case studies that feature complete training programs and sample exercises.

Section IV: Program Modifications for Clients with Special Considerations includes four chapters that explore considerations for clients with obesity, chronic disease, or musculoskeletal issues, as well as at various points in the lifespan, including youth, women during pregnancy, and older adults. These chapters detail how each disease, condition, injury, or stage in life impacts the exercise programming concepts learned in Section III.

Section V: Professional Responsibilities closes out the textbook with a chapter on the legal guidelines and business considerations that all personal trainers should be aware of throughout their careers. These include the use of important legal forms, record keeping, and risk management.

The true goal of this text is to provide an unparalleled, evidence-based resource to individuals interested in positively impacting the health and fitness of others by equipping them with the knowledge and skills needed to empower people to optimize their well-being and truly transform their lives.

We wish you good luck in your efforts and sincerely hope that this textbook serves you well as you prepare to become an ACE Certified Personal Trainer and remains a trusted resource throughout your career.

Sabrena Jo, MS
Director of Science and Research

Daniel J. Green
Senior Project Manager and Editor for
Publications and Content Development

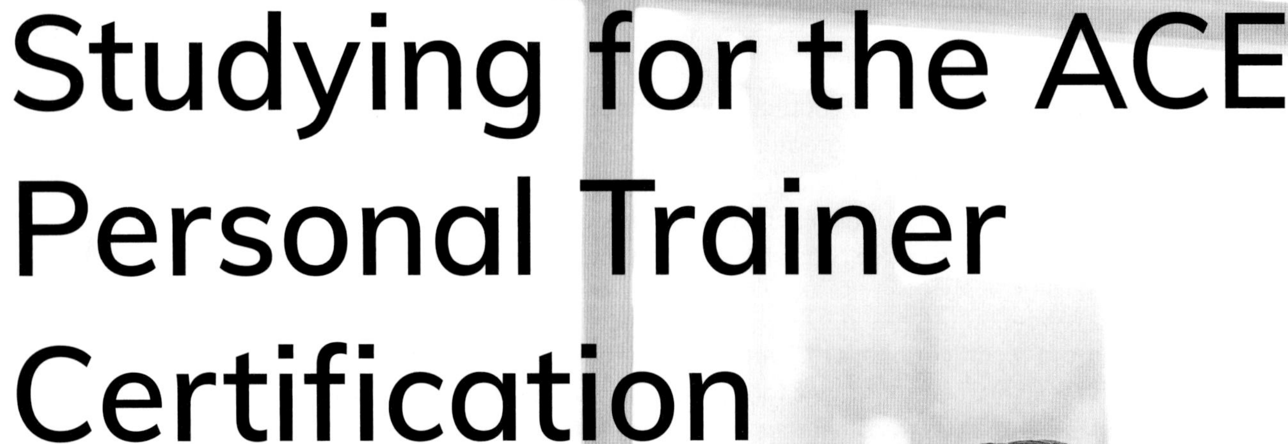

Studying for the ACE Personal Trainer Certification Exam

To help you on your journey to becoming an ACE Certified Personal Trainer, we have designed a comprehensive set of materials to not only guide you in your studies, but also serve as a trusted resource throughout your career.

The ACE Personal Trainer Study Program is divided into convenient modules to enable you to study more efficiently and effectively. The program includes this textbook, *The Exercise Professional's Guide to Personal Training Study Companion*, and the online ACE University.

ACE University

ACE University guides the study program for a self-study exam candidate and contains online study materials to support your understanding of the textbook content, including simulations that take you into a personal-training session to see important principles in action; video presentations that bring more complex topics to life to enhance your learning experience; and quizzes and interactive learning activities to help you assess your progress and understanding before you move from one chapter to the next.

ACE University also features an end-of-course exam review and practice tests with annotated responses to enhance learning. Finally, ACE University will help you stay on track by walking you through the study process and directing you when it is time to return to *The Exercise Professional's Guide to Personal Training* textbook or *Study Companion.*

To utilize ACE University, log in to your My ACE Account at www.ACEfitness.org/MyACE.

Course Outline and Time Commitment

The course outline is in the navigation bar of ACE University.

This is a self-paced, self-directed course that features an array of interactive resources to support you on your study journey. In preparation for your certification exam, we recommend that you complete all sections and take the associated quizzes until you pass each one consistently and can explain the reasoning for the correct answers. Before moving forward, we want you to feel confident with the material. You will find a sample course timeline in the course syllabus, located in ACE University, which can be modified based on the time you have available to dedicate to studying.

Important Tips and Study Support

The following eligibility requirements have been established for individuals to sit for the ACE Personal Trainer Certification examination:

- Must be at least 18 years of age
- Must hold a current adult CPR certificate and, if living in the U.S. or Canada, a current AED certificate* with live skills check

  * CPR and AED are both required in the U.S. and Canada. Candidates outside the U.S. and Canada are required to hold only current CPR due to differing laws regarding AED use by non-medical professionals in some countries. Candidates taking an ACE exam via computer-based testing must hold a current CPR/AED certificate prior to registration.

- Must have completed high school (or the equivalent)

For additional tips and resources, check out the ACE Answers web page at www.ACEfitness.org/ACEAnswers. ACE Answers offers a wide range of study support resources, including answers to commonly asked study questions, exam preparation blog articles, recorded videos, and lectures. You can also connect with ACE Answers and your peers at www.facebook.com/ACEFitnessAnswers.

SECTION I

Introduction

CHAPTER 1

Role and Scope of Practice for Personal Trainers

CHAPTER 2

The ACE Integrated Fitness Training® Model

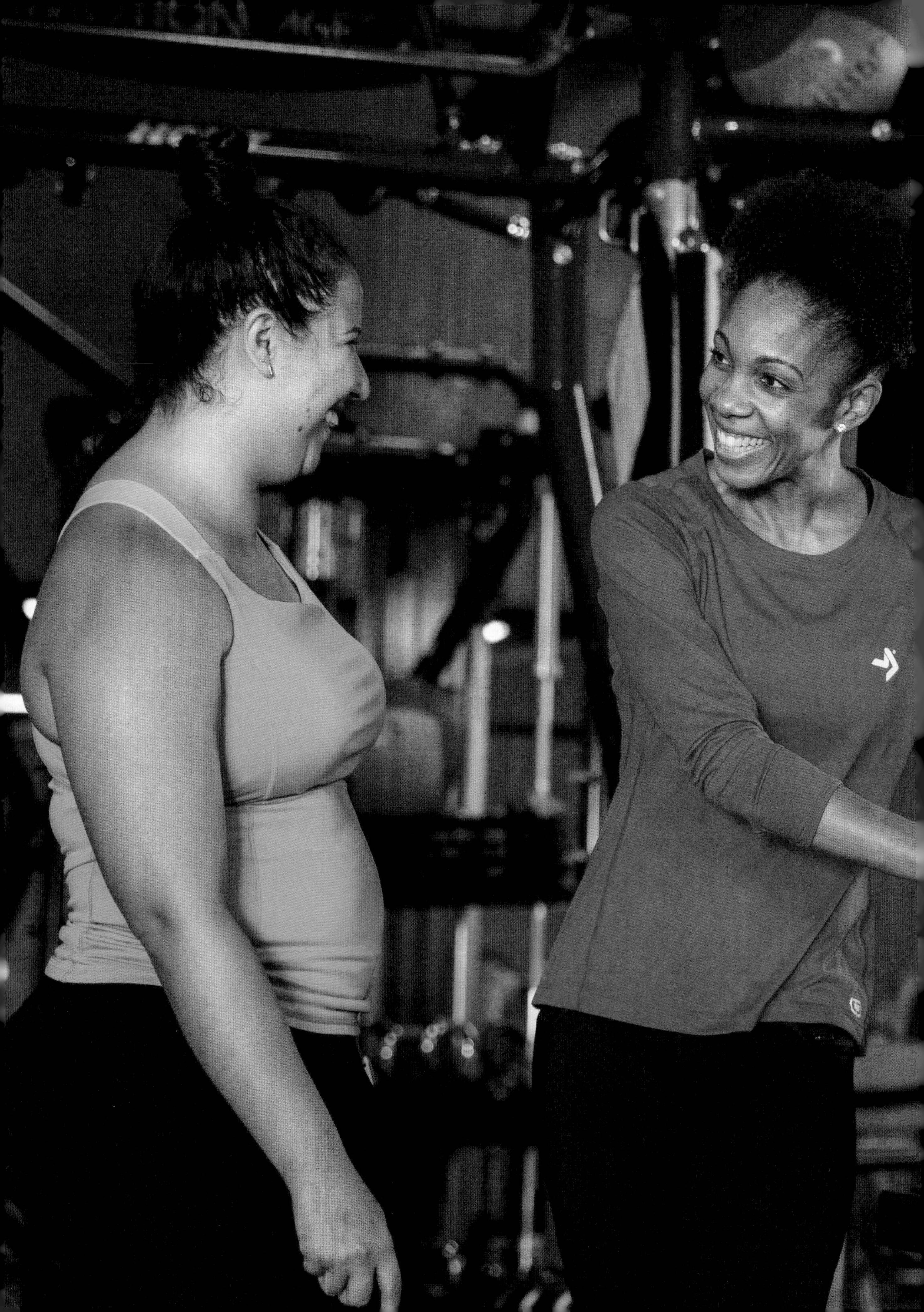

CHAPTER 1

Role and Scope of Practice for Personal Trainers

TODD GALATI, MA
Senior Director, Standards and Practice Advancement, American Council on Exercise; ACE Certified Personal Trainer, Medical Exercise Specialist, Health Coach, and Group Fitness Instructor

IN THIS CHAPTER

LEARNING OBJECTIVES:

Upon completion of this chapter, the reader will be able to:

- Define the health benefits associated with regular physical activity
- Explain the role and scope of the ACE Certified Personal Trainer
- Describe the similarities and differences among personal trainers and other professionals on the healthcare continuum
- Identify when and where to refer clients to other allied healthcare professionals
- List key factors for professional recognition and career development for personal trainers

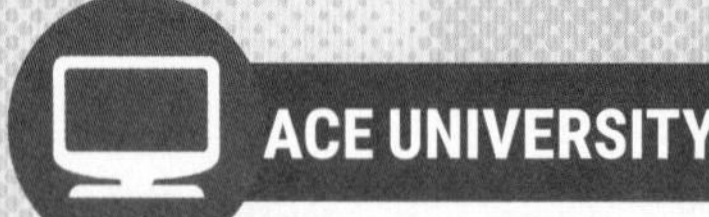

If your study program includes the ACE University, visit www.ACEfitness.org/MyACE and log in to your My ACE Account to take full advantage of the ACE Personal Trainer Study Program and online guided study experience.

A variety of media to support and expand on the material in this text is provided to facilitate learning and best prepare you for the ACE Personal Trainer Certification exam and a career as a personal trainer.

The health benefits associated with regular physical activity are well documented (Table 1-1). Ask most people if they would like to receive these life-enhancing health benefits and the response will be a resounding "Yes!" Yet, 10 years after the U.S. Department of Health & Human Services published the inaugural *Physical Activity Guidelines for Americans*, the 2018 *Guidelines* remind us that knowledge alone is not a catalyst for action [U.S. Department of Health & Human Services (USDHHS), 2018].

TABLE 1-1

Health Benefits Associated with Regular Physical Activity

Children and Adolescents
▸ Improved bone health (ages 3 through 17 years)
▸ Improved weight status (ages 3 through 17 years)
▸ Improved cardiorespiratory and muscular fitness (ages 6 through 17 years)
▸ Improved cardiometabolic health (ages 6 through 17 years)
▸ Improved cognition (ages 6 to 13 years)*
▸ Reduced risk of depression (ages 6 to 13 years)
Adults and Older Adults
▸ Lower risk of all-cause mortality
▸ Lower risk of cardiovascular disease mortality
▸ Lower risk of cardiovascular disease (including heart disease and stroke)
▸ Lower risk of hypertension
▸ Lower risk of type 2 diabetes
▸ Lower risk of adverse blood lipid profile
▸ Lower risk of cancers of the bladder, breast, colon, endometrium, esophagus, kidney, lung, and stomach
▸ Improved cognition*
▸ Reduced risk of dementia (including Alzheimer's disease)
▸ Improved quality of life
▸ Reduced anxiety
▸ Reduced risk of depression
▸ Improved sleep
▸ Slowed or reduced weight gain
▸ Weight loss, particularly when combined with reduced calorie intake
▸ Prevention of weight regain following initial weight loss
▸ Improved bone health
▸ Improved physical function
▸ Lower risk of falls (older adults)
▸ Lower risk of fall-related injuries (older adults)

Note: The Advisory Committee rated the evidence of health benefits of physical activity as strong, moderate, limited, or grade not assignable. Only outcomes with strong or moderate evidence of effect are included in this table.

*See Table 2-3 of the *Physical Activity Guidelines for Americans* (2nd ed.) for additional components of cognition and brain health.

Reprinted from U.S. Department of Health & Human Services (2018). *Physical Activity Guidelines for Americans* (2nd ed.) https://health.gov/paguidelines/second-edition/pdf/Physical_Activity_Guidelines_2nd_edition.pdf

Insufficient physical activity, tobacco use, poor nutrition, and excessive alcohol use are identified as common modifiable risk factors that can lead to **noncommunicable diseases (NCDs)** (Figure 1-1), with prolonged sitting/**sedentary** behaviors potentially one day joining this list (Dunstan, Thorp, & Healy, 2011). Deaths resulting from NCDs, otherwise known as chronic diseases, have surpassed communicable diseases as the greatest global health burden (Lozano et al., 2012), with the majority of deaths from NCDs resulting from **cardiovascular disease,** cancer, **diabetes,** and chronic respiratory diseases [World Health Organization (WHO), 2018a; Kochanek et al., 2017]. The WHO (2018a) estimates that chronic diseases are responsible for killing an estimated 41 million people annually, accounting for 71% of all deaths globally.

Numbers of this magnitude spread across all demographics, creating a need for policies, systems, and environmental changes that are inclusive and provide a greater opportunity for **health equity.** The WHO (2017) defines health equity as "the absence of avoidable or remediable differences among groups of people, whether those groups are defined socially, economically, demographically, or geographically." To truly affect chronic disease globally, health equity must be a priority for professionals across the full spectrum of healthcare in all communities.

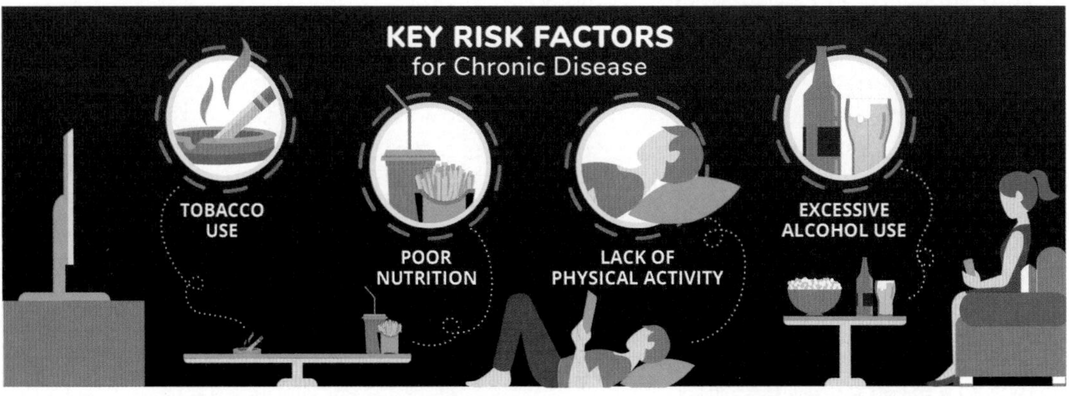

FIGURE 1-1
Risk factors that underlie all major noncommunicable diseases

Source: Centers for Disease Control and Prevention's National Center for Chronic Disease Prevention and Health Promotion

Physical inactivity was cited by Steven Blair (2009) as the greatest public health problem of the 21st century. The percentage of deaths attributed to low **cardiorespiratory fitness** was substantially higher than the percentages attributed to **obesity,** smoking, high **cholesterol,** and diabetes. More recently, researchers from the Cleveland Clinic conducted a retrospective study of 122,007 patients to assess the association between cardiorespiratory fitness and all-cause **mortality,** and to evaluate the relative benefit or harm of extreme cardiorespiratory fitness compared with modest levels of cardiorespiratory fitness. They found an inverse relationship between risk-adjusted all-cause mortality and cardiorespiratory fitness, where the adjusted mortality risk of lower cardiorespiratory fitness was greater than or equal to cardiovascular disease, diabetes, and smoking (Mandsager et al., 2018). In addition, Mandsager and colleagues (2018) found that individuals with extreme cardiorespiratory fitness, classified as cardiorespiratory fitness

>2 standard deviations above the mean for age and sex, had the lowest risk-adjusted all-cause mortality and that the benefits extended to patients who had **hypertension** or were 70 years or older. This research supports the findings reported by Blair (2009) and provides evidence supporting the importance of achieving and maintaining high levels of cardiorespiratory fitness (Mandsager et al., 2018). Unfortunately, these findings have not had a significant impact on physical-activity participation rates.

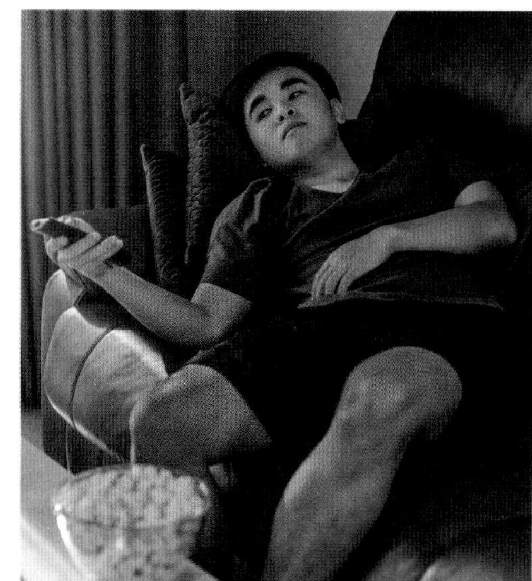

Researchers from the WHO found a nonsignificant change of 1.0% in levels of insufficient physical activity globally from 2001 (28.5%) to 2016 (27.5%) after analyzing pooled data from 358 surveys in 168 countries with more than 1.9 million total participants (Guthold et al., 2018). The prevalence of insufficient physical activity was found to be more than twice as high in high-income countries (36.8%) as in low-income countries (16.2%) in 2016, with insufficient physical activity increasing in prevalence by 5.2% (31.6% to 36.8%) in high-income countries from 2001 to 2016. In their interpretation of results, the researchers reported that if current trends continue, the 2025 global target of a 10% relative reduction in insufficient physical activity will not be met (Guthold et al., 2018).

Fortunately, leading health organizations are working collaboratively to provide actionable plans aimed at decreasing sedentary behaviors and increasing physical-activity levels. The *2018 Physical Activity Guidelines for Americans* provide a complete set of guidelines and examples of activities to improve cardiorespiratory fitness, muscular fitness, bone strength, balance, and **flexibility** in children, adults, older adults, women during pregnancy and the postpartum period, and adults with chronic diseases (USDHHS, 2018). The WHO (2018b) released the *Global Action Plan on Physical Activity 2018-2030: More Active People for a Healthier World*, a "systems-based" approach to reduce the global prevalence of physical inactivity in adults and adolescents by 2030 through 20 policy actions applicable to all countries to achieve four strategic objectives: create active societies, create active environments, create active people, and create active systems. The Prescription for Activity Task Force, comprised of industry leaders from all areas of the healthcare continuum, used the theory of change approach to strategic planning to produce a systems-change map detailing the pathway of change necessary in communities, care delivery, clinic-community integration, communications, informatics, funding and payment, and education and training to get 50% or more of Americans to achieve recommended levels of physical activity by 2035 (Bryant et al., 2017).

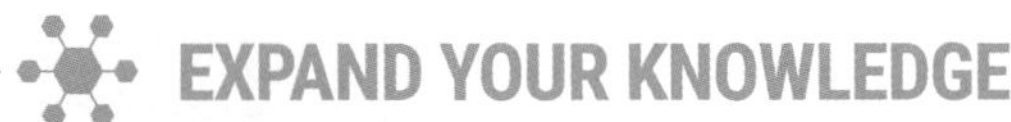

The Prescription for Activity Task Force

The Prescription for Activity (PfA) Task Force is comprised of volunteer national stakeholders from academic, healthcare, and community settings who gathered to examine the following questions:

- How can the healthcare industry mobilize people from communities across the United States to achieve recommended levels of physical activity—with a focus on those populations at greatest need?
- What steps might healthcare take to pursue the priorities and execute the strategies recommended by leading authorities such as the *Physical Activity Guidelines for Americans*, the American College of Sports Medicine's Exercise Is Medicine, the National Physical Activity Plan Healthcare Sector, and the U.S. Preventive Services Task Force?
- What steps would be required for clinical care and that which surrounds and supports it to become a force for a cultural shift leading to a healthier, more active U.S.?

The PfA Task Force developed a systems-change map illustrating how to mobilize healthcare to help more Americans achieve physical-activity guidelines, leading to better health outcomes and reductions in health disparities. The Ultimate Outcome of that map was as follows:

Culture Transformation:

Across diverse population groups within the U.S., being physically active is prioritized, feasible, and enjoyable.

As Measured By:

50% or more of Americans in every community, demographic, and age group achieve recommended levels of physical activity.

Target Year:

2035

The achievement of this outcome requires an ongoing focus on health equity, as the pursuit of a more physically active America, and the belief that every American must have an equal opportunity to achieve his or her best health, are fundamentally intertwined.

The PfA Task Force represents a tremendous opportunity for health and exercise professionals, who will be heavily involved in the community-level implementation of the goals set forth in the systems-change map. To see the full map, learn more about the PfA Task Force, and find out how you can get involved, visit www.prescriptionforactivity.org.

Even with well-established guidelines and action plans for physical activity, the majority of healthcare professionals have little or no formal education or practical experience in designing and leading exercise programs. Physicians give patients recommendations to exercise, but they generally do not provide specific instructions on how to exercise. ACE® Certified Personal Trainers, therefore, play a vital role on the healthcare continuum by designing and implementing effective exercise programs and coaching clients through health-related behavioral changes to help them achieve their goals for improved health and fitness. Throughout this textbook, opportunities to use a client-centered approach to personal training are presented. These features will help personal trainers identify when such an approach is likely to be most beneficial and will enable personal trainers to hone their skills.

Traditionally, the role of personal trainers was primarily focused on working with fitness enthusiasts in traditional fitness facilities. This role has changed due to the increasing number of adults and children who have **overweight** or obesity, are insufficiently active, and have related health issues stemming from physical inactivity. Personal trainers must now be prepared to work with clients ranging in age from youth to older adults and ranging in health and fitness status from physically inactive to athletic. Insufficient physical activity and the rising obesity epidemic have contributed to a positive outlook for personal training as a profession, especially for personal trainers who are prepared to coach clients to help them reach their fitness and health behavior goals.

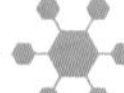

EXPAND YOUR KNOWLEDGE

The Future of Personal Training

The Bureau of Labor Statistics (BLS) of the U.S. Department of Labor (DOL) (2018), refers to professionals in the fitness industry as "fitness trainers and instructors," with personal trainers classified as "personal fitness trainers." The BLS (2018) describes the job role by stating that personal fitness trainers "design and carry out workout routines specific to the needs of their clients. They may work with individual clients or teach group classes. In larger facilities, personal trainers often sell their training sessions to gym members. They start by evaluating their clients' current fitness level, personal goals, and skills. Then, they develop personalized training programs for their clients to follow, and they monitor the clients' progress." The BLS (2018) further defines the nature of the job by stating that personal fitness trainers "work with an individual client or a small group. They may train in a gym or in clients' homes. Personal fitness trainers assess the clients' level of physical fitness and help them set and reach their fitness goals."

Expected Growth in Personal-training Jobs

According to the BLS (2018), employment of fitness trainers and instructors is projected to increase by 10% between 2016 and 2026. This expected increase is faster than the 7% average growth for all occupations combined and is attributed to a number of factors, including the following:

- Businesses and insurance providers supporting physical activity for employees
- Continued focus on physical activity to improve health and combat obesity
- Baby boomers continuing to be active to prevent injuries, illness, and chronic disease
- Older adults looking for low-impact exercise for relief from arthritis and other ailments

Personal trainers may work with apparently healthy clients, as well as individuals with chronic disease and other conditions who have obtained medical clearance if needed, helping them improve fitness and health. Experienced personal trainers with advanced education, training, and credentials will generally have the skills necessary to work with clients who have special needs for exercise programming following medical treatment for an injury or disease. In more clinical settings, the advanced exercise professional may work under the direction of a physician, **physical therapist,** or other rehabilitation professional, while in a club setting he or she may be more autonomous. In all situations, it is crucial for the exercise professional to stay within the boundaries of his or her education, certification, and legal **scope of practice,** and to work closely with each client's referring physician and other healthcare providers to ensure that the exercise program is complementary to their other treatments.

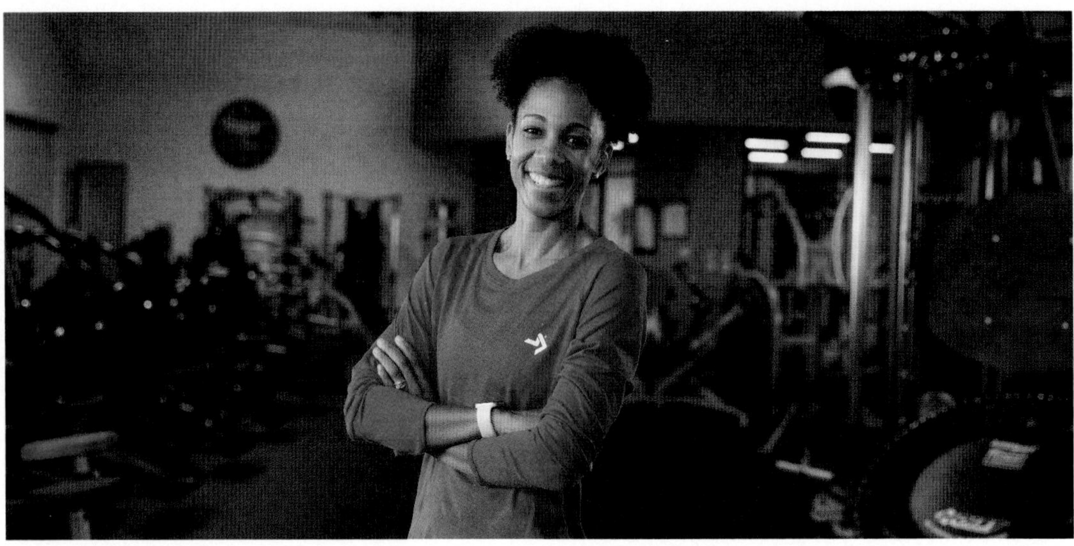

The ACE Personal Trainer Certification

The decision to pursue certification as a personal trainer is an important step in being recognized as a competent exercise professional. The ACE Personal Trainer Certification Program was developed to assess candidate competency in developing and delivering safe and effective exercise programs for individuals and groups who are apparently healthy or have medical clearance to exercise, as needed. Candidates who earn an ACE Personal Trainer Certification demonstrate that they meet or exceed the level of competency required to work as a professional personal trainer with minimal supervision. In the credentialing world, this threshold of professional competence is referred to as the "minimum competency" required for a person to work in a given profession. The primary purpose of a certification is always to protect the public from harm by assessing if the professional meets established levels of competence in the knowledge, skills, and abilities necessary to perform the job in a safe and effective manner. For personal trainers, earning a professional certification that is accredited by the National Commission for Certifying Agencies (NCCA), or a comparable certification program accreditor, can separate him or her from personal trainers who have not proven themselves to be at the same level of competence (see "Accreditation of Exercise Professional Certification Programs" on page 26).

Exercise professionals who earn the ACE Personal Trainer Certification are qualified to work as professional personal trainers with minimal supervision, developing and implementing personalized exercise programs that improve fitness and overall well-being for individuals and groups who are apparently healthy or have medical clearance to exercise. This does not mean that an ACE Certified Personal Trainer knows everything there is to know about personal training, just as successfully passing one's medical board exams does not mean that the physician knows everything there is to know about medicine. Instead, by earning an ACE Personal Trainer Certification, the professional has proven his or her competence in making safe and effective exercise-programming decisions in a variety of practical situations, while minimizing client risk and exposure to harm (e.g., physical, emotional, psychological, and financial).

DEFINING "SCOPE OF PRACTICE"

A scope of practice defines the legal range of services that professionals in a given field can provide, the settings in which those services can be provided, and the guidelines or parameters that must be followed. Many factors go into defining a scope of practice, including the education, training, and certifications or licenses required to work in a given field, the laws and organizations governing the specific profession, and the laws and organizations governing complementary professions within the same field. Most laws defining a profession are determined and regulated by state regulatory agencies, including licensure. As a result, the scope of practice for licensed practitioners can vary from state to state in a given profession. In addition, most professions have organizations that serve as governing bodies that set eligibility requirements to enter educational programs or sit for certification exams and establish codes for professional conduct and disciplinary procedures for professionals who break these codes.

The laws, rules, and regulations that govern a profession are established for the protection of the public. The laws governing a personal trainer's scope of practice and the ramifications faced by personal trainers who provide services that fall outside the defined scope are detailed in Chapter 16. The eligibility and certification requirements to work within this legal scope of practice are defined by the professional organizations that offer personal trainer certifications. These organizations also establish codes of ethical conduct and mandate that they are upheld by certified professionals and applicants in all actions related to personal training. It is crucial for practitioners in every industry to be aware of the scope of practice for their given profession, to ensure that they practice within the realm of the specific education, experience, demonstrated competency, and any regulatory requirements of their credential.

SCOPE OF PRACTICE FOR ACE CERTIFIED PERSONAL TRAINERS

Personal trainers as a collective group have a general scope of practice (Table 1-2). While this table provides general guidance, each professional must know what is within the specific scope of practice for his or her credential. The ACE Certified Personal Trainer scope of practice is presented in Figure 1-2. ACE Certified Personal Trainers must work within this defined scope of practice to provide effective services to their clients, gain and maintain support from the healthcare community, and avoid the legal ramifications of providing services outside their professional scope.

Personal trainers should never provide services that are outside their defined scope of practice. For example, a personal trainer may be asked nutrition questions by clients wanting to reduce weight and/or **body fat.** Personal trainers can help clients with their weight-loss goals by designing effective exercise programs that bring about positive **body composition** changes and helping them to adopt more healthful behaviors. This can include showing clients how to utilize the tools available at www.ChooseMyPlate.gov or educating them about the recommendations in the *Dietary Guidelines for Americans* to help them gain a better understanding of healthful foods and make better choices (U.S. Department of Agriculture, 2015). Clients who are looking for more detailed nutritional programming, such as meal plans, or other specific recommendations should be referred to a **registered dietitian (RD),** as these services are beyond the scope of practice of personal trainers and are in the legal domain of services provided by RDs in most states.

TABLE 1-2

General Scope of Practice for Personal Trainers

Actions outside Scope of Practice	Actions *within* Scope of Practice
Diagnosing illness or disease	▸ Following accepted guidelines for exercise programming for diseases and disorders as presented by the appropriate governing body (e.g., American College of Obstetricians and Gynecologists and American Diabetes Association) ▸ Assessing for exercise limitations ▸ Identifying potential risk factors through health screening and fitness assessment ▸ Referring clients to appropriate healthcare professionals as needed ▸ Adhering to guidance and limitations outlined in a medical release form provided by a client's physician or other healthcare professional
Prescribing diets or nutritional supplements	▸ Referring clients to a registered dietitian for meal planning or a specific diet plan ▸ Providing general information on healthy, evidence-based nutrition (e.g., *Dietary Guidelines for Americans*)
Treating injury or disease or rehabilitating clients following injury	▸ Using exercise programming to help clients improve overall health ▸ Helping clients adhere to advice from a physician or physical therapist ▸ Designing an exercise program after a client has been released from rehabilitation ▸ Referring clients to appropriate healthcare professionals as needed
Monitoring clinical progress for medically referred clients	▸ Documenting progress and reporting it to the appropriate healthcare professional or physician after receiving the client's permission to do so ▸ Following recommendations from a physician, physical therapist, registered dietitian, or other healthcare professional
Counseling clients	▸ Using coaching techniques to support clients through behavior change (e.g., increasing physical activity and adopting healthy eating habits) ▸ Providing general health and wellness information ▸ Referring clients to appropriate healthcare professionals as needed

To be most effective in their role on the healthcare continuum, personal trainers must have working knowledge of their unique areas of practice, where they overlap with other healthcare professions, and services that are outside their legal scope of practice.

For example, the same RD who can create specific meal plans for clients can also provide general guidelines about exercise to help them understand the important role that physical activity plays in improving health and creating a negative energy balance. However, if a client working with an RD wants a personalized exercise plan, he or she should be referred to a well-qualified personal trainer who holds an appropriate NCCA-accredited certification and is on the U.S. Registry of Exercise Professionals, if living in the U.S. (see page 27).

A personal trainer should *not* make recommendations that contradict those of the client's healthcare team. For example, if a client's physician's release has specific guidelines

FIGURE 1-2
The ACE Certified Personal Trainer Scope of Practice

The ACE Certified Personal Trainer is an exercise professional who has met all requirements of the American Council on Exercise to develop and implement personalized exercise programs that improve fitness and overall well-being for individuals and small groups who are apparently healthy or have medical clearance to exercise. The ACE Certified Personal Trainer realizes that personal training is a service industry focused on helping people enhance fitness and modify risk factors for chronic disease to improve health. As members of the allied healthcare continuum with a primary focus on prevention, ACE Certified Personal Trainers have a scope of practice that includes:

- Implementing a client-centered and evidence-based approach to personal training by providing personalized exercise programs and using behavior-change skills and strategies to coach clients to improved health and fitness
- Developing and implementing exercise programs that are safe, effective, and appropriate for individuals and small groups who are apparently healthy or have medical clearance to exercise
- Conducting health-history interviews and preparticipation health-screening with clients to determine the need for referral and identify contraindications for exercise
- Administering appropriate assessments for cardiorespiratory and muscular training based on the client's health history, current exercise, lifestyle factors, and goals utilizing research-substantiated and published protocols
- Coaching clients in setting and achieving realistic health, fitness, and behavior-change goals
- Teaching correct exercise methods and appropriate movement progressions and regressions through demonstration, explanation, and proper cueing and spotting techniques
- Empowering individuals to begin and adhere to their exercise programs using guidance, support, motivation, lapse- and relapse-prevention strategies, and effective feedback
- Designing structured exercise programs for one-on-one and small-group personal training
- Educating clients about fitness- and health-related topics to help them in adopting healthful behaviors that facilitate exercise program success
- Protecting client confidentiality according to the Health Insurance Portability and Accountability Act (HIPAA) and related regional, national, and international laws
- Always acting with professionalism, respect, and integrity
- Recognizing what is within the scope of practice and always referring clients to other healthcare professionals when appropriate
- Being prepared for emergency situations and responding appropriately if, and when, they occur

for exercise intensities, modalities, or exercises, the personal trainer must follow these guidelines when designing the client's exercise program. Importantly, if the personal trainer needs clarification about the physician's exercise guidelines, he or she should feel confident in reaching out to the physician's office with the client's written permission with any program-related queries. While the physician generally will not have the same knowledge about specific exercises as a personal trainer, the physician's guidelines will be based on the knowledge of the client's health, medications, ailments, injuries, and diseases, and *must* be followed for the health and safety of the client. Each state, province, and country has specific laws about the responsibilities of different healthcare professions. It is the responsibility of the personal trainer to learn and adhere to the laws in his or her geographical area, as well as adhere to the ACE Certified Personal Trainer scope of practice.

KNOWLEDGE, SKILLS, AND ABILITIES OF THE ACE CERTIFIED PERSONAL TRAINER

The ACE Personal Trainer Certification is designed for exercise professionals wanting to provide one-on-one and small-group exercise instruction to individuals who are apparently healthy or have a physician's clearance for exercise to help them reach their health and fitness goals. The certification program is continually evaluated to ensure that it is up to date with current research and industry standards. In addition, every five years a group of industry experts analyzes the specific job requirements for personal trainers to update the outline of tasks, knowledge, skills, and abilities necessary to perform the job of personal training effectively. After being validated by thousands of ACE Certified Personal Trainers, this outline is published as the ACE Personal Trainer Exam Content Outline, which serves as the blueprint for the ACE Personal Trainer Certification exam and provides a template for candidates preparing for the exam. It is also a written job description of the critical tasks performed by, and the knowledge, skills, and abilities required to be, an effective ACE Certified Personal Trainer.

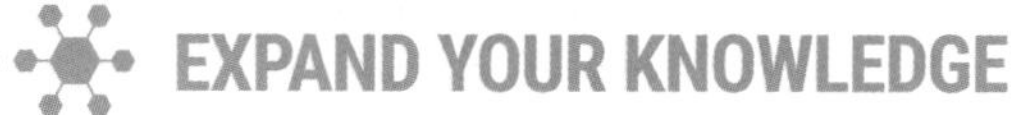

Using the Exam Content Outline as a Study Tool

The ACE Personal Trainer Exam Content Outline is a valuable tool for candidates preparing for the ACE Personal Trainer Certification Exam. It is the result of an in-depth job analysis conducted with a panel of personal-training subject matter experts. The results of this job analysis are validated via an industry-wide survey. The final result of this process is the ACE Personal Trainer Exam Content Outline, which is used in assembling each ACE Personal Trainer exam.

Candidates are encouraged to refer to this Exam Content Outline as they prepare for the ACE Personal Trainer exam, as it details the key concepts and competencies assessed by the exam. It does not provide the exact questions on an ACE exam; however, it does provide the main content "Domains" assessed by the exam and the percentage of questions that come from each Domain.

Each Domain is comprised of several "Tasks" that are essential for an exercise professional to perform competently in order to meet the required level of competence to earn the ACE Personal Trainer Certification. The percentages listed with each Domain represent the criticality of the tasks in the Domain, and the frequency with which a personal trainer will perform them.

The following steps should help you use the Exam Content Outline in preparing for the ACE Personal Trainer exam:

- Review the exam content Domains and their associated percentages. This will help you determine the relative weight of each Domain on the total examination.
- Review and understand each Task Statement. Each question on the ACE Personal Trainer exam is associated with one of the Task Statements, as they have been identified as the critical tasks a well-qualified personal trainer must perform consistently to provide safe and effective exercise programming.

- Review the Knowledge and Skill Statements associated with each Task. These describe the knowledge and skills in which an exercise professional must be competent to perform the essential tasks of an ACE Certified Personal Trainer.
- Refer back to the Exam Content Outline as you study to ensure that you have learned the knowledge and skills necessary to perform the essential Tasks of a well-qualified personal trainer.
- Refer back to the Exam Content Outline after completing the online practice tests to review the concepts and competencies covered in any Domains that have been identified as areas of focus as you continue your studies.

The ACE Personal Trainer Exam Content Outline can be found at www.ACEfitness.org/PTexamcontent.

Education and Experience

There is not a specific required course of study for individuals looking to enter the profession of personal training. To become an ACE Certified Personal Trainer, a candidate must show that he or she is able to apply the knowledge required to be a safe and effective personal trainer by passing the ACE Personal Trainer Certification exam. There are many paths to reaching this goal, including self-study using preparatory materials from ACE or other sources that cover the topics in the ACE Personal Trainer Certification Exam Content Outline, preparatory courses or workshops delivered live or online, educational internships, professional experience, trade schools, and college courses and degrees. Each candidate must select his or her own path based on time, financial resources, learning styles, and personal factors.

Preparation and Testing

The knowledge, skills, and abilities assessed by the ACE Personal Trainer Certification exam include developing and enhancing **rapport** with clients, establishing goals, coaching fitness- and health-related behavior change, collecting adequate health-history information and determining the appropriateness of referral, conducting appropriate assessments, designing and modifying exercise programs to help clients progress toward their goals, motivating clients to adopt and adhere to their exercise programs, and always acting in a professional manner while staying within the personal trainer's scope of practice. The ACE Integrated Fitness Training® Model is designed to help personal trainers competently navigate the process of working with clients, beginning with the initial meeting and continuing throughout the client–personal trainer relationship (see Chapter 2).

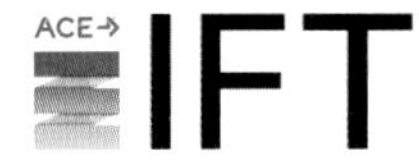

Exercise professionals interested in sitting for the ACE Personal Trainer Certification exam should download the *ACE Certification Candidate Handbook* from the ACE website (www.ACEfitness.org/getcertified/pdfs/Certification-Exam-Candidate-Handbook.pdf). This complimentary handbook explains how ACE certification exams are developed, what the candidate should expect, and the procedures for earning and maintaining an ACE certification. The handbook also includes explanations about the multiple-choice and client-scenario questions found on ACE certification exams, along with sample questions to help candidates understand the differences among *recall*, *application*, and *analysis* questions. In addition, the handbook provides candidates with test-taking strategies and a list of available study resources.

PROFESSIONAL RESPONSIBILITIES AND ETHICS

The primary purpose of professional certification programs is to protect the public from harm (e.g., physical, emotional, psychological, or financial) by ensuring that the public has access to, and a way to identify, well-qualified practitioners. Professionals who earn an ACE Personal Trainer Certification validate their capabilities and enhance their value to employers, clients, and other healthcare providers. This does not happen simply because the individual has a new title. This recognition is given because the ACE credential itself upholds rigorous standards established for assessing an individual's competence in making safe and effective exercise-programming decisions. ACE has established a professional code of ethics and disciplinary procedures, and ACE's four professional certifications have all received third-party accreditation from the NCCA, the gold standard for certification program accreditation in healthcare, fitness, health coaching, finance, and other industries.

To help ACE Certified Professionals understand the conduct expected from them as healthcare professionals in protecting the public from harm, ACE has developed the ACE Code of Ethics (see the Appendix). This code serves as a guide for ethical and professional practices for all ACE Certified Professionals. This code is enforced through the ACE Professional Practices and Disciplinary Procedures (https://www. ACEfitness.org/fitness-certifications/certified-code-of-ethics). All ACE Certified Professionals and candidates for ACE certifications must be familiar with, and comply with, the ACE Code of Ethics and ACE Professional Practices and Disciplinary Procedures.

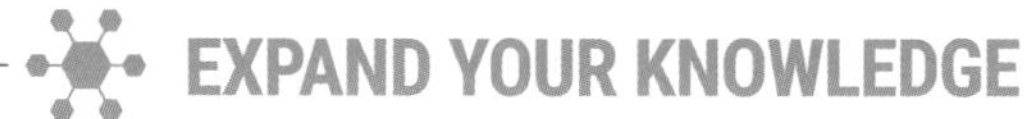

ACE Code of Ethics

The ACE Code of Ethics (see the Appendix) governs the ethical and professional standards to be followed by ACE Certified Professionals when working with clients, the public, or other health and exercise professionals. Every individual who registers for an ACE certification exam must agree to uphold the ACE Code of Ethics throughout the exam process and as a professional, should he or she earn an ACE certification. Exam candidates and ACE Certified Personal Trainers must have a comprehensive understanding of the code and the consequences and potential public harm that can come from violating each of its principles.

ACE Professional Practices and Disciplinary Procedures

The ACE Professional Practices and Disciplinary Procedures are intended to assist and inform ACE Certified Professionals, candidates for ACE certification, and the public about the ACE application and certification standards relative to professional conduct and disciplinary procedures. ACE may revoke or otherwise take action with regard to the application or certification of an individual in the case of:

- Ineligibility for certification
- Irregularity in connection with any certification examination
- Unauthorized possession, use, access, or distribution of certification examinations, score reports, trademarks, logos, written materials, answer sheets, certificates, certificant or applicant files, or other confidential or proprietary ACE documents or materials (registered or otherwise)

- Material misrepresentation or fraud in any statement to ACE or to the public, including, but not limited to, statements made to assist the applicant, certificant, or another to apply for, obtain, or retain certification
- Any physical, mental, or emotional condition of either temporary or permanent nature, including, but not limited to, substance abuse, which impairs or has the potential to impair competent and objective professional performance
- Negligent and/or intentional misconduct in professional work, including, but not limited to, physical or emotional abuse, disregard for safety, or the unauthorized release of confidential information
- The timely conviction, plea of guilty, or plea of *nolo contendere* ("no contest") in connection with a felony or misdemeanor that is directly related to public health and/or fitness instruction or education, and that impairs competent and objective professional performance

  These include, but are not limited to, rape, sexual abuse, actual or threatened use of a weapon of violence, or the prohibited sale, distribution, or possession with intent to distribute of a controlled substance.
- Failure to meet the requirements for certification or recertification

ACE has developed a three-tiered disciplinary process of review, hearing, and appeals to ensure fair and unbiased examination of alleged violation(s) of the Application and Certification Standards in order to (1) determine the merit of allegations and (2) impose appropriate sanctions as necessary to protect the public and the integrity of the certification process.

Certification Period and Renewal

ACE certifications are valid for two years from the date earned, expiring on the last day of the month. To renew certification for a new two-year cycle, ACE Certified Professionals must complete a minimum of 20 hours of ACE-approved continuing education credits (2.0 CECs) and maintain a current certificate in **cardiopulmonary resuscitation (CPR)** and, if living in North America, proper use of an **automated external defibrillator (AED).**

Continuing education is a standard requirement in healthcare to help ensure that professionals stay up to date with the latest research in their respective fields for the protection of the public. Given the dynamic nature of the fitness industry and the rapidly advancing research in exercise science, it is imperative for exercise professionals to complete continuing education on a regular basis. By completing continuing education, ACE Certified Professionals can stay current with the latest findings in exercise science and keep their services in line with the most recent guidelines for fitness and healthcare.

Client Privacy

Beginning with the initial health-history interview, clients will share confidential information with the personal trainer. Although the client–personal trainer relationship does not currently have the same legal requirements for confidentiality as patient–physician or patient–psychologist relationships, personal trainers should maintain that same level of security for each client's personal information. Failure to do so could prove detrimental for the client and the client–personal trainer relationship and may violate the ACE Code of Ethics and state or federal privacy laws.

To help prevent violations of client privacy, ACE Certified Professionals should become familiar with, and adhere to, the **Health Insurance Portability and Accountability Act (HIPAA),** which addresses the use and disclosure of individuals' protected health information. By following HIPAA regulations, personal trainers can maintain the confidentiality of each client's protected health information according to the same rules that govern most healthcare professions. More details about client privacy and keeping clients' protected health information secure can be found in Chapter 16 and the Appendix.

Safety

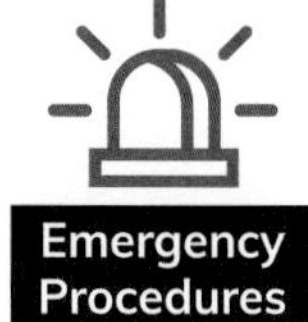

All exercise professionals should do what they can to minimize risk for everyone in the fitness facility. This includes having equipment that is properly spaced and in good working order; having racks, shelves, hooks, or other storage spots for portable equipment, including stability balls, dumbbells, and kettlebells; and ensuring that floors and equipment are cleaned, maintained, and free from clutter and moisture. Exercise professionals should also pay attention to the cleanliness of the facility, including the availability of wipes or other sterilizers for cleaning equipment following usage. An emergency plan, AED, and appropriate first-aid supplies are essential in the event an injury or incident occurs.

A personal trainer has additional client-specific risk-management responsibilities, beginning with the first meeting, when the personal trainer should conduct a health-history interview to determine whether the client requires a physician's referral prior to exercise or has limitations or **contraindications** for certain exercises. The personal trainer also needs to determine appropriate exercises and levels of intensity for initial exercise program design, as well as exercise program modifications. Then, by helping clients perform exercises in a safe and effective manner with proper progressions, the personal trainer can minimize the risk of injury and enhance the quality of service provided. Even with the best risk-management program, injuries and incidents can still occur. As such, ACE recommends that all ACE Certified Professionals carry professional liability insurance for protection in the event a client is injured during training (see Chapter 16).

Referral

It is important for healthcare professionals, including personal trainers, to understand their professional qualifications and boundaries, and to always refer clients who require services outside their scope of practice to the appropriately qualified healthcare professionals. Doing so ensures that clients are provided with appropriate care from well-qualified providers and prevents healthcare professionals from offering services that they do not have the education, training, credentials, and/or legal right to offer. Sometimes a personal trainer will need to investigate a bit further to determine if referral is warranted. For example, if a client wants to lose weight at a rate that is much faster than advisable for safe weight loss, the personal trainer can first explain healthy weight-loss rates and work with him or her to determine a safe and achievable goal. If the client is comfortable with this new goal, the personal trainer can design a program to help the client achieve it. However, if the client feels that he or she still wants to aim for the original weight-loss goal and timeline, the personal trainer should refer him or her to an RD, physician, or other appropriate healthcare professional.

Referrals can also come to the personal trainer from other health professionals. For example, a physician may provide a patient with exercise guidelines and then refer him or her to an ACE

Certified Personal Trainer for personalized exercise programming based on the physician's guidelines. In a situation like this, the personal trainer should provide the physician with a mutually agreed upon frequency of regular updates on the client's progress and program direction. It is always important for clients to be referred to the appropriate healthcare professional and for all health professionals involved to correspond regularly regarding each client's progress, provided they have the client's written permission to do so.

Supplements and Other Nutrition-related Concerns

Supplements are not regulated by the U.S. Food and Drug Administration (FDA) in the same way required for conventional food and drug products and the FDA is not authorized to evaluate supplements for effectiveness or safety before going to market. Unlike drugs, which need to be determined safe prior to going to market, supplements are deemed safe until proven unsafe. Therefore, their strength, purity, and effects are not guaranteed. Some supplements can cause adverse interactions and complications with other prescribed medications or congenital problems. Still, the supplement market constitutes a multibillion-dollar industry. The lure of this profitable revenue stream, coupled with consumer interest for a quick fix, leads some fitness facilities to sell nutritional supplements. It is not illegal for fitness facilities to sell commercial nutritional supplements, but it is irresponsible for them to provide supplement recommendations without staff that have the expertise and legal qualifications required to give such advice (e.g., RDs or physicians). Facilities selling dietary supplements are assuming liability risk in the event that a member has a negative reaction to a supplement recommended by a staff member who is not qualified (see Chapters 6 and 16).

Some personal trainers amass substantial knowledge about dietary supplements. However, they are no more qualified to recommend these supplements to clients than they are to recommend or prescribe medications. Unless a personal trainer also holds an appropriate nutrition-related credential, such as an RD or a physician, he or she does not have the expertise or legal qualifications necessary to recommend supplements. The ACE Position Statement on Nutrition Scope of Practice for Personal Trainers can be found in Chapter 6.

It is appropriate for personal trainers to educate themselves about supplements. Clients often ask personal trainers about supplements, thinking that supplements are necessary to achieve fitness, weight loss, or other goals. The personal trainer can help the client understand that fitness goals can be reached without supplements and that supplements can have negative and potentially harmful side effects. If a client insists on using dietary supplements, the personal trainer should refer the client to a qualified physician or RD for guidance.

Personal trainers not only can but *should* share general nonmedical nutrition information with their clients. Personal trainers provide an essential service to their clients, the industry, and the community at large when they are able to offer credible, practical, and relevant nutrition information to clients while staying within their professional scope of practice. It is within the scope of practice of all health and exercise professionals to share dietary advice endorsed or developed by the federal government, including the *Dietary Guidelines for Americans* (www.health.gov/dietaryguidelines) and the MyPlate recommendations (www.ChooseMyPlate.gov). It is essential that all ACE Certified Personal Trainers understand their nutrition-related scope of practice as defined in Chapter 6.

Ramifications of Offering Services Outside the Scope of Practice

To achieve their health and fitness goals, clients must adopt healthful behaviors that can include a regular exercise program, eating a more healthful diet, and initiating lifestyle changes to decrease stress. An ACE Certified Personal Trainer is qualified to help clients with comprehensive and personalized exercise programming needs, but the level of assistance the personal trainer can provide when it comes to nutrition, lifestyle, or post-rehabilitation programming can be confusing, especially to the newly certified personal trainer. The client scenarios in Table 1-3 are designed to provide personal trainers with a better understanding of services that are within and outside their scope of practice.

ACE Certified Professionals offering services that are within the legal realm of another healthcare profession are in violation of the ACE Code of Ethics and are at risk for potential legal ramifications. For example, if a client tells a personal trainer that he or she experiences muscle soreness following long training runs, the personal trainer can provide education about the benefits of massage, but cannot perform hands-on massage therapy for the client, as this would constitute the practice of massage without a license. All responses listed in Table 1-3 as "Inappropriate for an ACE Certified Personal Trainer" are examples of services that could result in an ACE Certified Personal Trainer facing legal ramifications, with possible prosecution for practicing other forms of medicine or healthcare without appropriate credentials.

TABLE 1-3

Appropriate Scope of Practice

Client Scenario	Inappropriate for an ACE Certified Personal Trainer	Appropriate for an ACE Certified Personal Trainer
Client stands with an exaggerated lordotic posture	Diagnosing the cause of the client's exaggerated lordosis	Implementing a core conditioning program to improve strength and flexibility imbalances in muscles acting on the hips and spine
Client wants to lose weight by trying the latest commercial diet	Helping the client to understand and implement the diet	Helping the client to make more healthful choices using the *Dietary Guidelines* and tools on www. ChooseMyPlate.gov
Client is cleared for exercise following physical therapy for rotator cuff impingement	Continuing with physical therapy exercises to treat shoulder impingement	Implementing exercises to improve shoulder stability and building on the work done in physical therapy
Client has tight iliotibial (IT) bands	Providing deep tissue massage to relieve tightness in the IT bands	Teaching the client self–myofascial release techniques for the IT bands using a foam roller
Client has soreness following a weekend tennis tournament	Recommending use of over-the-counter anti-inflammatory medications	Discussing proper techniques for performing light, dynamic stretching activities for the affected areas
Client tells you she is depressed due to problems with her spouse	Listening to the client and providing her with recommendations for improving the situation	Listening to the client with empathy and maintaining her confidentiality

The Healthcare Continuum

The healthcare continuum is composed of health professionals who are credentialed through certifications, registrations, and/or licensure and provide services to identify, prevent, and treat diseases and disorders. Physicians evaluate patients to diagnose ailments and implement treatment plans that can include medication, surgery, rehabilitation, or other actions. Physicians are assisted in their efforts by nurses, physician assistants, and other credentialed technicians. When ailments or treatment plans fall outside their areas of expertise, physicians refer patients to specialists for specific medical evaluations, physical or occupational therapy, psychological counseling, dietary planning, and/or exercise programming.

Physicians and nurses teach patients the importance of implementing their treatment plans. Physical therapists and **occupational therapists** lead patients through therapeutic exercise and teach them to perform additional exercises at home to facilitate rehabilitation. **Athletic trainers** primarily work with athletes to provide injury and illness prevention, emergency care, injury evaluation, and therapeutic exercises following injury. RDs assess nutritional needs and teach clients proper nutrition through meal plans, food-preparation methods, recipes, and implementation of specialized diets, especially in clinical settings. In addition to providing specialized care, healthcare professionals might also give patients or clients guidelines for general exercise (e.g., "try to walk up to 30 minutes per day, most days of the week"). However, few of them actually teach clients *how* to exercise effectively. This is where personal trainers hold a unique position on the healthcare continuum.

It is important that every personal trainer understands the role of exercise professionals in relation to the other members of the healthcare team (Figure 1-3). Each client will generally have a primary care physician who is responsible for his or her general medical care. If the

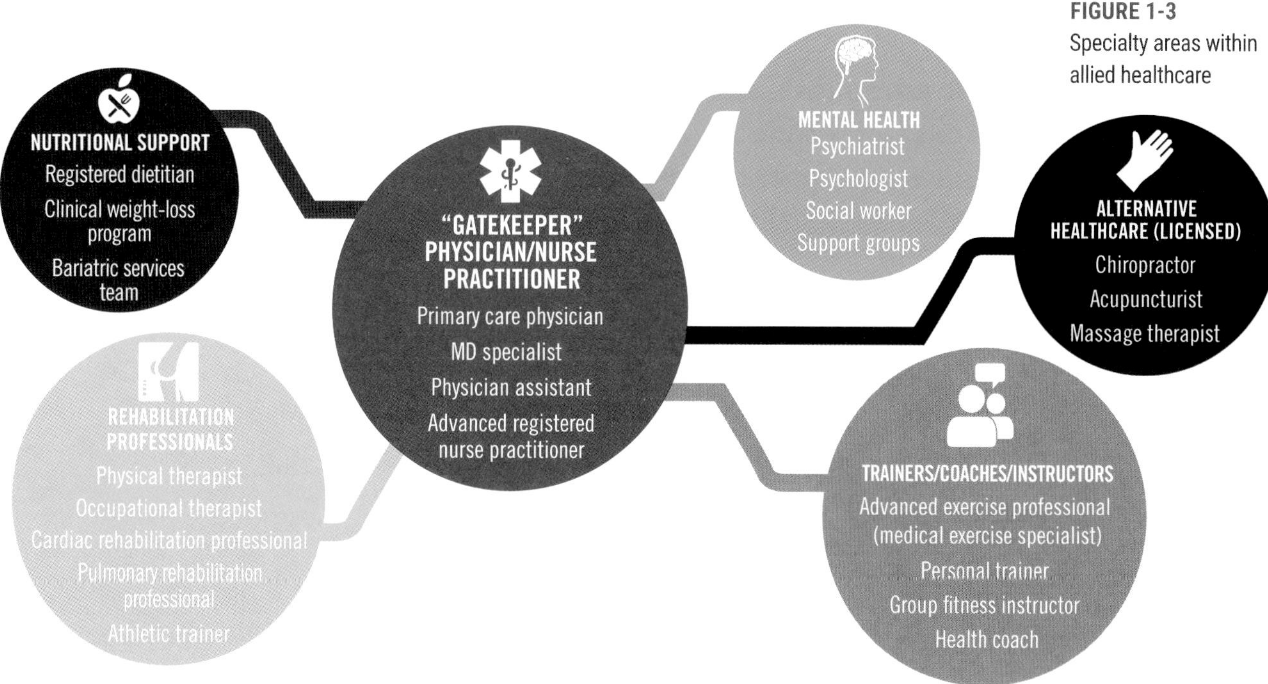

FIGURE 1-3
Specialty areas within allied healthcare

client is referred by his or her physician, the personal trainer should obtain written permission from the client to communicate with the referring physician to provide regular reports regarding the client's progress with the exercise program (see Chapter 16). Even when clients do not have a physician's referral, it is important for the personal trainer to maintain confidential records that include the client's program, progress, and health-history information.

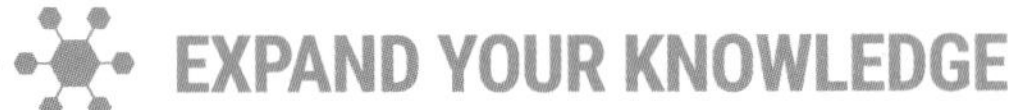

The Roles of Select Health, Wellness, and Exercise Professionals

While it is not necessary to memorize the details about each of the professionals listed here, understanding their roles will prove invaluable during a career as a personal trainer.

Acupuncturists

- Requirements for education and experience vary by state; a master's degree is the minimum requirement for national certification testing.
- The profession is regulated in most states.
- Acupuncturists stimulate specific points on the body using thin, sterile, stainless steel needles, electrical stimulation, acupressure, and other techniques to treat issues including chronic pain in the low-back, neck, and due to osteoarthritis.

Athletic Trainers

Athletic Trainer Certified (ATC):

- A baccalaureate-level degree with national certification
- The profession is regulated in most states.
- Responsibilities include injury prevention, emergency care, and therapeutic intervention; working with the team physician; and rehabilitation of injured players after athletic injury or post-surgery.

Chiropractors

Doctor of Chiropractic (DC):

- Post-baccalaureate degree program, typically four years in length
- A variety of different chiropractic philosophies and practices exist.
- DCs do not have prescription-writing or surgical privileges.

Dietitians

Registered Dietitian (RD) or Registered Dietitian Nutritionist (RDN):

- Requires a baccalaureate-level degree with clinical practicum and national certification testing
- Most states have laws regulating the practice of dietetics.
- Most RDs work in the treatment and prevention of disease in hospitals, health maintenance organizations, private practice, or other healthcare facilities.

Exercise Professionals

Exercise Professional:

- Specially trained in designing safe and effective personalized exercise programs, which may include personal training, group fitness instruction, or small-group training

- While a bachelor's degree is not required, many exercise professionals hold a degree in exercise science or a related discipline.
- The professional standard is current certification from a certification program accredited by the National Commission for Certifying Agencies (NCCA).

Exercise Physiologist:

- Allied health professional who holds an academic degree in exercise or applied physiology and is knowledgeable about the effects that exercise has on the musculoskeletal system, as well as on the cardiovascular and endocrine systems
- Trained to work with individuals with chronic diseases where exercise training has been shown to be of therapeutic benefit, including, but not limited to, cardiovascular disease, pulmonary disease, and metabolic disorders

Health Coaches

- Requirements for education, experience, and credentials vary by state and employer for this comparatively young profession.
- Allied health professional who helps clients identify and achieve desired health-behavior changes

Massage Therapists

- Requirements for education and experience vary by state; graduation from a 500-hour education program is required for national certification testing
- The profession is regulated in most states, with some regulation at the city and county levels.
- Massage therapists use touch to work on the muscles and other soft tissues to help release chronic muscle tension, relieve pain, reduce stress, and increase relaxation.

Medical Assistants

- Requirements for education and experience vary by state; typically, an associate-level degree with clinical practicum and national certification testing, though training can vary substantially and, in some cases, requires only a high-school diploma and on-the-job training.
- Blends administrative with clinical roles, mainly in outpatient clinics and medical offices

Mental Health Professionals

Psychiatrist:

- Medical doctor (MD) with post-graduate residency training in mental health care
- The only mental health professional who can prescribe medication

Psychologist–PhD or PsyD (doctor of psychology):

- Doctorate-level degree in psychology
- Psychologists receive specialized training in diagnosis, psychological assessment, psychotherapy, and research.
- Multiple subfields exist, including clinical, cognitive, community, counseling, developmental, educational, engineering, environmental, evolutionary, experimental, forensic, health, industrial/organizational, rehabilitation, school, and sports, among others.
- The scope of practice of a psychologist includes the diagnosis, prevention, treatment, and management of psychological problems and emotional and mental disorders of individuals and groups.

Clinical Social Worker—MSW (master's degree in social work) and LCSW (licensed clinical social worker) if psychotherapy is included within the scope of practice and state certification:

- Training programs require thousands of hours of direct clinical experience.
- Social workers help individuals and families in many capacities, including problem solving life situations and identifying community resources, as well as providing therapy for behavioral, emotional, and mental disorders such as anxiety and depression.

Licensed Professional Counselor (LPC) or Licensed Mental Health Counselor (LMHC):

- Baccalaureate- or master's-level degree in counseling or a related field, plus supervised clinical experience and a state certification, with variation by state
- Therapy is included within scope of practice.

Marriage and Family Therapist (MFT):

- Master's-level degree in most states, plus hundreds to thousands of hours of clinical experience, and licensure in some states
- Trained to assess, diagnose, and treat individuals, couples, families, and groups
- Therapy is included within scope of practice.

Nurses

Licensed Practical Nurse (LPN) or Licensed Vocational Nurse (LVN):

- Typically, an associate-level degree with clinical practicum

Registered Nurse (RN):

- Typically, an associate- or baccalaureate-level degree with clinical practicum and national certification testing, and licensure in all 50 states

Nurse Practitioner (NP):

- An advanced practice registered nurse with a graduate-level degree, typically requiring several years of practical clinical experience
- Able to prescribe some medications and practice somewhat independently, varying by state
- Nurse practitioners blend clinical expertise in diagnosing health conditions with emphasis on disease prevention and health management.

Doctorate of Nursing Practice (PhD or DNP):

- Doctoral degree in nursing

Occupational Therapists

Certified Occupational Therapy Assistant (COTA):

- Requires an associate-level degree with national certification
- The profession is regulated in most states.

Occupational Therapist Registered (OTR):

- Baccalaureate- or master's-level degree in an occupational therapy with national certification
- The profession is regulated in most states.
- OTRs treat injured or disabled individuals through the therapeutic use of everyday activities.

Doctor of Occupational Therapy (DrOT):

- A doctorate-level degree with a dissertation defense in occupational therapy

Physical Therapists

Physical Therapist (PT):

- A doctorate-level degree from an accredited physical therapist program required before taking the national licensure exam that allows them to practice; previously required only a bachelor's or master's degree
- PTs help injured people improve their movement and manage their pain, an important part of rehabilitation and treatment of individuals with chronic injury.

Physical Therapy Assistant (PTA):

- Have an associate-level degree and a national certification as a PTA.
- In some states, PTAs are required to have licensure to practice.

Doctor of Physical Therapy (DPT):

- A doctorate-level degree with a dissertation defense in physical therapy

Physicians

Doctor of Medicine (MD):

- Typically, four years of post-baccalaureate medical school and at least three years of postgraduate training upon completion of the degree, with licensure in all 50 states
- Able to prescribe medications and therapies
- May have admitting privileges at hospitals

Doctor of Osteopathy (DO):

- Same academic and clinical training as MDs, but also have instruction and practicum in osteopathic manipulation, which is the use of the hands to diagnose, treat, and prevent illness or injury

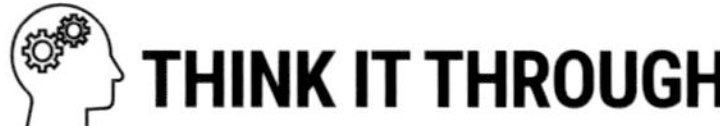

Developing Networking Skills

How comfortable are you with the notion, and actual process, of networking? Many people struggle when introducing themselves to strangers, actively promoting their services, and making those all-important professional connections. If this is an area of concern for you, how might you turn this hurdle into an opportunity? Do any of your clients or contacts work in healthcare? If so, you could ask them for advice, or even for a recommendation to talk with a healthcare professional near you.

Exercise Professionals in Allied Healthcare

Healthcare professionals recognize the important role that physical activity plays in improving and maintaining good health. Unfortunately, the lack of professional credentials held by some individuals working in the fitness industry has slowed the acceptance of exercise professionals as legitimate members of the allied healthcare team by some healthcare providers. As a result, ACE and other top professional fitness organizations have worked collaboratively to raise the standards of exercise professionals to better align with those seen in other allied health professions.

These efforts have been focused in the areas of certification program accreditation, establishing the United States Registry of Exercise Professionals, fitness facility standards for hiring exercise professionals who hold accredited certifications, and accreditation of exercise science academic programs.

ACCREDITATION OF EXERCISE PROFESSIONAL CERTIFICATION PROGRAMS

ACE and other top certification organizations in the fitness industry have earned third-party accreditation from the NCCA for their certification programs for exercise professionals. The NCCA is the accreditation body of the Institute for Credentialing Excellence (ICE) a nonprofit, 501(c)(3) organization that is a leading developer of standards for both certification and certificate programs. The NCCA *Standards for the Accreditation of Certification Programs*, developed and awarded by the credentialing industry, are considered the gold standard for certification program accreditation.

For a complete list of NCCA-accredited exercise professional certification programs, visit www.credentialingexcellence.org and search the NCCA Accredited Certification Programs directory under the Fitness and Wellness Industry.

The NCCA has reviewed and accredited the certification programs for most professions within allied healthcare. This includes the credentials for most nursing specialties, including nurse practitioners, oncology certified nurses, and nurse anesthetists, pharmacist specialties, RDs, occupational therapists, athletic trainers, acupuncturists, physician assistants, medical assistants, respiratory therapists, personal trainers, group fitness instructors, health coaches, and advanced exercise professionals. By earning NCCA accreditation for the ACE Personal Trainer, ACE Group Fitness Instructor, ACE Health Coach, and ACE Medical Exercise Specialist Certification programs, the American Council on Exercise has taken the professional and responsible steps necessary to help position ACE Certified Professionals as legitimate members of the healthcare continuum.

RECOGNITION FROM THE HEALTH AND FITNESS INDUSTRY

In the fitness industry, NCCA accreditation has become recognized as the third-party standard for accreditation of certifications for personal trainers and other exercise professionals, demonstrated by the following professional standards, guidelines, and recommendations:

- The Medical Fitness Association (2013), the professional membership organization for medically integrated health and fitness facilities, has made it a standard that medical fitness facilities hire exercise professionals who hold NCCA-accredited certifications.
- *ACSM's Health/Fitness Facility Standards and Guidelines* recommends that facilities hire only fitness directors, group exercise directors, program directors, personal trainers, exercise physiologists, and group exercise instructors who hold a certification from a nationally recognized certification program that has received third-party accreditation from an appropriate agency such as the NCCA [American College of Sports Medicine (ACSM), 2019].

In reference to the ACSM recommendation, the International Organization for Standardization (ISO) accreditation program for personnel certification bodies, titled ISO 17024, would be one other accreditation program for consideration.

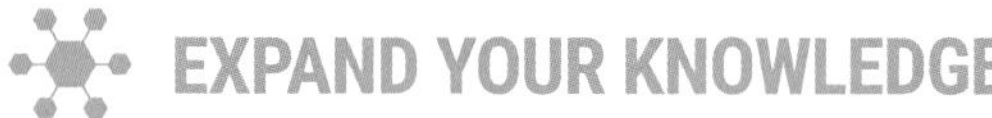

United States Registry of Exercise Professionals

The United States Registry of Exercise Professionals (USREPS) was established by the Coalition for the Registration of Exercise Professionals (CREP), a not-for-profit 501(c)(6) corporation comprised of organizations that offer NCCA-accredited certifications for exercise professionals. Coalition members are committed to advancing the exercise profession by securing recognition of exercise professionals registered on USREPS (www.usreps.org) for their distinct roles in medical, health, fitness, and sports performance fields. CREP is a primary advocate for exercise professionals who hold NCCA-accredited certifications on issues that pertain to regulation, access, and scope of work.

There are currently more than 175,000 well-qualified exercise professionals registered on USREPS. To be listed on USREPS, practitioners must hold a current NCCA-accredited exercise professional certification from a CREP member organization. USREPS is recognized internationally by the International Confederation of Registers for Exercise Professionals (ICREPs) (www.icreps.org) as the official registry of exercise professionals in the United States. ICREPs has created a global portability matrix to help exercise professionals earn any additional education or credentials they would need to join the registry and work in another ICREPs member country.

USREPS provides healthcare practitioners, insurance providers, policymakers, and employers a single source where they can find well-qualified exercise professionals in specific locations or verify multiple credentials from CREP member organizations held by an exercise professional. To stay on the registry, exercise professionals must maintain an NCCA-accredited certification from a CREP member organization.

RECOGNITION FROM THE EDUCATION COMMUNITY

The Commission on Accreditation of Allied Health Education Programs (CAAHEP)/Committee on Accreditation for the Exercise Sciences (CoAES) has established accreditations for two-year, four-year, and graduate-level academic programs in exercise science. The CAAHEP is the largest programmatic accreditor in the health sciences field. The CoAES was formed under the guidance and sponsorship of CAAHEP to establish standards that academic programs in kinesiology, physical education, and exercise science must meet to become accredited by CAAHEP (2013).

One of the primary outcomes assessed by the CAAHEP *Standards and Guidelines for the Accreditation of Educational Programs for Personal Fitness Training* is the students' performance on a national credentialing examination accredited by the NCCA. This recognition of NCCA-accredited personal trainer certifications as the standard for this outcome assessment is an important endorsement of the NCCA accreditation by the educational community. The ACE Personal Trainer Certification Program, with its NCCA accreditation, helps universities and colleges meet this outcome assessment standard for exercise science departments to earn accreditation from CAAHEP.

Career Development

It is important for every personal trainer to have a general idea of the career path that he or she wants to follow. Career paths can include becoming a fitness director or general manager of a fitness or wellness facility, opening a personal-training studio, opening a home-based personal-training business, or working part-time as a personal trainer. Career paths are personal. They

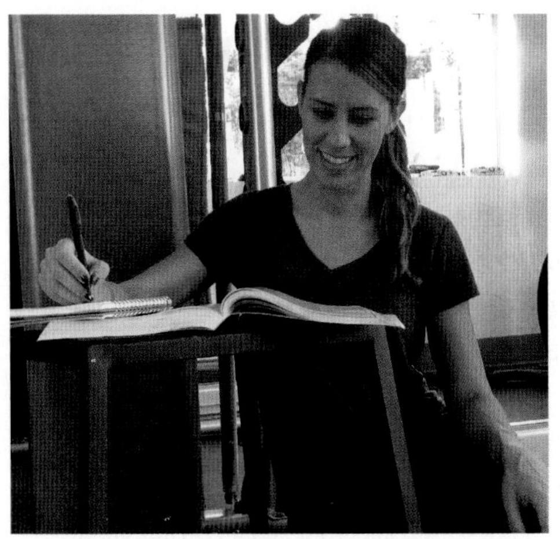

are based on the specific needs of the professional to meet his or her career objectives and must be balanced with other commitments.

Career paths should be viewed as guidelines to help exercise professionals reach career goals, with the flexibility to be modified as needed based on new clientele, changes in his or her personal life, industry recessions, and other important events. A career plan can help an exercise professional determine if continuing education or a new opportunity is in line with his or her goals. After setting a career plan, a personal trainer can use it as a template for researching and selecting continuing education to work toward his or her goals.

CONTINUING EDUCATION

ACE Certified Professionals are encouraged to select continuing education based on areas of interest, client needs, and desired career path. By completing continuing education in one or more areas of focus, a personal trainer can advance his or her career by becoming a specialist in areas such as weight management, youth fitness, sports performance, or senior fitness. This can help the personal trainer become recognized as an expert in a given field, attracting specific clientele and advancing his or her career. Factors that should be considered when selecting continuing education courses include checking if the course will be at the appropriate level for the exercise professional, seeing if the instructor has the appropriate qualifications to teach the course, learning if the course is approved by ACE for CECs or will have to be petitioned for CECs, and determining if the education provided is within the personal trainer scope of practice.

ACE Certified Professionals should select continuing education that will help advance their current knowledge, skills, and abilities, without being too advanced. The continuing education needs for a newly certified personal trainer and a personal trainer with 10 years of experience will be different. If these two professionals attend the same conference together, it would be beneficial for them to independently select sessions that meet their individual career paths and needs, rather than going to the same sessions and having the new personal trainer be overwhelmed by the advanced subject matter or the veteran not challenged by information that he or she already knows.

Continuing education should help the personal trainer work toward one or more career goals. For example, for a management-focused personal trainer, this could include taking business-management courses. It is also important for ACE Certified Professionals to stay current, as standards and guidelines are released based on new findings in exercise science and related healthcare research. A personal trainer can do this through continuing education courses or through his or her own research of the published scientific literature.

Specialization

Specialization is a great way for a personal trainer to become recognized as an expert for a particular type of training or client population. By gaining advanced knowledge and skills in a specialized area, a personal trainer can enhance the training services he or she provides to clients—and hopefully attract more clients seeking these specialty services. For example, a personal trainer who is interested in working with athletes might complete extensive continuing education in sports conditioning, possibly earning a specialty certificate in sports performance.

Areas of specialization should be selected by the personal trainer based on his or her desired career path, interests, and client base. The area of specialization should also fall within the scope of practice or provide the personal trainer with knowledge that is complementary to what he or she does within the scope of practice. For example, while a course on manual manipulations of the shoulder joint could be educational, it would provide therapeutic techniques that would be outside the defined scope of practice for personal trainers.

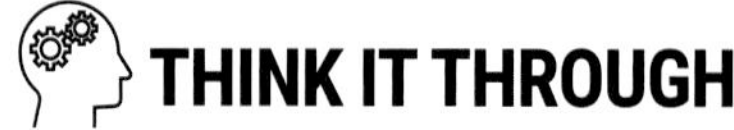

Finding a Niche

Although being able to effectively work with various types of clients can be rewarding for personal trainers, focusing on a certain population (e.g., youth, seniors, athletes, or individuals with obesity) can help personal trainers develop a niche, which gives them a competitive edge in the market. Which area of specialization would you most enjoy? If you decide to specialize, how would you approach getting the advanced continuing education required to become an expert in your area of specialization?

DEGREES

Having a degree in exercise science or a related field is not a requirement to earn an ACE Personal Trainer Certification or other NCCA-accredited personal-training certifications, but it can be helpful to the professional as he or she prepares for a certification exam. A majority of ACE Certified Professionals have four-year degrees, with many holding degrees in exercise science. Whether earned before or after becoming an ACE Certified Professional, a degree can prove helpful as personal trainers try to advance their careers into management or advanced positions within medical fitness or even education. For this reason, some personal trainers will decide years into their careers to earn a degree in exercise science, nutrition, business, or other subject area. Upon earning the degree, the personal trainer may advance his or her career, fulfill a personal goal, and earn ACE CECs for courses that provide education related to fitness and health.

NEW AREAS OF EXPERTISE WITHIN ALLIED HEALTHCARE

A personal trainer who wants to expand the services that he or she provides into another area of allied healthcare must earn the appropriate credentials to ethically and legally provide those services. This could include becoming a licensed massage therapist, earning a nutrition degree and becoming an RD, earning a doctorate in physical therapy and becoming a licensed physical therapist, going to medical school and becoming a medical doctor, or earning advanced exercise professional certifications. In these scenarios, the personal trainer earning the new credential will advance his or her career and expand the services that he or she can provide, becoming an advocate for exercise in his or her new professional arena.

ACE UNIVERSITY

If your study program includes the ACE University, visit www.ACEfitness.org/MyACE and log in to your My ACE Account to take full advantage of the ACE Personal Trainer Study Program and online guided study experience.

A variety of media to support and expand on the material in this text is provided to facilitate learning and best prepare you for the ACE Personal Trainer Certification exam and a career as a personal trainer.

SUMMARY

Understanding the ACE Certified Personal Trainer's scope of practice can be empowering, as it defines a unique profession dedicated to helping people improve their fitness, health, and quality of life through physical activity. Many of the professions in healthcare are devoted to *treating* disease, while a personal trainer primarily helps people *prevent* disease. In a society where almost two-thirds of the adult population has overweight and is insufficiently physically active, and youth are projected to possibly live shorter lives than their parents, the role that ACE Certified Personal Trainers play as part of the healthcare continuum has never been more important.

REFERENCES

American College of Sports Medicine (2019). *ACSM's Health/Fitness Facility Standards and Guidelines* (5th ed.). Champaign, Ill.: Human Kinetics.

Blair, S.N. (2009). Physical inactivity: The biggest public health problem of the 21st century. *British Journal of Sports Medicine*, 43, 1–2.

Bryant, C.X. et al. (2017). *Mobilizing Healthcare to Help More Americans Achieve Physical-activity Guidelines to Improve Outcomes and Reduce Health Disparities* [White Paper]. www.prescriptionforactivity.org

Bureau of Labor Statistics, U.S. Department of Labor (2018). *Occupational Outlook Handbook, Fitness Trainers and Instructors.* https://www.bls.gov/ooh/personal-care-and-service/fitness-trainers-and-instructors.htm

Commission on Accreditation of Allied Health Education Programs (2013). *Standards and Guidelines for the Accreditation of Educational Programs for Personal Fitness Training.* http://www.coaes.org/wp-content/uploads/2019/02/PFTStandards2013.pdf

Dunstan, D.W., Thorp, A.A., & Healy, G.N. (2011). Prolonged sitting: Is it a distinct coronary heart disease risk factor? *Current Opinion in Cardiology*, 26, 5, 412–419.

Guthold, R. et al. (2018). Worldwide trends in insufficient physical activity from 2001 to 2016: A pooled analysis of 358 population-based surveys with 1.9 million participants. *Lancet Global Health*, 6, 10, 1077–1086.

Kochanek, K.D. et al. (2017). *Mortality in the United States, 2016. NCHS Data Brief, No. 293.* Hyattsville, Md: National Center for Health Statistics.

Lozano, R. et al. (2012). Global and regional mortality from 235 causes of death for 20 age groups in 1990 and 2010: A systematic analysis for the Global Burden of Disease Study 2010. *The Lancet*, 380, 9859, 2095–2128.

Mandsager, K. et al. (2018). Association of cardiorespiratory fitness with long-term mortality among adults undergoing exercise treadmill testing. *JAMA Network Open*, 1, 6, e183605.

Medical Fitness Association (2013). *MFA's Standards & Guidelines for Medical Fitness Center Facilities* (2nd ed.). Monterey, Calif.: Healthy Learning.

U.S. Department of Agriculture (2015). *2015-2020 Dietary Guidelines for Americans* (8th ed.). www.health.gov/dietaryguidelines

U.S. Department of Health & Human Services (2018). *Physical Activity Guidelines for Americans* (2nd ed.). https://health.gov/paguidelines/second-edition/pdf/Physical_Activity_Guidelines_2nd_edition.pdf

World Health Organization (2017). *Health Systems: Equity.* www.who.int/healthsystems/topics/equity/en/

World Health Organization (2018a). *Noncommunicable Diseases.* https://www.who.int/news-room/fact-sheets/detail/noncommunicable-diseases

World Health Organization (2018b). *Global Action Plan on Physical Activity 2018-2030: More Active People for a Healthier World.* https://apps.who.int/iris/bitstream/handle/10665/272722/9789241514187-eng.pdf

SUGGESTED READINGS

American Council on Exercise (2018). *ACE Certification Candidate Handbook.* https://acewebcontent.azureedge.net/assets/certification/pdfs/Certification-Exam-Candidate-Handbook.pdf

American Council on Exercise (2018). *ACE Recertification Handbook.* https://acewebcontent.azureedge.net/assets/certification/pdfs/Recertification_Handbook_2018.pdf

U.S. Department of Health & Human Services (2003). *Summary of the HIPAA Privacy Rule.* https://www.hhs.gov/sites/default/files/privacysummary.pdf

ADDITIONAL RESOURCES

U. S. Registry of Exercise Professionals (USREPS)/ Coalition for the Registration of Exercise Professionals (CREP): www.usreps.org

Institute for Credentialing Excellence (ICE)/National Commission for Certifying Agencies (NCCA): www.credentialingexcellence.org

International Health, Racquet, and Sportsclub Association: www.ihrsa.org

Medical Fitness Association: www.medicalfitness.org

Medline Plus Reference on Drugs and Supplements (A service of the National Library of Medicine and National Institutes of Health): www.medlineplus.gov

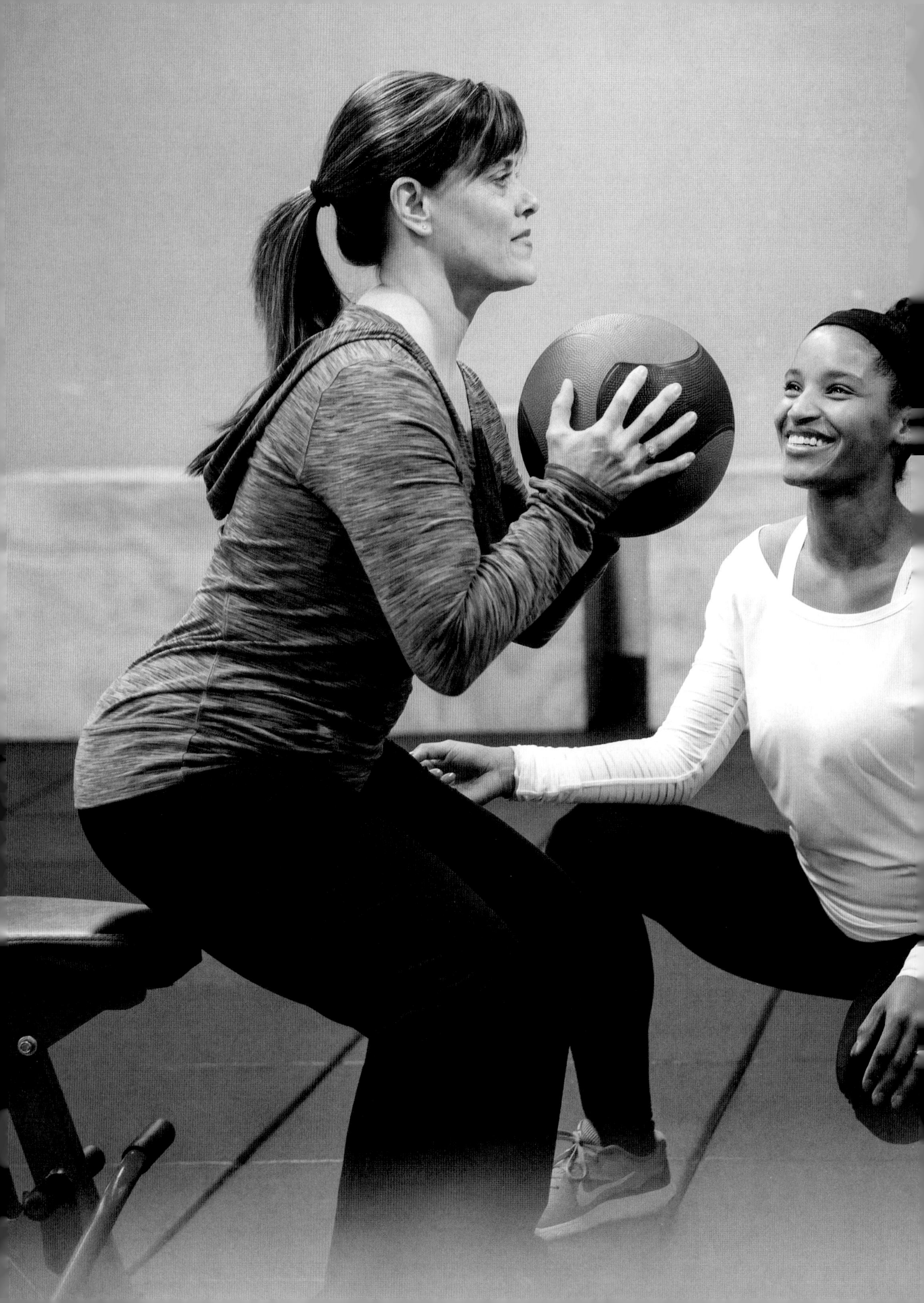

CHAPTER 2

The ACE Integrated Fitness Training® Model

TODD GALATI, MA

Senior Director, Standards and Practice Advancement, American Council on Exercise; ACE® Certified Personal Trainer, Medical Exercise Specialist, Health Coach, and Group Fitness Instructor

IN THIS CHAPTER

LEARNING OBJECTIVES:

Upon completion of this chapter, the reader will be able to:

- Discuss traditional versus contemporary training parameters
- Explain the function–health–fitness–performance continuum
- Demonstrate a basic understanding of the training components of the ACE Integrated Fitness Training Model
- Describe the ACE Mover Method™ and its application to personal training
- List key findings from research on the effectiveness of a personalized training program following the ACE Integrated Fitness Training Model versus a standardized training program

ACE UNIVERSITY

If your study program includes the ACE University, visit www.ACEfitness.org/MyACE and log in to your My ACE Account to take full advantage of the ACE Personal Trainer Study Program and online guided study experience.

A variety of media to support and expand on the material in this text is provided to facilitate learning and best prepare you for the ACE Personal Trainer Certification exam and a career as a personal trainer.

During the past 30 years, personal training has evolved from an occupation focused largely on improving the fitness of clients who are often already fit to a profession that plays a key role on the healthcare continuum by helping an aging and increasingly inactive and **overweight** population to improve function, health, fitness, and quality of life through exercise and related health-behavior changes. As a result, personal trainers must now be prepared to work with a diverse population of clients with a varied list of unique health issues that can often be improved by regular physical activity.

Fortunately, exercise science research and industry guidelines have kept pace with this increased demand, providing specialized evidence-based programming options for a variety of health issues. ACE Certified Personal Trainers can put these concepts into action by developing personalized programs that help clients enhance function for **activities of daily living (ADL)**; lose weight to positively affect metabolic function; develop good movement patterns to avoid injury and improve postural fitness; enhance **cardiorespiratory fitness** to improve heart health, longevity, endurance, and performance; and increase muscular development to bolster strength, **balance, speed,** and **power.**

At the same time, advancements in health coaching and behavioral science have resulted in knowledge, skills, and abilities that personal trainers can apply to help build client **self-efficacy** and fuel exercise program **adherence.** This has led to advances in personal training that have shifted the focus from more traditional training parameters to greater emphasis on contemporary training parameters, resulting in a client-centered approach to exercise programming to effectively address each client's needs and goals (Table 2-1).

TABLE 2-1
Traditional Training Parameters versus Contemporary Training Parameters

Traditional Training Parameters	Contemporary Training Parameters	
Cardiorespiratory (aerobic) fitness Muscular endurance Muscular strength Flexibility	Health-behavior change Postural (kinetic chain) stability Kinetic chain mobility Movement efficiency Core conditioning Balance Cardiorespiratory (aerobic and anaerobic) fitness	Metabolic markers (ventilatory thresholds) Muscular endurance Muscular strength Flexibility Agility, coordination, and reaction time Speed and power

Exercise professionals are well aware that the benefits of exercise include improved health, fitness, mood, weight management, stress management, and other health-related parameters. The *Physical Activity Guidelines for Americans* reinforce these positive benefits by acknowledging that regular exercise is a critical component of good health and that individuals can reduce their risk of developing **chronic disease** by staying physically active and

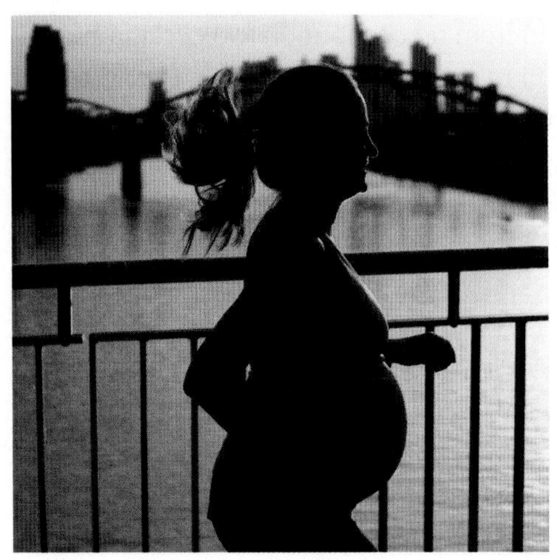

participating in structured exercise on a regular basis (U.S. Department of Health & Human Services, 2018).

The second edition of the *Physical Activity Guidelines for Americans* expand on the previous edition by providing key guidelines for preschool-aged children, children and adolescents, adults, older adults, women during pregnancy and the postpartum period, adults with chronic health conditions, and adults with disabilities. The key guidelines suggest that adults should move more and sit less throughout the day. For substantial health benefits, adults should do at least 150 minutes a week of moderate-intensity cardiorespiratory physical activity, 75 minutes a week of vigorous-intensity aerobic physical activity, or an equivalent combination of the two (U.S. Department of Health & Human Services, 2018). In addition, adults should participate in muscle-strengthening activities of at least moderate intensity, involving all major muscle groups, on two or more days per week (U.S. Department of Health & Human Services, 2018). While the latest *Guidelines* endorse exercise as a means to achieving good health, they do not provide specific instructions for *how* to exercise.

The American College of Sports Medicine (ACSM, 2018) publishes general evidence-based recommendations for cardiorespiratory exercise (noted as cardiovascular endurance exercise in its publication) and muscular-training exercise (noted as resistance training it its publication). While these guidelines provide broad ranges for exercise frequency, intensity, time, type, volume, pattern, and progression (FITT-VP), they do not provide specific instructions for *how* to exercise. In addition, there are exercise guidelines for many specific groups, including youth, older adults, women during pregnancy and the postpartum period, and people who have **obesity, hypertension, hyperlipidemia, osteoporosis,** and a variety of other chronic disease conditions and health considerations (see Chapters 12 through 15). These guidelines are based on medical and scientific research, are published by the governing body for each respective group, and provide specific exercise recommendations to help individuals engage in activity safely and effectively in order to improve their health and quality of life.

So how does a personal trainer pull it all together? How does a novice or even an experienced personal trainer know what type of initial exercise program is appropriate for each client, if and when fitness assessments are beneficial, how to address foundational movement, balance, or postural issues, and how to progress or modify a program based on observed and reported feedback? To address these questions and more, the American Council on Exercise® (ACE) developed the ACE Integrated Fitness Training (ACE IFT®) Model to provide personal trainers with a systematic and comprehensive approach to training that integrates exercise programming and progressions with a client-centered approach to facilitate health-behavior changes, while also improving posture, movement, **flexibility,** balance, core function, cardiorespiratory fitness, and **muscular fitness** (**muscular strength** and **muscular endurance**). To gain an understanding of the ACE IFT Model, it is helpful to first review the full continuum of human movement and fitness.

Function–Health–Fitness–Performance Continuum

The function–health–fitness–performance continuum is based on the premise that human movement and fitness can progress and regress along a spectrum that starts with developing or reestablishing basic functional movements and extends to performing highly advanced and specialized motions and physical work seen in athletics (Figure 2-1). Each individual is at a unique point on this continuum based upon factors that include health status and physical limitations; frequency, intensity, and types of physical activities; and any participation in, and goals for, athletic performance. Both lifecycle and lifestyle factors can influence where an individual currently falls on the continuum.

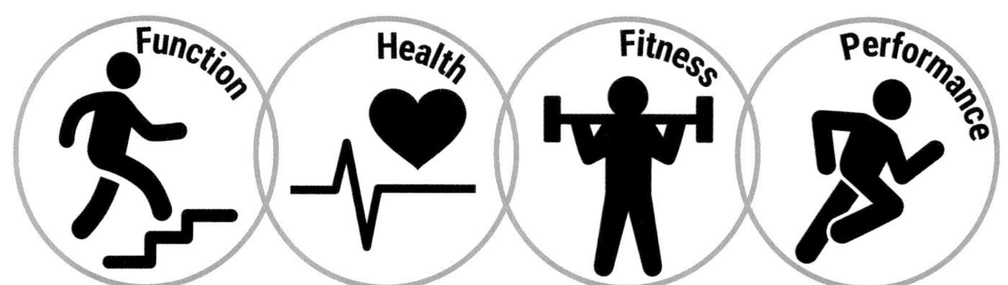

FIGURE 2-1 The function–health–fitness–performance continuum

Lifecycle factors include infant and child development, adolescent and pubescent growth spurts, adulthood, pregnancy, and aging. Early child development is focused primarily on gaining the strength, **stability,** and balance to perform basic human functional movements like holding one's head up, rolling over, sitting, crawling, standing, and eventually taking first steps. As children grow, their movements help them to build healthier bodies and develop the fitness to jump, climb, and run longer and faster. As adolescents and teens, human development includes considerable skeletal growth and muscular development. This developmental progression helps people progress from low-functioning infants to young adults who have good health, fitness, and even some performance-related skills and abilities. Unfortunately, far too often lifestyle factors (e.g., smoking, excessive alcohol consumption, poor nutrition, and inadequate sleep and physical activity) disrupt natural human development, resulting in individuals regressing along the continuum to where they are less fit, are at risk for, or have, chronic disease and other health issues, and may even have impaired functional movement.

While the function–health–fitness–performance continuum is not a training method, personal trainers can utilize this concept to understand that clients ebb and flow along this continuum based on the lifecycle and lifestyle factors that are impacting, positively or negatively, their opportunities for, and participation in, physical activity. Personal trainers can help clients progress along this continuum by meeting them where they are and providing personalized exercise programs and coaching based on each client's current health, fitness, and goals.

A personal trainer working with a client who has difficulties performing ADL should first establish goals aimed at helping the client improve basic functional movements. If a client has been insufficiently active for an extended period or is at risk for health issues, the personal trainer should provide the client with personalized programming that improves both health and functional movements. Personal trainers working with clients who have adequate functional movements and health can help them to improve fitness and, if appropriate, incorporate performance-related exercises.

Introduction to the ACE Integrated Fitness Training Model

Meeting each client's personalized needs can be a welcome challenge for an experienced personal trainer—and at the same time a potentially confusing and frustrating endeavor for a newly certified exercise professional. While the function–health–fitness–performance continuum provides a suggested sequence for training clients ranging from physically inactive to performance-oriented, it does not address the individual components of fitness and how they fit together.

The ACE IFT Model is a comprehensive system for exercise programming that pulls together the multifaceted training parameters required to be a successful personal trainer. It organizes the latest exercise science and health-behavior research into a systematic approach to designing, implementing, and modifying exercise programs based on the unique abilities, needs, and goals of each individual. Since its launch in 2010, the ACE IFT Model has evolved to incorporate new evidence-based practices in fitness assessments, exercise programming, and coaching skills. It has also evolved, based on user feedback, into a model that is just as robust in terms of science, content, and comprehensive programming, while being simplified in its presentation and terminology.

The ACE IFT Model has two training components:

- Cardiorespiratory Training
- Muscular Training

Each training component has three phases that are named to accurately reflect the training focus of each phase (Figure 2-2). The two training components of the ACE IFT Model are structured based on evidence-based exercise programming and progressions, and associated fitness and functional assessments, that produce physiological adaptations to exercise that improve function, health, fitness, and performance. The training components are independent

FIGURE 2-2
ACE Integrated Fitness Training Model

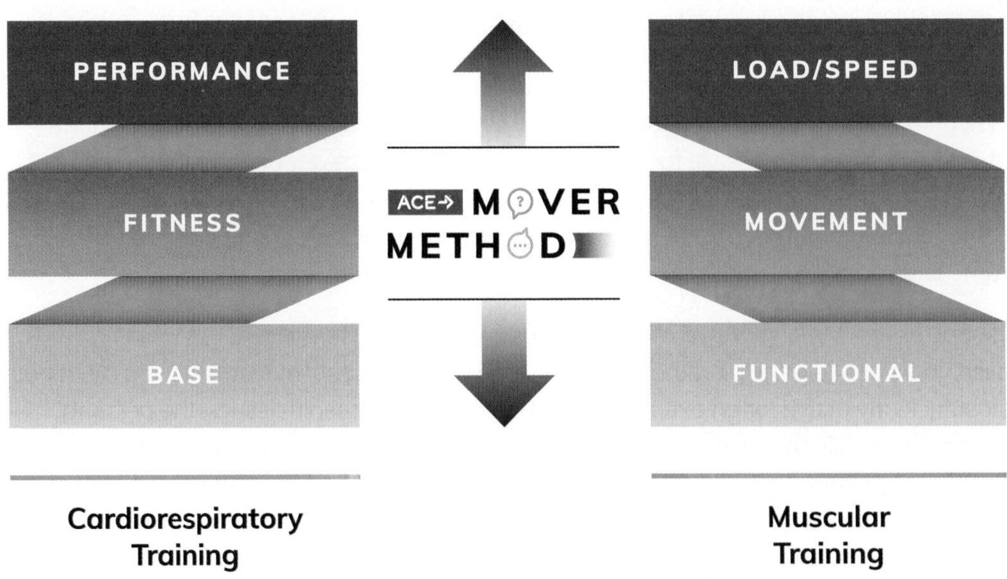

of each other, allowing for the integration of any Cardiorespiratory Training phase with any Muscular Training phase to meet the personalized health and fitness goals of each client. This adaptable programming allows the ACE IFT Model to be used with everyone from **previously physically inactive** clients who have limited exercise experience to high-performance endurance athletes who have poor postural stability and seasoned weight lifters who have low cardiorespiratory fitness.

The ACE IFT Model also provides exercise professionals with tools and methods to help clients make fitness-related behavior changes that facilitate physical-activity participation and adherence to make lasting improvements in health and well-being. The ACE IFT Model is introduced here and detailed further in Chapters 8 through 11.

A CLIENT-CENTERED APPROACH TO PERSONAL TRAINING

The greatest impact that personal trainers can regularly have on the lives of their clients is to help them to positively change health-related behaviors and establish positive relationships with exercise. For this reason, the client–personal trainer relationship is the foundation of the ACE IFT Model. It is built upon **rapport,** trust, and **empathy,** with the personal trainer serving as a "coach" to the client throughout his or her physical activity and health behavior-change journey. This approach starts with realizing that the "client" is the first person in the client–personal trainer relationship. Clients are paying the personal trainer for an important service: to guide them through a personalized journey to improve health and fitness and to reach their unique goals.

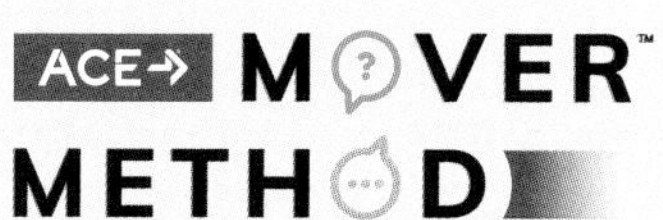

Introducing the ACE Mover Method Philosophy and ACE ABC Approach™

A key element of using the ACE IFT Model to empower clients to make behavioral changes to improve their health, fitness, and overall quality of life is the adoption of the ACE Mover Method, which is founded on the following tenets:

- Each professional interaction is client-centered, with a recognition that clients are the foremost experts on themselves.
- Powerful open-ended questions and active listening are utilized in every session with clients.
- Clients are genuinely viewed as resourceful and capable of change.

ACE→ ABC APPROACH™

Exercise professionals can easily apply the ACE Mover Method through the ACE ABC Approach:

- Ask open-ended questions
- Break down barriers
- Collaborate

Every client–personal trainer interaction offers an opportunity to utilize coaching skills to help build rapport while positioning the client as an active partner in his or her behavior-change journey. Asking questions leads to the identification of goals and options for breaking down barriers, which in turn leads to collaborating on next steps. The ACE Mover Method provides the foundational skills for communicating effectively with clients, but it is not the equivalent of a health coaching certification. Personal trainers should work in concert with other professionals, such as health coaches and **registered dietitians** and other allied health professionals whenever appropriate, to take a team approach to improving their clients' health and wellness.

Step 1 of this process involves asking powerful questions to identify what the client hopes to accomplish by working with an exercise professional and what, if any, physical activities the client enjoys. Open-ended questions are the key to sparking this discussion.

Step 2 involves asking more questions to discover what potential barriers may get in the way of the client reaching his or her specific goals. Questions like "What do you need to *start* doing now to move closer to your goals?" and "What do you need to stop doing that will enable you to reach your goals?" can be very revealing.

Step 3 is all about collaboration as the client and exercise professional work together to set **SMART goals** and establish specific steps to take action toward those goals. Allowing the client to lead the discussion of how to monitor and measure progress empowers him or her to take ownership of their personal behavior-change journey.

Throughout this textbook, look for ACE Mover Method features to learn more about effective strategies for employing a client-centered approach to personal training.

Clients want to know that their personal trainer cares about them. This is similar to what individuals seek when hiring the services of other professionals who have an impact on their quality of life, and it is at the heart of a client-centered approach to personal training. From physicians to financial planners, people will continue to work with the same professional if they can see that the professional truly cares about them and their health, whether it be physical or financial. Clients should already have a belief that the personal trainer they hire has the knowledge, skills, and abilities to help them reach their goals. With rare exception, they do not care to hear *all* the science, training methods, and other health-related information that the personal trainer knows. Instead, they want to hear that their personal trainer is invested in them. Successful personal

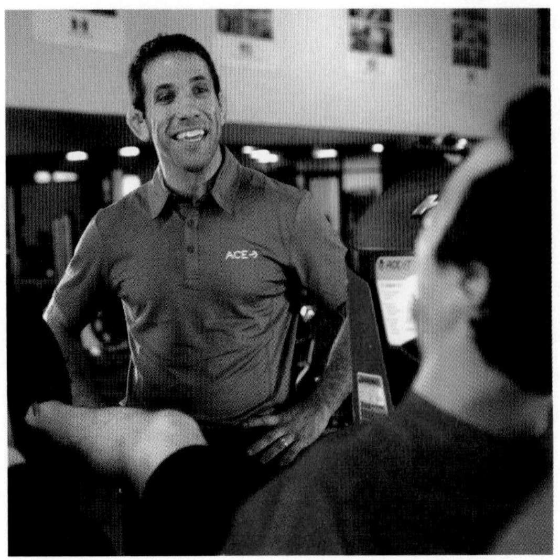

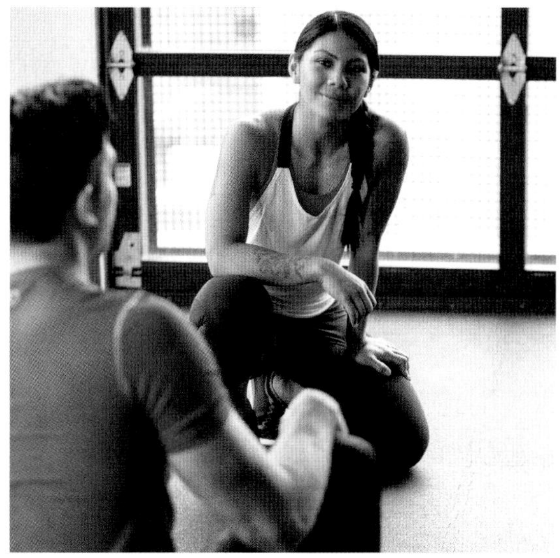

trainers keep the conversation focused on the client. They have paid for the session, so it is their time.

Building rapport is a critical component of a client-centered approach, as this process promotes open communication, develops trust, and fosters the client's desire to participate in an exercise program. Rapport should be developed early through open communication and initial positive experiences with exercise, and then enhanced through behavioral strategies that help build long-term adherence. The components of, and techniques for, open communication, rapport development, and the facilitation of program adherence that are part of a client-centered approach to personal training are presented in Chapters 3 through 5.

A primary goal of every personal-training session should be to have the client wanting to return for the next session. Starting with the first session, the personal trainer should include exercise programming that provides an appropriate level of challenge for the client at that time. Exercises and intensities should provide an adequate yet achievable level of challenge, and progressions should be appropriately matched to the gains that the client has made since the last session.

Fitness assessments, once thought to be a mandatory starting point for any exercise program, are not actually necessary for many clients. This should not be confused with health screening, which should be conducted with each client to determine if he or she has any limitations for, or should receive medical clearance prior to, exercise participation (see Chapter 5). Before conducting a fitness assessment with a client, it is important to determine if the assessment is necessary to help the client reach his or her goals, and if the client is interested in completing the fitness assessment.

The ACE IFT Model provides personal trainers with the option to either conduct evidence-based fitness assessments or lead clients through early sessions that incorporate exercise programming that delivers appropriate movement and fitness challenges while also providing the personal trainer with valuable feedback about a client's current postural stability, joint **mobility,** functional movement, balance, cardiorespiratory fitness, and muscular fitness. Early training sessions that include exercises that provide "assessment" information can be the key to success for many clients by helping them to get moving right away. They also provide the personal trainer with useful information to help him or her modify each client's program during subsequent sessions to build on that success. Exercises and exercise sequences that can be used for both training sessions and client assessments using the ACE IFT Model are presented, along with evidence-based fitness assessments, in Chapters 7 through 11.

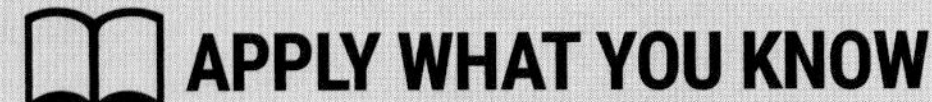

APPLY WHAT YOU KNOW

Facilitating Behavior Change

Applying behavior-change strategies in the design and delivery of comprehensive exercise programs that help clients reach their unique fitness and wellness goals is a primary function performed by successful personal trainers. Some of the key steps that facilitate fitness-related health-behavior change include:

- Implementing strategies for developing and enhancing rapport
- Identifying each client's readiness to change behavior and stage of behavior change (see Chapter 3)
- Creating a caring, supportive climate in which a client's motivation can flourish
- Fostering exercise adherence by creating positive exercise experiences that build self-efficacy
- Determining the need for, and appropriate selection and timing of, assessments and reassessments
- Designing, leading, and modifying exercise programs based on each client's current health and fitness status, needs, and goals
- Fostering a sense of self-reliance to empower clients to take ownership of their lifestyle changes
- Utilizing appropriate strategies to help clients transition from one stage of behavior change to the next
- Implementing **relapse**-prevention strategies
- Helping clients transition from **extrinsic motivation** to **intrinsic motivation**
- Establishing realistic short- and long-term goals to prevent discouragement and/or burnout, providing multiple opportunities for success and promoting adherence
- Factoring a client's external stressors into total fatigue to avoid training plateaus and prevent **overtraining syndrome**
- Empowering clients by helping them increase self-efficacy and knowledge to train on their own
- Supporting clients in making physical activity a life-long habit

CARDIORESPIRATORY TRAINING

The ACE IFT Model provides a systematic approach to cardiorespiratory training that can help move a client all the way from being physically inactive to training for a personal record in an event like a half marathon. While this will not be a training goal of most previously physically inactive individuals, having an organized system of training that can allow for long-term progression is empowering for personal trainers because it provides them with strategies for training the entire spectrum of clientele—from the physically inactive person to the competitive athlete.

The Cardiorespiratory Training component of the ACE IFT Model is divided into three phases, each with a title that defines its training focus (Figure 2-3).

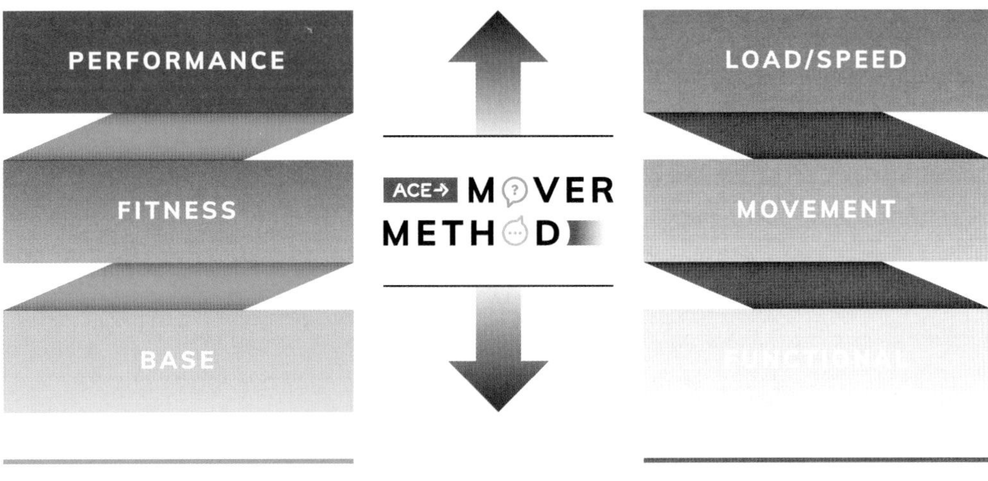

FIGURE 2-3
ACE IFT Model Cardiorespiratory Training phases

An overview of the primary objectives of Base, Fitness, and Performance Training follows, with detailed information about cardiorespiratory assessments and programming associated with each training phase presented in Chapter 8.

Base Training

Base Training is focused on developing an initial aerobic base in clients who have been insufficiently active. This should not be confused with the "aerobic-base training" that is performed by endurance athletes as the foundation of their offseason training. Instead, it is focused on getting people to move consistently to establish basic cardiorespiratory endurance to improve health, energy, mood, and caloric expenditure and to serve as a foundation for progressing to Fitness Training.

Any client who is not consistently performing moderate-intensity cardiorespiratory exercise for bouts of at least 20 minutes on at least three days per week should begin with Base Training. The initial cardiorespiratory exercise performed should be of an appropriate duration and intensity that the client can tolerate. Personal trainers can learn about their clients' current cardiorespiratory exercise participation during the investigation stage of the client–personal trainer relationship (see Chapter 5). No cardiorespiratory assessments are recommended during the Base Training phase, since many of the clients who start in this phase will be unfit and may have difficulty completing an assessment of this nature.

A client who has been physically inactive for an extended period might only be able to initially perform five minutes of continuous cardiorespiratory exercise at a moderate or low-to-moderate intensity. In a scenario of this nature, the personal trainer should give the client positive feedback for completing the five-minute exercise bout, remind the client that bouts of physical activity of any length are beneficial in reducing health risks, and document the total time completed. This would serve as the client's baseline cardiorespiratory fitness data and the starting point for Cardiorespiratory Training progressions to build an aerobic base.

Regardless of the initial duration, the goal for all clients in Base Training is to create early positive exercise experiences to help clients become regular exercisers while gradually increasing exercise duration and frequency until the client is performing cardiorespiratory exercise three to five days per week for a duration of 20 minutes or more. The easiest method for monitoring intensity with clients during Base Training is to use the **talk test.** If the client can perform the exercise and talk comfortably, he or she is likely below the **first ventilatory threshold (VT1).** By exercising below VT1, clients should be exercising at a moderate intensity classified by a **rating of perceived exertion (RPE)** of 3 to 4 (0 to 10 scale) (see Chapter 8).

Fitness Training

Fitness Training is focused on enhancing the client's aerobic efficiency by progressing the program through increased duration of sessions, increased frequency of sessions when possible, and the integration of exercise performed at and above VT1 (see Table 2-2, page 45). The inclusion of cardiorespiratory exercise performed at and above VT1 allows personal trainers to blend moderate-intensity exercise (below VT1) with moderate to vigorous-intensity exercise (at or above VT1 to just below VT2; RPE = 5 to 6 on the 0 to 10 scale) in a client's program to create variety and facilitate physiological adaptations leading to greater cardiorespiratory fitness levels. Both new and existing clients who can consistently perform moderate-intensity physical activity for bouts of 20 minutes or more on at least three days per week can perform Fitness Training. As with Base Training, the initial Fitness Training program should be performed at an appropriate duration, intensity, and frequency for the client based on his or her current level of exercise participation.

Personal trainers can incorporate intervals into exercise programs for clients with Fitness Training goals to add variety to individual sessions and to introduce more intense training stimuli to elicit desired physiological adaptations to exercise. Personal trainers should keep in mind each client's current cardiorespiratory fitness level when selecting interval intensities and durations to ensure that the increased challenge is appropriate for the client. By providing clients with intervals that offer increased yet achievable challenges, personal trainers can help their clients simultaneously increase fitness and self-efficacy.

Individual goals for Fitness Training will vary greatly among clients. Those looking to improve fitness and overall health can benefit from increased exercise frequency, duration, and the introduction of intervals. Clients with goals for longer endurance events, such as completing a 10K run or a half marathon, will need to include some exercise sessions of longer duration to reach the total exercise duration required to complete the event. Personal trainers can help each client work toward his or her unique goals by manipulating training variables and then adjusting them regularly based on the client's progress, recovery, challenges, and timeline. Many clients will spend years focused on various cardiorespiratory goals within Fitness Training, while those with endurance performance–oriented goals should be progressed to Performance Training.

Performance Training

Individuals who progress to Performance Training will have goals that are focused on success in endurance sports and events. This may include achieving a personal record in a cycling, swimming, or rowing event, running a local marathon in a time that qualifies them for a national-level event, or finishing top-five at a state or national championship. In these examples, the training programs will progress beyond the parameters of fitness to focus on performance through increased speed, power, and endurance.

Performance Training requires adequate training volume to prepare clients to comfortably complete their events. This is only the first step, as clients focused on Performance Training will have goals that go far beyond simply finishing an event. To help them achieve higher-level performance goals, personal trainers will want to continue building on the moderate- and vigorous-intensity exercise in their programs while integrating intervals that push clients up to and beyond the **second ventilatory threshold (VT2)**, where efforts are of very high intensity (RPE = 7 to 10 on the 0 to 10 scale) and short duration.

Personal trainers can help clients advance their endurance performance by designing programs that include periodized training plans with each day's training focused on specific variables such as distance, recovery, increased speed, or improved power. Periodized training plans allow personal trainers to manipulate key training variables, including total training volume, as well as frequency and duration of intervals performed both between VT1 and just below VT2 and at or above VT2, to help each client reach his or her unique performance goals. As a client's total weekly training time increases, a greater percentage of his or her training time will typically be at moderate intensities to accommodate the increased training volume and to allow for recovery from higher-intensity interval-training sessions.

Table 2-2 provides a summary of the three phases of Cardiorespiratory Training.

TABLE 2-2
Cardiorespiratory Training

Base Training	▸ Focus on moderate-intensity cardiorespiratory exercise (RPE = 3 to 4), while keeping an emphasis on enjoyment. ▸ Keep intensities below the talk-test threshold (below VT1). ▸ Increase duration and frequency of exercise bouts. ▸ Progress to Fitness Training when the client can complete at least 20 minutes of cardiorespiratory exercise below the talk test threshold.
Fitness Training	▸ Progress cardiorespiratory exercise duration and frequency based on the client's goals and available time. ▸ Integrate vigorous-intensity (RPE = 5 to 6) cardiorespiratory exercise intervals with segments performed at intensities below, at, and above VT1 to just below VT2.
Performance Training	▸ Progress moderate- and vigorous-intensity cardiorespiratory exercise. ▸ Program sufficient volume for the client to achieve goals. ▸ Integrate near-maximal and maximal intensity (RPE = 7 to 10) intervals performed at and above VT2 to increase aerobic capacity, speed, and performance. ▸ Periodized training plans can be used to incorporate adequate training time below VT1, from VT1 to just below VT2, and at or above VT2.

Note: RPE = Rating of perceived exertion (0 to 10 scale); VT1 = First ventilatory threshold; VT2 = Second ventilatory threshold

MUSCULAR TRAINING

The Muscular Training component of the ACE IFT Model provides a systematic approach to training that starts with helping clients to improve poor postural stability and **kinetic chain** mobility, and then incorporates programming and progressions to help people train for general fitness, strength, body building, and athletic performance. While many clients will not progress to training for athletic performance, using a training model that provides the personal trainer with the knowledge and tools to work with clients across a broad spectrum of movement skills and challenges is empowering.

The ACE IFT Model Muscular Training component is divided into three phases, each with a title that defines its training focus (Figure 2-4).

FIGURE 2-4
ACE IFT Model Muscular Training phases

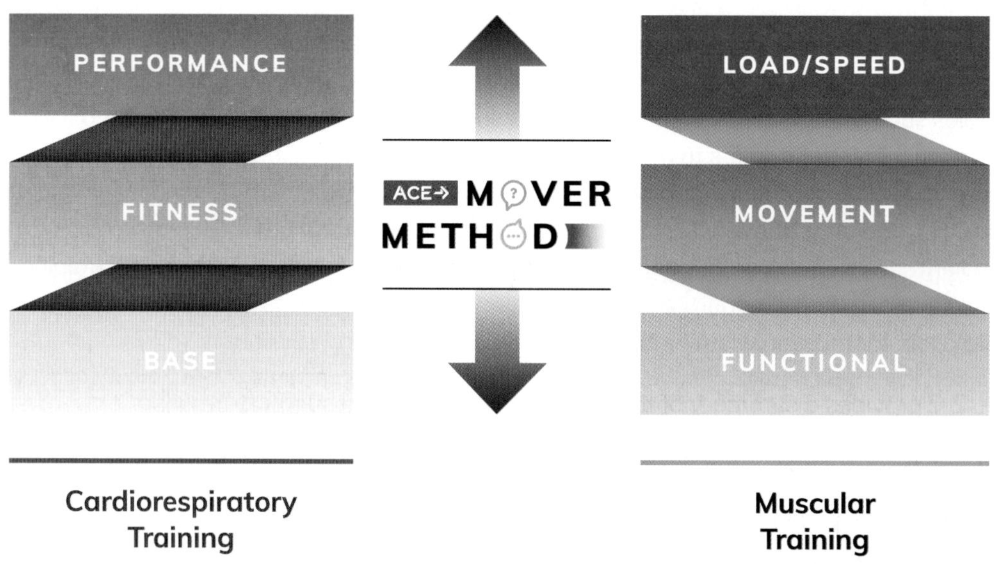

An overview of the primary objectives of Functional, Movement, and Load/Speed Training follows, with detailed information about muscular fitness assessments and programming associated with each training phase presented in Chapters 9 through 11.

Functional Training

Functional Training focuses on the Muscular Training goals of establishing, or in many cases reestablishing, postural stability and kinetic chain mobility through the introduction of exercise programs that improve joint function through improved muscular endurance, flexibility, core function, **static balance,** and **dynamic balance.** This basic muscular function is typically gained as part of normal child development. Unfortunately, physical inactivity coupled with an increasingly technology-driven world has resulted in more adults having compromised posture, balance, and muscular function.

Exercise selection for Functional Training will focus on core and balance exercises that improve the strength and function of the muscles responsible for stabilizing the spine and

center of gravity (COG) during static positions and dynamic movements. Exercises for Functional Training will initially use primarily body-weight resistance. As clients progress to Movement Training and Load/Speed Training, it is important to still include Functional Training exercises in their workouts. These can be included as part of either the warm-up or cool-down, or by incorporating progressions that increase the challenge of the Functional Training exercises by increasing the resistance or balance challenges.

Movement Training

The primary focus of Movement Training is on helping clients develop good movement patterns without compromising postural or joint stability. Movement Training focuses on the five primary movement patterns (Figure 2-5):

- **Bend-and-lift movements:** These movements are performed throughout the day as a person sits, stands, or squats down to lift an object off the floor.
- **Single-leg movements:** These movements involve single-leg balance and movement as performed during walking or going up and down stairs. In addition, lunging movements are performed when a person steps forward to reach down with one hand to pick up something small off the floor.

FIGURE 2-5
Five primary movement patterns

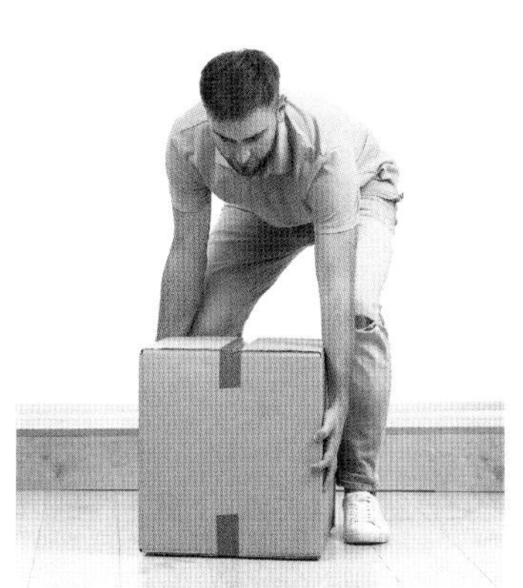

a. Bend-and-lift movement

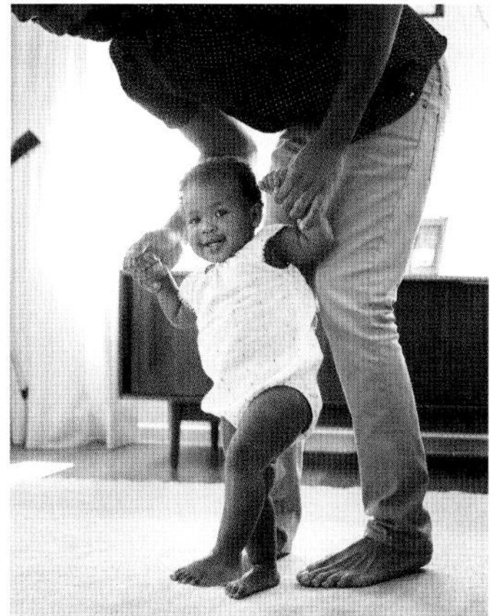

b. Single-leg movement

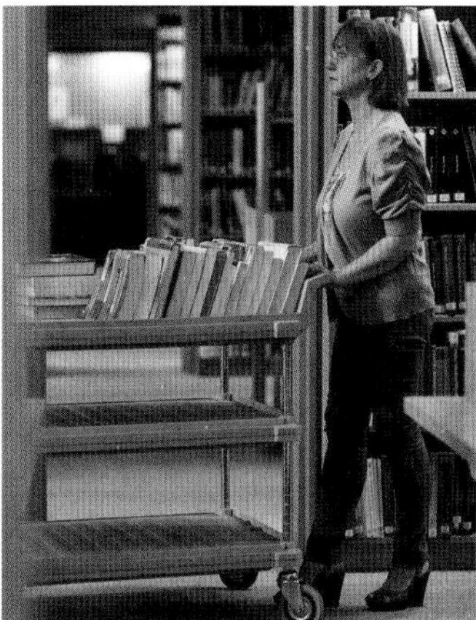

c. Pushing movement

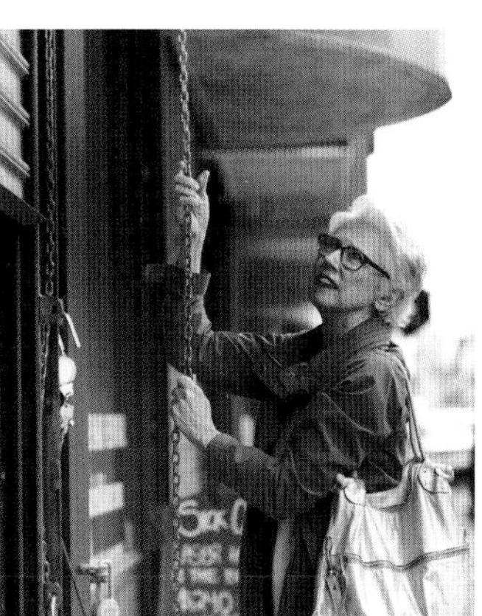

d. Pulling movement

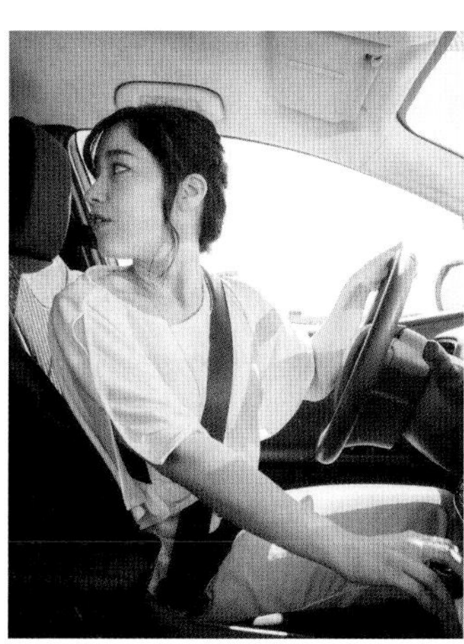

e. Rotational movement

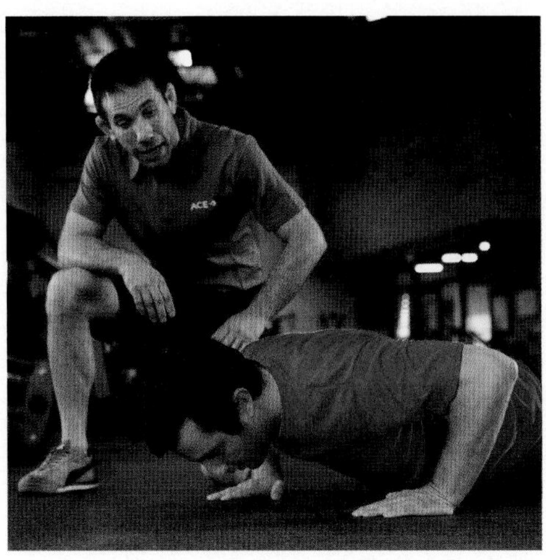

- **Pushing movements:** These upper-body movements occur in four primary directions: forward (e.g., when pushing open a door), overhead (e.g., lifting something to a high shelf), **lateral** (e.g., lifting one's torso when getting up from a side-lying position), and downward (e.g., pushing oneself up and out of the side of a swimming pool).
- **Pulling movements:** These movements occur during exercises like a seated row or pull-up, or when pulling open a door.
- **Rotational movements:** These movements often occur in the torso as force transfers from the legs to the arms (e.g., throwing a ball) or during twisting movements like a dancer performing pirouettes or a golfer striking a ball.

Movement Training exercises should emphasize the proper sequencing of movements and control of the body's COG throughout the normal **range of motion (ROM)** being performed. Personal trainers should integrate Functional Training exercises into Movement Training programs to help clients maintain and improve postural stability and kinetic chain mobility, as they are essential for performing the five primary movement patterns well (see Table 2-3, page 50). One option for including Functional Training exercises is to add them to the warm-up to prepare the body for the more rigorous movements that follow. Body-weight exercises are often used initially during Movement Training, with external resistance introduced typically to build muscular endurance with an emphasis on controlled motion. Personal trainers should make sure that clients can perform the five primary movement patterns well before adding external loads to the movement patterns to decrease the risk of injury that can result from loading poorly executed movements.

Load/Speed Training

The broad focus of Load/Speed Training is on applying external loads to movements that create a need for increased force production that results in muscular adaptations. Loads can be applied through resistance training, **high-intensity interval training (HIIT),** speed work, **plyometrics,** power lifting, and other sport-specific resistance (e.g., using swim training paddles or pedaling large gears while cycling uphill).

As with Movement Training, Load/Speed Training should integrate Functional Training exercises to help clients maintain and enhance postural stability and kinetic chain mobility to adequately support the increased workloads and force production (see Table 2-3, page 50). Load/Speed Training also integrates the five primary movements that are the focus of Movement Training, with the emphasis being on loading the movements through different planes of motion, angles, speeds, and combined movements [e.g., lunge with a rotation (Figure 2-6) and kettlebell swing (Figure 2-7)].

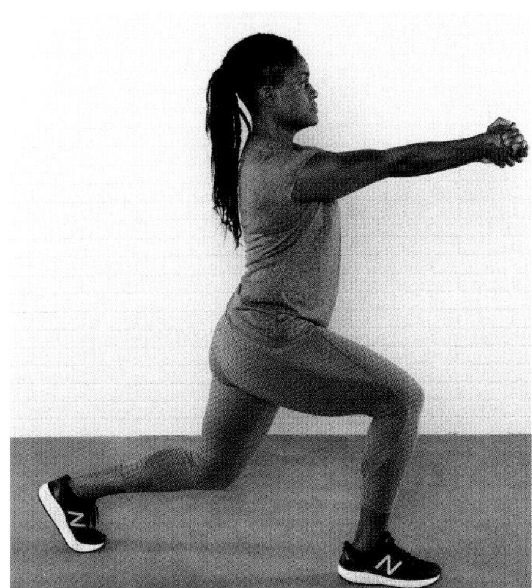
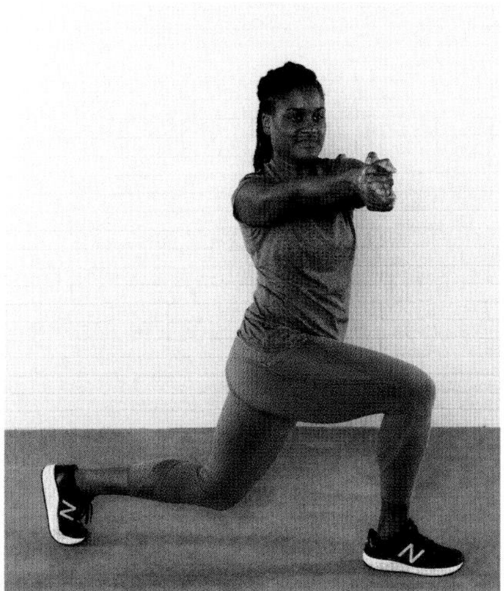

FIGURE 2-6
Lunge with rotation

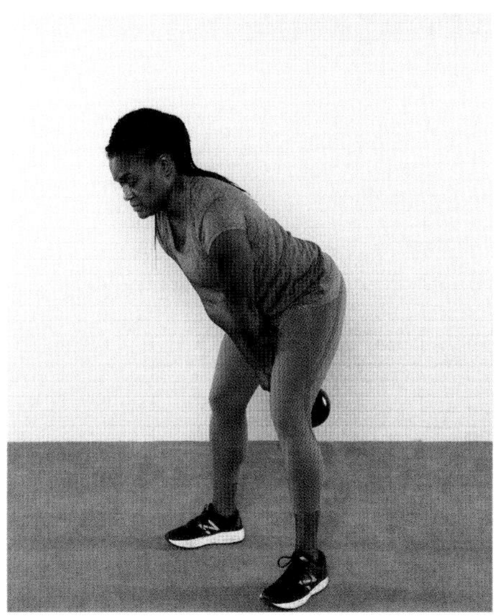
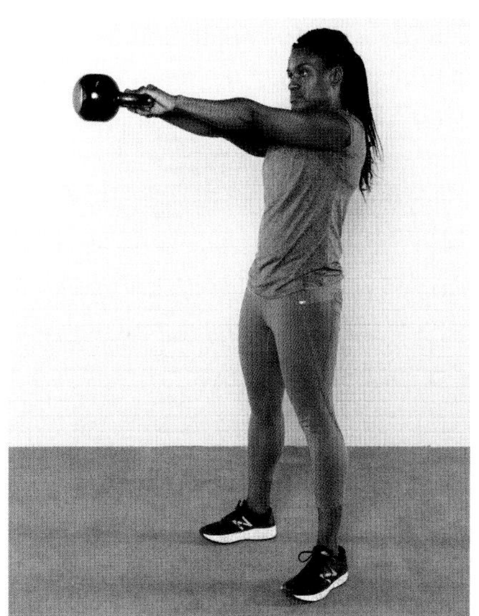

FIGURE 2-7
Kettlebell swing

Clients can have a variety of individual goals that are reached through Load/Speed Training. Fitness-related goals for this type of training include muscular strength, muscular endurance, muscle **hypertrophy,** and positive changes in **body composition.** Personal trainers can help clients reach their fitness-related Load/Speed Training goals by designing exercise programs for each client that incorporate appropriate muscular-training variables, including exercise selection and the frequency and intensity with which each exercise is performed.

Clients who have athletic performance goals can benefit from training that builds speed, **agility, quickness,** and power. Before advancing to training for athletic performance goals, clients should consistently exhibit good postural stability, kinetic chain mobility, and movement patterns. They should also have a good foundation of muscular strength to produce and control the force generated during athletic performance–focused exercises and drills. Exercise selection for clients with athletic performance goals can include power lifting, plyometrics, speed work, and drills for agility, **coordination,** and quickness.

Table 2-3 provides a summary of the three phases of Muscular Training.

TABLE 2-3
Muscular Training

Functional Training	▸ Focus on establishing/reestablishing postural stability and kinetic chain mobility. ▸ Exercise programs should improve muscular endurance, flexibility, core function, and static and dynamic balance. ▸ Progress exercise volume and challenge as function improves.
Movement Training	▸ Focus on developing good movement patterns without compromising postural or joint stability. ▸ Programs should include exercises for all five primary movement patterns in varied planes of motion. ▸ Integrate Functional Training exercises to help clients maintain and improve postural stability and kinetic chain mobility.
Load/Speed Training	▸ Focus on application of external loads to movements to create increased force production to meet desired goals. ▸ Integrate the five primary movement patterns through exercises that load them in different planes of motion and combinations. ▸ Integrate Functional Training exercises to enhance postural stability and kinetic chain mobility to support increased workloads. ▸ Programs should focus on adequate resistance training loads to help clients reach muscular strength, endurance, and hypertrophy goals. ▸ Clients with goals for athletic performance will integrate exercises and drills to build speed, agility, quickness, and power.

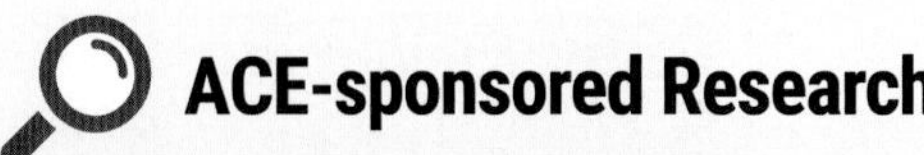

Effectiveness of the ACE Integrated Fitness Training Model

In a randomized trial, Dalleck and colleagues compared the effectiveness of two exercise training programs for improving cardiorespiratory fitness, muscular fitness, and cardiometabolic health (Dalleck et al., 2016). Participants were randomized into one of two training programs: (1) an ACE IFT Model personalized training program, and (2) a standardized training program designed according to current American College of Sports Medicine guidelines (ACSM, 2018). Each training program was 13 weeks in length, with weeks 1 through 3 focused on cardiorespiratory training and weeks 4 through 13 including both cardiorespiratory training and muscular training.

The standardized training group performed cardiorespiratory exercise at an intensity based on a percentage of their **heart-rate reserve (HRR),** progressing from 40 to 45% HRR in week 1 to 60 to 65% HRR in weeks 9 through 13. Each participant in the ACE IFT Model group received a personalized exercise program based on **heart rate (HR)** at their unique ventilatory thresholds (VT1 and VT2), with exercise intensity progressing from HR <VT1 in week 1 to HR >VT2 in weeks 9 through 13. Both groups performed cardiorespiratory exercise three days per week, starting with 25 minutes per session in week 1 and progressing to 50 minutes per session in weeks 9 through 13. The muscular training program for the standardized training group was comprised of two sets of 12 repetitions on a resistance training machine circuit of traditional exercises performed three days per week. The ACE IFT Model group performed a muscular training circuit comprised of two sets of 12 repetitions of multijoint/multiplanar exercises using free weights and machine modalities that allowed for free motion during exercise.

Baseline and follow-up assessment results revealed that when compared to the standardized training group, the ACE IFT Model personalized training group had significantly ($p<0.05$) greater beneficial changes in **body-fat percentage, fat-free mass, $\dot{V}O_2max$, systolic blood pressure, diastolic blood pressure,** right and left leg stork-stand performance, bench press at five-repetition maximum (5-RM), and leg press (5-RM). Additionally, 100% of individuals in the ACE IFT Model training group experienced positive improvements in $\dot{V}O_2max$ (i.e., all individuals were responders), which was significantly ($p<0.05$) greater than the 64.3% of individuals in the standardized training group who showed positive improvements in $\dot{V}O_2max$ (Figure 2-8).

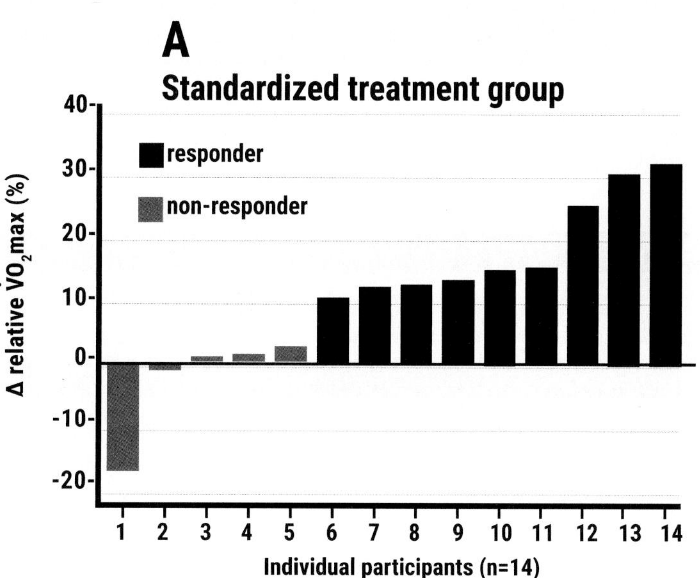

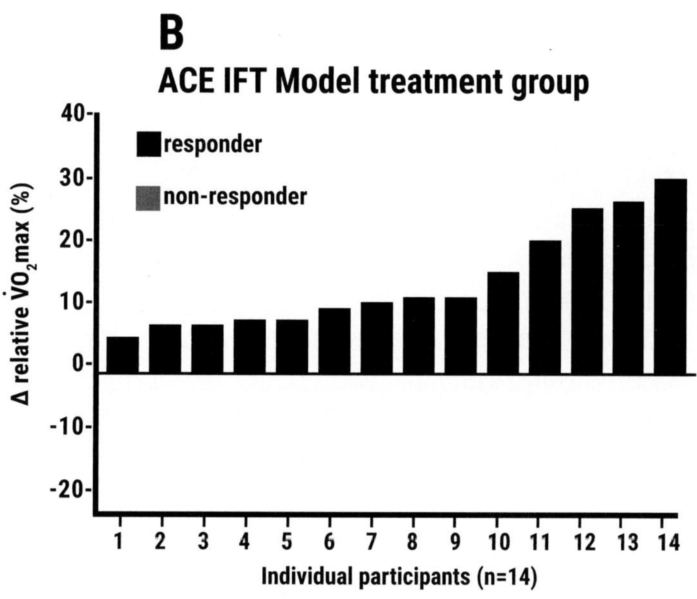

FIGURE 2-8
Individual variability in relative $\dot{V}O_2max$ response (% change) to exercise training in the standardized (A) and ACE IFT Model (B) treatment groups

Interestingly, the remaining 35.7% of individuals in the standardized training group experienced undesirable changes in $\dot{V}O_2max$ and were categorized as non-responders to cardiorespiratory exercise training. The ACE IFT Model personalized training group also had significantly more individuals elicit favorable responses (i.e., responders) in cardiometabolic, anthropometric, muscular, and neuromotor outcome measurements when compared to the standardized training group (Table 2-4).

TABLE 2-4

Cardiometabolic, Anthropometric, and Muscular and Neuromotor Exercise Responders

	Responders in the "Standardized" Group (%)	Responders in the "ACE IFT Model" Group (%)
Cardiometabolic responders		
Systolic BP	42.9	100
HDL cholesterol	50.0	100
Triglycerides	85.7	85.7
Blood glucose	42.9	92.9
Anthropometric responders		
Waist circumference	78.6	92.9
Percent body fat	78.6	100
Muscular and neuromotor responders		
Right-leg stork stand	78.6	100
Left-leg stork stand	85.7	92.9
5-RM bench press	64.3	100
5-RM leg press	64.3	100

Note: BP = Blood pressure; HDL = High-density lipoprotein; 5-RM = 5-repetition maximum

Conclusions

- Personalized exercise programming using the ACE IFT Model elicited significantly greater improvements in $\dot{V}O_2max$, muscular fitness, and key cardiometabolic risk factors when compared to standardized exercise programming following 13 weeks of exercise training.
- The ACE IFT Model personalized training group had significantly increased training responsiveness compared to the standardized exercise training group, with 100% of the participants favorably responding to the training stimulus.
- Dalleck et al. (2016) concluded that "these novel findings are encouraging and underscore the importance of personalized exercise programming to enhance training efficacy and limit training unresponsiveness."

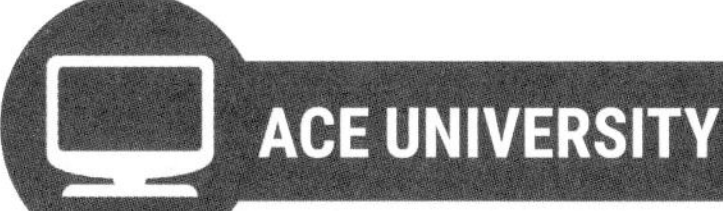

If your study program includes the ACE University, visit www.ACEfitness.org/MyACE and log in to your My ACE Account to take full advantage of the ACE Personal Trainer Study Program and online guided study experience.

A variety of media to support and expand on the material in this text is provided to facilitate learning and best prepare you for the ACE Personal Trainer Certification exam and a career as a personal trainer.

SUMMARY

Successful personal trainers consistently demonstrate excellent communication skills and teaching techniques, while understanding the physiological needs and unique considerations of their clients. The ACE IFT Model is built upon and advanced by current exercise and behavioral science, and the effectiveness of the Model has been validated through peer-reviewed research (Dalleck et al., 2016). Personal trainers can use the ACE IFT Model to provide clients with evidence-based exercise programs that are personalized for each client's unique health, fitness, and goals.

REFERENCES

American College of Sports Medicine (2018). *ACSM's Guidelines for Exercise Testing and Prescription* (10th ed.). Philadelphia: Wolters Kluwer.

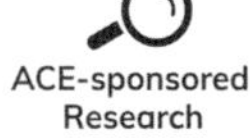

Dalleck, L.C. et al. (2016). Does a personalized exercise prescription enhance training efficacy and limit training unresponsiveness? A randomized controlled trial. *Journal of Fitness Research*, 5, 3, 15–27.

U.S. Department of Health & Human Services (2018). *Physical Activity Guidelines for Americans* (2nd ed.). www.health.gov/paguidelines/

SUGGESTED READING

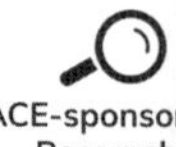

Dalleck, L.C. et al. (2016). *ACE-SPONSORED RESEARCH: Does the ACE Integrated Fitness Training® Model Enhance Training Efficacy and Responsiveness?* https://www.acefitness.org/education-and-resources/professional/certified/research-special-issue-2017/6307/ace-sponsored-research-does-the-ace-integrated-fitness-training-sup-sup-model-enhance-training?authorScope=118

SECTION II

A Client-centered Approach to Personal Training

CHAPTER 3
Basics of Behavior Change

CHAPTER 4
Effective Communication, Goal Setting, and Teaching Techniques

CHAPTER 5
Preparticipation Health Screening

CHAPTER 6
Nutrition for Health and Fitness

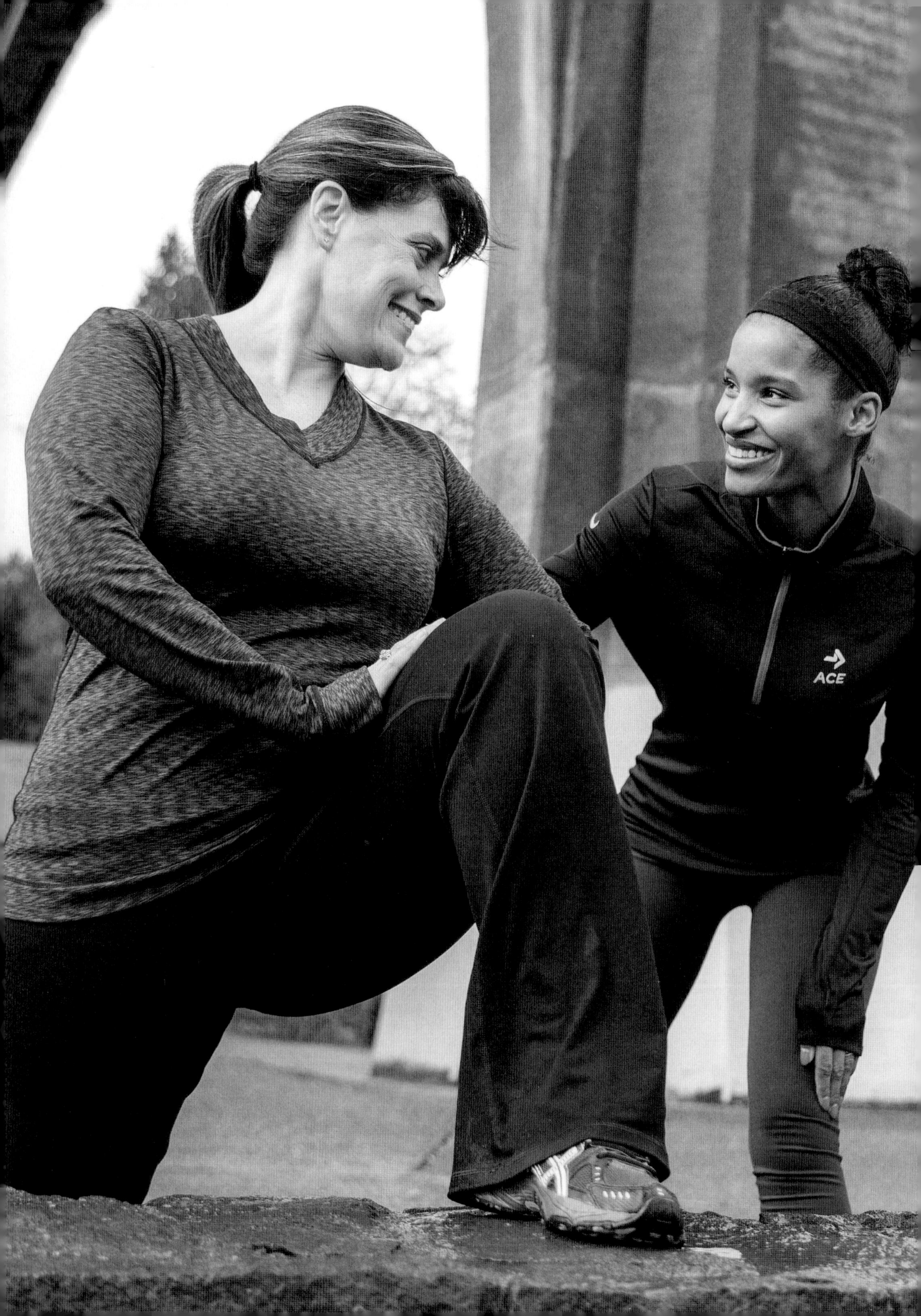
ACE

CHAPTER 3

Basics of Behavior Change

SABRENA JO, MS
Director of Science and Research, American Council on Exercise; ACE Certified Personal Trainer, Health Coach, and Group Fitness Instructor

IN THIS CHAPTER

LEARNING OBJECTIVES:

Upon completion of this chapter, the reader will be able to:

- Identify common behavioral theory models
- Explain self-determination theory and strategies that may be used to support its framework when working with clients
- Describe the transtheoretical model of behavior change and its component stages
- Implement basic strategies founded on common behavioral theory models to help clients adopt and maintain physical-activity behaviors
- Identify principles of behavior change and how they may affect clients who are embarking on a new physical-activity program for the first time or clients who are already engaged in a physically active lifestyle
- Implement basic strategies to decrease the likelihood of client dropout by taking into account adherence-related factors

ACE UNIVERSITY

If your study program includes the ACE University, visit www.ACEfitness.org/MyACE and log in to your My ACE Account to take full advantage of the ACE Personal Trainer Study Program and online guided study experience.

A variety of media to support and expand on the material in this text is provided to facilitate learning and best prepare you for the ACE Personal Trainer Certification exam and a career as a personal trainer.

With only 23.5% of adults in the United States meeting both aerobic activity and muscle-strengthening guidelines, it is clear that exercise professionals, including personal trainers, have a significant challenge in helping people initiate—and then stick with—exercise programs (Centers for Disease Control and Prevention, National Center for Health Statistics, 2018). If it were as simple as educating people about the important health benefits of regular exercise that prompted them to be more **physically active,** it is likely that more of the population would lead active lifestyles, as there have been widespread public health campaigns geared toward spreading this message for decades. However, information alone is often not enough to prompt individuals to commit to regular exercise, nor is hiring a personal trainer if the client–personal trainer relationship is not founded on **rapport,** mutual trust, and an understanding of the client's **readiness to change.** As indicated in the ACE Integrated Fitness Training® (ACE IFT®) Model (see Chapter 2), a critical component in helping clients achieve success is incorporating the ACE Mover Method™ philosophy. The ACE Mover Method is an integral part of the ACE IFT Model. This unique philosophy allows personal trainers to adopt a client-centered approach to training clients, which is critical to the clients' success. Every opportunity with a client is an opportunity to build a positive and meaningful relationship through utilizing a few key coaching skills, such as those emphasized in the ACE ABC Approach™. It is through the lens of the ACE Mover Method philosophy and the skills mastered in the ACE ABC Approach that personal trainers will gather vital information from clients by asking powerful, open-ended questions and actively listening to them to collaborate and design a truly personalized exercise program.

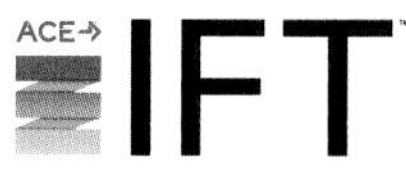

It is increasingly evident that a successful personal trainer does more than design exercise programs and teach proper movement techniques. To optimally support clients, an effective personal trainer must also be skilled in coaching people in the process of adopting and adhering to health-related behavior change, while promoting the conditions in which motivation flourishes. This focus on applying the ACE Mover Method, through techniques such as the ACE ABC Approach, is detailed throughout several chapters of the textbook, and is what sets ACE® Certified Personal Trainers apart in the industry. Personal training involves far more than programming sets, repetitions, and exercise duration; at its core, it is about motivating clients to adopt and adhere to behavior changes to positively impact their health, fitness, and overall quality of life.

Behavioral Theory Models

There is no simple formula to predict why some people adopt healthy behaviors and others do not. Behavior change, in general, is complicated by the following factors (2018 Physical Activity Guidelines Advisory Committee, 2018):

- Environmental influences (e.g., physical and social) are important determinants of health behavior change.
- Behavior change is an ongoing process, rather than a single event, and the factors that influence it change over time.
- Behavioral intention and action are not the same.

Different factors influence initiating a behavior change and maintaining that change over time. Despite this complexity, personal trainers must be able to effectively work with real people and the unique challenges, characteristics, and considerations that come with each individual. A personal trainer's objective should go beyond solely designing a great workout. Instead, the goal should be to empower each client to adopt a life-long habit of regular physical activity. To provide guidance in supporting health behavior change, numerous models and theories have been developed. These research-supported frameworks examine various factors affecting health behaviors, including people's beliefs about their health, their beliefs about their ability to change, and their readiness to make a change. Each of the following models has relevance for personal trainers.

HEALTH BELIEF MODEL

The **health belief model** states that people's ideas and underlying emotions about illnesses, prevention, and treatments may influence health behaviors and decisions about changing (or not changing) health behaviors (Rosenstock, 1966). The outcome variable of interest is the decision to change, so the model is especially applicable to people in the early stages of change, where they are still weighing the pros and cons. The model states that at least four variables influence a person's decision to change. The first two involve a person's beliefs about a health threat. The second two reflect the person's beliefs about the health behavior that could reduce the threat (Sears, Brehm, & Bell, 2014) (Figure 3-1).

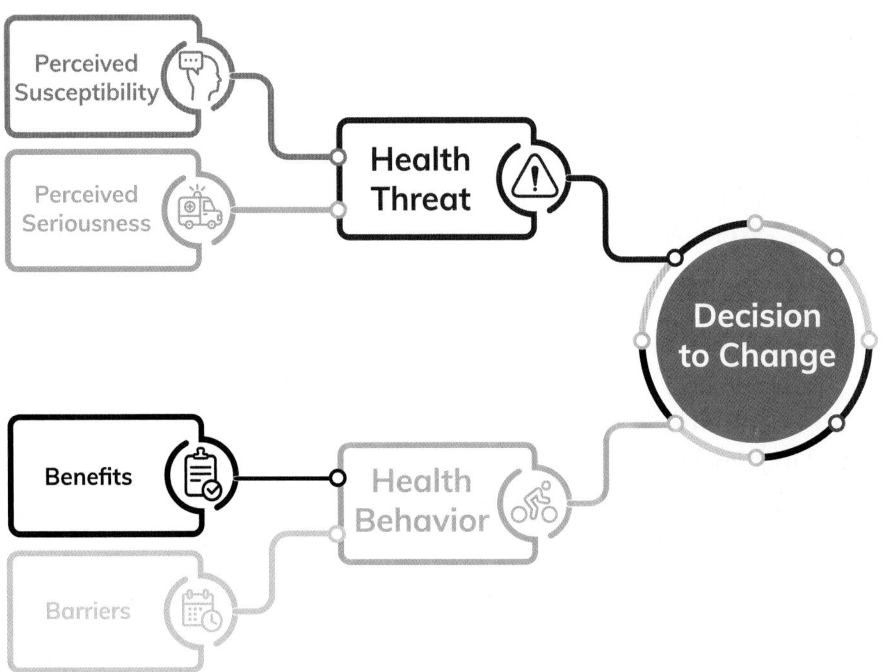

FIGURE 3-1
The health belief model

The belief in the health threat has two components, **perceived susceptibility** to an illness and **perceived seriousness** of the illness. Perceived susceptibility refers to people's perceptions of how likely they are to develop the illness. Perceived seriousness refers to people's perceptions regarding the short- and long-term severity of the illness. Health screenings that indicate a potential problem sometimes motivate behavior change because they may alter people's perceptions of susceptibility. For example, people who have not thought much about what they eat may become more aware of their eating habits if they hear their **blood pressure** is high. They may suddenly feel more susceptible to **hypertension** and feel motivated to prevent its development through beneficial health-behavior change, perhaps by improving their food choices and exercising.

The second set of variables relates to perceptions of the health behavior. People may perceive both benefits and barriers to taking action with a specific health behavior. Beliefs about benefits may include how effective the person thinks a health behavior would be in preventing or treating an illness. Beliefs about barriers or drawbacks of a health behavior might include how difficult implementing the new behavior would be and the negative effects associated with doing so. If people feel susceptible to high blood pressure, but do not believe that limiting fast-food intake would help very much or be easy enough to do long-term, they would be unlikely to change the amount of fast food they eat. Addressing health beliefs is especially important for clients in the early stages of behavior change. The personal trainer should always discuss with clients their beliefs about health concerns and behavior change and correct misperceptions with accurate information. Good information will help clients weigh the pros and cons of behavior change and hopefully form intentions to modify their lifestyles.

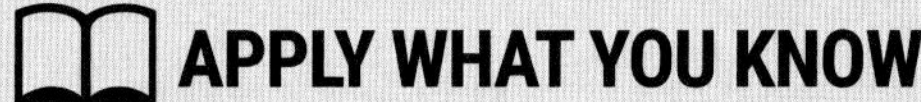

The Health Belief Model in Action

When working with a client who has been recently diagnosed with having the **metabolic syndrome (MetS),** a personal trainer can consider the constructs of the health belief model in evoking the client's motivation to change. For example, through a collaborative conversation, the personal trainer may reinforce the notion of perceived susceptibility by clarifying the client's understanding of his or her diagnosis, discussing the conditions that make up MetS, and exploring the client's family history, which can increase his or her risk of developing **cardiovascular disease** and **type 2 diabetes.**

To address perceived seriousness, the personal trainer can explore the client's understanding of the health risks associated with MetS, adding relevant information and correcting misunderstandings as appropriate. Then, together the client and personal trainer can explore lifestyle changes that can help to control and reduce the risk for negative health consequences, such as hypertension and **heart disease.** If the client is open to a discussion about nutrition and is seeking guidance about dietary strategies, the personal trainer can explain, with permission from the client, the benefits of a healthful diet, including increased consumption of fruits and vegetables and decreased sodium intake, for controlling blood pressure. The personal trainer can then prompt the client to consider ways in which he or she feels most inclined to go about making such dietary changes. Barriers to implementing dietary changes should be as low as possible, so the personal trainer should strategize with the client to devise realistic goals and plans. This discussion should not be overwhelming, but rather should empower the client, evoking newfound motivation to make a dietary change.

An interesting exception to the health belief model is that sometimes people coping with serious illnesses, such as cancer or heart disease, may be at greatest risk of *not* engaging in health-promoting behavior, despite feeling susceptible to a serious illness. This holds true even if they believe in the value of the health behavior. People facing such challenges may become psychologically and physically worn down by their disease, medical regimens, and financial costs. They may lose hope, become socially isolated, and be less likely to engage in positive health behaviors. The lived experience of illness over time can alter perceptions of the benefits and barriers for health behaviors. Thus, personal trainers must realize that the process of making decisions about health behaviors is dynamic and complex.

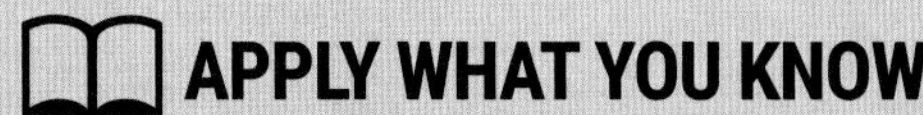

APPLY WHAT YOU KNOW

Case Study: Health Belief Model

The following case study is an example of how the health belief model explains behavior. A personal trainer is approached by a 39-year-old **physically inactive** man who is nearly 100 pounds (45 kg) **overweight.** His father recently died at age 65 of a stroke due to complications related to uncontrolled hypertension (a disease for which lifestyle modification is a major component of management). This individual is very busy with his family and job, but knows that if he does not take action, he may develop a disease similar to the one that took his father's life. As the personal trainer talks to this person, it becomes clear that even though he knows he should exercise, making a change has not yet become a priority in his life and he is not prepared to make a commitment to an exercise program.

According to the health belief model, there are numerous reasons why this individual is not ready to start an exercise program. Despite his high perception of the seriousness of, and susceptibility to, developing a lifestyle-related disease, he does not have any noticeable symptoms of a disease state. In fact, he says he feels fine, only complaining of a lack of energy to make it through a typical day. This should signal to the personal trainer that this individual may need a cue to action to help him get started. It is likely that this individual has not had a recent physical exam, and this may be a good place to start. He could receive information during a physical that would serve as motivation to get started on making a change. His numerous comments about his busy life and his feelings of being overwhelmed by how much weight he has gained should serve as important cues that he perceives many barriers to successfully participating in an exercise program. When the client decides he is ready to begin an exercise program, it will be crucial for the personal trainer to create a plan that is flexible and simple to start and maintain. If the personal trainer presents program options that require a huge time commitment and schedule reorganization, this individual may be immediately turned off. Instead, the personal trainer needs to set him up to succeed, providing something on which to build (e.g., starting with small, achievable steps).

SELF-DETERMINATION THEORY

People pursue activities and goals in which they are naturally interested or from which they believe they will benefit. The type of motivation involved with those pursuits is likely to determine whether they stick with or discontinue them. This is the crux of

self-determination theory, which posits that different types of motivation (i.e., intrinsic versus extrinsic) influence the extent to which a person will seek out new activities and persevere at a given task (Deci & Ryan, 2008).

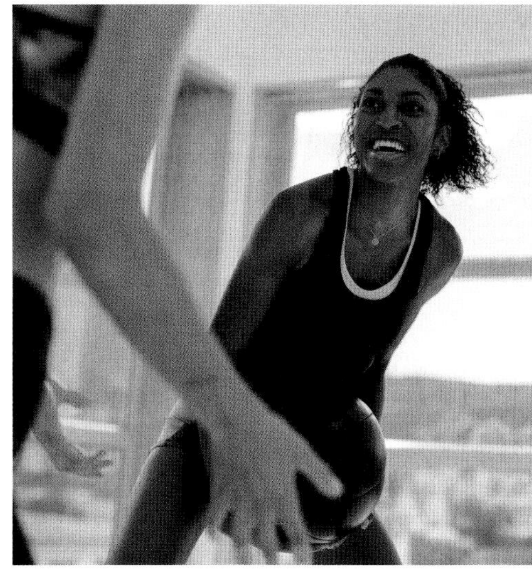

Motivation

People generally do not like to be told what to do unless they have actively sought and asked for advice. People like to feel that they have choices, and that they can make decisions about behavior according to their own wishes and in accordance with their own values and goals. Self-determination theory examines two basic types of motivation: **autonomous motivation** and **controlled motivation.** Autonomous motivation means that people feel as if they are behaving of their own free will. They are doing something because they want to do it. To be autonomously motivated to the fullest extent is known as having **intrinsic motivation.** Controlled motivation, on the other hand, means people are doing something because they feel pressured by demands from external forces.

These two types of motivation feel very different to people. It is critically important that personal trainers respect a client's **autonomy** and start from the understanding that while the personal trainer may be an expert on exercise program design and implementation, ultimately the client is the expert on him- or herself, and lasting change will happen only when the client is ready and has decided that it should.

In the exercise context, to be intrinsically motivated means that a person is engaged in an exercise activity for the inherent pleasure and experience that comes from the engagement itself. Having more intrinsic participation motives or goals associated with exercise, such as social engagement, challenge, and skill development, is associated with greater exercise participation (Teixeira et al., 2012). People who are intrinsically motivated report being physically active because they truly enjoy it. Such involvement in an activity is associated with positive attitudes and emotions (e.g., happiness, freedom, and relaxation), maximal effort, and persistence when faced with barriers (Ryan & Deci, 2000).

While many people truly enjoy being physically active, very few (if any) adults are completely intrinsically motivated. Fundamental goals of personal trainers include maximizing client enjoyment and engagement, while also being careful not to expect that their clients will always demonstrate intrinsic motivation.

The reality is that most adults experience some amount of controlled motivation, which involves the engagement in exercise for any benefit other than for the joy of participation. Controlled motivation often results in people being physically active because of some external factor (e.g., lose weight, be healthy, make their spouse happy, look good, or meet new people) and may lead to feelings of tension, guilt, or pressure related to participation (Ryan & Deci, 2000).

Most everyone falls somewhere on the continuum between controlled and autonomous motivation. Instead of feeling like they need to make their clients more intrinsically motivated, personal trainers may strive to enhance the feelings of enjoyment and accomplishment that come with program participation.

In their work in developing self-determination theory, researchers Ryan and Deci (2000) reported that people have innate psychological needs, and when those needs are met, the conditions are favorable for supporting intrinsic motivation. The three needs they identified are **competence,** autonomy, and **relatedness.** Competence relates to the self-perception that a person can successfully perform a task, which is enhanced when he or she receives positive performance **feedback** (see Chapter 4). Receiving negative feedback, on the other hand, diminishes the perception of competence and may thwart intrinsic motivation. Along with competence, a sense of autonomy is important for intrinsic motivation such that an individual must feel that his or her behavior is self-determined and not coerced or controlled. Lastly, social environments that promote relatedness, or a belongingness and connectedness with others, are contexts in which intrinsic motivation may flourish.

Personal trainers can create environments wherein their clients' basic psychological needs are met by (1) creating opportunities for mastery experiences through offering appropriately challenging exercises and consistent positive feedback (promoting competence), (2) including the client in aspects of goal setting and program design (promoting autonomy), and (3) encouraging a sense of camaraderie among the client and others in the fitness setting (promoting relatedness) (Figure 3-2). Encouraging client ownership and continued involvement in the exercise program design will further facilitate the development of intrinsic motivation by enhancing client self-sufficiency. Many personal trainers are afraid to teach their clients to be independent because they fear that their services will no longer be needed. In reality, failing to build client independence is related to less-motivated clients who may ultimately be more likely to drop out (Higgins et al., 2014).

FIGURE 3-2
Creating an environment that supports intrinsic motivation

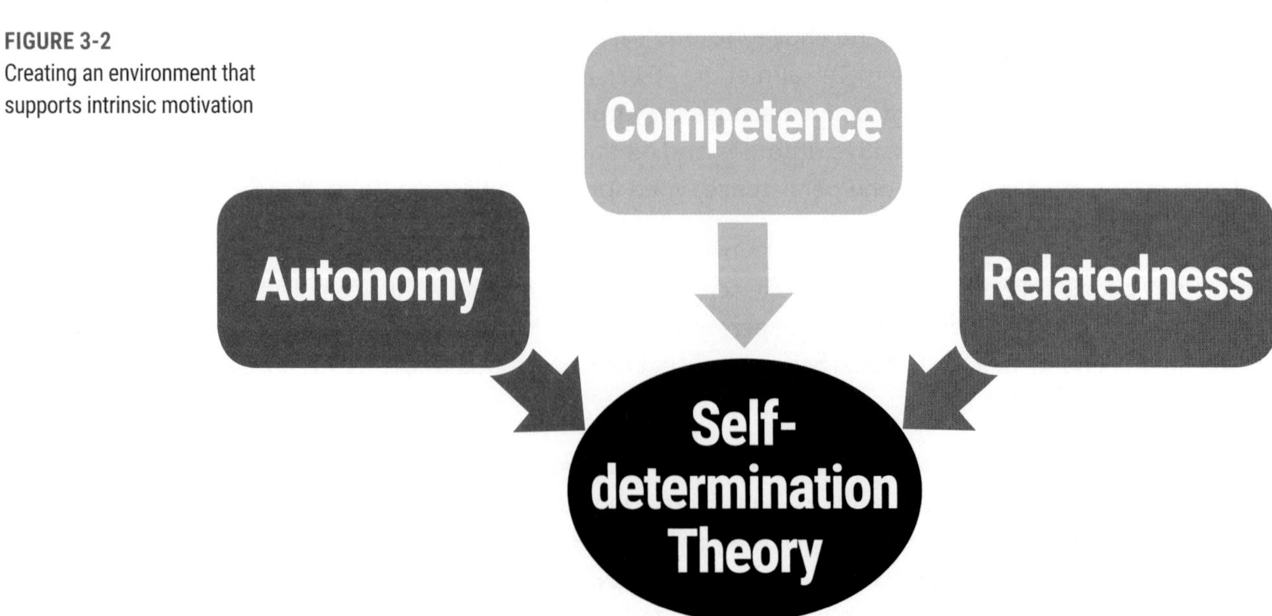

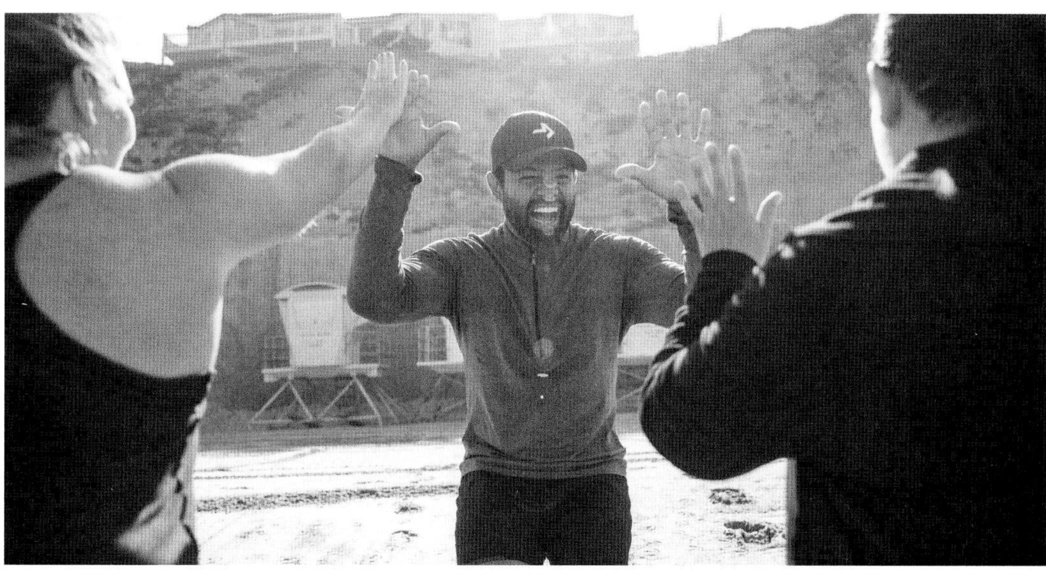

Motivational Climate in the Exercise Setting

Research on motivational climate in the exercise setting indicates that an exerciser's self-determination for physical activity is low when motivated by external factors (e.g., to please others or gain a reward) and, conversely, is high when motivated by internal factors (e.g., enjoyment and self-care) (Ng et al., 2012). Further, it has been shown that supportive others, such as personal trainers, can play a critical role in fostering the development of increased self-determined motivation (Ryan & Deci, 2000).

Similar to how individuals' perceptions influence their belief about the actions they take for health, so too do perceptions about their environment affect the efforts they put forth in the exercise setting. Seminal research suggests that environments can be perceived by participants as either task-involving or ego-involving (Nicholls, 1984). Task-involving climates promote a focus on individual effort and improvement where everyone is made to feel valued and welcomed and cooperation is fostered among everyone in the setting. Ego-involving climates, on the other hand, highlight the most skilled or fit participants among a group and rivalry is encouraged to the point where members may feel embarrassed if they do not know how to use a piece of equipment or perform an exercise correctly. Perhaps not surprisingly, participants who exercise in task-involving climates report having higher self-esteem, feeling more competent and autonomous, feeling a greater sense of relatedness to others, and experiencing more enjoyment, versus ego-involving climates where they report greater physical exhaustion and higher anxiety (Reinboth & Duda, 2006; Vazou, Ntoumanis, & Duda, 2006; Reinboth & Duda, 2004). Research on a separate aspect of climate—the extent to which it is perceived as caring—has also shown psychological benefit. That is, a caring climate wherein physical-activity participants perceive the setting to be a safe and supportive environment that fosters a sense of belonging and where participants feel their exercise leaders have genuine concern for their well-being is associated with higher enjoyment, greater commitment to the activity, and higher empathic concern for others (Brown, Fry & Moore, 2017; Brown & Fry, 2014; Brown & Fry, 2013; Brown & Fry, 2011).

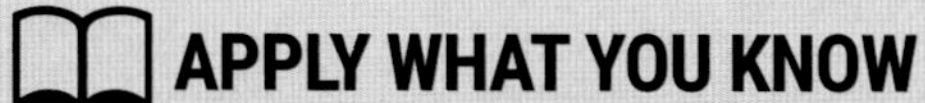

APPLY WHAT YOU KNOW

Creating a Caring, Task-involving Climate

In combination, the research described on page 67 suggests that creating a caring and task-involving climate may provide significant psychological benefits to clients through increased enjoyment, social interactions, and feelings of competence. The following describes strategies that may be used specifically by personal trainers.

- Personal trainers may foster a caring, task-involving climate by emphasizing **process goals** (e.g., making it to the gym four times this week) rather than **outcome goals**. (e.g., losing 10 pounds) (see Chapter 4). Further, encouraging clients to focus on the intrinsic rewards associated with exercise (e.g., feeling better and having more energy) versus extrinsic rewards (e.g., getting in shape for swimsuit season) will help personal trainers put the focus more on process goals. De-emphasizing outcome goals may also be helpful because clients have less control over the rate at which their bodies respond to exercise (e.g., pounds lost per week). However, the improved mood that goes along with being physically active may happen immediately.
- Being careful not to compare clients to others is another important aspect of creating a caring, task-involving climate. Instead of offering information such as, "Compared to people your age, you should be completing 20 push-ups," a personal trainer may reframe the conversation to, "Over the next four weeks, we could aim to increase your push-ups by one repetition per set at each workout. How does that sound to you?"
- Personal trainers have a unique opportunity to celebrate the accomplishments of their clients each time they meet. For example, a personal trainer could make positive, encouraging remarks about milestones such as completing more repetitions, lifting heavier weight, performing an exercise with greater ease, or making it into the gym more frequently. Positive feedback is critical, as clients may not be aware of their progress, especially if their focus has been on outcome goals that surface more slowly. These types of statements demonstrate that clients are cared for and valued by the personal trainer, bolstering the caring environment.
- To promote feelings of belonging and relatedness, personal trainers may consider introducing their clients to other members of the gym before or after their sessions. Going a step further and encouraging clients and other members to cheer each other on when physical-activity and fitness milestones are reached is another effective option for fostering a caring, task-involving climate. Lastly, one of the most important roles of the personal trainer is to provide genuine warmth and acceptance to all clients, taking extra steps to enhance rapport and help the client feel supported. In this way, personal trainers may fulfill the "supportive others" role, which is critical in the development of client self-determined motivation.

Social-support Strategies

How can **social support** be employed to help clients? One way is to suggest that they seek support from others on an ongoing basis. The following are social-support strategies personal trainers can suggest to clients:

- Find an enjoyable and reliable exercise partner. This strategy could be applied in personal-training sessions (if the personal trainer is comfortable and skilled at conducting sessions with more than one person) or for workouts when the client is not with the personal trainer. If partners are not readily available in the exercise setting, look to community agencies or programs offered by organizations such as churches, social groups, or universities.
- Ask friends and family members to be encouraging and positive about the exercise program. Find out if they have a similar interest in becoming more physically active and invite them to join in the program.
- Ask for reminders from friends and family members about physical-activity goals or appointments.
- Set up fun “contests” with a friend that base rewards on meeting process goals, such as meeting at the park for a scheduled walk 10 times without an absence. The main objective is to use accountability to someone else as a motivational tool for encouraging more consistent exercise participation, which may ultimately empower the client to become more accountable to him- or herself.
- Add a social element to the exercise program. For example, arrive at an exercise session a little early if it affords the opportunity to chat with other members.
- Find an enjoyable activity that is based on being physically active with a group or club such as dancing, bowling, or hiking.

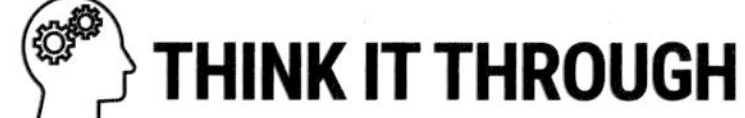

Promoting Social Connectedness

What strategies will you use to help clients connect with others to enhance their social relatedness and sense of belonging?

TRANSTHEORETICAL MODEL OF BEHAVIOR CHANGE

An important factor in the successful adoption of any exercise program is the client’s readiness to make a change. This individual readiness for change is the focus of a well-accepted model examining health behaviors called the **transtheoretical model of behavior change (TTM)** (Prochaska & DiClemente, 1984). More commonly called the **stages-of-change model,** the TTM is important for personal trainers to understand when promoting the adoption of exercise programs. Not everyone is necessarily eager to begin exercising, which is an important concept to keep in mind when attempting to design and implement personalized exercise programs (Morgan, 2001; Marcus et al., 2000). Succeeding at making a behavior change is not a simple task. To better delineate the process of starting and maintaining a behavior change, the TTM is separated into four components:

- Stages of change
- Processes of change
- Self-efficacy
- Decisional balance

Stages of Change

The first component of the TTM is made up of the five stages of behavioral change (Figure 3-3). These stages can be related to any health behavior, but in the physical-activity context the stages are as follows:

- The **precontemplation** stage is the stage during which people are physically inactive and are not even intending to begin an activity program. They do not see physical activity as relevant in their lives and may even discount the importance or practicality of being physically active.
- The **contemplation** stage consists of people who are still inactive but are thinking about becoming more active in the near future (within the next six months). They are starting to consider physical activity as important and have begun to identify the implications of being inactive. However, they are ambivalent about change and are still weighing the pros and cons of becoming physically active.

FIGURE 3-3
Stages of behavior change

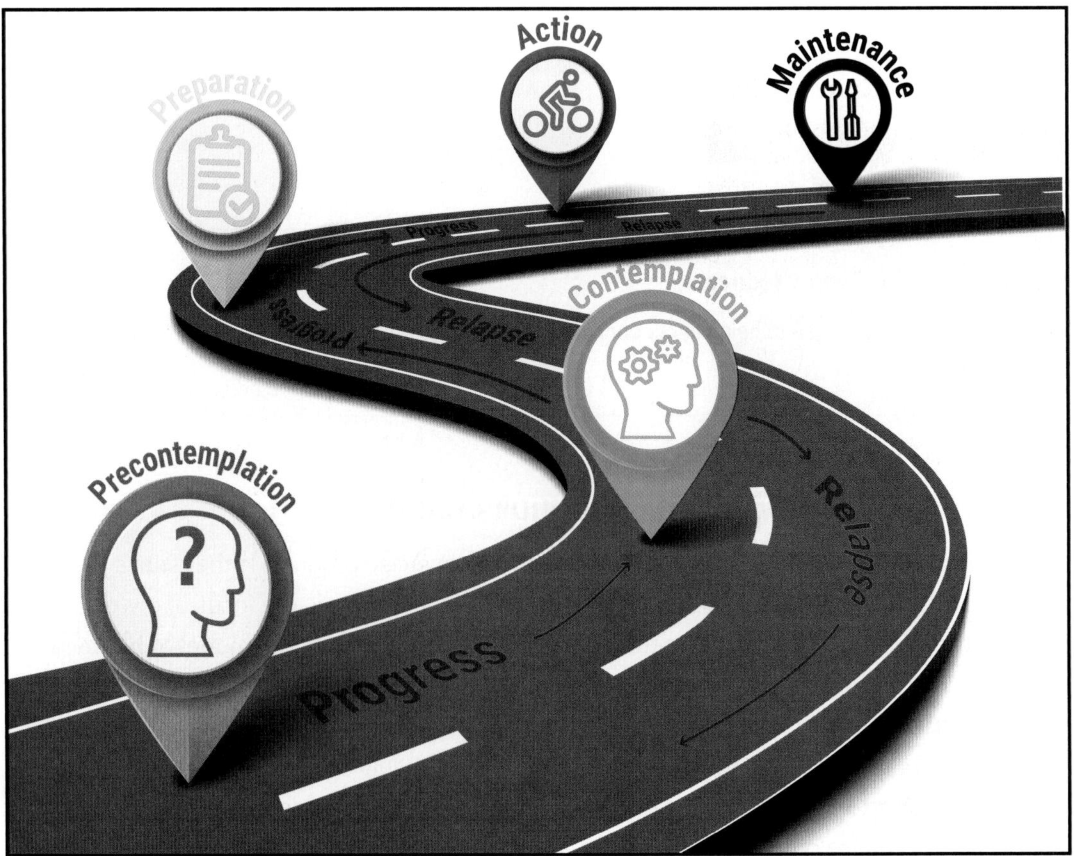

- The **preparation** stage is marked by some engagement in physical activity, as individuals are mentally and physically preparing to adopt an activity program. Activity during the preparation stage may be a sporadic walk, or even a periodic visit to the gym, but it is inconsistent. People in the preparation stage are ready to adopt and live an active lifestyle.
- The **action** stage is comprised of people who are engaging in regular physical activity but have been doing so for less than six months.
- The **maintenance** stage is marked by regular physical-activity participation for longer than six months.

Processes of Change

The second component of the TTM is likely the most important for personal trainers to understand, as it entails the processes of change that people use to move through the stages. Each stage transition has a unique set of processes and is based on specific individual decisions and mental states, including individual readiness and motivation. In reality, there is no established "correct" way to progress through the stages of change, nor is it a linear process. For example, individuals may vacillate between precontemplation and contemplation for years. Further, when a client moves from one stage to the next is not always clear. Personal trainers may gauge generally where a client is on the behavior-change continuum and then use the interventions specified in Table 3-1 to help him or her advance to the next stage. By asking clients **open-ended questions** (questions that cannot be answered with only a few words, or a "yes" or "no") and listening to their answers

TABLE 3-1

The Stages of Behavioral Change

Stage	Traits	Goals	Strategies
Precontemplation	▸ Unaware or under-aware of the problem, or believe that it cannot be solved	▸ Increase awareness of the risks of maintaining the status quo and of the benefits of making a change ▸ Focus on addressing something relevant to them ▸ Have them start thinking about change	▸ Validate lack of readiness to change and clarify that this decision is theirs ▸ Encourage reevaluation of current behavior and self-exploration, while not taking action ▸ Explain and personalize the inherent risks ▸ Utilize general sources, including media, Internet, and brochures, to increase awareness ▸ Explore the client's personal values
Contemplation	▸ Aware of the problem and weighing the benefits versus risks of change ▸ Have little understanding of how to go about changing	▸ Collaboratively explore available options ▸ Support cues to action and provide basic structured guidance upon request from the client and with permission	▸ Validate lack of readiness to change and clarify that this decision is theirs ▸ Encourage evaluation of the pros and cons of making a change ▸ Identify and promote new, positive outcome expectations and boost self-confidence

Continued on the next page

TABLE 3-1 *(continued)*

Stage	Traits	Goals	Strategies
Preparation	▸ Seeking opportunities to engage in the target behavior	▸ Co-create an action plan with frequent positive feedback and reinforcements on their progress	▸ Verify that the individual has the underlying skills for behavior change and encourage small steps toward building self-efficacy ▸ Identify and assist with problem-solving obstacles ▸ Assist the client in identifying social support and establishing goals
Action	▸ Desire for opportunities to maintain activities ▸ Changing beliefs and attitudes ▸ High risk for lapses or returns to undesirable behavior	▸ Establish the new behavior as a habit through motivation and adherence to the desired behavior	▸ Use behavior-modification strategies ▸ Empower clients to restructure cues and social support toward building long-term change ▸ Increase awareness of inevitable lapses and bolster self-efficacy in coping with lapses ▸ Support clients in establishing systems of accountability and self-monitoring
Maintenance	▸ Empowered, but desire a means to maintain adherence ▸ Good capability to deal with lapses	▸ Maintain support systems ▸ Maintain interest and avoid boredom or burnout	▸ Reevaluate strategies currently in effect ▸ Plan for contingencies with support systems, although this may no longer be needed ▸ Reinforce the need for a transition from external to internal rewards ▸ Plan for potential lapses ▸ Encourage reevaluation of goals and action plans as needed

(see "Motivational Interviewing" on page 107), a personal trainer may identify the current stage of change and tailor his or her approach accordingly.

It is important to understand the processes behind clients' desire to change and to maintain change. This necessitates being aware that people rely on different **cognitions** and strategies based on the specific stage they are in to move forward and progress through the stages of change. The processes presented in Table 3-2 can be categorized as either **cognitive** processes (which result in new ways of thinking that reinforce motivation to change) or behavioral processes (which support the behavior-change process), both of which influence an individual's progress through the stages of change (Sears, Brehm, & Bell, 2014).

Cognitive processes result in new ways of thinking and reinforce a client's motivation to change. Some examples of clients' cognitive processes include:

- Receiving information on the benefits of changing a specific behavior (e.g., physical activity can be good for mental health, not just weight loss)
- Having an emotional change of heart to ignite a drive for change (e.g., being influenced by a close relative with cardiovascular disease to reevaluate one's own dietary habits)

- Considering how one's behavior affects others (e.g., how being a positive role model for engaging in physical activity affects a child's perception of being physically active)
- Developing a self-image based on one's own vision, values, and goals for life (e.g., being a leader by demonstrating an active lifestyle and incorporating walking meetings)
- Connecting with like-minded people who may positively influence one's feelings about a certain behavior (e.g., joining a fitness challenge at a gym where a person is an active member)

Behavioral processes, on the other hand, involve action-oriented learning where clients experience the behaviors and adopt those that work for them (e.g., making a commitment to write down a behavior in a journal). Behavioral processes may also use cues to encourage behavior (see "Operant Conditioning" on page 82). Additional examples of behavioral processes include:

- Using substitutions that replace old risky health behaviors with new health-promoting behaviors (e.g., packing a healthy lunch instead of relying on fast food)
- Recruiting and nurturing social-support systems (e.g., talking to one's family about why sleep is important to you and asking for their support with setting a new schedule)
- Creating personalized rewards (e.g., rewarding oneself with a new pair of running shoes when a certain mile threshold is reached)

TABLE 3-2
Processes of Change

Processes of Change	Description
Consciousness raising	Finding and learning new facts, ideas, and tips that support healthy behavior change
Dramatic relief	Experiencing negative emotions because the negative behavior (e.g., being physically inactive or eating fast food) is perceived to be problematic, then feeling relief from deciding to change
Self-reevaluation	Realizing behavior change is an important part of one's identity as a person
Environmental reevaluation	Realizing how the behavior influences the environment, especially the person's social environment
Self-liberation	Deciding to change and experiencing a new belief in the ability to change
Helping relationships	Seeking and using social support for behavior change
Counter-conditioning	Substituting healthier behaviors and cognitions for the unhealthy behavior
Reinforcement management	Increasing rewards for healthy behavior change and decreasing rewards for unhealthy behavior
Stimulus control	Removing reminders and cues to engage in unhealthy behaviors and replacing them with reminders/cues for healthy behavior
Social liberation	Taking advantage of opportunities to be with people who model the new behavior, noticing the social norms that reinforce the new behavior

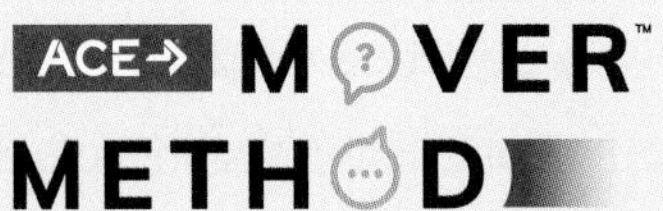

The Healthy Eating Contemplator

A client you have been working with for the past eight months is now in the maintenance stage of change for participating in regular physical activity. While she has been successful with implementing and adhering to an exercise program that includes meeting with you twice per week, attending one group exercise class per week, and accumulating 7,000 steps five days per week, she mentions to you that she is not making any changes to improve her nutrition. Also, she makes it clear that she understands the importance of eating a healthier diet but is not planning on making a change right now, though she does intend to do so within the next six months.

ACE ABC APPROACH

The following is an example of how the ACE ABC Approach can be used to work with clients who may be in the contemplation stage of change for a health-related goal.

Ask: Asking powerful open-ended questions to find out what eating a healthier diet means to the client will spark a discussion about client expectations and food preferences.

Personal Trainer: You mentioned being interested in eating a healthier diet. What does eating healthier mean to you?

Client: I have not put a lot of thought into the specifics yet, but I know the amount of fast food, soda, and candy I eat throughout the week cannot be good for me and is not helping me with my overall goals of wanting to lose weight and improve my fitness.

Break down barriers: At this point in the conversation, more open-ended questions can be used to discover what potential obstacles may get in the way of working toward the goal. The following questions can be used to prompt the client to share more about what may hold her back from making dietary changes.

Personal Trainer: The amount of fast food and sugary foods and beverages you eat is a concern for you. Have you tried adopting healthier eating habits in the past? How were you able to be successful and what, if anything, prevented you from reaching your goals?

Client: Yes. The amount of fast food and unhealthy snacking I am doing is a concern for me, and I see how it is getting in the way of my goals. I have made many attempts at eating better over the years and have been successful with planning out my meals and snacks, but only for a short period before I am right back to eating out and refilling my snack drawer at work with unhealthy foods. Being busy at work, feeling stressed, and not knowing enough about cooking seems to hold me back. Planning ahead is one thing that helps me, but I don't have enough time to get serious about my nutrition right now.

Personal Trainer: You have learned a lot about what works and does not work from your previous experience and you do not have time to get serious about nutrition now. What do you have time for?

Client: Well, I know the reason I eat out so much is that it is convenient, and the main reason I don't bring food to work is because I don't know enough healthy options and don't want to just eat the same thing every day. At this point, I could start looking into healthy lunch and snack options that are easy to prepare and are accessible. I also could see if the places where I currently eat have any healthier food choices, since I am already going there anyway.

Collaborate: Working together with the client on goals and solutions is the next step of this discussion. Now that the client has mentioned potential barriers (e.g., inconvenience) and suggested some potential options for moving forward, it is time to decide on the next steps. The following question can be used to prompt the progression to goal setting.

Personal Trainer: Now that we know what you mean by eating healthier, that planning out your meals has helped you in the past, and that being busy at work leads you to seek convenient food choices over healthy choices, how would you like to move forward?

Client: Looking to see if the regular fast food places I visit have any healthier options seems like a good place to start. If I know what options are the healthiest, I can make better decisions without having to make any major changes.

Personal Trainer: What can you do within the next week to get started?

Client: I will spend one hour visiting the websites of the three main places I like to eat and making a list of healthy alternatives for each place. I will keep the list in the notes section of my phone and when I am ready to make a healthier choice I will already know what I want.

From this sample interaction, you can see how the ACE ABC Approach allows the client and personal trainer to work together in a nonjudgmental way by the personal trainer meeting the client where she is and letting her decide what next steps are right for her. Ultimately, the client was in control and decided on an action without the personal trainer telling her what she should or should not do. This leads into the next steps for the personal trainer, as there is now something specific to follow up with the client about in the next session.

Self-efficacy

The third component of the TTM is **self-efficacy** (the degree to which an individual believes he or she can successfully perform a given behavior). The concept was originally described by Albert Bandura as part of his groundbreaking **social cognitive theory,** which posited that as people learn behaviors, they are influenced by (1) cognitive and personal factors (such as knowledge, outcome expectations, and attitudes), (2) behavioral factors (including skills, practice, self-evaluation, and self-efficacy), and (3) environmental factors (such as social norms, community influences, behavior reinforcement, and observational learning) (Bandura, 1986). In

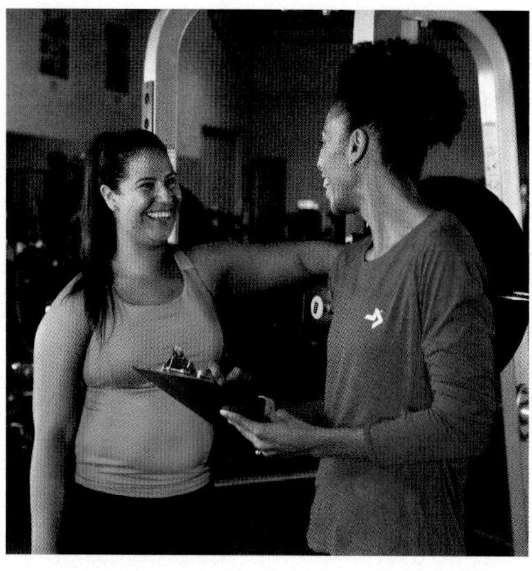

other words, according to social cognitive theory, how people think about things exerts a strong influence on their behaviors. Social cognitive theory supports the importance of having positive outcome expectations, goal setting, self-monitoring behavior, prompting intention formation (helping clients make a decision to change), and planning, which are all important practices for personal trainers to embrace.

Self-efficacy in the exercise context is the belief in one's own capabilities to successfully engage in an exercise program. Self-efficacy is an important component of exercise-related behavior change because it is strongly related to program adoption and maintenance. In fact, research points to self-efficacy as the strongest, most consistent psychological correlate of physical-activity behavior (Higgins et al., 2014).

There is a circular relationship between self-efficacy and behavior change, such that a person's self-efficacy is related to whether he or she will participate in an activity, and a person's participation in activity influences his or her self-efficacy level. Therefore, self-efficacy acts as both a determinant and an outcome of behavior change. Additionally, there is a reliable relationship between self-efficacy for activity and stage of behavior change, such that those in the precontemplation and contemplation stages have significantly lower levels of self-efficacy than individuals in the action and maintenance stages. This is a logical relationship, as those in the precontemplation and contemplation stages are not yet engaging in physical activity, which may be reflective of the belief that they do not have the ability or knowledge required to be active, while those in the action and maintenance stages are engaged in regular activity programs, thus demonstrating a belief in the ability to be regularly active.

The relationship between stage of change and self-efficacy implies that by increasing self-efficacy, a person may progress through the stages more efficiently. This is critical for people in the contemplation and preparation stages, as they are thinking about or wanting to be physically active and working toward the point where they can be regularly active, but still have some doubts about achieving that goal. By specifically focusing on increasing these individuals' levels of self-efficacy, a personal trainer may be best able to support them in progressing to the action stage more quickly.

Because self-efficacy is a subjective perception of one's own ability to succeed, it is difficult to quantify. To develop an understanding of a client's self-efficacy regarding exercise participation, a personal trainer may ask questions about the sources of self-efficacy information. Specifically, through conversation, a personal trainer can gain knowledge about a client's previous experience with exercise, feelings and emotions associated with starting a new program, expectations and apprehensions related to program involvement (e.g., physiological, psychological, and environmental), and potential barriers for program **adherence.** As client self-efficacy will continually change, personal trainers can help clients leverage increases in self-efficacy and collaborate with clients to make program modifications when self-efficacy levels decrease. In general, by being aware of self-efficacy levels, personal trainers will be better able to foster motivation in their clients and help them create positive self-belief.

How does a person develop self-efficacy? Personal history of physical activity during adulthood is a clear correlate of current physical-activity status (Bauman et al., 2012). This means that an individual who has had past success in adopting and maintaining a physical-activity program will have higher self-efficacy regarding his or her ability to be active in the future. It also means that those individuals with no exercise experience may have much lower self-efficacy regarding their ability to engage in an exercise program. Therefore, it is essential to provide beginners with positive exercise experiences very early in their programs. This can be as simple as creating short-term success by designing a workout that the client will master and that will demonstrate growth and achievement. In fact, this should be the case for the program in general, as each workout should build on previous accomplishments.

Sources of Self-efficacy

Personal trainers can use the following six sources of self-efficacy to help influence client self-efficacy levels and promote exercise adoption and continued adherence (Warner et al., 2014; Bandura, 1997).

- **Past performance experience** is an influential source of self-efficacy information. Personal trainers may ask clients about their previous experiences with exercise, fitness facilities, and personal trainers. These previous experiences will strongly influence their current self-efficacy levels.
- **Vicarious experience** is important for a client who is new to exercise and who has little previous personal experience with a supervised program. The observation or knowledge of someone else who is successfully participating in a similar program—or has done so in the past—can increase one's self-efficacy. This is particularly true if the person being observed is perceived by the client to be similar to him- or herself (e.g., age, **chronic** illness status, sex, and/or fitness level).
- **Verbal persuasion** typically occurs in the form of feedback and encouragement from teachers. Statements from others are most likely to influence self-efficacy if they come from a credible, respected, and knowledgeable source. Different clients will require different amounts of verbal encouragement and statements of belief. Being aware of how much feedback a client needs and then providing that verbal support is an important motivational tool for personal trainers.
- **Physiological state appraisals** related to exercise participation are important because a client may experience **emotional arousal,** pain, or fatigue. The types of appraisals clients make about their physiological states may lead to judgments about their ability to participate successfully. It is important to help clients evaluate appraisals of their physiological states to create positive interpretations. By teaching clients to appropriately identify muscle fatigue, soreness, and tiredness, as well as the implications of these states, personal trainers can help clients view the "feelings" of working out in a more positive light.
- **Emotional state and mood appraisals** of program participation can also influence self-efficacy. Negative mood states and emotional beliefs associated with exercise,

such as fear, anxiety, anger, and frustration, are related to reduced levels of self-efficacy and lower levels of participation. On the other hand, positive mood states and emotional beliefs, including mastery, are related to higher levels of self-efficacy. Hence, giving encouraging coaching cues and tailoring client programs that are sufficiently challenging, yet simply mastered, contribute to elevated moods and positive emotional states.

- **Imaginal experiences** refer to the imagined experiences (positive or negative) of exercise participation. It is important to understand a client's preconceived notion of what exercise will be like, as this information will influence actual self-efficacy levels. The personal trainer may encourage positive imagined experiences by asking open-ended questions such as, "How do you imagine you'll feel when you reach your goal of being able to walk on the treadmill for 20 minutes without stopping?"

With this information, the personal trainer will be better able to design and deliver a program that sets up the client for success. In an exercise program, self-efficacy levels will influence the types of tasks an individual wants to engage in, how hard they will try, and if they will persist. Specifically, people with high self-efficacy will choose challenging tasks, set goals, and display a commitment to master those tasks. They will display maximal effort to reach their goals and will even increase their effort when challenges arise. Highly self-efficacious clients tend to work hard to overcome obstacles and recover from setbacks, and ultimately, are much more likely to adhere to a program (Bauman et al., 2012).

On the other hand, people with low self-efficacy will be more likely to choose non-challenging tasks that are non-threatening and easy to accomplish. They will display minimal effort to protect themselves in the face of a challenge—since failing when not working hard will be a lesser blow to their self-efficacy than failing when doing their best—and, if faced with too many setbacks, are more likely to give up and drop out of the program (Bandura, 1994).

Decisional Balance

The final of the four components of the TTM is **decisional balance,** which refers to the evaluation of pros and cons about adopting and/or maintaining an activity program. Individuals in the precontemplation and contemplation stages of change perceive more cons (e.g., sweating, sore muscles, time, cost, unwanted physical changes, and boredom) related to being regularly active than pros. The cons that prevent an individual from being active may be real or perceived. As people progress through the stages of change, the balance of pros and cons shifts, such that people in the action and maintenance stages perceive more pros about being active than cons. The behavior of people in these later stages reflects this change in decisional balance. The decisional balance worksheet presented in Figure 3-4 can be used to help clients weigh the perceived benefits against the potential costs involved with making a physical activity–related behavior change. While this worksheet is a valuable tool to help personal trainers and clients work together to clarify benefits as well as to examine potential barriers or obstacles, it is important that personal trainers do not become overly reliant on worksheets. The most effective approach is for personal trainers to use worksheets in conjunction with effective communication and observation skills to build a complete understanding of client needs to inform the development of appropriate programming.

Instructions:

- Work with the client to document the gains and potential losses that he or she might experience when making a lifestyle change.
- Identify and list the recommended implementation strategies needed to achieve the gains and list coping strategies that can be used to deal with the potential losses or obstacles associated with the change.

DECISIONAL BALANCE WORKSHEET

Perceived gains associated with adopting desired behaviors	Perceived losses associated with adopting desired behaviors
1. ______	1. ______
2. ______	2. ______
3. ______	3. ______
4. ______	4. ______
Strategies to maximize potential for achieving gains	**Strategies to minimize potential of perceived losses**
1. ______	1. ______
2. ______	2. ______
3. ______	3. ______
4. ______	4. ______

FIGURE 3-4
Decisional balance worksheet

The natural shift in decisional balance that occurs as people progress through the stages of change suggests that influencing clients' perceptions about being active may help encourage them to start an activity program. When working on shifting decisional balance, it is important to remember the processes of change related to moving from one stage to the next. For example, when working with individuals in the precontemplation and contemplation stages of change, it is important to emphasize a wide variety of benefits of being physically active and avoid refuting the cons they perceive about exercise. Often, the cons that non-exercisers perceive about physical activity are a result of misinformation and/or lack of experience. **Motivational interviewing** skills (see Chapter 4) are often helpful when working with individuals who are in these initial two stages to help them put into their own words reasons for making a behavior change, if and when they are ready to do so. Additionally, it is important that the discussed benefits are both short- and long-term. For example, emphasizing only the long-term health benefits of an activity program can be overwhelming and may make those benefits seem unattainable. Focusing on the short-term benefits, such as increased energy and mastery of the exercise itself, will give the client something to look forward to experiencing or accomplishing immediately.

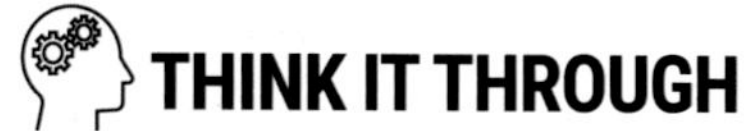

Tailoring the Approach to the Current Stage of Change

Review the following examples of individuals in each of the stages of change. How would you respond in each of these scenarios?

Precontemplation: You are having a discussion with your uncle, who is questioning how anyone can make a living by helping people exercise. Your uncle is physically inactive and thinks that exercise is for people who take aerobics classes or for bodybuilder types who are looking to bulk up. He views exercise as completely irrelevant to his life. Your initial thought is to argue with your uncle and to tell him that he is completely misinformed, but this would be counterproductive. How would you educate your uncle without lecturing or arguing with him?

Contemplation: You receive a phone call at the gym from a woman who saw an advertisement for a free trial week. She says that she does not currently work out and that she has never exercised in a gym before. She seems very apprehensive and nervous on the phone and says that she is not sure if she will like it, but that she knows she needs to be more active. She asks if there is any programming for beginners and if someone will be available to help her if she comes in, as she does not know what she is doing. How would you respond? What is the most appropriate course of action for working with this potential client?

Preparation: You are approached by a member at the gym who comes in a few times a month and goes through a basic workout. He tells you that he wants to be more consistent, but that he is having a difficult time finding the motivation. He says that he is not sure what he needs to be doing and that he needs help. How would you respond to this club member to best enhance his motivation for lasting lifestyle change?

Action: You have a client who has been consistently training three days a week for two months. She is seeing great results and loves her workouts. She is always happy to come in and never misses an appointment. The client has two children and, with the school year coming to an end, knows her schedule will change. She really wants to continue to train. You encourage the client by telling her how great she has done, reminding her how much she has accomplished. The two of you then talk about the challenges she will face trying to stick to her workouts when her children are out of school. How will you help your client adjust to her new schedule?

Maintenance: A long-time client has lost more than 60 pounds (27 kg) over the past year and feels great. He rarely misses an appointment and has reached his goals and loves being physically active. He has even started taking his family for hikes on the weekends. You understand, however, that this state of consistency may not last forever, so you plan a session with the client to evaluate the program and set new goals. How would you manage this meeting and what topics would you discuss to help him anticipate and overcome potential obstacles to continued success?

Lapse and Relapse

Because moving along the behavior-change continuum is not necessarily a linear process, it should not be a surprise if clients move back into an earlier stage on the continuum, even after maintaining a behavior for years. In fact, **relapse** (the return of an original behavior, such as being physically inactive, after many **lapses,** or slips in a program) can occur during any stage of the TTM, including maintenance. Lapses from regular physical-activity participation are common and should be planned for and expected. From unplanned events and schedule changes to vacations and illnesses, there are countless things that can trigger such a lapse.

An important strategy for dealing with a lapse is to address it before it happens through conversation with a client. Personal trainers may inform their clients about the likelihood of a relapse and prepare them in advance, so that they are able to get back on track with their activity programs soon after experiencing one. Typically, clients will face one or more barriers, such as a lack of time or finances, scheduling conflicts, support issues, or dissatisfaction with the program, so it is important to develop strategies to counter attrition before adherence problems arise. Collaborating with clients on what to do in those situations, rather than telling them what to do, will help them draw upon their own unique skills and resources during stressful, busy, or difficult times.

Another key to dealing with lapses and preventing relapse is to enhance social support. Personal trainers can offer support outside of the training session, whether in the form of a phone call, email, text message, or social media platform. Further, personal trainers may explore with clients enhanced support at home, as it is important to get family members and/or friends involved to some degree when a client is embarking on a behavior-change plan. In fact, evidence suggests that adherence to an exercise program is increased when an exerciser has support from his or her spouse or immediate family members, either by joint participation or by demonstration of a positive attitude toward participation (Greaves et al., 2011). In general, the individuals supporting a client must understand the commitment the client has made to being physically active.

Similar to the techniques described earlier for creating a caring, task-involving climate, personal trainers may create a support system within the exercise environment, which can be accomplished by maximizing opportunities for group involvement and social interaction and making clients feel as though they belong and are part of a team of people who have common interests and goals. Further, clients can be encouraged to engage with each other outside of the gym by registering for upcoming events (e.g., fun run or 5K walk) or interacting on social media forums (e.g., private Facebook group created for clients). Ultimately, feeling connected to others who are physically active reduces the likelihood that a client will relapse to a pattern of sporadic activity and/or **sedentary** behavior.

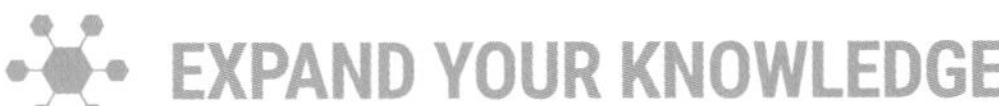

Willpower

Understanding willpower may help personal trainers empathize with clients and help better prepare them to avoid a relapse into physically inactive and/or sedentary habits. Willpower is the ability to ignore temporary pleasure or discomfort to pursue a longer-term goal, and it is a biological function. It is a mind-body response, not a virtue. Anyone using willpower for long periods or for multiple tasks will have less resolve to make better choices. A review of the literature on self-control and decision-making abilities has shown that willpower is inherently limited (Hagger et al., 2010). That is, self-control depletes willpower in much the same way that exercise temporarily depletes physical power. Researchers have found that in experiments where people exert their willpower on one occasion, they have difficulty doing so a second time (Hagger et al., 2010). This effect was discovered with a variety of self-control tasks, such as avoiding tempting foods, suppressing emotions, and sticking with challenging problems.

Using willpower is essentially relying on one's rational side to control or dictate what the emotional side wants—and it is not really a fair fight, as emotions are a more powerful driver of decisions than reason. If clients set too many goals or have goals that are too large and imposing, they can, by force of will, maintain things for a short period. At the first sign of trouble, however—when they get stuck in traffic on the way home from work or have extra responsibilities in dealing with family matters—their resolve crumbles, and they get too worn out to maintain the new, difficult behaviors.

Given that willpower is inherently limited, clients should have strategies to conserve it. Planning for moments of diminished self-control reinforces willpower when it is needed most. For example, when a client makes food choices when he or she is hungry or tired, the choices made are often of poorer nutritional quality. A better strategy is to organize meals for the day in advance when the client has higher resolve. Another effective strategy for conserving willpower is to think in advance about how to deal with specific obstacles before they arise. In a study on exercise and self-regulation, investigators found that people who wrote in a journal about how they would handle barriers to exercise were more likely to stick with an exercise program (Sniehotta et al., 2005). Another study found that journaling in advance about overcoming barriers helped people succeed at a challenging self-control task, even after a previous task had depleted their willpower (Webb & Sheeran, 2003).

Principles of Behavior Change

As most exercise professionals are active themselves, they sometimes have difficulty relating to the challenges of getting started from a **previously physically inactive** state. This is part of the reason why it is important for personal trainers to understand and apply the theoretical constructs detailed in the previous section in their work with clients. The main benefit of using such models and theories is that they properly address exercise as a health behavior. As mentioned before, the adoption of physical activity is a complicated process that requires replacing unhealthy, inactive behaviors with healthy, active behaviors. It is the personal trainer's job to provide guidance and support to help clients change their behaviors by positively influencing their attitudes, motives, emotions, and performance. The process of behavioral change is a gradual progression that requires effort, dedication, and commitment, as well as an understanding of the following factors that influence behavior.

OPERANT CONDITIONING

Operant conditioning is the process by which behaviors are influenced by their **consequences.** More specifically, it examines the relationship between **antecedents,** behaviors, and consequences (Martin & Pear, 2010). Operant conditioning examines the **behavior chains** that lead to the engagement of certain behaviors and the avoidance of others, taking into account the consequences associated with each behavior.

In an exercise program, the goal is to increase healthy behaviors in clients' lives. According to the principle of operant conditioning, behaviors are strengthened when they are reinforced. In the personal-training context, using **positive reinforcements** means that positive or healthy behaviors have consequences that are going to increase the likelihood of the behavior happening again. At the most basic level with a new client, a positive behavior is simply showing up to the gym. If the success of this behavior (which can be a real victory for a new exerciser) is ignored by the personal trainer, the likelihood of it happening again will decrease. However, if the client is verbally rewarded for showing up and is further rewarded with a positive, pleasant, and supportive workout experience, then the behavior has been positively reinforced and the likelihood of it happening again has been increased. As personal trainers, the opportunity to trigger lasting change is always present, and the basic principle of operant conditioning can serve as a good reminder of the influence personal trainers have with each client they encounter.

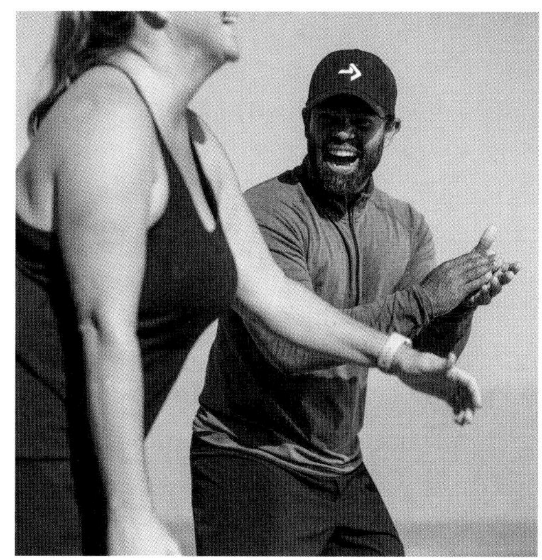

Antecedents

Part of the learning experience is realizing the consequences of specific behaviors under certain conditions. Antecedents help in this process, as they are stimuli that precede a behavior and often signal the likely consequences of the behavior. An example of an ineffective antecedent is a man looking at the clock and realizing he is late for his workout. This would lead to the behavior of rushing out the door and speeding to the gym, where he is able to complete only part of his scheduled training appointment.

Antecedents can be manipulated in the environment to maximize the likelihood of desirable behaviors. This type of influence by antecedents on behavior is called **stimulus control,** which is a valuable tool in behavior modification. For example, a client who frequently leaves the office late and is therefore late for his workout is getting only half of his scheduled workout time. To help with this problem, he sets an alarm on his computer for the days of his workouts to remind himself 15 minutes before it is time to leave. This reminder triggers him to prepare to leave his office and head to the gym—resulting in a full workout session.

APPLY WHAT YOU KNOW

Stimulus Control

An effective option for helping clients with behavior change is stimulus control. As previously discussed, stimulus control refers to adjusting the environment to increase the likelihood of healthy behaviors. Simple and effective stimulus-control strategies may include choosing a gym that is in the direct route between home and work; keeping a gym bag in the car that contains all the required items for a workout; having workout clothes, socks, and shoes laid out for early-morning workouts; and writing down workout times as part of a weekly schedule. A less obvious, but very important stimulus-control technique is for personal trainers to encourage their clients to surround themselves with other people who have similar health and fitness goals. By associating with people who are also interested in being active, clients will naturally develop support systems for behavior change. The overall goal of stimulus control is to make being physically active as convenient as possible.

Consequences

The most important component of operant conditioning is what happens after a behavior is executed. The consequence following a behavior will influence its future occurrence. Consequences fall under the categories of presentation, non-occurrence, or removal of a positive or aversive stimulus. Positive reinforcement is the presentation of a positive stimulus that increases the likelihood that the behavior will reoccur in the future. **Negative reinforcement,** which also increases the likelihood that a behavior will reoccur in the future, consists of the removal or avoidance of negative stimuli following a behavior. In other words, the removal of something negative that once followed a behavior makes a person more likely to perform the behavior again. For example, if a client associates muscular training with muscle soreness (a negative stimulus) from previous high-intensity workouts that were not appropriate for his experience level, he is not likely to want to participate in muscular-training activities again in the future. However, if the personal trainer creates an initial muscular-training program at a low level of intensity without progressing too quickly, soreness may be avoided (avoidance of the negative stimulus). This will increase the likelihood that the client will adhere to the program. **Extinction** occurs when a positive stimulus that once followed a behavior is removed and the likelihood that the behavior will reoccur is decreased. **Punishment** also decreases the likelihood of the behavior reoccurring and consists of an aversive stimulus following a behavior.

COGNITIONS AND BEHAVIOR

As reflected in the health belief model, self-determination theory, and TTM, a person's exercise behavior is influenced by how he or she thinks about exercise and about succeeding in an exercise program. Not only should personal trainers understand what their clients think about exercise participation, but they should also support clients in becoming more aware of their own thoughts, or cognitions.

Replacing Irrational Thoughts

Each person has a unique way of viewing the world and interpreting events. Most people understand this concept on a basic level but may sometimes operate on the assumption that their personal judgments are an accurate perception of reality without realizing that they may not be perceiving the whole picture. Some clients may suffer from **cognitive distortions** (Figure 3-5) that reinforce irrational and potentially harmful thought patterns that interfere with their well-being (Burns, 1999). The personal trainer may help a client recognize and replace irrational cognitions with healthier, more productive and factual thinking by asking the client to answer questions such as the following:

- What is the evidence for and against this thought?
- What would I tell a friend in this same situation (as opposed to what I tell myself)?
- What is the worst that could realistically happen? How bad would that be?
- Is it really true that I must, should, ought to, have to...?
- Are there any other possible responses besides blaming myself?
- Is there any conceivable way to look at this positively?

- Is thinking this way helping the situation, myself, or others, or only making it worse?
- How have I effectively managed or tolerated these situations in the past?

Going through the process of answering these questions may help clients to check, challenge, and change their own words, through which they are better able to understand why their irrational thoughts may be impeding progress or unnecessarily skewing their perceptions about physical activity in a negative way.

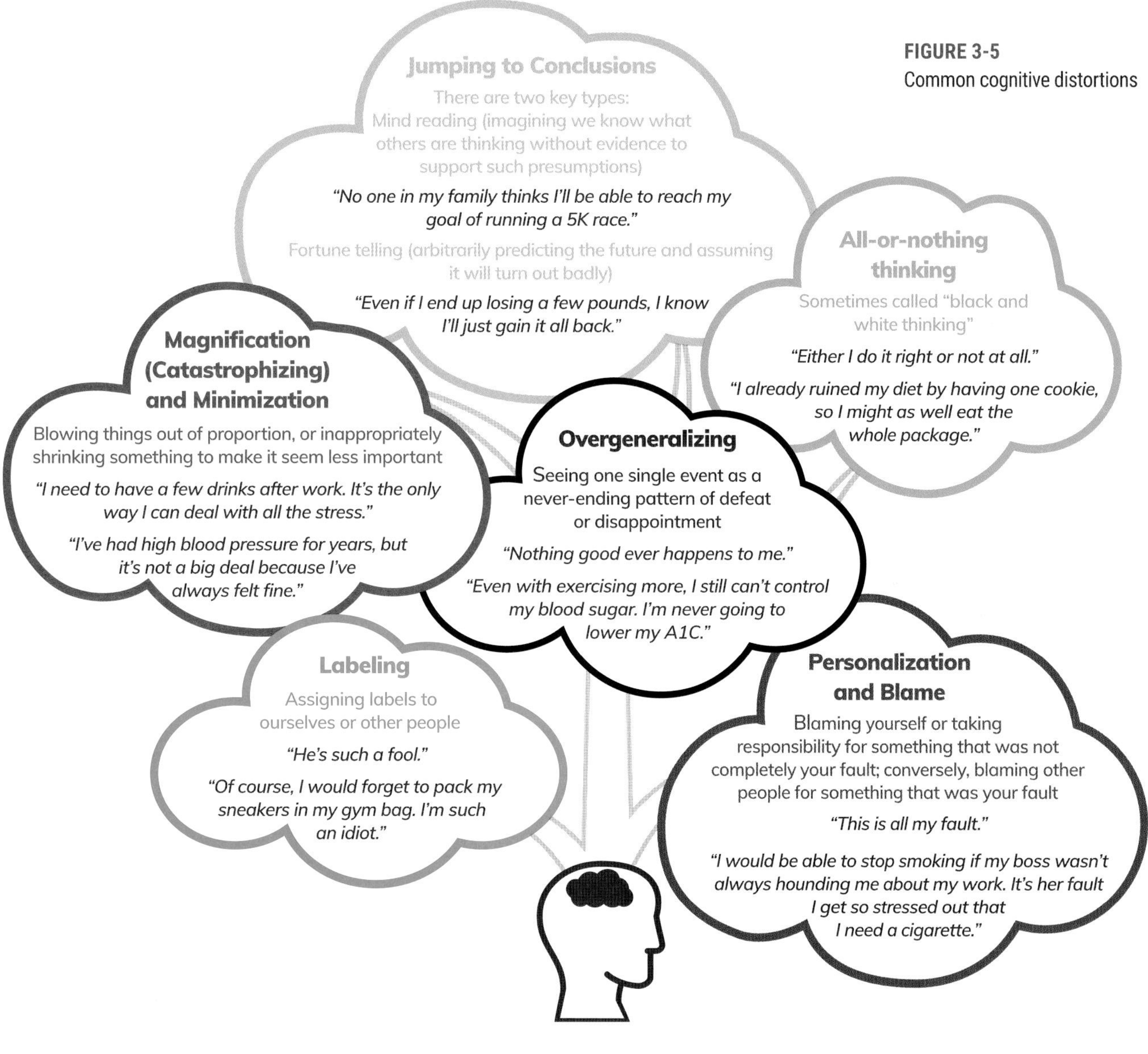

FIGURE 3-5
Common cognitive distortions

THINK IT THROUGH

Reflecting on Your Own Behavior-change Strategies

Think about your own daily routine and how you may already be using principles of behavior change in your own life. Are there any techniques you can encourage your clients to use to improve their chances for success at sustained healthy lifestyle change?

Goal Setting

Goal setting is one of the most widely used and straightforward behavior-change strategies. However, it is often used ineffectively. People tend to set goals and then get started on the program, quickly forgetting about the goals. Goal setting, to be maximally effective, must be a collaborative process between the client and personal trainer and included as a regular part of the exercise-program planning. Personal trainers can help clients remain aware of what they are working toward and what it will take to get there. Additionally, the goals should be written following the **SMART goal** guidelines (specific, measurable, attainable, relevant, and time-bound) (see Chapter 4). Personal trainers may assist clients through the goal-setting process and help them understand how to set effective and appropriate goals.

Self-monitoring

Self-monitoring is one of the cognitive processes of self-regulation, which describes an individual's evaluation of his or her thoughts and feelings and how that information is then used to shape goals and behaviors. Self-regulation encompasses self-control and involves resisting impulsive behavior and making choices that align with one's values and vision.

As clients progress and adhere to their behavior-change plans, the personal trainer can utilize open-ended questions such as "What's helping you stay in this stage?" "What else could support you in your continued success?" and "What are your high-risk temptations?" These types of questions enable clients to acknowledge how far they have come, while also recognizing potential barriers and further reinforcing the habits they have cultivated, rather than relying on willpower alone. It is worth noting that problem solving often evolves naturally from self-monitoring, as clients become aware of the situations that move them toward, or steer them further away from, their specific goals. Through self-monitoring, clients can articulate new action steps and adjust plans as needed to promote continued progress.

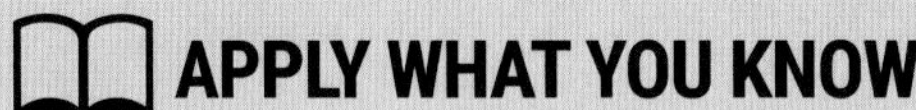

Behavioral Interventions

There are several pieces of information that personal trainers need to obtain when working with a new client. The first one is past activity experience and the client's feelings and perceptions about that experience. In other words, how might past experiences with exercise influence the current experience? In this discussion, the personal trainer can identify client apprehensions, comfort zones, and abilities and should be able to get a pretty good idea of the client's current exercise-specific self-efficacy level.

A personal trainer should also seek information about the client's social-support network. If the client does not have a support network that embraces and encourages an active lifestyle, he or she will face many more obstacles to achieving long-term program adherence. Everything from family and friend physical-activity levels to work environment is relevant and important in designing an appropriate program. Some of this information will be easily gathered in initial meetings and some of it will surface over time as the client–personal trainer relationship is better established (see Chapter 4).

Personal trainers should also identify clients' attitudes, opinions, and beliefs about physical activity and then make efforts to help guide client decisional balance and self-efficacy. Almost all new exercisers have misconceptions about being physically active. It is up to the personal trainer to teach the truths about living an active lifestyle. This is best done through a continual process of education, experience, and trust development that provides logical information to help dispute irrational beliefs and foster the creation of a rational and realistic view of fitness.

In other words, each training session is an opportunity for the personal trainer to empower the client to make lasting changes (see Chapter 4). It is critical that initial program experiences build mastery and positive emotional states. Clients must believe early on that they can do it. If doubt lingers for an extended period, the client may lose confidence and drop out. Personal trainers must treat each client as an individual and address the unique goals, needs, attitudes, and beliefs of each person.

Lastly, personal trainers and clients should collaborate on effective goal setting from the very beginning. This requires the personal trainer to explore goal-setting techniques and self-monitoring strategies. Personal trainers should empower their clients to take their physical-activity experiences into their own hands.

Physical Activity and Adherence

For the purposes of a personal trainer, exercise adherence refers to a client's voluntary and regular active involvement in an exercise program. Most people know that being physically active has many health benefits and have even started an exercise program at some time in their lives. Yet, existing approaches may not be effective for getting people to stick with a program. Unfortunately, the solution is not simple. There are many factors related to exercise that influence adherence and dropout (e.g., environment, support, leadership, and knowledge). Because there is no exact formula for helping people continue with a program, it is up to personal trainers to combine their communication, behavior-change, and program-design skills to create well-rounded exercise programs that not only get people fit and healthy, but that also create an exercise experience that is positive and valued by the clients. The potential determinants for physical activity can be broken down into three categories:

- Personal attributes
- Environmental factors
- Physical-activity factors

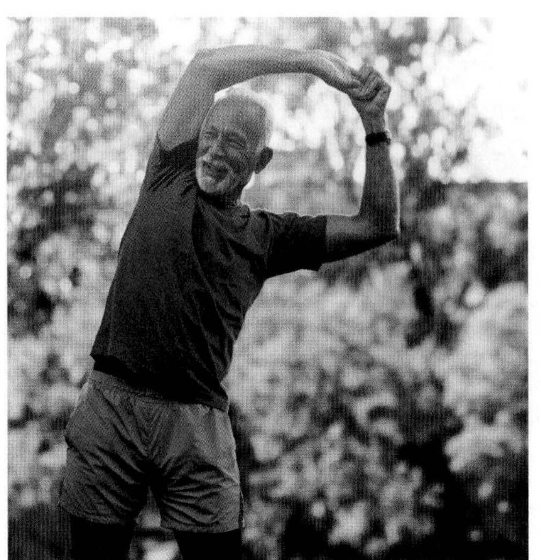

Having a general understanding of these factors can help prepare personal trainers for the various challenges that clients may face during participation in an exercise program.

PERSONAL ATTRIBUTES

Demographic Variables

Adherence to physical-activity programs has been consistently related to education, income, age, and sex [Centers for Disease Control and Prevention (CDC), 2013]. Specifically, lower levels of activity are seen with increasing age, fewer years of education, and lower income. Age, however, has been shown to be unrelated to adherence levels when examined in supervised exercise settings. Since personal trainers are directly involved with supervised fitness programs, this is particularly relevant, because when exercise sessions are conducted under the guidance of exercise professionals, adherence levels are increased among various age groups (Lowry et al., 2013; Dorgo et al., 2011). Regarding sex, men demonstrate higher and more consistent activity adherence rates than women (CDC, 2013). Demographic variables always occur concurrently, so it can be difficult to understand the specific effects of one demographic variable versus another. Nevertheless, the general trends are apparent and consistent.

Health Status

Individuals who suffer from chronic illness, such as heart disease and **diabetes,** typically exercise less than those who are healthy (Newsom et al., 2012). In their review on health behavior change following chronic illness, Newsom and colleagues (2012) reported that although physical limitations may be a mitigating factor for reduced physical activity, it may also be that common misconceptions still exist that those with **chronic disease** should not exercise. The researchers also stated that given the clear benefits of increased physical activity for individuals with chronic conditions, their findings suggest an important shortcoming in efforts to improve health behavior following diagnosis. Clinicians working together with clients/patients to set health-related goals may be an effective strategy to support change for those newly diagnosed with a chronic illness. Developing a referral network with local healthcare providers can place exercise professionals on the front lines of helping individuals with chronic disease see the value in engaging in safe and effective exercise (see Chapter 1).

Physical-activity History

Physical-activity history is an important and influential personal attribute variable (Bauman et al., 2012). Therefore, it is important that personal trainers gather physical-activity history information from their clients. This information can help in the development of the current program, as client preferences should be considered, and it will also give the personal trainer a good idea of the challenges that the client may face in adhering to the program.

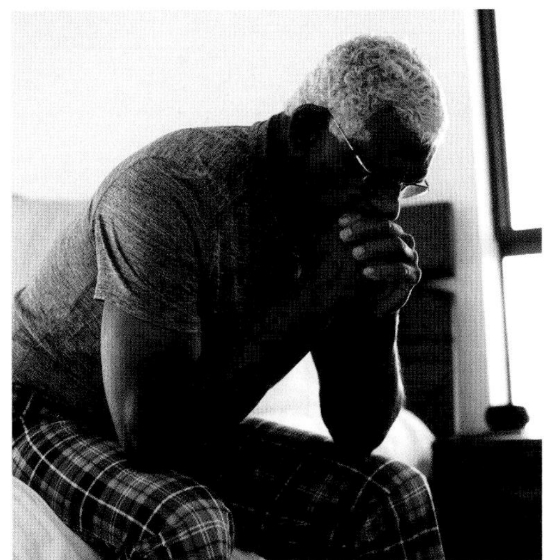

Psychological Traits

Difficulty managing negative thoughts and moods has been shown to be a barrier to lifestyle interventions involving physical activity. That is, mood may affect adherence to physical activity, with lower levels of depression, stress, and anxiety and **negative affect** predicting adherence, while higher levels of stress, depression, and anger predict attrition (Burgess, Hassmen, & Pumpa, 2017).

Not enjoying a physical-activity program can also negatively influence adherence. Working with clients to create an exercise program that is enjoyable, sustainable, and fits into their lifestyles is crucial because enjoyment levels can often be turned around with careful attention and creative, personalized strategies (Burgess, Hassmen, & Pumpa, 2017).

Knowledge, Attitudes, and Beliefs

Individuals have a wide variety of knowledge, attitudes, and beliefs about starting and sticking with an exercise program. Modifying the way a person thinks and feels about exercise has been shown to influence his or her intentions regarding being physically active. As described earlier in the section on the health belief model, health perception, which is a knowledge, attitude, and belief variable, has been linked to adherence, such that those who perceive their health to be poor are unlikely to start or adhere to an activity program. **Locus of control** is another variable in this category, as a belief in personal control over health outcomes is a consistent predictor of physical activity among healthy adults (Cobb-Clark, Kassenboehmer, & Schurer, 2014). Finally, the variable of perceived barriers, such as lack of time, consistently demonstrates a negative association with physical-activity program adherence (Martinez-Ramos et al., 2015).

A client's beliefs and expectations about self-progress play a huge role in adherence and affect the success of a physical-activity program. In a review of the determinants of adherence to a lifestyle intervention in adults with **obesity,** researchers found that when physical activity was undertaken only in the pursuit of weight loss, and when the weight was not lost at a satisfactory rate, individuals felt disheartened and lost motivation to continue (Burgess, Hassmen, & Pumpa, 2017). Thus, personal trainers should be careful when discussing weight-loss expectations with individuals and ensure that unrealistic goals do not increase the likelihood of attrition. Discussing the physical and psychological health benefits of long-term lifestyle change will help steer clients toward collaborating on goals based on health and quality of life as opposed to a time-limited weight-loss focus, which is difficult to control.

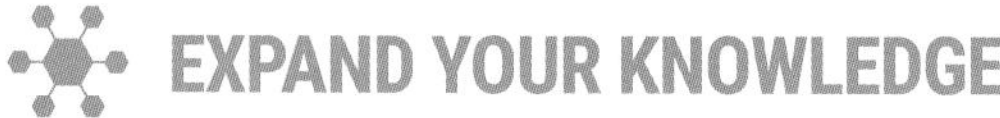

Locus of Control

A person's explanations for why things happen may influence his or her efforts when embarking on a behavior-change program. Most people tend to attribute their own behavior to the situation while attributing others' behaviors to personality. This makes sense, as individuals have considerable information about their own thoughts and behaviors, while the information they have about another person is limited to what they observe. For example, a personal trainer may have a client who frequently misses appointments. The personal trainer might assume this behavior is caused by the client's personality traits, perhaps concluding that the client is disorganized or lacking in self-control. On the other hand, the client, who has more information about his or her own behavior, might attribute the frequently missed sessions to a difficult situation, perhaps an unpredictable work schedule or overwhelming family demands.

Individual clients also may tend to emphasize either internal or external causes for their own health and behavior. Locus of control is the extent to which people think things happen for internal versus external reasons (Rotter, 1966). In the example above, the client who is frequently missing appointments might attribute the behavior to internal causes and decide he or she is disorganized or unreliable. Alternatively, the client might attribute the behavior to external causes, such as the work or family situation. External causes can include other people—a boss who makes excessive and unpredictable demands or a babysitter who is unreliable. Sometimes people attribute their behaviors to simple bad luck, fate, or another external cause.

In general, people with more of an internal locus of control, who have a stronger sense of control over their lives and who tend to attribute events and outcomes to internal factors such as effort and ability, may be more likely to exhibit positive health behaviors, such as exercising regularly. On the other hand, those with a more external locus of control, and particularly people who believe health is primarily a matter of luck, may be less likely to exercise or seek health information (Grotz et al., 2011).

In conversations with clients who seem to exhibit an external locus of control, personal trainers can empower the clients to view the behavior-change plan as being achievable and under the clients' control. For example, when a client starts explaining why he or she cannot find time to exercise, the personal trainer can intently listen and collaborate with the client to start with small, "easy" changes. In addition, personal trainers can support clients in viewing challenges that arise as a function of (sometimes) controllable and changeable factors, rather than personal failings. This can be difficult, but emphasizing past successes and highlighting personal strengths can prove powerful in terms of building client self-efficacy and internal locus of control over time.

ENVIRONMENTAL FACTORS

Access to Facilities

Access to facilities most commonly refers to facility location. When fitness facilities are conveniently located near a person's home or work, he or she is more likely to adhere to the program. However, low access to affordable facilities and limited space available for physical activity in the home are also commonly reported concerns (Venditti et al., 2014). Personal trainers may ask their clients about these issues to understand how convenient (or inconvenient) it is for them to access locations or facilities in which to be physically active.

Time

Lack of time is arguably the most common reason reported for not engaging in physical activity, as people perceive that they simply do not have enough time to be physically active. Finding balance among life's usual obligations, such as work and family routines, while still devoting time to health and physical activity, may be difficult (Martinez-Ramos et al., 2015). The perception of not having enough time to be active may reflect not being interested in or enjoying the activity, or not being committed to the activity program. Personal trainers may encourage their clients to change their perception of time availability through the use of goal setting, time management, and prioritizing. Further, personal trainers should consider implementing time-efficient exercise sessions [e.g., **reduced-exertion high-intensity interval training (REHIT)**; see Chapter 11] or collaborating with clients about opportunities to be physically active throughout their day. If a client considers health and physical activity to be top priorities, it is likely that he or she will find the time to be active.

Social Support

A positive correlation between social support from family and friends and physical-activity behavior has been found (Scarapicchia et al., 2017). It is difficult for a client to maintain an exercise program if he or she does not have support from others. When support is broken down into specific types, support from a spouse is shown to be an important and reliable predictor of program adherence. Further, the presence of an active partner may bolster motivation for, and adherence to, physical activity (Hull et al., 2010). Social support is also a critical topic for personal trainers and clients to discuss. If a client is lacking support from family and friends, personal trainers must be proactive in creating and establishing a support network for the client.

PHYSICAL-ACTIVITY FACTORS

Intensity

Of utmost importance in exercise and physical-activity programming is client enjoyment. Initially, clients may find it more tolerable and enjoyable to engage in low-intensity activities. There is emerging research, however, that suggests that **high-intensity interval training (HIIT)** may be more palatable to exercisers (both beginning and advanced) than one might naturally imagine (Astorino & Vella, 2018; Olney et al., 2018). A reduced time commitment coupled with the dynamic nature of HIIT are possible contributors to the reported similar or higher enjoyment levels in comparison with prolonged moderate-intensity cardiorespiratory exercise. Further, evidence has shown that HIIT can effectively improve **insulin** sensitivity, blood pressure, and **body composition** in adults, and these improvements are comparable to those resulting from continuous, long-duration, moderate-intensity cardiorespiratory exercise with effects more likely occurring in adults with overweight and obesity (2018 Physical Activity Guidelines Advisory Committee, 2018) (see Chapters 8 and 11 for details on how to safely and effectively program HIIT for a variety of clients).

Injury

There is a reliable association between physical activity and injury, such that the higher the dose of physical activity, the higher the risk for developing an activity-related injury (Knapik et al., 2011). Dose is determined by the frequency, duration, and intensity of the activity. Runners, for example, who run 40 miles (64 km) per week are more likely to be injured than those who run 15 miles (24 km) per week (2018 Physical Activity Guidelines Advisory Committee, 2018). Accordingly, even the most active and committed clients will experience adherence challenges when injured. Too much physical activity introduced too soon in a client's program will increase his or her risk for injury and subsequent dropout, so personal trainers must be diligent in designing programs that take into account appropriate progression (see Chapters 8 and 11 for details on program design using the ACE IFT Model).

PROGRAM DESIGN

A significant part of a personal trainer's job is exercise program design. The personal trainer must have the ability to design a personalized, safe, and effective physical-activity program for each client. A personal trainer must also be able to design a program with regard to each client's personal preferences, schedule, experience, apprehensions, and constraints (e.g., money, access, and time). If a personal trainer does not create customized programs, he or she will be unable to build a stable business that is based on promoting long-term adherence to physical activity.

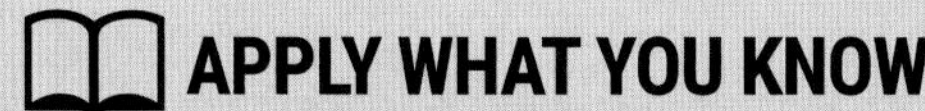

APPLY WHAT YOU KNOW

Increasing the Enjoyment Factor

What is it about a program that keeps a client coming back? Sometimes even the most comprehensive and carefully designed programs do not lead to program adherence. What is missing? An important concept to ponder is the type of experience the program creates for the client. The toughest competition for a client's time does not involve other facilities, personal trainers, or coaches. The real competition is the couch, family time, technology, friends, work, and so on. The exercise program must have enough value in the client's life for it to take priority over other demands so that long-term adherence occurs. How do the program, facility, and people involved make the client feel? Is the program *fun?* Do clients enjoy the experience of being involved in the program? If personal trainers create an environment where people want to be, they will attract and retain more clients. Creating enjoyable, positive experiences for clients will help ensure that they look forward to continually returning and, as a result, progressing toward their goals.

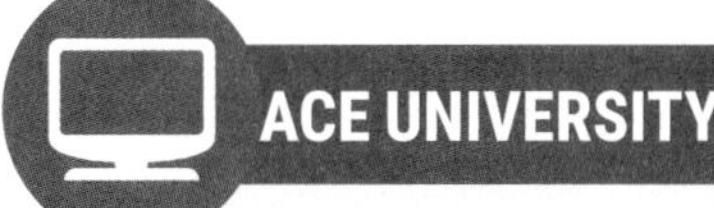

If your study program includes the ACE University, visit www.ACEfitness.org/MyACE and log in to your My ACE Account to take full advantage of the ACE Personal Trainer Study Program and online guided study experience.

A variety of media to support and expand on the material in this text is provided to facilitate learning and best prepare you for the ACE Personal Trainer Certification exam and a career as a personal trainer.

SUMMARY

Helping clients make changes in their physical-activity behaviors is a challenging and ongoing process. It requires a personal trainer to excel at communication, rapport building, and program design. A firm understanding of the models and theories of behavioral change will provide personal trainers with the knowledge, skills, and abilities required to support their clients in enacting lasting lifestyle changes. Further, taking into account clients' personal, environmental, and physical-activity factors related to adherence and incorporating that knowledge into personalized program design will increase the likelihood of clients successfully achieving their health and fitness goals and maintaining physical activity throughout life.

REFERENCES

2018 Physical Activity Guidelines Advisory Committee (2018). *2018 Physical Activity Guidelines Advisory Committee Scientific Report*. Washington, D.C.: U.S. Department of Health & Human Services.

Astorino, T.A. & Vella, C.A. (2018). Predictors of change in affect in response to high intensity interval exercise (HIIE) and sprint interval exercise (SIE). *Physiology & Behavior*, 196, 211–217.

Bandura, A. (1997). *Self-efficacy: The Exercise of Control*. New York, NY: Freeman.

Bandura, A. (1994). Self-efficacy. In: Ramachaudran, V.S. (Ed.) *Encyclopedia of Human Behavior* (Vol. 4; pp. 71–81). New York: Academic Press.

Bandura, A. (1986). *Social Foundations of Thought and Action: A Social Cognitive Theory*. Englewood Cliffs, N.J.: Prentice-Hall.

Bauman, A.E. et al. (2012). Correlates of physical activity: Why are some people physically active and others not? *Lancet*, 10, 258–271.

Brown, T.C. & Fry, M.D. (2014). Motivational climate, staff members' behaviors, and members' psychological well-being at a national fitness franchise. *Research Quarterly for Exercise & Sport*, 85, 208–217.

Brown, T.C. & Fry, M.D. (2013). Association between females' perceptions of college aerobics class motivational climates and their responses. *Women & Health*, 53, 843–857.

Brown, T.C. & Fry, M.D. (2011). Helping members commit to exercise: Specific strategies to impact the climate at fitness centers. *Journal of Sport Psychology in Action*, 2, 70–80.

Brown, T.C., Fry, M.D., & Moore, W.G. (2017). A motivational climate intervention and exercise-related outcomes: A longitudinal perspective. *Motivation Science*, 3, 4, 337–353.

Burgess, E., Hassmen, P., & Pumpa, K.L. (2017). Determinants of adherence to lifestyle intervention in adults with obesity: A systematic review. *Clinical Obesity*, 7, 3, 123–135.

Burns, D.D. (1999). *Feeling Good: The New Mood Therapy* (revised edition). New York: Wm. Morrow & Co.

Centers for Disease Control and Prevention, National Center for Health Statistics (2018). *National Health Interview Survey (NHIS), Early Release of Selected Estimates Based on Data From the 2017 National Health Interview Survey*. https://www.cdc.gov/nchs/nhis/releases/released201806.htm#7

Centers for Disease Control and Prevention (2013). Adult participation in aerobic and muscle-strengthening physical activities—United States, 2011. *Morbidity and Mortality Weekly Report*, 62, 17, 326–330.

Cobb-Clark, D.A., Kassenboehmer, S.C., & Schurer, S. (2014). Healthy habits: The connection between diet, exercise, and locus of control. *Journal of Economic Behavior & Organization*, 98, 1–28.

Deci, E.L. & Ryan, R.M. (2008). Facilitating optimal motivation and psychological well-being across life's domains. *Canadian Psychology*, 49, 1, 14–23.

Dorgo, S. et al. (2011). Comparing the effectiveness of peer mentoring and student mentoring in a 35-week fitness program for older adults. *Archives of Gerontology & Geriatrics*, 52, 3, 344–349.

Greaves, C. et al. (2011). Systematic review of reviews of intervention components associated with increased effectiveness in dietary and physical activity interventions. *BMC Public Health*, 11, 119.

Grotz, M. et al. (2011). Health locus of control and health behavior: Results from a nationally representative survey. *Psychology, Health, & Medicine*, 16, 2, 129–140.

Hagger, M.S. et al. (2010). Ego depletion and the strength model of self-control: A meta-analysis. *Psychological Bulletin*, 136, 4, 495–525.

Higgins, T.J. et al. (2014). Physical activity interventions differentially affect exercise task and barrier self-efficacy: A meta-analysis. *Health Psychology*, 33, 8, 891–903.

Hull, E.E. et al. (2010). Influence of marriage and parenthood on physical activity: A 2-year prospective analysis. *Journal of Physical Activity and Health*, 7, 5, 577–583.

Knapik, J.J. et al. (2011). Association between ambulatory physical activity and injuries during United States Army basic combat training. *Journal of Physical Activity and Health*, 8, 496–502.

Lowry, R. et al. (2013). Obesity and other correlates of physical activity and sedentary behaviors among U.S. high school students. *Journal of Obesity*, DOI: 10.1155/2013/276318.

Marcus, B.H. et al. (2000). Physical activity behavior change: Issues in adoption and maintenance. *Health Psychology*, 19, 32–41.

Martin, G. & Pear, J. (2010). *Behavior Modification: What It Is and How to Do It* (9th ed.). Englewood Cliffs, N.J.: Prentice-Hall.

Martinez-Ramos, E. et al. (2015). Prolonged sitting time: Barriers, facilitators and views on change among primary healthcare patients who are overweight or moderately obese. *PLoS ONE*, 10, 6, 1–21.

Morgan, W.P. (2001). Prescription of physical activity: A paradigm shift. *Quest*, 53, 336–382.

Newsom, J.T. et al. (2012). Health behavior change following chronic illness in middle and later life. *The Journals of Gerontology*, 67B, 3, 279–288.

Ng, J.Y.Y. et al. (2012). Self-determination theory applied to health contexts: A meta-analysis. *Perspectives on Psychological Science*, 7, 325–340.

Nicholls, J.G. (1984). Achievement motivation: Concepts of ability, subjective experience, task choice, and performance. *Psychological Review*, 91, 328–348.

Olney, N. et al. (2018). Comparison of acute physiological and psychological responses between moderate-intensity continuous exercise and three regimes of high-intensity interval training. *Journal of Strength & Conditioning Research*, 32, 8, 2130–2138.

Prochaska, J.O. & DiClemente, C.C. (1984). *The Transtheoretical Approach: Crossing Traditional Boundaries of Therapy*. Homewood, Ill.: Dow Jones/Irwin.

Reinboth, M. & Duda, J.L. (2006). Perceived motivational climate, need satisfaction, and indices of well-being in team sports: A longitudinal perspective. *Psychology of Sport & Exercise*, 7, 269–286.

Reinboth, M. & Duda, J.L. (2004). The motivational climate: Perceived ability and athletes' psychological and physical wellbeing. *The Sport Psychologist*, 18, 237–251.

Rosenstock, I.M. (1966). Why people use health services. *Milbank Memorial Fund Quarterly*, 44, 94–127.

Rotter, J.B. (1966). Generalized expectancies of internal versus external control of reinforcements. *Psychological Monographs*, 80, 1–28.

Ryan, R.M. & Deci, E.L. (2000). Self-determination theory and the facilitation of intrinsic motivation, social development, and well-being. *American Psychologist*, 55, 68–78.

Scarapicchia, T.M.F. et al. (2017). Social support and physical activity participation among healthy adults: A systematic review of prospective studies. *International Review of Sport & Exercise Psychology*, 10, 1, 50–83.

Sears, S.R., Brehm, B.A., & Bell, K. (2014). Understanding behavior change: Theoretical models. In: Brehm, B.A. *Psychology of Health and Fitness*. Philadelphia: F.A. Davis.

Sniehotta, F.F. et al. (2005). Long-term effects of two psychological interventions on physical exercise and self-regulation following coronary rehabilitation. *International Journal of Behavioral Medicine*, 12, 244–255.

Teixeira, P. et al. (2012). Exercise, physical activity, and self-determination theory: A systematic review. *International Journal of Behavioral Nutrition and Physical Activity*, 13, 78.

Vazou, S., Ntoumanis, N., & Duda, J.L. (2006). Predicting young athletes' motivational indices as a function of their perceptions of the coach- and peer-created climate. *Psychology of Sport & Exercise*, 7, 3, 215–233.

Venditti, E.M. et al. (2014). Short and long-term lifestyle coaching approaches used to address diverse participant barriers to weight loss and physical activity adherence. *International Journal of Behavior, Nutrition, & Physical Activity*, 11, 16, 1–23.

Warner, L. M. et al. (2014). Sources of self-efficacy for physical activity. *Health Psychology*, 33, 11, 1298–1308.

Webb, T.L. & Sheeran, P. (2003). Can implementation intentions help to overcome ego-depletion? *Journal of Experimental Psychology*, 39, 279–286.

SUGGESTED READINGS

American Council on Exercise (2019). *The Professional's Guide to Health and Wellness Coaching*. San Diego: American Council on Exercise.

Brown, T.C. & Fry, M.D. (2011). Helping members commit to exercise: Specific strategies to impact the climate at fitness centers. *Journal of Sport Psychology in Action*, 2, 70–80.

Fortier, M., Guerin, E., & Segar, M.L. (2016). Words matter: Reframing exercise is medicine for the general population to optimize motivation and create sustainable behavior change. *Applied Physiology of Nutrition & Metabolism*, 41, 1212–1216.

Teixeira, P. et al. (2012). Exercise, physical activity, and self-determination theory: A systematic review. *International Journal of Behavioral Nutrition and Physical Activity*, 13, 78.

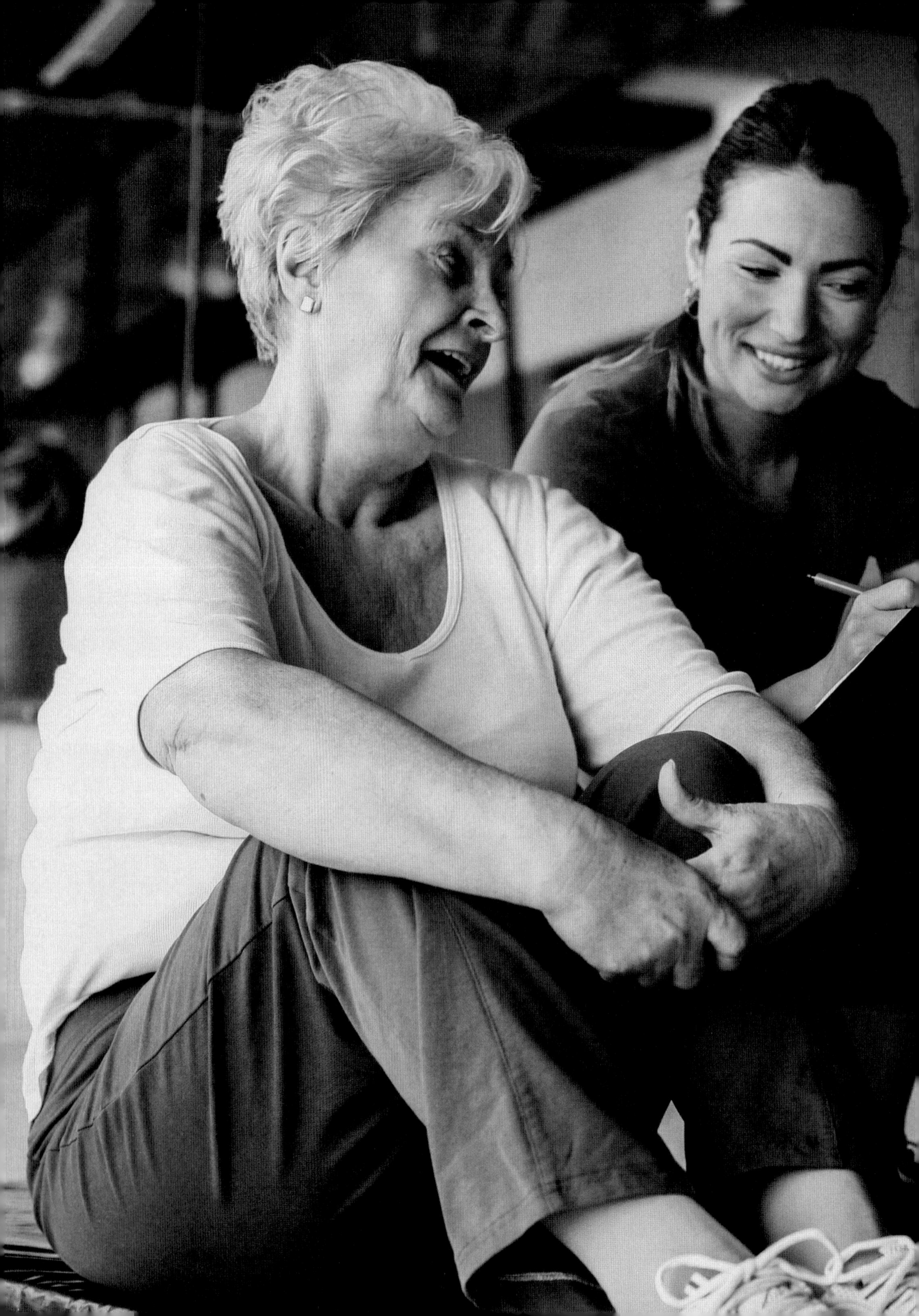

CHAPTER 4

Effective Communication, Goal Setting, and Teaching Techniques

SABRENA JO, MS
Director of Science and Research, American Council on Exercise; ACE® Certified Personal Trainer, Health Coach, and Group Fitness Instructor

IN THIS CHAPTER

LEARNING OBJECTIVES:

Upon completion of this chapter, the reader will be able to:

- Identify the stages of the client–personal trainer relationship
- Implement practices to enhance client–personal trainer rapport, including respecting cultural differences, using effective verbal and nonverbal communication techniques, and maintaining professional boundaries
- Apply strategies for effective client–personal trainer relationship building in the investigation stage utilizing active listening and motivational interviewing skills
- Support clients in the implementation of their physical-activity and exercise plans through effectively collaborating on and setting goals, generating ideas and discussing options, and evaluating their programs
- Educate clients on self-monitoring techniques to improve program adoption and adherence
- Employ effective teaching techniques during exercise sessions to enhance client learning and promote the safe and effective execution of exercises

ACE UNIVERSITY

If your study program includes the ACE University, visit www.ACEfitness.org/MyACE and log in to your My ACE Account to take full advantage of the ACE Personal Trainer Study Program and online guided study experience.

A variety of media to support and expand on the material in this text is provided to facilitate learning and best prepare you for the ACE Personal Trainer Certification exam and a career as a personal trainer.

ACE Certified Personal Trainers powerfully influence their clients' lives when they support them through changing their habits and help them establish a positive relationship with exercise. A personal trainer can have an immediate positive impact on a client's health by first creating enjoyable exercise experiences—that ultimately lead to exercise **adherence**—and then gradually progressing the exercise plan by applying program-design strategies that produce results. Through effective communication, skillful goal-setting, and proactive coaching skills, personal trainers may support physical-activity adoption and adherence, along with implementing comprehensive exercise programs that help clients reach their unique health and fitness goals.

Stages of the Client–Personal Trainer Relationship

The early days of the client–personal trainer relationship can be thought of as consisting of four stages, each requiring somewhat different communication skills on the part of the personal trainer (Figure 4-1). When personal trainers meet new clients for the first time, they begin by breaking the ice and building **rapport,** which refers to a relationship marked by mutual understanding and trust. The rapport stage begins with first impressions, so it is important that personal trainers present themselves in an approachable, professional manner from day one, using both effective verbal and nonverbal communication skills. Rapport continues to build over time, and the longer personal trainers and clients work together, the more they come to understand one another. An early, mutual experience of trust and respect sets the stage for the client–personal trainer relationship.

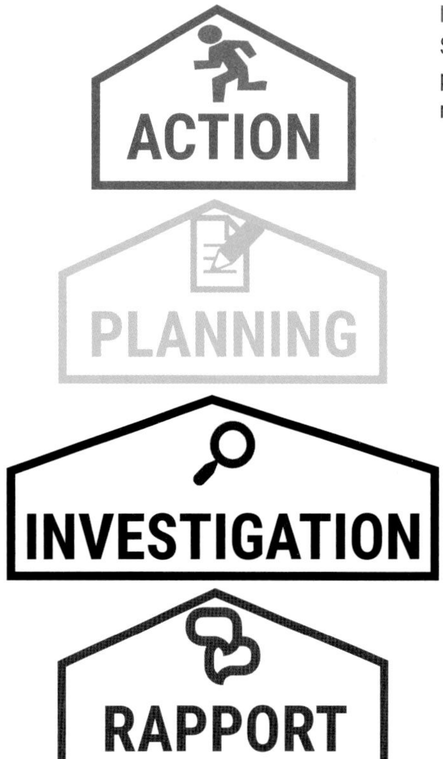

FIGURE 4-1
Stages of the client–personal trainer relationship

Together, the client and personal trainer enter the investigation stage next, where the focus is on discussing the client's health, fitness, and lifestyle information, any available test results, physician recommendations, and the client's goals and exercise history. During this stage, **active listening** and utilizing the skills of **motivational interviewing** help the personal trainer understand the client and elicit as much helpful information as possible while evoking a client's motivation (e.g., values and goals) for changing his or her level of activity.

Next, the client–personal trainer relationship progresses to the planning stage, during which the personal trainer designs an exercise program in partnership with the client, drawing upon effective verbal and nonverbal communication skills. At this point, clients are ready to begin working out, signaling the beginning of the action stage of the client–personal trainer relationship. The ability to effectively teach new motor skills becomes essential.

It is important to remember that while these stages describe the traditional progression of the client–personal trainer relationship, they often overlap and recur. For example, rapport building continues throughout the duration of the client–personal trainer relationship. Similarly, personal trainers frequently reinvestigate client data as they review workout records and assessment results, and then update the exercise plan and teach new skills accordingly. Personal trainers who complete only a single session with clients may go through all the stages during that session. Excellent communication skills are essential during all these stages.

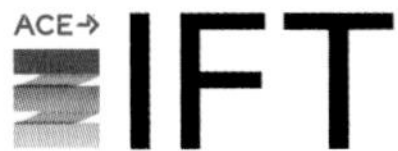

At this point in your studies, you have come across the ACE Integrated Fitness Training® (ACE IFT®) Model, ACE Mover Method™, ACE ABC Approach™, and now the four stages of the client–personal trainer relationship. While it is important to remember these concepts, it is imperative that the practical application of this information is not lost when taking a client-centered approach to personal training.

Beginning with the ACE Mover Method, keep each interaction client-centered, use active listening, ask **open-ended questions,** and recognize that clients are the experts on themselves and are resourceful and capable of change. This works best when rapport has been established, which is the first stage of the client–personal trainer relationship. Next, the three steps of the ACE ABC Approach can be thought of as skills for effective communication and the drivers for empowering clients to make behavioral changes throughout the life of the professional relationship. The ACE ABC Approach may be used the most during the rapport and investigation stages of the client–personal trainer relationship, but one should always be coaching and communicating effectively regardless of the stage of the relationship. As the relationship progresses to planning, this is where the ACE IFT Model is used to develop an effective exercise program, taking into consideration what was learned about values, motivation, goals, activity history, interests, and medical history during the rapport and investigation stages. Once an exercise program is created and an initial training focus is determined, the relationship is ready to progress to action. To truly stay client-centered, it is important not to lose sight of how the various concepts tie together to deliver a client-centered personal-training experience.

Rapport Stage

Empathy and rapport evolve over time from good communication between the personal trainer and client. Research suggests that the time spent establishing a good working relationship enhances adherence to behavior-change programs (Ryan et al., 2011). Personal trainers develop empathy with a client when they put themselves in the client's position. While one person may never truly understand what it is like to be another person, the client usually appreciates the personal trainer's willingness to try to understand. Personal trainers' attempts to understand are conveyed through active listening with an open, nonjudgmental mind as they ask questions and try to paraphrase, reflect, and summarize what they are hearing.

During the rapport stage, the personal trainer sets the scene for establishing mutual understanding and trust. Most people have a "gut response," or first impression, when meeting another person. Many factors influence clients' first impressions of a personal trainer, including the personal trainer's physical appearance, facial expressions, attire, and self-confidence. Although the first opportunity to build rapport occurs instantly during the first client–personal

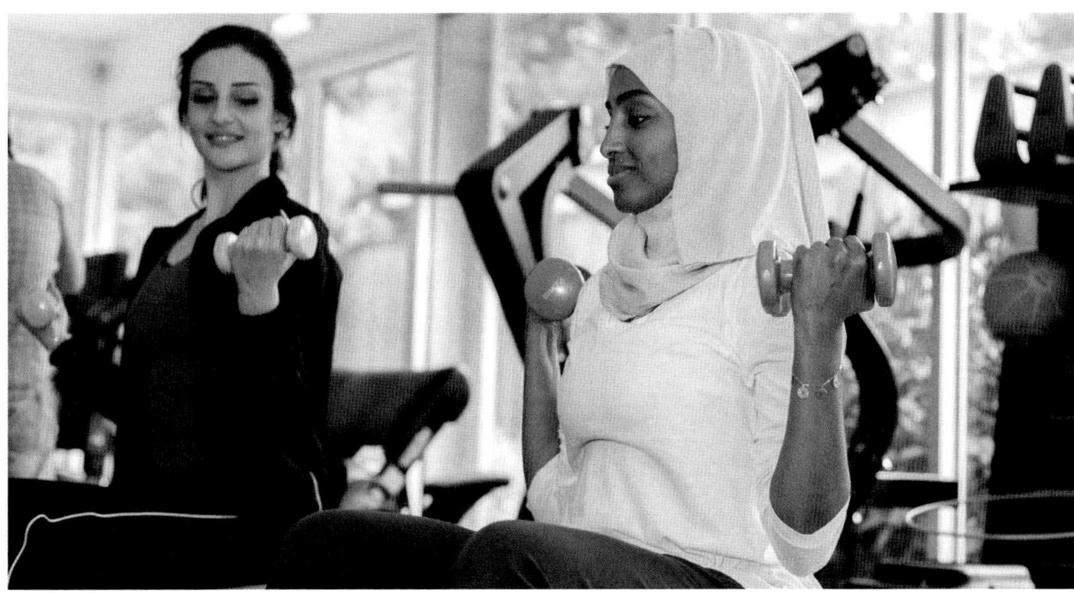

trainer meeting, it is useful to consider the rapport-building process a continual task that endures throughout the client–personal trainer relationship. Rapport continues to develop through good verbal and nonverbal communication, as personal trainers work to create a climate of respect and trust.

CULTURAL COMPETENCE

Personal trainers who have had little difficulty developing rapport with clients similar to themselves may find it takes a little more effort to build trust with people who differ from themselves in terms of age, gender, race, ethnicity, size, socioeconomic status, educational background, ability, and fitness level. Personal trainers can improve their rapport-building ability by learning as much as possible about each client, and by trying to better understand clients different from themselves. Personal trainers who work with people from different backgrounds can develop **cultural competence** by taking time to learn about clients' beliefs, attitudes, values, and lifestyles. Cultural competence can be defined as the ability to communicate and work effectively with people from different cultures.

Training programs for cultural competence for healthcare providers typically focus on communication skills. Culturally competent workers have the ability to recognize social and cultural differences that may exist between providers and clients and adapt their communication styles accordingly (Teal & Street, 2009). Providers are encouraged to elicit and understand clients' perspectives and individualize recommendations based on client input. Many medical schools have incorporated training programs in cultural competence and **person-centered care** into their classes.

Ethnicity and race have been the most studied factors in terms of cultural competence training. While little research exists on racial and ethnic discrimination in the fitness industry, one can assume that this service sector would be vulnerable to America's national ethos. Research in healthcare suggests that ethnic minorities, who often work with providers of different ethnic backgrounds, rate the quality of healthcare more negatively than whites (Macintosh et al., 2013).

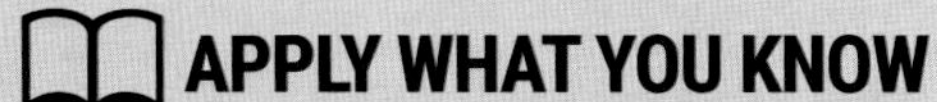

Increasing Your Cultural Competence

You can increase your cultural competence in several ways. Begin by acknowledging your own biases regarding people of other backgrounds, including ethnic background, race, sex, gender, sexual orientation, age, socioeconomic level, size, and physical ability. For example, some people may hold the idea that older adults are frail, people with **obesity** are lazy, or that men are less communicative than women. People who are not fluent in English may be perceived as less intelligent than native speakers. Uncoordinated people who learn motor skills slowly may be perceived as inferior to athletes.

Personal trainers who are working with clients from an unfamiliar demographic can learn about clients' beliefs, attitudes, and lifestyles by talking to others who work with similar groups and reading any information they can find about that group. It is important to know, for example, that some older people and some cultural groups may believe that asking questions is rude and indicates that the speaker has been unclear. Many people pretend they agree with and understand a health or exercise professional, when in fact they may not agree or understand at all (Wright, Frey, & Sopory, 2007). Sometimes, people say they have been performing their exercise programs when in fact they have not been doing so, simply to appear in a good light.

Once you have thought about your own biases and learned more about other groups, you should be careful not to form new stereotypes. Work to understand each individual client using active listening skills and by treating each client with dignity and respect.

FIRST IMPRESSIONS

Positive first impressions provide a great start for the rapport-building process. Clients perceive positive experiences when they are characterized by a sense of caring, respect, clear communication, and professionalism on the part of the personal trainer. When clients perceive that their concerns are taken seriously and their questions are carefully considered and clearly answered, they are more likely to come away with a positive impression of the personal trainer. Meeting in an environment that is clean and organized also facilitates a good first meeting between a client and a personal trainer.

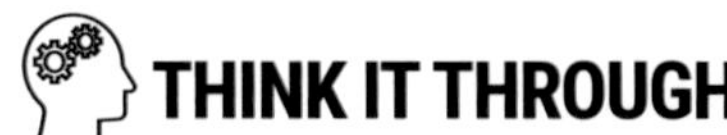

The Customer Experience

Think about a recent encounter you had with someone working in a service industry. Did you walk away with a strong first impression, either positive or negative? What elements of the interaction made you feel that way? What could the individual have done differently to provide you the best possible customer experience?

VERBAL AND NONVERBAL COMMUNICATION

Verbal communication is only a small part of the messages people send when they interact with others. People pay attention to much more than words in their effort to decipher messages and understand social situations. While people hear each other's words, they seek to verify verbal content by evaluating the speaker's appearance, facial expressions, body language, and tone of voice. If someone's words ("I am glad to meet you") and body language (e.g., lack of eye contact, disinterested facial expression, and turned-away body position) do not match, people generally trust body language over verbal content (Ambady & Weisbuch, 2010).

When speaking with clients, the personal trainer should speak clearly and use language that is easily understood by clients, without talking down to them. It is certainly appropriate to use exercise science vocabulary, but the personal trainer should be sure to define terms that may be unfamiliar to clients. Verbal content can be enhanced with visual information that illustrates concepts (e.g., pictures, diagrams, and charts). Exercise demonstrations may accompany verbal explanations.

Nonverbal communication has many components, including:

- **Voice quality:** A weak, hesitant, or soft voice does not inspire client confidence. On the other hand, a loud, tense voice tends to make people nervous. Developing a voice that is firm and confident communicates professionalism.
- **Eye contact:** Direct, friendly eye contact shows clients they are the center of the personal trainer's attention, whether the personal trainer is listening or talking. When a listener looks away while a person is speaking, the speaker feels as though he or she is not being heard. Similarly, when a speaker looks away, the listener does not feel important; the speaker does not seem to care about the listener's reaction.
- **Facial expression:** Facial expressions convey emotion but work best when the emotion is sincere (most clients can sense an artificial smile). As personal trainers work with clients, their faces should display the concern, thoughtfulness, and/or enjoyment they are feeling.
- **Hand gestures:** Use of hand gestures varies from culture to culture. In general, people are most comfortable when a speaker uses relaxed, fluid hand gestures while explaining something. When listening, a personal trainer's hands should be comfortably resting. Fidgeting hands, clenched fists, abrupt gestures, and finger pointing may be distracting to clients.
- **Body position:** An open, well-balanced, erect body position communicates confidence. A body posture that is leaning or stooped suggests fatigue and boredom, while a rigid, hands-on-hips stance may be interpreted as aggressive. When the personal trainer and client are seated together in discussion, the personal trainer may also want to mirror the body positioning of the client for enhanced engagement.

Throughout the session, the personal trainer should remain cognizant of the client's nonverbal communication, adjusting the flow of the conversation when necessary. This type of awareness and recognition is a skill that requires practice and will improve with experience. Table 4-1 lists common body language that the personal trainer may observe when working with a client. If any of these are encountered, the personal trainer should take the opportunity to evaluate how he or she may re-engage the

TABLE 4-1
Common Body Language Indicators

Body Language	Potential Meaning
Crossed arms	Anger, defiance, or disinterest (unless the client is cold)
Feet pointed toward the door Repeatedly looking at a watch	Bored or anxious to leave
Biting lip	Tension or trepidation
Cracking knuckles	Comforting habit
Use of a barrier (such as a purse, backpack, or briefcase)	Personal space is being invaded

client in the session. Often, a simple question such as "How are you feeling about this?" communicates to the client that the coach has a genuine interest in his or her comfort and well-being, and desires to adjust the conversation according to his or her preferences.

In addition to body language, many other behaviors serve as forms of communication. For example, when the personal trainer is late for an appointment, this communicates a lack of respect to the client. A lack of professionalism and attentiveness is communicated when the personal trainer interrupts an appointment to make a phone call or perform other tasks.

PROFESSIONAL BOUNDARIES

Having strong rapport and engagement with clients can sometimes develop into a double-edged sword if personal trainers fail to maintain professional distance from their clients. When personal trainers and clients work together for an extended period of time, it is normal for each to experience a feeling of friendliness toward the other. However, the professional effectiveness of personal trainers is undermined when they become too personally involved with their clients.

Personal involvement occurs when the personal trainer becomes very close friends with the client or enters into a romantic relationship. It is difficult to maintain a client–personal trainer relationship once this has occurred. In fact, the client–personal trainer relationship should cease immediately if a romantic relationship has developed. In general, personal trainers should express genuine concern for clients. When clients start chatting about intimate issues, personal trainers should keep their distance and work to redirect the conversation to more professional topics.

Maintaining professional boundaries also comes into play when coaching clients on movement techniques. Personal trainers should be careful not to put their hands on clients unless they have first asked and then received permission to do so (e.g., asking a client if it is acceptable to touch his or her arms for spotting purposes during an overhead shoulder exercise). In addition, texting and interacting on social media is a topic for discussion early in the client–personal trainer relationship, as communication on social platforms and personal messaging should be kept professional. Personal trainers should provide options for using these forms of communication for connecting professionally with clients and then work with the clients to come up with an agreed-upon plan. For example, some clients may prefer texting over emails, while others might not want to connect electronically at all and would prefer a phone call when communicating outside of scheduled training sessions.

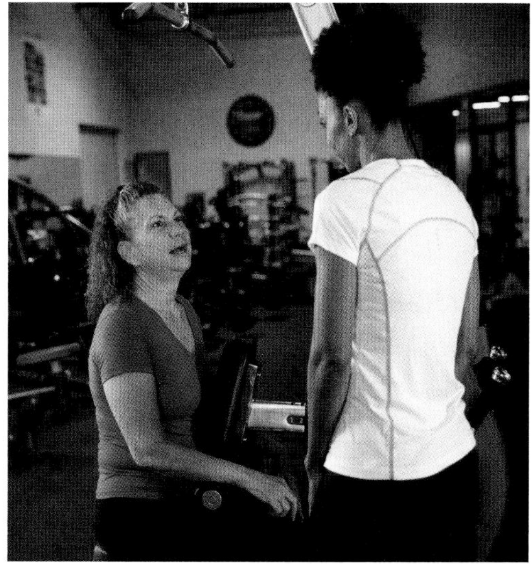

DEALING WITH DIFFICULT CLIENTS

Building rapport can take more effort when clients are reluctant to begin exercising, are afraid of getting injured, or are depressed and anxious about their health. Some clients may have had bad experiences that led them to develop prejudices against athletes, physical educators, and individuals who are physically active and therefore may initially be critical of information coming from a personal trainer. Some individuals may have less trust in people who appear to be different from them. Nevertheless, personal trainers who behave professionally and try to understand their clients often win the hearts and trust of even the most reluctant clients.

Personal trainers who encounter resistance from their clients may be able to ask clarifying questions to better understand clients' perspectives about exercise and what they see as barriers, challenges, and discomforts, as well as what they see as the value/benefit of being more active. Further, a personal trainer who senses distrust from a client might explain his or her background working with clients with similar injuries, health problems, or whatever a particular client's concern might be. Displaying certifications and other credentials could also bolster the client's perception of the personal trainer's level of expertise. Ultimately, however, personal trainers must keep in mind that they are there to support their clients and, through effective communication skills, help evoke their motivation to change if and when they are ready to do so.

Investigation Stage

Rapport continues to build during the investigation stage, as personal trainers gather information and elicit insights from their clients. Much of this information is very personal in nature, including medical concerns, fitness-assessment results, body weight, and exercise history. Clients may be somewhat embarrassed and uneasy discussing this information with someone they have just met. Clients who sense that the personal trainer is a professional who has their best interests at heart are likely to be more honest and comfortable during the investigation stage.

GATHERING INFORMATION

Many personal trainers ask clients to complete forms such as the **lifestyle and health-history questionnaire** (see Figure 5-4, pages 150–153). Taking time to review this form with clients can help the personal trainer clarify questions and elicit more information.

Personal trainers should use the investigation stage not only to learn about a client's current health and fitness levels, but also to understand a client's exercise likes and dislikes and their reasons for exercising. Personal trainers should ask clients about their previous experiences with physical activity to uncover factors that furthered or disrupted exercise adherence. A personal trainer who listens carefully to clients' descriptions of past experiences can learn a great deal about clients' personal preferences, such as whether they like to exercise alone or with a friend, in the morning or at the end of the day, or at moderate or vigorous intensities. What has worked (or not worked) in previous exercise programs may work (or not work) again. Careful attention can help personal trainers read between the lines of fitness forms, while good listening skills help their understanding of the emotions behind the stories that clients tell.

APPLY WHAT YOU KNOW

Identifying a Client's Readiness for Change

Success in personal training requires skill in understanding behavioral change and how to facilitate lifestyle changes. Adopting healthy behavior is a complex process, and several theories have been developed to explain factors affecting lifestyle change. One such model is the **transtheoretical model of behavior change (TTM)**—also called the **stages-of-change model**—which is detailed in Chapter 3. This model begins with identifying a client's readiness to change using a readiness to change questionnaire (Figure 4-2), which provides a good indication of when an individual is ready to adopt healthy behaviors. Personal trainers should never assume that because someone purchases personal-training sessions, he or she is actually committed and ready to change his or her behavior. Instead, the personal trainer should utilize the insight gleaned to enhance the exploratory process. The person may simply be appeasing a significant other, using gifted sessions before they expire, or have been pressured into starting an exercise program after a doctor's stern recommendation.

FIGURE 4-2
Readiness to change questionnaire

	YES	NO
Are you looking to change a specific behavior?	☐	☐
Are you willing to make this behavioral change a top priority?	☐	☐
Have you tried to change this behavior before?	☐	☐
Do you believe there are inherent risks/dangers associated with not making this behavioral change?	☐	☐
Are you committed to making this change, even though it may prove challenging?	☐	☐
Do you have support for making this change from friends, family, and loved ones?	☐	☐
Besides health reasons, do you have other reasons for wanting to change this behavior?	☐	☐
Are you prepared to be patient with yourself if you encounter obstacles, barriers, and/or setbacks?	☐	☐

ACTIVE LISTENING

Active listening occurs when the personal trainer listens to a client carefully, empathetically, and with an open mind, trying to put him- or herself in the client's shoes. Engaging communication occurs most easily in quiet, private spaces that limit distraction.

Some personal trainers tend to believe that because they get paid to give advice, the more they say, the better. They love to talk about exercise and health and equate information delivery with performance and clients getting their money's worth. Unfortunately, this focus on talking can interfere with good communication if the personal trainer always dominates discussions with clients and interrupts clients before they are finished speaking.

Active listening takes a great deal of attention and skill. People may pretend to listen so as not to appear rude but may only hear part of what the speaker says, tuning out parts they find uninteresting, offensive, or hard to understand. Instead of listening carefully, the listener is often busy formulating arguments, forming judgments about the speaker, or thinking about what to say next. Sometimes the listener is simply daydreaming and thinking about other things. Listeners are often preoccupied with themselves and their own thoughts.

Strategies personal trainers can use for effective communication and active listening are described in the motivational interviewing section that follows. Importantly, when a client perceives that a personal trainer is engaged through asking salient questions and offering thoughtful responses, communication flourishes and rapport continues to build.

MOTIVATIONAL INTERVIEWING

Occasionally, personal trainers may find themselves working with clients who are not ready to commit to an exercise program. They may have been pushed into trying a personal-training session by a friend or family member, or they may be ambivalent about change. While it is tempting to forge ahead and tell these clients what they should be doing, the personal trainer's advice may be wasted on clients who have not yet made a commitment to exercise. Unless a client has made a decision to change, his or her exercise attempts are likely to be short-lived. A more beneficial approach is to discuss why clients feel unable to become more active.

Motivational interviewing, which was originally designed for therapists working in addiction-counseling programs, is designed to show supportive concern while challenging a client's current behavior (Miller & Rollnick, 2013; Goldstein, DePue, & Kazura, 2008), but it can also be used by personal trainers discussing physical activity with their clients. Motivational interviewing may help clients feel the need to become more active and make a decision to start exercising. Motivational interviewing refers to a method of speaking with people in a way that motivates them to make a decision to change their behavior. Although motivational interviewing is not based on the TTM, there is a natural fit between the two, as the process of motivational interviewing parallels the **contemplation** stage of change, given that the client is ready to explore his or her **ambivalence** about behavior change (see Chapter 3).

In the common **directing style** of communication, the personal trainer takes charge of the conversation and advises a client on what to do, telling him or her how to best proceed by offering advice and specific direction. In contrast, motivational interviewing employs a **guiding style** of communication in which the personal trainer encourages, supports, and assists the client in the process of change. Motivational interviewing emphasizes establishing rapport, reducing resistance, and eliciting a client's own rationale for change, or **change talk.** The aims of the process are to support people as they resolve their ambivalence toward behavior change, decide to make a change, and then persevere with the new behavior. Miller and Rollnick (2013) note that confrontational, forceful, guilt-ridden, and authoritarian approaches are largely ineffective and contraindicated in motivational interviewing.

APPLY WHAT YOU KNOW

Using the Importance Ruler

For clients who are weighing the pros and cons of committing to a behavior change, personal trainers may find it beneficial to evoke change talk through the use of scaling questions. One such specific tool is called the "importance ruler." The personal trainer may ask, "On a scale of 1 to 10, with 1 being not important at all and 10 being extremely important, how important is it to you to make this change?" The key to this technique is the follow-up question after the client provides a number: "What led you to choose a 7 and not a 5?" The answer will nearly always come as some formulation of change talk. On the other hand, if the personal trainer asks, "Why did you choose a 7 and not a 9?" **sustain talk** (i.e., reasons for sustaining the current unwanted behavior) will ensue. Thus, when using this question, personal trainers should always ask why the client chose a higher number on the ruler, rather than a lower number. See the ACE Mover Method feature that follows for an example of how this technique can be effectively used with a client.

Use the steps below to practice the importance ruler conversation with a client, friend, or family member.

1. Find out one lifestyle change the person wants to make.
2. Ask the person to rate the importance of this change:

   On a scale of 1 to 10, how important is it for you to make this change? ____

   What makes you a ____ instead of a ____? (Remember to use a higher number on the ruler rather than a lower number.)
3. Give a short verbal summary of what you heard the person say.

As a client moves through ambivalence and develops an increasing commitment to change, this tool can help gauge the client's perceived importance of the change. The information gleaned from this short conversation may give the personal trainer valuable insight into the client's reasons for wanting to change that could lead him or her toward making the decision to change.

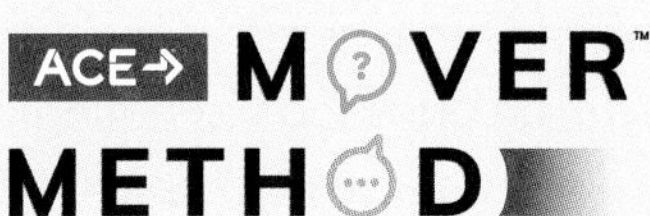

Using the Importance Ruler to Partner on Change

You have been working with a client for three months. At the end of a recent session, she mentions that working with you has been a step in the right direction, but she knows there is more she could be doing to improve her lifestyle. She tells you that she would like to increase her physical-activity levels throughout the day, especially at work, and make better food choices.

ACE ABC APPROACH

The ACE Mover Method for clients expressing a desire to change may begin with the use of a scaling tool such as the importance ruler to initiate the ACE ABC Approach. The following example illustrates the proper use of this technique.

Personal Trainer: You mentioned wanting to improve upon your current lifestyle by being more physically active during the day and eating better. On a scale of 1 to 10, with 10 being most important, how important is it to you to make these changes?

Client: At this point in my journey, I would say that I am at a 6.

Personal Trainer: That's great! Why a 6 and not a 3?

Client: I'd say I'm a 6 and not a 3 because I have already started making changes, like working with a personal trainer. Also, I have explored options for increasing my activity levels and I'm more aware of my food choices. Ultimately, I want to have more energy and look better and feel better!

Ask: Asking powerful open-ended questions helps to evoke further change talk from the client and allows you to work together with the client to identify specific steps the client would like to take.

Personal Trainer: You have already made some positive changes and are exploring additional options. Of all the choices you have been considering, what do you think you would enjoy the most?

Client: I've wanted to sign up for a lunchtime boot-camp class that is held in the park across from where I work. I can see them working out from the window in our break room and they always look like they're having fun, laughing, and working hard at the same time. It reminds me of being on a team, which is something I enjoyed when I was younger.

Break down barriers: Discuss with the client what obstacles may get in her way of achieving this goal of participating in a lunchtime activity.

Personal Trainer: Joining a boot-camp class at work sounds like a great way to become more active and being part of a team will give you a sense of joy that you had when you were younger. Are there any barriers that could prevent you from joining the class?

Client: The main thing preventing me from committing to this is that I am so hungry by lunch that it's hard for me to focus on anything but eating. The funny thing is that for the past three weeks, I've been keeping exercise clothes in my car in case I decide, "Today is the day to get started."

Collaborate: Working together with the client on goals and solutions is the next step of this conversation. Encourage the client to use her expertise to create next steps and overcome barriers.

Personal Trainer: In the past, you have not exercised on your lunch break because you're hungry, but joining the boot-camp class would be something you would enjoy. What options can you think of for managing your hunger and still achieving this goal?

Client: I don't have to wait until my lunch break to eat. I see plenty of my coworkers eating throughout the day. I think that with a little planning I could figure out some ways to eat before the class begins.

Personal Trainer: How will you move forward?

Client: I think my first step this week should be to check with human resources to find out about signing up for the class. Once I am enrolled, I will plan to bring my lunch to work one day next week, eat before boot camp, and try the class. Thinking about my schedule for next week, Wednesday would be the right day to get started.

Using a scaling question to direct a conversation into the ACE Mover Method provides coaching opportunities during any point of a personal-training session. Recognizing and acting upon these opportunities will not only improve rapport with your clients, but also increase client adherence, **self-efficacy,** and enjoyment of the fitness journey.

The "spirit" of motivational interviewing is rooted in four key interconnected components: collaboration, acceptance, compassion, and evocation (Table 4-2). A set of conversational skills comprised of asking open-ended questions, offering **affirmations, reflective listening,** and **summarizing** (referred to as **OARS**) is a key aspect of motivational interviewing (Table 4-3). Throughout the process, the personal trainer partners with the client to elicit the client's own motivation and wisdom, leaving the decision to change up to the client.

The spirit of motivational interviewing and OARS are put into practice throughout the following overlapping processes (Miller & Rollnick 2013):

- **Engaging:** All relationships begin with engagement. In this step, personal trainers talk with their clients to understand their perspectives in a nonjudgmental way. Key components of engaging include developing rapport and building a helpful connection and working relationship.
- **Focusing:** The process of engaging leads the client to express areas on which he or she would like to focus. A direction toward one or more goals usually emerges. Focusing is a collaborative process wherein the client's goals are clarified and the direction the client wants to move is determined.

- **Evoking:** After a focus on a particular change is identified, the personal trainer elicits the client's own motivations for change. Evoking is prompting the client to voice his or her arguments for change (change talk) and is considered the heart of motivational interviewing. If a client expresses reasons why he or she cannot make a change (sustain talk), the personal trainer redirects the conversation back to change talk.
- **Planning:** During the planning process, the client and personal trainer collaborate on how to execute change. Personal trainers help clients talk through their goals, identify resources to achieve those goals, and set up ways to evaluate how well the plan worked after it is enacted.

TABLE 4-2
Spirit of Motivational Interviewing

Component	Definition	Importance
Collaboration	The personal trainer functions as a partner in collaboration with the client, based on the recognition that people are the undisputed experts on themselves. Collaboration allows the client's ideas to be integrated into how the behavior change should occur.	The activation of the client's self-expertise is a key condition for change to occur. When the goal is for the client to change, the personal trainer cannot do it alone—a partnership is necessary.
Acceptance	The personal trainer values the inherent worth and potential of every client through empathy, honoring individual autonomy and affirming a person's strengths and efforts. Acceptance involves respecting the client's decisions about whether and how the behavior change should occur.	Acceptance is the essence of the person-centered approach wherein the client's absolute worth is recognized, autonomy to choose his or her own way is emphasized, empathy to understand the client's perspective is practiced, and the client's strengths and efforts are positively acknowledged and affirmed.
Compassion	The personal trainer demonstrates compassion when he or she deliberately pursues the welfare and best interests of the client, giving priority to the client's needs.	It is critical that the personal trainer avoids evoking his or her own goals and values during a motivational interviewing conversation. Compassion allows the trust engendered between the client and personal trainer to be honest and well-deserved.
Evocation	The personal trainer elicits the client's own motivation for a particular change, instead of telling the client why he or she should change.	Through conversation, the personal trainer evokes and strengthens the client's motivations for change. This approach recognizes that clients already have within them the positive arguments for change and that these motivations are likely to be more persuasive than whatever argument the personal trainer could provide. Notably, people talk themselves into changing and are typically resistant to being told what to do.

Source: Miller, W.R. & Rollnick, S. (2013). *Motivational Interviewing: Helping People Change* (3rd ed.). New York, N.Y.: The Guildford Press.

TABLE 4-3

OARS: The Core Communication Skills of Motivational Interviewing

Skill	Definition	Importance	Examples
Asking open-ended questions	Open-ended questions are queries asked in a way that allow a client to reflect and elaborate. These are the opposite of closed questions, which typically require short phrases or one-word answers (e.g., "yes" or "no").	Asking open-ended questions allows the personal trainer to understand the client's internal frame of reference, drawing out motivations and clear directions for change. Closed questions, on the other hand, result in short answers that are not as helpful for collaboration.	"Why is it important to you to get more physical activity into your day?" "What would you gain by exercising more?" "How can I help you with being more physically active?"
Offering affirmations	When the personal trainer makes a statement valuing a positive client attribute or behavior, he or she is demonstrating the skill of affirming.	A personal trainer mind-set that "accentuates the positive" in clients by looking for strengths, productive behaviors, and good intentions enhances the client's ability for volitional change and growth. This counters the idea that people will change if you make them feel bad enough.	"Clearly, you've spent some time thinking about exercise and have even tried a few workouts on your own." "You really tried hard this week!" "Your intention was good, even though it didn't turn out exactly as you planned."
Reflective listening	Reflective listening is the skill of active listening whereby the personal trainer seeks to understand the client's feelings by offering reflections as guesses about the client's statements. Once a reflective statement is given, the client has a chance to either confirm or correct what the personal trainer reflected.	Reflective listening focuses on a client's own narrative, rather than asserting the personal trainer's understanding of it. Reflections are statements, versus questions, and are more likely to encourage continued exploration. Repeated questions may make the client feel like he or she is being interrogated, which may evoke defensiveness rather than openness. Thus, following open-ended questions with reflections helps break up a stream of continuous queries.	"You're frustrated that your efforts at exercising aren't getting the results you want." "Family time spent being physically active outdoors is enjoyable for you." "You're worried that it's too hard to lose weight."

TABLE 4-3 *(continued)*

Skill	Definition	Importance	Examples
Summarizing	When a personal trainer reflects two or more statements said by a client, he or she is summarizing. This is essentially a longer version of reflective listening.	Summaries help clients reflect on the various experiences they have expressed and invite further exploration. They give clients an opportunity to hear their statements collected together in a way that may present the whole picture of a problem, versus only one or two elements (as is typical in reflecting).	"Your roommates always have junk food in the house and you're concerned that you won't be able to resist snacking on it when you're hungry." "Your past experiences with physical activity have left you feeling anxious about your abilities and you feel this ultimately leads you to quit a new exercise program after the first few workouts." "After you take a yoga class, you feel relaxed and also happy that you did something good for yourself."

Note: OARS = Open-ended questions, affirmations, reflective listening, and summarizing

Source: Miller, W.R. & Rollnick, S. (2013). *Motivational Interviewing: Helping People Change* (3rd ed.). New York, NY: The Guildford Press.

Given that many personal trainers are accustomed to sharing their expertise by providing instructions and recommendations, implementing a guiding style of communication may prove challenging at first. Generally, such eagerness to offer advice and propose solutions involves the best of intentions, in that personal trainers want to help clients improve their health and fitness. This tendency—known as the **righting reflex**—relies heavily on directing individuals to "fix" what seems to be wrong with them in an effort to set them on a better path (Miller & Rollnick, 2013). However, the reality is that such an approach is often ineffective and may even prove counterproductive, particularly among clients who want to change but are hesitant to do so because they see both the advantages and disadvantages of doing so. Miller and Rollnick (2013) state: "If you are arguing for change and your client is arguing against it, you've got it exactly backward."

It is important to note that while motivational interviewing may seem simple, it is not easy. As such, becoming adept at motivational interviewing takes training and practice. While this chapter provides a very brief introduction to motivational interviewing, personal trainers seeking more in-depth information are encouraged to consider enrolling in a motivational interviewing training program or seeking out other professional education to build and refine this complex set of skills, including two ACE resources: *The Professional's Guide to Health and Wellness Coaching* (ACE, 2019) and *Coaching Behavior Change* (ACE, 2014).

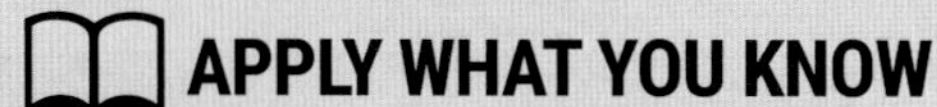

APPLY WHAT YOU KNOW

Practice Using Open-ended Questions

Miller and Rollnick (2013) recommend that individuals first learning motivational interviewing use the following five open-ended questions to practice their skills.

1. Why do you want to make this change?
2. How might you go about making this change?
3. What are the three best reasons for you to do it?
4. How important is it to you to make this change?

After receiving answers from each of these questions, reflect back and summarize the client's response. Then, ask:

5. What do you think you will do?

Go through this process with three clients, friends, family members, or coworkers and reflect on the experience. What did you learn? What worked well? How might you incorporate this into your personal-training sessions?

RESPONDING TO DIFFICULT DISCLOSURES

Personal trainers are sometimes unsure of how to respond when clients share information that is very sad, such as a disclosure of a client's serious illness or the illness or death of someone close to the client. Often, a short response is all that is required, such as "I'm so sorry," "That must have been very hard," or "I can only imagine how difficult that must have been for you and your family." The personal trainer should follow the client's lead as to whether he or she wants to say anything more on a topic or not. If the situation affects exercise program design in any way, the personal trainer can turn the conversation back to the practical details. For example, "Now that your mother has moved in with you and your family, what is the best time for you to get to the fitness center?" If clients reveal medical information that causes concern, they should be referred to their healthcare providers for medical clearance (see Chapter 5). If a medical condition places a client outside of the personal trainer's **scope of practice** and expertise, the client should be referred to someone with the necessary training and experience (see Chapter 1).

Sometimes personal trainers hear information that worries or even alarms them. For example, a personal trainer may suspect a client is suffering from **depression,** an **eating disorder,** or another serious health problem. In such cases, personal trainers should follow referral procedures that encourage the client to seek professional help (see Chapter 5). Personal trainers may also wish to share their concerns (while maintaining the confidentiality of the client) with their supervisors or a colleague to confirm their referral plan (see Chapter 16).

Planning Stage

The planning stage of the client–personal trainer relationship should be viewed as a give-and-take opportunity in terms of communication. While personal trainers move into a more active role during this stage, they must continue to listen to clients' responses to their ideas and suggestions and also elicit input from the client. Client adherence often improves when clients actively partner with personal trainers in the process of exercise program design. The planning stage generally moves through the following steps:

- Setting goals
- Generating and discussing alternatives
- Formulating a plan
- Evaluating the exercise program

SETTING GOALS

Setting goals is an important process for initial and continued behavioral change. It is an integral part of all exercise programs. The best thing about goal setting is that it is relatively simple to employ and extremely effective when done properly. Goal setting must be used systematically and should be an active part of the program to maximize adherence. The following are a few key considerations to keep in mind during the goal-setting process:

- **Avoid setting too many goals:** Keep the number of goals manageable and attainable so that the client is not overwhelmed with all that he or she needs to accomplish.
- **Avoid setting negative goals:** If the client wants to set a goal of not missing any workouts, the personal trainer should help the client reframe this goal in a positive way: "I will attend every scheduled workout session." Setting negative goals puts the focus on the behavior that should be avoided, not the behavior to be achieved. It is important that the client is thinking about achievement, not avoidance.
- **Set short- and long-term goals, as well as process and performance goals:** Clients should be achieving short-term successes in each workout.
- **Include the client in the process:** For a client to optimize success in attaining a desired outcome—to achieve one's vision of what life will be like after a behavior change has been made—it is important that the client's values inform the development of his or her goals. Thus, collaboration between the client and personal trainer during the goal-setting process will strongly influence the potential success of client achievement.
- **Revisit the goals on a regular basis:** This is the most important thing that a personal trainer can do to maximize the effectiveness of the goal-setting process. Goals need regular adjusting and should be consistently used as a tool to help direct attention and effort, and to promote persistence.

Goal-setting Theory

Goal-setting theory grew out of work done by psychologists Edwin Locke and Gary Latham. They were especially interested in the relationship between goal setting and achievement in work settings, but their theory has been applied in many other contexts over the past 50 years.

According to goal-setting theory, goals affect people's performance, or inspire behavioral change, through four primary mechanisms (Locke & Latham, 2002):

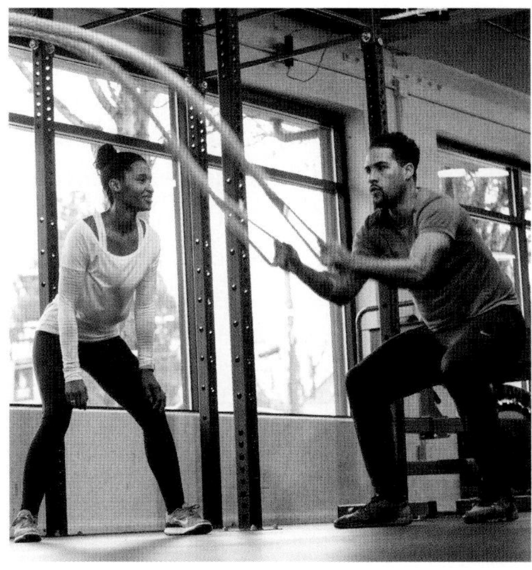

- **Directed attention:** Goals help people direct their thoughts and behaviors toward the activities necessary to move toward their goals. In a personal-training context, this might mean that a goal of becoming more physically active would influence daily movement breaks and other associated health behaviors, like allowing time in the weekly schedule to pursue recreation activities that involve physical exertion.
- **Mobilized effort:** In general, goals increase the effort people will expend to achieve the goals. Goal-setting theory states that challenging goals elicit more effort, at least in the short term. However, it is important that ambitious goals be seen as both positive and achievable, or clients are likely to give up. For this reason, in personal training, it may be particularly helpful to work with clients to develop both short- and long-term goals.
- **Persistence:** Clients trying to reach goals generally persist longer in their target behaviors. For example, tight deadlines lead to more work productivity. The application to personal training is that challenging goals rooted in the client's own personal motivations stimulates them to persist through difficulties.
- **Strategy:** Goal setting stimulates clients to look for and use strategies that will help them attain goals.

These four mechanisms are easily understood when comparing hypothetical clients with vague versus specific goals, assuming the specific goals are realistic. For example, consider a client with a goal to "get in shape" versus a client with a goal to "walk 30 minutes a day, five days per week." Without well-established goals, clients are less clear on the direction of their behavior-change plans, will show less effort and persistence in their programs, and will be unclear regarding which strategies will be most helpful in the process of lifestyle change. Setting **SMART goals,** as described in the following section, helps clients and personal trainers establish clear, well-defined goals that will foster client success.

Goal setting varies in its effect on a person's behavior depending upon a number of variables. Goal-setting theory lists a number of goal moderators that personal trainers can consider as they work with clients to set helpful goals (Locke & Latham, 2002).

- **Goal commitment:** The stronger a client's personal commitment to a goal, the more effective the goal will be in motivating behavior change. As predicted by **self-determination theory** (see Chapter 3), people generally set more ambitious goals and work harder toward the goals if the goals are perceived to be freely chosen and personally meaningful.

- **Goal importance:** The more important the client considers the goal and the more he or she views the goal as being in alignment with his or her values, the more motivating the goal.
- **Self-efficacy:** The higher a person's self-efficacy with regard to the behaviors needed for reaching a goal, the more likely he or she will be to persist in the face of difficulty.
- **Feedback:** Clients who receive **feedback** on their progress toward a goal are more likely to continue pursuing that goal. This can be accomplished through check-ins during personal-training sessions and/or via daily self-monitoring of goal progress through the use of apps or wearable devices.
- **Task complexity:** As the complexity of goals increases, individuals will need more strategies for achieving the goal. As such, personal trainers can collaborate with clients to establish both **process goals** and **performance goals** (also called performance goals).

SMART Goals

Clients often express fairly general exercise-related goals, such as wanting to "get in better shape" or "lose some weight." The personal trainer should help clients define goals in more specific and measurable terms so that progress can be evaluated. Effective goals are commonly said to be SMART goals, which means they are:

- **Specific:** Goals must be clear and unambiguous, stating precisely what should be accomplished.
- **Measurable:** Goals must be trackable so that clients can see whether they are making progress.
- **Attainable:** Goals should be realistically achievable by the individual client. The achievement of goal reinforces commitment to the program and encourages the client to continue exercising.
- **Relevant:** Goals must be pertinent to the particular interests, needs, and abilities of the individual client.
- **Time-bound:** Goals must contain estimated timelines for completion. Clients should regularly monitor progress toward goals.

The personal trainer should err on the conservative side of goal setting in terms of what might be realistically achieved by the client, particularly in the early stages of the behavior-change process. Lofty goals feel good and sound inspirational, but clients are soon disappointed when progress is slow (Moore et al., 2011; Nackers, Ross, & Perri, 2010). Fitness indicators that may demonstrate change include those listed in Table 4-4. These indicators may be incorporated into SMART goals, depending upon a client's specific interests.

The personal trainer should be sure to include process goals as well as performance goals. A process goal is something a client does, such as completing a certain number of workouts per week. A performance goal is something achieved, like weight loss or a resistance lifted on a strength-training machine. Clients often reach process goals before noticeable changes occur in terms of weight loss or improved performance and should be reminded of the importance of these successes. More suggestions for setting goals are presented in Table 4-5.

TABLE 4-4
Fitness Indicators for SMART Goal Setting

Fitness Indicator	Notes for Goal Setting
Emotional health indicators	Clients may have measurable improvements in mood, energy level, and sleep quality, and fewer feelings of stress and irritability following exercise.
Resting heart rate	Many personal trainers have their clients measure resting heart rate, either first thing in the morning or before falling asleep at night. Clients new to exercise often experience a decrease in resting heart rate after a few months of exercise.
Heart rate during a given submaximal workload	Clients performing cardiorespiratory exercise are also likely to experience a decrease in exercise heart rate during exercise performed at a standard workload on a piece of equipment that is similar to the type of exercise that was performed during fitness testing. The submaximal load or loads must be identical each time the client is tested.
Muscular strength and endurance	Gains in muscular strength and endurance occur fairly quickly during the first few months of an exercise program. A client's gains in terms of the amount of resistance used or the number of repetitions performed are easily measured.
Walking test	Measuring fitness improvement with some sort of timed walking test usually yields positive results if clients have been walking as part of their exercise programs for several weeks.
Flexibility	Flexibility is very slow to improve and should only be included in the assessment if the exercise program includes regular stretching or range-of-motion exercise.
Balance	Balance measures show the most improvement for adults participating in some sort of balance-training program, which are becoming increasingly popular, especially among older adults.
Skill level	Clients participating in an activity that requires skill (e.g., rock climbing, tennis, and golf) will be pleased to see improvements in their motor-skill levels. Skill improvement may be measured via motor-skill tests or activity/game performance.
Medical indicators, such as resting blood pressure, blood lipid levels, or blood sugar levels	If any of these are the focus of clients' exercise programs, clients should have these measures taken at regular intervals as established by their healthcare providers. These variables may be affected by many other factors, including diet or changes in body weight, and these factors should be taken into consideration when evaluating exercise results.
Body weight	Body weight is easily measured, but is a poor indicator of body-composition changes. Body weight may remain unchanged even though positive changes in body composition are occurring, or it may change by several pounds or kilograms due to changes in hydration. Nevertheless, clients on a weight-reduction program who are more than a few pounds or kilograms overweight will probably see a decrease in weight. Clients should work for slow and consistent weight loss, which is more likely to yield long-term weight-loss maintenance.
Body size	Clients who have a goal to lose only a few pounds may not see much change in scale weight. Body-composition changes (fat loss with an increase in muscle mass) may still lead to a change in body size. Lean tissue, because of its greater density, takes up less space than fat tissue. Many people are happy when a waistband on a skirt or pair of pants fits more loosely. Many personal trainers encourage clients to watch for changes in the way their clothes fit.
Body composition	If body composition is measured, the same test should be used consistently. Some personal trainers record circumferences or skinfolds without predicting body composition. Changes in these measures may be indicative of fat loss or increases in muscle size.

TABLE 4-5

How to Set Health and Fitness Goals That Motivate Clients for Long-term Adherence

- Listen carefully to understand what clients hope to accomplish with an exercise program.
- Help them define specific, measurable goals.
- Suggest additional goals that clients may not have thought of, such as feeling more energetic and less stressed.
- Break large goals (reachable in six months or more) into small goals (reachable in three to six months) and even weekly goals (such as completing a certain number of exercise sessions).
- Include many process goals, such as the completion of exercise sessions. In other words, simply completing workouts accomplishes a goal.
- Record goals and set up a record-keeping system to record workouts and track progress toward goals.
- Be sure clients understand what types of exercise will help them reach their health and fitness goals.
- Reevaluate and revise goals and exercise recommendations periodically to prevent discouragement if large goals are not being met.

Reprinted with permission from Brehm, B.A. (2004). *Successful Fitness Motivation Strategies.* Champaign, Ill.: Human Kinetics, page 11.

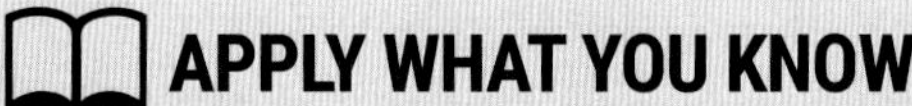

APPLY WHAT YOU KNOW

Goal-generating Questions for Clients

- What are your short-term goals (three to six months) and long-term goals (beyond six months)?
- What could hinder your fitness program (e.g., work schedules, commute times, and child care/activities)?
- What motivates you?
- What things are most important to you? How will a healthy lifestyle complement or support this?
- What kinds of exercise programs have you tried in the past?
- What did you like most and least about your previous exercise programs?
- What types of exercise or activities do you currently enjoy?
- What is your favorite exercise or activity?
- How will you integrate exercise into your life?
- How much time do you have to commit to exercise?
- What kind of support (e.g., family and friends) do you have to help you change your lifestyle?
- What is something you are good at now? Did you know you were good at it before you did it for the first time?
- When was the last time you exercised regularly (at least three times per week) and how long did it last? Why did you stop?

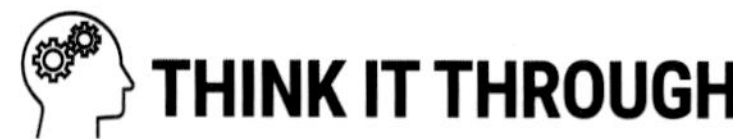

THINK IT THROUGH

Setting Effective Goals

Your new client comes to you with a goal of "losing a few pounds and having more energy to play with her grandkids throughout the day." How might you help her structure her goal in a way that best facilitates long-term success?

GENERATING IDEAS AND DISCUSSING OPTIONS

Once goals have been clarified, the client and personal trainer are ready to generate and discuss various ways of achieving these goals. The personal trainer should remember that, although it may not have been formally stated, the ultimate goal for every client is adherence to the exercise program. Similarly, the personal trainer hopes that the client will find the exercise program achievable and rewarding, so that the client continues working with the personal trainer, and more importantly, develops a lifelong habit of regular physical activity.

A number of variables influence client adherence, as described in Chapter 3, and these should be taken into consideration as the client and personal trainer explore options for working toward the established goals. For example, one of the most common causes of exercise dropout is that clients perceive the exercise program as too time-consuming. If a client has dropped out of programs for this reason in the past, it makes sense for the personal trainer to encourage a fairly modest exercise program that may necessitate some goal adjustment but will be preferable to an ambitious program that is never performed.

When clients are only going to be working with a personal trainer for one session or a few sessions, the exercise program design must be simple enough that a client can perform the program on his or her own. When a long-term client–personal trainer relationship is anticipated, the program can be more complex, as the personal trainer will be providing ongoing guidance. As the client and personal trainer work together to evaluate options, the personal trainer should encourage the client to take the lead in determining what seems realistic, especially in terms of time commitment and scheduling.

FORMULATING A PLAN

Personal trainers should consider all the information gathered during the investigation stage, current research for exercise program design, and the client's goals, and then collaborate with the client on next steps for achieving those goals (see Chapters 8 through 11). This is an excellent opportunity to use a client-centered approach. Clients should feel empowered throughout the planning process, as they are the expert on their goals, needs, and exercise preferences. Once a plan is mutually agreed upon, it should be written down and a copy should be given to the client. The plan should include all the information that the client needs to get started.

The personal trainer should also take this opportunity to help the client feel prepared to begin an exercise program. Many clients appreciate advice on what to wear, where to go, and any other tips on facility etiquette and customs that might help them feel more comfortable in a new environment. Personal trainers often fail to realize how intimidating a fitness facility can be to a newcomer. Offering some guidance—especially if a client will be exercising on his or her own—can be extremely valuable in helping clients to feel both comfortable and competent as they engage in physical activity.

EVALUATING THE EXERCISE PROGRAM

Exercise program evaluation occurs regularly, as the client and personal trainer review exercise records at their sessions together and discuss what is working and what needs to change. Clients may also be reassessed periodically to measure progress toward goals. The exercise program should be evaluated in terms of both exercise challenge and adherence. Programs can be modified as necessary to provide a more realistic or challenging stimulus. If adherence is faltering, the client and personal trainer should discuss what is causing problems and revise the exercise program design as necessary.

Action Stage

Once the exercise program design is complete, the client is ready to begin exercising. In many cases, the program is a combination of exercise completed by clients on their own (for example, taking a walk twice a week at home) and exercise performed with the personal trainer instructing and supervising. The personal trainer can enhance client success in many ways during the action stage.

SELF-MONITORING APPROACHES

In addition to a specific written exercise plan, the personal trainer may give the client—or better yet, design with the client's input—a system for recording exercise sessions, including any relevant data the personal trainer and client wish to track. Examples include mobile apps for tracking physical activity or electronic systems at fitness centers that record the exercise, resistance, repetitions, and sets of a muscular-training workout, and/or the time, intensity, heart rate, and so forth for cardiorespiratory exercise. The world of mobile apps is constantly evolving, so personal trainers should do their best to stay up-to-date on the latest options and understand the various features of the more popular apps, as clients often have questions in this area.

Research has shown that self-monitoring is one of the most effective ways to support behavioral change, including exercise program adherence and improved eating behaviors (Olander et al., 2013; Burke, Wang, & Sevick, 2011). Self-monitoring systems help in two ways. First, they increase client self-awareness. Self-monitoring acts as a mirror to give clients a more objective view of their behaviors. Second, self-monitoring systems may enhance client–personal trainer communication. As the personal trainer reviews the workout record, questions about what is working and what is not working will arise, leading to productive discussions between personal trainers and their clients.

EFFECTIVE TEACHING TECHNIQUES

Personal trainers often find themselves in the role of teacher. Personal trainers teach motor skills such as correct lifting techniques for muscular training, how to use exercise machines, and how to perform **flexibility** exercises. Depending upon their training and expertise, personal trainers may coach sports drills, teach yoga postures, or explain post-rehabilitation exercises. Personal trainers may also teach clients about information in the **cognitive domain,** such as explaining health problems, how physical activity affects physiological variables, and how to prevent injury. Understanding how people learn most effectively can help personal trainers provide sound instruction to diverse groups of clients.

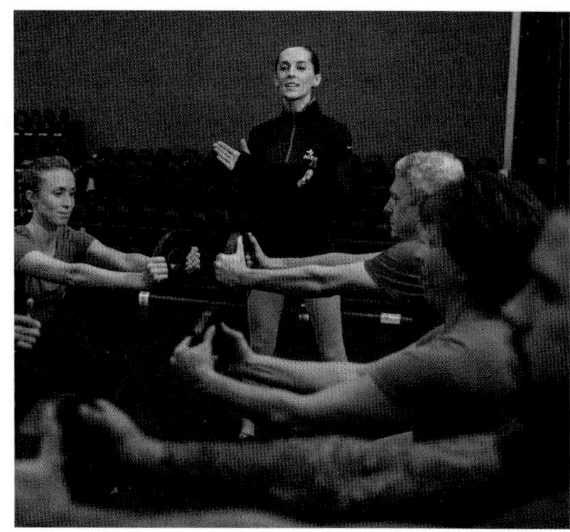

Stages of Learning

Many researchers have developed models to describe the stages of **motor learning.** One classic model popular in the exercise science literature divides motor learning into three stages: cognitive, associative, and autonomous (Fitts & Posner, 1967). This model works well for the types of motor skills that personal trainers tend to teach, since clients are usually building onto motor skills they already know (e.g., walking, cycling, and lifting). In such cases, explaining the upcoming skill is helpful. As clients try to understand the new skill, they are said to be in the **cognitive stage of learning.** Neuroscientists have demonstrated that different brain activity occurs when new motor skills are first being learned, as compared to the brain activity demonstrated once the motor skill has become more established (Rosenkranz, Kacar, & Rothwell, 2007). Personal trainers introducing a new motor skill can almost "see" clients thinking about what to do. Movements in this stage are often uncoordinated and jerky. In this stage of learning, personal trainers should use the "tell, show, do" teaching technique—as described in a following section—and provide ample opportunity for practice. This stage of learning occurs most frequently in the early stages of the client–personal trainer relationship. The personal trainer should be careful at this stage not to overwhelm clients by teaching them too many new or complex motor skills.

In the **associative stage of learning,** clients begin to master the basics and are ready for more specific feedback that will help them refine the motor skill. So that clients do not learn the skill incorrectly, personal trainers must balance the giving of appropriate feedback without providing too much information that might overwhelm the learning (see "Providing Feedback" on page 125).

In the **autonomous stage of learning,** clients are performing motor skills effectively and naturally, and the personal trainer is doing less teaching and more observing. Once some skills are learned, the personal trainer may decide to teach progressions or introduce new exercises or routines, and the process begins all over again.

Personal trainers working with athletes and clients trying to master complex motor skills, such as skiing and other sports skills, may find the Fitts and Posner model (1967) less helpful. Some research suggests that too much explanation and cognitive work may actually interfere with learning complex motor skills (Renshaw et al., 2010). Personal trainers working with athletes should talk with coaches and consult with other resources to learn how to devise training programs that address the needs specific to each sport and enhance each client's personal performance.

Learning Styles

Clients learn in many different ways. People gather information through their senses (primarily visual, auditory, and kinesthetic), and process the information in their muscles and nervous systems, including the many areas of the brain. People usually have a preference for gathering information with one pathway over others, although most people use a combination of pathways. The personal trainer can identify which pathway a client prefers by observing actions during learning situations and by listening for clues in language (Table 4-6). Using a combination of visual, auditory, and kinesthetic approaches gives a client more information to enhance learning and understanding. All three techniques may be used to introduce a new skill, but once a personal trainer learns what works best for each client, he or she should emphasize the preferred learning style.

TABLE 4-6
Preferred Learning Style Indicators

	Visual	Auditory	Kinesthetic*
Client actions	▸ Watches intently ▸ Prefers reading	▸ Listens carefully ▸ Prefers hearing	▸ Touches or holds ▸ Prefers to be spotted
Client statement	▸ "Oh, I see" ▸ "Let me see that again"	▸ "Yeah, I hear you" ▸ "Say that one more time"	▸ "I feel that" ▸ "This does not feel right"
Strategy	▸ Demonstrations	▸ Question and answer	▸ Hands-on supervision

*Personal trainers should request a client's permission before employing kinesthetic learning techniques that involve touching.

Clients who prefer auditory learning may like a lot of explanation and ask many questions. Visual learners learn by watching and appreciate longer demonstrations with less talking, while kinesthetic learners learn by doing, needing to feel the movement before catching on. Personal trainers may simply ask their clients how they prefer to learn new information and then implement teaching strategies that address their clients' preferred learning styles.

The pace of teaching should also be modified for each client, as clients should feel successful in their mastery of new exercises. Success improves self-efficacy, which means that clients will continue to exert the effort required to meet new challenges. While some clients catch on to new skills quickly, others do so more slowly and require a great deal of patience and support on the part of the personal trainer.

"Tell, Show, Do"

Motor learning is the process of acquiring and improving motor skills. Many adult clients are quite self-conscious in the motor-skill domain, especially if they have had little experience with sports and physical activity. Personal trainers with a strong background in physical education and sport are often surprised at the lack of motor ability they see in many adult clients. Motor skills are taught most effectively if the following points are kept in mind:

- **Remind beginners that it takes time and practice to improve motor skills:** Physical education specialists have noted that many people tend to believe that good coordination and athletic ability are something with which a person is born

(Rink, 2004). While ability in the motor-skills domain certainly varies from person to person, motor skills are more strongly related to practice and experience than strictly to natural ability. It is important for people new to physical activity to understand that motor-skill improvement takes a great deal of practice—and that the people they see in the fitness center have often been performing similar movement patterns and choreography for years. The same holds true for athletes in every sport.

Many clients new to exercise feel self-conscious participating in a personal-training session. They may feel out of place, awkward, and clumsy. The personal trainer must help new clients feel supported and cared for in the exercise environment (see Chapter 3). Importantly, personal trainers must select exercises that are appropriate for the client's current ability level to help build self-efficacy through successful performance.

- **Introduce new skills slowly and clearly:** "Tell, show, do" illustrates a good way to introduce a new skill. The personal trainer should begin with a very short explanation of what he or she is going to do and why. Explanations should be short and clear. Safety information should be emphasized, along with guidelines for preventing injury. Skills should be explained in terms of what the skill is accomplishing or why it is important.

  A personal trainer may often combine the telling and showing phases of skill introduction, demonstrating while explaining the skill. When describing certain movements, the personal trainer should focus on explaining the goal of the movement rather than giving distracting details about limb position (Wulf, Shea, & Lewthwaite, 2010). For example, a personal trainer would not teach someone how to use an elliptical trainer by describing when to bend and straighten the knees. Instead, the personal trainer would emphasize moving the pedals around in a smooth, steady motion. The personal trainer should demonstrate the skill accurately and allow clients time to watch.

  Teaching muscular-training exercises or exercise positions does require some explanation of limb position for safety and effectiveness. For example, when teaching lat pull-downs (see Figure 9-39, page 372), the personal trainer might ask the client to avoid pulling the bar behind the neck, as this could place the shoulders at risk. These descriptions should be brief and simple.

- **Allow clients the opportunity for focused practice:** Once the personal trainer has "told and shown," the client is ready to "do," or perform the motor skill. People learn more quickly when they focus on performing the motor skill without being distracted by talking or listening. The personal trainer should observe the client's practice and prepare to give helpful feedback, as well as to elicit feedback from the client.

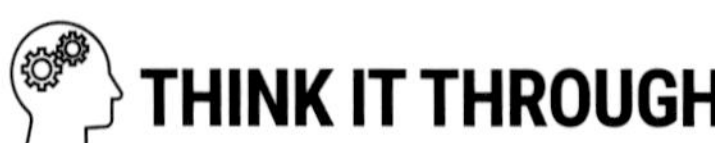

Tell, Show, Do

Use the "tell, show, do" method to teach a friend, family member, or client an exercise he or she has never performed before. Ask the client for feedback on the experience and brainstorm ways to improve this aspect of your training sessions.

Providing Feedback

Providing clients with information about their progress and performance in an exercise program is one of the most important roles of a personal trainer. This information is called feedback. Learning is virtually non-existent without feedback, because if clients do not know how they are doing, they do not have a reason to make adjustments and change their behaviors. The type of feedback that provides information on progress can be referred to as **knowledge of results** and without it, persistence suffers as people may become frustrated and give up. Feedback also helps in the goal-setting process. Both **intrinsic feedback** and **extrinsic feedback** can contribute to knowledge of results and provide information about progress toward goal attainment.

Extrinsic feedback is the reinforcement, error correction, and encouragement that personal trainers give to their clients. Intrinsic feedback is information that the clients provide themselves based on their own sensory systems (e.g., what they feel, see, or hear). While extrinsic feedback is always important in the exercise environment, long-term program adherence is highly dependent on the client's ability to provide his or her own feedback. It is important for personal trainers to not give too much feedback. As client motivation, self-efficacy, and ability develop, personal trainers should allow their clients more opportunity to provide themselves feedback by tapering off the amount of external feedback provided.

Whether a client is achieving goals and experiencing success or falling short of desired performance levels, it is up to the personal trainer to help the client use feedback to adjust and reestablish goals for continued motivation and program participation (Teixeira et al., 2012).

During an exercise session, once a client has tried a new skill, the personal trainer should respond by giving helpful feedback. The feedback should do three things:

- Provide reinforcement for what was done well
- Correct errors
- Motivate clients to continue practicing and improving

The correcting of errors, which may be seen as the more "negative" point, should be sandwiched between reinforcement and motivation (Coker, Fischman, & Oxendine, 2006). For example, "Your breathing and timing were just right on the first four lifts. Remember to keep breathing, even as the exercise starts to feel harder. You'll find the work easier now that you are learning how to breathe correctly."

The personal trainer should limit feedback to a few simple points and avoid overloading the client with information. The personal trainer should decide which errors are the most important to correct first, which typically include those that involve safety, occur earliest in the movement sequence, or are fundamental in some other way. Feedback should be phrased positively, pointing out what the clients should do. For example, a personal trainer might say "Remember to breathe," rather than "Don't hold your breath."

Sometimes personal trainers can provide helpful feedback by touching clients to indicate where they are supposed to feel the movement, or to help them achieve the correct body

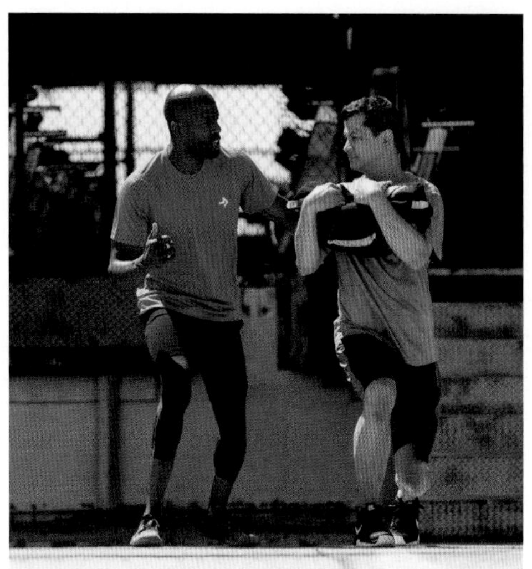

position. Some clients are uncomfortable being touched or may misinterpret physical contact. Personal trainers should discuss their training methods early in the client–personal trainer relationship, explain the purpose of any physical contact, and always ask clients for permission for this type of contact.

Modeling

It is important for personal trainers to model the healthful lifestyle guidance they are providing to their clients. First, it is good for business, since it enhances a personal trainer's credibility (Maguire, 2008). Personal trainers must promote the notion, and genuinely believe, that physical fitness and regular exercise are important and deliver benefits that are worth the cost—the financial cost of personal training and the cost of the time and energy the client must put into the exercise program. If personal trainers are not personally passionate about physical activity, they will lack persuasive power and authenticity. Similarly, personal trainers should model other healthful lifestyle attributes, such as not smoking and following a generally healthful diet.

Second, when personal trainers model a healthful lifestyle, clients see that it can be done and it gives them confidence that they can do it, too. Cultivating a healthful lifestyle is not easy in a culture that has engineered physical activity out of daily living. If a personal trainer cannot achieve a physically active lifestyle, who can?

In addition to serving as role models themselves, personal trainers can increase clients' motivation to exercise and self-confidence in their ability to stick to a regular exercise program by exposing clients to role models similar to the clients themselves. For example, a client who is older and coping with the joint pain of **arthritis** may not see the personal trainer as a realistic model if the personal trainer is young and pain-free. But if the personal trainer can arrange for a friend, client, or colleague who is more similar to the client to attend a session or simply work out while the client is nearby, this can provide a more suitable model for the client. People who see people like themselves exercising will develop more confidence in their own exercise abilities (Ashford, Edmunds, & French, 2010).

Personal trainers should model not only healthful behaviors, but good attitudes as well. Especially important is the modeling of exercise for positive reasons, as opposed to negative reasons that might promote negative body image or disordered eating and unhealthy exercise behavior (DiBartolo et al., 2007). For example, personal trainers should promote the attitude that physical activity can feel good, reduce stress, and lead to wonderful health and fitness improvements. Underlying this positive perspective is the notion that exercise offers a diverse array of benefits, all of which can meaningfully enhance a client's life.

EXPAND YOUR KNOWLEDGE

Using Behavioral Contracts

Behavioral contracting is an effective behavior-modification strategy. In behavioral contracting for lifestyle change, the client and personal trainer set up a system of rewards for adopting a new behavior. This tool is most effective when the rewards are outlined by, and meaningful to, the client. If the rewards are not meaningful, the client may not find them to be worth pursuing. Behavioral contracting works differently for each individual and personal trainers have to be careful not to push certain rewards on clients. Additionally, behavioral contracting is most effective when it is used consistently. Once certain goals are met, contracts need to be reconstructed throughout the duration of program participation.

Contracts typically spell out the behavior the client is expected to perform based on what the client has expressed interest in doing. Behavior-change contracts may be motivational for some clients, but they can also be problematic. Some personal trainers have found that contracts that set behavioral expectations too high may instill a sense of frustration and of feeling overwhelmed in some clients, especially when high expectations are not achieved. Ultimately, a personal trainer's role is to support clients in being accountable to themselves, as opposed to being accountable to the personal trainer, as this is key for lasting behavior change.

Behavior-change contracts that offer **extrinsic motivation** for exercise may be helpful for getting clients started (Figure 4-3). People who exercise to achieve an external reward, such as a free personal-training session or movie passes, are said to be extrinsically motivated. People who exercise because they enjoy the activity or because exercise feels good are said to have **intrinsic motivation** (see Chapter 3). Most people exercise for both intrinsic and extrinsic reasons. Research shows that people who exercise regularly for extended periods of time often do so because of intrinsic motivation (Teixeira et al., 2012).

FIGURE 4-3
Sample behavioral contract

I Will: (Do what) ____

(When) ____

(How often)____

(How much)____

How confident am I that I will do this? ______ (on a scale of 1 to 10, with 1 being not at all confident and 10 being completely confident)

If I successfully make this positive lifestyle change by ______, I will reward myself with _____

____

____.

If I fail to successfully make this positive lifestyle change, I will forfeit this reward.

I, ______________________________, have reviewed this contract and I agree to discuss the experience involved in accomplishing or not accomplishing this health-behavior improvement with ________________________ on ____________.

Signed (Client): ____

Signed (Personal trainer):____

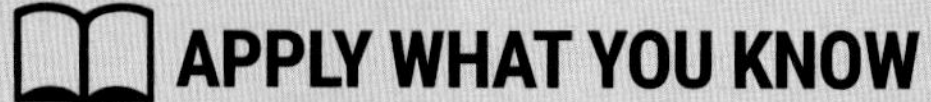

Incorporating Effective Communication and Teaching Techniques into Daily Interactions with Clients

Personal trainers can continue to build productive relationships with clients throughout their daily interactions by using the following techniques.

- Personal trainers should periodically reinforce their credentials through attending conferences and taking continuing education courses to further develop effective communication skills and teaching techniques in order to best support their clients.
- Personal trainers should prepare for each personal-training session by cultivating a mindful presence. Instead of rushing into a new session preoccupied with other matters, personal trainers should take a few minutes to review the materials on upcoming clients, set goals for the upcoming session, and prepare to focus mindfully on the next client. A mindful presence means keeping one's awareness in the present moment with an open, nonjudgmental attitude. This allows personal trainers to listen effectively and put fresh energy and undivided attention into each session.
- Personal trainers should ask clients for feedback on their own performance. Client feedback may be obtained from a feedback form that is either returned directly to the personal trainer or to the personal trainer's supervisor, or through an open-ended question, such as "What did you enjoy most about the training session today?" or "What can I do differently to best support you in our next session?" Client feedback can be helpful as personal trainers evaluate their communication and teaching skills.
- Personal trainers should use electronic communication channels with discretion. Both clients and personal trainers should give clear direction on how they prefer to be contacted. Many clients do not wish to receive email every day reminding them to exercise, although they may not mind a reminder of an upcoming personal-training session. Personal trainers may wish to let clients contact them at a work telephone number, but not on their mobile or home telephone numbers. In addition, personal trainers who allow clients access to their Internet pages, such as Facebook, should be sure to maintain such pages in a professional manner and establish clear boundaries.
- Personal trainers should try to make training fun in an effort to support clients developing a positive, lifelong habit of regular physical activity. While certain stages of the client–personal trainer relationship tend to be more focused and perhaps more serious, personal trainers should do what they can to make sessions fun and enjoyable. This may include incorporating purposeful games into the exercise program design. Some clients are more open to humor in the form of games, funny stories, or jokes than others, though playfulness should never "cross the line" or detract from the personal-training activities and the client's expressed goals for the client–personal trainer partnership.

ACE UNIVERSITY

If your study program includes the ACE University, visit www.ACEfitness.org/MyACE and log in to your My ACE Account to take full advantage of the ACE Personal Trainer Study Program and online guided study experience.

A variety of media to support and expand on the material in this text is provided to facilitate learning and best prepare you for the ACE Personal Trainer Certification exam and a career as a personal trainer.

SUMMARY

Successful personal trainers consistently demonstrate excellent communication skills and teaching techniques throughout the various stages of the client–personal trainer relationship. During the rapport stage, personal trainers begin to establish trust and understanding with their clients. In the investigation stage, personal trainers use active listening and effective verbal and nonverbal communication skills to gather information from clients so that they may provide support in strengthening motivation to change. In the planning stage, personal trainers use both good listening and teaching skills to design an exercise program in partnership with the client. During the action stage, personal trainers use effective, personalized teaching techniques to help clients learn motor skills and increase self-confidence.

Personal trainers who work with clients who differ from themselves can benefit from developing cultural competence and learning about their clients' beliefs, attitudes, and lifestyles. Personal trainers must become adept at developing strong collaborative partnerships with clients while maintaining professional boundaries. They must also learn to provide helpful direction to clients through all the stages of learning and incorporate effective communication and teaching techniques into their daily interactions with clients. An effective client–personal trainer relationship is an ever-evolving, dynamic journey of collaboration.

REFERENCES

Ambady, N. & Weisbuch, M. (2010). Nonverbal behavior. In: Fiske, S.T., Gilbert, D.T. & Lindzey, G. (Eds.). *Handbook of Social Psychology*. New York: McGraw-Hill.

American Council on Exercise (2019). *The Professional's Guide to Health and Wellness Coaching*. San Diego: American Council on Exercise.

American Council on Exercise (2014). *Coaching Behavior Change*. San Diego: American Council on Exercise.

Ashford, S., Edmunds, J., & French, D.P. (2010). What is the best way to change self-efficacy to promote lifestyle and recreational physical activity? A systematic review and meta-analysis. *British Journal of Health Psychology*, 15, 2, 265–288.

Brehm, B.A. (2004). *Successful Fitness Motivation Strategies*. Champaign, Ill.: Human Kinetics.

Burke, L.E., Wang, J., & Sevick, M.A. (2011). Self-monitoring in weight loss: A systematic review of the literature. *Journal of the American Dietetic Association*, 111, 1, 92–102.

Coker, C.A., Fischman, M.G., & Oxendine, J.B. (2006). Motor skill learning for coaching and performance. In: Williams, J.M. (Ed.) *Applied Sport Psychology*. New York: McGraw-Hill.

DiBartolo, P.M. et al. (2007). Are there "healthy" and "unhealthy" reasons for exercise? Examining individual differences in exercise motivations using the Function of Exercise Scale. *Journal of Clinical Sport Psychology*, 1, 2, 93–120.

Fitts, P.M. & Posner, M.I. (1967). *Human Performance*. Belmont, Calif.: Brooks/Cole.

Goldstein, M.G., DePue, J., & Kazura, N.A. (2008). Models for provider-patient interaction and shared decision making. In: Shumaker, S.A., Ockene, J.A., & Riekert, K.A. (Eds.) *The Handbook of Health Behavior Change* (3rd ed.). New York: Springer.

Locke, E.A. & Latham, G.P. (2002). Building a practically useful theory of goal setting and task motivation: A 35-year odyssey. *American Psychologist*, 57, 9, 705–717.

Macintosh, T. et al. (2013). Socially-assigned race, healthcare discrimination and preventive healthcare services. *PLoS One*, 8, 5, e64522.

Maguire, J.S. (2008). The personal is professional: Personal trainers as a case study of cultural intermediaries. *International Journal of Cultural Studies*,11, 2, 211–229.

Miller, W.R. & Rollnick, S. (2013). *Motivational Interviewing: Helping People Change* (3rd ed.). New York: Guilford.

Moore, S.D. et al. (2011). Outcome expectations and realizations as predictors of weight regain among dieters. *Eating Behaviors*, 12, 1, 60–63.

Nackers, L.M., Ross, K.M., & Perri, M.G. (2010). The association between rate of initial weight loss and long-term success in obesity treatment: Does slow and steady win the race? *International Journal of Behavioral Medicine*, 17, 161–167.

Olander, E.K. et al. (2013). What are the most effective techniques in changing obese individuals' physical activity self-efficacy and behaviour: A systematic review and meta-analysis. *International Journal of Behavioral Nutrition and Physical Activity*, 3, 10, 29.

Renshaw, I. et al. (2010). A constraints-led perspective to understanding skill acquisition and game play: A basis for integration of motor learning theory and physical education praxis. *Physical Education & Sport Pedagogy*, 15, 2, 117–138.

Rink, J.E. (2004). It's okay to be a beginner: Teach a motor skill, and the skill may be learned. *Journal of Physical Education, Recreation, and Dance*, 75, 6, 31–35.

Rosenkranz, K., Kacar, A., & Rothwell, J.C. (2007). Differential modulation of motor cortical plasticity and excitability in early and late phases of human motor learning. *Journal of Neuroscience*, 27, 44, 12058–12066.

Ryan, R.M. et al. (2011). Motivation and autonomy in counseling, psychotherapy, and behavior change: A look at theory and practice. *The Counseling Psychologist*, 39, 2, 193–260.

Teal, C.R. & Street, R.L. (2009). Critical elements of culturally competent communication in the medical encounter: A review and model. *Social Science & Medicine*, 68, 3, 533–543.

Teixeira, P.J. et al. (2012). Exercise, physical activity, and self-determination theory: A systematic review. *International Journal of Behavioral Nutrition and Physical Activity*, 9, 78.

Wright, K.B., Frey, L., & Sopory, P. (2007). Willingness to communicate about health as an underlying trait of patient self-advocacy: The development of the willingness to communicate about health (WTCH) measure. *Communication Studies*, 58, 1, 35–52.

Wulf, G., Shea, C., & Lewthwaite, R. (2010). Motor skill learning and performance: A review of influential factors. *Medical Education*, 44, 75–84.

SUGGESTED READINGS

American Council on Exercise (2019). *The Professional's Guide to Health and Wellness Coaching*. San Diego: American Council on Exercise.

Brehm, B.A. (2014). *Psychology of Health and Fitness*. Philadelphia: F.A. Davis.

Miller, W.R. & Rollnick, S. (2013). *Motivational Interviewing: Helping People Change* (3rd ed.). New York: Guilford.

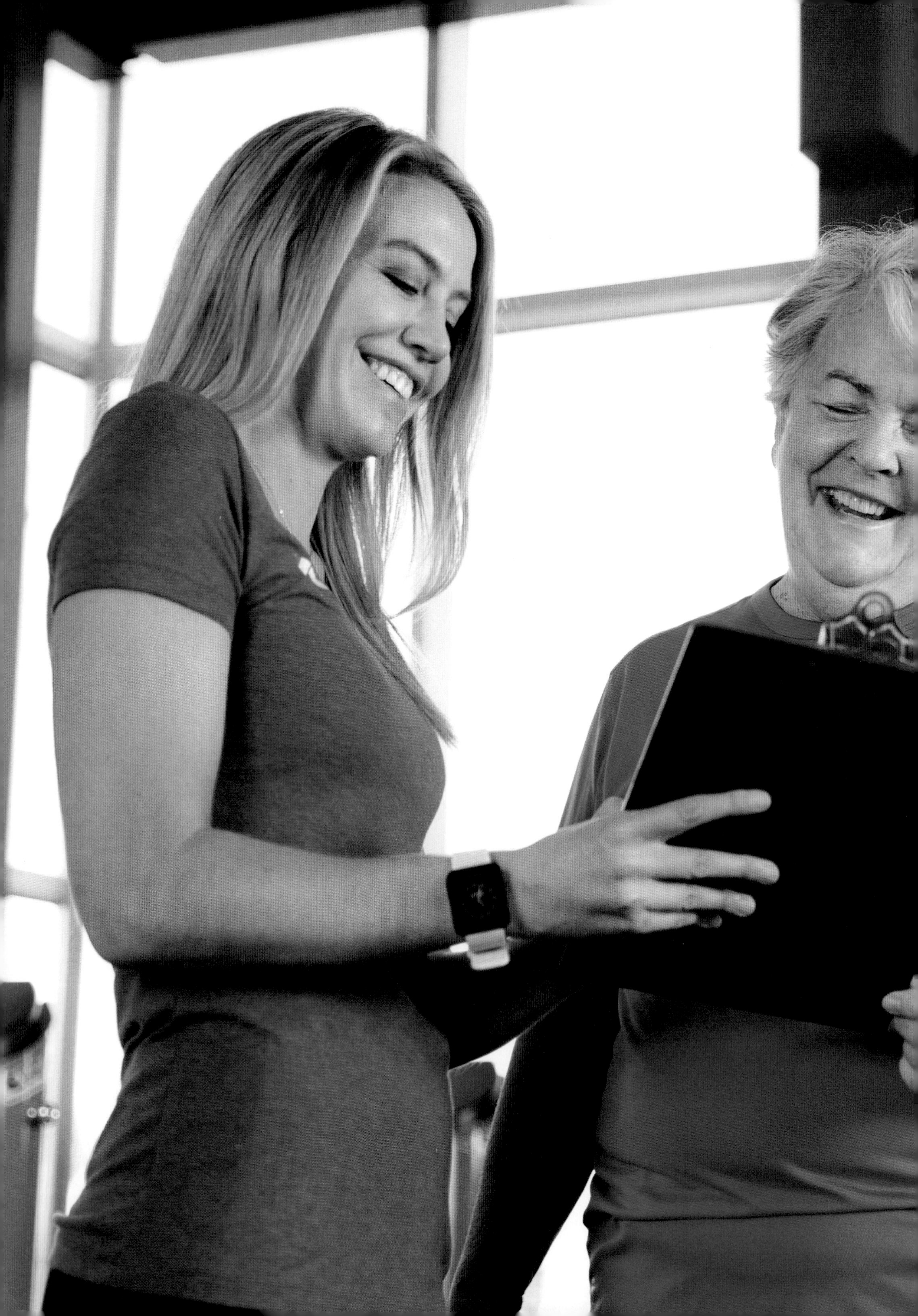

CHAPTER 5

Preparticipation Health Screening

SABRENA JO, MS
Director of Science and Research, American Council on Exercise; ACE Certified Personal Trainer, Health Coach, and Group Fitness Instructor

IN THIS CHAPTER

LEARNING OBJECTIVES:

Upon completion of this chapter, the reader will be able to:

- Administer exercise preparticipation health screening for clients
- Recognize scenarios in which a client should receive further evaluation from a qualified healthcare professional prior to engaging in increased physical activity
- Identify additional forms that must be completed by a client to ensure a successful exercise experience
- Explain the effects of select medications on resting and exercise heart rates

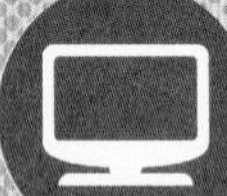

ACE UNIVERSITY

If your study program includes the ACE University, visit www.ACEfitness.org/MyACE and log in to your My ACE Account to take full advantage of the ACE Personal Trainer Study Program and online guided study experience.

A variety of media to support and expand on the material in this text is provided to facilitate learning and best prepare you for the ACE Personal Trainer Certification exam and a career as a personal trainer.

Prior to designing and implementing a formal exercise program, an ACE® Certified Personal Trainer must first develop initial **rapport** with a client in order to determine his or her individual needs, goals, and interests. This is established through effective communication skills, as described in Chapters 3 and 4. A thorough preparticipation health screening is part of the initial client–personal trainer interaction to help ensure that the client is physically and mentally ready to embark on a structured exercise program. This information, in combination with the client's stated goals and any chosen assessments, can then be used to develop a personalized exercise routine based on the guidelines set forth in the ACE Integrated Fitness Training® Model (see Chapters 8 through 11).

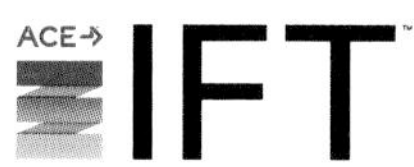

Inherent Health Risks with Exercise

Research demonstrates the positive impact that exercise and physical activity have on reducing a person's risk for developing cardiovascular, pulmonary, and metabolic diseases, as well as certain types of cancer, **anxiety, depression,** and premature death [American College of Sports Medicine (ACSM), 2018; U.S. Department of Health & Human Services, 2018]. While exercise and physical activity promote numerous physiological, psychological, and emotional benefits, there are some inherent risks. In general, moderate levels of exercise and physical activity do not provoke dangerous cardiovascular or musculoskeletal events in healthy individuals, but there is an increased risk for harm in individuals who are unhealthy presenting with exertional signs and symptoms suggestive of a disease, or who have been diagnosed with an existing cardiovascular, metabolic, or renal disease and plan on performing vigorous to near-maximal-intensity exercise (ACSM, 2018). Individuals with underlying **cardiovascular disease (CVD)** performing unaccustomed vigorous physical activity are at the greatest risk for activity-associated **acute myocardial infarction (AMI)** and **sudden cardiac death (SCD).**

The risk of exercise-related AMI and SCD is highest among individuals with underlying CVD who perform a level of physical activity to which they are not accustomed. That said, it is important to note that the risk of an adverse cardiovascular event during exercise is extremely low for asymptomatic individuals, even when exercising at a vigorous intensity.

Further consideration should be given when assessing an individual's risk as to whether the exercise program may be self-directed or should be conducted under the supervision of a personal trainer. With self-directed exercise, a standard questionnaire is completed by the individual with little to no feedback from the personal trainer. These questionnaires are designed to provide information regarding existing risks for participation in activity and the need for medical clearance beforehand. A preparticipation health screening *must* be performed on all new participants, regardless of age, upon entering a facility that offers exercise equipment or services. The screening procedure should be valid, simple, cost-efficient, time-efficient, and appropriate for the target population.

Preparticipation Health Screening

The ACSM preparticipation guidelines are designed to remove any unnecessary barriers to becoming more physically active (ACSM, 2018). Risk-factor profiling or classification is not part of the exercise preparticipation health-screening process because supporting evidence is lacking for the presence of risk factors without underlying disease increasing the risk for activity-related cardiovascular events and screening must not become a barrier to participation. Further, the guidelines note that when an individual becomes more physically active, his or her risks decline. The new health-screening process is based on three factors that have been identified as important risk modulators of exercise-related cardiovascular events:

- The individual's current level of physical activity
- Diagnosed cardiovascular, metabolic, or renal disease and/or the presence of signs or symptoms of cardiovascular, metabolic, or renal disease
- The desired exercise intensity

This screening protocol makes general recommendations for medical clearance, leaving the specifics—such as the need for medical exams or exercise tests—up to the discretion of the healthcare provider.

The goal of this process is to identify individuals:

- Who should receive medical clearance before initiating an exercise program or increasing the frequency, intensity, and/or volume of their current program
- With clinically significant disease(s) who may benefit from participating in a medically supervised exercise program
- With medical conditions that may require exclusion from exercise programs until those conditions are resolved or better controlled

Figure 5-1 presents the preparticipation health-screening algorithm, while an exercise preparticipation checklist is presented in Figure 5-2. This algorithm shows that medical clearance is needed only under the following circumstances, with regular exercise defined as performing planned, structured physical activity for at least 30 minutes at moderate intensity on at least three days/week for at least the past three months:

- **For those who do not exercise regularly:** If a client has cardiovascular, metabolic, or renal disease, or signs or symptoms that suggest he or she does, then medical clearance is necessary.
- **For regular exercisers:** If a client has signs or symptoms suggestive of cardiovascular, metabolic, or renal disease, he or she should discontinue exercise and seek medical clearance. If a client has a known history of cardiovascular, metabolic, or renal disease and has a desire to progress to vigorous-intensity aerobic exercise, medical clearance is recommended.

While the identification of the signs and symptoms referenced in this algorithm may be within the **scope of practice** of most personal trainers, interpretation of those same signs and symptoms should be made only by qualified healthcare professionals within the context in which they appear (ACSM, 2018):

- Pain; discomfort (or other **angina** equivalent) in the chest, neck, jaw, arms, or other areas that may result from **myocardial ischemia**
- Shortness of breath at rest or with mild exertion **(dyspnea)**
- **Orthopnea** (dyspnea in a reclined position) or **paroxysmal nocturnal dyspnea** (onset is usually two to five hours after the beginning of sleep)
- Dizziness, or **syncope,** most commonly caused by reduced perfusion to the brain
- Ankle **edema**
- **Palpitations** or **tachycardia**

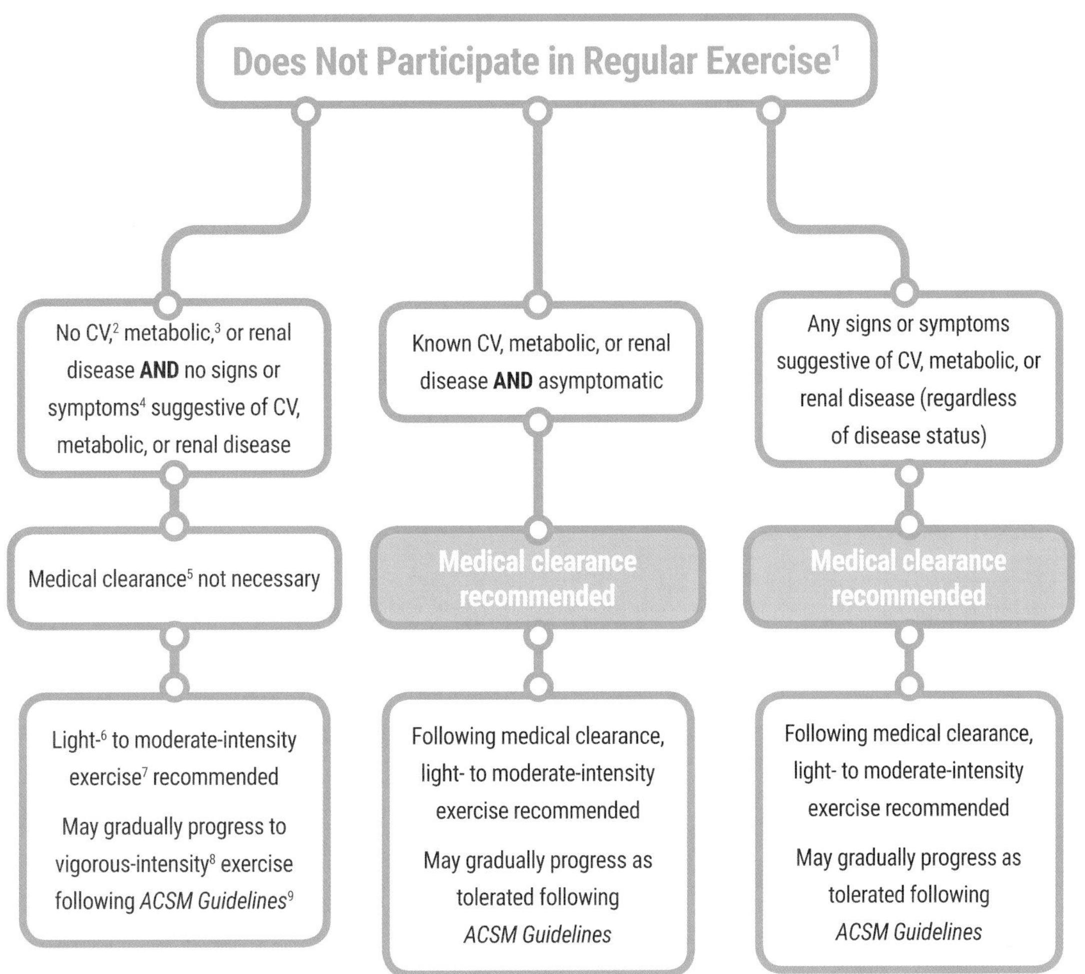

FIGURE 5-1
The American College of Sports Medicine's preparticipation health-screening algorithm

[1] **Exercise participation** Performing planned, structured physical activity for at least 30 minutes at moderate intensity on at least 3 days/week for at least the past 3 months

[2] **Cardiovascular disease** Cardiac, peripheral vascular, or cerebrovascular disease

[3] **Metabolic disease** Type 1 and 2 diabetes mellitus

[4] **Sign and symptoms** At rest or during activity. Includes pain, discomfort in the chest, neck, jaw, arms, or other areas that may result from ischemia; shortness of breath at rest or with mild exertion; dizziness or syncope; orthopnea or paroxysmal nocturnal dyspnea; ankle edema; palpitations or tachycardia; intermittent claudication; known heart murmur; unusual fatigue or shortness of breath with usual activities

[5] **Medical clearance** Approval from a healthcare professional to engage in exercise

[6] **Light-intensity exercise** 30–39% HRR or $\dot{V}O_2R$, 2–2.9 METs, RPE 9–11, an intensity that causes slight increases in HR and breathing

[7] **Moderate-intensity exercise** 40–59% HRR or $\dot{V}O_2R$, 3–5.9 METs, RPE 12–13, an intensity that causes noticeable increases in HR and breathing

[8] **Vigorous-intensity exercise** ≥60% HRR or $\dot{V}O_2R$, ≥6 METs, RPE ≥14, an intensity that causes substantial increases in HR and breathing

[9] **ACSM Guidelines** *ACSM's Guidelines for Exercise Testing and Prescription*, 10th edition

Note: CV = Cardiovascular; HRR = Heart-rate reserve; $\dot{V}O_2R$ = Oxygen uptake reserve; METs = Metabolic equivalents; RPE = Rating of perceived exertion; HR = Heart rate; ACSM = American College of Sports Medicine

Reprinted with permission from American College of Sports Medicine (2018). *ACSM's Guidelines for Exercise Testing and Prescription* (10th ed.). Philadelphia: Wolters Kluwer.

Continued on the next page

FIGURE 5-1
(*continued*)

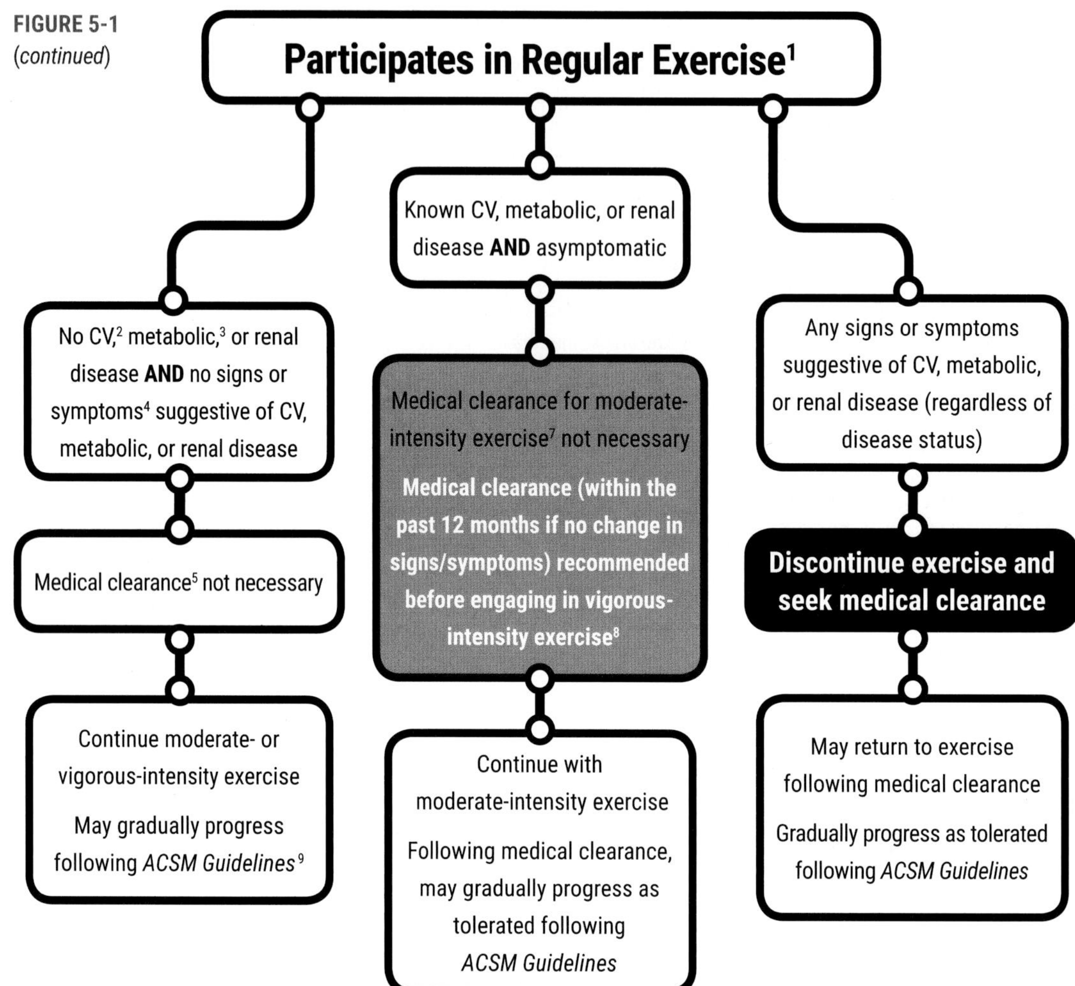

[1] **Exercise participation** Performing planned, structured physical activity for at least 30 minutes at moderate intensity on at least 3 days/week for at least the past 3 months

[2] **Cardiovascular disease** Cardiac, peripheral vascular, or cerebrovascular disease

[3] **Metabolic disease** Type 1 and 2 diabetes mellitus

[4] **Sign and symptoms** At rest or during activity. Includes pain, discomfort in the chest, neck, jaw, arms, or other areas that may result from ischemia; shortness of breath at rest or with mild exertion; dizziness or syncope; orthopnea or paroxysmal nocturnal dyspnea; ankle edema; palpitations or tachycardia; intermittent claudication; known heart murmur; unusual fatigue or shortness of breath with usual activities

[5] **Medical clearance** Approval from a healthcare professional to engage in exercise

[6] **Light-intensity exercise** 30–39% HRR or $\dot{V}O_2R$, 2–2.9 METs, RPE 9–11, an intensity that causes slight increases in HR and breathing

[7] **Moderate-intensity exercise** 40–59% HRR or $\dot{V}O_2R$, 3–5.9 METs, RPE 12–13, an intensity that causes noticeable increases in HR and breathing

[8] **Vigorous-intensity exercise** ≥60% HRR or $\dot{V}O_2R$, ≥6 METs, RPE ≥14, an intensity that causes substantial increases in HR and breathing

[9] **ACSM Guidelines** *ACSM's Guidelines for Exercise Testing and Prescription,* 10th edition

Note: CV = Cardiovascular; HRR = Heart-rate reserve; $\dot{V}O_2R$ = Oxygen uptake reserve; METs = Metabolic equivalents; RPE = Rating of perceived exertion; HR = Heart rate; ACSM = American College of Sports Medicine

Reprinted with permission from American College of Sports Medicine (2018). *ACSM's Guidelines for Exercise Testing and Prescription* (10th ed.). Philadelphia: Wolters Kluwer.

EXERCISE PREPARTICIPATION HEALTH-SCREENING QUESTIONNAIRE FOR EXERCISE PROFESSIONALS

Assess your client's health needs by marking all *true* statements.

Step 1

SYMPTOMS

Does your client experience:

☐ chest discomfort with exertion
☐ unreasonable breathlessness
☐ dizziness, fainting, blackouts
☐ ankle swelling
☐ unpleasant awareness of a forceful, rapid, or irregular heart rate
☐ burning or cramping sensations in your lower legs when walking short distances

If you **did** mark any of these statements under the symptoms, **STOP,** your client should seek medical clearance before engaging in or resuming exercise. Your client may need to use a facility with a **medically qualified staff**.

If you **did not** mark any symptoms, continue to steps 2 and 3.

Step 2

CURRENT ACTIVITY

Has your client performed planned, structured physical activity for at least 30 minutes at moderate intensity on at least 3 days per week for at least the past 3 months?

Yes ☐ No ☐

Continue to Step 3.

Step 3

MEDICAL CONDITIONS

Has your client had or does he or she currently have:

☐ a heart attack
☐ heart surgery, cardiac catheterization, or coronary angioplasty
☐ pacemaker/implantable cardiac defibrillator/rhythm disturbance
☐ heart valve disease
☐ heart failure
☐ heart transplantation
☐ congenital heart disease
☐ diabetes
☐ renal disease

Evaluating Steps 2 and 3:

- If you **did not mark any of the statements in Step 3,** medical clearance is not necessary.
- If you marked Step 2 **"yes"** and **marked any of the statements in Step 3,** your client may continue to exercise at light to moderate intensity without medical clearance. Medical clearance is recommended before engaging in vigorous exercise.
- If you marked Step 2 **"no"** and **marked any of the statements in Step 3,** medical clearance is recommended. Your client may need to use a facility with a **medically qualified staff.**

FIGURE 5-2
Exercise preparticipation health-screening questionnaire for exercise professionals

Reprinted with permission from American College of Sports Medicine (2018). *ACSM's Guidelines for Exercise Testing and Prescription* (10th ed.). Philadelphia: Wolters Kluwer.

- **Intermittent claudication** (pain sensations or cramping in the lower extremities during exercise that is associated with inadequate blood supply)
- Known heart murmur
- Unusual fatigue or shortness of breath with usual activities

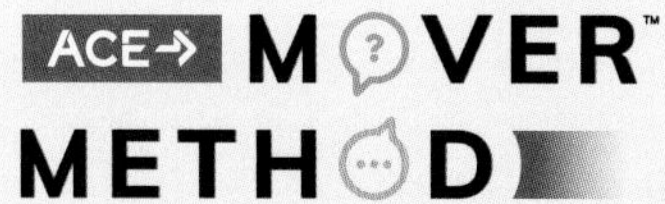

The Excited New Client in Need of Medical Clearance

Today, during an initial meeting with your new client Nathaniel, he lets you know that he is excited to begin a structured exercise program and that he has been looking forward to working with a personal trainer.

ACE ABC APPROACH™

Following is an example of how using the ACE ABC Approach™ to coaching can facilitate the preparticipation health-screening process.

Ask: Asking powerful open-ended questions will help you learn more about Nathaniel's goals and what he would like to accomplish by working with a personal trainer.

Personal Trainer: Thank you for letting me know how excited you are to get started working together. How would you describe your health and fitness journey up to this point?

Client: Well, I used to enjoy hiking, lifting weights, and even doing martial arts, but it's been a long time since I did any of those things. Over the past two months, I started walking two days per week for 10 or 15 minutes to try to manage my diabetes.

Personal Trainer: Managing your diabetes is important to you. How do you envision me helping to support your goals?

Client: Yes, it is imperative that I manage my diabetes. I need help figuring out a structured physical-activity program that is consistent and includes different types of activities, so I don't get bored. I want to make sure that I keep my diabetes under control by improving my diet and moving more. If I could get back to a point where I felt like being active more than two days per week, that would be great!

Break down barriers: At this point in the conversation, asking more open-ended questions could help to uncover the potential barriers that might prevent Nathaniel from participating in a structured, consistent program.

Personal Trainer: Structure, consistency, and variety are important to you, and you also want to make sure your diabetes stays under control. You mentioned earlier that you enjoyed hiking, lifting weights, and martial arts. What changed? How come you no longer do those activities?

Client: I'm not 100% sure why I stopped. It seems like I just started slowing down and finding reasons not to exercise. Then I started gaining weight, and the more I put on, the less I felt like doing.

Personal Trainer: You lost momentum. What did you learn from that experience? Are there any specific obstacles you think might disrupt your momentum this time?

Client: That's a nice way to put it. I think the main obstacles I'll face will be my work schedule, my "non-exercise"-related habits, and the difficulty of starting something new. Even finding the time to walk for 15 minutes twice per week is sometimes challenging, but I'm pretty motivated right now to get myself moving. I try to encourage myself by remembering how good I feel after my walks.

Personal Trainer: Reminding yourself of that fantastic post-walk feeling is a great strategy. What else?

Client: I think I need a plan that makes it easy to schedule activity as part of my day. It's easy to get wrapped up in my job, so I forget to get up and move. Maybe it will help if I put activity breaks in my calendar. Having regularly scheduled sessions with you before or after work will also help me to be accountable.

Personal Trainer: Adopting a consistent and varied exercise program is exciting for you, and you've come up with some great ideas for how to overcome potential obstacles. Part of my job is to make sure I do everything possible to create safe and effective programs for you, so it is crucial to know if you are on any medications for your diabetes or if you have discussed your plans for increasing your physical activity with your doctor.

Client: No meds at the moment. I hope if I keep walking and get my diet figured out I won't ever have to be on them. I haven't seen my doctor in a little over a year. The last time we talked, she told me about the benefits of being more active, but I was not ready to get started at that time. I think she would like the idea of me exercising. Do I need to ask her?

Collaborate: Working together on goals is the next step now that barriers and solutions for adopting healthier behaviors have been identified. Also, because this client is not currently physically active, and he presents with diabetes, it is vital to ensure that he has received clearance from his doctor before setting or working on any exercise-related goals.

Personal Trainer: The more your doctor knows about how you are managing your diabetes, the better equipped she is to help you. By discussing your plans with your doctor before we start working together, it allows her to communicate any limitations, restrictions, or guidelines. This will help to ensure that any plan we create for you will be safe and effective and that everyone on your healthcare team is on the same page. Are you open to the idea of contacting your doctor?

Client: I am, yes. Thank you. I like the idea of us all working together. It's probably a good idea for me to connect with my doctor anyway, since I have not seen her in over a year.

Personal Trainer: I want to be clear that asking you to see your doctor before we can work together is by no means a way of saying I don't want to help you. It is just the opposite. I want to see you get the right kind of help so that I can do what I do best when we work together: give you a great physical-activity experience that is enjoyable and helps you manage your diabetes. What can you do within the next week to get started?

Client: I will contact my doctor's office this week to make them aware of my plans to increase my physical activity. I am not sure if they will clear me for exercise over the phone or want me to come in for an appointment. Either way, I will work with my doctor to make sure she supports my goals and to see if she has any recommendations. Also, I want to make sure I am ready to start working with you once my doctor signs off, so I will keep walking twice a week. This way, I'll be set to go once I hear back from my doctor!

Personal Trainer: Great! I will provide you with a medical release form that your doctor can sign and make sure we have everything we need to get started. Please let me know when you have the form filled out and we will get our first training session scheduled. I look forward to hearing back from you soon.

The preparticipation health-screening process is an important initial step to take with clients, as it provides an opportunity to build rapport, get to know each other, learn about past exercise experience and health history and determine if medical clearance is needed before beginning a formal exercise program. The ACE ABC Approach can be used throughout the screening process to gather all the pertinent information in a way that feels like a conversation and not an interview.

Addressing the need for medical clearance while also supporting the client's enthusiasm and readiness to get started is important, as you do not want the requirement for medical clearance to be a barrier to becoming more physically active.

RESISTANCE TRAINING

Current evidence is insufficient regarding cardiovascular complications during low-to-moderate intensity resistance training to warrant formal prescreening recommendations (ACSM, 2018). Limited data are available on the topic, but it appears that the risk of complications is low.

SELF-GUIDED SCREENING

Preparticipation health screening for individuals wanting to initiate an exercise program may be conducted using the **Physical Activity Readiness Questionnaire for Everyone (PAR-Q+)** form (Figure 5-3). This form is evidence-based and was developed with a goal of reducing unnecessary barriers to exercise. The PAR-Q+ can be used as either a self-guided screening tool or as an additional element of screening for use by personal trainers seeking additional client information.

This important screening document is regularly updated and revised and there are different versions depending on the clientele with whom you are working. The PAR-Q+ and ePARmed-X+ (for clients who have had a positive response to the PAR-Q+ or have been referred to use this more comprehensive form by a healthcare professional) were created to reduce barriers for all individuals to become more physically active. These forms are updated on a regular basis and publicly available at www.eparmedx.com.

2020 PAR-Q+

The Physical Activity Readiness Questionnaire for Everyone

The health benefits of regular physical activity are clear; more people should engage in physical activity every day of the week. Participating in physical activity is very safe for MOST people. This questionnaire will tell you whether it is necessary for you to seek further advice from your doctor OR a qualified exercise professional before becoming more physically active.

GENERAL HEALTH QUESTIONS

Please read the 7 questions below carefully and answer each one honestly: check YES or NO.	**YES**	**NO**
1) Has your doctor ever said that you have a heart condition ☐ **OR** high blood pressure ☐?	☐	☐
2) Do you feel pain in your chest at rest, during your daily activities of living, **OR** when you do physical activity?	☐	☐
3) Do you lose balance because of dizziness **OR** have you lost consciousness in the last 12 months? Please answer **NO** if your dizziness was associated with over-breathing (including during vigorous exercise).	☐	☐
4) Have you ever been diagnosed with another chronic medical condition (other than heart disease or high blood pressure)? **PLEASE LIST CONDITION(S) HERE:** ______	☐	☐
5) Are you currently taking prescribed medications for a chronic medical condition? **PLEASE LIST CONDITION(S) AND MEDICATIONS HERE:** ______	☐	☐
6) Do you currently have (or have had within the past 12 months) a bone, joint, or soft tissue (muscle, ligament, or tendon) problem that could be made worse by becoming more physically active? Please answer **NO** if you had a problem in the past, but it **does not limit your current ability** to be physically active. **PLEASE LIST CONDITION(S) HERE:** ______	☐	☐
7) Has your doctor ever said that you should only do medically supervised physical activity?	☐	☐

If you answered NO to all of the questions above, you are cleared for physical activity.
Please sign the PARTICIPANT DECLARATION. You do not need to complete Pages 2 and 3.

- Start becoming much more physically active – start slowly and build up gradually.
- Follow Global Physical Activity Guidelines for your age (https://apps.who.int/iris/handle/10665/44399).
- You may take part in a health and fitness appraisal.
- If you are over the age of 45 yr and NOT accustomed to regular vigorous to maximal effort exercise, consult a qualified exercise professional before engaging in this intensity of exercise.
- If you have any further questions, contact a qualified exercise professional.

PARTICIPANT DECLARATION

If you are less than the legal age required for consent or require the assent of a care provider, your parent, guardian or care provider must also sign this form.

I, the undersigned, have read, understood to my full satisfaction and completed this questionnaire. I acknowledge that this physical activity clearance is valid for a maximum of 12 months from the date it is completed and becomes invalid if my condition changes. I also acknowledge that the community/fitness center may retain a copy of this form for its records. In these instances, it will maintain the confidentiality of the same, complying with applicable law.

NAME ______ DATE ______

SIGNATURE ______ WITNESS ______

SIGNATURE OF PARENT/GUARDIAN/CARE PROVIDER ______

If you answered YES to one or more of the questions above, COMPLETE PAGES 2 AND 3.

Delay becoming more active if:

- You have a temporary illness such as a cold or fever; it is best to wait until you feel better.
- You are pregnant - talk to your health care practitioner, your physician, a qualified exercise professional, and/or complete the ePARmed-X+ at www.eparmedx.com before becoming more physically active.
- Your health changes - answer the questions on Pages 2 and 3 of this document and/or talk to your doctor or a qualified exercise professional before continuing with any physical activity program.

 1 / 4
01-11-2019

FIGURE 5-3
The Physical Activity Readiness Questionnaire for Everyone

Continued on the next page

FIGURE 5-3
(continued)

2020 PAR-Q+

FOLLOW-UP QUESTIONS ABOUT YOUR MEDICAL CONDITION(S)

1. Do you have Arthritis, Osteoporosis, or Back Problems?
If the above condition(s) is/are present, answer questions 1a-1c — If **NO** ☐ go to question 2

1a.	Do you have difficulty controlling your condition with medications or other physician-prescribed therapies? (Answer **NO** if you are not currently taking medications or other treatments)	YES ☐ NO ☐
1b.	Do you have joint problems causing pain, a recent fracture or fracture caused by osteoporosis or cancer, displaced vertebra (e.g., spondylolisthesis), and/or spondylolysis/pars defect (a crack in the bony ring on the back of the spinal column)?	YES ☐ NO ☐
1c.	Have you had steroid injections or taken steroid tablets regularly for more than 3 months?	YES ☐ NO ☐

2. Do you currently have Cancer of any kind?
If the above condition(s) is/are present, answer questions 2a-2b — If **NO** ☐ go to question 3

2a.	Does your cancer diagnosis include any of the following types: lung/bronchogenic, multiple myeloma (cancer of plasma cells), head, and/or neck?	YES ☐ NO ☐
2b.	Are you currently receiving cancer therapy (such as chemotheraphy or radiotherapy)?	YES ☐ NO ☐

3. Do you have a Heart or Cardiovascular Condition? This includes Coronary Artery Disease, Heart Failure, Diagnosed Abnormality of Heart Rhythm
If the above condition(s) is/are present, answer questions 3a-3d — If **NO** ☐ go to question 4

3a.	Do you have difficulty controlling your condition with medications or other physician-prescribed therapies? (Answer **NO** if you are not currently taking medications or other treatments)	YES ☐ NO ☐
3b.	Do you have an irregular heart beat that requires medical management? (e.g., atrial fibrillation, premature ventricular contraction)	YES ☐ NO ☐
3c.	Do you have chronic heart failure?	YES ☐ NO ☐
3d.	Do you have diagnosed coronary artery (cardiovascular) disease and have not participated in regular physical activity in the last 2 months?	YES ☐ NO ☐

4. Do you currently have High Blood Pressure?
If the above condition(s) is/are present, answer questions 4a-4b — If **NO** ☐ go to question 5

4a.	Do you have difficulty controlling your condition with medications or other physician-prescribed therapies? (Answer **NO** if you are not currently taking medications or other treatments)	YES ☐ NO ☐
4b.	Do you have a resting blood pressure equal to or greater than 160/90 mmHg with or without medication? (Answer **YES** if you do not know your resting blood pressure)	YES ☐ NO ☐

5. Do you have any Metabolic Conditions? This includes Type 1 Diabetes, Type 2 Diabetes, Pre-Diabetes
If the above condition(s) is/are present, answer questions 5a-5e — If **NO** ☐ go to question 6

5a.	Do you often have difficulty controlling your blood sugar levels with foods, medications, or other physician-prescribed therapies?	YES ☐ NO ☐
5b.	Do you often suffer from signs and symptoms of low blood sugar (hypoglycemia) following exercise and/or during activities of daily living? Signs of hypoglycemia may include shakiness, nervousness, unusual irritability, abnormal sweating, dizziness or light-headedness, mental confusion, difficulty speaking, weakness, or sleepiness.	YES ☐ NO ☐
5c.	Do you have any signs or symptoms of diabetes complications such as heart or vascular disease and/or complications affecting your eyes, kidneys, **OR** the sensation in your toes and feet?	YES ☐ NO ☐
5d.	Do you have other metabolic conditions (such as current pregnancy-related diabetes, chronic kidney disease, or liver problems)?	YES ☐ NO ☐
5e.	Are you planning to engage in what for you is unusually high (or vigorous) intensity exercise in the near future?	YES ☐ NO ☐

 2 / 4
11-01-2019

2020 PAR-Q+

FIGURE 5-3
(continued)

6.	**Do you have any Mental Health Problems or Learning Difficulties?** This includes Alzheimer's, Dementia, Depression, Anxiety Disorder, Eating Disorder, Psychotic Disorder, Intellectual Disability, Down Syndrome If the above condition(s) is/are present, answer questions 6a-6b — If **NO** ☐ go to question 7	
6a.	Do you have difficulty controlling your condition with medications or other physician-prescribed therapies? (Answer **NO** if you are not currently taking medications or other treatments)	YES ☐ NO ☐
6b.	Do you have Down Syndrome **AND** back problems affecting nerves or muscles?	YES ☐ NO ☐
7.	**Do you have a Respiratory Disease?** This includes Chronic Obstructive Pulmonary Disease, Asthma, Pulmonary High Blood Pressure If the above condition(s) is/are present, answer questions 7a-7d — If **NO** ☐ go to question 8	
7a.	Do you have difficulty controlling your condition with medications or other physician-prescribed therapies? (Answer **NO** if you are not currently taking medications or other treatments)	YES ☐ NO ☐
7b.	Has your doctor ever said your blood oxygen level is low at rest or during exercise and/or that you require supplemental oxygen therapy?	YES ☐ NO ☐
7c.	If asthmatic, do you currently have symptoms of chest tightness, wheezing, laboured breathing, consistent cough (more than 2 days/week), or have you used your rescue medication more than twice in the last week?	YES ☐ NO ☐
7d.	Has your doctor ever said you have high blood pressure in the blood vessels of your lungs?	YES ☐ NO ☐
8.	**Do you have a Spinal Cord Injury?** This includes Tetraplegia and Paraplegia If the above condition(s) is/are present, answer questions 8a-8c — If **NO** ☐ go to question 9	
8a.	Do you have difficulty controlling your condition with medications or other physician-prescribed therapies? (Answer **NO** if you are not currently taking medications or other treatments)	YES ☐ NO ☐
8b.	Do you commonly exhibit low resting blood pressure significant enough to cause dizziness, light-headedness, and/or fainting?	YES ☐ NO ☐
8c.	Has your physician indicated that you exhibit sudden bouts of high blood pressure (known as Autonomic Dysreflexia)?	YES ☐ NO ☐
9.	**Have you had a Stroke?** This includes Transient Ischemic Attack (TIA) or Cerebrovascular Event If the above condition(s) is/are present, answer questions 9a-9c — If **NO** ☐ go to question 10	
9a.	Do you have difficulty controlling your condition with medications or other physician-prescribed therapies? (Answer **NO** if you are not currently taking medications or other treatments)	YES ☐ NO ☐
9b.	Do you have any impairment in walking or mobility?	YES ☐ NO ☐
9c.	Have you experienced a stroke or impairment in nerves or muscles in the past 6 months?	YES ☐ NO ☐
10.	**Do you have any other medical condition not listed above or do you have two or more medical conditions?** If you have other medical conditions, answer questions 10a-10c — If **NO** ☐ read the Page 4 recommendations	
10a.	Have you experienced a blackout, fainted, or lost consciousness as a result of a head injury within the last 12 months **OR** have you had a diagnosed concussion within the last 12 months?	YES ☐ NO ☐
10b.	Do you have a medical condition that is not listed (such as epilepsy, neurological conditions, kidney problems)?	YES ☐ NO ☐
10c.	Do you currently live with two or more medical conditions?	YES ☐ NO ☐

PLEASE LIST YOUR MEDICAL CONDITION(S) AND ANY RELATED MEDICATIONS HERE: ______________________________

____

GO to Page 4 for recommendations about your current medical condition(s) and sign the PARTICIPANT DECLARATION.

 3/ 4
11-01-2019

Continued on the next page

FIGURE 5-3
(continued)

2020 PAR-Q+

If you answered NO to all of the FOLLOW-UP questions (pgs. 2-3) about your medical condition, you are ready to become more physically active - sign the PARTICIPANT DECLARATION below:

- It is advised that you consult a qualified exercise professional to help you develop a safe and effective physical activity plan to meet your health needs.
- You are encouraged to start slowly and build up gradually - 20 to 60 minutes of low to moderate intensity exercise, 3-5 days per week including aerobic and muscle strengthening exercises.
- As you progress, you should aim to accumulate 150 minutes or more of moderate intensity physical activity per week.
- If you are over the age of 45 yr and **NOT** accustomed to regular vigorous to maximal effort exercise, consult a qualified exercise professional before engaging in this intensity of exercise.

If you answered **YES** to **one or more of the follow-up questions** about your medical condition:
You should seek further information before becoming more physically active or engaging in a fitness appraisal. You should complete the specially designed online screening and exercise recommendations program - the **ePARmed-X+ at www.eparmedx.com** and/or visit a qualified exercise professional to work through the ePARmed-X+ and for further information.

Delay becoming more active if:

You have a temporary illness such as a cold or fever; it is best to wait until you feel better.

You are pregnant - talk to your health care practitioner, your physician, a qualified exercise professional, and/or complete the ePARmed-X+ **at www.eparmedx.com** before becoming more physically active.

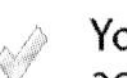
Your health changes - talk to your doctor or qualified exercise professional before continuing with any physical activity program.

- You are encouraged to photocopy the PAR-Q+. You must use the entire questionnaire and NO changes are permitted.
- The authors, the PAR-Q+ Collaboration, partner organizations, and their agents assume no liability for persons who undertake physical activity and/or make use of the PAR-Q+ or ePARmed-X+. If in doubt after completing the questionnaire, consult your doctor prior to physical activity.

PARTICIPANT DECLARATION

- All persons who have completed the PAR-Q+ please read and sign the declaration below.
- If you are less than the legal age required for consent or require the assent of a care provider, your parent, guardian or care provider must also sign this form.

I, the undersigned, have read, understood to my full satisfaction and completed this questionnaire. I acknowledge that this physical activity clearance is valid for a maximum of 12 months from the date it is completed and becomes invalid if my condition changes. I also acknowledge that the community/fitness center may retain a copy of this form for records. In these instances, it will maintain the confidentiality of the same, complying with applicable law.

NAME ______________________ DATE ______________________

SIGNATURE ______________________ WITNESS ______________________

SIGNATURE OF PARENT/GUARDIAN/CARE PROVIDER ______________________

For more information, please contact
www.eparmedx.com
Email: eparmedx@gmail.com

Citation for PAR-Q+
Warburton DER, Jamnik VK, Bredin SSD, and Gledhill N on behalf of the PAR-Q+ Collaboration. The Physical Activity Readiness Questionnaire for Everyone (PAR-Q+) and Electronic Physical Activity Readiness Medical Examination (ePARmed-X+). Health & Fitness Journal of Canada 4(2):3-23, 2011.

The PAR-Q+ was created using the evidence-based AGREE process (1) by the PAR-Q+ Collaboration chaired by Dr. Darren E. R. Warburton with Dr. Norman Gledhill, Dr. Veronica Jamnik, and Dr. Donald C. McKenzie (2). Production of this document has been made possible through financial contributions from the Public Health Agency of Canada and the BC Ministry of Health Services. The views expressed herein do not necessarily represent the views of the Public Health Agency of Canada or the BC Ministry of Health Services.

Key References
1. Jamnik VK, Warburton DER, Makarski J, McKenzie DC, Shephard RJ, Stone J, and Gledhill N. Enhancing the effectiveness of clearance for physical activity participation; background and overall process. APNM 36(S1):S3-S13, 2011.
2. Warburton DER, Gledhill N, Jamnik VK, Bredin SSD, McKenzie DC, Stone J, Charlesworth S, and Shephard RJ. Evidence-based risk assessment and recommendations for physical activity clearance; Consensus Document. APNM 36(S1):S266-s298, 2011.
3. Chisholm DM, Collis ML, Kulak LL, Davenport W, and Gruber N. Physical activity readiness. British Columbia Medical Journal. 1975;17:375-378.
4. Thomas S, Reading J, and Shephard RJ. Revision of the Physical Activity Readiness Questionnaire (PAR-Q). Canadian Journal of Sport Science 1992;17:4 338-345.

 4/ 4
11-01-2019

Note: The blood-pressure threshold mentioned in question 4b does not align with current guidelines. Please adhere to the recommendations presented in Chapter 13 when working with clients.

PATIENTS IN CARDIAC REHABILITATION AND MEDICAL FITNESS FACILITIES

Personal trainers working with clients with known CVD in clinical settings, such as cardiac rehabilitation and medical fitness facilities, should use a more in-depth screening tool than the ones presented in the previous sections (ACSM, 2018). Specifically, it is recommended they use the risk-stratification criteria from the American Association of Cardiovascular and Pulmonary Rehabilitation (AACVPR) (www.aacvpr.org/Portals/0/Registry/AACVPR%20Risk%20Stratification%20Algorithm_June2012.pdf).

> It is imperative that the client's personal physician be made aware of any signs or symptoms suggestive of **coronary artery disease** that may have been discovered as a result of the preparticipation health screening or during an ongoing exercise program.

Additional Forms

Once the preparticipation health-screening process has been completed, the need for outside referral has been determined (yes or no), and the client is cleared for exercise, an appropriate program can then be developed.

Beyond the initial PAR-Q+ or preparticipation health screening, there are several important forms that personal trainers should review, keep accessible, and utilize as needed with their clients. These forms include an agreement to participate (see Figure 16–1, page 753), an informed consent, or "assumption of risk," form (see Figure 16–2, pages 754–756), as well as the following:

Lifestyle and health-history questionnaire (Figure 5–4)

- This form collects more detailed medical and health information beyond the preparticipation health screening, including the following:
  - Past and present exercise and physical-activity information
  - Medications and supplements
  - Recent or current illnesses or injuries, including **chronic** or **acute** pain
  - Surgery and injury history
  - Family medical history
  - Lifestyle information (related to nutrition, stress, work, sleep, etc.)

Medical release (Figure 5-5)

- This form provides the personal trainer with the client's medical information and explains physical-activity limitations and/or guidelines as outlined by his or her physician. *Deviation from these guidelines must be approved by the client's personal physician.*

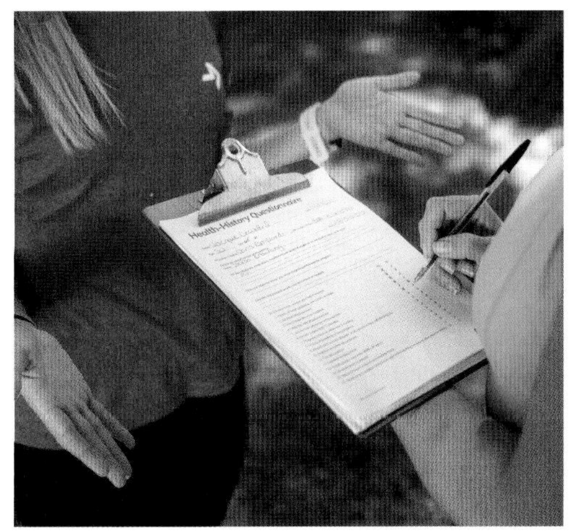

FIGURE 5-4
Sample lifestyle and health-history questionnaire

Name: ______________________ Date: ________ Date of birth: ________

Medical Information

1. How would you describe your present state of health?
   ☐ Very well ☐ Healthy ☐ Unhealthy ☐ Unwell ☐ Other: ______________
2. List current medications, how often you take them, and dosages (include prescriptions and over-the-counter medications). ______________________
3. Do you take all of your medications as they have been prescribed by your healthcare provider? ☐ Yes ☐ No
   If not, please share why (e.g., cost, side effects, or feeling as though they are unnecessary). ______________
4. Do you take any vitamin, mineral, or herbal supplements? ☐ Yes ☐ No
   If yes, list type and amount per day: ______________
5. When was the last time you visited your physician? ______________
6. Have you ever had your cholesterol checked? ☐ Yes ☐ No
   Date of test: ________ What were the results? ______________
   Total cholesterol: ______ High-density lipoprotein (HDL): ______ Low-density lipoprotein (LDL): ______
   Triglycerides: ______
7. Have you ever had your blood sugar checked? ☐ Yes ☐ No
   What were the results? ______
8. Please check any that apply to you and list any important information about your condition:

☐ Allergies (Specify: ________)
☐ Amenorrhea
☐ Anemia
☐ Anxiety
☐ Arthritis
☐ Asthma
☐ Celiac disease
☐ Chronic sinus condition
☐ Constipation
☐ Crohn's disease
☐ Depression
☐ Diabetes
☐ Diarrhea
☐ Disordered eating
☐ Gastroesophageal reflux disease (GERD)
☐ High blood pressure
☐ Hypoglycemia
☐ Hypo/hyperthyroidism
☐ Insomnia
☐ Intestinal problems
☐ Irritability
☐ Irritable bowel syndrome (IBS)
☐ Menopausal symptoms
☐ Osteoporosis
☐ Premenstrual syndrome (PMS)
☐ Polycystic ovary syndrome (PCOS)
☐ Pregnant
☐ Skin problems
☐ Ulcer
☐ Major surgeries: ______________
☐ Past injuries: ______________
☐ Describe any other health conditions that you have: ______________

FIGURE 5-4
(continued)

Family History

1. Has anyone in your immediate family been diagnosed with the following?

☐ Heart disease	If yes, what is the relation? ________	Age of diagnosis: ____
☐ High cholesterol	If yes, what is the relation? ________	Age of diagnosis: ____
☐ High blood pressure	If yes, what is the relation? ________	Age of diagnosis: ____
☐ Cancer	If yes, what is the relation? ________	Age of diagnosis: ____
☐ Diabetes	If yes, what is the relation? ________	Age of diagnosis: ____
☐ Osteoporosis	If yes, what is the relation? ________	Age of diagnosis: ____

Nutrition

1. What are your dietary goals? ____________________

2. Have you ever followed a modified diet? ☐ Yes ☐ No

   If yes, describe: ____________________

3. Are you currently following a specialized eating plan (e.g., low-sodium or low-fat)? ☐ Yes ☐ No

   If yes, what type of eating plan? ____________________

4. Why did you choose this eating plan? ____________________

   Was the eating plan prescribed by a physician? ☐ Yes ☐ No

   How long have you been on the eating plan? ________

5. Have you ever met with a registered dietitian or attended diabetes education classes? ☐ Yes ☐ No

   If no, are you interested in doing so? ☐ Yes ☐ No

6. What do you consider to be the major issues with your nutritional choices or eating plan (e.g., eating late at night, snacking on high-fat foods, skipping meals, or lack of variety)? ____________________

   ____

   ____

7. How many glasses of water do you drink per day? ____ 8-ounce glasses

8. What do you drink other than water? List what and how much per day. ____________________

9. Do you have any food allergies or intolerance? ☐ Yes ☐ No

   If yes, what? ____________________

10. Who shops for and prepares your food? ☐ Self ☐ Spouse ☐ Parent ☐ Minimal preparation

11. How often do you dine out? ____ times per week

12. Please specify the type of restaurants for each meal:

    Breakfast: ____________ Lunch: ____________

    Dinner: ____________ Snacks: ____________

Continued on the next page

FIGURE 5-4
(*continued*)

13. Do you crave any foods? ☐ Yes ☐ No

If yes, please specify: ____________________

Substance-related Habits

1. Do you drink alcohol? ☐ Yes ☐ No

If yes, how often? ________ times per week Average amount? ________

2. Do you drink caffeinated beverages? ☐ Yes ☐ No

If yes, average number per day: ____________

3. Do you use tobacco? ☐ Yes ☐ No

If yes, how much (cigarettes, cigars, or chewing tobacco per day)? ____________________

Physical Activity

1. Do you currently participate in any structured physical activity? ☐ Yes ☐ No

If so, please describe:

________ minutes of cardiorespiratory activity, ________ times per week

________ muscular-training sessions per week

________ flexibility-training sessions per week

________ minutes of sports or recreational activities per week

List sports or activities you participate in: ____________________

2. Do you engage in any other forms of regular physical activity? ☐ Yes ☐ No

If yes, describe: ____________________

3. Have you ever experienced any injuries that may limit your physical activity? ☐ Yes ☐ No

If yes, describe: ____________________

4. Do you have any physical-activity restrictions? If so, please list: ____________________

____

____

5. What are your honest feelings about exercise/physical activity? ____________________

____

____

6. What are some of your favorite physical activities? ____________________

____

____

FIGURE 5-4
(continued)

Occupational

1. Do you work? ☐ Yes ☐ No

   If yes, what is your occupation? ____________________

   If you work, what is your work schedule? ____________________

2. Describe your activity level during the work day: ____________________

Sleep and Stress

1. How many hours of sleep do you get at night? ________
2. Rate your average stress level from 1 (no stress) to 10 (constant stress) ________
3. What is most stressful to you? ____________________
4. How is your appetite affected by stress? ☐ Increased ☐ Not affected ☐ Decreased

Weight History

1. What is your present weight? ________ ☐ Don't know
2. What would you like to do with your weight? ☐ Lose weight ☐ Gain weight ☐ Maintain weight
3. What was your lowest weight within the past 5 years? ________
4. What was your highest weight within the past 5 years? ________
5. What do you consider to be your ideal weight (the sustainable weight at which you feel best)? ________ ☐ Don't know
6. What are your current waist and hip circumferences? ________ Waist ________ Hip ☐ Don't know
7. What is your current body composition? ________% body fat ☐ Don't know

Goals

1. On a scale of 1 to 10, how likely are you to adopt a healthier lifestyle (1 = very unlikely; 10 = very likely)? ________
2. Do you have any specific goals for improving your health? ☐ Yes ☐ No If yes, please list them in order of importance.

   ____

   ____

3. Do you have a weight-loss goal? ☐ Yes ☐ No

   If yes, what is it? ____________________

4. Why do you want to lose weight?

   ____

   ____

FIGURE 5-5
Sample medical release form

Date ____________

Dear Doctor:

Your patient, ________________________________, wishes to start a personalized training program. The activity will involve the following:

(type, frequency, duration, and intensity of activities)

If your patient is taking medications that will affect his or her exercise capacity or heart-rate response to exercise, please indicate the manner of the effect (raises or lowers exercise capacity or heart-rate response):

Type of medication(s) ____

Effect(s) ____

Please identify any recommendations or restrictions that are appropriate for your patient in this exercise program:

____

____

____

Thank you.
Sincerely,

Fred Fitness
Personalized Gym
Address
Phone

__________________________ has my approval to begin an exercise program with the recommendations or restrictions stated above.

Signed____Date__________

Phone___________________________________

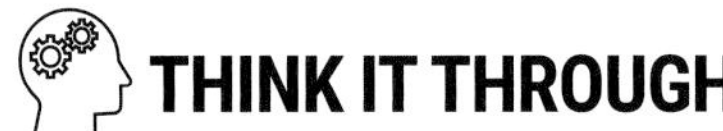

Application of Legal Forms

Training clients requires carefully gathering information about lifestyle, goals, physical-activity history, and health history, conditions, or concerns. After reviewing all of the sample forms presented in this chapter, decide which ones you will use and how you will adapt them to your own practice. Be sure to have all of the forms you plan to use in your practice reviewed by a legal professional in your area. Protecting your clients and yourself from the risks associated with exercise is a prudent and necessary part of doing business as a personal trainer.

Medications

Medication or substance (e.g., caffeine and nicotine) use is another important topic to review when discussing health history. These substances alter the biochemistry of the body and may affect a client's ability to perform or respond to exercise. The properties of these drugs must be understood by the personal trainer and discussed with the client. When designing and supervising an exercise program, it is important to realize that many substances, over-the-counter medications, and prescription drugs affect the heart's response to exercise. There are hundreds of thousands of different drugs on the market and each may be referred to by the manufacturer's brand name (e.g., Inderal) or by the scientific generic name (e.g., propranolol). Table 5-1 lists select medications and substances that may affect a person's response to exercise. To use the table, consult the client, the client's physician, or a medical reference to find the correct category for the medication. Then, refer to the general category under which each drug is grouped, such as **beta blockers, antihistamines,** or **bronchodilators.** The drugs in each group are thought to have a similar effect on most people, although individual responses will vary.

A particular response is usually dose dependent; the larger the dose, the greater the response. An important factor to consider in this dose-related response is the time when the medication is taken. As medications are metabolized, their effects diminish. If a personal trainer has any questions concerning a client's medications, it is essential that the personal trainer discuss them with the client and his or her physician.

If you or the client are concerned about the effects of a medication and its impact on exercise, a medical clearance form can be utilized to seek clarification and recommendations. The following are some of the most common categories of medications of which personal trainers should be aware.

ANTIHYPERTENSIVES

High blood pressure, or **hypertension,** is common in modern society, and there are many medications used for its treatment. Most antihypertensives primarily affect one of four different sites: the heart, to reduce its force of contraction; the peripheral blood vessels, to open or dilate them to allow more room for the blood; the brain, to reduce the sympathetic nerve outflow; or the kidneys, to reduce blood volume by excreting more fluid. The site that the medication acts on helps to determine its effect on the individual as well as any potential side effects. The following are common antihypertensives.

TABLE 5-1
Effects of Select Substances on Heart-rate Response

Medications	Resting HR	Exercise HR	Exercise Capacity	Comments
Beta blockers	↓	↓	↓ $\dot{V}O_2$max with acute and ↑ with chronic administration	Dose-related response
Angiotensin II receptor blockers (ARBs) and calcium channel blockers (CCBs)	↓ or ↔	↓ or ↔	↔	
Other antihypertensives*	↑, ↔, or ↓	↑, ↔, or ↓	Usually ↔	Many antihypertensive medications are used. Some may decrease, a few may increase, and others do not affect HR. Some exhibit variable and dose-related responses.
Antihistamines	↑	↔	↔ performance and endurance	
Antidepressants and antianxiety medications	↑ or ↔	↑ or ↔		
Stimulants	↑	↑	↑ or ↔ endurance and performance	
Caffeine	↑	↑ or ↔	↑ endurance	
Bronchodilators	↔	↔	↔ $\dot{V}O_2$max; ↑ or ↔ in individuals with COPD	
Alcohol	↔	↔	↓ performance and $\dot{V}O_2$max	Exercise prohibited while under the influence; effects of alcohol on coordination increase possibility of injuries
Nicotine-replacement therapy	↑	↑	↔ or ↓	
Nonsteroidal anti-inflammatory drugs (NSAIDs)			↔ or ↑ performance	

↑ = increase; ↔ = no significant change; ↓ = decrease; HR = Heart rate; $\dot{V}O_2$max = Maximal oxygen uptake; COPD = Chronic obstructive pulmonary disease

* Many antihypertensive medications can cause positional hypotension, meaning the blood pressure drops when changing positions (sitting to standing). Therefore, a client may become dizzy if he or she moves too fast after performing abdominal work on the floor.

Note: Many medications are prescribed for conditions that do not require clearance. Do not forget other indicators of exercise intensity (e.g., client's appearance or rating of perceived exertion).

This table in not intended to be an exhaustive list of all medications and their effects on heart rate. For more information on this topic, refer to American College of Sports Medicine (2018). *ACSM's Guidelines for Exercise Testing and Prescription* (10th ed.). Philadelphia: Wolters Kluwer.

Beta Blockers

Beta-adrenergic blocking agents, or beta blockers, are commonly prescribed for a variety of cardiovascular and other disorders. These medications block beta-adrenergic receptors and limit **sympathetic nervous system** stimulation. In other words, they block the effects of **catecholamines** (**epinephrine** and **norepinephrine**) throughout the body, and reduce resting, exercise, and maximal heart rates. This reduction in **heart rate (HR)** requires modifying the method used for determining exercise intensity. Using **rating of perceived exertion** or the **talk test** versus **target heart rate,** for example, would be appropriate for ensuring a safe and effective cardiorespiratory exercise intensity for someone on beta blockers.

Calcium Channel Blockers

Calcium channel blockers prevent calcium-dependent contraction of the smooth muscles in the arteries, causing them to dilate, which lowers **blood pressure (BP).** These agents also are used for angina and heart dysrhythmias (rapid or irregular HR). There are several types of calcium channel blockers on the market, and their effect on BP and HR depends on the specific agent. Notice in Table 5-1 that calcium channel blockers may increase, decrease, or have no effect on the HR. Therefore, while it is important to know the general effects of a category of medication, remember that individual responses can vary.

Angiotensin-converting Enzyme Inhibitors

Angiotensin-converting enzyme (ACE) inhibitors block an enzyme secreted by the kidneys, preventing the formation of a potent hormone (angiotensin II) that constricts blood vessels. If this enzyme is blocked, the vessels dilate and BP decreases. ACE inhibitors should not affect HR but will cause a decrease in BP at rest and during exercise.

Angiotensin II Receptor Antagonists

Angiotensin II receptor antagonists (or blockers) are a newer class of antihypertensive agents. These drugs are selective for angiotensin II (type 1 receptor). Angiotensin II receptor antagonists are well tolerated, and do not adversely affect blood lipid profiles or cause "rebound hypertension" after discontinuation.

Diuretics

Diuretics are medications that increase the excretion of water and **electrolytes** through the kidneys. They are usually prescribed for high BP, or when a person is accumulating too much fluid, as occurs with congestive heart failure. They have no primary effect on the HR, but they can cause water and electrolyte imbalances, which may lead to dangerous cardiac **arrhythmias.** Because diuretics can compromise hydration status and decrease blood volume, they may predispose an exerciser to **dehydration.** A client taking diuretics needs to maintain adequate fluid intake before, during, and after exercise, especially in a warm, humid environment. Diuretics are sometimes used by athletes to try to lose weight for sport. This is a dangerous practice that should not be condoned by a responsible personal trainer.

BRONCHODILATORS

Asthma medications, also known as bronchodilators, relax or open the air passages in the lungs, allowing better air exchange. There are many different types, but the primary action of each is to stimulate the sympathetic nervous system. Bronchodilators increase exercise capacity in persons limited by **bronchoconstriction** but otherwise have minimal effect on resting and exercise HRs and BPs.

COLD MEDICATIONS

Sympathomimetic drugs are compounds that mimic the activity of the sympathetic nervous system (e.g., increase BP and HR) and are often found in medications that treat allergic rhinitis, nasal congestion, and asthma (see above section). For example, decongestants act directly on the smooth muscles of the blood vessels to stimulate **vasoconstriction.** In the upper airways, this constriction reduces the volume of the swollen tissues and results in more air space. Vasoconstriction in the peripheral vessels may raise BP and increase HR both at rest and possibly during exercise.

Antihistamines block the histamine receptor, which is involved with the mast cells and the allergic response. These medications do not have a direct effect on the HR or BP, but they do produce a drying effect in the upper airways and may cause drowsiness.

Most cold medications are a combination of decongestants and antihistamines and may have combined effects. However, they are normally taken in low doses and have minimal effect on exercise capacity.

ACE UNIVERSITY

If your study program includes the ACE University, visit www.ACEfitness.org/MyACE and log in to your My ACE Account to take full advantage of the ACE Personal Trainer Study Program and online guided study experience.

A variety of media to support and expand on the material in this text is provided to facilitate learning and best prepare you for the ACE Personal Trainer Certification exam and a career as a personal trainer.

SUMMARY

Information gathered through a careful preparticipation health screening helps personal trainers design exercise programs that are personalized to meet the unique needs and goals of each client. As discussed in Chapters 3 and 4, effective communication and interviewing skills are helpful during the initial meetings with clients when private health information and feelings and experiences regarding physical activity and exercise are shared for the first time. The information obtained from the preparticipation health screening and additional forms reviewed in this chapter is essential for working with clients to help them safely achieve their health, physical-activity, and/or fitness goals.

REFERENCES

American College of Sports Medicine (2018). *ACSM's Guidelines for Exercise Testing and Prescription* (10th ed.). Philadelphia: Wolters Kluwer.

Chisholm, D.M. et al. (1975). Physical activity readiness. *British Columbia Medical Journal*, 17, 375–378.

Jamnik, V.K. et al. (2011). Enhancing the effectiveness of clearance for physical activity participation: Background and overall process. *Applied Physiology, Nutrition, and Metabolism*, 36, Suppl. 1, S3–S13.

Thomas, S., Reading, J., & Shephard, R.J. (1992). Revision of the Physical Activity Readiness Questionnaire (PAR-Q). *Canadian Journal of Sport Science*, 17, 4, 338–345.

U.S. Department of Health & Human Services (2018). *Physical Activity Guidelines for Americans* (2nd ed.). www.health.gov/paguidelines

Warburton, D.E.R. et al. (2011). Evidence-based risk assessment and recommendations for physical activity clearance; Consensus Document. *Applied Physiology, Nutrition, and Metabolism*, 36, 51, S266–S298.

SUGGESTED READINGS

American Council on Exercise (2019). *The Professional's Guide to Health and Wellness Coaching*. San Diego: American Council on Exercise.

Moore, G.E., Durstine, J.L., & Painter, P.L. (Eds). (2016). *ACSM's Exercise Management for Persons with Chronic Disease and Disabilities* (4th ed.). Champaign, Ill.: Human Kinetics.

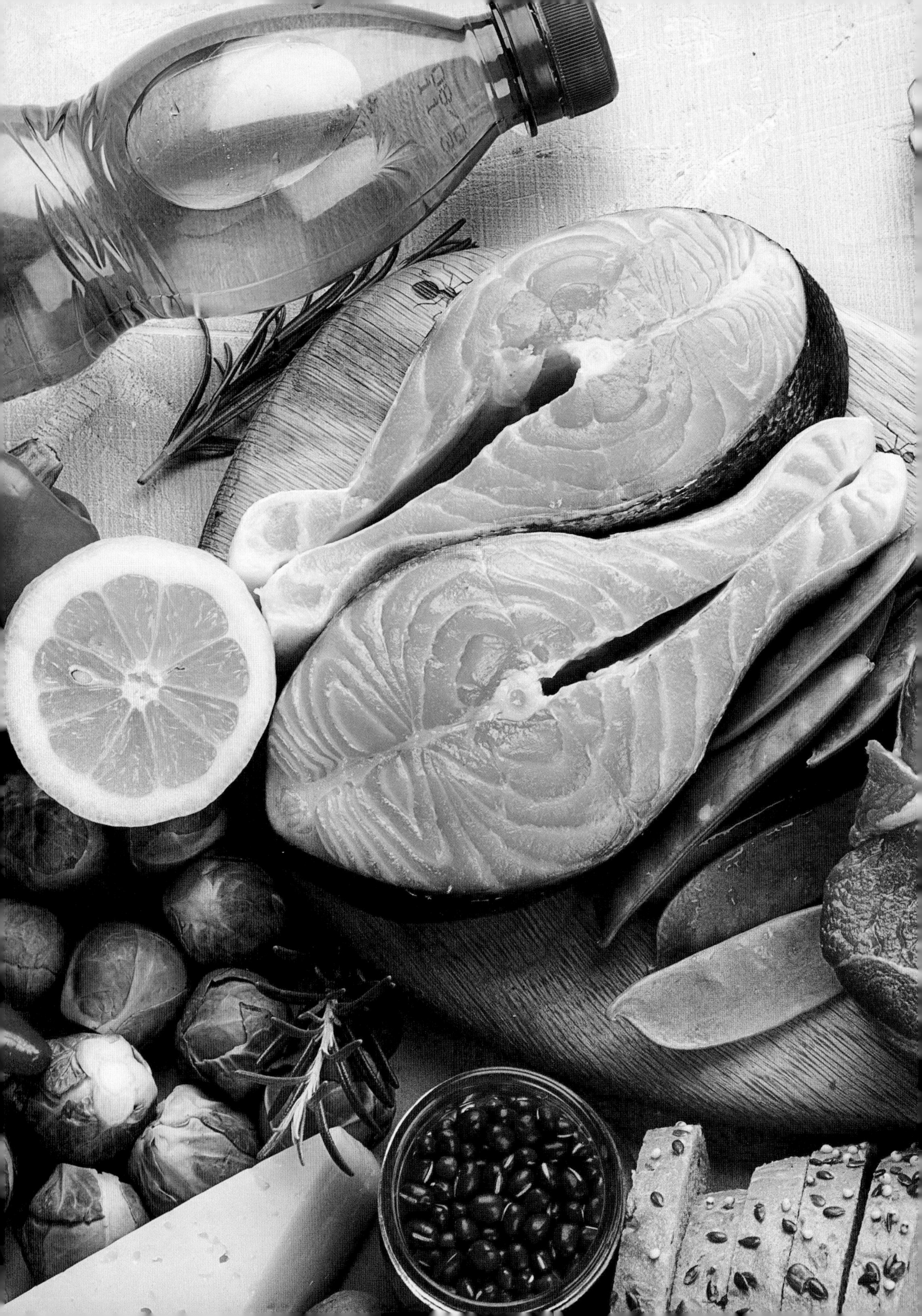

CHAPTER 6

Nutrition for Health and Fitness

NATALIE DIGATE MUTH, MD, MPH, RDN, FAAP, FACSM, CSSD
Board-certified Pediatrician and Obesity Medicine Physician; Registered Dietitian Nutritionist; W.E.L.L. Clinic Director, Children's Primary Care Medical Group; Adjunct Assistant Professor of Community Health Sciences, UCLA Fielding School of Public Health

IN THIS CHAPTER

LEARNING OBJECTIVES:

Upon completion of this chapter, the reader will be able to:

- Explain what is within a personal trainer's scope of practice as it relates to nutrition
- Discuss the current *Dietary Guidelines for Americans* and other evidence-based eating patterns
- Dissect a nutrition label to determine the total number of calories; calories from fat, protein, and carbohydrate; and overall nutritional value of a product
- Outline practical strategies within a personal trainer's scope of practice to improve client food literacy
- Explain proper fueling and hydration principles for before, during, and after exercise
- Discuss nutritional supplements with clients while staying within scope of practice

ACE UNIVERSITY

If your study program includes the ACE University, visit www.ACEfitness.org/MyACE and log in to your My ACE Account to take full advantage of the ACE Personal Trainer Study Program and online guided study experience.

A variety of media to support and expand on the material in this text is provided to facilitate learning and best prepare you for the ACE Personal Trainer Certification exam and a career as a personal trainer.

ACE® Certified Personal Trainers enjoy the rewarding opportunity to help clients not only improve their fitness but also adopt healthful nutrition habits. The federal government's *Dietary Guidelines for Americans* and MyPlate provide a foundation upon which personal trainers can help clients optimize their nutrition and overall health. In addition, use of these resources and tools provides an opportunity to incorporate nutrition into sessions with clients while staying within **scope of practice.**

ACE Position Statement on Nutrition Scope of Practice for Personal Trainers

It is the position of the American Council on Exercise (ACE) that personal trainers not only can but should share general nonmedical nutrition information with their clients.

In the current climate of an epidemic of **obesity,** poor nutrition, and physical inactivity, paired with a multibillion-dollar diet industry and a strong interest among the general public in improving eating habits and increasing physical activity, personal trainers are well positioned to partner with clients in the journey to live healthier lifestyles. Personal trainers provide an essential service to their clients, the industry, and the community at large when they are able to offer credible, practical, and relevant nutrition information to clients while staying within their professional scope of practice.

Ultimately, an individual personal trainer's scope of practice as it relates to nutrition is determined by state policies and regulations, education and experience, and competencies and skills. While this implies that the nutrition-related scope of practice may vary among personal trainers, there are certain actions that are within the scope of practice of all personal trainers.

For example, it is within the scope of practice of all personal trainers to share evidence-based dietary guidelines and resources, such as those endorsed or developed by the federal government, especially the *Dietary Guidelines for Americans* (www.health.gov/dietaryguidelines) and the MyPlate recommendations (www.ChooseMyPlate.gov). Personal trainers who have earned a certification accredited by the National Commission for Certifying Agencies (NCCA) that provides basic nutrition information, such as those provided by ACE, and those who have undertaken nutrition continuing education, should also be prepared to discuss:

- Principles of healthy nutrition and food preparation
- Food to be included in the balanced daily diet
- Essential **nutrients** needed by the body
- Actions of nutrients on the body
- Effects of deficiencies or excesses of nutrients
- How nutrient requirements vary through the lifecycle
- Principles of pre- and post-workout nutrition and hydration
- Information about nutrients contained in foods or supplements

Personal trainers who do not feel comfortable sharing this information are strongly encouraged to complete continuing education to further develop nutrition competency and skills and to develop relationships with **registered dietitians (RDs)** or other qualified health professionals who can provide this information as requested by clients. Working with health coaches—or even becoming an ACE Certified Health Coach—may be particularly fruitful, as health coaches can provide much-needed support and guidance around the behavioral aspects of making and sustaining dietary changes. It is within the personal trainer's scope of practice to distribute and disseminate information or programs that have been developed by an RD or medical doctor. Note that some RDs may elect to use the newer title of registered dietitian nutritionist (RDN) and that there is no difference between the two credentials.

The actions that are outside the scope of practice of personal trainers include, but may not be limited to, the following:

- Personalized nutrition recommendations or meal planning other than that which is available through government guidelines and recommendations, or has been developed and endorsed by an RD or physician
- Nutritional assessment to determine nutritional needs and nutritional status, and to recommend nutritional intake
- Specific recommendations or programming for nutrient or nutritional intake, caloric intake, or specialty diets
- Nutritional counseling, education, or advice aimed to prevent, treat, or cure a disease or condition, or other acts that may be perceived as **medical nutrition therapy**
- Development, administration, evaluation, and consultation regarding nutritional care standards or the nutrition care process
- Recommending, prescribing, selling, or supplying nutritional supplements to clients
- Promotion or identification of oneself as a "nutritionist" or "dietitian"

Engaging in these activities can place a client's health and safety at risk and possibly expose the personal trainer to disciplinary action and litigation. To ensure maximal client safety and compliance with state policies and laws, it is essential that the personal trainer recognize when it is appropriate to refer to an RD or physician. ACE recognizes that some fitness and health clubs encourage or require their employees to sell nutritional supplements. If this is a condition of employment, ACE suggests that personal trainers:

- Obtain complete scientific understanding regarding the safety and efficacy of the supplement from qualified healthcare professionals and/or credible resources. Note: Generally, the Office of Dietary Supplements (www.ods.od.nih.gov), the National Center for Complementary and Alternative Medicine (www.nccam.nih.gov), and the Food and Drug Administration (www.FDA.gov) are reliable places to go to examine the validity of the claims as well as risks and benefits associated with taking a particular supplement. Since the sites are from trusted resources and in the public domain, personal trainers can freely distribute and share the information contained on these sites.
- Stay up-to-date on the legal and/or regulatory issues related to the use of the supplement and its individual ingredients
- Obtain adequate insurance coverage should a problem arise

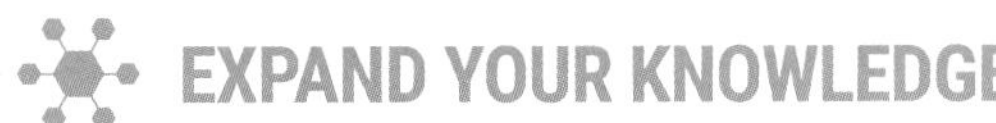

Deepening Skills in Facilitating Behavior Change

The Academy of Nutrition and Dietetics notes that the most effective strategies for facilitating health- and nutrition-related behavior change include **cognitive behavioral therapy, motivational interviewing,** self-monitoring, financial rewards, goal setting, problem solving, and social support (Spahn et al., 2010). Many of these client-centered skills are in the toolbox of ACE Certified Personal Trainers and are presented in previous chapters of this textbook. However, exercise professionals who wish to further position themselves as trusted partners for clients seeking sustainable health behavior changes are encouraged to explore continued learning opportunities to further develop applied coaching knowledge and skills.

In addition to attending quality continuing education workshops, conferences, and webinars, personal trainers may consider earning a specialty certification, such as becoming an ACE Behavior Change Specialist (www.acefitness.org/fitness-certifications/specialty-certifications/behavior-change.aspx). This specialized program teaches elevated communication skills and key tools to facilitate behavior change and support clients in creating a foundation for a healthy lifestyle. Additionally, personal trainers may consider earning an additional certification, such as becoming an ACE Certified Health Coach (www.ACEfitness.org/fitness-certifications/health-coach-certification), in order to provide additional support and services to further optimize clients' health and well-being. This certification program equips professionals with evidence-based behavior-change principles and practical skills along with an in-depth understanding of the impact of lifestyle behaviors (e.g., sleep, stress, exercise, nutrition, and substance use) on the prevention and management of **chronic diseases** in order to empower clients to enact meaningful and lasting lifestyle changes.

Inherently, personal trainers work with clients with varying levels of nutritional knowledge, informed and influenced by numerous sources, such as popular media, education, family members, culture, other health and exercise professionals, and their own lived experiences. As such, in addition to deepening their own knowledge and skills, it is imperative that personal trainers seek opportunities to work collaboratively with other qualified professionals, such as RDs (see page 195) and certified health coaches in order to most optimally support each unique client in his or her personal behavior-change journey.

Dietary Reference Intakes and Acceptable Macronutrient Distribution Ranges

In determining the types and amounts of foods to recommend, the *Dietary Guidelines* rely heavily on the latest scientific evidence as well as established reference intakes for specific nutrients for individuals across age and sex. In fact, much of the information contained within the 2015-2020 *Dietary Guidelines for Americans* (8th ed.) [U.S. Department of Agriculture (USDA), 2015] is based upon **Dietary Reference Intakes (DRIs)** published by the National Academy of Medicine, formerly the Institute of Medicine (IOM, 2006). DRI is a generic term used to refer to four types of reference values:

- **Recommended Dietary Allowance (RDA)**: The RDA represents the level of intake of a nutrient that is adequate to meet the known needs of practically all healthy persons. If the level is at or above the RDA, then the client almost certainly consumes a sufficient amount (since the RDA covers 97 to 98% of the population).

- **Estimated Average Requirement (EAR)**: The EAR is the adequate intake in 50% of an age- and sex-specific group. If a person's intake falls well below the EAR, it is likely that person does not consume enough of the nutrient. If the level is between the EAR and the RDA, then it is likely the client consumes enough of the nutrient (50%+ likelihood).
- **Tolerable Upper Intake Level (UL)**: This is the maximal intake that is unlikely to pose a risk of adverse health effects to almost all individuals in an age- and sex-specific group. Comparing a person's usual intake of a nutrient to the UL helps to determine whether he or she is at risk of nutrient toxicity. The UL is set so that even the most sensitive people should not have an adverse response to a nutrient at intake levels near the UL. Thus, many people who have intakes above the UL may never experience a nutrient toxicity, though it is difficult to assess which clients may be most and least at risk for a nutrient overdose.
- **Adequate Intake (AI)**: The AI is a recommended nutrient intake level that, based on research, appears to be sufficient for good health. If the nutrient in question has not been adequately studied and too little information is available to determine an EAR (a level good enough for 50% of the population), then it is also not possible to determine an RDA (a level good enough for 97 to 98% of the population). In these cases, the AI is published. If a client's intake is at or exceeds the AI, then it is very likely that he or she consumes enough of the nutrient to prevent deficiency. If intake is below the AI, then it is possible (but not certain) that the client is deficient in that nutrient.

DRIs for specific nutrients are available at www.nationalacademies.org. In addition, personal trainers may access the DRI interactive calculator available at http://fnic.nal.usda.gov/fnic/interactiveDRI/ to determine recommended nutrient needs based on sex, age, height, weight, and activity level.

In addition to the DRIs, the IOM has established a range, known as the **Acceptable Macronutrient Distribution Range (AMDR),** for the percentage of **calories** that should come from **carbohydrates, protein,** and **fat** for both optimal health and reduction of chronic disease risk. While many weight-loss diets purport success based on variations from these recommendations, strong evidence supports that it is not the relative proportion of **macronutrients** that determines long-term weight-loss success, but rather calorie content and whether a person can maintain the intake over time.

Select daily nutritional goals by sex and age for the macronutrients are shown in Table 6-1.

The *Dietary Guidelines* and The National Academies of Sciences, Engineering, and Medicine offer a number of tables that are excellent resources for personal trainers. Be sure to visit www.health.gov/dietaryguidelines and http://nationalacademies.org/hmd/~/media/Files/Report%20Files/2019/DRI-Tables-2019/6_DRIValues_Summary.pdf?la=en and familiarize yourself with the many valuable tools you can share with clients. While it is not necessary to commit each table to memory, it is beneficial to make general observations and consider how you would apply the content in real-world settings.

TABLE 6-1

Daily Nutritional Goals for Age-Sex Groups Based on Dietary Reference Intakes and Dietary Guidelines Recommendations*

	Source of Goal[A]	Female 14–18	Male 14–18	Female 19–30	Male 19–30	Female 31–50	Male 31–50	Female 51+	Male 51+
Calorie level(s) assessed		1,800	2,200, 2,800, 3,200	2,000	2,400, 2,600, 3,000	1,800	2,200	1,600	2,000
Macronutrients									
Protein, g	RDA	46	52	46	56	46	56	46	56
Protein, % kcal	AMDR	10–30	10–30	10–35	10–35	10–35	10–35	10–35	10–35
Carbohydrate, g	RDA	130	130	130	130	130	130	130	130
Carbohydrate, % kcal	AMDR	45–65	45–65	45–65	45–65	45–65	45–65	45–65	45–65
Dietary fiber, g	14g/1,000 kcal	25.2	30.8	28.0	33.6	25.2	30.8	22.4	28.0
Added sugars, % kcal	DGA	<10%	<10%	<10%	<10%	<10%	<10%	<10%	<10%
Total fat, % kcal	AMDR	25–35	25–35	20–35	20–35	20–35	20–35	20–35	20–35
Saturated fat, % kcal	DGA	<10%	<10%	<10%	<10%	<10%	<10%	<10%	<10%
Linoleic acid, g	AI	11	16	12	17	12	17	11	14
Linolenic acid, g	AI	1.1	1.6	1.1	1.6	1.1	1.6	1.1	1.6

* Refer to http://health.gov/dietaryguidelines/2015/guidelines/appendix-7/ for information about the needs for children and adolescents.

[A] RDA = Recommended Dietary Allowance; AMDR = Acceptable Macronutrient Distribution Range; DGA = 2015-2020 *Dietary Guidelines* recommended limit; 14 g fiber per 1,000 kcal = basis for AI for fiber; AI = Adequate Intake

Reprinted from United States Department of Agriculture (2015). 2015-2020 *Dietary Guidelines for Americans* (8th ed.). www.health.gov/dietaryguidelines

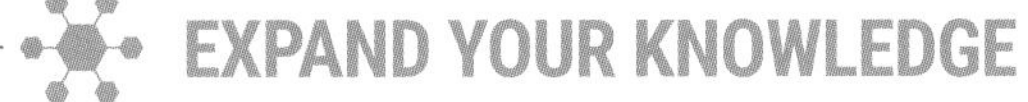

Finding Credible Sources of Nutrition Information

While the *Dietary Guidelines for Americans* and MyPlate form the foundation of both this chapter and the ACE Certified Personal Trainer's scope of practice as it relates to nutrition, these are not the only credible resources. As noted in the following section, the *Dietary Guidelines* are sometimes influenced by political pressure and are therefore criticized for being potentially biased. To broaden their understanding of dietary recommendations, personal trainers may want to familiarize themselves with other credible resources, including the following:

- Academy of Nutrition and Dietetics (www.eatright.org)
- Canada's Dietary Guidelines for Health Professionals and Policy Makers (https://food-guide.canada.ca/en/guidelines/)
- Harvard University's Healthy Eating Plate (www.hsph.harvard.edu/nutritionsource/healthy-eating-plate/)

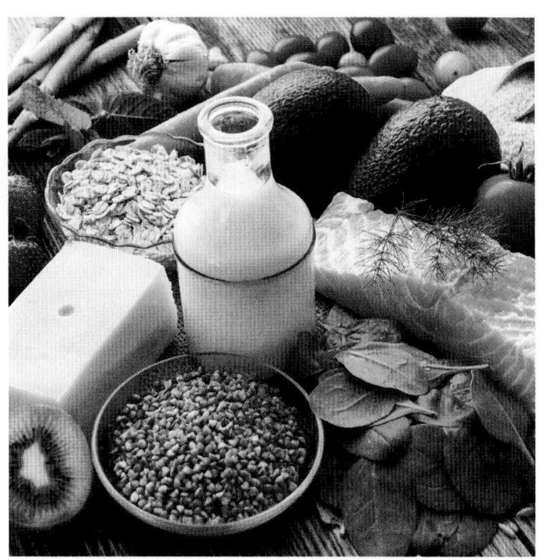

Dietary Guidelines

Every five years, a panel of nutrition experts from a variety of fields, such as dietetics, medicine, and public health, update the *Dietary Guidelines* through a rigorous process, including a review of the nutrition-related scientific literature and a series of meetings over several years. This committee of experts develops a report that is made available to the public and federal agencies for comment (the scientific report of the 2015 Dietary Guidelines Advisory Committee is available at https://health.gov/dietaryguidelines/2015-scientific-report/). Ultimately, the report is reviewed and edited before it is approved by Congress and becomes the federal government's official nutrition advice for Americans. Once published, the document is intended to be used by health professionals and government officials to develop educational materials and design and implement nutrition-related programs. It is within the scope of practice of the personal trainer to use and disseminate the information contained within the *Dietary Guidelines*, as well as its associated tools and resources.

Though the development of the *Dietary Guidelines* is influenced by political pressures, efforts are made to ultimately publish scientifically supported evidence for optimal nutrition for the generally healthy population. As such, the *Dietary Guidelines* generally reflect the best evidence on how to eat for optimal health for Americans aged two and older, including those at increased risk of chronic disease.

The 2015-2020 *Dietary Guidelines for Americans* offer five big-picture recommendations that are key to good nutrition. An overview of these five key recommendations, how they pertain to personal trainers, and how this information can best be used to support clients in achieving their nutrition goals are provided here. In addition, readers are referred to www.health.gov/dietaryguidelines for a full review of the report.

KEY GUIDELINE 1: FOLLOW A HEALTHY EATING PATTERN ACROSS THE LIFESPAN

All food and beverage choices matter. Choose a healthy eating pattern at an appropriate calorie level to help achieve and maintain a healthy body weight, support nutrient adequacy, and reduce the risk of chronic disease.

The 2015-2020 *Dietary Guidelines for Americans* make a point to emphasize overall eating patterns more so than individual nutrients, recognizing that the overall nutritional value of a person's diet is more than "the sum of its parts." The main components of a healthy eating pattern include:

- A variety of vegetables from five subgroups—dark green, red and orange, legumes (beans and peas), starchy, and other

- Fruit
- Grains, primarily whole grains
- Fat-free or low-fat dairy, including milk, yogurt, cheese, and/or fortified soy products
- A variety of foods rich in protein, including seafood, lean meats and poultry, eggs, legumes (beans and peas), nuts, seeds, and soy products
- Limited amounts of **saturated fats** (less than 10% of calories), **trans fat** (as low as possible), added sugars (less than 10% of calories), and sodium (less than 2,300 mg per day). If alcohol is consumed, it should be consumed in moderation, defined as up to one drink per day for women and two drinks per day for men. One drink is equivalent to 12 ounces of beer, 5 ounces of wine, or 1.5 ounces of hard liquor.

The three types of healthy eating patterns discussed at most length in the *Dietary Guidelines* are the **Healthy U.S.-Style Eating Pattern,** the **Healthy Mediterranean-Style Eating Pattern,** and the **Healthy Vegetarian Eating Pattern.**

The Healthy U.S.-Style Eating Pattern is based on the types and proportions of foods Americans typically consume, but in nutrient-dense forms and appropriate amounts. It is designed to meet nutrient needs while not exceeding calorie requirements and while staying within limits for overconsumed dietary components.

The Healthy Mediterranean-Style Eating Pattern is adapted from the Healthy U.S.-Style Eating Pattern, modifying amounts recommended from some food groups to more closely reflect eating patterns that have been associated with positive health outcomes in studies of Mediterranean-style diets. The Healthy Mediterranean-Style Eating Pattern contains more fruits and seafood and less dairy, meats, and poultry than does the Healthy U.S.-Style Eating Pattern. The pattern is similar to the Healthy U.S.-Style Eating Pattern in nutrient content, with the exception of providing less calcium and vitamin D.

The Healthy Vegetarian Eating Pattern is adapted from the Healthy U.S.-Style Pattern, modifying amounts recommended from some food groups to more closely reflect eating patterns reported by self-identified **vegetarians** in the National Health and Nutrition Examination Survey (NHANES). Based on a comparison of the food choices of these vegetarians to nonvegetarians in NHANES, amounts of soy products (particularly tofu and other processed soy products), legumes, nuts and seeds, and whole grains were increased, and meat, poultry, and seafood were eliminated (USDA, 2015). Dairy and eggs were included because they were consumed by the majority of these vegetarians. This pattern can be **vegan** if all dairy choices are comprised of fortified soy beverages (soy milk) or other plant-based dairy substitutes. This pattern is similar in meeting nutrient standards to the Healthy U.S.-Style Eating Pattern, but somewhat higher in calcium and **fiber** and lower in vitamin D.

Each of these patterns provides notable health benefits and can be consumed at varying calorie levels based on individual needs. They can also be adapted to meet cultural and personal preferences. In fact, moderate to strong evidence shows that these healthy eating patterns are associated with reduced risk of chronic diseases such as **cardiovascular disease, type 2 diabetes,** obesity, and some cancers (USDA, 2015). In all, the most important components of a healthy eating pattern include high intakes of vegetables and fruits and low intakes of processed meats and poultry, sugar-sweetened beverages (e.g., soda), and refined grains (e.g., processed "junk food" like chips).

MyPlate and MyPlate Daily Food Plan Checklists

While the *Dietary Guidelines* describe these three types of eating patterns, many of the most robust tools available from the federal government to help translate recommendations into action are based on the Healthy U.S.-Style Eating Pattern. For example, the MyPlate recommendations aim to translate the *Dietary Guidelines* into a simple image that people can use to guide nutrition choices. MyPlate simplifies the government's nutrition messages into an easily understood and implemented graphic—a dinner plate divided into four sections: fruits, vegetables, protein, and grains, accompanied by a glass of nonfat milk (to represent calcium-rich foods) (Figure 6-1). The goal is to influence Americans to eat a more balanced diet by encouraging people to make half their plate vegetables and fruits. Free downloadable educational materials to share with clients are available on the MyPlate website (www.ChooseMyPlate.gov).

FIGURE 6-1
MyPlate graphic

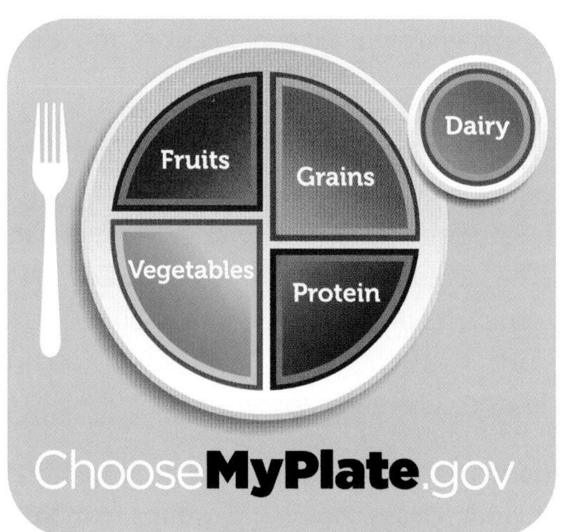

The MyPlate Daily Food Plan Checklists offer a good place to start when working with clients to identify daily calorie and nutrient needs. At www.ChooseMyPlate.gov/MyPlatePlan, consumers can input their age, sex, height, weight, and physical-activity level to get a personalized eating plan to meet calorie needs. Users are categorized into one of 12 different energy levels (from 1,000 to 3,200 calories per day) and are given the recommended number of **servings** to eat from each of the five food groups.

NIH Body Weight Planner

The goal of a dietary intervention to decrease weight is to create a caloric deficit so that fewer calories are consumed than are expended. With about 3,500 calories in a pound of fat, a 500- to 1,000-calorie deficit each day through decreased food intake and increased physical activity leads to about a 1- to 2-pound (0.45 to 0.9 kg) weight loss per week, at least at first. While predicting weight loss based on the equation of 3,500 calories per pound is useful early on in weight loss, as an individual loses weight, metabolism (and thus energy expenditure) changes and the equation becomes less accurate and overpredicts weight loss. While these calculations can help empower clients to take action, it is important to remember that weight management involves a complex interplay among environmental, behavioral, genetic, and hormonal factors (see Chapter 12).

The NIH Body Weight Planner (https://www.niddk.nih.gov/bwp), a tool initially developed and validated by researchers at the Massachusetts Institute of Technology in partnership with the National Institutes of Health, more accurately accounts for these metabolic changes. It approximates that for every 10-calorie decrease in daily caloric intake, the average adult with **overweight** will lose about 1 pound (0.45 kg). Half of the weight will be lost by one year and 95% of the weight change will occur by three years (Hall et al., 2011). For example, a woman who decreases her daily caloric consumption from 2,200 calories to 2,000 calories would lose about 20 pounds (9.1 kg), with the first 10 pounds (4.5 kg) lost within one year of the lowered caloric intake, and about 10 more pounds (4.5 kg) lost by the end of three years, assuming she maintains the reduction in caloric intake. If she had created a 500-kcal deficit each day, she would lose 25 pounds (11.4 kg) in the first year and about 25 more pounds (11.4 kg) by the end of three years.

Simply enter a client's age, sex, weight, height, current physical-activity level, goal weight, planned activity level, and goal time frame and the NIH Body Weight Planner determines the caloric needs to maintain the current weight, reach a goal weight in a specified amount of time, and sustain the new body weight based on planned physical-activity levels.

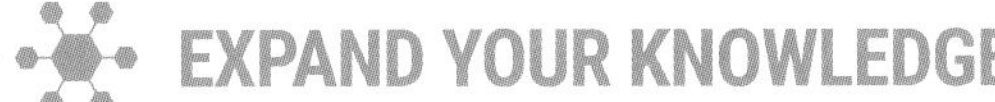

What Is More Important for Weight Loss: Exercise or Nutrition?

Many people wonder which is more effective for achieving weight-loss goals, increasing caloric expenditure through exercise or decreasing caloric intake through diet modification. Ultimately, both approaches can lead to weight loss and the most effective method is the one to which clients will adhere. Often, clients begin a weight-loss journey by decreasing caloric intake because the required behavior changes are perceived to be more doable than increasing physical activity. Others find increasing caloric expenditure to be the best starting point. When looking at the various components of a weight-loss program, both calorie reduction and physical activity play vital roles and the combination of these factors can lead to energy expenditure exceeding energy intake. Also, the combined effects of exercise and decreased caloric intake can lead to achieving weight-loss goals in a shorter period of time (Fayh et al., 2013). A randomized clinical trial compared the effects of achieving a 5% reduction in weight through diet or diet plus exercise on cardiovascular parameters of individuals with obesity. Interestingly, during this study, both groups reached the weight-loss goal, showing that making only dietary changes may lead to weight loss. However, the diet plus exercise group achieved a 5% reduction of weight in an average of 66 days compared to 80 days for the dietary intervention–only group, suggesting that that the combination of diet and exercise is more efficient for reaching weight-loss goals (Fayh et al., 2013).

Also, the *2018 Physical Activity Guidelines for Americans* suggest that exercise is essential when making a lifestyle change because it increases the caloric deficit to speed weight loss and is crucial for maintaining weight loss (U.S. Department of Health & Human Services, 2018). Importantly, regular physical activity provides health benefits regardless of how body weight changes over time and helps to reduce **abdominal fat** (or **visceral fat**) and preserve muscle mass during weight-loss efforts.

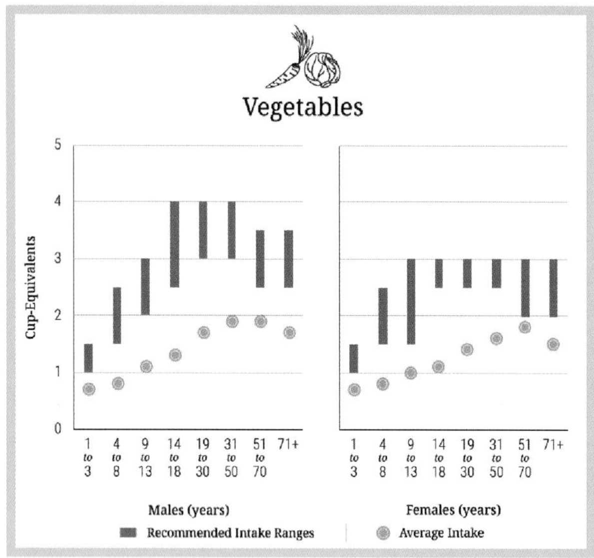

FIGURE 6-2
Vegetables

Reprinted from United States Department of Agriculture (2015). *2015-2020 Dietary Guidelines for Americans* (8th ed.). www.health.gov/dietaryguidelines

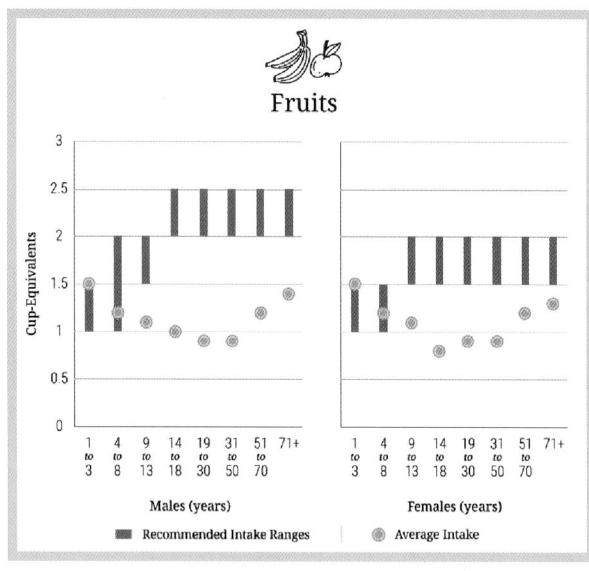

FIGURE 6-3
Fruits

Reprinted from United States Department of Agriculture (2015). *2015-2020 Dietary Guidelines for Americans* (8th ed.).www.health.gov/dietaryguidelines

KEY GUIDELINE 2: FOCUS ON VARIETY, NUTRIENT DENSITY, AND AMOUNT

To meet nutrient needs within calorie limits, choose a variety of nutrient-dense foods across and within all food groups in recommended amounts.

The *Dietary Guidelines* suggest that Americans are most likely to meet nutrient needs and manage weight by choosing nutrient-dense foods, which provide high levels of vitamins, minerals, and other nutrients that may have health benefits relative to caloric content. Categories of nutrient-dense foods include vegetables, fruits, grains, dairy, protein foods, and oils.

Vegetables

Vegetables are an important contributor to a healthy eating pattern. Vegetables are classified into five subgroups—dark green, red and orange, legumes (beans and peas), starchy, and other. While all subgroups are high in nutrients overall, some groups contain higher amounts of certain nutrients. For example, dark green vegetables are highest in vitamin K, while red and orange vegetables are high in vitamin A, legumes contain the most fiber, and starchy vegetables are highest in potassium. The *Dietary Guidelines* advise Americans to eat vegetables from all of the subgroups. Current vegetable intake compared to recommended intake is shown in Figure 6-2.

Fruits

Whole fruits, including fresh, frozen, canned, and dried forms, provide key nutrients, including dietary fiber, potassium, and vitamin C. Note that dried and canned fruits and fruit juices "count" as fruits, but are more calorie-dense than fresh and frozen fruits and thus should be consumed with attention to **portion** sizes. The *Dietary Guidelines* advise that no more than half of fruit should come from fruit juice and that juice that is less than 100% fruit is considered to be a "sugary drink" (and should be avoided, although the *Guidelines* come short of saying that directly, and instead note that added sugars can be accommodated as long as they do not exceed 10% of total calorie intake per day, while staying within calorie recommendations). Current fruit intake compared to recommended intake is shown in Figure 6-3.

Grains

Grains include foods such as rice, oatmeal, and popcorn, as well as products that contain grains like bread, cereals, crackers, and pasta. Grains can either be refined or whole. Refined grains are heavily processed and provide limited nutritional value (essentially, through processing, all of the nutrients are removed and then four B vitamins and iron are added back, thus creating "enriched grains"). Whole grains contain the entire grain kernel and provide health and nutritional value, including fiber, iron, zinc, manganese, folate, magnesium, copper, **thiamin, niacin,** vitamin B6, phosphorus, selenium, **riboflavin,** and vitamin A. Whole grains include foods such as brown rice, quinoa, and oats. The majority of grain consumption should come from whole grains. When choosing foods, it is easiest to identify whole-grain products by looking at the ingredient list on the nutrition label. "Whole grain" should be the first ingredient, or the second after water. Whole grains contain 16 grams of whole grain per 1 ounce-equivalent. Foods that are partly whole grain also can contribute to grain needs and should contain at least 8 grams of whole grain per 1 ounce-equivalent. Examples of "1 ounce-equivalent" include a slice of bread, half a cup of pasta or rice, 1 cup of cereal, or one tortilla. Current grain intake compared to recommended intake is shown in Figure 6-4.

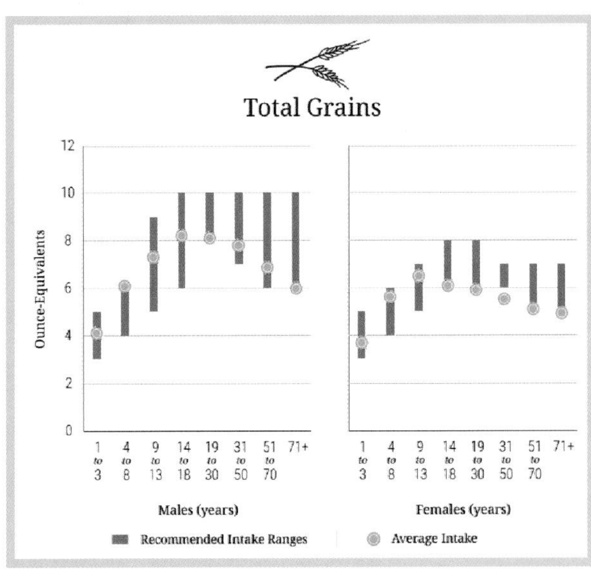

FIGURE 6-4
Grains

Reprinted from United States Department of Agriculture (2015). *2015-2020 Dietary Guidelines for Americans* (8th ed.). **www.health.gov/dietaryguidelines**

Dairy

The dairy group includes milk, yogurt, cheese, and fortified soy beverages. Dairy products are high in calcium, phosphorus, vitamin A, vitamin D (usually through fortification), riboflavin, vitamin B12, protein, potassium, zinc, choline, magnesium, and selenium. The *Dietary Guidelines* do not consider plant "milk," such as coconut, almond, rice, and hemp, as dairy because their overall nutritional value is not similar to dairy and soy milk, though they do contain calcium.

The *Dietary Guidelines'* emphasis on milk products also has been a source of debate and controversy. While milk products are not necessary to meet nutrient needs, they do contain many nutrients, including calcium, vitamin D, and potassium—all nutrients consumed in inadequate amounts by much of the population. Moderate evidence suggests that milk intake improves bone health in children and adolescents and contributes to decreased risk of cardiovascular disease, type 2 diabetes, and **hypertension** in adults (USDA, 2015). The *Dietary Guidelines* suggest that adults should aim for 3 cups per day of milk, children older than three should consume 2.5 cups, and children ages two to three should consume 2 cups. However, the *Dietary Guidelines* also acknowledge that the Healthy Mediterranean-Style Eating Plan, which is low in dairy products, is comparable in nutritional value to the Healthy U.S.-Style Eating Plan. The current dairy intake compared to recommended intake in the Healthy U.S.-Style Eating Pattern is shown in Figure 6-5.

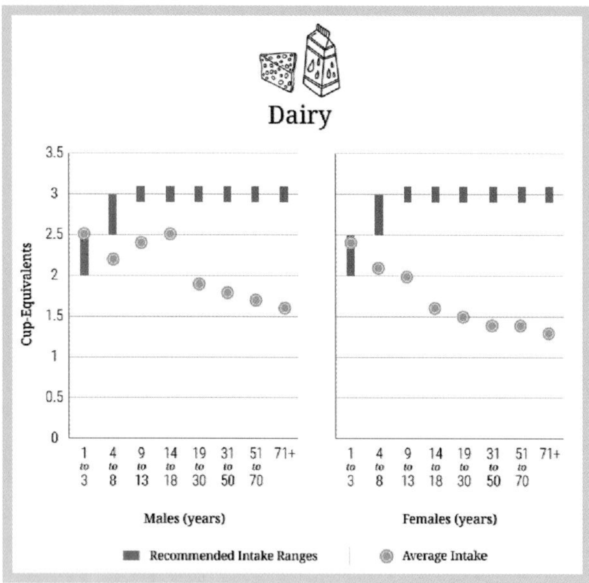

FIGURE 6-5
Dairy

Reprinted from United States Department of Agriculture (2015). *2015-2020 Dietary Guidelines for Americans* (8th ed.). www.health.gov/dietaryguidelines

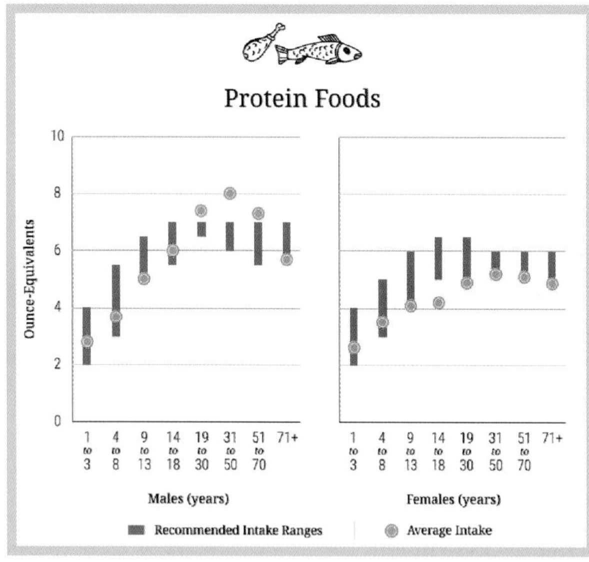

FIGURE 6-6
Protein foods

Reprinted from United States Department of Agriculture (2015). *2015-2020 Dietary Guidelines for Americans* (8th ed.). www.health.gov/dietaryguidelines

Protein Foods

Protein foods include a diversity of foods from plant and animal sources, including the following subgroups: seafood; meats, poultry, and eggs; and nuts, seeds, and soy products. Legumes and peas also are considered protein foods in addition to being included in the vegetables group. Additionally, many dairy products are high in protein. Protein foods are high in nutrients, such as niacin, vitamin B12, vitamin B6, riboflavin, selenium, choline, phosphorus, zinc, copper, vitamin D, and vitamin E. Some subgroups contain higher levels of specific nutrients than others. For example, meat provides the most zinc; poultry the most niacin; seafood the most vitamin B12, vitamin D, and **omega-3 fatty acids**; eggs the most choline; seeds the most vitamin E; and meat, poultry, and seafood the most heme iron, which is better absorbed than plant sources of iron. Current protein intake compared to recommended intake is shown in Figure 6-6.

Due to the increasing evidence supporting the health benefits of seafood, the *Dietary Guidelines* recommend that adults consume 8 or more ounces of seafood per week [equivalent to about 250 mg per day of the omega-3 fatty acids eicosapentaenoic acid (EPA) and docosahexaenoic acid (DHA)], comprising about 20% of total recommended protein intake. The *Dietary Guidelines* state that the benefit of consuming high levels of omega-3 fatty acids contained in seafood outweighs the risks of increased mercury intake, though individuals should aim to consume a mix of different types of seafood to decrease mercury exposure. The benefits and recommended intake also hold true for pregnant and breastfeeding women. Pregnant women, however, should be especially cautious to choose seafood that is low in mercury and avoid tilefish, shark, swordfish, and king mackerel.

Oils

Oils are fats that contain a high percentage of **monounsaturated fats** and **polyunsaturated fats** and are liquid at room temperature. Oils are not a food group; however, the *Dietary Guidelines* recognize them as an important part of a healthy eating pattern because they contain essential **fatty acids** and vitamin E. Commonly consumed plant oils include canola, corn, olive, peanut, safflower, soybean, and sunflower oils. Oils are naturally

FIGURE 6-7
Oils

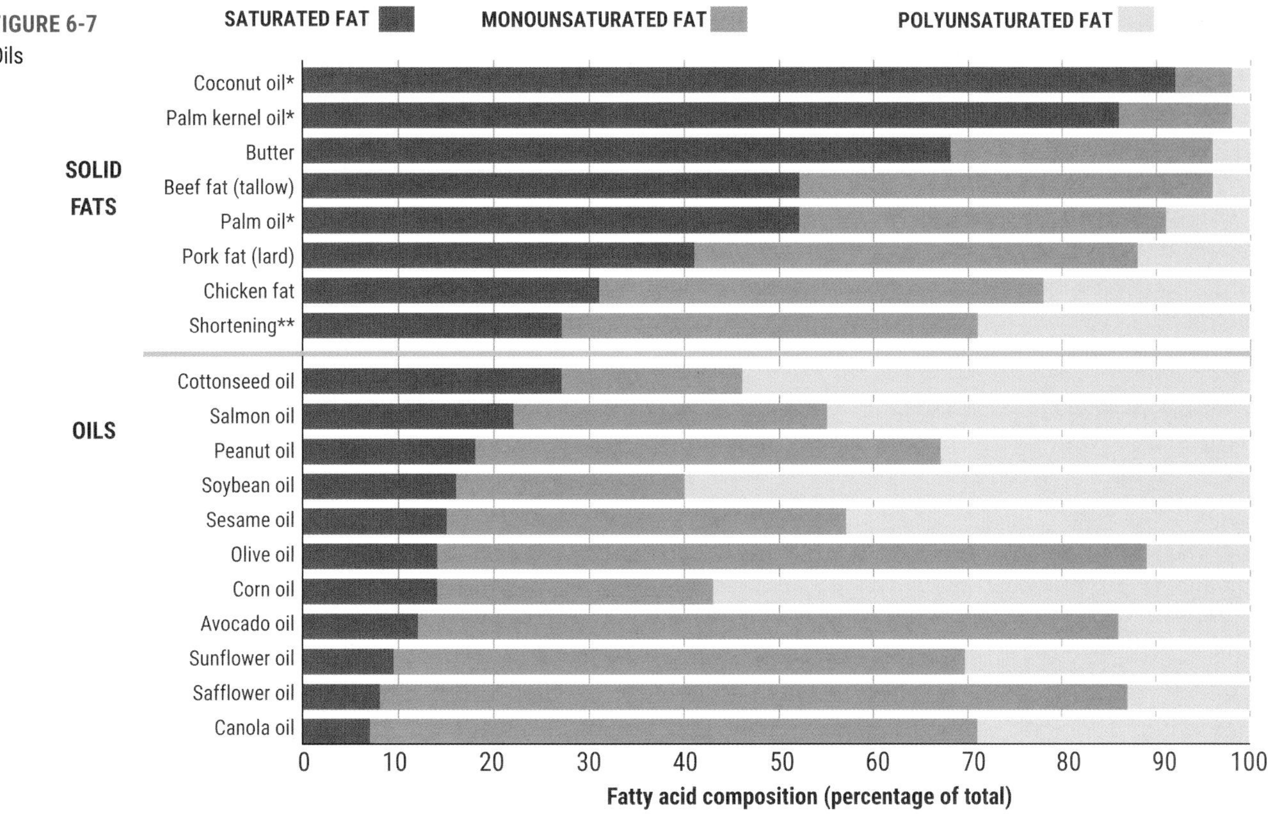

* Coconut, palm kernel, and palm oil are called oils because they come from plants. However, they are solid or semi-solid at room temperature due to their high content of short-chain saturated fatty acids. They are considered solid fats for nutritional purposes.

** Shortening may be made from partially hydrogenated vegetable oil, which contains trans fatty acids.

Reprinted from United States Department of Agriculture (2015). *2015-2020 Dietary Guidelines for Americans* (8th ed.). www.health.gov/dietaryguidelines

present in olives, nuts, avocados, and seafood. Tropical plant oils such as coconut, palm kernel, and palm oil are not included in the oils category due to their high saturated fat content. Americans are advised to consume about 5 teaspoons of oil per day for a 2,000-calorie diet. The nutritional composition of commonly consumed oils is shown in Figure 6-7.

Limits on Calories that Remain

The recommended food patterns are intended to meet nutritional needs while staying within calorie limits. For most people who follow the *Dietary Guidelines*, few calories will remain for "other purposes" (i.e., added sugars, added refined starches, solid fats, more than the recommended amounts of nutrient-dense foods, and alcohol).

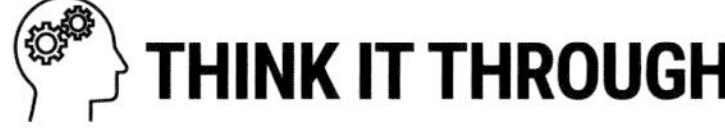

Assessing Nutritional Intake

- Record your nutritional intake for two weekdays and one weekend day.
- Assess how your intake compares to the recommendations. Which food group recommendations are you meeting? Which are you exceeding? Where are you falling short?
- What changes might you make to improve your nutrition? What are you already doing well?

TABLE 6-2

The Many Ways to Say Sugar

Agave syrup
Anhydrous dextrose
Brown sugar
Cane juice
Confectioner's powdered sugar
Corn sweetener
Corn syrup
Corn syrup solids
Crystal dextrose
Dextrin
Dextrose
Evaporated corn sweetener
Fructose
Fruit juice concentrate
Fruit nectar
Glucose
High-fructose corn syrup
Honey
Invert sugar
Lactose
Liquid fructose
Malt syrup
Maltose
Maple syrup
Molasses
Nectar
Pancake syrup
Raw sugar
Sucrose
Sugar
Sugar cane juice
Trehalose
Turbinado sugar
White granulated sugar

KEY GUIDELINE 3: LIMIT CALORIES FROM ADDED SUGARS AND SATURATED FATS AND REDUCE SODIUM INTAKE

Consume an eating pattern low in added sugars, saturated fats, and sodium. Cut back on foods and beverages higher in these components to amounts that fit within healthy eating patterns.

The *Dietary Guidelines* urge Americans to pay attention to—and limit—consumption of foods with low to no nutritional value, especially those that are, or may be, harmful to health such as added sugars, saturated fat, and sodium. New to the 2015-2020 *Dietary Guidelines* compared to previous editions, dietary cholesterol is no longer noted as a nutrient to limit, as it is likely not harmful to health for most people.

Added Sugars

Natural sugars include fruit sugar (**fructose**) and milk sugar (**lactose**). However, most sugars in the typical American diet are added sugars, which can come in many different forms (Table 6-2). While the body metabolizes natural and added sugars in the same way, most foods high in added sugars have very little nutritional value. These added sugars contribute about 270 calories per day, or more than 13% of the total calories in the American diet. The most commonly consumed food products containing these added sugars are sugar-sweetened beverages and snacks and sweets. The *Dietary Guidelines* recommend that Americans consume no more than 10% of calories from added sugars, while staying within calorie limits. Noncaloric sweeteners may be used to reduce caloric intake in the short term, but their long-term value for helping to lose weight and maintain weight loss is still unclear. The primary sources of these added sugars for Americans ages 2 and older are shown in Figure 6-8.

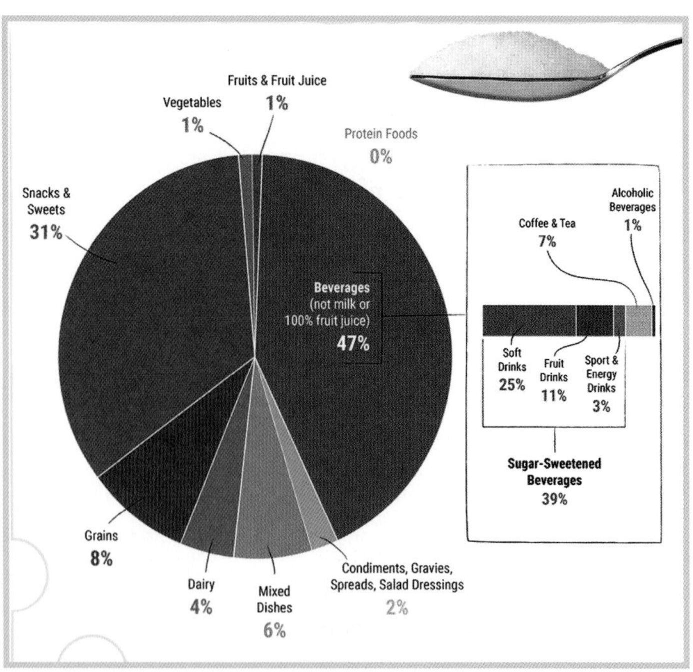

FIGURE 6-8
Food category sources of added sugars in the U.S. population ages 2 years and older

Reprinted from United States Department of Agriculture (2015). *2015-2020 Dietary Guidelines for Americans* (8th ed.). www.health.gov/dietaryguidelines

Saturated Fats

The types of fatty acids consumed play a more significant role in health than the amount of fat consumed. "Solid fats" include saturated fats and trans fats. A high intake of saturated fat is associated with increased total and **low-density lipoprotein (LDL)** cholesterol—both of which increase the risk of cardiovascular disease. The *Dietary Guidelines* recommend a diet containing <10% of total calories from saturated fat. Major sources of saturated fat for Americans include full-fat cheese, pizza, grain-based desserts, dairy-based desserts, fried foods, sausage, franks, bacon, and ribs. Evidence suggests that the health benefits are best when saturated fat is replaced with foods higher in polyunsaturated and monounsaturated fats, such as most types of vegetable oils. Salmon, tuna, and other fatty fish and many types of nuts and seeds, such as flaxseeds, are high in polyunsaturated fat. The scientific understanding of saturated fats continues to emerge, and there is debate about whether saturated fats are as harmful to health as was previously believed. That said, the *Dietary Guidelines* do not hedge and report that strong and consistent evidence shows that replacing saturated fats with polyunsaturated fats is associated with decreased total and LDL cholesterol and decreased risk of cardiovascular events such as heart attacks and cardiovascular disease–related deaths (USDA, 2015). The primary sources of saturated fat for Americans ages 2 and older are shown in Figure 6-9.

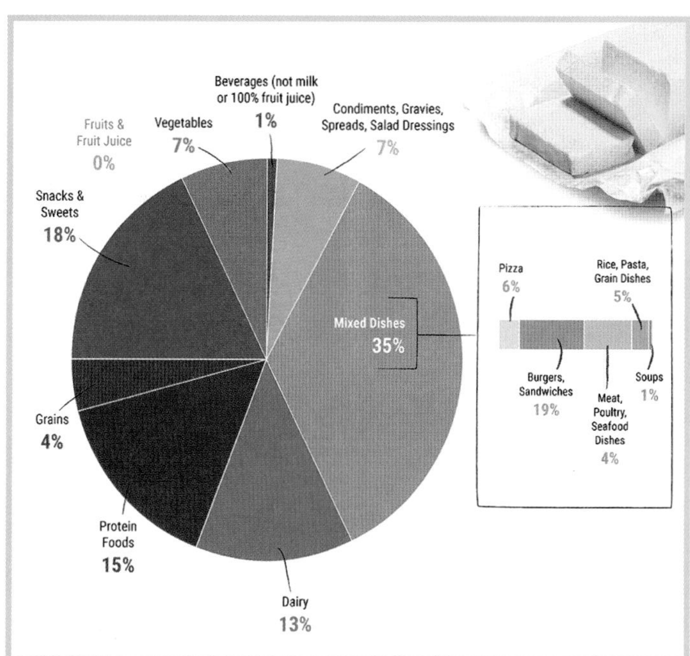

FIGURE 6-9
Food category sources of saturated fats in the U.S. population ages 2 years and older

Reprinted from United States Department of Agriculture (2015). *2015-2020 Dietary Guidelines for Americans* (8th ed.). www.health.gov/dietaryguidelines

Trans Fats

Trans fats are found naturally in dairy and meat products ("ruminant trans fats"), but the majority of intake comes from processed foods ("artificial trans fats"). Artificial trans fats increase LDL cholesterol and contribute to increased cardiovascular disease risk. Trans fats are required by law to be listed on the food label, although foods that contain <0.5 grams of trans fat per serving are allowed to claim "0 grams" of trans fat. Consumers can identify these foods by looking on the ingredient list for the words "partially hydrogenated." Americans should consume as little artificial trans fats as possible.

Sodium and the Dietary Approaches to Stop Hypertension Eating Plan

Sodium intake is associated with high levels of blood pressure for some people. Maintaining a normal blood pressure decreases the risk of cardiovascular disease, **congestive heart failure,** and kidney disease. The estimated intake of sodium per day for the average American is 3,440 mg, far more than the recommended amount of <2,300 mg for lower-risk populations and 1,500 mg for higher-risk individuals (i.e., those who have elevated cholesterol or hypertension—about 50% of adults). In fact, fewer than 15% of Americans meet sodium goals. This is at least in part due to the fact that sodium is ubiquitous in the food supply, especially in canned, processed, and restaurant-prepared dishes. Added table salt also contributes significantly to daily intake. The primary sources of sodium for Americans ages 2 and older are shown in Figure 6-10.

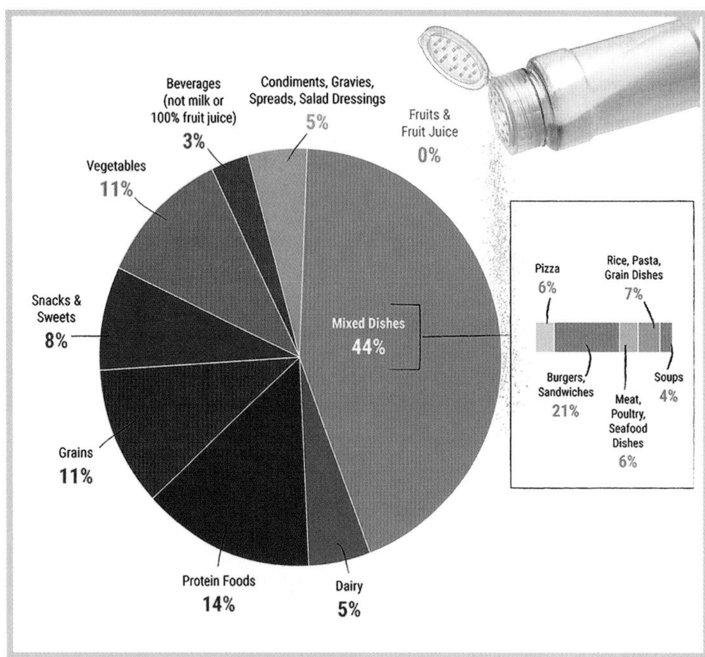

FIGURE 6-10
Food category sources of sodium in the U.S. population ages 2 years and older

Reprinted from United States Department of Agriculture (2015). *2015-2020 Dietary Guidelines for Americans* (8th ed.). www.health.gov/dietaryguidelines

The personal trainer can help clients decrease sodium intake by collaborating to set goals to:

- Read nutrition labels and pay attention to sodium content
- Consume more fresh foods and fewer processed foods
- Eat more home-prepared meals and add little table salt or sodium-containing seasonings
- When eating out, ask that salt not be added
- Reduce calorie intake (since most foods also contain sodium)

In addition, individuals with hypertension are advised to follow the low-sodium **Dietary Approaches to Stop Hypertension (DASH) eating plan** to optimize health and decrease blood pressure. The DASH eating plan is low in saturated fat, cholesterol, and total fat. The staples are whole grains, fruits, vegetables, and legumes. Fish, poultry, lean meats, nuts, and other unsaturated fats as well as low-fat dairy products are also encouraged. Consequently, it is rich in potassium, magnesium, calcium, protein, and fiber. Red meat, sweets, and sugar-containing beverages are very limited. Thus, it is low in saturated and total

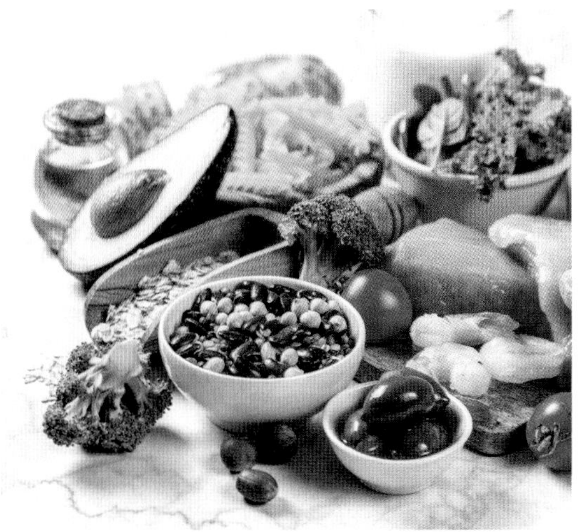

fat and cholesterol. The DASH eating plan recommends that men drink two or fewer and women drink one or fewer alcoholic beverages per day. While developed to reduce blood pressure, the DASH eating plan can be adopted by anyone regardless of whether the person has elevated blood pressure. In fact, some studies suggest that the eating plan may also reduce cardiovascular disease risk by lowering total cholesterol and LDL cholesterol in addition to lowering blood pressure (reviewed in Eckel et al., 2014).

The DASH eating plan lowers **systolic blood pressure (SBP)** by about 5 to 6 mmHg and **diastolic blood pressure (DBP)** by 3 mmHg when compared to a typical American diet of the 1990s. This effect on blood pressure holds true across ages, sex, and ethnicity for individuals with blood pressures 120–159/80–95 mmHg (Eckel et al., 2014). Several variations of the DASH eating plan have been studied with even more pronounced results. For example, when 10% of calories from carbohydrates were replaced with an equal number of calories from protein or unsaturated fat, SBP decreased by an additional 1 mmHg compared to the standard DASH eating plan in both hypertensive and nonhypertensive individuals. When looking at only hypertensive individuals, SBP decreased by 3 mmHg compared to the standard DASH eating plan (Eckel et al., 2014).

Note that certain populations, such as individuals participating in intensive physical activity in hot and humid environments, need sufficient sodium intake to replace sodium lost in fluid. The AI for sodium in people nine to 50 years old is 1,500 mg per day and the UL is 2,200 to 2,300 mg per day. Most athletes will meet sodium needs with a sodium intake within this range, although making recommendations regarding the timing and amount of sodium replacement is outside the scope of the *Dietary Guidelines*.

KEY GUIDELINE 4: SHIFT TO HEALTHIER FOOD AND BEVERAGE CHOICES

Choose nutrient-dense foods and beverages across and within all food groups in place of less healthy choices. Consider cultural and personal preferences to make these shifts easier to accomplish and maintain.

While the *Dietary Guidelines* advocate an overall healthy and balanced nutrition pattern that is low in added sugars and sodium, the reality is that most Americans eat nothing like the eating patterns recommended by the *Dietary Guidelines*, as shown in Figure 6-11. By making shifts in dietary patterns, Americans can achieve and maintain a healthy body weight, meet nutrient needs, and decrease the risk of chronic disease.

Overall, the *Dietary Guidelines* advise that Americans shift their eating patterns to:

- Consume more vegetables
- Consume more fruits
- Consume more whole grains and fewer refined grains

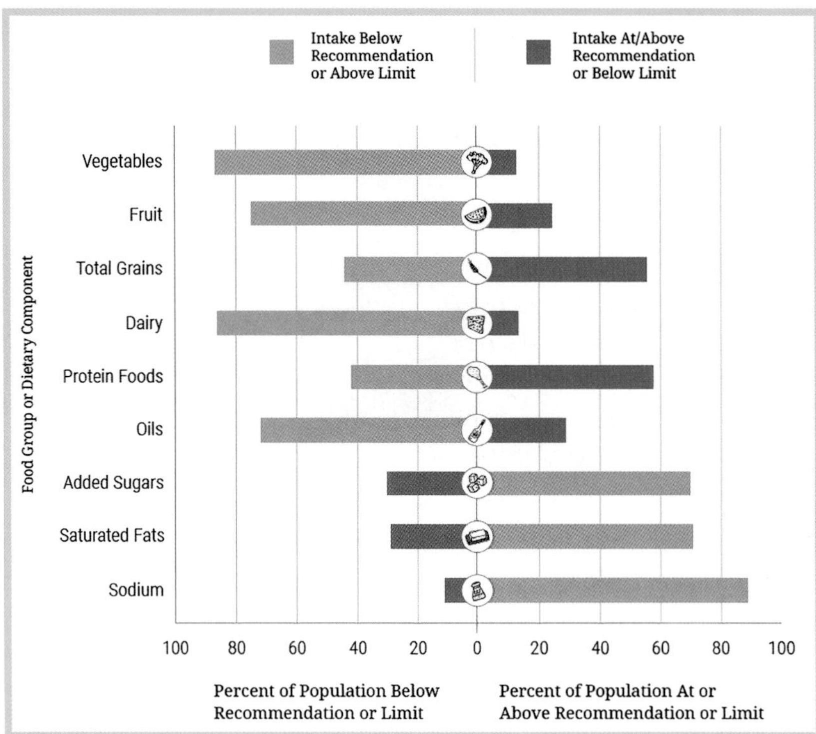

FIGURE 6-11
Dietary intakes compared to recommendations. Percent of the U.S. population ages 1 year and older who are below, at, or above each dietary goal or limit

Reprinted from United States Department of Agriculture (2015). *2015-2020 Dietary Guidelines for Americans* (8th ed.). www.health.gov/dietaryguidelines

- Consume more dairy products
- Increase variety in protein food choices and choose more nutrient-dense foods. That is, eat more seafood in place of meat, poultry, or eggs and use legumes or nuts and seeds in mixed dishes instead of some meat or poultry. Men and teenage boys should consume less protein, especially meat, poultry, and eggs.
- Exchange solid fats for oils
- Reduce added sugar consumption to less than 10% of calories per day
- Reduce saturated fat intake to less than 10% of calories per day
- Reduce sodium intake

Examples of how these shifts might play out in a daily eating plan include:

- Shift from high-calorie snacks (such as tortilla chips with cheese dip) to nutrient-dense snacks (carrots with hummus dip)
- Shift from fruit products with added sugars (fruit-filled cereal bar) to whole fruit (apple)
- Shift from refined grains (white bread) to whole grains (whole-wheat bread)
- Shift from snacks high in sodium (meat and cheese sticks) to unsalted snacks (unsalted cashews)
- Shift from solid fats (butter in a frying pan) to oils
- Shift from beverages with added sugars (soda) to no-sugar-added beverages (seltzer water)

The *Dietary Guidelines* also note that roughly 20% of Americans meet the *Physical Activity Guidelines for Americans* (U.S. Department of Health & Human Services, 2018) and 30% engage in no leisure-time physical activity (USDA, 2015). Most people would benefit from moving more and sitting less, even if for only a few minutes at a time.

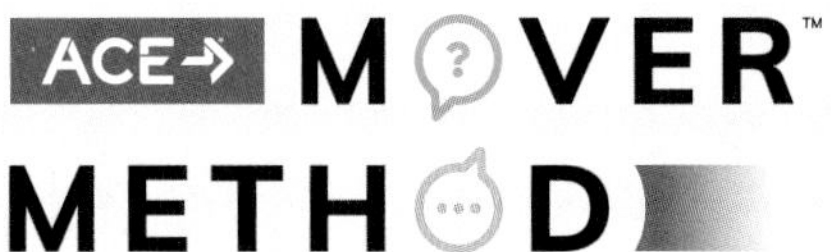

The New Client Recently Diagnosed with Hypertension

During the warm-up portion of an exercise session, your new client shares with you his results from a recent doctor's appointment. His doctor informed him that because his blood pressure has been above 130/80 mmHg at his last three visits, he has been diagnosed as having hypertension. His doctor did not prescribe any medication but instead discussed diet, weight loss, and increased physical activity to promote healthy lifestyle change. The client tells you that he is interested in increasing his physical-activity levels and improving his diet to manage his new diagnosis but that dietary changes will be the hardest for him to initiate and maintain.

ACE ABC APPROACH

The following is an example of how the ACE ABC Approach™ can be used to explore this client's concerns around nutrition.

Ask: Use powerful open-ended questions to discover how the client believes lifestyle changes will improve his high blood pressure.

Personal Trainer: You mentioned that exercise and diet changes are important to the management of your blood pressure and that making changes to your diet would be the biggest challenge for you. What is the best possible outcome you can achieve by making these lifestyle changes?

Client: By changing my activity and nutrition habits, I am hoping to keep my blood pressure under control, avoid taking medication, and improve my overall quality of life.

Break down barriers: At this point in the conversation, you can drill down more deeply into the potential barriers that may get in the way of these goals by asking another open-ended question.

Personal Trainer: You want to make these changes to manage your blood pressure, avoid medication, and improve your quality of life. What obstacles do you think might get in the way of these goals?

Client: It will be easy for me to add more physical activity into my life because I enjoy it and now, with the news about my blood pressure and knowing exercise can help, I am motivated. Eating better, on the other hand, is not something I am looking forward to. My doctor gave me a printout detailing something called the DASH eating plan and it's clear that I am not eating enough fruits and vegetables. I want to eat more, but I don't see how I can add this into my routine.

Personal Trainer: Tell me more about how many fruits and vegetables you eat currently and how that compares to what you know about the DASH eating plan.

Client: I don't eat fruits and vegetables daily. I eat about one to two pieces of fruit per week and occasionally have vegetables. On the printout my doctor gave me, it says that to follow the DASH eating plan I need to eat four to five servings of fruit and vegetables per day. That's a lot more produce than I eat currently. I don't know if I can do that.

Collaborate: Work together with the client on next steps and solutions to barriers to decide which options are best moving forward.

Personal Trainer: You're not concerned with your ability to add more exercise to your life, and you are feeling overwhelmed by the amount of fruits and vegetables recommended as part of the DASH eating plan, but you would like to eat more. What action step could you see yourself taking within the next month to increase the amount of fruits and vegetables you eat?

Client: Over the next month I would like to work my way up to eating fruits and vegetables daily by finding convenient ways to add them to my diet. The form I received from my doctor says I should eat four to five servings of fruits and vegetables per day and I would like to work my way toward that.

Personal Trainer: I can provide you with some additional resources that will help you to know more about convenient ways to integrated fruits and vegetables into a regular part of your eating plan if you think that would be helpful.

Client: I would appreciate that. Right now, I eat fruits and vegetables a few times a week, not daily. It's not that I don't like them; it just seems like more work to prepare them than the foods I regularly eat.

Personal Trainer: From the information that I shared with you, is there something you can do to get started within the next week?

Client: This week, I can take the list you gave me to my grocery store and pick one fruit and one vegetable to eat daily using the servings suggestions on the list.

The ACE ABC Approach is used in this scenario to find out what the client wants to accomplish and why, identify potential barriers, and plan on next steps. The client in this scenario wants to make a change and the personal trainer is guiding him toward action without telling the client what he should or should not be doing. The client remains in control of what goals are meaningful and how he would like to work toward them.

KEY GUIDELINE 5: SUPPORT HEALTHY EATING PATTERNS FOR ALL

Everyone has a role in helping to create and support healthy eating patterns in multiple settings nationwide, from home to school to work to communities.

The *Guidelines* charge all sectors of society to play an active role in the movement to make the United States healthier by developing coordinated partnerships, programs, and policies to support healthy eating. Food and activity behaviors are best viewed in the context of a **socio-ecological model.** The USDA (2015) describes this model as an approach that emphasizes the development of coordinated partnerships, programs, and policies to support healthy eating and active living.

In this framework, interventions should extend well beyond providing traditional education to individuals and families about healthy choices, and should help build skills, reshape the environment, and reestablish social norms to facilitate individuals' healthy choices (Figure 6-12).

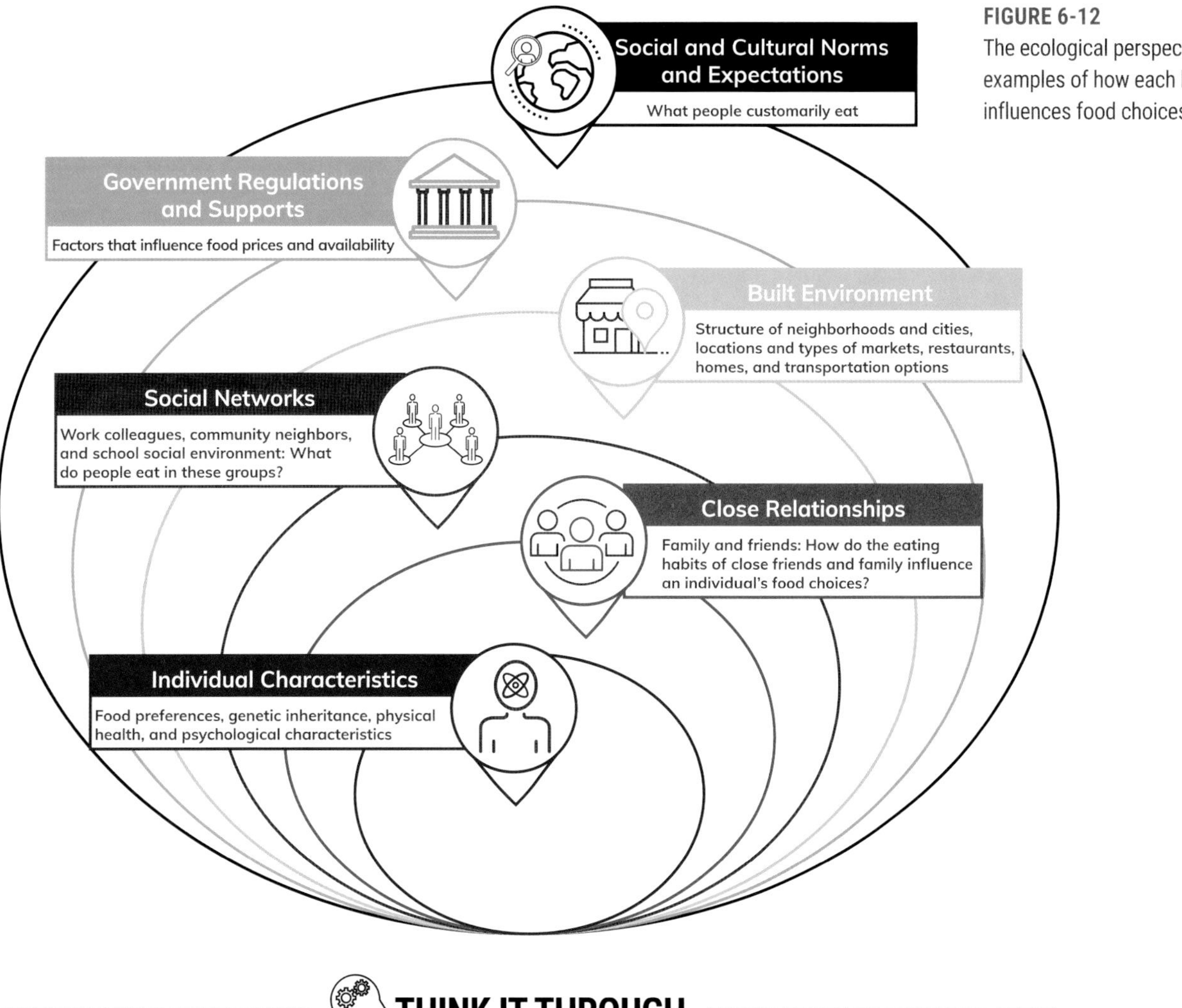

FIGURE 6-12
The ecological perspective, with examples of how each level influences food choices

THINK IT THROUGH

The Ecological Perspective

Taking an ecological perspective facilitates the understanding of many types of health behaviors, including eating behaviors (Sallis & Owen, 2015).

Consider your own eating behaviors. Using an ecological perspective, list supports and barriers at each level that influence your behavior. How might taking into consideration high-level factors like community design and public policies influence your work as personal trainer?

Personal trainers can best "meet people where they are" to understand individual choices and motivators by paying particular attention to:

- **Food access:** Access to healthy, safe, and affordable food choices is influenced by several factors, including proximity to grocery stores, financial resources, transportation, and neighborhood resources such as average income and availability of public transportation.

- **Household food insecurity:** This occurs when access to nutritious and safe food is limited or uncertain. Food insecurity affects a family's ability to obtain food and make healthy choices and can worsen stress and chronic disease risk.
- **Acculturation:** Acculturation involves moving toward a typical American eating plan from what is often a more nutritious eating pattern of the home country. The recommended eating pattern is flexible to accommodate traditional and cultural foods. Individuals and families are encouraged to maintain their traditional healthy eating and physical-activity patterns and avoid adopting less healthy behaviors (USDA, 2015).

The most effective interventions are multifaceted, using a combination of strategies to impact behavior change, and also multilevel in that they function across the various aspects of the socio-ecological model. An impactful intervention might include a combination of changes across one or more of the following domains:

- **Home:** Develop skills in meal planning and cooking. Limit screen time at home and build in time for family physical activity.
- **School:** Commit to offering only healthy meals and snacks; provide nutrition labels and calorie and nutrient information in cafeterias; reach out to parents about making healthy changes at home; increase the amount and quality of nutrition education and school gardens; commit to support physical-activity programs, high-quality physical education, and active play.
- **Worksite:** Offer health and wellness programs, including nutritional counseling, active breaks, and flexible schedules that allow for physical activity and walking meetings. Provide stand-up desks to decrease sitting time.
- **Community:** Support shelters, food banks, farmers markets, community gardens, and walkable communities.
- **Food retail:** Reach out to consumers about making healthy changes; increase access to healthy and affordable food options.

Several specific strategies personal trainers can employ to support clients in shifting eating patterns to improve health and more closely resemble the recommended intakes include the following:

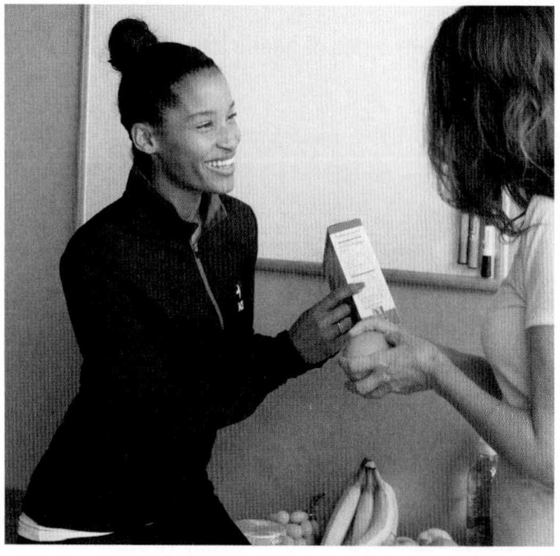

- Partner with individuals to increase awareness of the foods and beverages that make up their own or their family's eating patterns and identify areas where they can make small changes that align with the *Dietary Guidelines*, such as modifying recipes or food selections.
- Enhance self-efficacy with skills like gardening, cooking, meal planning, and label reading.
- Explore ways that individuals can model healthy eating behaviors for friends and family.

- Co-create plans to help clients limit screen time and time spent being sedentary and increase physical activity.

Food Labels

For people to make healthy nutrition decisions, they first have to be able to understand which nutrients contribute to a healthy diet, and second, know which foods contain those nutrients. While the bulk of a healthy diet is made up of whole, unprocessed foods that do not carry food labels, there are processed or prepared foods (e.g., low-fat milk and milk products) that can be part of a healthy diet and do have food labels. The food label, a required component of nearly all packaged foods, can help people turn knowledge into action. It can also be a source of confusion and misunderstanding.

HISTORY AND PRESENT STATE OF FOOD LABELING

It was not until the early 1970s, when consumers faced a boom in production of processed foods, that nutrition labels were included on packaged foods. As an increasing number of foods arrived on grocery store shelves, many of which made nutrition claims, the Food and Drug Administration (FDA) proposed regulations in 1972 to require food labels on packaged foods that added nutrients or made nutrition claims. The labels would be voluntary for foods without claims. The first nutrition labels contained basic nutrition information, including calories, protein, carbohydrate, and fat, as well as the RDA for protein and several vitamins and minerals. Inclusion of sodium, saturated fat, and polyunsaturated fat was optional (Food and Nutrition Board, 2010).

As more products arrived on shelves and consumers became increasingly interested in reviewing food labels, food manufacturers responded with a plethora of ambiguous claims touting nutritional value and health benefits, even though FDA regulations had long prohibited mention of disease prevention or health promotion on food labels. Though companies could not explicitly state or imply that a food's nutrient properties could help to prevent, cure, or treat any disease or symptom, ambiguous nutrition claims designed to catch consumers' attention (such as "extremely low in saturated fat") became commonplace. The FDA policy helped to protect consumers against potentially harmful claims. However, it also limited manufacturers' ability to advertise the benefits of foods that provided legitimate health benefits, such as foods that were high in fiber. In 1984, the National Cancer Institute and Kellogg's launched a food-labeling campaign on a high-fiber cereal box linking the high-fiber intake to a possible reduction in some cancers. In the absence of regulatory action, other food manufacturers followed suit, leading to a frenzy of nutrition and health claims on food labels (Food and Nutrition Board, 2010).

In 1990, congress passed the Nutrition Labeling and Education Act (NLEA), which gave the FDA the authority to require nutrition labeling on most food packages and specified the information and nutrients that must be included on the label. It also required specific criteria for approved health claims. The FDA's stated goal in developing the label criteria was to (1) minimize confusion, (2) help consumers choose healthier diets, and (3) provide an incentive to companies to improve the nutritional value of their products. The Nutrition Facts panel with which most of today's consumers are familiar was mandated in 1993. Though trans fats were not initially included on the nutrition label, their inclusion was required by 2003 if the product contained more than 0.5 grams of trans fat per serving. This regulation drastically decreased the amount of trans fats used in food production (Food and Nutrition Board, 2010).

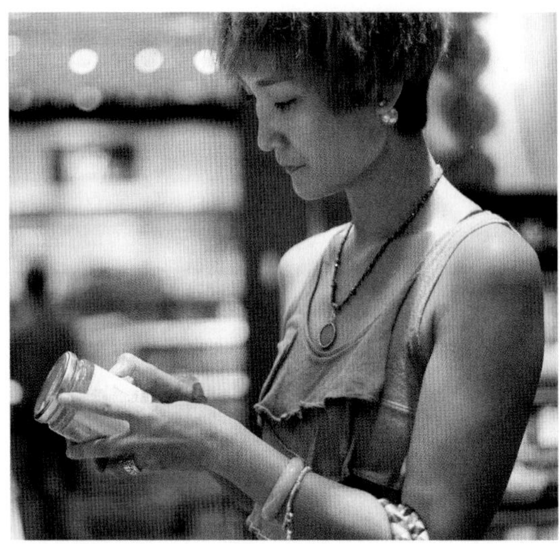

In 2016, the FDA introduced a new Nutrition Facts label. The new label includes a few design changes, including increased font size and bold type for "calories" and "serving size" and the actual amount, in addition to **percent daily value (PDV)** of vitamin D, calcium, iron, and potassium. Content changes to the label include the addition of "added sugars" in grams and a PDV for added sugars. Vitamin D and potassium are required additions to the label, while vitamins A and C no longer must be included. Calcium and iron are still required. "Calories from fat" is no longer required, as the type of fat is more important than the amount. Daily values for some nutrients, such as sodium, dietary fiber, and vitamin D, are updated based on new DRIs from the National Academy of Medicine. Finally, the new label includes updates to serving sizes. Law requires that serving sizes be based on amounts of food and beverages that people commonly consume, not what they should consume. Because people are eating larger portions, the new label includes a serving size as a larger amount. For instance, a serving of ice cream used to be 1/2 cup but is now 2/3 cup. It is important for personal trainers to recognize this change and that the serving size is not a recommendation of how much to eat. (In many cases, people should eat less than one serving of a food.) The number of servings per container has long been a source of confusion. Now, packages that are between one and two servings will be required to be labeled as one serving since people commonly consume the whole package in one sitting. For larger package sizes, manufacturers must include two column labels to include the amounts per serving and amounts per package.

Health Claims

The issue of whether or not to allow health claims was addressed by the NLEA. Claims that can be used on food and **dietary supplement** labels include **health claims, nutrient content claims,** and **structure/function claims.**

Health claims describe a relationship between a food or food component and the prevention or treatment of a disease or health-related condition. To be included on a nutrition label, health claims must be authorized by the FDA or be based on an authoritative statement of a scientific body of the federal government or the National Academies of Science, after notification to the FDA. A listing of currently allowed health claims is available at https://www.fda.gov/Food/LabelingNutrition/ucm2006876.htm.

Qualified health claims are allowed on product labels if there is emerging evidence for a relationship between a food or food component and decreased risk of a disease or health condition, but the scientific evidence is not conclusive. The statement must include a qualifying statement saying that the evidence supporting the claim is limited.

Nutrient content claims imply health benefits by describing the level of a nutrient in a product using terms like "free," "high," or "low," or compared to another product using terms like "more," "reduced," and "lite." A product can be labeled as "healthy" if it has "healthy" levels of total fat, saturated fat, cholesterol, and sodium. A listing of nutrient content claims is available at https://www.fda.gov/food/food-labeling-nutrition/nutrient-content-claims.

Structure/function claims are regulated by the **Dietary Supplement Health and Education Act (DSHEA).** They typically apply to supplements and do not need to be preapproved by the FDA. These types of claims relate a nutrient or dietary ingredient to normal human structure or function, such as "calcium builds strong bones," or describe a benefit related to addressing a nutrient deficiency. It must state a disclaimer that the FDA has not evaluated the claim and that the supplement is not intended to treat, cure, or prevent any disease.

Front-of-Package Labeling

Since 1987, when the American Heart Association first developed the "Heart Guide Initiative" to tag foods that were the most heart healthy, organizations from PepsiCo and General Mills to grocery stores, nonprofits, and academic groups have implemented front-of-package (FOP) labeling to communicate with consumers. While intended to help consumers make healthier choices, the multiple and varied labels have been confusing and, in many cases, misleading. This issue came to public attention in 2009 when a popular sugar-sweetened cereal, along with macaroni and cheese, ice cream, and fruit roll-ups, were given a SmartChoice FOP label. In anticipation of potential regulation on FOP labeling systems, Congress mandated the IOM to develop a two-part report on FOP labeling (Food and Nutrition Board, 2012; Food and Nutrition Board, 2010). The IOM committee concluded that "It is time for a fundamental shift in strategy, a move away from systems that mostly provide nutrition information without clear guidance about its healthfulness, and toward one that encourages healthier food choices through simplicity, visual clarity, and the ability to convey meaning without written information. An FOP system should be standardized and it also should motivate food and beverage companies to reformulate their products to be healthier and encourage food retailers to prominently display products that meet this standard" (Food and Nutrition Board, 2012). The report advised a labeling system that is based on calories, saturated and trans fat, sugar, and salt. As of the time of this writing, no action has been taken.

READING THE NUTRITION LABEL

While the nutrition label provides a large amount of useful nutrition information, it can also be a source of confusion for many consumers. A personal trainer can play an important role in helping consumers effectively use the nutrition label to guide them in making healthy choices.

A Stepwise Approach

A personal trainer can assist clients in dissecting the food label (Figure 6-13) by taking a stepwise approach. Start from the top with the serving size and the number of servings per container. In general, serving sizes are standardized so that consumers can compare similar products. All of the nutrient amounts listed on the food label are for one serving, so it is

FIGURE 6-13
Nutrition facts label

Nutrition Facts

1	8 Servings Per Container	
	Serving Size	**2/3 cup (55g)**
2	**Amount Per Serving**	
	Calories	**230**
		% Daily Value*
3	**Total Fat** 8g	**10%**
4	Saturated Fat 1g	**5%**
5	*Trans* Fat 0g	**0%**
6	**Cholesterol** 0mg	**0%**
7	**Sodium** 160mg	**7%**
8	**Total Carbohydrate** 37g	**13%**
9	Dietary Fiber 4g	**14%**
	Total Sugars 12g	
10	Includes 10g Added Sugars	**20%**
11	**Protein** 3g	
12	Vitamin D 2mcg	10%
	Calcium 260mg	20%
	Iron 8mg	45%
	Potassium 235mg	6%

* The % Daily Value (DV) tells you how much a nutrient in a serving of food contributes to a daily diet. 2,000 calories a day is used for general nutrition advice.

1 Serving Size
The label presents serving sizes as the amount that most people actually consume in a sitting. This is not necessarily the same as how much one should eat per serving. All of the nutrition information on the label is based on one serving. If you eat twice the serving size shown here, multiply the nutrient and calorie values by two.

2 Calories
The number of calories listed represents the total calories from fat, carbohydrate, and protein (manufacturers are allowed to round this value to the nearest 5- or 10-calorie increment). 100 calories per serving is considered moderate, while 400 calories or more per serving is considered high. A 5'4", 138-lb active woman needs about 2,200 calories each day. A 5'10", 174-lb active man needs about 2,900 calories.

3 Total Fat
Fat is calorie-dense and, if consumed in large portions, can increase the risk of weight problems. While once vilified, most fat, in and of itself, is not bad. Adults should consume 20 to 35% of total calories from fat.

4 Saturated Fat
Saturated fat is part of the total fat in food. It is listed separately because it plays an important role in raising blood cholesterol and your risk of heart disease. Eat less than 10% of total calories from saturated fat.

5 Trans Fat
Trans fat works a lot like saturated fat, except it is worse. This fat starts out as a liquid unsaturated fat, but then food manufacturers add some hydrogen to it, turning it into a solid saturated fat (that is what "partially hydrogenated" means when you see it in the food ingredients). They do this to increase the shelf-life of the product, but in the body the trans fat damages the blood vessels and contributes to increasing blood cholesterol and the risk of heart disease. Individuals should consume as little trans fat as possible.

6 Cholesterol
Many foods that are high in cholesterol are also high in saturated fat, which can contribute to heart disease. Dietary cholesterol itself likely does not cause health problems.

Daily Value
Daily Values are listed based on a 2,000-calorie daily eating plan. Your calorie and nutrient needs may be a little bit more or less based on your age, sex, and activity level (see https://fnic.nal.usda.gov/fnic/interactiveDRI/). For saturated fat, trans fat, sodium, and added sugars, choose foods with a low % (5% or less) Daily Value. For dietary fiber, vitamins, and minerals, your Daily Value goal is to reach 100% of each.

Ingredients: *This portion of the label lists all of the foods and additives contained in a product, in descending order by weight.*

Allergens: *This portion of the label identifies which of the most common allergens may be present in the product.*

(More nutrients may be listed on some labels)

mcg = micrograms (1,000 mcg = 1 mg)
mg = milligrams (1,000 mg = 1 g)
g = grams (about 28 g = 1 ounce)

7 Sodium
You call it "salt," the label calls it "sodium." Either way, it may add up to high blood pressure in some people. So, keep your sodium intake low—less than 2,300 mg each day.

8 Total Carbohydrate
Carbohydrates are in foods like bread, potatoes, fruits, and vegetables, as well as processed foods. Carbohydrate is further broken down into dietary fiber and sugars. Consume foods high in fiber often and those high in sugars, especially added sugars, less often. Adults should consume 45 to 65% of total calories from carbohydrates.

9 Dietary Fiber
There are two kinds of dietary fiber: soluble and insoluble. Fruits, vegetables, whole-grain foods, beans, and peas are all good sources and can help reduce the risk of heart disease and cancer. Individuals should try to eat 14 grams of dietary fiber for every 1,000 calories consumed.

10 Sugars
Too much sugar contributes to weight gain and increased risk of diseases like diabetes and fatty liver disease. Foods like fruits and dairy products contain natural sugars (fructose and lactose), but also may contain added sugars. It is recommended to consume no more than 10% of total calories from added sugar, or a total of 50 g per day based on a 2,000-calorie eating plan.

11 Protein
To limit saturated fat, eat small servings of lean meat, fish, and poultry. Use skim or low-fat milk, yogurt, and cheese. Try vegetable proteins like beans, grains, and cereals. Adults should consume 10 to 35% of total calories from protein.

12 Vitamins and Minerals
Your goal here is 100% of each for the day. Don't count on one food to do it all. Let a combination of foods add up to a winning score.

important to determine how many servings are actually being consumed to accurately assess nutrient intake.

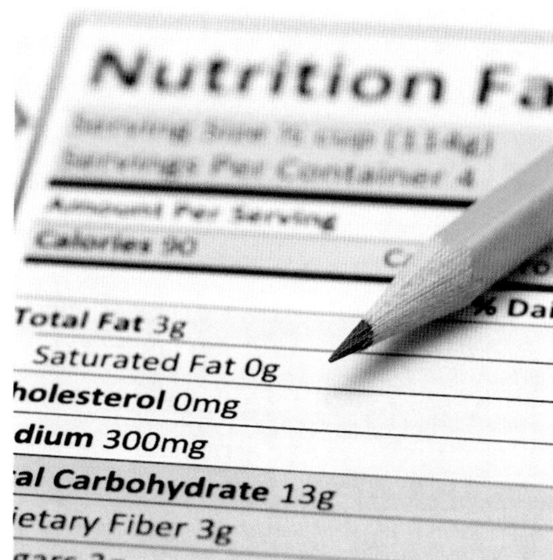

Next, attention should be given to the total calories, which indicate how much energy a person gets from a particular food. Americans tend to consume too many calories, without meeting daily nutrient requirements. This part of the nutrition label is the most important factor for weight control. In general, 40 calories per serving is considered low, 100 calories is moderate, and 400 or more calories is considered high [U.S. Food & Drug Administration (FDA), 2004].

The next two sections of the label note the nutrient content of the food product. Ideally, intake of saturated and trans fat and sodium should be minimized, and adequate amounts of fiber should be consumed, along with vitamins and minerals, especially vitamin D, potassium, calcium, and iron. The food label includes the total amount of sugars (natural and added), as well as the amount of added sugars.

The PDVs are listed for key nutrients to make it easier to compare products (just make sure that the serving sizes are similar), evaluate nutrient content claims (does 1/3 reduced-sugar cereal really contain less carbohydrate than a similar cereal of a different brand?), and make informed dietary tradeoffs (e.g., balance consumption of a high-fat product for lunch with lower-fat products throughout the rest of the day). In general, 5% daily value or less is considered low, while 20% daily value or more is considered high (FDA, 2004).

The footnote at the bottom of the label reminds consumers that all PDVs are based on a 2,000-calorie diet. Individuals who need more or fewer calories should adjust recommendations accordingly. For example, 3 grams of fat provides 5% of the recommended amount for someone on a 2,000-calorie diet, but 7% for someone on a 1,500-calorie diet.

Legislation also requires food manufacturers to list all potential food **allergens** on food packaging. The most common food allergens are fish, shellfish, soybean, wheat, egg, milk, peanuts, and tree nuts. This information usually is included near the list of ingredients on the package. Clearly, this information is especially important to clients with food allergies. For clients who follow a gluten-free diet, this is also an easy way to identify if wheat is a product ingredient.

Clients should carefully review the ingredients list. Note that the ingredient list is in decreasing order of substance weight in the product. That is, the ingredients that are listed first are the most abundant ingredients in the product. The ingredient list is useful to help identify whether or not the product contains trans fat, solid fats, added sugars, whole grains, and refined grains.

- **Trans fat:** Although trans fat is included in the "fat" section of the nutrition label, if the product contains <0.5 grams per serving, the manufacturer does not need to claim it.

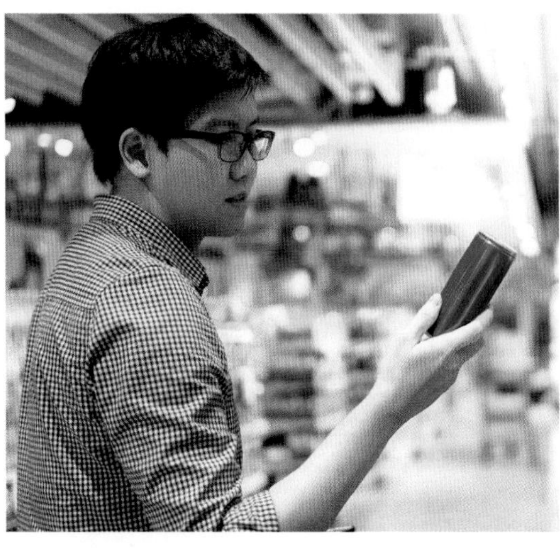

However, if a product contains "partially hydrogenated oils," then the product contains trans fat.

- **Solid fats:** If the ingredient list contains beef fat, butter, chicken fat, coconut oil, cream, hydrogenated oils, palm kernel oils, pork fat (lard), shortening, or stick margarine, then the product contains solid fats.
- **Added sugars:** Ingredients signifying added sugars are listed in Table 6-2. In many cases, products contain multiple forms of sugar.
- **Whole grains:** To be considered 100% whole grain, the product must contain all of the essential parts of the original kernel—the bran, germ, and endosperm. When choosing products, the whole grain should be the first or second ingredient. Examples of whole grains include brown rice, buckwheat, bulgur (cracked wheat), millet, steel-cut oats, popcorn, quinoa, rolled oats, whole-grain sorghum, whole-grain triticale, whole-grain barley, whole-grain corn, whole oats/oatmeal, whole rye, whole wheat, and wild rice.
- **Refined grains:** Refined grains are listed as "enriched." If the first ingredient is an enriched grain, then the product is not a whole grain. This is one way to understand whether or not a "wheat bread" is actually whole wheat or a refined product.

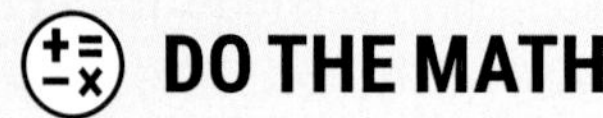

DO THE MATH

Nutrition Label Sample Problem

Using the nutrition label from Figure 6-13, determine (1) the number of calories per container; (2) the calories from carbohydrate, protein, and fat per serving; and (3) the percentage of calories from carbohydrate, protein, and fat.

1. 230 calories per serving x 8 servings per container = 1,840 calories per container
2. *Carbohydrate:* 37 grams carbohydrate per serving x 4 calories per gram = 148 calories per serving from carbohydrate

   Protein: 3 grams protein per serving x 4 calories per gram = 12 calories per serving from protein

   Fat: 8 grams fat per serving x 9 calories per gram = 72 calories per serving from fat

   Note that the label rounds the 232 calories calculated in question 2 to 230 calories.
3. *Carbohydrate:* 148 calories from carbohydrate/230 calories = 64% carbohydrate

   Protein: 12 calories from protein/230 calories = 5% protein

   Fat: 72 calories from fat/230 calories = 31% fat

Food Safety and Selection

An important but often underestimated key to healthy eating is to avoid foods contaminated with harmful bacteria, viruses, parasites, and other microorganisms. About one in six Americans, or 48 million people, become sick each year from foodborne illness, 128,000 are hospitalized, and approximately 3,000 die (Centers for Disease Control and Prevention, 2011). Special populations most at risk include pregnant women, infants and young children, older adults, and people who are immunocompromised. The majority of foodborne illnesses are preventable with a few simple precautions (Table 6-3). Refer to www.fightbac.org, www.foodsafety.gov, or www.cdc.gov/foodsafety for more information.

TABLE 6-3

Steps to Safe Food Handling

To avoid microbial foodborne illness:
▸ Clean hands, food contact surfaces, and fruits and vegetables. Meat and poultry should not be washed or rinsed.
▸ Separate raw, cooked, and ready-to-eat foods while shopping, preparing, or storing foods.
▸ Cook foods to a safe temperature to kill microorganisms [bacteria grow most rapidly between the temperatures of 40 and 140° F (4 and 60° C)]. Pregnant women should eat only certain deli meats and frankfurters that have been reheated to steaming hot.
▸ Refrigerate perishable food promptly (within two hours) and defrost foods properly. Eat refrigerated leftovers within three or four days.
▸ Avoid raw (unpasteurized) milk or any products made from unpasteurized milk, raw or partially cooked eggs, or foods containing raw eggs, raw or undercooked meat and poultry, unpasteurized juice, and raw sprouts. This is especially important for infants and young children, pregnant women, older adults, and those who are immunocompromised.

Reprinted from U.S. Department of Agriculture (2015). 2015-2020 *Dietary Guidelines for Americans* (8th ed.). www.health.gov/dietaryguidelines

Clients can employ the following tips while grocery shopping to reduce the risk of foodborne illness:

- Check produce for bruises and feel and smell for ripeness.
- Look for a "sell-by" date for breads and baked goods, a "use-by" date on some packaged foods, an "expiration date" on yeast and baking powder, and a "packaged date" on canned and some packaged foods.
- Make sure packaged goods are not torn and cans are not dented, cracked, or bulging.
- Separate fish and poultry from other purchases by wrapping them separately in plastic bags.
- Pick up refrigerated and frozen foods last. Make sure all perishable items are refrigerated within one hour of purchase.

Practical Considerations for Personal Trainers

While much of the buzz around nutrition often relates to individual ingredients or a proportion of calories from specific macronutrients, there is an increasing movement toward an overall healthy eating pattern based on the consumption of more whole foods. In order to assist clients in translating the most current evidence and recommendations into practical and sustainable nutrition changes while keeping within scope of practice, personal trainers can offer further support, guidance, and resources in the following ways.

PROVIDING GROCERY STORE TOURS

The average grocery store in America has about 40,000 products from which to choose. For this reason, grocery shopping can be an overwhelming and confusing experience for many clients. The traditional guidance to stick to the perimeter of the store can help narrow the choices, and as such this advice has been dispensed by health educators and health agencies for quite some time. The outer aisles are usually where most of the whole, fresh foods are located, with the exception of whole grains, beans, and legumes, which are commonly found in the center aisles. Aside from these items, the majority of foods that are located in the center aisles of the store are highly processed and nutrient-deficient. For clients seeking further support and guidance navigating the plethora of options, personal trainers may opt to expand their offerings to provide grocery store tours, which have been found to be an effective strategy for helping clients learn healthier shopping and eating practices (Nikolaus et al., 2016).

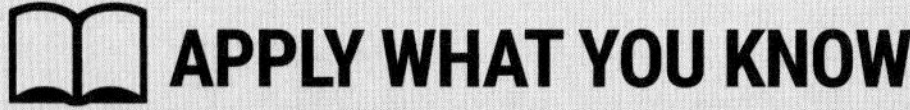

Eating Healthy on a Budget

It is estimated that approximately 32% of working families in the U.S. may not have enough money to meet basic needs (Roberts, Povich, & Mather, 2012). Specifically, as of 2018 the USDA reported that 11.8% of Americans were food insecure, a percentage that rises disproportionately for households with children and people of color (Coleman-Jensen et al., 2018). Personal trainers will likely work with individuals for which healthy eating is impacted by financial limitations and should therefore be prepared to support individuals in understanding and navigating options. This may include, but is not limited to:

- Supporting clients in accessing additional support as needed through established programs, such as the Supplemental Nutrition Access Program
- Providing resources upon client request, such as a list of local food pantries
- Collaboratively brainstorming money-saving shopping tips, such as buying in bulk, using coupons, purchasing generic or store brands, and considering frozen over fresh produce when most economical

COLLABORATING WITH REGISTERED DIETITIANS

As discussed earlier in the chapter, the issues, questions, and controversies that surround nutrition are numerous and quite nuanced. Personal trainers should strive to provide clients with the facts and allow for a personalized approach to nutrition, referring them to an RD when needed. Issues that would indicate the need for a referral include, but are not limited to, disordered eating, multiple chronic disease states, client request for meal planning, or a need for detailed nutrition information beyond the scope of practice of a personal trainer. Personal trainers can expand their referral networks by visiting http://www.eatright.org/find-an-expert. It is advised that personal trainers attend local nutrition-related events and conferences and develop community resources through collaboration with other health and exercise professionals.

Fueling Before, During, and After Exercise

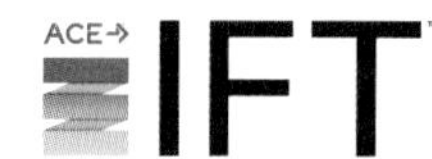

Creating and implementing safe and effective exercise programs for clients can be accomplished effectively through the guidelines set forth in the ACE Integrated Fitness Training® Model, which include asking important questions during the initial interview, selecting appropriate assessments, developing programs that are informed by the results of those assessments, and progressing clients as appropriate.

Physically active individuals need the right types and amounts of food before, during, and after exercise to maximize the amount of energy available to fuel optimal performance and minimize the amount of gastrointestinal distress. Sports nutrition strategies should address three exercise stages: pre-exercise, during exercise, and post-exercise (Figure 6-14).

FIGURE 6-14
Sports nutrition strategies

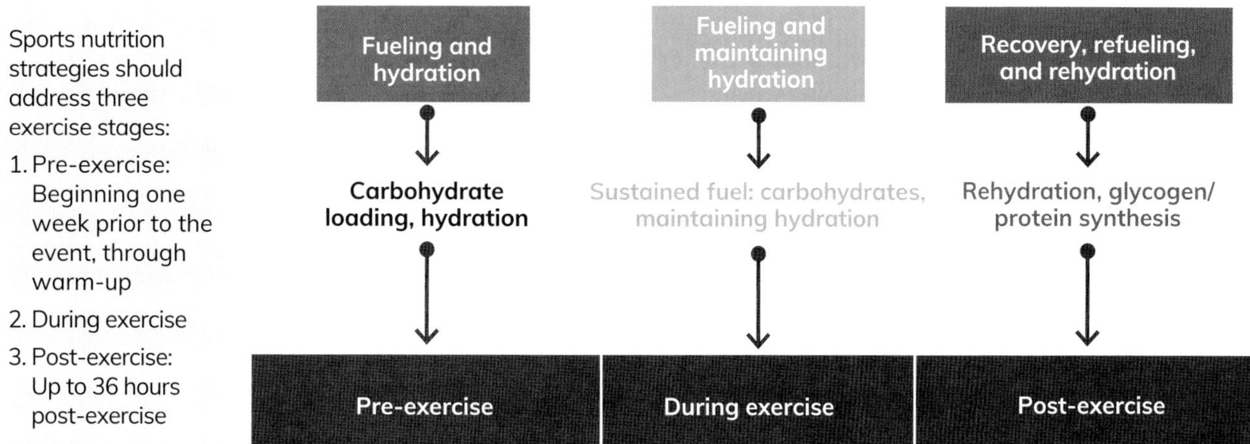

PRE-EXERCISE FUELING

The two main goals of a pre-exercise snack are to (1) optimize **glucose** availability and **glycogen** stores and (2) provide the fuel needed to support exercise performance. Keeping this in mind, in the days up to a week before a strenuous endurance effort, an athlete should consider what nutritional strategies might set the stage for optimal performance. For example,

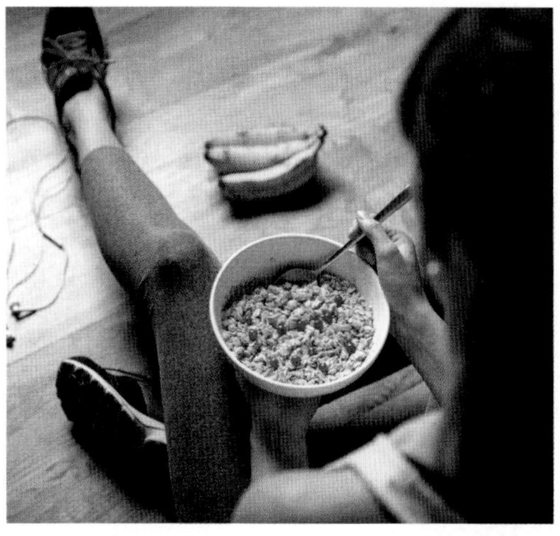

an individual preparing for a long endurance event might consider the pros and cons of **carbohydrate loading.** On the day of the event or an important training session, the athlete should aim to eat a meal about four to six hours prior to the workout to minimize gastrointestinal distress and optimize performance. Four hours after eating, the food will already have been digested and absorbed; now liver and muscle glycogen levels are increased. To translate this into an everyday, practical recommendation, athletes who plan to work out for an extended duration in the early afternoon should be certain to eat a wholesome, carbohydrate-rich breakfast. Those who exercise in the early morning may benefit from a carbohydrate-rich snack before going to bed.

Some research also suggests that eating a relatively small carbohydrate- and protein-containing snack (e.g., 50 grams of carbohydrate and 5 to 10 grams of protein) 30 to 60 minutes before exercise helps increase glucose availability near the end of long-duration workout and helps to decrease exercise-induced protein catabolism (Kreider et al., 2010). The exact timing and size of the snack for peak performance will vary by individual and type of exercise. As a general rule, individuals should try out any snacks or drinks with practice sessions and workouts prior to relying on them to help athletic performance during competition. In general, a pre-exercise or pre-workout meal or snack should be:

- Relatively high in carbohydrate to maximize blood glucose availability (*Note:* Although no DRIs exist for pre-exercise carbohydrate intake, most credible sources recommended 1.0 to 4.5 g of carbohydrate per kg of body weight, depending on the type of food and the time of the exercise or event.)
- Relatively low in fat and fiber to minimize gastrointestinal distress and facilitate gastric emptying
- Moderate in protein
- Approximately 400 to 800 calories—an amount that should fuel the exercise without causing noticeable sluggishness or fullness
- Well-tolerated by the individual

FUELING DURING EXERCISE

The goal of during-exercise fueling is to provide the body with the essential nutrients needed by muscle cells and to maintain optimal blood glucose levels. During a prolonged endurance effort, such as a marathon, an athlete is at risk of "hitting the wall"—a phenomenon often occurring around mile 20 of a marathon. This is when extreme fatigue sets in due to depleted carbohydrate stores. However, there are gradations on the physical demands of exercise based on the duration of the exercise session. Exercise lasting less than one hour can be adequately fueled with existing glucose and glycogen stores. No additional carbohydrate-containing drinks or foods are necessary. When exercise lasts longer than one hour, blood glucose levels begin to dwindle. After one to three hours of continuous moderate-intensity exercise (65 to 80% $\dot{V}O_2max$), muscle glycogen stores may become depleted. If no glucose is consumed, the blood glucose levels drop, resulting in further depletion of muscle and liver glycogen stores. When this happens, regardless of the athlete's mental toughness or desire to maintain intensity, performance falters. To maintain a ready energy supply during a prolonged, moderate-to-vigorous, continuous exercise session (>60 minutes), athletes should consume glucose-containing beverages and snacks. Athletes should consume 30 to 60 grams of carbohydrate per hour of training (Rodriguez, Di Marco, & Langley, 2009). This is especially important for prolonged exercise and exercise in extreme heat, cold, or high altitude; for athletes who did not consume adequate amounts of food or drink prior to the training session; and for athletes who did not carbohydrate load or who restricted energy intake for weight loss.

Carbohydrate consumption during prolonged exercise should begin shortly after the initiation of the exercise. The carbohydrates will be more effective if the 30 to 60 grams per hour are consumed in small amounts in 15- to 20-minute intervals rather than as a large **bolus** after two hours of exercise (Rodriguez, Di Marco, & Langley, 2009). Some experts believe that adding protein to carbohydrate during exercise will help to improve performance, but the evidence is inconclusive.

POST-EXERCISE REPLENISHMENT

The main goal of post-exercise fueling is to replenish glycogen stores and facilitate muscle repair. The average client training at moderate intensities every few days does not need any aggressive post-exercise replenishment. Normal dietary practices following exercise will facilitate recovery within 24 to 48 hours, but athletes following vigorous training regimens, especially those who will participate in multiple training sessions in a single day (e.g., triathletes or athletes participating in training camp for a team sport), will benefit from strategic refueling. Studies show that the best post-workout meals include mostly carbohydrates accompanied by some protein (Kreider et al., 2010). Refueling should begin within 30 minutes after exercise and be followed by a high-carbohydrate meal within two hours (Kreider et al., 2010). The carbohydrates replenish the used-up energy that is normally stored as glycogen in muscle and liver. The protein helps to rebuild the muscles that were fatigued with exercise. A carbohydrate intake of 1.5 g/kg of body weight in the first 30 minutes after exercise and then every two

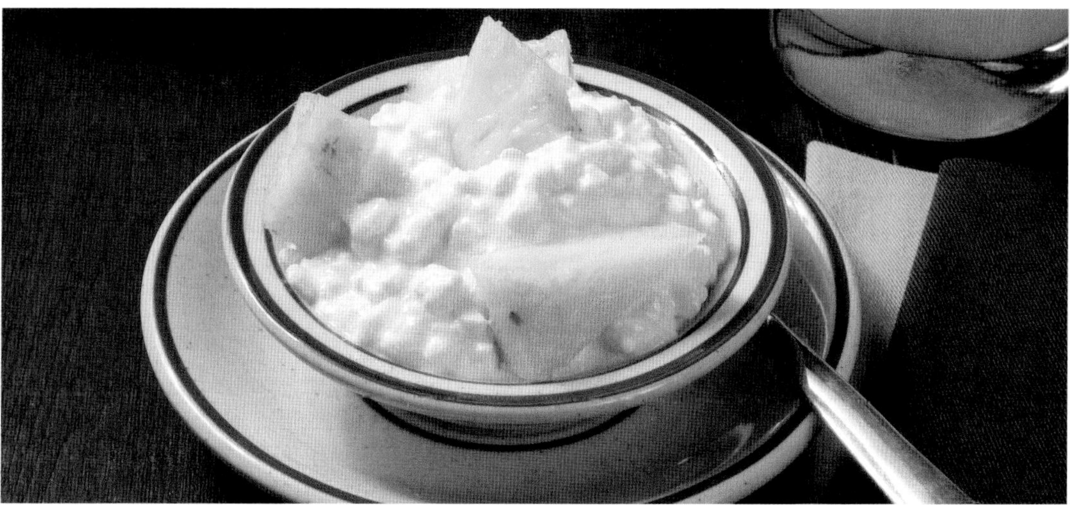

hours for four to six hours is recommended (Rodriguez, Di Marco, & Langley, 2009). After that, the athlete can resume his or her typical, balanced diet. Of course, the amount of refueling necessary depends on the intensity and duration of the training session. A long-duration, low-intensity workout may not require such vigorous replenishment.

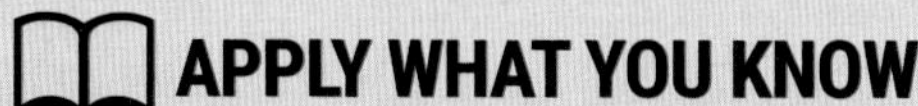

Post-workout Snack and Meal Ideas

In the several hours following a prolonged and strenuous workout, consuming snacks and meals high in carbohydrate with some protein can set the stage for optimal glycogen replenishment and subsequent performance. Here are a few snack and meal ideas that fit the bill:

Snack 1: In the first several minutes after exercise, consume 16 oz of Gatorade or other sports drink, a power gel such as a Clif Shot or GU, and a medium banana. This quickly begins to replenish muscle carbohydrate stores. *Carbohydrates: 73 g; Protein: 1 g; Calories: 296*

Snack 2: After cooling down and showering, grab another quick snack such as 12 oz of orange juice and 1/4 cup of raisins. *Carbohydrates: 70 g; Protein 3 g; Calories: 292*

Small meal appetizer: Enjoy a spinach salad with tomatoes, chickpeas, green beans, and tuna and a whole-grain baguette. *Carbohydrates: 70 g; Protein: 37 g; Calories: 428*

Small meal main course: Replenish with whole-grain pasta with diced tomatoes. *Carbohydrates: 67 g; Protein: 2 g; Calories: 276*

Dessert: After allowing ample time for the day's snacks and meals to digest, finish your refueling program with one cup of frozen yogurt and berries. *Carbohydrates: 61 g; Protein: 8 g; Calories: 276*

Fluid and Hydration Before, During, and After Exercise

When it comes to fluid balance during exercise, it seems like the proverbial double-edged sword: Drinking too little can lead to **dehydration**—a scary condition exercisers have been cautioned against in every text, handout, and presentation on fluid replacement. However, drinking too much plain water—out of fear of not drinking enough—could lead to **hyponatremia** (i.e., low sodium in the blood), a condition less well known and understood, but equally frightening. Here is the good news: the body is very good at handling and normalizing large variations in fluid intake. For this reason, severe hyponatremia and dehydration are rare and generally affect very specific high-risk populations during specific types of activities [i.e., anyone exercising at a low to moderate intensity for an extended period of time (generally four hours or more) while consuming too much water may be at risk]. Both conditions are highly preventable. To prevent dehydration and hyponatremia, the goal is to drink just the right amount of fluid and/or **electrolytes** before, during, and after exercise to maintain a state of **euhydration,** which is a state of "normal" body water content—the perfect balance between "too much" and "not enough" fluid intake (Table 6-4).

TABLE 6-4

Fluid Replacement Recommendations Before, During, and After Exercise

	Fluid	Comments
Before Exercise	▸ Drink 5–7 mL/kg (0.08–0.11 oz/lb) at least 4 hours before exercise (12–17 ounces for a 154-lb individual)	▸ If urine is not produced or is very dark, drink another 3–5 mL/kg (0.05–0.08 oz/lb) two hours before exercise. ▸ Sodium-containing beverages or salted snacks will help retain fluid.
During Exercise	▸ Monitor individual body-weight changes during exercise to estimate sweat loss. ▸ Composition of fluid should include 20–30 mEq/L of sodium, 2–5 mEq/L of potassium, and 5–10% of carbohydrate.	▸ Prevent a >2% loss in body weight. ▸ Amount and rate of fluid replacement depends on individual sweating rate, environment, and exercise duration.
After Exercise	▸ Consumption of normal meals and beverages will restore euhydration. ▸ If rapid recovery is needed, drink 1.5 L/kg (23 oz/lb) of body weight lost.	▸ Goal is to fully replace fluid and electrolyte deficits. ▸ Consuming sodium will help recovery by stimulating thirst and fluid retention.

Reprinted with permission from American College of Sports Medicine (2018). *ACSM's Guidelines for Exercise Testing and Prescription* (10th ed.). Philadelphia: Wolters Kluwer.

HYDRATION BEFORE EXERCISE

Most people begin exercise euhydrated with little need for a rigorous prehydration regimen. However, if fewer than eight to 12 hours have elapsed since the last intense training session or fluid intake has been inadequate, the individual may benefit from a prehydration program.

Some clients may try to hyperhydrate with glycerol-containing solutions that act to expand the extra- and intra-cellular spaces. While glycerol may be advantageous for certain individuals who meet specific criteria, glycerol is unlikely to be advantageous for those who will experience no to mild dehydration during exercise (loss of <2% body weight) and glycerol use may in fact contribute to increased risk of hyponatremia (van Rosendal et al., 2010).

HYDRATION DURING EXERCISE

The goal of fluid intake during exercise is to prevent performance-diminishing or health-altering effects from dehydration or hyponatremia. A personal trainer can share the following guidelines with clients:

- **Aim for a 1:1 fluid replacement to fluid loss ratio:** Ideally, exercisers should consume the same amount of fluid as they lose in sweat. An easy way to assess post-exercise hydration is to compare pre- and post-exercise body weight. The goal is to avoid weight loss greater than 2%. There is no one-size-fits-all recommendation, though if determining individual needs is not feasible, clients should aim to drink 0.4 to 0.8 L/h (8 to 16 oz/h), with the higher rate for faster, heavier individuals in a hot and humid environment and the lower rate for slower, lighter individuals in a cool environment (Sawka et al., 2007). Because people sweat at varying rates and exercise at different intensities, this range may not be appropriate for everyone. However, when individual assessment is not possible, this recommendation works for most people.

- **Drink fluids with sodium during prolonged exercise sessions:** If an exercise session lasts longer than two hours or a client is participating in an event that stimulates heavy sweat (and consequently, sodium) losses, then the client should consider consuming a sports drink that contains elevated levels of sodium. In one study, researchers did not find a benefit from sports drinks that contain only the 18 mmol/L (or 100 milligrams per 8 oz) of sodium typical of most sports drinks and thus concluded that higher levels would be needed to prevent hyponatremia during prolonged exercise (Almond et al., 2005). Table 6-5 presents the sodium content of some popular drinks. The IOM recommends that people exercising for prolonged periods in hot environments consume sports drinks that contain 20 to 30 mEq/L (0.5 to 0.7 g/L) of sodium to stimulate thirst and replace sweat losses and 2 to 5 mEq/L (0.8 to 2.0 g/L) of potassium to replace sweat losses (Rodriguez, Di Marco, & Langley, 2009). Alternatively, exercisers can consume extra sodium with meals and snacks prior to a lengthy exercise session or a day of extensive physical activity. Additional sodium or supplementation with salt tablets seems to be unnecessary based on the limited research on this topic (Hew-Butler et al., 2006; Speedy et al., 2002).
- **Drink carbohydrate-containing sports drinks to reduce fatigue:** Individuals exercising for longer than one hour should also consume carbohydrate with fluids. With prolonged exercise, muscle glycogen stores become depleted and blood glucose becomes a primary fuel source. To maintain performance levels and prevent fatigue, individuals should choose drinks and snacks that provide about 30 to 60 grams of rapidly absorbed carbohydrate for every hour of training. As long as the carbohydrate concentration is about 6 to 8%, it will have little effect on gastric emptying (Rodriguez, Di Marco, & Langley, 2009).

Sports drinks play an important role in replenishing fluids, glucose, and sodium lost during moderate-to-vigorous exercise lasting more than one hour. Although sports drinks

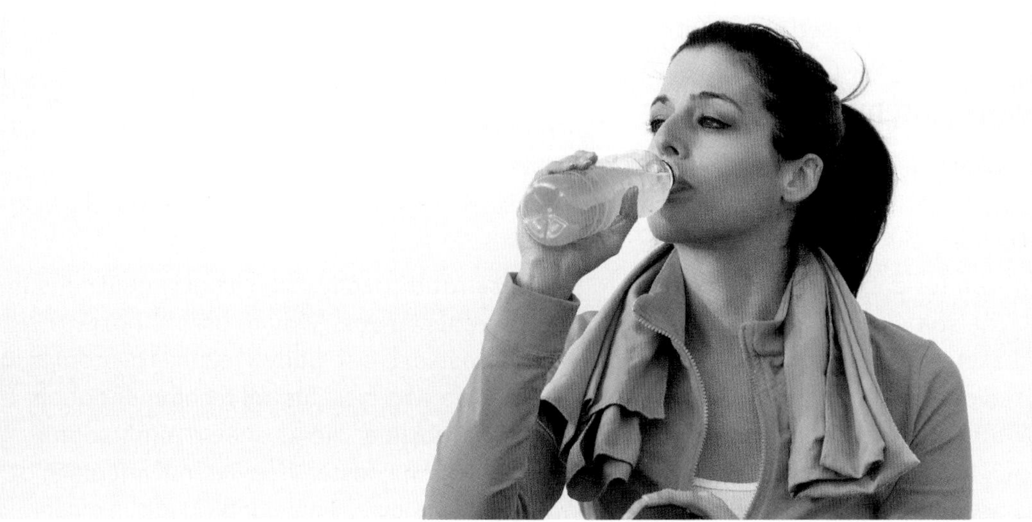

may not completely protect against hyponatremia, they serve an important purpose in endurance exercise. Table 6-5 provides nutritional information for some of the most popular sports drinks.

TABLE 6-5
Evaluating Sports Drinks

Beverage	Serving Size (oz)	Calories (kcal)	Sodium (mg)	Carbohydrate (g)	Carbohydrate Concentration (%)	Sugars (g)
Gatorade Thirst Quencher	12	80	160	22	6.2%	21
Gatorade Endurance formula	12	90	300	22	6.2%	13
Pedialyte*	12	35	370	9	2.5%	9
Powerade	12	78	150	21	5.9%	20.4
Propel	12	0	162	0	0%	0
Ultima	12	0	59	0	0%	0
Zico Coconut Water	12	36	50	8	2.2%	6.4

*Although Pedialyte is not marketed as a sports drink, it is sometimes used by athletes as such.

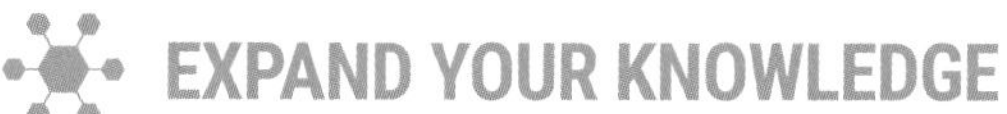

Endurance Training and Hydration Status

Past headlines shared the unlikely but real tragedy of the 28-year-old novice Boston Marathon runner who suffered severe hyponatremia and later died en route to the hospital, as well as the story of the 24-year-old elite runner who collapsed from dehydration while exploring desolate trails in the Grand Canyon's summer heat without sufficient water. In all, a scattering of half marathon and marathon deaths have drawn attention to the safety concerns of these endurance challenges.

Underlying heart conditions, dehydration, and hyponatremia most often are the causes of death during races in young athletes. Sadly, it turns out that not many runners are paying serious attention to hydration. In one study, a whopping 65% of the athletes studied were "not at all" concerned about keeping themselves hydrated (Brown et al., 2011). This nonchalance can come at a cost. Drinking too little can lead to dehydration, which results from a sweat rate that exceeds fluid replenishment. Exercising at very high intensities, exercising in humid conditions, and low fluid intake all increase the likelihood of dehydration. Dehydration, along with high exercise intensity, hot and humid environmental conditions, poor fitness level, incomplete heat **acclimatization,** and a variety of other factors can all raise body temperature and together lead to heat stroke.

While dehydration is a serious concern, individuals should also be aware that drinking too much—out of fear of not drinking enough—could lead to hyponatremia, a less well-known and less understood but equally frightening condition characterized by a low blood sodium level. Exertional hyponatremia results from excessive intake of low-sodium fluids during prolonged endurance activities—that is, drinking a greater volume of fluid than the volume lost in sweat—and possibly, to a lesser extent, from inappropriate fluid retention.

A study of 488 Boston Marathon runners published in the *New England Journal of Medicine* found that 13% (22% of women and 8% of men) had hyponatremia, and 0.6% had critical hyponatremia, at the end of the race. Runners with hyponatremia were more likely to be of low **body mass index,** consume fluids at every mile (and more than 3 liters total throughout the race), finish the race in more than four hours, and gain weight during the run. The greatest predictor of hyponatremia was weight gain, which researchers attributed to excessive fluid intake (Almond et al., 2005). Importantly, hyponatremia is not limited to runners. Anyone exercising at a low to moderate intensity for an extended period of time (generally four hours or more) while consuming too much water can be at risk.

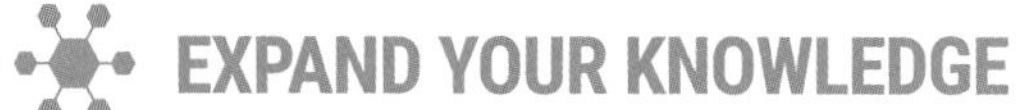

Myth: Drinking Fluids Before and During Exercise Causes Gastrointestinal Distress

Rationale: Since blood flow is diverted away from the gastrointestinal system during exercise, fluids consumed before or during exercise will just sit around sloshing in the stomach during the workout.

The science: It is true that gastric emptying, or the speed with which the stomach empties its contents into the **small intestine,** slows down during exercise. This is largely because exercise-induced sympathetic stimulation diverts blood flow from the gastrointestinal (GI) system to the heart, lungs, and working muscles. As a result, individuals sometimes experience stomach cramps along with a variety of other uncomfortable GI issues such as reflux, heartburn, bloating, gas, nausea, and vomiting. It turns out, though, that good hydration with the right fluids can help increase gastric emptying and lead to reduced GI problems with exercise. Gastric emptying is maximized when the amount of fluid in the stomach is high. On the other hand, high-intensity exercise (>80% $\dot{V}O_2$max), dehydration, **hyperthermia,** and consumption of high-energy (>8% carbohydrate), **hypertonic** drinks (like juices and some soft drinks) slow gastric emptying.

A personal trainer can recommend the following practical tips to prepare the gut for exercise or competition (Brouns & Beckers, 1993):

- Get acclimatized to heat.
- Stay hydrated.
- Practice drinking during training to improve competition-day comfort.
- Avoid eating too much before and during exercise.
- Avoid high-energy, hypertonic food and drinks before (within 30 to 60 minutes) and after exercise. Limit protein and fat intake before exercise.
- Ingest a high-energy, high-carbohydrate diet.
- Avoid high-fiber foods before exercise.
- Limit **nonsteroidal anti-inflammatory drugs (NSAIDs)** such as ibuprofen and naproxen, alcohol, caffeine, antibiotics, and nutritional supplements before and during exercise, as they can cause GI discomfort. The client should experiment during training to identify his or her triggers.
- Urinate and defecate prior to exercise.
- Consult a physician if GI problems persist, especially abdominal pain, diarrhea, or bloody stool.

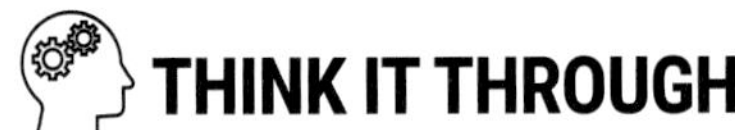

Hydration during Endurance Exercise

Individuals who perform extended endurance activities, such as those lasting an hour or longer, can benefit from drinking fluids containing sodium and carbohydrate. What would you say to a client who wants to know the best approach for hydration during a prolonged endurance running event?

POST-EXERCISE HYDRATION

Following exercise, the client should aim to correct any fluid imbalances that occurred during the exercise session. This includes consuming water to restore hydration, carbohydrates to replenish glycogen stores, and electrolytes to speed rehydration. If the client will have at least 12 hours to recover before the next strenuous workout, rehydration with the usual meals and snacks and water should be adequate. The sodium in the foods will help retain the fluid and stimulate thirst. If rehydration needs to occur quickly, the clients should drink about 1.5 L of fluid for each kilogram (or 0.70 L of fluid for each pound) of body weight lost (Sawka et al., 2007). This will be enough to restore lost fluid and also compensate for increased urine output that occurs with rapid consumption of large amounts of fluid. A severely dehydrated athlete (>7% body weight loss) with symptoms (nausea, vomiting, or diarrhea) may need intravenous fluid replacement and should seek medical attention immediately. Those at greatest risk of hyponatremia should be careful not to consume too much water following exercise and instead should focus on replenishing sodium.

Nutritional Supplements

The Dietary Supplement and Health Education Act (DSHEA) dictates supplement production, marketing, and safety guidelines. The following are the highlights of the legislation. Personal trainers and their clients must be aware that savvy product manufacturers and marketing experts have found ingenious ways to get around some of the rules.

- A dietary supplement is defined as a product (other than tobacco) that functions to supplement the diet and contains one or more of the following ingredients: a vitamin, mineral, herb or other botanical, **amino acid,** a nutritional substance that increases total dietary intake, metabolite, constituent, or extract, or some combination of these ingredients.
- Safety standards provide that the Secretary of the Department of Health & Human Services may declare that a supplement poses imminent risk or hazard to public safety. A supplement is considered **adulterated** if it, or one of its ingredients, presents a "significant or unreasonable risk of illness or injury" when used as directed, or under normal conditions. It may also be considered adulterated if too little information is known about the risk of an unstudied ingredient.
- Supplement labels cannot include claims that the product diagnoses, prevents, mitigates, treats, or cures a specific disease. Instead, they may describe the supplement's effects on the "structure or function" of the body or the "well-being" achieved by consuming the substance. Unlike other health claims, these nutritional support statements are not approved by FDA prior to marketing the supplement.

- Supplements must contain an ingredient label, including the name and quantity of each dietary ingredient. The label must also identify the product as a "dietary supplement" (FDA, 1995).

Many clients experiment with various herbs and supplements. The websites of the FDA (www.fda.gov) and the National Institutes of Health Office of Dietary Supplements (www.ods.od.nih.gov) provide reputable, up-to-date information about numerous supplements and herbs that personal trainers can reference. If a client is also on medications, there is risk for drug-supplement interactions, and it is important to recommend that the client disclose and discuss this with a doctor, pharmacist, or highly qualified RD.

Personal trainers should endeavor to provide clients with evidence-based educational resources on the effectiveness of various nutritional supplements. This will ensure clients are able to make informed decisions and fully understand how consumption of these products will impact their health, performance, and training. Personal trainers should take a conservative approach to discussing supplements, always being mindful of their scope of practice.

A critical issue that must be initially addressed pertaining to nutritional supplements is safety. In the scientific literature, when no side effects have been reported, this has been interpreted to mean that the nutritional supplement in question is safe for the length of time and dosages evaluated (Kerksick et al., 2018). Nutritional supplements found to have sound theoretical rationale with the majority of available research in relevant populations using appropriate dosing regimens demonstrating their safety are placed into the category of "strong evidence to support efficacy and apparently safe" (Kerksick et al., 2018).

NUTRITIONAL SUPPLEMENTS WITH STRONG EVIDENCE TO SUPPORT EFFICACY AND APPARENT SAFETY

Creatine

It has been suggested that the most effective supplement available to fitness enthusiasts to increase high-intensity exercise performance and muscle mass is creatine monohydrate (Kerksick et al., 2018). Indeed, there is a mountain of scientific literature demonstrating that creatine supplementation increases skeletal muscle mass during exercise training.

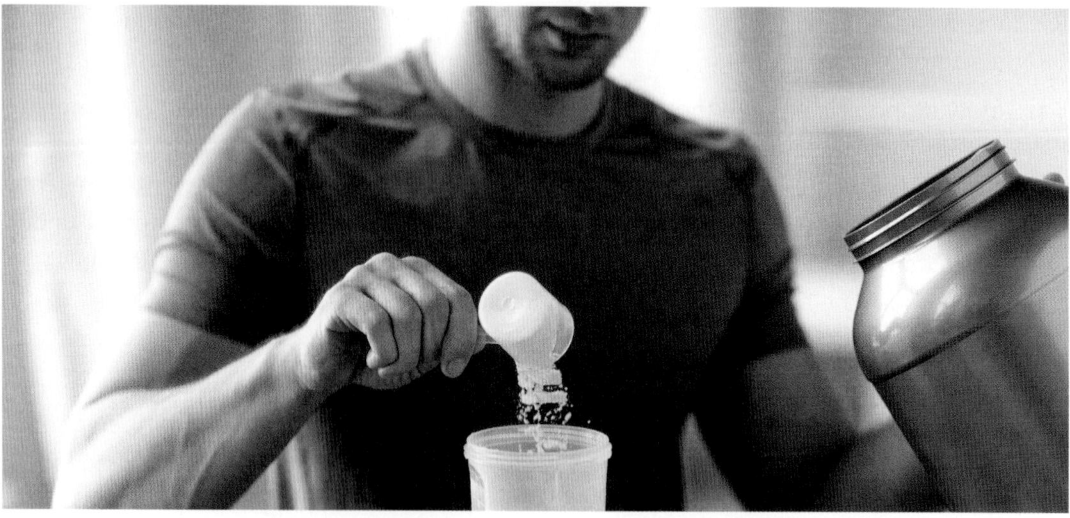

Moreover, the long-term safety of creatine monohydrate has been well-established. Creatine is an essential substrate for the **phosphagen energy system** and involved in **adenosine triphosphate (ATP)** regeneration during high-intensity exercise. As such, creatine supplementation has also been shown to result in an enhanced ability to match cellular ATP production and demand during high-intensity and repeated bouts of intense exercise. Creatine supplementation can increase creatine storage in skeletal muscle with a loading phase (20 to 25 grams/day for five to seven days), followed by a maintenance dose of 3 to 5 grams/day.

Caffeine

Caffeine is a natural stimulant found in coffee, tea, and also many nutritional supplements. There is robust scientific evidence demonstrating that caffeine ingestion serves as effective **ergogenic** aid for **aerobic** and **anaerobic** exercise performance. Caffeine ingested orally is quickly absorbed into the bloodstream and peaks within 30 to 60 minutes. Caffeine mechanistically effects the **central nervous system,** primarily by antagonism of adenosine receptors, which results in enhanced mood, reduced perception of pain, and increased attention. At the skeletal muscle level, caffeine ingestion promotes enhanced sodium/potassium pump activity, greater calcium release from the **sarcoplasmic reticulum,** and increased **fat oxidation/glycogen sparing**. Overall, it has been recommended that a dosage of ~3 to 6 mg/kg of body weight of caffeine ingested 30 to 60 minutes prior to exercise will increase work capacity, time to exhaustion, and reduced perceived effort during endurance exercise (Naderi et al., 2016).

Post-exercise Carbohydrate Ingestion

This is a classic nutritional recommendation for recreational enthusiasts and athletes alike. After prolonged and exhaustive endurance-related exercise, the most important factor determining the timeframe to recovery is muscle glycogen replenishment (Ivy, 2004). It has been well established for quite some time that post-exercise carbohydrate ingestion is critical to synthesis of muscle glycogen. More recently, both the precise timing of carbohydrate ingestion and optimal carbohydrate dosage have become better understood (Beelen et al., 2010). Post-exercise muscle glycogen replenishment occurs in two phases—a rapid rate that persists for 30 to 60 minutes after exercise cessation and a considerably reduced rate (60 to 90%) in the time period afterward. There is also evidence for a dose-response relationship between post-exercise dosage of carbohydrate ingestion and the rate of muscle glycogen resynthesis. For example, it has been shown that administration of 1.2 grams/kg/hour of carbohydrate increased muscle glycogen content 150% more than 0.8 grams/kg/hour. However, ingestion of 1.6 grams/kg/hour provided no further increase in muscle glycogen content. Importantly, eating carbohydrates in smaller amounts over time is more effective at restoring muscle glycogen than eating one or two larger amounts less frequently. In summary, to optimize muscle glycogen repletion post-exercise, it has been recommended to ingest 1.2 grams/kg/hour of carbohydrate at 15- to 30-minute intervals immediately upon exercise termination (Beelen et al., 2010).

Protein Supplementation

Many people use protein supplements to boost protein intake and ensure consumption of a particular protein type or amino acid. To aid in efficient **digestion** and **absorption,** most protein supplements are sold as **hydrolysates,** which are short amino-acid chains of partially digested protein. **Whey** and **casein** tend to be the most popular.

Whey, the liquid remaining after milk has been curdled and strained, is a high-quality protein that contains all of the **essential amino acids.** There are three varieties of whey—whey protein powder, whey protein concentrate, and whey protein isolate—all of which provide high levels of the essential and **branched-chain amino acids (BCAAs),** vitamins, and minerals. Whey powder is 11 to 15% protein and is used as an additive in many food products. Whey concentrate is 25 to 89% protein, while whey isolate is 90+% protein; both forms are commonly used in supplements. Notably, while the isolate is nearly pure whey, the proteins can become denatured during the manufacturing process, decreasing the supplements' usefulness. Unlike the other whey forms, the isolate is lactose-free (Hoffman & Falvo, 2004). Studies of whey protein have found that whey offers numerous health benefits, including increased muscle **hypertrophy** and muscular strength (when combined with muscular training) and bone growth (Hayes & Cribb, 2008).

Casein, the source of the white color of milk, accounts for 70 to 80% of milk protein. Casein exists in what is known as a **micelle,** a compound similar to a soap sud that has a water-averse inside and water-loving outside. This property allows the protein to provide a sustained slow release of amino acids into the bloodstream, sometimes lasting for hours. Some studies suggest that combined supplementation with casein and whey offers the greatest muscular strength improvements following a 10-week intensive muscular-training program (Kerksick et al., 2006).

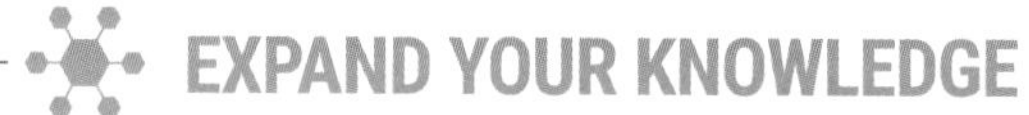

Is There a Need for Protein Supplementation?

Supplemental protein use is a common practice among both recreational exercisers and athletes striving to enhance gains in strength and muscle mass following workouts and is often a controversial topic (Morton et al., 2018). Many Americans consume more protein than the current recommendations for protein intake call for, which includes an AMDR of 10 to 35% for adults 19 and older (USDA, 2015) and an RDA of 0.8 g/kg/day (IOM, 2006). The needs for athletes are 1.2 to 2.0 g/kg/day (Academy of Nutrition and Dietetics, American College of Sports Medicine, and Dietitians of Canada, 2016), with specific needs for optimal adaptation being based on experience level, nutrient needs, athletic goals, and training and competition timing within a periodized program.

So, is supplemental protein needed? According to a systematic review of 49 studies presented by Morton et al. (2018), protein supplementation may augment resistance-training adaptations. The following observations about protein supplementation were made:

- Supplementation augments increases in **one-repetition maximum (1-RM)** strength and **fat-free mass (FFM).**
- Supplementation is more effective in resistance-trained individuals compared to novices but is less effective with increasing chronological age.
- The benefits do not increase with intakes above 1.6 g/kg/day.
- The current RDA may not be enough to maximize strength and FFM with resistance training.
- Resistance training alone is the more important stimulus, and timing of intake plays a minor, if any, role in influencing gains.

Sodium Bicarbonate

It is well known that recovery from **cellular acidosis** is paramount in order to restore the capacity to regenerate ATP from both the phosphagen system and **glycolysis.** Muscle **buffering capacity** can be augmented by nutritional strategies. Indeed, alkalizing agents have been studied extensively for their potential to enhance performance by attenuating the extent to which metabolic acidosis contributes to fatigue during high-intensity exercise performance (Peart et al., 2012). One such alkalizing substance that has been found to improve recovery by increasing the muscle buffering capacity is sodium bicarbonate. The mechanism by which sodium bicarbonate ingestion mediates an ergogenic effect is by promoting removal of protons from the **skeletal muscle milieu.** Given the fact that increased concentrations of proton molecules within the muscle cell are detrimental to skeletal muscle performance, it should be recognized that an increased rate of removal from the skeletal muscle environment will result in a more rapid recovery. This in turn will permit a better performance of subsequent high-intensity exercise bouts.

The main drawback to using sodium bicarbonate is that some individuals experience gastrointestinal distress with its ingestion. Accordingly, it has been recommended to first purposefully experiment with the sodium bicarbonate–loading protocols to maximize the alkalizing effects and minimize the risk of potential symptoms. The recommended dosage and timeframe for sodium bicarbonate ingestion is 0.2 to 0.4 grams/kg with 1 liter of fluids at 60 to 120 minutes pre-exercise (Peart et al., 2012). Sodium bicarbonate can be ingested either in capsule form or in a flavored beverage.

β-alanine

The amino acid β-alanine is naturally occurring and found in foods such as fish and meat. β-alanine is also a precursor and rate-limiting molecule for synthesis of carnosine. Carnosine itself is found in skeletal muscle and has numerous important physiological functions, including calcium, **enzyme,** and pH regulation. Therefore, β-alanine supplementation has been heavily studied given its potential mechanistic ergogenic benefits. The case for β-alanine supplementation appears to be quite clear. In a meta-analysis, it was reported that performance of high-intensity exercise lasting between 60 and 240 seconds benefited from β-alanine supplementation (Hobson et al., 2012). In terms of the most efficacious dosage, 3 to 6 grams per day of β-alanine for a duration of four to 10 weeks has been recommended (Naderi et al., 2016). Beyond that timeframe, a maintenance dosage of 1.2 grams per day of β-alanine has been suggested (Naderi et al., 2016).

NUTRITIONAL SUPPLEMENTS WITH LITTLE TO NO EVIDENCE TO SUPPORT EFFICACY AND/OR APPARENT SAFETY

A myth can be defined as an untrue explanation for a natural phenomenon. Unfortunately, numerous myths remain pervasive and well-engrained throughout the fitness industry, in particular as it pertains to various nutritional supplements. In this section are a list of nutritional supplements with little to no evidence to support efficacy and/or safety.

Glutamine

Glutamine is an amino acid that is used in the biosynthesis of proteins. It was originally suggested that glutamine supplementation might simulate protein synthesis and thereby promote enhanced muscular performance. However, more recent research has found glutamine supplementation does not benefit muscular performance and, therefore, it has been concluded that there is insufficient scientific evidence to support glutamine supplementation for increases in **lean body mass** and/or muscular performance (Kerksick et al., 2018).

Arginine

Arginine is an amino acid that is used in the biosynthesis of proteins. In the body, arginine changes into the potent **vasodilator** nitric oxide. Given that nitric oxide is known to promote **vasodilation** and enhance skeletal muscle blood flow, it has been suggested that arginine supplementation may increase exercise performance (Alvares et al., 2011). However, the majority of the other published scientific literature regarding arginine supplementation have not reported a beneficial ergogenic result (Kerksick et al., 2018).

Carnitine

Carnitine is an ammonium compound produced by the liver and kidneys. It serves as a transporter of long-chain fatty acids into the **mitochondria** to be oxidized for energy production and therefore plays a key role in the regulation of **lipid** metabolism. Accordingly, both scientists and sport nutritionists alike have entertained the notion that supplementation could increase the **bioavailability** of carnitine and enhance overall capacity for lipid metabolism. Nevertheless, to date, the majority of research findings on carnitine supplementation reports it does not significantly alter total muscle carnitine content, enhance lipid metabolism, improve exercise performance, and/or elicit weight loss in individuals with overweight or obesity (Kerksick et al., 2018).

Chronic Use of Antioxidants

It has been conventional wisdom that antioxidant supplementation may benefit exercise performance by countering the increase in **free radicals** associated with exercise because of the long- and well-established link between cell damage and free radicals. Several key studies (Teixeira et al., 2009; Gomez-Cabrera et al., 2008; Close et al., 2006) questioned the effectiveness of the antioxidant supplementation strategy altogether, as it has been demonstrated that antioxidant supplementation hampers favorable exercise training adaptations and interferes with the recovery process.

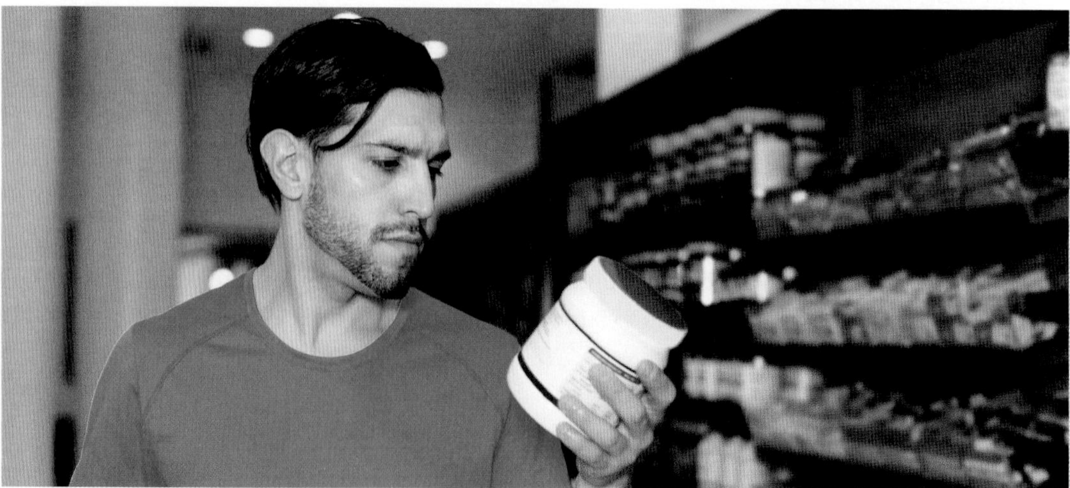

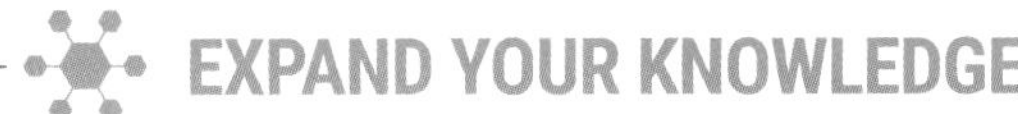

EXPAND YOUR KNOWLEDGE

Supplement Labels

The FDA does not closely regulate dietary supplements and provides no guarantee that the nutrients and ingredients contained in a supplement label are actually what exists in the product. However, the FDA does have some rules for supplement labeling.

When it comes to supplements, the nutrition label is referred to as a Supplement Fact panel. Items that must be listed in the Supplement Fact panel include:

- Names and quantities of dietary ingredients, serving size, and servings per container
- Total calories, total fat, saturated fat, added sugars, cholesterol, sodium, total carbohydrate, dietary fiber, sugars, protein, vitamin D, potassium, calcium, and iron when present in measurable amounts
- Any vitamin, mineral, or other nutrient added to the product for the purpose of supplementation, or if a claim is made about them
- Percent daily values for all ingredients for which the FDA has established daily values (except for protein and when supplements are intended for children less than four years of age)

In addition to the Supplement Fact panel, supplement packaging must include the name of the dietary supplement, the amount of the supplement, the ingredient list, and the name and location of the manufacturer, packer, or distributor.

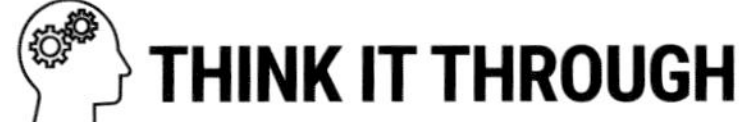

THINK IT THROUGH

Discussing Supplements with Clients

Recommending supplements to clients is outside of the personal trainer's scope of practice. However, personal trainers should be prepared to discuss information about the safety and efficacy of supplements, as well as supplement regulation, as can be found within trusted resources and in the public domain. When discussing supplements with clients, it is critical that the information provided does not come across as an endorsement and that a referral is made to a qualified medical professional or RD when considering supplements. How would you respond to a client asking for specific supplement recommendations without advising or endorsing, while making a referral at the same time?

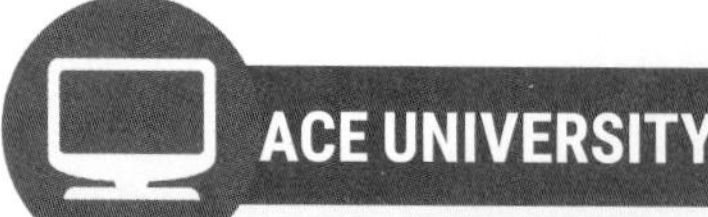

If your study program includes the ACE University, visit www.ACEfitness.org/MyACE and log in to your My ACE Account to take full advantage of the ACE Personal Trainer Study Program and online guided study experience.

A variety of media to support and expand on the material in this text is provided to facilitate learning and best prepare you for the ACE Personal Trainer Certification exam and a career as a personal trainer.

SUMMARY

An individual's health is greatly influenced by the foods he or she consumes. While each nutrient plays a specific role in the body's well-being, it is the balance among these different nutrients that allows for most optimal functioning and prevention of chronic diseases. The *Dietary Guidelines* emphasize a movement away from a focus on specific nutrients toward an overall healthy eating pattern. Personal trainers are ideally positioned to not only support and spread this message, but also to use the nutrition tools and tips to empower clients to translate recommendations into real and practical nutrition changes.

Ultimately, by having a firm understanding of the *Dietary Guidelines* and its associated tools, personal trainers can incorporate nutrition education based upon these resources into their work while simultaneously staying within scope of practice and safely maximizing impact.

REFERENCES

Academy of Nutrition and Dietetics, Dietitians of Canada, and American College of Sports Medicine (2016). Position of the Academy of Nutrition and Dietetics, Dietitians of Canada, and the American College of Sports Medicine: Nutrition and athletic performance. *Journal of the Academy of Nutrition and Dietetics*, 116, 3, 501–528.

Almond, L. et al. (2005). Hyponatremia among runners in the Boston Marathon. *New England Journal of Medicine*, 352, 15, 1550–1556.

Alvares, T.S. et al. (2011). L-arginine as a potential ergogenic aid in healthy subjects. *Sports Medicine*, 41, 233–248.

American College of Sports Medicine (2018). *ACSM's Guidelines for Exercise Testing and Prescription* (10th ed.). Philadelphia: Wolters Kluwer.

Beelen, M. et al. (2010). Nutritional strategies to promote postexercise recovery. *International Journal of Sport Nutrition and Exercise Metabolism*, 20, 515–532.

Brouns, F. & Beckers, E. (1993). Is the gut an athletic organ? Digestion, absorption and exercise. *Sports Medicine*, 15, 242–257.

Brown, S. et al. (2011). Lack of awareness of fluid needs among participants at a midwest marathon. *Sports Health: A Multidisciplinary Approach*, 3, 5, 451–454.

Centers for Disease Control and Prevention (2011). *CDC Estimates of Foodborne Illness in the United States*. www.cdc.gov/foodborneburden/PDFs/FACTSHEET_A_FINDINGS_updated4-13.pdf

Close, G.L. et al. (2006). Ascorbic acid supplementation does not attenuate post-exercise muscle soreness following muscle-damaging exercise but may delay the recovery process. *The British Journal of Nutrition*, 95, 976–981.

Coleman-Jensen, A. et al. (2018). *Household Food Security in the United States in 2018*. https://www.ers.usda.gov/webdocs/publications/90023/err256_summary.pdf?v=0

Eckel R.H. et al. (2014). 2013 AHA/ACC guideline on lifestyle management to reduce cardiovascular risk: A report of the American College of Cardiology/American Heart Association Task Force on Practice Guidelines. *Journal of the American College of Cardiology*, 63, 25 Pt B, 2960–2984.

Fayh, A.P.T. et al. (2013). Effects of 5% weight loss through diet or diet plus exercise on cardiovascular parameters of obese: A randomized clinical trial. *European Journal of Nutrition*, 52, 1443–1450.

Food and Nutrition Board (2012). *Front-of-Package Nutrition Rating Systems and Symbols: Promoting Healthier Choices*. Washington, D.C.: National Academies Press.

Food and Nutrition Board (2010). *Examination of Front-of-Package Nutrition Rating Systems and Symbols: Phase 1 Report*. Washington, D.C.: National Academies Press.

Gomez-Cabrera, M.C. et al. (2008). Oral administration of vitamin C decreases muscle mitochondrial biogenesis and hampers training-induced adaptations in endurance performance. *The American Journal of Clinical Nutrition*, 87, 142–149.

Hall, K.D. et al. (2011). Quantification of the effect of energy imbalance on bodyweight. *The Lancet*, 378, 9793, 826–837.

Hayes, A. & Cribb, P.J. (2008). Effect of whey protein isolate on strength, body composition, and muscle hypertrophy during resistance training. *Current Opinions in Clinical Nutrition and Metabolic Care*, 11, 40–44.

Hew-Butler, T.D. et al. (2006). Sodium supplementation is not required to maintain serum sodium concentrations during an Ironman triathlon. *British Journal of Sports Medicine*, 40, 3, 255–259.

Hobson, R.M. et al. (2012). Effects of β-alanine supplementation on exercise performance: A meta-analysis. *Amino Acids*, 43, 25–37.

Hoffman, J.R. & Falvo, M.J. (2004). Protein: Which is best? *Journal of Sports Science and Medicine*, 3, 118–130.

Institute of Medicine (2006). *Dietary Reference Intakes: The Essential Guide to Nutrient Requirements*. Washington, D.C.: National Academies Press.

Ivy, J.L. (2004). Regulation of muscle glycogen repletion, muscle protein synthesis and repair following exercise. *Journal of Sports Science and Medicine*, 3, 131–138.

Kerksick, C.M. et al. (2018). ISSN exercise & sports nutrition review update: Research & recommendations. *Journal of the International Society of Sports Nutrition*, 15, 38.

Kerksick, C.M. et al. (2006). The effects of protein and amino acid supplementation on performance and training adaptations during ten weeks of resistance training. *Journal of Strength and Conditioning Research*, 20, 3, 643–653.

Kreider, R.B. et al. (2010). ISSN exercise & sport nutrition review: Research & recommendations. *Journal of the International Society of Sports Nutrition*, 7, 7.

Morton, R.W. et al. (2018). A systematic review, meta-analysis and meta-regression of the effect of protein supplementation on resistance training-induced gains in muscle mass and strength in healthy adults. *British Journal of Sports Medicine*, 52, 376–384.

Naderi, A. et al. (2016). Timing, optimal dose and intake duration of dietary supplements with evidence-based use in sports nutrition. *Journal of Exercise Nutrition & Biochemistry*, 20, 1–12.

Nikolaus, C.J. et al. (2016). Grocery store (or supermarket) tours as an effective nutrition education medium: A systematic review. *Journal of Nutrition, Education and Behavior*, 48, 8, 544–554.e1.

Peart, D.J. et al. (2012). Practical recommendations for coaches and athletes: A meta-analysis of sodium bicarbonate use for athletic performance. *Journal of Strength and Conditioning Research*, 26, 1975–1983.

Roberts, B., Povich, D., & Mather, M. (2012). *The Working Poor Family Project, Policy Brief: Low-Income Working Families: The Growing Economic Gap.* http://www.workingpoorfamilies.org/wpcontent/uploads/2013/01/Winter-2012_2013-WPFP-Data-Brief.pdf

Rodriguez, N.R., Di Marco, N.M., & Langley, S. (2009). American College of Sports Medicine position stand: Nutrition and athletic performance. *Medicine & Science in Sports & Exercise*, 41, 709–731.

Sallis, J.F. & N. Owen. (2015). Ecological models of health behavior. In: Glanz, K. (Ed.) *Health Behavior: Theory, Research, and Practice* (5th ed.). Hoboken, N.J.: John Wiley & Sons.

Sawka, M.N. et al. (2007). American College of Sports Medicine position stand: Exercise and fluid replacement. *Medicine & Science in Sports & Exercise*, 39, 2, 377–390.

Spahn J.M. et al. (2010). State of the evidence regarding behavior change theories and strategies in nutrition counseling to facilitate health and food behavior change. *Journal of the American Dietetic Association*, 110, 6, 879–891.

Speedy, D.B. et al. (2002). Oral salt supplementation during ultradistance exercise. *Clinical Journal of Sport Medicine*, 12, 5, 279–284.

Teixeira, V.H. et al. (2009). Antioxidants do not prevent postexercise peroxidation and may delay muscle recovery. *Medicine and Science in Sports and Exercise*, 41, 1752–1760.

U.S. Department of Agriculture (2015). *2015-2020 Dietary Guidelines for Americans* (8th ed.) www.health.gov/dietaryguidelines

U.S. Department of Health & Human Services (2018). *Physical Activity Guidelines for Americans* (2nd ed.). www.health.gov/paguidelines/

U.S. Food & Drug Administration (2004). *How to Understand and Use the Nutrition Facts Label.* www.fda.gov/Food/IngredientsPackagingLabeling/LabelingNutrition/ucm274593.htm#calories

U.S. Food and Drug Administration (1995). *Dietary Supplement Health and Education Act of 1994.* https://ods.od.nih.gov/About/DSHEA_Wording.aspx

van Rosendal, S.P. et al. (2010). Guidelines for glycerol use in hyperhydration and rehydration associated with exercise. *Sports Medicine*, 40, 2, 113–129.

SUGGESTED READING

U.S. Department of Agriculture (2015). *2015-2020 Dietary Guidelines for Americans* (8th ed.). www.health.gov/dietaryguidelines

SECTION III

Assessments, Programming, and Progressions

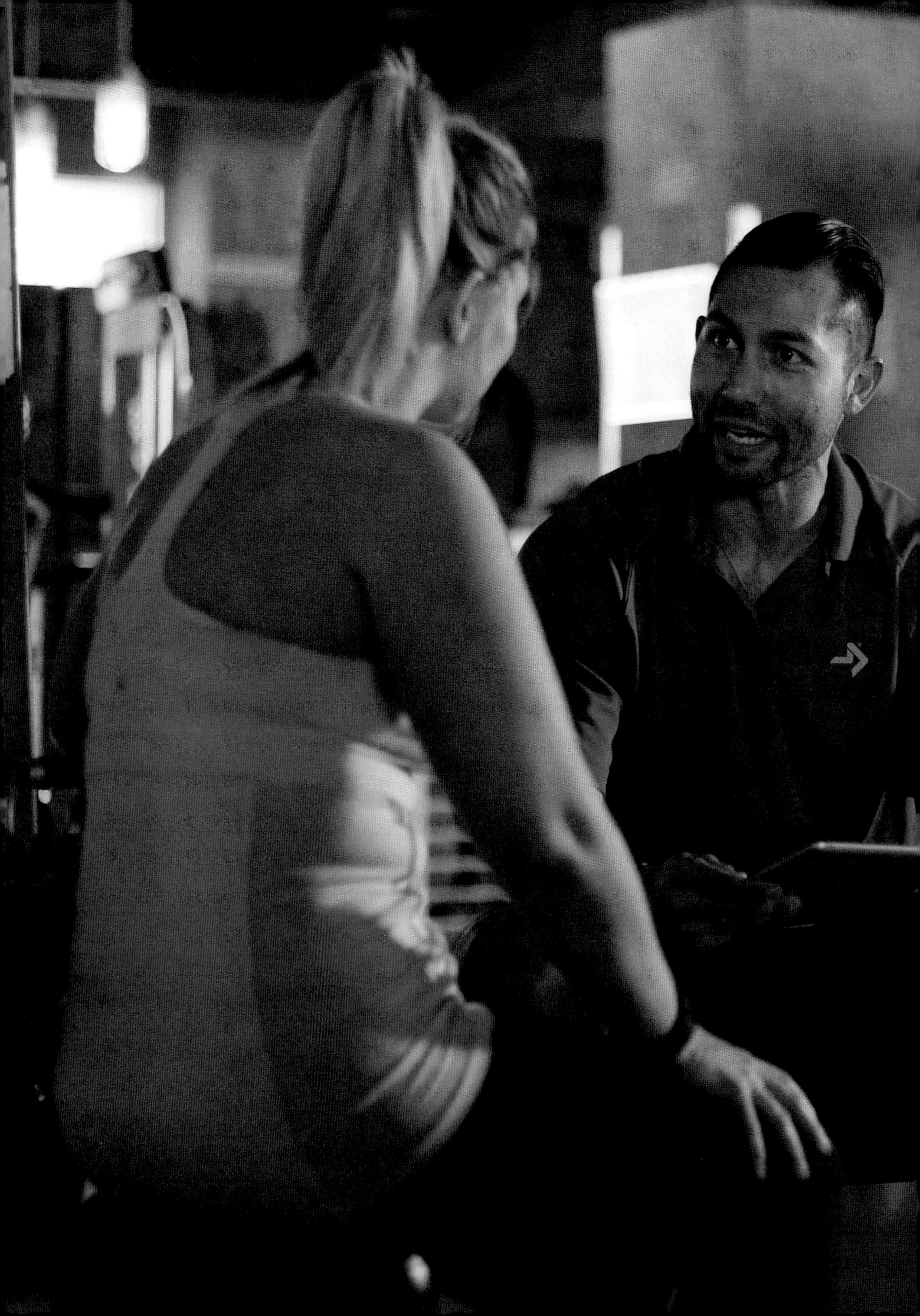

CHAPTER 7

Resting Assessments and Anthropometric Measurements

JAMES S. SKINNER, PhD
Senior Advisor for Exercise Science, American Council on Exercise; Professor Emeritus, Indiana University; Former President, American College of Sports Medicine

IN THIS CHAPTER

LEARNING OBJECTIVES:

Upon completion of this chapter, the reader will be able to:

- Explain the need for proper sequencing of assessments taken at rest
- Describe how to measure heart rate and blood pressure at rest and the conditions under which they should be measured
- Identify the various methods to estimate body composition and explain the advantages and disadvantages of each
- Explain the practical reasons for using body mass index, as well as its limitations for estimating overweight and obesity
- Identify anatomical landmarks and assessment protocols associated with various circumference measurements

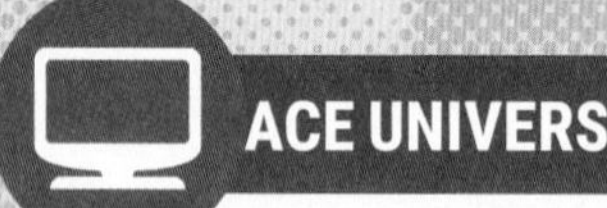

If your study program includes the ACE University, visit www.ACEfitness.org/MyACE and log in to your My ACE Account to take full advantage of the ACE Personal Trainer Study Program and online guided study experience.

A variety of media to support and expand on the material in this text is provided to facilitate learning and best prepare you for the ACE Personal Trainer Certification exam and a career as a personal trainer.

It has been standard practice to conduct physiological assessments at the beginning of the client–personal trainer relationship. Traditionally, these baseline assessments are conducted in an effort to:

- Identify areas of health/injury risk for potential referral to the appropriate healthcare professional(s)
- Collect baseline data that can be used to develop a personalized cardiorespiratory and muscular training program and allow for comparison of subsequent evaluations
- Educate clients about their present physical condition and health risks by comparing their results to normative data for age and sex
- Motivate clients by helping them establish realistic goals

Sequencing Assessments

There is debate over the timing and specific modalities that are chosen during an initial assessment. The justification for assessments in this initial session is based on the long-standing notion that some, if not all, assessments need to be conducted at the beginning of the client–personal trainer relationship to collect baseline information from which personalized programming can be developed. ACE® Certified Personal Trainers need to be aware that not all clients need or desire a complete fitness assessment from the start. In fact, assessments may demotivate some individuals, as they may feel uncomfortable, intimidated, overwhelmed, or embarrassed by their current physical condition, their inadequacies in performing the assessment protocols, or even by the fear of the results. Proper assessment selection can mitigate some of these considerations. There is also the argument that some clients will be motivated after an assessment, once they realize what their health and fitness status is and what could be done to make improvements. Chapters 8 and 10 detail a variety of physiological assessments that can be performed, as well as the populations that likely would benefit from such assessments. Regardless of the assessments selected and how the assessment timelines are structured, personal trainers should remember that a preparticipation health screening *must* be included (see Chapter 5).

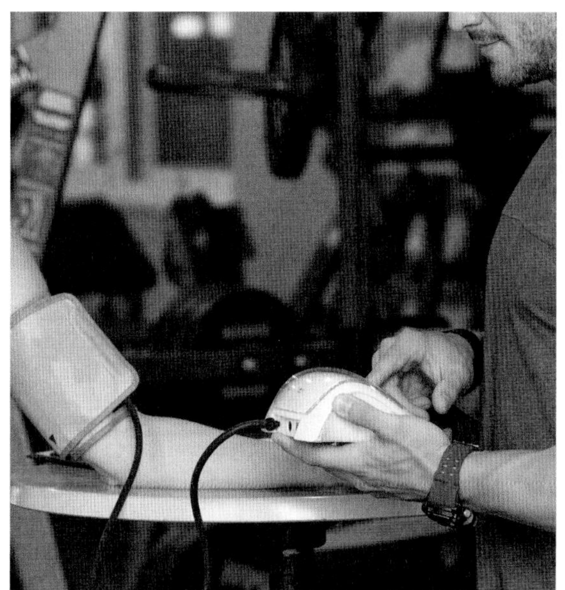

Savvy personal trainers must have a good understanding of the client's needs, determine the appropriate assessment battery, and then create a suitable timeline for when the assessments will be conducted (if at all). It is important to understand each client's needs and goals and to be empathetic when evaluating the relevance and timing of assessments.

APPLY WHAT YOU KNOW

Building Self-efficacy by Choosing the Right Assessments

Many new clients will begin a program with very low **self-efficacy** for exercise ability and program success. As a personal trainer, what are you doing to combat this issue from the very start? Because past performance experience is a critical source of self-efficacy information, each early experience should be focused on creating success and building confidence. A mistake many exercise professionals make is to schedule an entire session of assessments. Put yourself in the client's place: How do assessments make you feel? When a person is new to exercise and/or has **obesity**, what is the likely result of the assessments? Ultimately, each client should leave the first session feeling successful and looking forward to the next. Determine which assessments (if any) are necessary and conduct only those assessments [see Chapters 8 and 10 for information on selecting appropriate assessments in conjunction with the ACE Integrated Fitness Training® (ACE IFT®) Model]. In some cases, a personal trainer may elect to collect all the assessment information needed by simply observing a client's movement techniques during an introductory workout session. Decisions regarding assessment administration (and whether or not to conduct them) may positively affect **rapport** and help build client self-efficacy, enjoyment, success, and program **adherence**.

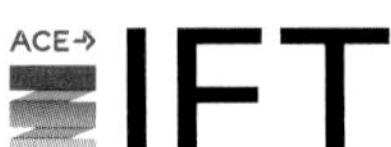

The assessments that merit consideration generally include the following:

- Resting vital signs [**heart rate (HR), blood pressure (BP),** height, and weight]
- Static posture and movement assessments (see Chapter 10)
- Joint **flexibility** and muscle length (see Chapter 10)
- Balance and core function (see Chapter 10)
- **Cardiorespiratory fitness** (see Chapter 8)
- **Body composition** and **anthropometry**
- **Muscular fitness** (**muscular endurance** and **muscular strength**) (see Chapter 10)
- Skill-related parameters (**agility, coordination, power, reactivity,** and **speed**) (see Chapter 10)

Table 7-1 presents a suggested template that personal trainers can follow when sequencing assessments relevant to clients' needs, preferences, and desires. However, personal trainers should perform assessments only after they have reviewed their client's preparticipation health-screening questionnaire (see Figure 5-2, page 141) and conducted an initial interview to identify important program variables based on readiness to change behavior, stage of behavioral change, and general goals (see Chapters 3 and 4).

Physiological influences on an assessment must be considered when establishing the assessment sequence and timeline for a client. For example, resting BP and HR should be measured before any exertion to avoid recording a value that is artificially high and

TABLE 7-1
Sample Assessment Sequence

1st session—Preparticipation health screening
▸ ACSM exercise preparticipation health-screening questionnaire and algorithm ▸ Physical Activity Readiness Questionnaire for Everyone (PAR-Q+) ▸ Lifestyle and health-history questionnaire ▸ Medical clearance if necessary ▪ Medical release form ▸ Resting measures and vital signs ▪ Heart rate, blood pressure, height, and weight
1st or 2nd session
▸ Static postural assessment (frontal, sagittal, and transverse views) ▸ Static balance ▪ Unipedal stance test ▸ Movement assessments (squat, step-up, shoulder-push stabilization, standing row, and thoracic spine mobility) ▸ Joint flexibility and muscle length ▪ Thomas test ▪ Passive straight-leg raise ▪ Shoulder flexion/extension assessment
Weeks 1–8
▸ Cardiorespiratory fitness assessments if necessary (client is in, or ready to progress to, the Fitness or Performance Training phases of the ACE Integrated Fitness Training Model) ▪ Talk test or submaximal talk test for VT1 ▪ VT2 assessment ▸ Core function ▪ McGill's torso muscular endurance test battery ▸ Body composition and anthropometry if necessary ▸ Muscular fitness ▪ Muscular endurance (push-up and body-weight squat) ▪ Muscular strength [1-RM testing (bench-press, squat, or estimated)]
Week 9 and beyond
▸ Skill-related assessments ▪ Dynamic balance (Y balance test) for athletic populations and clients with sport-related goals ▪ Muscular power (vertical jump assessment) ▪ Speed, agility, and quickness (T-test)

Note: VT1 = First ventilatory threshold; VT2 = Second ventilatory threshold; 1-RM = One-repetition maximum

does not reflect the resting state. Body composition should be estimated before activity to avoid either underestimation of fat stores from **dehydration,** or overestimation of fat stores due to **vasodilation** in surface vessels associated with **thermoregulation.** Although an optimal sequence of assessments for cardiorespiratory and muscular fitness is yet to be established, if performing various assessments within the same session, it is suggested that BP and HR are permitted to return to baseline values and that the sequence of assessments should be organized to avoid repeatedly stressing the same muscle group. Additionally, any follow-up assessments should be performed in the same sequence as the original assessments [American College of Sports Medicine (ACSM), 2018]. Significant gains in strength during the initial one to four weeks of training may be associated with neurological adaptations rather than a change in muscle physiology. Therefore, any assessment of strength performed in the early weeks may not reflect the true state before training.

Professionalism as a personal trainer includes management of the assessment environment and gaining experience in properly conducting assessments. Personal trainers must embody the highest level of professionalism by being fully prepared when conducting assessments and integrating the following (ACSM, 2018):

- Distribution of instructions in advance of assessments that clearly outline the client's responsibilities (e.g., clothing, eating and hydration recommendations, and abstaining from certain products such as stimulants)
- Obtaining a signed **informed consent** from the client, a document required from both ethical and legal standpoints (see Figure 16-2, pages 754–756). This document must ensure that the client knows and understands the purposes, protocols, and risks associated with assessments and exercise. The personal trainer must allow the client the opportunity to ask questions pertaining to the assessment protocol(s).
- Organization of all necessary documentation forms, data sheets, and assessment tables
- Communication and demonstration skills, clearly explaining the assessments, sequence, and instructions in a calm, confident manner
- Calibration and proper working condition of all exercise equipment
- Environmental control, ensuring room temperature is ideally between 68 and 72° F (20 to 22° C) with a relative humidity below 60% and adequate airflow. Additionally, the assessment environment should be quiet and private to reduce anxiety.

Cardiovascular Assessments at Rest

HEART RATE

The pulse rate (which in most people is identical to the HR) can be measured at any point on the body where an artery's pulsation is close to the surface. The following are some common sites where the pulse can be felt or palpated:

- **Radial artery:** The radial artery is on the **ventral** aspect of the wrist on the side of the thumb (Figure 7-1). **Palpation** of the pulse at the radial artery can be performed by both clients and personal trainers. In fact, intermittent palpation of the radial pulse, first by the client, followed by the personal trainer, can help ensure accurate assessment of HR.
- **Carotid artery:** The carotid artery is located in the neck, **lateral** to the trachea. It is more easily palpated when the neck is slightly extended (Figure 7-2). Clients often

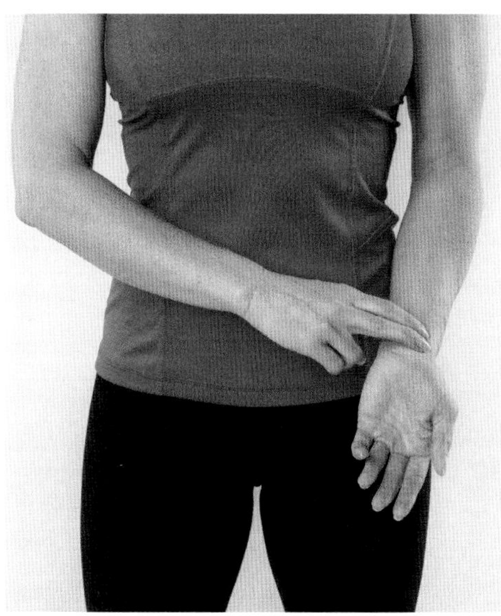

FIGURE 7-1
Taking the pulse at the radial artery

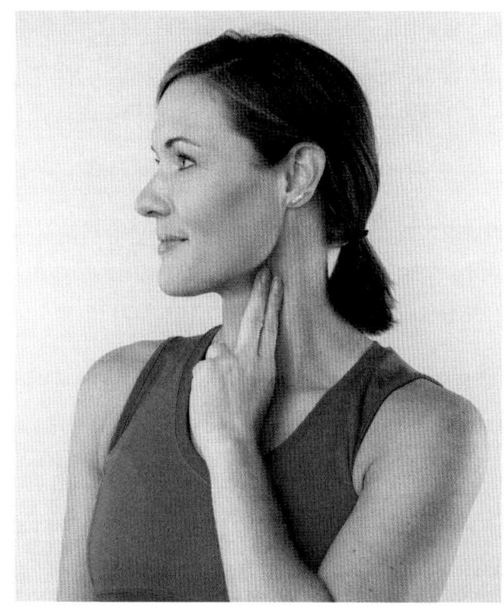

FIGURE 7-2
Taking the pulse at the carotid artery

have an easier time finding their pulse at the carotid artery, which makes it an ideal anatomical location for self-assessment of HR during exercise. Note: Personal trainers and clients should not push too hard on the carotid artery, as this may evoke a **vasovagal response** that actually slows down the HR.

It is also possible to auscultate the heartbeat using a stethoscope placed over the chest. HR is recorded in beats per minute (bpm) (e.g., 65 bpm). Note: When palpating the client's pulse, if the personal trainer feels any irregularity in the rate or rhythm of the pulse, it is recommended that the client contact his or her personal physician.

HR is a valid indicator of work intensity or stress on the body during exercise. However, because so many factors can influence resting HR and their effects can vary greatly from one person to another, resting HR is less valid. Lower resting and submaximal HRs may indicate higher fitness levels, since cardiovascular adaptations to cardiorespiratory exercise increase **stroke volume (SV),** thereby reducing HR. Conversely, higher resting and submaximal HRs may indicate lower physical fitness.

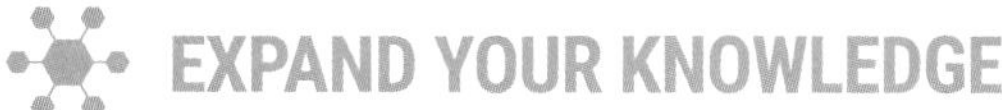

Factors Affecting Resting Heart Rate

While the research literature is clear that submaximal exercise HRs will be lower with endurance training, the response of **resting heart rate (RHR)** is less clear. Part of the confusion might be the result of cross-sectional comparisons, where highly trained endurance athletes are compared to untrained individuals; the athletes generally have RHR values that are 15 to 30 bpm lower than those of their untrained counterparts. In longitudinal studies, where untrained individuals have been endurance-trained for varying periods of time, the findings are mixed (Wilmore et al.,1996).

RHR is influenced by many factors, including fitness, fatigue, genetics, body composition, drugs and medication, alcohol, caffeine, and stress.

A traditional classification system exists to categorize RHR:

- Sinus bradycardia (slow HR): RHR <60 bpm
- Normal sinus rhythm: RHR 60 to 100 bpm
- Sinus tachycardia (fast HR): RHR >100 bpm

Average RHR is approximately 60 to 70 bpm in males and 72 to 80 bpm in females. The higher values found in women are attributed in part to smaller heart chamber size (less blood ejected per beat) and lower **hemoglobin** levels (less oxygen per unit of blood).

The following are some key notes about RHR:

- Knowing a client's RHR provides insight into his or her potential for developing the **overtraining syndrome,** as any elevation in RHR >5 bpm over the client's normal RHR that remains over a period of days is a good reason to reduce or taper the intensity and total volume of exercise.
- Certain drugs, medications, and supplements can directly affect RHR. Individuals should abstain from consuming non-prescription stimulants or depressants for a minimum of 12 hours prior to measuring RHR.
- Body position affects RHR. Standing or sitting positions elevate HR more than **supine** or **prone** positions due to the involvement of postural muscles and the effects of gravity.
- **Digestion** increases RHR. The processes of **absorption** and digestion require energy, necessitating the delivery of additional blood to the **gastrointestinal tract,** while blood flow to other parts of the body are not changed.
- Environmental factors can affect RHR. Noise, as well as high and low temperatures, can place additional stress on the body, increasing HR as the body attempts to respond.
- Psychological or emotional stress can affect RHR. Sharing of personal information or thinking about stressful situations (e.g., arguments with others or problems at work or at home) can cause the RHR to rise.

Keep in mind that true RHR is measured just before the client gets out of bed in the morning. Therefore, in most personal-training environments, the personal trainer's assessment of RHR is not a measure of true RHR.

- Clients should be resting comfortably for several minutes or more in a quiet, restful environment before obtaining RHR.
- RHR may be measured indirectly by placing the fingertips on a pulse site (palpation) or directly by listening through a stethoscope (**auscultation**).
- Place the tips of the index and middle fingers (not the thumb, which has a pulse of its own) over the artery and lightly apply pressure.
- To determine RHR, count the number of beats for 30 or 60 seconds and then correct that score to bpm, if necessary.
- When measuring by auscultation, place the bell of the stethoscope to the left of the client's sternum just above or below the nipple line. (It is important to be respectful of the client's personal space.)
- Clients may also measure their own RHR before rising from bed in the morning and report it to the personal trainer.

BLOOD PRESSURE

BP is defined as the outward force exerted by the blood on the vessel walls. It is generally recorded as two numbers (e.g., 120/80 mmHg). The **systolic blood pressure (SBP)** is the higher number and represents the pressure created by the heart as it pumps blood into circulation via ventricular contraction (**systole**). This represents the greatest pressure during one cardiac cycle. The **diastolic blood pressure (DBP)** is the lower number and represents the pressure that is exerted on the artery walls as blood remains in the arteries during the filling phase of the cardiac cycle or between beats when the heart relaxes (**diastole**). It is the lowest pressure during one cardiac cycle.

BP is measured within the arterial system. Pressures in that system will vary depending on where they are taken. When a person is standing, the pressure at the feet is higher because of gravity (i.e., the weight of the blood is greatest at the lowest level and there is more blood in the lower arteries). Likewise, the pressure at the head is lower. Because one wants to know the pressures in the heart, BP is measured at a location that is on the same level as the heart itself. The standard site of measurement is the brachial artery (Figure 7-3), given its easy accessibility and proximity to the heart.

BP is measured indirectly by listening to the **Korotkoff sounds**; these are sounds made from vibrations as blood moves along the walls of the vessel. These sounds are present only when there is some degree of wall deformation. If the vessel has unimpeded blood flow, no vibrations are heard. However, under pressure of a BP cuff, vessel deformity facilitates hearing these sounds. This deformity is created as the air bladder within the cuff is inflated, restricting the flow of blood.

When the pressure in the cuff is higher than the pressure in the heart during contractions, the brachial artery collapses and blood flow through the cuff is blocked. As the air is slowly released from the bladder, blood begins to flow past the compressed area, creating turbulent flow and vibration along the vascular wall, producing the onset of tapping Korotkoff sounds, corresponding to SBP.

As the pressure in the cuff is reduced to the point where there is no deformation of the arterial wall, this represents the pressure in the arteries during relaxation or diastole. This is

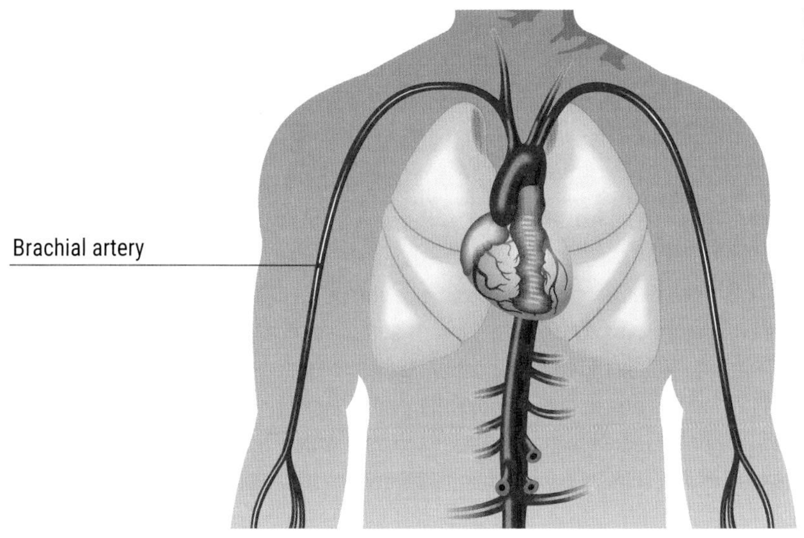

FIGURE 7-3
Brachial artery

the DBP. DBP is indicated by a significant muffling of sound and the disappearance of sound (Figure 7-4). Typically, in adults with normal BP, the disappearance of sound is recorded as DBP. In children and adults with the disappearance of sound occurring below 40 mmHg, but who appear healthy, the first sign of significant muffling may be used.

The classification of BP for adults is presented in Table 7-2. Refer to Chapter 13 for recommendations for working with clients who are at risk for, or who have been diagnosed with, hypertension.

FIGURE 7-4
Korotkoff sounds

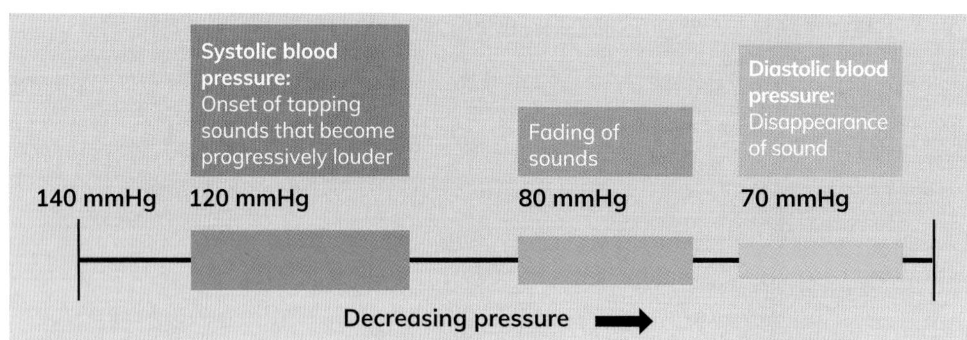

TABLE 7-2
Categories of Blood Pressure in Adults*

Category	SBP		DBP
Normal	<120 mmHg	and	<80 mmHg
Elevated	120–129 mmHg	and	<80 mmHg
Hypertension			
Stage 1	130–139 mmHg	or	80–89 mmHg
Stage 2	≥140 mmHg	or	≥90 mmHg

Note: SBP = Systolic blood pressure; DBP = Diastolic blood pressure

*Individuals with SBP and DBP in two different categories should be designated to the higher BP category. BP is based on an average of two or more careful readings obtained on two or more occasions.

Reprinted with permission from Whelton, P.K. et al. (2017). 2017 ACC/AHA/AAPA/ABC/ACPM/AGS/APhA/ASH/ASPC/NMA/PCNA guideline for the prevention, detection, evaluation, and management of high blood pressure in adults: A report of the American College of Cardiology/American Heart Association Task Force on Clinical Practice Guidelines. *Journal of the American College of Cardiology*, Nov 7. pii: S0735-1097 (17) 41519-1.

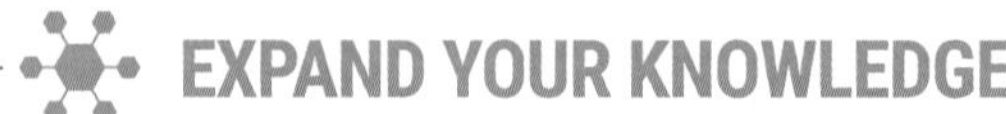

EXPAND YOUR KNOWLEDGE

Accuracy of Blood Pressure Machines

Clients sometimes ask about the BP machines found at pharmacies and personal BP monitors used at home. While these monitors can provide useful information, the results may not be accurate. As an example, readings obtained from wrist BP monitors are usually higher and less accurate than readings from the arm. Compared to readings obtained by auscultation, one study (Ringrose et al., 2017) found that home monitors provided SBP or DBP readings that were not accurate within 5 mmHg 69% of the time. Inaccurate readings within 10 mmHg and 15 mmHg were found 29% and 7% of the time, respectively.

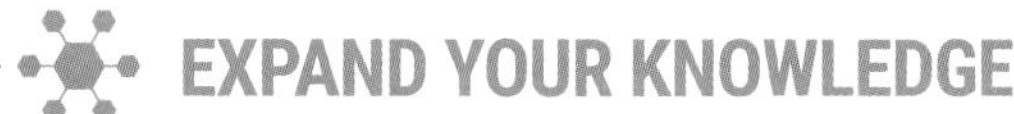

Blood Pressure and Cardiovascular Disease

A positive correlation exists between elevated BP and the risk of cardiovascular events [e.g., **myocardial infarction** or **stroke**]. For individuals 40 to 70 years old, each 20 mmHg increase in resting SBP or each 10 mmHg increase in resting DBP above normal doubles the risk of **cardiovascular disease** (ACSM, 2018). A difference of 15 mmHg or more between arms increases the risk of **peripheral vascular disease** and **cerebral vascular disease** and is associated with a 70% risk of dying from **heart disease** (McManus & Mant, 2012). If the personal trainer discovers an abnormal BP reading, it is prudent to recommend that clients visit their personal physician.

BP can be reduced with medication or certain behavioral modifications (e.g., exercise, diet, weight loss, sodium restriction, smoking cessation, and stress management). For those with elevated BP (120–129/<80 mmHg), BP can be realistically reduced with lifestyle interventions. For those with true clinical **hypertension** (see Table 7-2), it is likely that their personal physicians will want to treat the hypertension with medication and lifestyle interventions. The personal trainer can provide guidance and motivation on appropriate lifestyle-modification practices.

Anthropometric Measurements and Body Composition

Body composition refers to the relative proportions of lean tissue and fat tissue. **Lean body mass** is composed of muscles, **connective tissue,** bones, blood, nervous tissue, skin, and organs. For the most part, lean mass is metabolically active tissue that allows the body to perform work. A certain amount of **body fat** is necessary for insulation and thermoregulation, **hormone** production, cushioning of vital organs, and maintenance of certain body functions; this is called **essential body fat.** For men, this is between 2 and 5%, while it is between 10 and 13% for women. The remainder of body fat is stored throughout the body in **adipose** tissue, either under the skin (**subcutaneous fat**) or inside the body cavity surrounding the visceral organs (**visceral fat**), which acts as a readily available source of energy or to cushion and protect vital organs. Just as lean tissue contributes to athletic performance, an appropriate percentage of body fat also can be associated with successful athletic performance.

Many people can lose weight or body fat easily for short periods of time but are unsuccessful at long-term weight management. Regular exercise is a key component not only in effective weight loss, but also in maintaining a healthy weight. Personal trainers must consider their own skill level, protocol accuracy, and equipment availability, as well as the client's personal concerns, when determining the most appropriate method to assess body composition and body shape/size. Personal trainers may also opt to use more than one method (e.g., skinfold, BMI, and abdominal circumference).

MEASUREMENT OF LEAN AND FAT TISSUE

It is important to differentiate between **overweight** and **overfat.** Overweight is defined as excess body weight relative to a person's height. Since only height and weight are factored into the equation, excess body weight could be attributed to either fat mass or lean tissue. Overfat, a more accurate depiction of body composition, indicates an excess amount of body fat.

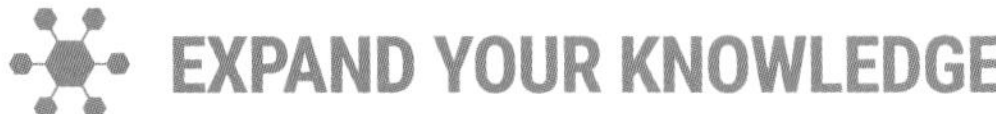

Body-composition Assessment

Assessment of body composition may be of great interest to some clients and may be a primary reason for eliciting the services of a personal trainer. However, it is important to note that if a client has extreme obesity, some of the body-composition assessment techniques will be inaccurate and contraindicated. In such cases, it may be more appropriate to utilize only BMI and circumference measurements (see pages 234–243).

Although there are many methods for assessing body composition, some are impractical in a fitness setting given the expense and expertise needed to operate the equipment [e.g., **hydrostatic weighing, air displacement plethysmography** (e.g., Bod-Pod), **bioelectrical impedance analysis (BIA), total body electrical conductivity (TOBEC),** and **dual-energy X-ray absorptiometry (DXA)**] (Table 7-3). Less-sophisticated BIA and **near-infrared interactance,** as well as skinfold techniques, are often available in fitness centers but are less accurate.

TABLE 7-3
Body-composition Assessments

Method	Description
Bioelectrical impedance analysis (BIA)* Whole-body BIA machines are found primarily in laboratory settings. Less-sophisticated BIA devices are sometimes found in fitness settings.	BIA measures electrical signals as they pass through fat, lean mass, and water in the body. In essence, this method assesses leanness, but calculations can be made based on this information. BIA accuracy is based primarily on the sophistication of the machine and the validity of the prediction algorithms. Many fitness centers utilize BIA due to the simplicity of use. Optimal hydration is necessary for accurate results.
Air displacement plethysmography (ADP) Example: Bod Pod (or Pea Pod for children) Marketed for the fitness setting, but it is cost-prohibitive for most facilities	The Bod Pod is an egg-shaped chamber that measures the amount of air that is displaced when a person sits in the machine. Two values are needed to determine body fat: air displacement and body weight. ADP has a high accuracy rate but the equipment is expensive.
Dual-energy x-ray absorptiometry (DXA)* Typically found in clinical settings; may be found in exercise physiology departments at colleges and universities	DXA ranks among the most accurate and precise methods. DXA is a whole-body scanning system that delivers a low-dose x-ray that reads bone and soft-tissue mass. DXA has the ability to identify regional body-fat distribution.

TABLE 7-3 *(continued)*

Method	Description
Hydrostatic weighing (i.e., underwater weighing) The gold standard: Many methods of body-fat assessment are based on calculations derived from hydrostatic weighing. May be found in exercise physiology departments at colleges and universities	This method measures the amount of water a person displaces when completely submerged, thereby indirectly measuring body fat via body density. It is generally not practical in a fitness-center setting due to the size of the apparatus and the complexity of the technique required for accurate measurements, which involves the individual going down to the bottom of a tank, exhaling all air from the lungs (expiratory reserve volume), and then holding the breath until the scale settles and records an accurate weight. The assessment must then be repeated to ensure reliability.
Magnetic resonance imaging (MRI) Found in hospitals and diagnostic centers	MRI uses magnetic fields to assess how much fat a person has and where it is deposited. Since MRIs are located in clinical settings, using an MRI solely for calculation of body fat is not practical.
Near-infrared interactance (NIR)* Example: Futrex Found in fitness settings	NIR uses a fiber optic probe connected to a digital analyzer that indirectly measures tissue composition (fat and water). Typically, the biceps are the assessment site. Calculations are then plugged into an equation that includes height, weight, frame size, and level of activity. This method is relatively inexpensive and fast, but generally not as accurate as other techniques.
Skinfold measurement Very commonly used in fitness settings	Skinfold calipers are used to "pinch" a fold of skin and fat. Several sites on the body are typically measured. The measurements are plugged into an equation that calculates body-fat percentage.
Total body electrical conductivity (TOBEC) Found in clinical and research settings	TOBEC uses an electromagnetic force field to assess relative body fat. Much like the MRI, it is impractical and too expensive for the fitness setting.

*These body-composition assessment techniques are not accurate when used with obese clients.

HYDROSTATIC WEIGHING

Hydrostatic weighing, also called underwater weighing, is considered the benchmark for measuring body composition. When compared with cadaver assessments, there is only a 1.5 to 2.0% margin of error. The concept behind hydrostatic weighing is based on the Archimedes Principle, which provides the following equation:

$$\text{Density} = \text{Mass}/\text{Volume}$$

This technique measures the amount of water displaced when a person is completely submerged and exhales all available air from the lungs [leaving only the **residual volume (RV)** and a small volume of air in the gastrointestinal tract]. Given that a pound of fat takes up more space than a pound of muscle because it is less dense, it will therefore displace more water. The body is weighed on an underwater scale. As water buoyancy (i.e., the counterforce of water) reduces body weight significantly, and air and fat mass increase buoyancy, their respective contributions to underwater weight have to be determined. To minimize error with this protocol, the RV should be measured in water. This volume can be 100 to 200 mL lower underwater than out of the water due to the noncompressible nature of water that helps compact the lungs. Given the costs, equipment, and expertise needed to accurately measure RV, mathematical calculations are often used to estimate RV; this may introduce a margin of error of 300 to 400 mL. For every 100 mL error in estimation of RV, the percent body fat error changes by 0.7%. Therefore, the final error may be as much as 2.1% to 2.8% (0.7%/100 mL x 3 or 4).

Hydrostatic weighing is not a practical approach for the standard fitness center. The apparatus is expensive and takes up a lot of room, assessment takes a considerable amount of time and expertise, and many people feel uncomfortable remaining submerged underwater after they have exhaled all available air from their lungs. This evaluation tool is often found in elite clinical settings and in many colleges and universities.

SKINFOLD MEASUREMENTS

One of the most widely used methods to estimate body fat incorporates the measurement of select subcutaneous adipose tissue sites (Gibson, Wagner, & Heyward, 2019). Given the ease of administration and low cost, skinfold measurements are still considered the most practical assessment tool for measuring body composition in the fitness setting. Measuring skinfold thickness is a practical and reasonably accurate way to estimate percent body fat if performed properly by a trained technician who uses a high-quality skinfold caliper (ACSM, 2018). The assessment is based on the principle that subcutaneous fat is proportional to total body fat. Because this proportion varies with sex, age, race or ethnicity, and other factors (ACSM, 2018), one must use the prediction equation that was developed on the same population as the person being evaluated.

While some skinfold protocols demonstrate similar accuracy to the more expensive techniques, the margin of error increases when personal trainers are unfamiliar with identifying exact skinfold locations or when they lack experience or technique in correctly locating and grasping the correct skinfold site. Considering how critical a body-composition score can be to a client's psyche and motivational levels, it is extremely important that personal trainers demonstrate strong skills and reliability when assessing body composition.

The assessment of body composition can be quite invasive. It is important for personal trainers to conduct these assessments in a private area to put the client at ease. Clients should be instructed on appropriate attire to promote easy access to measurement sites. The personal trainer should act as a professional and be competent in the chosen method. Assessment accuracy is improved by proper hydration, so it is important to instruct the client not to exercise prior to the assessment and to maintain adequate hydration throughout the day.

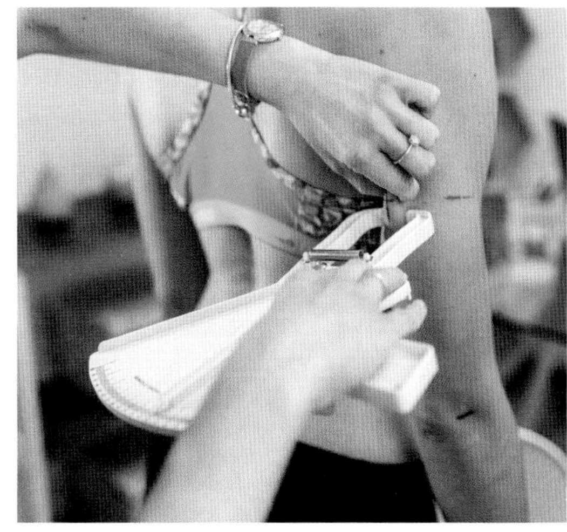

Subcutaneous body fat can be measured using a device called a skinfold caliper. If a personal trainer plans to use a caliper, it is mandatory that the caliper has a constant tension, regardless of how far apart the heads are. For that reason, inexpensive calipers costing $10 to $25 that use a spring that has more tension the more it is stretched will be inaccurate, especially with clients with obesity. Harpenden and Lange calipers cost $250 to $400 but are much more accurate.

In an average person, approximately 50% of body fat is distributed just below the skin. If a client has obesity, more than 50% of the body fat will be located in the internal cavities and the assumption upon which the equations are based (i.e., that 50% is subcutaneous) may not be valid. In addition, it is more difficult to grasp skinfolds with a lot of fat, which could also affect the accuracy of the measurements.

Skinfold formulas are derived from calculations based on extensive research derived from hydrostatic weighing. In general, the skinfold caliper method produces a measurement that is ±3.5% of that obtained in hydrostatic weighing. Further measurement error can range higher if the personal trainer is inexperienced or uses poor technique, if the client has obesity or is extremely thin, or if the caliper is of poor quality or is not properly calibrated (ACSM, 2018). Before conducting skinfold measurements, personal trainers must familiarize themselves with the exact site locations and proper grasping technique.

While the accuracy of skinfold measurements in estimating percentage body fat may not be adequate, the technique can be useful. For example, if personal trainers are experienced and skilled, such that they can reliably measure a given skinfold, changes over time can be accurately tracked. During subsequent reassessments following a program of exercise and/or dietary changes, body composition may change due to a loss of body fat and/or an increase in lean tissue. Between measurements, clients may notice changes in the way their clothes fit. These subjective observations will be motivating to the client. Objective reassessments of body composition will be especially important for a client who has not noticed any significant change on the bathroom scale. Clients may need to be reminded that as lean mass increases and body fat decreases, the scale cannot differentiate between the two. Table 7-4 presents the standard values for percentage body fat.

TABLE 7-4

Standard Values for Percentage Body Fat

	Age (years)				
Percentile (Men)	**20–29**	**30–39**	**40–49**	**50–59**	**60+**
90	7.9	12.4	15.0	17.0	18.1
80	10.5	14.9	17.5	19.4	20.2
70	12.6	16.8	19.3	21.0	21.7
60	14.8	18.4	20.8	22.3	23.0
50	16.6	20.0	22.1	23.6	24.2
40	18.6	21.6	23.5	24.9	25.6
30	20.7	23.2	24.9	26.3	27.0
20	23.3	25.1	26.6	28.1	28.8
10	26.6	27.8	29.2	30.6	31.2
Percentile (Women)	**20–29**	**30–39**	**40–49**	**50–59**	**60+**
90	15.1	15.5	16.8	19.1	20.2
80	16.8	17.5	19.5	22.3	23.3
70	18.4	19.2	21.7	24.8	25.7
60	19.8	21.0	23.7	26.7	27.5
50	21.5	22.8	25.5	28.4	29.2
40	23.4	24.8	27.5	30.1	30.8
30	25.5	26.9	29.5	31.8	32.6
20	28.2	29.6	31.9	33.9	34.4
10	33.5	33.6	35.1	36.1	36.6

Reprinted with permission from The Cooper Institute, Dallas, TX. For more information: www.cooperinstitute.org.

ANTHROPOMETRIC MEASUREMENTS

Anthropometric measurements are easy to administer, require minimal equipment, and provide fundamental data, including body weight, height, and their associations, as indicated by BMI. These measurements also provide information on the circumferences of various parts of the body. Together, these data present information on body size and body shape. Also, it is useful to compare initial values obtained to those recorded after the implementation of lifestyle modifications. BMI, waist circumference, and WHR are typically used to classify overweight and obesity and the risks of obesity-related diseases. However, their purpose is not to measure body fatness or obesity. These indices are commonly used because of their associations with morbidity and mortality rates, as well as because of their low cost and simplicity.

Common goals for many clients initiating an exercise program are to positively modify numerous anthropometric and body-composition measurements. Given both the widespread prevalence of obesity and the fact that excessive fat mass is associated with a myriad of unhealthy conditions, this is an admirable target. Regrettably, clients frequently establish goals that are incongruent with what the scientific literature suggests are likely to occur with exercise training. In a client-centered approach, it is critical for the personal trainer to understand and convey how much various anthropometric and body-composition parameters are realistically going to change in the coming months. Without this knowledge, attainable anthropometric and body-composition goals for the exercise program cannot be established and it is highly probable that clients will become disenchanted with the program when they fall short of lofty goals.

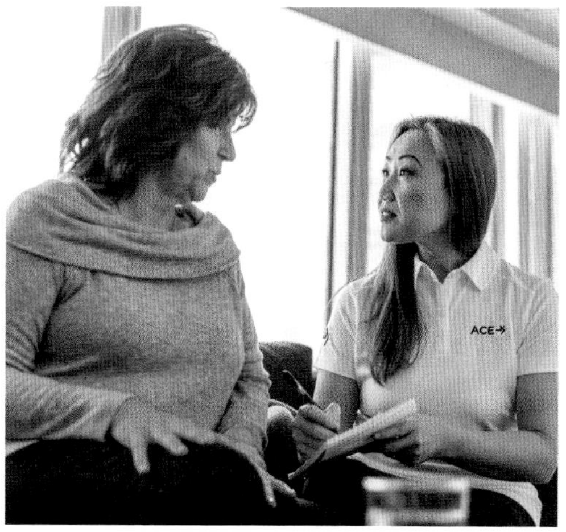

Exclusive ACE-sponsored research has examined training responsiveness to the ACE IFT Model for a variety of anthropometric and body-composition parameters in younger and older adults (Montano et al., 2018; Nolan et al., 2018; Dalleck et al., 2016). The expected change and timeline for key anthropometric and body composition outcomes measures are summarized in Table 7-5. Personal trainers can apply these research findings when collaborating with clients on setting attainable and realistic exercise program goals.

ACE-sponsored Research

Acknowledging a client's enthusiasm and desire to change while also providing information to shape realistic expectations is an essential aspect of the client–personal trainer relationship. Having conversations about what anthropometric and body-composition changes can be expected in a given amount of time is crucial for client safety, motivation, and adherence, and for setting attainable goals that will lead to long-term success.

Clients may express a desire to achieve an exercise-related goal within a time frame that is not realistic. Often, these goals and the motivation to achieve them are sparked by upcoming events (e.g., a reunion, wedding, or vacation), and the client is excited, motivated, and ready to get started. Working together to uncover specific goals and agreed-upon realistic expectations while supporting the client's motivation and current readiness to change will create the ideal environment for a productive and meaningful personal-training experience.

TABLE 7-5

The Expected Change and Timeline for Key Anthropometric and Body-composition Measures

Health Outcome	Expected Change	Timeline
Body fat (%)	↓ 2.7–5.9	2–3 months
Waist Circumference (cm)	↓ 1.9–3.3	2–3 months

Sources: Montano, E.E. et al. (2018). Do younger and older adults experience similar adaptations to individualized exercise training? *Journal of Exercise Physiology Online*, 21, 6, 41-59; Nolan, P.B. et al. (2018). The effect of detraining after a period of training on cardiometabolic health in previously sedentary individuals. *International Journal of Environmental Research and Public Health*, 15, 10; Dalleck, L.C. et al. (2016). Does a personalized exercise prescription enhance training efficacy and limit training unresponsiveness? A randomized controlled trial. *Journal of Fitness Research*, 5, 3, 15–27.

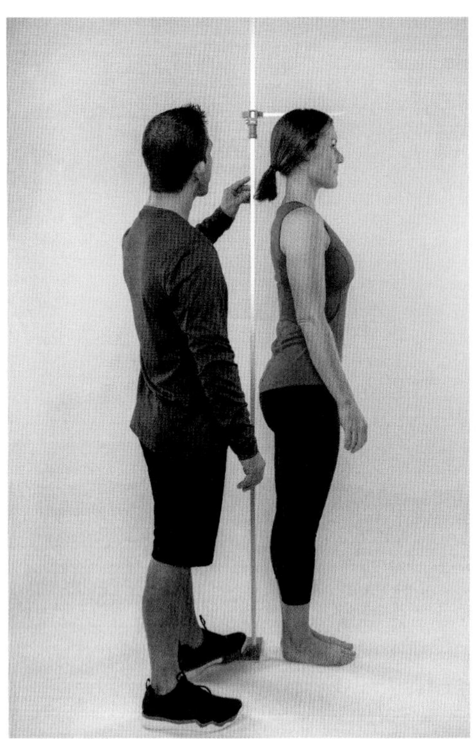
FIGURE 7-5
Free-standing stadiometer

Height, Weight, and Body Mass Index

Height is the vertical distance between the soles of the feet and the top of the head. This is generally measured using a **stadiometer,** a piece of equipment with a ruler and a sliding horizontal board that rests on top of the head. Some stadiometers are part of a weighing scale so that both measures can be done at the same time, while others are free-standing or mounted on a wall (Figure 7-5).

To measure height, clients stand on a hard surface, remove their shoes and socks, and stand up straight directly underneath the drop-down horizontal headboard. If using a wall-mounted stadiometer, clients stand with the back of their feet, calves, buttocks, upper back, and the back of their head in contact with the wall. With the mass distributed evenly across both feet and the arms hanging freely to the sides, the movable headboard is brought down until it touches the topmost part of the head, pressing firmly enough to compress the hair.

Weight is the maximal force exerted by the person on a weight scale, while wearing lightweight clothing and standing erect with weight evenly distributed across both feet. Assuming the availability of an accurate and reliable weight scale, ask clients to remove any "heavy" items from their pockets (e.g., keys, cell phone, or wallet) and to remove any heavy items of clothing (e.g., shoes, jackets, or sweaters). Record the time of day and the client's state (e.g., level of hydration and recent food consumption), as this will be useful when making comparisons with results from later assessments.

Body weight is made up of bone, lean tissue (primarily muscle), and fat. The relation between height and weight gives no indication of the density of the bones, or of the amount of muscle and fat and their relative contribution to the overall weight. While BMI provides objective, easily obtained information, it does not estimate actual body composition. As a result, BMI can incorrectly categorize some individuals. For example, individuals who are extremely muscular or have large frames can score high on the BMI charts, resulting in a label of "overweight" or even "obese," while older adults with decreased lean tissue, lower **bone density,** and excess body fat may score "normal." See below for the equation to determine BMI:

$$\text{BMI} = \text{Weight (kg)/Height}^2\text{ (m) or } \frac{\text{Weight (lb)}}{\text{Height}^2\text{ (in)}} \times 703$$

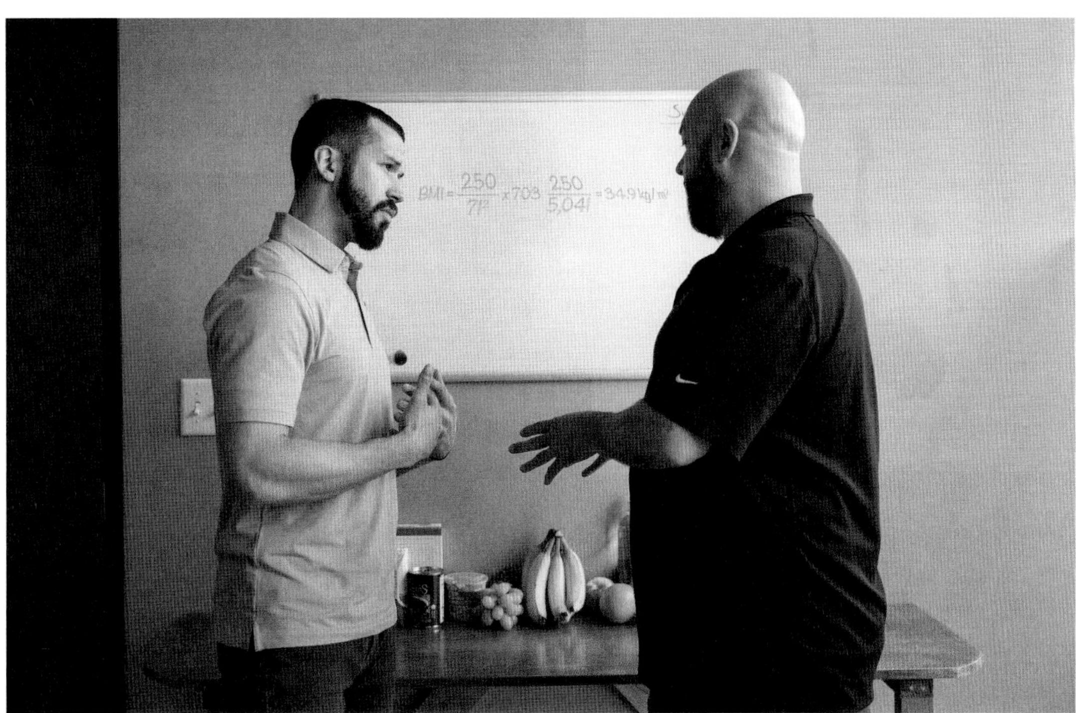

As BMI increases, so do health risks for several preventable causes of premature death including stroke, heart disease, certain types of cancer, **type 2 diabetes,** and heart disease. It is estimated that, worldwide, 39% (1.9 billion) of adults (aged 18 and over) have overweight and 13% (650 million) have obesity (WHO, 2018), with the American population estimated at 39.8% obesity (CDC, 2017). Further, 41 million children under the age of five have overweight or obesity and 340 million children and adolescents aged five to 19 years old have overweight or obesity (WHO, 2018), with 18.5% of American youth estimated as having overweight or obesity (CDC, 2017). A BMI of 25 kg/m^2 or greater increases a person's risk for cardiovascular disease, metabolic syndrome, hypertension, and type 2 diabetes. Table 7-6 is a BMI reference chart that can be used to discuss the health risks of having overweight or obesity and to set long-term weight-loss goals for clients.

TABLE 7-6

Classification of Overweight and Obesity by Body Mass Index (BMI)

	BMI (kg/m^2)	Obesity Class
Underweight	<18.5	—
Normal	18.5–24.9	—
Overweight	25.0–29.9	—
Obesity	30.0–34.9	I
	35.0–39.9	II
Extreme Obesity	≥40.0	III

Note: Increased waist circumference also can be a marker for increased risk, even in persons of normal weight.

Source: National Heart, Lung, and Blood Institute (2019). *Classification of Overweight and Obesity by BMI, Waist Circumference, and Associated Disease Risks.* https://www.nhlbi.nih.gov/health/educational/lose_wt/BMI/bmi_dis.htm

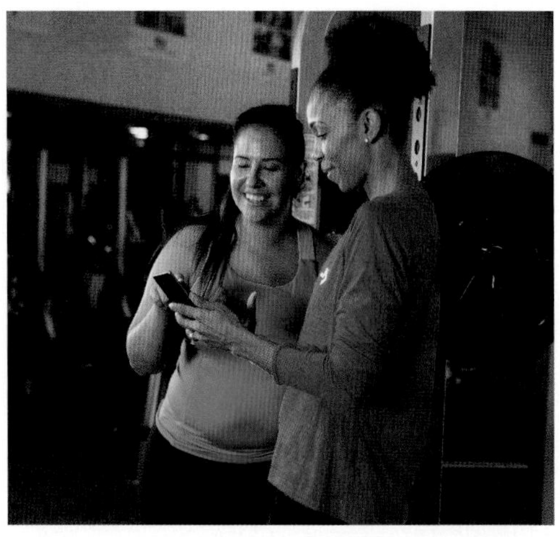

Calculating BMI is quick and inexpensive. BMI charts are used by many healthcare agencies to assess body mass and associated risks. If BMI charts are the *only* method of assessing body structure, the results could be misinterpreted and many individuals could be misclassified. A simple observation of the client that contradicts with his or her BMI category should make the personal trainer question the label and, in these situations—when warranted and if welcomed by the client—proceed with a body-composition assessment to gain a more accurate indicator of disease risk.

Online BMI calculators are available where an individual can simply key in his or her height and weight and be given the BMI, including one on ACE's website (www.ACEfitness.org/calculators). The Centers for Disease Control and Prevention (CDC) website has a BMI calculator specifically for children and teens (www.cdc.gov/healthyweight/bmi/calculator.html).

APPLY WHAT YOU KNOW

Why Is BMI a Poor Estimate of Fatness?

Women tend to have less muscle mass, lower bone density, and/or more body fat than men. Therefore, looking at BMI alone does not provide a good indication of body composition. Jackson et al. (2002) studied the relation between BMI and measured percent body fat in a sample of 655 black and white men and women who ranged in age from 17 to 65 years and had BMI values from about 17 to 47 kg/m^2. For the same BMI, females had 10% higher levels of body fat than males.

With age, there is a loss of muscle. If people were to lose muscle but gain fat, such that their body weight was the same, measuring BMI would give no indication of what changes in body composition had occurred. Standing height also tends to decrease with age. If there are minimal changes in body weight, BMI at the shorter heights would increase by 1.5 kg/m^2 in men and 2.5 kg/m^2 in women (Srikanthan, Seeman, & Karlamangla, 2009).

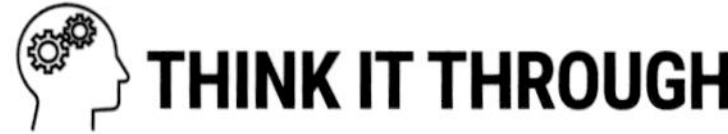

THINK IT THROUGH

Weight Categories and Body-composition Assessment

An active, well-muscled client has recently participated in his employer's wellness fair. Based on his weight and height measurements, he tells you that he falls into the "overweight" category. However, according to the body-composition assessment you have conducted with him, he is considered healthy and does not meet the criteria for having overweight. How would you explain this discrepancy to your client?

Managing Expectations

During an initial consultation with a highly motivated new client, the client mentions that he has been making some health-related changes over the past year but has not been able to achieve his goals. The client shares that his 20-year high school reunion is in three months and he would like to lose 40 pounds (18 kg) to look and feel his best.

Working with clients expecting specific changes within a time frame that may not be realistic can be challenging. However, it is the responsibility of the personal trainer to work with each client to set clear and realistic expectations.

ACE ABC APPROACH™

Here is an example of how the ACE ABC Approach™ may be applied in this scenario.

Ask: Asking powerful open-ended questions during this initial session will help the personal trainer find out what the client hopes to accomplish by working with a personal trainer and assess what additional information the client may need to achieve his goals.

Personal Trainer: You have been making healthy changes over the past year but have not noticed the results you wanted. What specifically are you hoping to achieve by working with a personal trainer?

Client: I want to lose 40 pounds (18 kg) before my high-school reunion in three months. I've already lost 10 pounds (4.5 kg) in the past year but I 'd like to lose 40 pounds (18 kg) more to get closer to my high-school weight.

Personal Trainer: Losing weight is a priority for you. What is your current understanding of a healthy approach to weight loss?

Client: I know that losing weight is not easy and that there is a relationship between physical activity, nutrition, and weight loss. Based on my experience over the past year, I had to work hard to lose small amounts of weight. I am not sure how much weight I can lose before my reunion but thought my best shot would involve working with a personal trainer.

Personal Trainer: Thank you for sharing that with me. You are correct, losing weight can be challenging, and how much activity you do and what you eat is essential to meeting that goal. There are other factors to keep in mind when it comes to weight loss, and I'd like to share these with you if it's ok to go into that in more detail.

Client: Yes, please.

Personal Trainer: One key characteristic of successful weight loss is that it occurs steadily and gradually at a rate of about 1 to 2 pounds (0.5 to 0.9 kg) per week through ongoing lifestyle changes. We have about 12 weeks to work together before your reunion, which means we can set a realistic goal of losing 12 to 24 pounds (5.5 to 10.9 kg) within your target time frame. Does that make sense?

Client: Yeah, it does. Even though I would like to lose 40 pounds (18 kg) in 12 weeks, it would be more realistic for me to set a goal of losing 12 to 24 pounds (5.5 to 10.9 kg). That's not bad. I've already lost 10 pounds (4.5 kg), and if I could lose 24 (10.9 kg) more before my reunion, I would feel good about that!

Break down barriers: Personal trainers can empower the client to overcome potential barriers by asking open-ended questions to learn about previous challenges and potential obstacles that could stand in the client's way.

Personal Trainer: You mentioned that you were successful at losing 10 pounds (4.5 kg) in the past year. Would you tell me more about that experience?

Client: I had to work hard. I increased the number of calories I burned by becoming more physically active throughout the day and I began a regular exercise routine. I was consistent for four months, and that is when the weight came off. I was eating better by taking lunch and healthy snacks to work. I was doing a good job, and then I started to get burned out and lost my motivation. My schedule at work changed and I began commuting during high traffic times. The healthy choices I was making started to decrease as I became busier, and I went back to eating whatever was convenient.

Personal Trainer: It sounds like consistency and motivation were key factors to your initial success. What lessons did you learn that could help you achieve your goals this time?

Client: I realized that I need to make a more realistic schedule for both eating and exercise. I got overwhelmed last time trying to do too much too soon. Now I am comfortable with my new work schedule, I already have a gym membership, and I'm hiring a personal trainer. My upcoming reunion has motivated me.

Collaborate: Working together with the client on goals and solutions is the next step and allows the client to continue building his exercise and lifestyle-change program.

Personal Trainer: You've learned a lot from your past attempt. To be successful, you recognize that you have to be consistent with physical activity and nutrition, but in a way that does not overwhelm you. Being as specific as you can be, what will you do to move forward?

Client: I'd like to meet with you three times per week starting this week, and I have a buddy at work who works my same shift, and we are going to walk for 30 minutes Monday through Friday. I'll also take lunch with me to work two days per week by bringing leftovers from dinner, and I can leave some healthy snacks and water bottles in my car. That way, when I'm stuck in traffic, I'll have some options other than stopping for fast food.

This interaction is an example of how a personal trainer can use the ACE ABC Approach to set clear expectations with a client who initially has a goal that may not be realistic or safe. In this scenario, the personal trainer acknowledges the client's enthusiasm, asks for permission before sharing relevant information, and then follows up by making sure the client understands what was shared. This strategy is known as elicit-provide-elicit, and it is a client-centered approach to sharing information with a client. Ultimately, the client and personal trainer arrive at a realistic goal, and the ACE ABC Approach allows the client to decide on his next steps.

Circumference Measurements

Circumference measurements are sometimes good predictors of health problems (e.g., waist circumference is correlated with the risk of developing heart disease). In addition, an overall body assessment may motivate some clients when they see changes in their body dimensions. In the case of excess body fat, clients may be inspired by a decline in circumference measurements, while individuals who are interested in muscular **hypertrophy** may be motivated by increases in circumference. However, some clients will be demotivated to begin an exercise program if they are self-conscious or may discontinue a program if measurement changes are smaller than they hoped.

When taking circumference measurements, accuracy is important. Therefore, the personal trainer must use precise anatomical landmarks for taking each measurement. In addition, procedures must be followed in accordance with established guidelines:

- When measuring body circumferences, it is important to measure precisely and consistently.
- All measurements should be made with a non-elastic, yet flexible tape.
- The tape should be snug against the skin's surface without pressing into the subcutaneous layers. Clients being assessed should wear thin, form-fitting materials that allow for accurate measurements.
- Personal trainers should rotate through the battery of sites, initially measuring each site only once.
- Duplicate measurements should be taken at each site. If recorded values are not within 5 mm, it is necessary to remeasure. Personal trainers should wait 20 to 30 seconds between measurements to allow the skin and subcutaneous tissue to return to their normal positions.

Many of the assessments measuring body size and proportions can be used in conjunction with body-composition assessment. Protocols are basically the same for all anthropometric assessments:

- These assessments should be performed prior to exercise.
- The personal trainer should explain the procedure for each assessment and ensure that the client is comfortable with the proposed measurement sites.
- Each measurement must be performed using the precise landmarks.
- The personal trainer should record values on the assessment form and then evaluate and classify the client's measurements using normative data.
- Personal trainers should discuss health and fitness concerns related to abnormal readings and educate clients on strategies to reduce personal risk and improve overall health.

When taking circumference measurements, it is important to be consistent in terms of both location and technique so that the baseline values can be used to track progress later in a client's training program (ACSM, 2018):

- *Abdominal circumference:* With the client standing upright with arms at the sides, feet together, and abdomen relaxed, a horizontal measure is taken at the height of the iliac crest, typically level with the umbilicus (Figure 7-6).

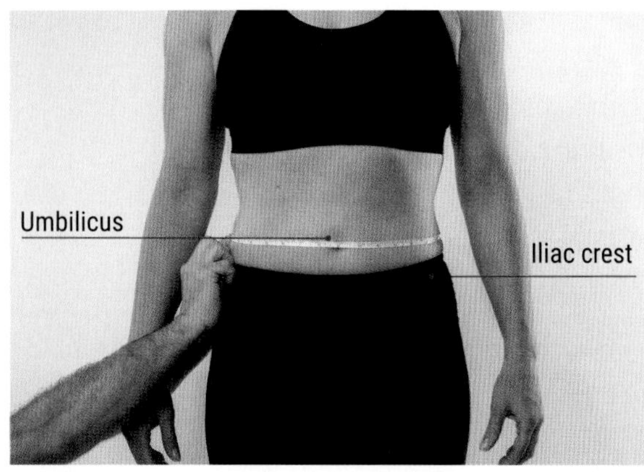

FIGURE 7-6
Abdominal circumference

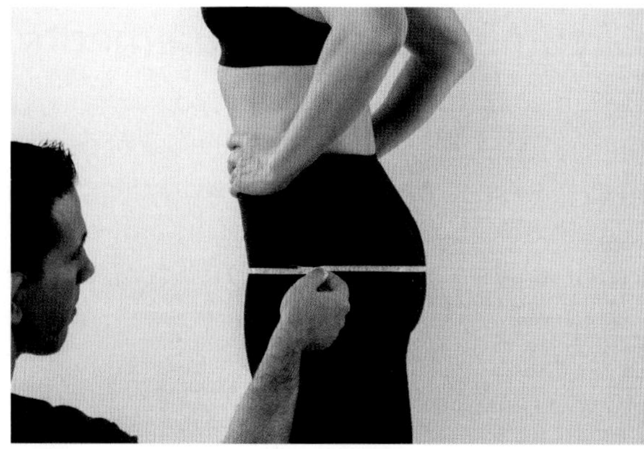

FIGURE 7-7
Hip circumference

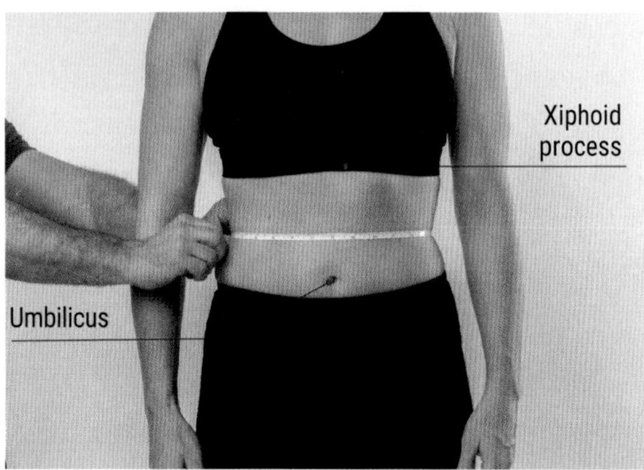

FIGURE 7-8
Waist circumference

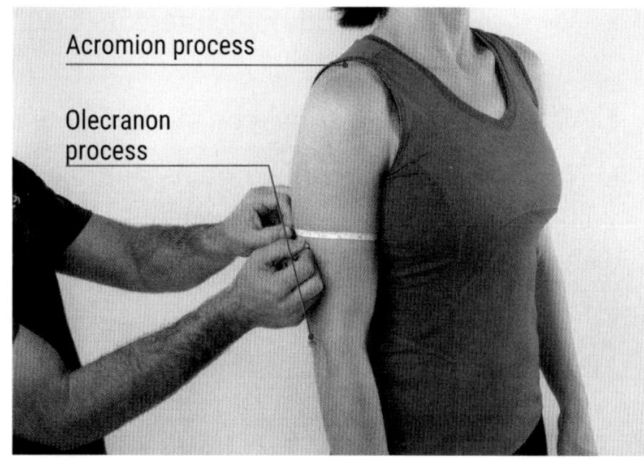

FIGURE 7-9
Biceps circumference

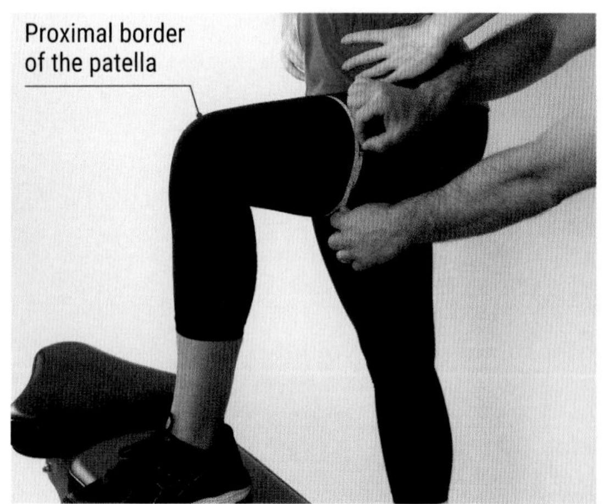

FIGURE 7-10
Midthigh circumference

- *Hip circumference:* With the client standing erect and the feet together, a horizontal measure is taken at the maximal circumference of the buttocks (Figure 7-7).
- *Waist circumference:* With the client standing upright with arms at the sides, feet together, and abdomen relaxed, a horizontal measure is taken at the narrowest part of the torso (above the umbilicus and below the xiphoid process) (Figure 7-8).
- *Biceps circumference:* With the client standing upright with arms hanging freely at the sides and the hands facing the thighs, a horizontal measure is taken midway between the acromion and olecranon process (Figure 7-9).
- *Midthigh circumference:* With the client standing with one foot on a bench so the knee is flexed at 90 degrees, a measure is taken midway between the inguinal crease (i.e., the crease between the torso and the thigh) and the proximal border of the patella, perpendicular to the tibia (Figure 7-10).

WAIST CIRCUMFERENCE

For every 1-inch (2.5-cm) increase in waist circumference in men, the following associated health risks are found (Janssen et al., 2004):

- BP increases by 10%
- Blood **cholesterol** level increases by 8%
- **High-density lipoprotein (HDL)** decreases by 15%
- **Triglycerides** increase by 18%
- Metabolic syndrome risk increases by 18%

Cerhan et al. (2014) looked at a much larger cohort and found similar increases in risk for all-cause mortality among men and women.

Table 7-7 presents the risk categories associated with various waist circumferences for men and women.

TABLE 7-7

Criteria for Waist Circumference in Adults

	Waist Circumference	
Risk Category	**Females**	**Males**
Very low	<27.3 in (<70 cm)	<31.2 in (<80 cm)
Low	27.3–34.7 in (70–89 cm)	31.2–38.6 in (80–99 cm)
High	35.1–42.5 in (90–109 cm)	39.0–46.8 in (100–120 cm)
Very high	>42.9 in (>110 cm)	>46.8 in (>120 cm)

Reprinted with permission from Bray, G.A. (2004). Don't throw the baby out with the bath water. *American Journal of Clinical Nutrition*, 70, 3, 347–349.

WAIST-TO-HIP RATIO

As mentioned previously, excess body fat poses significant disease risks. The location of the fat deposits may even be a better indicator of disease risk (Jensen et al., 2013).

The **waist-to-hip ratio (WHR)** helps differentiate individuals with **android** body-fat patterns (masculine- or apple-shape) from those who have **gynoid** body-fat patterns (feminine- or pear-shape). Those who are apple-shaped carry excess fat in the abdominal area, while pear-shaped individuals carry excess fat in the hips and thighs. Though any extra fat weight can be detrimental to a person's health, those who are android and have a high WHR are at a greater health risk. Visceral fat is located inside the body around the viscera and contributes to android fat distribution. Excess visceral fat is unhealthy because it has been associated with **insulin resistance,** many types of inflammation in the body, and the production of blood lipids. There is a strong correlation between excess visceral fat and a number of disease risks, including type 2 diabetes, **hypercholesterolemia,** and hypertension.

To determine a client's WHR, the waist measurement is divided by the hip measurement. Table 7-8 illustrates the relative risk ratings for WHRs.

TABLE 7-8

Waist-to-Hip Circumference Ratio Norms for Men and Women

		RISK			
	Age	Low	Moderate	High	Very High
Men	20–29	<0.83	0.83–0.88	0.89–0.94	>0.94
	30–39	<0.84	0.84–0.91	0.92–0.96	>0.96
	40–49	<0.88	0.88–0.95	0.96–1.00	>1.00
	50–59	<0.90	0.90–0.96	0.97–1.02	>1.02
	60–69	<0.91	0.91–0.98	0.99–1.03	>1.03
Women	20–29	<0.71	0.71–0.77	0.78–0.82	>0.82
	30–39	<0.72	0.72–0.78	0.79–0.84	>0.84
	40–49	<0.73	0.73–0.79	0.80–0.87	>0.87
	50–59	<0.74	0.74–0.81	0.82–0.88	>0.88
	60–69	<0.76	0.76–0.83	0.84–0.90	>0.90

Reprinted with permission from Gibson, A.L., Wagner, D.R., & Hayward, V.H. (2019). *Advanced Fitness Assessment and Exercise Prescription* (8th ed.). Champaign, Ill.: Human Kinetics.

Using Circumference Measurements to Motivate Clients

Daniel J. Green, Senior Project Manager & Editor for Publications and Content Development, American Council on Exercise

From early 2017 to early 2018, I completed a project focused on adhering to the federal *Dietary Guidelines* (U.S. Department of Agriculture, 2015) and *Physical Activity Guidelines* (U.S. Department of Health & Human Services, 2018) for a full year. To monitor my progress, I worked with my doctor and personal trainer to collect baseline data that we then tracked over the course of the project. We monitored everything from BP and cholesterol to cardiorespiratory and muscular fitness. In addition, we conducted a series of circumference measurements: hip, waist, abdomen, biceps, and midthigh, as well as WHR.

While all of the data were valuable and provided insight into the results of my efforts, I found the changes in my circumference measures to be particularly helpful, especially when my motivation suffered as I reached weight plateaus or struggled to make significant progress in my strength and endurance performance. In addition to the fact that certain circumference measurements are predictors of health problems, the changing numbers served as a reminder that despite any physical or psychological struggles I faced (and there were many), my body was changing as a result of the changes in my lifestyle (Figure 7-11). Yes, I felt better and my clothes fit more comfortably, but having measurable, trackable data was extremely valuable in keeping me motivated and on track.

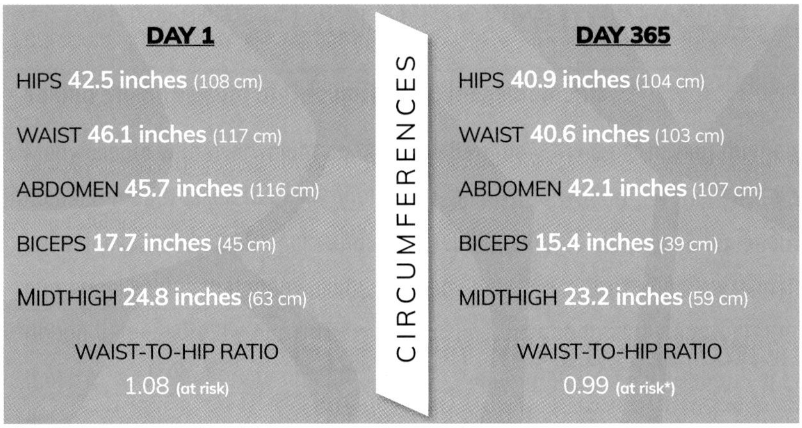

CIRCUMFERENCES

DAY 1	DAY 365
HIPS 42.5 inches (108 cm)	HIPS 40.9 inches (104 cm)
WAIST 46.1 inches (117 cm)	WAIST 40.6 inches (103 cm)
ABDOMEN 45.7 inches (116 cm)	ABDOMEN 42.1 inches (107 cm)
BICEPS 17.7 inches (45 cm)	BICEPS 15.4 inches (39 cm)
MIDTHIGH 24.8 inches (63 cm)	MIDTHIGH 23.2 inches (59 cm)
WAIST-TO-HIP RATIO 1.08 (at risk)	WAIST-TO-HIP RATIO 0.99 (at risk*)

FIGURE 7-11
The results of one year of lifestyle change

* <0.95 is the target

For tips on using a client-centered approach for clients making a lifestyle change, visit https://www.acefitness.org/education-and-resources/lifestyle/blog/6915/8-lessons-learned-from-a-year-of-lifestyle-change?authorScope=118

APPLY WHAT YOU KNOW

Taking the Stress out of Circumference Measurements

Many clients with overweight and obesity find the process of having their circumference measurements taken to be an unpleasant and demotivating experience. To help alleviate their uneasiness, personal trainers should consider using an alternative technique that eliminates the numerical values that many clients find so upsetting. For example, personal trainers can use a ribbon to measure the circumferences, cutting the ribbon at the appropriate lengths. Then, when these measurements are repeated later in the program (and the ribbons are noticeably shorter), personal trainers and their clients have a clear visual representation of the progress made.

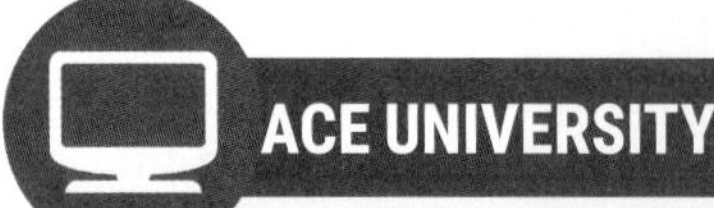

If your study program includes the ACE University, visit www.ACEfitness.org/MyACE and log in to your My ACE Account to take full advantage of the ACE Personal Trainer Study Program and online guided study experience.

A variety of media to support and expand on the material in this text is provided to facilitate learning and best prepare you for the ACE Personal Trainer Certification exam and a career as a personal trainer.

SUMMARY

Assessments are an integral part of any client-centered personal-training program. When selected thoughtfully and conducted properly, assessments can provide valuable health, fitness, and performance information for the personal trainer to use in exercise program design, implementation, and monitoring. Assessment information is also important for goal setting, determining disease risks, and developing rapport with the client. Not all assessments are suitable for all clients. It is up to the personal trainer to work with the client to decide the timing and most beneficial series of assessments for each individual client. Periodic reassessments are also important to evaluate progress and continue to foster the client–personal trainer relationship.

REFERENCES

American College of Sports Medicine (2018). *ACSM's Guidelines for Exercise Testing and Prescription* (10th ed.). Philadelphia: Wolters Kluwer.

Bray, G.A. (2004). Don't throw the baby out with the bath water. *American Journal of Clinical Nutrition*, 70, 3, 347–349.

Bray, G.A. & Gray, D.S. (1988). Obesity: Part I: Pathogenesis. *Western Journal of Medicine*, 149, 429–441.

Centers for Disease Control and Prevention (2017). *Prevalence of Obesity Among Adults and Youth: United States, 2015-2016*. NCHS Data Brief No. 288. https://www.cdc.gov/nchs/data/databriefs/db288.pdf

Cerhan, J.R. et al. (2014). A pooled analysis of waist circumference and mortality in 650,000 adults. *Mayo Clinic Proceedings*, 89, 3, 335–345.

Dalleck, L.C. et al. (2016). Does a personalized exercise prescription enhance training efficacy and limit training unresponsiveness? A randomized controlled trial. *Journal of Fitness Research*, 5, 3, 15–27.

Gibson, A.L., Wagner, D.L., & Heyward, V.H. (2019). *Advanced Fitness Assessments and Exercise Prescription* (8th ed.). Champaign, Ill.: Human Kinetics.

Jackson, A.S. et al. (2002). The effect of sex, age and race on estimating percentage body fat from body mass index: The Heritage Family Study. *International Journal of Obesity & Related Metabolic Disorders*, 26, 6, 789–796.

Janssen, I. et al. (2004). Waist circumference and health risk. *American Journal of Clinical Nutrition*, 79, 379–384.

Jensen, M.D. et al. (2013). 2013 AHA/ACC/TOS guideline for the management of overweight and obesity in adults: A report of the American College of Cardiology/American Heart Association Task Force on Practice Guidelines and The Obesity Society. *Journal of the American College of Cardiology*. DOI: 10.1016/j.jacc.2013.11.004

McManus R.J. & Mant J. (2012). Do differences in blood pressure between arms matter? *Lancet*, 10, 379, 872–873.

Montano, E.E. et al. (2018). Do younger and older adults experience similar adaptations to individualized exercise training? *Journal of Exercise Physiology Online*, 21, 6, 41-59.

National Heart, Lung, and Blood Institute (2019). *Classification of Overweight and Obesity by BMI, Waist Circumference, and Associated Disease Risks*. https://www.nhlbi.nih.gov/health/educational/lose_wt/BMI/bmi_dis.htm

Nolan, P.B. et al. (2018). The effect of detraining after a period of training on cardiometabolic health in previously sedentary individuals. *International Journal of Environmental Research and Public Health*, 15, 10.

Ringrose, J. et al. (2017). An assessment of the accuracy of home blood pressure monitors when used in device owners. *American Journal of Hypertension*, 30, 7, 683–689.

Srikanthan P., Seeman, T.E., & Karlamangla, A.S. (2009). Waist-hip-ratio as a predictor of all-cause mortality in high-functioning older adults. *Annals of Epidemiology*, 19, 10, 724–731.

U.S. Department of Agriculture (2015). *2015-2020 Dietary Guidelines for Americans* (8th ed.). www.health.gov/dietaryguidelines

U.S. Department of Health & Human Services (2018). *Physical Activity Guidelines for Americans* (2nd ed.). www.health.gov/paguidelines/

Whelton P.K. et al. (2018). 2017 ACC/AHA/AAPA/ABC/ACPM/AGS/APhA/ASH/ASPC/ NMA/PCNA Guideline for the Prevention, Detection, Evaluation, and Management of High Blood Pressure in Adults: A Report of the American College of Cardiology/American Heart Association Task Force on Clinical Practice Guidelines. *Journal of the American College of Cardiology*, 71, 19, e127-e248.

Wilmore J.H. et al. (1996). Endurance exercise training has a minimal effect on resting heart rate: The HERITAGE study. *Medicine & Science in Sports & Exercise*, 28, 7, 829–835.

World Health Organization (2018). *Obesity and Overweight*. https://www.who.int/news-room/fact-sheets/detail/obesity-and-overweight

ACE-sponsored Research

SUGGESTED READINGS

American College of Sports Medicine (2019). *ACSM's Health/Fitness Facility Standards and Guidelines* (5th ed.). Champaign, Ill.: Human Kinetics.

American College of Sports Medicine (2018). *ACSM's Guidelines for Exercise Testing and Prescription* (10th ed.). Philadelphia: Wolters Kluwer.

American Council on Exercise (2019). *The Professional's Guide to Health and Wellness Coaching*. San Diego, Calif.: American Council on Exercise.

Heyward, V.H. & Wagner, D. (2004). *Applied Body Composition Assessment*. Champaign, Ill.: Human Kinetics.

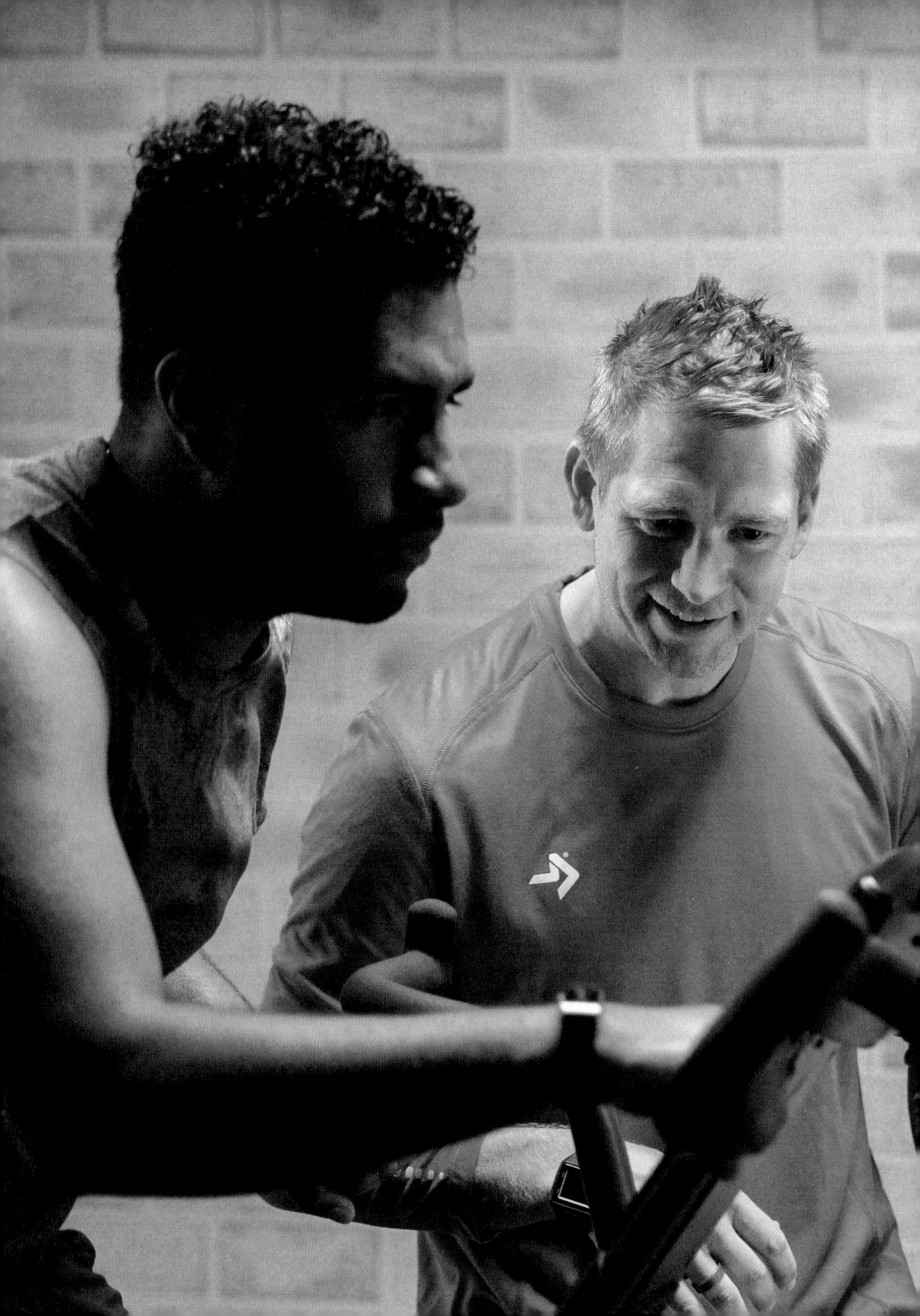

CHAPTER 8

Cardiorespiratory Training: Physiology, Assessments, and Programming

LANCE C. DALLECK, PhD
Professor of Exercise and Sport Science, Western Colorado University

IN THIS CHAPTER

LEARNING OBJECTIVES:

Upon completion of this chapter, the reader will be able to:

- Identify the acute and chronic physiological responses to cardiorespiratory training
- Recognize key environmental considerations for cardiorespiratory training
- Explain the procedures for ventilatory threshold assessment
- Evaluate the results of cardiorespiratory fitness assessments and apply them to cardiorespiratory programming
- Identify key programming considerations for limiting sedentary time
- List the three phases of the ACE Integrated Fitness Training (ACE IFT®) Model for Cardiorespiratory Training
- Design personalized Cardiorespiratory Training programs for clients ranging from physically inactive individuals to endurance athletes utilizing assessment and programming tools from each phase of the ACE IFT Model

ACE UNIVERSITY

If your study program includes the ACE University, visit www.ACEfitness.org/MyACE and log in to your My ACE Account to take full advantage of the ACE Personal Trainer Study Program and online guided study experience.

A variety of media to support and expand on the material in this text is provided to facilitate learning and best prepare you for the ACE Personal Trainer Certification exam and a career as a personal trainer.

Humans are designed to move. Since emerging as a distinct species, humans moved to secure food, escape from dangerous situations, attract mates, and do a variety of other activities that allowed the species to thrive. In the small groups of hunter-gatherers that still exist, everyday levels of physical activity are extraordinarily high (Lightfoot, 2013; Pontzer et al., 2012). The so-called "diseases of civilization" (e.g., **heart disease**, **diabetes,** and many cancers) are very uncommon in these groups (Pijl, 2011). Since physical movement is essential for human survival, the organ systems involved in energy metabolism (i.e., the muscular and cardiorespiratory systems) function best when subjected to regular physical challenges. Physical activity leads to improvements in work capacity (e.g., **cardiorespiratory fitness**), a sense of well-being, and overall health, as well as a reduction in chronic disease. However, the obligatory need for physical activity is very low in modern society. Most people can do their jobs and feed themselves with a minimum of exertion. Accordingly, the need for people to structure their lives in a way that intentionally includes either higher levels of physical activity or even any exercise at all has risen dramatically.

Anatomical Systems

It is paramount for personal trainers to have a working knowledge of the anatomy and physiology that underpins cardiorespiratory training, which is also commonly referred to as aerobic training and cardiovascular training. Indeed, knowledge of the cardiovascular and respiratory systems provides insight into the acute responses to different exercise and recovery conditions in both physically inactive and trained clients. Moreover, numerous chronic adaptations to cardiorespiratory training occur within the cardiovascular and respiratory systems, including larger maximal cardiac output values, plasma volume expansion, increased strength and endurance of the respiratory muscles, and reduced blood pressure. Overall, an understanding of basic cardiorespiratory anatomy and physiology, coupled with how these systems respond to different acute and chronic exercise stimuli, will enhance the ability of personal trainers to design and implement safe and effective cardiorespiratory training programs for their clients.

CARDIOVASCULAR SYSTEM

The cardiovascular, or circulatory, system is a closed-circuit system composed of the heart, blood vessels, and blood. Blood continuously travels a circular route through the heart into the **arteries,** then to the **capillaries,** into the **veins,** and back to the heart. Together with the respiratory system, the heart and blood vessels deliver oxygen and nutrients to the body's tissues while also removing waste, such as carbon dioxide and metabolic by-products.

Blood, the fluid component of the cardiovascular system, links the internal environment of the body to the external environment by transporting materials between the two environments as well as among the various cells and tissues. The liquid component of blood, called **plasma,** is responsible for carrying **hormones,** plasma proteins, food materials (e.g., **carbohydrates, amino acids,** and **lipids**), **ions** (e.g., sodium, chloride, and bicarbonate), and gases (e.g., oxygen, nitrogen, and carbon dioxide) throughout the body. The portion of the blood that is not plasma contains the formed elements, which include red blood cells, various types of white blood cells, and **platelets.**

Given that blood "feeds" virtually all tissues, its primary function is transportation. In addition, the cardiovascular system plays an important role in temperature regulation and acid–base balance.

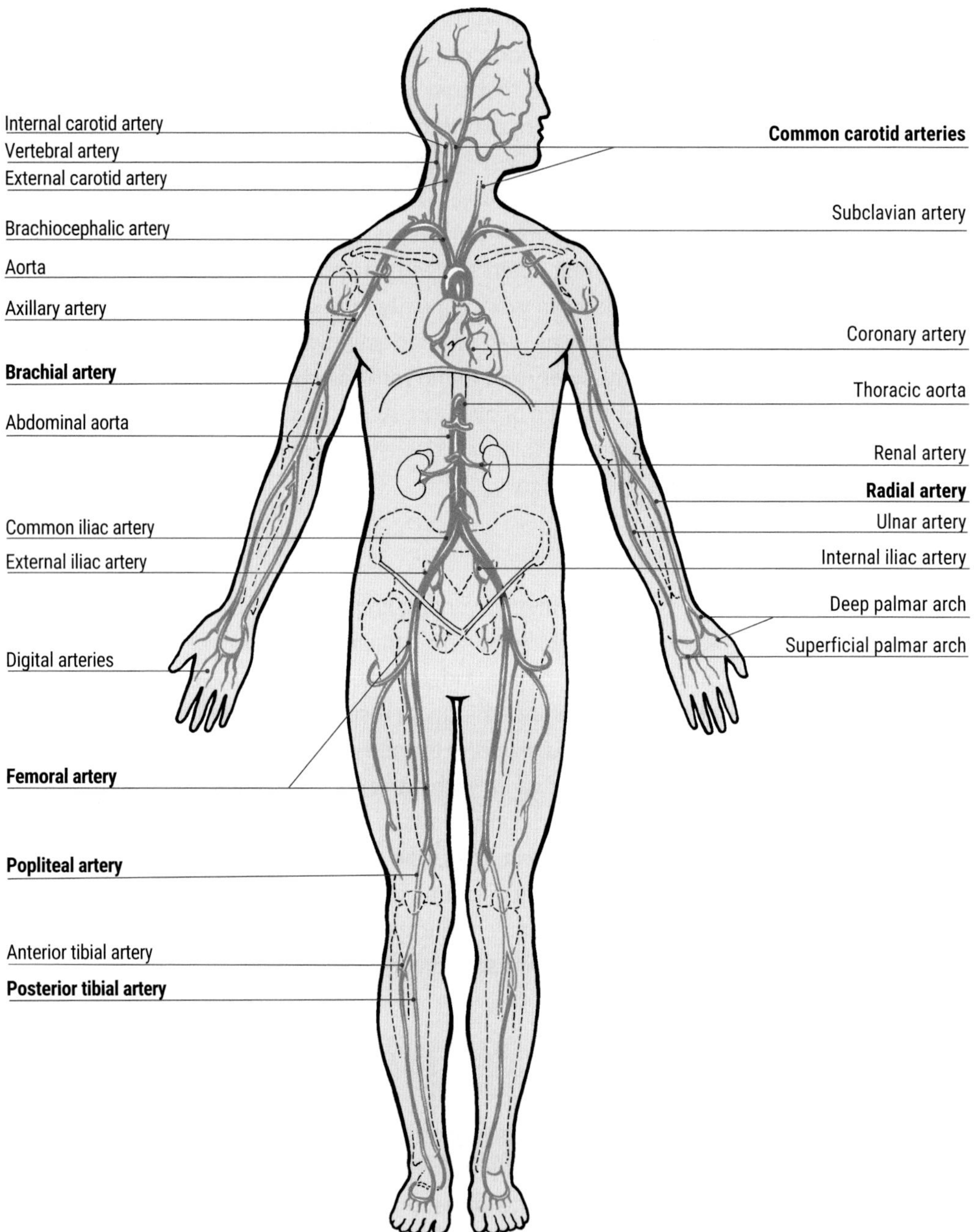

FIGURE 8-1a
Major arteries of the body (anterior view)

Blood is transported throughout the body via blood vessels. The categories of blood vessels include the following:

- Arteries and **arterioles,** which carry oxygen-rich blood away from the heart
- Capillaries, which provide sites for gas, nutrient, and waste exchange between the blood and tissues
- **Venules** and veins, which return oxygen-poor blood to the heart

As blood leaves the heart to nourish the body, it is carried by the arteries (Figure 8-1a). Large arteries, such as the **aorta** and its major branches, are thick and elastic and are passively stretched as the blood is ejected from the heart. **Arteriosclerosis** (i.e., hardening of the arteries and narrowing of the arteries due to plaque accumulation), which is

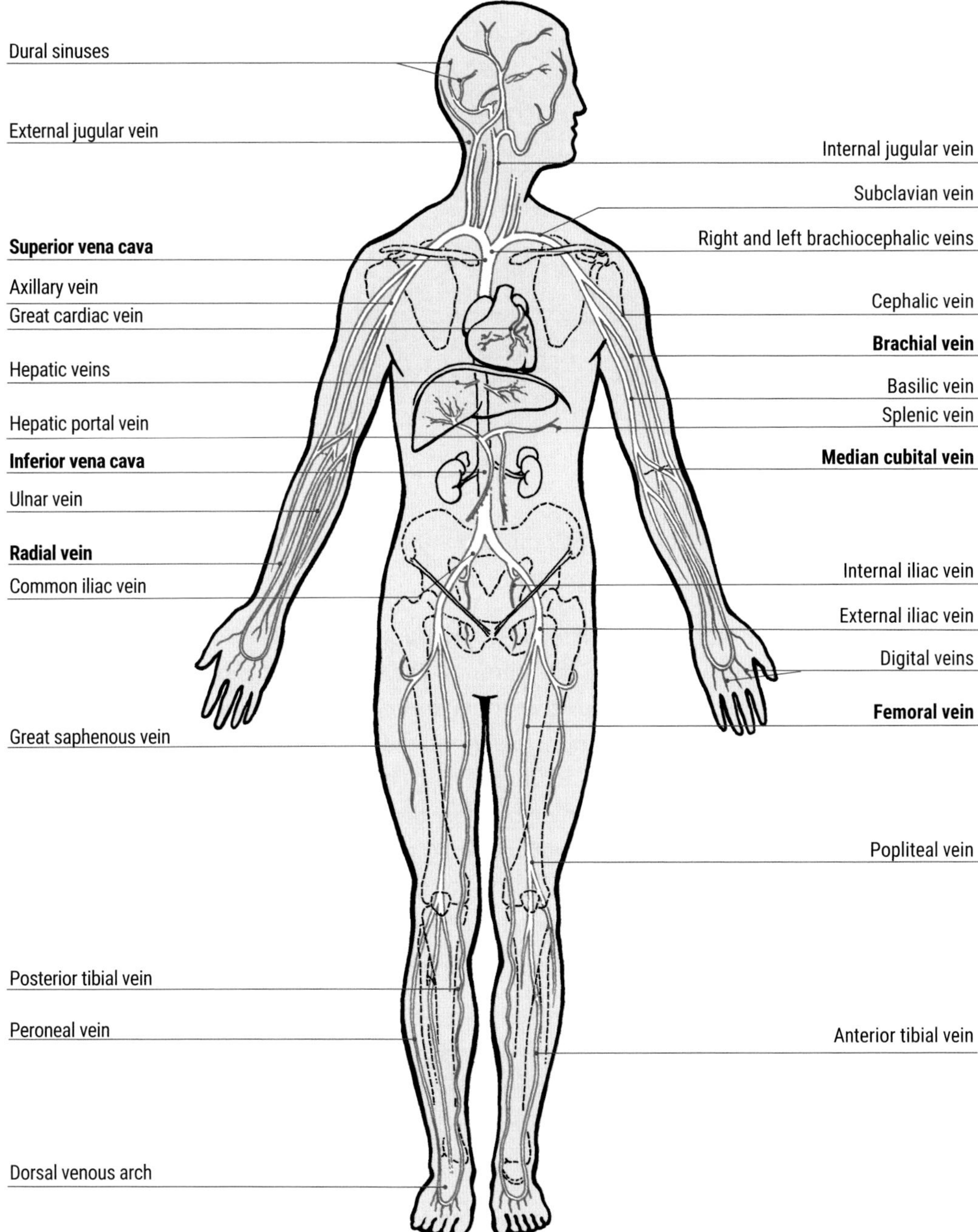

FIGURE 8-1b
Major veins of the body (anterior view)

commonly seen in older adults, contributes to arterial rigidity and decreases the arteries' ability to expand. This condition gives way to an increase in **blood pressure (BP),** which is commonly associated with aging. As arteries lead away from the heart, they branch extensively to form a "tree" of smaller, microscopic vessels called arterioles. Eventually, the arterioles develop into "beds" of much smaller structures, the capillaries. Capillaries have extremely thin walls, and, consequently, allow the exchange of materials between the blood and the **interstitial fluid** between the cells. Blood passes from the capillary beds to small venous vessels called venules. As venules lead back to the heart, they increase in size and become veins (Figure 8-1b). The walls of veins are thinner and less elastic than arterial walls. Commonly found inside the veins of the lower limbs are valves that allow blood to flow in only one direction—toward the heart. Blood leaving the major veins—the

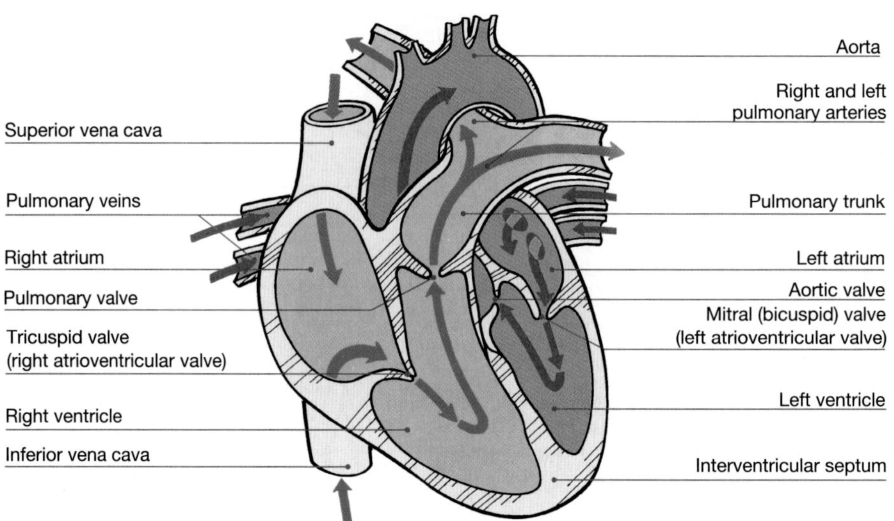

FIGURE 8-2
Structure of the heart and flow of blood within it

superior and inferior vena cava—empties directly into the heart, where it is transported to the lungs to pick up a fresh supply of oxygen.

The heart serves as a pump, pushing the blood throughout the body. It is located between the lungs and lies just left of center, behind the sternum. The adult heart is approximately the size of a closed fist. It is divided into four chambers and is often considered two pumps in one, as the right two chambers are responsible for pulmonary circulation and the left two chambers are responsible for systemic circulation. The chambers of the heart consist of two atria and two **ventricles.** The atria are small and located superior to the ventricles, which make up the bulk of the heart. The right **atrium** and the right ventricle form the right pump, while the left atrium and left ventricle combine to form the left pump (Figure 8-2). The right and left sides of the heart are separated by a muscular wall, called the interventricular septum, which prevents the mixing of blood from the two sides of the heart.

To function as a pump, the heart must have both receiving and propulsion chambers, as well as valves, which direct blood flow through the heart. Blood movement within the heart is from the atria (the receiving chambers) to the ventricles (the propulsion chambers) and from the ventricles to the arteries. Backward movement of blood within the heart is prevented by four one-way valves.

The right and left atrioventricular valves connect the right and left atria with the right and left ventricles, respectively. Backflow from the arteries into the ventricles is prevented by the pulmonary semilunar valve (right ventricle) and the aortic semilunar valve (left ventricle).

The right side of the heart receives blood that is partially depleted of its oxygen content and contains an elevated level of carbon dioxide after having passed through the cells. This blood is then pushed into the lungs, where it releases its carbon dioxide in exchange for oxygen. This is called the **pulmonary circuit.** The left side of the heart receives newly oxygenated blood from the lungs and pumps it to the various tissues of the body through the **systemic circuit.** The specific pathway of blood through the heart starts as venous blood (blood coming back to the heart through the veins). All the blood from the venous system enters the right atrium first. From there, blood enters the right ventricle, which pumps it to the lungs through the pulmonary arteries (the exception to arteries carrying oxygen-rich blood). In the lungs, the blood picks up a fresh supply of oxygen and gives off carbon dioxide. The oxygenated blood returns from the lungs to the left atrium through the pulmonary veins (the exception to veins carrying oxygen-poor blood). From the left atrium, blood enters the left ventricle, and is then pumped through the aorta to the rest of the body (except for the lungs).

The **cardiac cycle** is the period from the beginning of one heartbeat to the beginning of the next. The right and left sides of the heart perform their pumping actions simultaneously. In other words, when the heart beats, both atria contract together to empty the blood into the ventricles.

Approximately 0.1 seconds after the atria contract, both ventricles contract to deliver blood to the pulmonary and systemic circuits. The repeating phases of contraction and relaxation are called systole and diastole. Systole refers to the contraction phase of the cardiac cycle, during which blood leaves the ventricles, while diastole refers to the relaxation phase of the cardiac cycle, during which blood fills the ventricles.

RESPIRATORY SYSTEM

The structures of the respiratory system make it possible for the body to exchange gases between the external environment and the tissues. Specifically, the respiratory system provides a means to replace oxygen and remove carbon dioxide from the blood. In addition, it makes speech possible and plays an important role in the regulation of the acid–base balance during exercise. The respiratory system is made up of the nose, nasal cavity, **pharynx, larynx,** trachea, **bronchi,** and lungs. Together, these structures form a group of passages that filter air and transport it into the lungs, where gas exchange occurs within microscopic air sacs called **alveoli** (Figure 8-3).

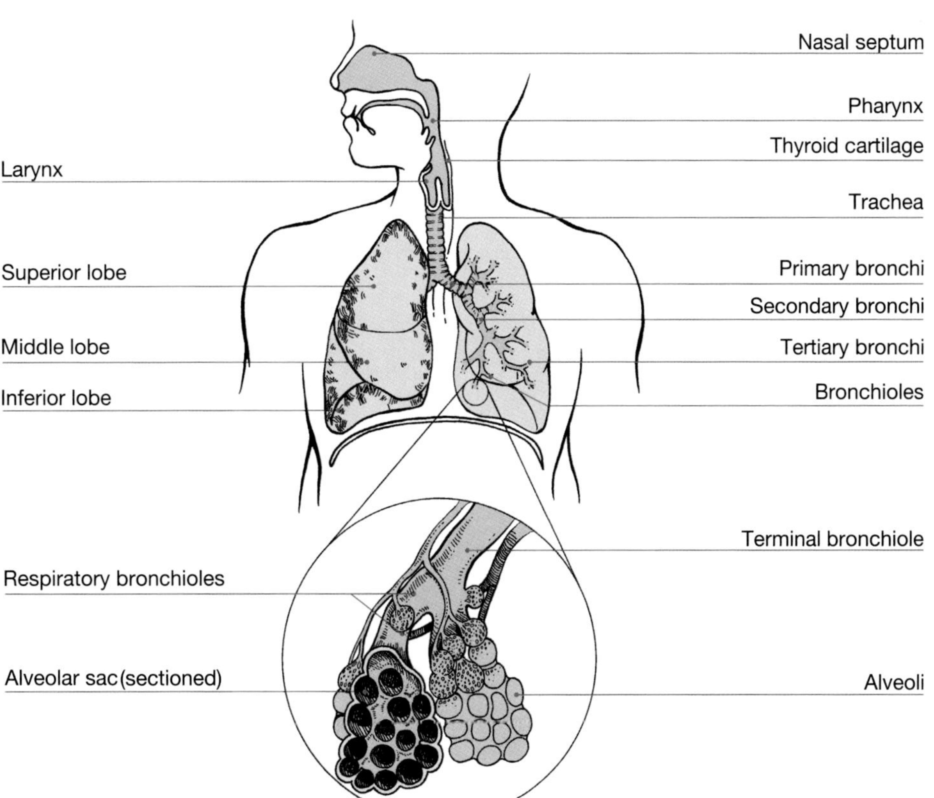

FIGURE 8-3
Upper and lower respiratory pathways

Air enters the respiratory system through both the nostrils and the mouth. The air is warmed and passed through the pharynx (throat), and then the larynx (the area of the "Adam's apple"). Humans normally breathe approximately 5 to 6 liters of air per minute through the nose when at rest, but use the mouth as the primary passageway for air when ventilation is increased to approximately 20 to 30 liters per minute during exercise. From the larynx, air travels through the trachea (windpipe), which extends to the fifth or sixth thoracic vertebrae, where it divides into two smaller branches: the right and left primary bronchi. The primary bronchi divide into smaller secondary bronchi, one for each lobe of the lung. The secondary bronchi then branch into many tertiary bronchi that repeatedly branch further, resulting in tiny **bronchioles.** The bronchioles continue to branch to form terminal bronchioles, which ultimately divide into even smaller respiratory bronchioles that end in clusters of alveoli (i.e., thin-walled air sacs).

The lungs contain approximately 300 million alveoli, which provide an enormous surface area for gas exchange. It is estimated that the total surface area available for diffusion in the human lung is about the size of a tennis court.

The lungs are encased within the rib cage. These paired, cone-shaped structures house the primary, secondary, and tertiary bronchi, as well as the various bronchioles and alveoli. The two lungs are separated by a space called the **mediastinum,** which contains several important organs, including the heart, aorta, esophagus, and part of the trachea. The lungs rest on top of the most important muscle of **inspiration,** the **diaphragm,** which is the only skeletal muscle considered essential for life. When the diaphragm contracts, it forces the abdominal contents downward and forward, while the external intercostals (groups of muscles that run between the ribs) lift the ribs outward (Figure 8-4). This action reduces the pressure in the membranes surrounding the lungs and, in turn, causes the lungs to expand. This expansion allows airflow into the lungs. At rest, the diaphragm and external intercostals perform most

FIGURE 8-4
Diaphragm and intercostal muscles

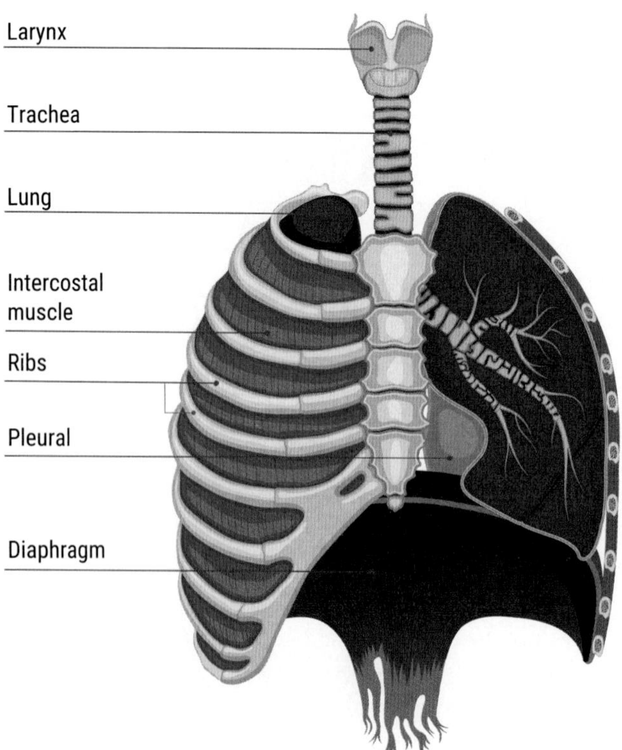

of the work of inspiration. However, during physical activity, accessory muscles of inspiration are recruited, including the pectoralis minor, scalenes, and sternocleidomastoid. By assisting the diaphragm and external intercostals in the effort to further increase the volume of the **thorax,** these muscles aid in inspiration. **Expiration** occurs passively during normal, quiet breathing, requiring no assistance from muscle action. However, during exercise, expiration becomes active. Important muscles of expiration, such as the rectus abdominis, internal obliques, serratus posterior, and internal intercostals, are activated to help pull the rib cage downward and force air from the lungs by squeezing the abdominal organs upward against the diaphragm.

The muscles of respiration adapt to regular exercise training, as do the locomotor skeletal muscles. Regular endurance exercise increases the oxidative capacity of respiratory muscles, which improves respiratory muscle endurance. This is important because respiratory muscles have been shown to fatigue with exercise, adversely affecting the ability to breathe during both moderate- and high-intensity activities. Improving respiratory muscle endurance enhances exercise performance at various intensities.

Physiology of the Cardiorespiratory System

Cardiorespiratory fitness is defined as the capacity of the heart and lungs to deliver blood and oxygen (O_2) to the working muscles during exercise. A person's capacity to perform cardiorespiratory exercise depends largely on the interaction of the cardiovascular and respiratory systems as they provide O_2 to be transported in the blood to the active cells so that carbohydrates and **fatty acids** can be converted to **adenosine triphosphate (ATP)** to fuel muscular activity. These two systems are also important for the removal of metabolic waste products, such as carbon dioxide (CO_2) and **lactate,** and for the dissipation of heat produced by metabolic processes. There are three basic processes that must interact to provide adequate blood and nutrients to the tissues:

- Getting O_2 into the blood—a function of **pulmonary ventilation** coupled with the O_2-carrying capacity of the blood
- Distributing blood flow and delivering O_2 to the active tissues—a function of **cardiac output**
- Extracting O_2 from the blood to complete the metabolic production of ATP—a function of localizing the extraction of O_2 from the delivery of cardiac output to the active muscles and the oxidative **enzymes** located within the active cells

OXYGEN-CARRYING CAPACITY

The O_2-carrying capacity of blood is determined primarily by two variables: (1) the ability to adequately ventilate the alveoli in the lungs and (2) the **hemoglobin (Hb)** concentration of the blood. Pulmonary ventilation is a function of both the rate and depth (**tidal volume**) of breathing. At the onset of exercise, both tidal volume and breathing rate increase. This increase in ventilation volume brings more O_2 into the lungs, where it can be transferred into the blood. Because air flows in and out of the alveoli via the same bronchial tubes, it is particularly important to maintain an adequate tidal volume during even heavy exercise so that the gas concentrations in the alveoli can be effectively exchanged. If this does not happen, and the O_2 concentration in the alveoli is too low and the CO_2 concentration is too high, the tendency for the gases to move in the desired direction (O_2 from alveoli to pulmonary capillaries or CO_2 from pulmonary capillaries to alveoli) is reduced. Normally, respiration does not limit exercise performance in healthy individuals. However, individuals with **emphysema** (degradation of the alveoli) or **asthma** (constriction of the breathing passages) cannot move enough air through their lungs to adequately aerate the alveoli and thereby oxygenate the blood. As a result, the blood leaving the lungs is not sufficiently loaded with O_2 and exercise capacity is diminished. Additionally, because the brain is very sensitive to the CO_2 concentration in the blood, a failure to adequately ventilate the lungs will result in elevated blood CO_2 concentration, with the result being that the exerciser will feel an urgent need to stop exercising.

Hemoglobin is a protein in red blood cells that is specifically adapted to bond with (i.e., carry) O_2 molecules (Figure 8-5). When O_2 enters the lungs, it diffuses through the pulmonary membranes into the bloodstream, where it binds to Hb. The O_2 is then carried within the bloodstream throughout the body. Individuals with low Hb concentrations (i.e., **anemia**) cannot carry as much O_2 in their blood as individuals with normal Hb concentrations. For example, in people with anemia (i.e., less than 12 g of Hb per 100 mL of blood), the blood's O_2-carrying capacity is severely limited, and they fatigue very easily. In the warmer, more acidic, and lower O_2 environment of the exercising muscles, Hb reverses its tendency to bind with O_2 and releases it to the tissues. In most healthy individuals, the O_2-carrying capacity of the blood is not a limiting factor in the performance of cardiorespiratory exercise.

FIGURE 8-5
Molecules of oxygen (O_2) bind to the protein hemoglobin in red blood cells

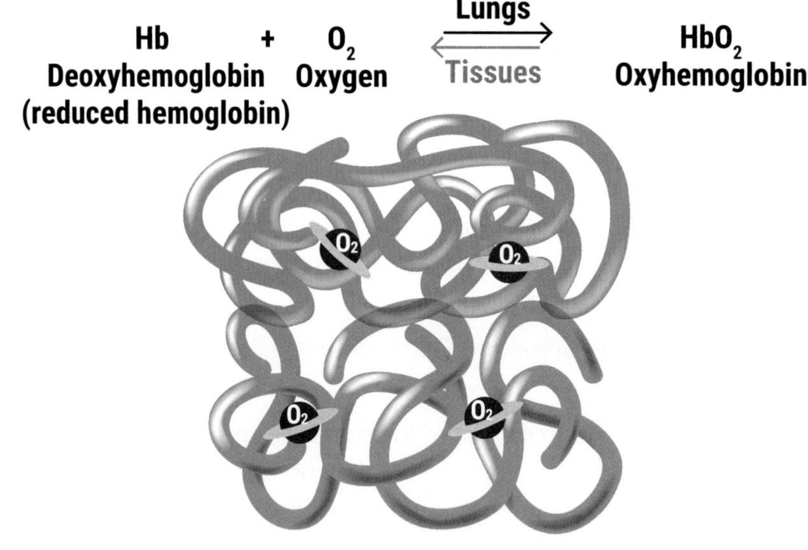

OXYGEN DELIVERY

Probably the most important factor in cardiorespiratory fitness is the delivery of blood to the active cells, which is a function of cardiac output, and the distribution of more blood to active areas (e.g., muscles) and less blood to inactive areas (e.g., digestive system). Cardiac output is the product of **heart rate (HR)** (in beats per minute) and **stroke volume (SV)** (in liters), or the quantity of blood pumped per heartbeat:

$$\text{Cardiac output} = \text{HR} \times \text{SV}$$

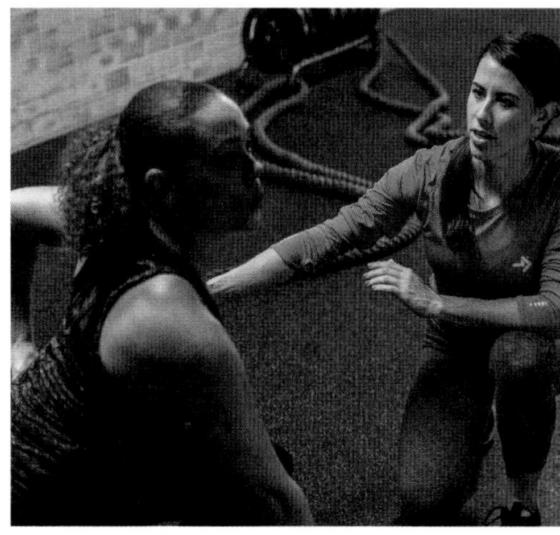

At rest, cardiac output averages approximately 5 liters (1.3 gallons) per minute. During maximal exercise, this number normally increases to 20 to 25 liters per minute (~5 to 6.5 gallons) and can increase to up to 30 to 40 liters (~8 to 10.5 gallons) per minute in highly trained individuals. The increase in cardiac output is brought about by increases in both HR and SV. HR generally increases in a linear fashion up to maximal levels, while SV increases up to approximately 40 to 50% of an individual's maximal capacity and then plateaus. Stroke volume increases, in part, as a result of the enlargement of the left ventricle due to chronic cardiorespiratory training, which is limited by the capacity of the ventricle's chamber to increase. The increase in SV is brought about by increases in both venous return and in the contractile force of the heart (represented as the **ejection fraction,** or the percentage of the **end-diastolic volume** that is ejected with each contraction of the heart). The ejection fraction is normally 50 to 60% at rest and increases to 60 to 80% during exercise. Equally important is the ability of the circulation to selectively increase the percentage of the increased cardiac output that is delivered to the exercising muscles and to actually decrease blood flow to the **viscera.** This means that the increased cardiac output is used very efficiently. This redistribution of blood flow is accomplished by active **vasoconstriction** in the viscera and inactive muscles and active **vasodilation** in the active muscles (regulated by **metabolites** produced in the active muscles). In individuals with **cardiovascular disease (CVD),** the ejection fraction may be reduced after the loss of heart muscle tissue following a **myocardial infarction** or heart failure. In individuals with **ischemia** during exercise (i.e., inadequate blood flow to the heart because of narrowed coronary arteries), the ejection fraction may be normal at rest and then decrease with exercise. This is because ischemic tissue (i.e., tissue receiving too little blood flow to restore ATP aerobically) loses much of its contractility. An everyday situation that most people would recognize is sleeping on one's arm. The tingling feeling and inability to move the arm properly (as a result of lack of blood flow to the arm due to body position) is comparable to what happens to the heart tissue when myocardial ischemia occurs.

OXYGEN EXTRACTION

The third important factor in determining cardiorespiratory fitness is the extraction of O_2 from the blood at the cellular level for the **aerobic** production of ATP. The amount of O_2 extracted is largely a function of muscle-fiber type and the availability of specialized oxidative enzymes. For example, **slow-twitch muscle fibers** (**type I muscle fibers**) are specifically adapted for O_2 extraction and utilization due to their high levels of oxidative enzymes. This enhances aerobic production of ATP in the **mitochondria** of the cells. One of the most important adaptations to training is an increase in the number and size of the mitochondria, with a corresponding increase in the levels of oxidative enzymes used to aerobically produce ATP.

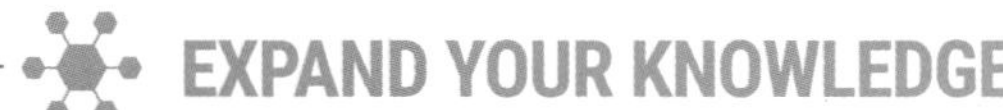

Understanding the Ventilatory Response to Exercise

During exercise, higher intensities increase respiratory rates, resulting in larger volumes of air moving into and out of the lungs. This volume of air, called **minute ventilation ($\dot{V}_E$)**, reflects the body's metabolism and defines the volume of air moved through the lungs on a minute-by-minute basis. As exercise intensity progressively increases, so too does the amount of air moving into and out of the respiratory tract, representing a linear relationship. As the intensity of exercise continues to increase, there is a point at which ventilation starts to increase in a nonlinear fashion [i.e., the **first ventilatory threshold (VT1)**]. This point where ventilation deviates from the progressive linear increase corresponds with (but is not identical to) the development of muscle and blood acidosis. Blood buffers, which are compounds that help to neutralize acidosis, work to reduce the muscle fiber acidosis. This leads to an increase in CO_2, which the body attempts to eliminate with the increase in ventilation (Figure 8-6).

- Lactic acid manufactured within muscle cells dissociates into lactate$^-$ + hydrogen (H^+).
- The blood's bicarbonate buffer (predominantly $NaHCO_3$) dissociates into sodium (Na^+) + HCO_3^-.
- H^+ and HCO_3^- combine to form H_2CO_3 (carbonic acid), which is transported to the lungs and dissociated into H_2O and CO_2, both of which are removed from the body during expiration, increasing $\dot{V}_E$.
- Na^+ and lactate combine to form Na-lactate, some of which enters the mitochondria within the muscle cell for energy use, some of which is shuttled to the heart tissue for energy use, and some of which is shuttled to the liver for reconversion back to usable forms of energy.

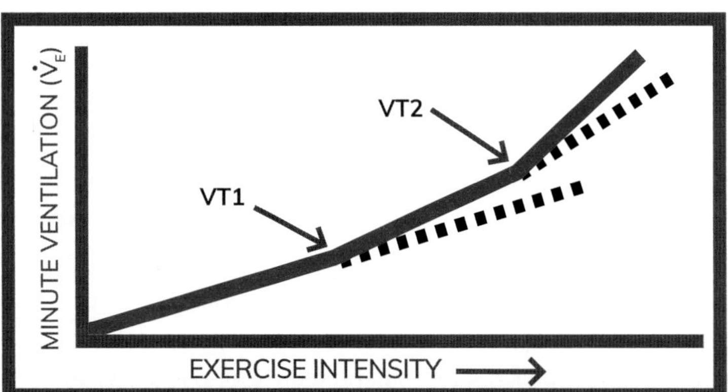

FIGURE 8-6
Ventilatory response to increasing exercise intensity

Note: VT1 = First ventilatory threshold; VT2 = Second ventilatory threshold

Physiological Adaptations to Acute and Chronic Cardiorespiratory Exercise

MUSCULAR SYSTEM

The organ systems stressed during physical activity and exercise adapt in a way that is very specific to the type of exercise performed. The muscle fibers that are recruited to perform exercise are the only ones stimulated to adapt. During low-intensity endurance exercise, this usually means adaptations in the type I muscle fibers (i.e., the slow-twitch muscle fibers).

These adaptations involve increasing the size and number of mitochondria within the cell to augment aerobic ATP generation (Figure 8-7). There is also a growth of more capillaries around the recruited muscle fibers, which enhances the delivery of oxygenated blood to the muscle fibers. If the recruitment is near the upper limit of a given muscle fiber's capacity to generate force, there may also be adaptations in the contractile mechanism (i.e., the **actin** and **myosin** filaments), leading to **hypertrophy** of those muscle fibers. During higher-intensity exercise, the **type II muscle fibers** (i.e., the **fast-twitch muscle fibers**) may also be recruited. They adapt primarily by increasing the number of **anaerobic** enzymes so that anaerobic energy production will be enhanced. With increased training intensity, there may also be an increase in the contractile proteins, resulting in hypertrophy of the muscle fibers.

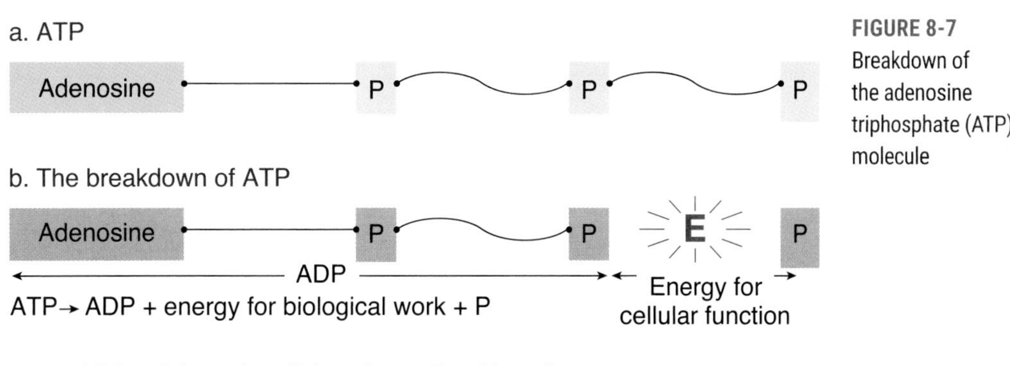

FIGURE 8-7
Breakdown of the adenosine triphosphate (ATP) molecule

CARDIOVASCULAR SYSTEM

Due to the expansion of blood volume that occurs with endurance training, the heart muscle will hypertrophy, enlarging its chambers and becoming a bigger and stronger muscle that is able to deliver a higher cardiac output to the muscles. These adaptations are primarily in the form of a larger SV, as **maximal heart rate (MHR)** does not increase with training. This increase in SV is due to chamber enlargement, greater amounts of chamber filling (end-diastolic volume), and greater chamber emptying (ejection fraction) of the heart with each beat. There is also some evidence that the redistribution of the cardiac output to the active muscles (via vasodilation) may improve after training, thus making the increase in cardiac output more effective in terms of delivering O_2 where it is needed.

RESPIRATORY SYSTEM

Although somewhat less adaptable than the heart and circulatory system, the muscles of the respiratory system will adapt as exercise is performed regularly to allow for increased ventilation of the alveoli, which is where the cardiovascular system interfaces with the respiratory system (see Figure 8-4). The muscles involved in respiration span the thorax and abdomen and include the following:

- The diaphragm, which is the body's key breathing muscle, and the external intercostals used during passive (resting) inspiration

- The group of muscles that pull the rib cage upward (e.g., sternocleidomastoid, scalene, pectoralis minor, and portions of the serratus anterior) during active (exercise) inspiration
- The group of muscles that pull the rib cage downward (e.g., abdominals, serratus posterior, and internal intercostals) during active expiration

Both the strength and fatigue resistance of the respiratory muscles improve with training, allowing greater ventilation for longer periods than existed before training. This stronger musculature may lead to an increase in tidal volume, which delivers more O_2 to the alveoli and reduces the relative amount of respiratory dead space (i.e., air trapped in the bronchial tubes that never reaches the alveoli) at high breathing frequencies, thus making ventilation more efficient.

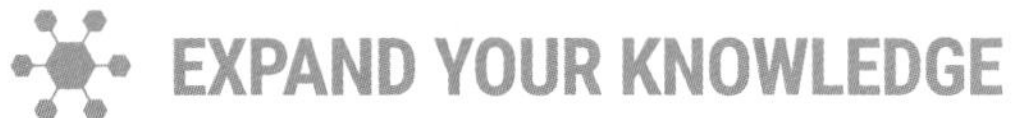

Sedentary Behavior versus Physical Inactivity

Sedentary behavior refers to too much sitting, while **physical inactivity** signifies too little exercise. For example, an individual can be considered active according to the current physical-activity guidelines, but still spend too much time sitting in front of the TV (Owen et al., 2011). This is known as the "active couch potato" phenomenon. This term might describe, for example, an office worker who participates in group exercise classes for 45 minutes every lunch break throughout the work week, but who spends the remainder of the day seated at his or her desk. Researchers are increasingly interested in whether or not individuals who fall within the active couch potato category are at increased risk for health problems (Katzmarzyk & Lee, 2012). Indeed, it has been reported that total sedentary time was consistently associated with various unfavorable cardiometabolic biomarkers (e.g., **insulin resistance** and elevated blood **triglycerides**), even after adjusting for physical-activity time (Brocklebank et al., 2015).

The fact that sedentary behavior and physical inactivity are two distinct health domains has important ramifications for ACE® Certified Personal Trainers. If clients are to achieve optimal health, personal trainers should provide guidance on reducing sedentary time.

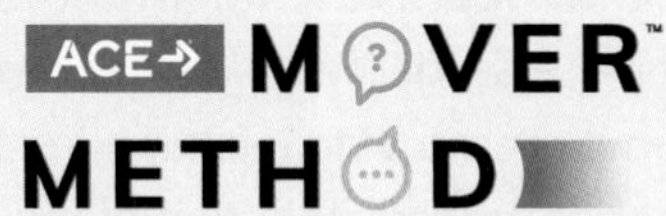

The Active Couch Potato

During a recent meeting with a client, she lets you know that she is concerned with the progress she is making. Over the past year, she has been consistently attending group exercise classes for 45 minutes on her lunch breaks, including both moderate-intensity cardiorespiratory training and muscular training. While she was initially losing weight and feeling more fit, she is no longer getting the same results. In addition, she shares that during a recent doctor's appointment she brought up these challenges and was told by her doctor that even though she has maintained her physical-activity levels over the past year, she is still doing too much sitting. Her doctor told her that her total sedentary time might put her at risk for cardiometabolic conditions such as insulin resistance and elevated triglycerides. The client requested a meeting with you to establish some new goals to address her sedentary behaviors.

ACE→ ABC APPROACH

The following is an example of how the ACE Mover Method™ and the ACE ABC Approach™ can be used to explore the differences between physical inactivity and sedentary behavior, while empowering a client to move forward with actionable steps for decreasing sitting time.

Ask: Asking powerful open-ended questions during this exploratory conversation can help you confirm what the client already knows about the differences between sedentary behavior and physical inactivity. The following is an example of an initial question to ask:

Personal Trainer: In your perfect vision of your future self, what would you like to see different about your lifestyle to address the sedentary behaviors your doctor mentioned?

Client: For the past year, I thought I was doing enough to manage my health, but in speaking with my doctor I realized that even though I have become more physically active, I have not made significant changes to my overall lifestyle. At this point, I want to find ways to add more movement to my day-to-day life to reduce my total sedentary time.

Break down barriers: Ask more open-ended questions to find out what obstacles might get in the way of the client decreasing sitting time.

Personal Trainer: What is currently preventing you from adding more movement to your daily routine?

Client: I'm just so busy with my home life and my career. I'm always looking for reasons to relax, whether I'm at home or work. For me, this means sitting down. I honestly don't know if I have the time to add more movement into my day.

Collaborate: Working together with the client on goals and solutions is the next step now that the client has expressed her wants (to reduce sedentary behaviors) and barriers (lack of time).

Personal Trainer: I'm sure there was a time when it seemed like you were too busy to add 45 minutes of exercise to your daily work schedule and now you have maintained this goal for a year.

Client: That's a good point. There was a time when I thought I could never add working out during lunch to my schedule, but here I am. I thought it was enough, but according to my doctor, it's not.

Personal Trainer: On one hand, you feel you are doing enough, but on the other hand, you are surprised that your doctor said you need to do more to protect your long-term health. What options do you have available for moving more throughout your day?

Client: I do have a standing desk at work that I have only used a few times. Perhaps I could set up a plan for using it more. Maybe I could also get in more walking throughout my day during other breaks.

Personal Trainer: Those are both excellent ideas! The good news is that bouts of physical activity, of any length, can lead to health benefits. Being as specific as possible, how will you move forward?

Client: Starting tomorrow, I will stand for 10 minutes each hour throughout my day and I will determine some steps I can take to bring life back into the abandoned garden I have in my yard. I'll use alarms on my phone to remind me to stand each hour or to take an activity break.

The difference between sedentary behavior and physical inactivity is an important distinction. In this scenario, the client has incorporated an exercise routine into her day and spends 45 minutes being active. However, the remainder of her waking hours are being spent sitting. The ACE ABC Approach can be used to guide clients toward any change they are wanting to make, including decreasing sitting time, to work toward optimal health.

TIME REQUIRED FOR INCREASES IN CARDIORESPIRATORY FITNESS

Cardiorespiratory adaptations to exercise begin with the first exercise bout but are usually not readily measurable for a couple of weeks. **Maximal oxygen uptake ($\dot{V}O_2$max)**, which is the traditional standard marker of the cardiorespiratory fitness-training effect, increases with training, but reaches a peak and plateaus within about six months (Foster, Porcari, & Lucia, 2008). However, changes in **ventilatory threshold (VT),** a significant marker of metabolism that permits prediction of **lactate threshold** from the $\dot{V}_E$ response during progressive exercise, may continue for years. This change is attributed primarily to capillary growth and increased mitochondrial density (size and number) in the active muscles (Figure 8-8). To support these cardiorespiratory adaptations, the capacity of the muscle to store additional **glycogen** increases and the ability to mobilize and use fatty acids as a fuel source is also enhanced. This ability increases for some time beyond the primary increase in $\dot{V}O_2$max.

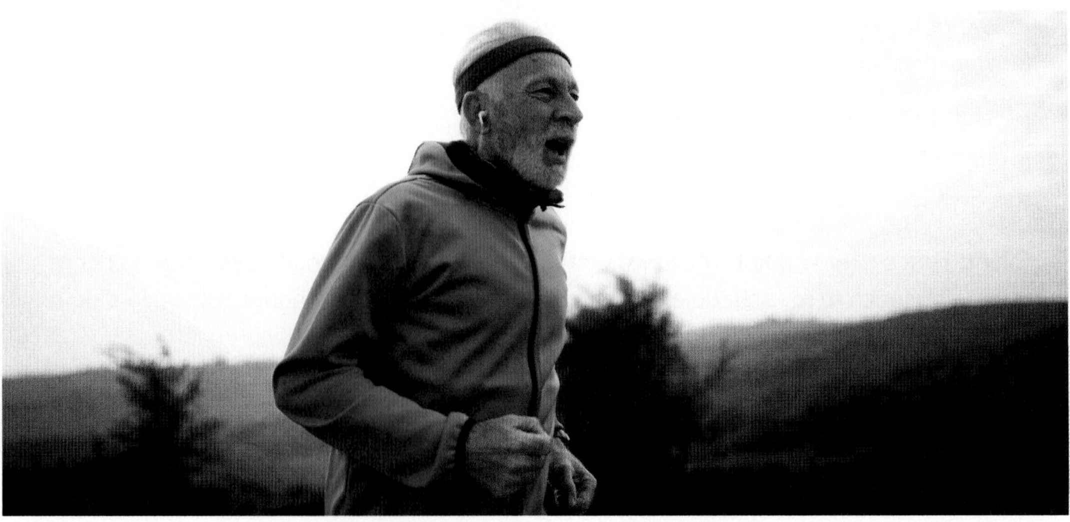

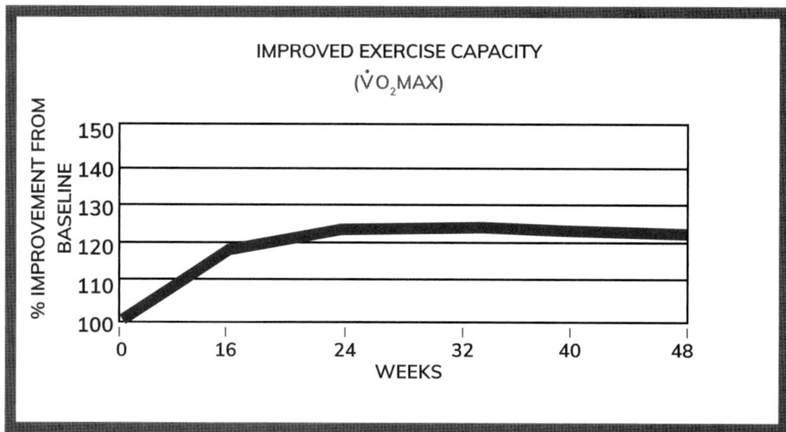

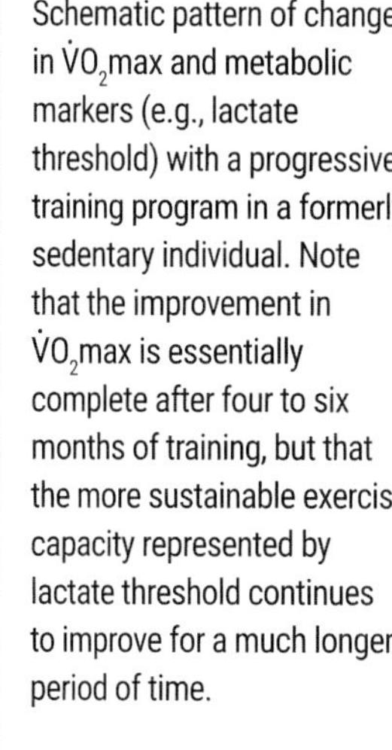
FIGURE 8-8
Schematic pattern of changes in $\dot{V}O_2$max and metabolic markers (e.g., lactate threshold) with a progressive training program in a formerly sedentary individual. Note that the improvement in $\dot{V}O_2$max is essentially complete after four to six months of training, but that the more sustainable exercise capacity represented by lactate threshold continues to improve for a much longer period of time.

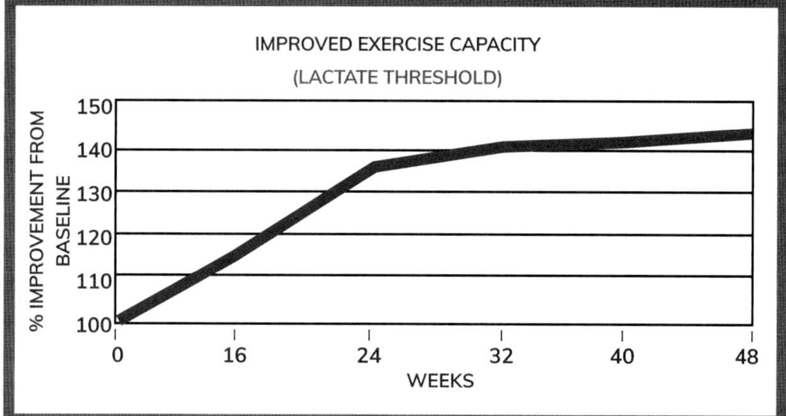

PHYSIOLOGICAL ADAPTATIONS TO STEADY-STATE AND INTERVAL-BASED EXERCISE

The primary adaptations to exercise training typically occur during steady-state exercise at moderate intensity. The term **steady state** refers to an intensity of exercise where the energy and physiological demands of the exercise bout are met by the intake and delivery of O_2 to the physiological systems in the body. At steady state, the rate of **oxygen uptake ($\dot{V}O_2$),** HR, cardiac output, ventilation, blood lactate concentration, and body temperature reach stable (although elevated) levels after a short period of exercise. Exercise duration is primarily limited by the willingness to continue (psychological) or by the availability of O_2, muscle glycogen, and/or blood **glucose** (physiological). When an exercise bout begins or exercise intensity changes, the body takes between 45 seconds and three to four minutes to achieve steady state. The time needed to achieve this level, sometime referred to as a "second wind," varies according to several factors, including fitness level (more fit individuals achieve steady state faster) and exercise intensity (when working at higher intensities, people require longer periods to achieve steady state).

There are several studies suggesting that **high-intensity interval training (HIIT)** (a few rounds of high-intensity exercise alternated with lower-intensity recovery periods) promotes similar or greater improvements in $\dot{V}O_2$max and fitness than steady-state exercise (Bacon et al., 2013). While this may prove to be a more time-efficient method of training, the appropriateness of this training modality must always be considered for deconditioned or at-risk clients. Research on HIIT also demonstrates additional adaptations beyond the cardiorespiratory benefits that include anaerobic adaptations to improve an individual's tolerance for the buildup of lactate (lactate threshold) that may continue to increase long after $\dot{V}O_2$max adaptations have reached their maximal extent (Laursen et al., 2002; Stepto et al., 1998). This adaptation enhances one's ability to sustain higher intensities of exercise for longer periods (Foster, Porcari, & Lucia, 2008).

A universal principle of training is that it is necessary to progressively perform higher intensities of exercise to effectively challenge or overload the cardiorespiratory system. Since muscle fibers that are not recruited are not likely to adapt, it is probable that there is little or no adaptation of type II muscle fibers during moderate-intensity cardiorespiratory training, whereas there would be with higher-intensity training. Generally, these intensities are not sustained through steady-state exercise. The overload on the heart to deliver blood to the exercising muscles during higher-intensity or non-steady-state exercise likely provokes adaptations that allow SV to increase to levels that are not achievable with lower-intensity steady-state training. These adaptations are probably attributable to large increases in venous blood return that occur with very high-intensity exercise that increases end-diastolic volume (i.e., chamber filling).

Environmental Considerations when Exercising

One of the many demands that sustained physical exertion places on the body is increased heat production. Contracting skeletal muscles produce large amounts of heat, and the body must regulate internal temperature by making adjustments in the amount of heat that is lost. In fact, metabolism often rises 20 to 25 times above resting levels during intense cardiorespiratory exercise by elite athletes, resulting in a potential increase in body temperature of 1° C every five to seven minutes (McArdle, Katch, & Katch, 2019).

The importance of body-temperature regulation is related to the critical processes of metabolism. That is, enzymes that regulate metabolic pathways are greatly influenced by changes in body temperature. An increase in body temperature >104° F (40° C) may be damaging to the protein structure of enzymes, eventually resulting in cellular destruction. A decrease in body temperature below 93.2° F (34° C) may cause a slowed metabolism and abnormal cardiac function. Thus, it is clear that body temperature must be carefully regulated.

An important concept should be kept in mind regarding temperature regulation: within the body, temperature may vary. There is a gradient (i.e., difference) between deep body temperature, such as the area surrounding internal organs, and shell (or skin) temperature. Thus, when referring to body temperature, an emphasis should be placed on using specific, descriptive terms (i.e., core temperature or skin temperature).

The body's temperature regulatory center is located in the **hypothalamus** in the brain. Receptors in the core and the skin send information to the hypothalamus about temperature changes within the body and the environment, respectively. During a bout of sustained submaximal exercise in a cool/moderate environment (i.e., low humidity and room temperature), muscular contraction produces heat in amounts directly proportional to exercise intensity. The venous blood draining from the exercising muscle carries excess heat throughout the body's core. Thermal core receptors signal the hypothalamus that the core temperature is rising, which directs the nervous system to commence sweating and increase blood flow to the skin. These processes increase body-heat loss and minimize the increase in body temperature (Figure 8-9).

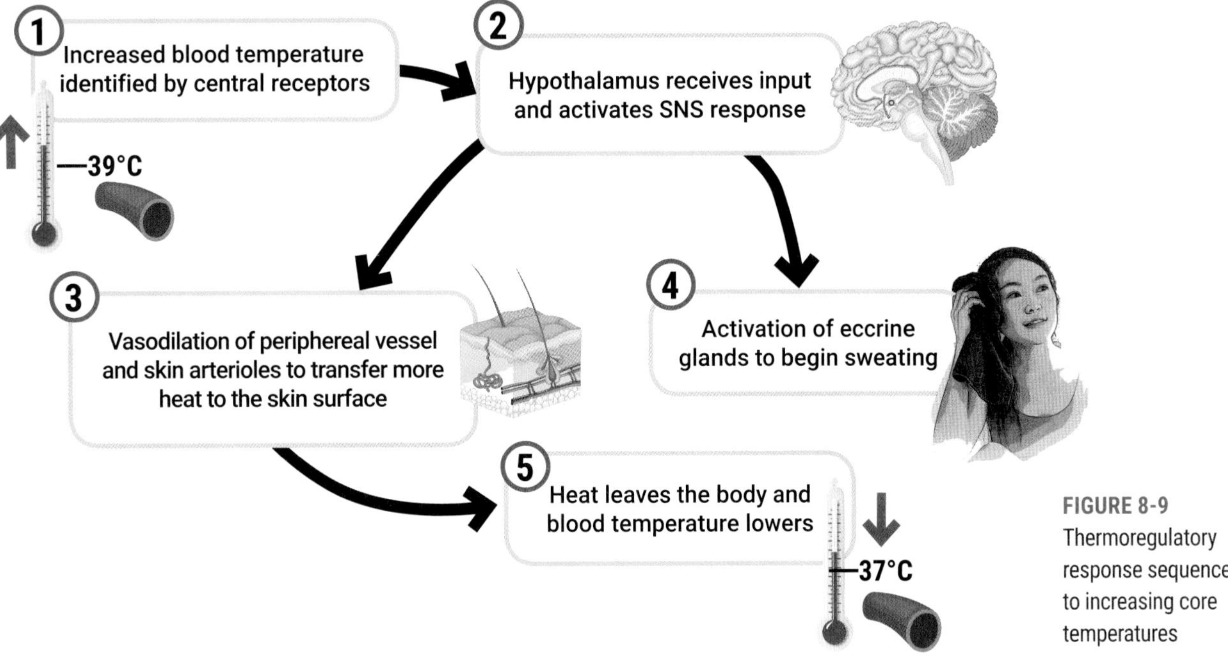

FIGURE 8-9
Thermoregulatory response sequence to increasing core temperatures

Source: Porcari, J.P., Bryant, C.X., & Comana, F. (2015). *Exercise Physiology.* Philadelphia: F.A. Davis Company.

Heat can be gained or lost (transferred) with **radiation, conduction,** and **convection.** This transfer is always from the area of high to low temperature. **Evaporation,** the main mechanism during exercise, involves only the loss of heat.

- Radiation is heat lost or gained in the form of infrared rays, which involves the transfer of heat from the surface of one object to another without any physical contact (e.g., the sun's rays transferring heat to the earth's surface).
- Conduction is the transfer of heat from the surface of the warmer object in contact with the surface of a cooler object (e.g., the transfer of heat from the body to a metal chair while a person is sitting on it).
- Convection is a form of conduction wherein heat is transferred to or from air or water molecules in contact with the body. As water or air molecules are warmed or cooled and moved away from the skin (such as in forced convection when the wind from a fan blows over the skin), cooler molecules replace them.
- Evaporation occurs when heat is transferred from the body to water on the surface of the skin (e.g., sweat). When this water accumulates sufficient heat, it is converted to a gas (water vapor), removing heat from the body as it vaporizes.

Figure 8-10 illustrates the balance between heat gain and heat loss via these mechanisms, while Figure 8-11 depicts heat balance during exercise.

At rest, the body relies predominantly on conduction, convection, and radiation for thermoregulation. During sustained exercise in a moderate environment, these mechanisms play minor roles in heat loss due to the small temperature gradient between the skin and the room. As environmental temperature and exercise intensity increase, the extent of heat loss due to conduction, convection, and radiation are further reduced due to a decrease in the skin-to-room temperature gradient. Thus, the body relies on evaporation as the primary means of losing heat during exercise (Table 8-1).

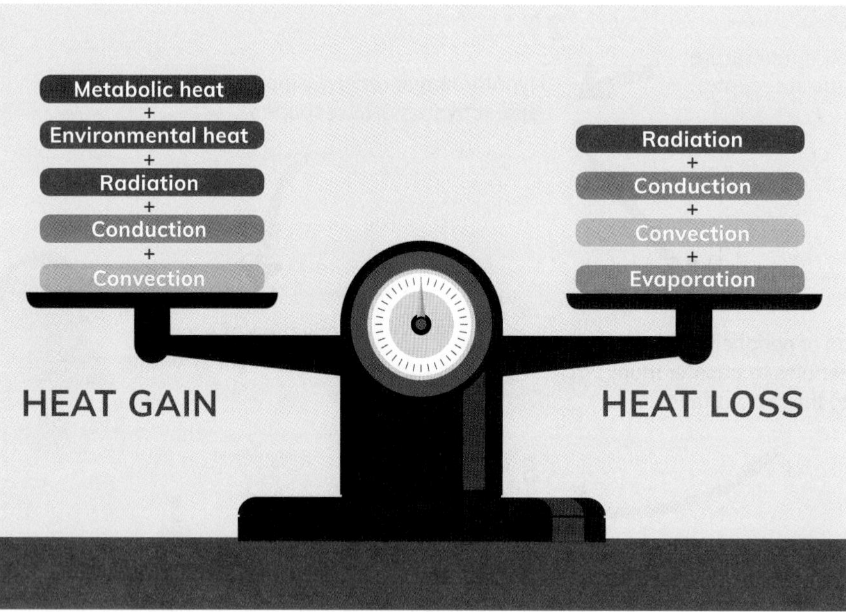

FIGURE 8-10
The balance between heat gained from internal metabolic processess and from external environmental factors and heat lost by radiation, conduction, convection, and evaporation

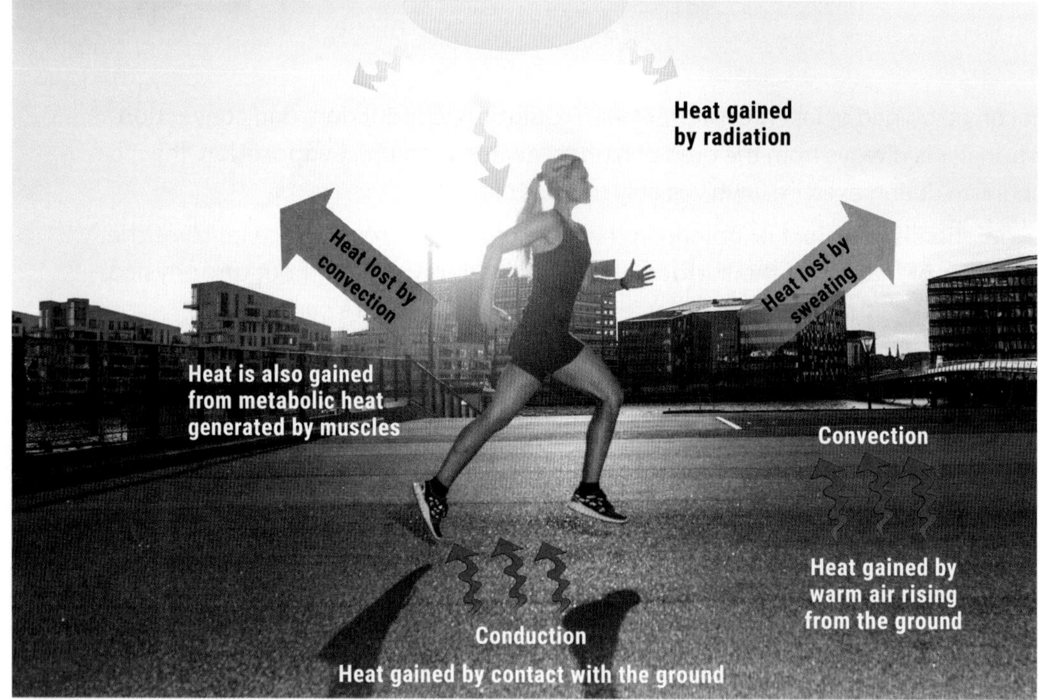

FIGURE 8-11
The complex interaction between the body's mechanisms for heat balance during exercise and environmental conditions

TABLE 8-1
Mechanisms of Thermoregulation

Thermoregulatory Mechanism	Rest	Exercise
Conduction and convection	20% of total	10–15% of total
Radiation	55–60% of total	5% of total
Evaporation	20% of total	80% of total
Excretion/lungs*	5–10% of total	<2% of total

*300 mL in mucus membranes

Source: Porcari, J.P., Bryant, C.X., & Comana, F. (2015). *Exercise Physiology*. Philadelphia: F.A. Davis Company.

EXERCISING IN THE HEAT

Exercising in the heat poses a signification threat to individuals if they do not take adequate precautions. The danger of heat overload is compounded if people are not adequately hydrated prior to starting exercise, wear excessive clothing, or have **overweight** or **obesity.** For example, heat-induced problems are very common in football in the late summer, when a number of issues combine to increase risk. The weight of the football padding adds to the external work that the person has to do. This added work increases the amount of heat build-up, sweating, and **dehydration.** The football padding also makes it difficult to dissipate the heat, as the heat gets trapped beneath the padding and helmet and evaporation cannot occur. A similar phenomenon occurs in people with overweight or obesity, as body fat lies over the muscles and effectively traps the heat from escaping.

Considerable metabolic heat is produced during exercise. To reduce this internal heat load, blood is brought to the skin surface through **peripheral vasodilation** to be cooled. When the sweat glands secrete water onto the skin, it is evaporated (when relative humidity is low), serving to cool the underlying blood, which then returns to the interior of the body to lower the core temperature. If environmental conditions are favorable, these mechanisms will adequately prevent the body temperature from rising by more than about 2 to 3° F, even during heavy exercise. There is some evidence that during prolonged exercise there is a "stop now" temperature for most people. The value will be slightly different from person to person but is approximately 104° F (40° C). Heat injuries usually occur when heat loss is compromised, as when wearing heavy clothing, or when the heat-sensing mechanism fails (as with amphetamine use). There is evidence that in the presence of heat injuries, the ability to turn off heat production is compromised even after exercise is stopped (Rae et al., 2008).

During exercise in the heat, however, dissipating internal body heat is more difficult, and external heat gained from the environment may significantly add to the total heat load. This results in a higher HR than normal at any level of exercise. For example, if a man walks at 3 miles per hour and his HR is 125 beats per minute (bpm), walking at the same speed in the heat may result in a HR of 135 to 140 bpm. Thus, exercisers (regardless of the type of exercise performed) will have to decrease their absolute workload in the heat to stay within their target HR zones.

This elevated HR comes about primarily for two reasons. First, as the body tries to cool down, the high degree of vasodilation in the vessels supplying the skin reduces venous return of blood to the heart while simultaneously maintaining blood flow to the exercising muscles, and SV declines. The heart attempts to maintain cardiac output by elevating HR. Second, sweating results in a considerable loss of body water. If lost fluids are not replenished, dehydration eventually results, and blood volume declines. This reduced blood volume also decreases venous return to the heart, leading to a higher HR to maintain cardiac output.

A hot, humid environment is the most stressful environment for exercising. When the air contains a large quantity of water vapor, sweat will not evaporate readily. Since the evaporative process is the most efficient mechanism for cooling the body, adequate cooling may not occur in humid conditions. Under these conditions, **heat exhaustion** and **heat stroke** become dangerous possibilities. Heat exhaustion usually develops in non-acclimatized individuals and is typically a result of inadequate circulatory adjustments to exercise coupled with fluid loss. Heat stroke is a complete failure of the heat-regulating mechanisms, with the core temperature exceeding 104° F (40° C). Both conditions require immediate medical attention. Symptoms of heat exhaustion and heat stroke, as well as recommendations for addressing these conditions, are presented in Table 8-2.

TABLE 8-2
Heat Exhaustion and Heat Stroke

	Signs and Symptoms	Recommendations
Heat Exhaustion	Weak, rapid pulse Low blood pressure Headache Nausea Dizziness General weakness Paleness Cold, clammy skin Profuse sweating	Stop exercising Move to a cool, ventilated area Lie down and elevate feet 12–18 inches (30–46 cm) Give fluids Monitor temperature
Heat Stroke	Hot, dry skin Bright red skin color Rapid, strong pulse Labored breathing Elevated body core temp (>104° F or 40° C)	Stop exercising Remove as much clothing as feasible Try to cool the body immediately in any way possible (wet towels, ice packs/baths, fan, alcohol rubs) Give fluids Transport to emergency room immediately

Figure 8-12 combines measures of heat and humidity into a simple-to-use heat index that provides guidelines regarding when exercise can be safely undertaken, and when it should be avoided.

Personal trainers should share the following tips with clients before they consider exercising in the heat:

- **Begin exercising in the heat gradually:** Becoming acclimated to exercising in the heat takes approximately nine to 14 days. Start by exercising for short periods of time each day.
- **Always wear lightweight, well-ventilated clothing:** Wear light-colored clothing if exercising in the sun, as white reflects heat better than other colors.
- **Never wear impermeable or nonbreathable garments:** The notion that wearing rubber suits or nonbreathable garments adds to weight loss is a myth, as the change in weight is due to fluid loss, not fat loss. Wearing impermeable clothing is a dangerous practice that could lead to significant heat stress and heat injury.
- **Replace body fluids as they are lost:** It is important to realize that the thirst mechanism is not sensitive enough to prompt someone when to drink. Therefore, drink fluids at regular intervals while exercising. Frequent consumption of small amounts of fluid to minimize sweat-related weight loss is the best practice. While there are many commercially available sports drinks, rehydration with water is adequate except under extreme conditions where greater than 3% of a person's body weight is lost. Fluid intake recommendations for before, during, and after exercise are presented in Table 8-3.

FIGURE 8-12
Heat index chart

ACTUAL THERMOMETER READING (°F) (°C GIVEN IN PARENTHESES)

Equivalent or Effective Temperature* (°F) (°C given in parentheses)

Relative Humidity	70 (21)	75 (24)	80 (27)	85 (29)	90 (32)	95 (35)	100 (38)	105 (41)	110 (43)	115 (46)	120 (49)
0	64 (18)	69 (21)	73 (23)	78 (26)	83 (28)	87 (31)	91 (33)	95 (35)	99 (37)	103 (39)	107 (42)
10	65 (18)	70 (21)	75 (24)	80 (27)	85 (29)	90 (32)	95 (35)	100 (38)	105 (41)	111 (44)	116 (47)
20	66 (19)	72 (22)	77 (25)	82 (28)	87 (31)	93 (34)	99 (37)	105 (41)	112 (44)	120 (49)	130 (54)
30	67 (19)	73 (23)	78 (26)	84 (29)	90 (32)	96 (36)	104 (40)	113 (45)	123 (51)	135 (57)	148 (64)
40	68 (20)	74 (23)	79 (26)	86 (30)	93 (34)	101 (38)	110 (43)	123 (51)	137 (58)	151 (66)	
50	69 (21)	75 (24)	81 (27)	88 (31)	96 (36)	107 (42)	120 (49)	135 (57)	150 (66)		
60	70 (21)	76 (24)	82 (28)	90 (32)	100 (38)	114 (46)	132 (56)	149 (65)			
70	70 (21)	77 (25)	85 (29)	93 (34)	106 (41)	124 (51)	144 (62)				
80	71 (22)	78 (26)	86 (30)	97 (36)	113 (45)	136 (58)					
90	71 (22)	79 (26)	88 (31)	102 (39)	122 (50)						
100	72 (22)	80 (27)	91 (33)	108 (42)							

*Combined index of heat and humidity and what it feels like to the body

How to Use Heat Index

1. Locate temperature across top
2. Locate relative humidity down left side
3. Follow across and down to find Equivalent or Effective Temperature
4. Determine Heat Stress Risk on chart at right

Note: This heat index chart is designed to provide general guidelines for assessing the potential severity of heat stress. Individual reactions to heat will vary. In addition, studies indicate that susceptibility to heat disorders tends to increase among children and older adults. Exposure to full sunshine can increase heat index values by up to 15° F.

Effective Temperature (°F) (°C given in parentheses)	Heat Stress Risk with Physical Activity and/or Prolonged Exposure
90–105 (32–41)	Heat cramps or heat exhaustion possible
106–130 (41–54)	Heat cramps or heat exhaustion likely Heat stroke possible
131–151 (54–66)	Heat stroke highly likely

TABLE 8-3

Fluid Replacement Recommendations Before, During, and After Exercise

	Fluid	Comments
Before Exercise	Drink 5–7 mL/kg (0.08–0.11 oz/lb) at least 4 hours before exercise (12–17 oz for 154-lb individual).	If urine is not produced or very dark, drink another 3–5 mL/kg (0.05–0.08 oz/lb) before exercise. Sodium-containing beverages or salted snacks will help retain fluid.
During Exercise	Monitor individual body-weight changes during exercise to estimate weight loss. Composition of fluid should include 20–30 mEq/L of sodium, 2–5 mEq/L of potassium, and 5–10% of carbohydrate.	Prevent a >2% loss in body weight. Amount and rate of fluid replacement depends on individual sweating rate, environment, and exercise duration.
After Exercise	Consumption of normal meals and beverages will restore euhydration. If rapid recovery is needed, drink 1.5 L/kg (23 oz/lb) of body weight lost.	Goal is to fully replace fluid and electrolyte deficits. Consuming sodium will help recovery by stimulating thirst and fluid retention.

Reprinted with permission from American College of Sports Medicine (2018). *ACSM's Guidelines for Exercise Testing and Prescription* (10th ed.). Philadelphia: Wolters Kluwer.

Recording daily body weight is an excellent way to prevent accumulative dehydration. For example, if 5 pounds (2.3 kg) of body water is lost after cardiorespiratory exercise, this water should be replaced before exercising again the next day. If lost water has not been regained, exercise should be curtailed until the body is adequately rehydrated.

Air movement is critical for adequate cooling. Even in cool conditions, if there is limited air movement (e.g., exercising on an indoor cycle, treadmill, or other equipment), the microclimate next to the body can become the same temperature as the body (~100° F, or 38° C), and saturated with water vapor from sweat (just like exercising in the tropics). This microclimate will reduce heat loss and may put the exerciser at risk of a heat injury. Maintaining good air movement around the exerciser allows the microclimate to be better regulated and facilitates heat loss.

EXERCISING IN THE COLD

The major problems encountered when exercising in the cold are associated with an excessive loss of body heat, which can result in **hypothermia** and/or **frostbite.** When the skin or blood temperature drops, the thermoregulatory center activates mechanisms that conserve body heat and increase heat production. There are three primary ways in which the body avoids excessive heat loss: **peripheral vasoconstriction, nonshivering thermogenesis,** and **shivering.**

Peripheral vasoconstriction is the narrowing of the arterioles (due to sympathetic stimulation), which reduces the blood flow to the shell of the body, thus decreasing the amount of body heat lost to the environment. When altering skin blood flow is not enough to prevent heat loss, nonshivering thermogenesis is increased. This involves stimulation of the metabolism (as directed by the **sympathetic nervous system**) to increase internal heat production. Shivering is the next bodily process that occurs if peripheral vasoconstriction and nonshivering thermogenesis are not adequate in preventing heat loss. Shivering is a rapid, involuntary cycle of contraction and relaxation of skeletal muscles, which can increase the body's rate of heat production by four to five times.

The two major cold stressors are air and water. The effects of cold air are compounded by wind. As wind increases, so do convective heat loss and the rate of body cooling. An index based on the cooling effect of wind is windchill, which refers to the cooling power of the environment (Figure 8-13). As windchill increases, so does the risk of freezing body tissues. Water, on the other hand, is actually more detrimental than air in terms of heat loss. In general, the body loses heat four times faster in water than it does in air of the same temperature. This rate can be increased even more if the cold water is moving around the individual (e.g., in a current) due to increased heat loss through convection. A body immersed in cold water [59° F (15° C)] for prolonged periods can experience extreme hypothermia and even death.

Additionally, the cold can cause a generalized vasoconstriction that can increase **peripheral resistance** and BP. This may cause problems in people who are hypertensive or who have heart disease. Following exercise, chilling can occur quickly if the body surface is wet with

FIGURE 8-13
Windchill factor chart

	ACTUAL THERMOMETER READING (°F) (°C GIVEN IN PARENTHESES)											
Estimated wind speed (in mph) (km/h given in parentheses)	50 (10)	40 (4)	30 (-1)	20 (-7)	10 (-12)	0 (-18)	-10 (-23)	-20 (-29)	-30 (-34)	-40 (-40)	-50 (-46)	-60 (-51)
	Equivalent or Effective Temperature* (°F) (°C given in parentheses)											
Calm	50 (10)	40 (4)	30 (-1)	20 (-7)	10 (-12)	0 (-18)	-10 (-23)	-20 (-29)	-30 (-34)	-40 (-40)	-50 (-46)	-60 (-51)
5 (8)	48 (9)	37 (3)	27 (-3)	16 (-9)	6 (-14)	-5 (-21)	-15 (-26)	-26 (-32)	-36 (-38)	-47 (-44)	-57 (-49)	-68 (-56)
10 (16)	40 (4)	28 (-2)	16 (-9)	4 (-16)	-9 (-23)	-24 (-31)	-33 (-36)	-46 (-43)	-58 (-50)	-70 (-57)	-83 (-64)	-95 (-71)
15 (24)	36 (2)	22 (-6)	9 (-13)	-5 (-21)	-18 (-28)	-32 (-36)	-45 (-43)	-58 (-50)	-72 (-58)	-85 (-65)	-99 (-78)	-112 (-80)
20 (32)	32 (0)	18 (-8)	4 (-16)	-10 (-23)	-25 (-32)	-39 (-39)	-53 (-47)	-67 (-55)	-82 (-63)	-96 (-71)	-110 (-79)	-124 (-87)
25 (40)	30 (-1)	16 (-9)	0 (-18)	-15 (-26)	-29 (-34)	-44 (-42)	-59 (-51)	-74 (-59)	-88 (-67)	-104 (-76)	-118 (-83)	-133 (-92)
30 (48)	28 (-2)	13 (-11)	-2 (-19)	-18 (-28)	-33 (-36)	-48 (-44)	-63 (-53)	-79 (-62)	-94 (-70)	-109 (-78)	-125 (-87)	-140 (-96)
35 (56)	27 (-3)	11 (-12)	-4 (-20)	-20 (-29)	-35 (-37)	-51 (-46)	-67 (-55)	-82 (-63)	-98 (-72)	-113 (-81)	-129 (-89)	-145 (-98)
40 (64) [Wind speeds greater than 40 mph (64 km/h) have little additional effect.]	26 (-3)	10 (-12)	-6 (-21)	-21 (-29)	-37 (-38)	-53 (-47)	-69 (-56)	-85 (-65)	-100 (-73)	-116 (-82)	-132 (-91)	-146 (-99)
	GREEN				YELLOW				RED			
	LITTLE DANCER (for properly clothed person). Maximal danger of false sense of security.				**INCREASING DANGER** Danger for freezing of exposed flesh				**GREAT DANGER**			

sweat and heat loss continues. There are documented cases of runners who ran in a cold environment, got sweaty, slowed from fatigue, and developed clinical hypothermia (increased heat losses from sweat and air movement coupled with decreased heat production from a reduced exercise intensity).

Personal trainers should share the following tips with clients before they consider exercising in a cold environment.

- **Wear several layers of clothing:** That way, garments can be removed or replaced as needed. As exercise intensity increases, remove outer garments. Then, during periods of rest, warm-up, cool-down, or low-intensity exercise, put them back on. A head covering is also important, because considerable body heat radiates from the head.
- **Allow for adequate ventilation of sweat:** Sweating during heavy exercise can soak inner garments. If evaporation does not readily occur, the wet garments can continue to drain the body of heat during rest periods, when retention of body heat is extremely important. In particularly cold outdoor environments, if there is any meaningful wind, it is better to begin an exercise bout going into the wind and finish with the wind at one's back. If the opposite happens, the exerciser can become quite sweaty when moving with the wind, and then have to return with wet clothing against the wind while facing increased heat losses from convection and evaporation.
- **Wear breathable clothing:** Select garment materials that allow the body to give off body heat during exercise and retain body heat during inactive periods. Cotton is a good choice for exercising in the heat because it readily soaks up sweat and allows evaporation. For those same reasons, however, cotton is a poor choice for exercising in the cold. Wool is an excellent choice when exercising in the cold because it maintains body heat even when wet. Newer synthetic materials (e.g., polypropylene) are also excellent choices, as they wick sweat away from the body, thereby preventing heat loss. When windchill is a problem, nylon materials are good for outerwear. Synthetic materials like Gore-Tex, although much more expensive than nylon, are probably the best choice for outerwear because they can block the wind, are waterproof, and allow moisture to move away from the body.
- **Replace body fluids in the cold, just as in the heat:** Fluid replacement is also vitally important when exercising in cold air. Large amounts of water are lost from the body during even normal respiration, and this effect becomes magnified when exercising.
- **Monitor body weight:** Because sweat losses may not be as obvious as when exercising in the heat, monitoring of body weight over several days is recommended.

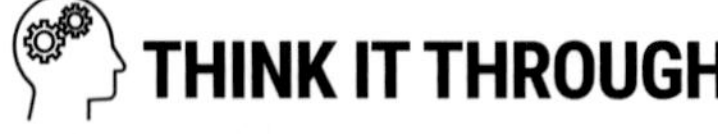

Minimizing the Risks of Exercising in the Cold

During the winter months, many exercisers become less physically active because of frigid outdoor conditions. However, there are ways to minimize the discomfort and risk of exercising in the cold. How would you educate a client about simple strategies to make exercising in the cold more accessible?

EXERCISING AT HIGHER ALTITUDES

At moderate (5,000–8,000 feet) to high altitudes (8,000–14,000 feet), the relative availability (i.e., **partial pressure**) of O_2 in the air is reduced (Figure 8-14). Because there is less pressure to drive the O_2 molecules into the blood as it passes through the lungs, the O_2 carried in the blood is reduced. Therefore, a person exercising at high altitude will not be able to deliver as much O_2 to the exercising muscles and exercise intensity will have to be reduced (e.g., the person will have to walk or run more slowly) to keep the HR in a target zone. Typically, the negative effect of altitude on performance is greatest on about the third day at altitude. The first phase of **acclimatization** takes place in approximately two weeks, although it may take several months to fully acclimatize. Even after acclimatization, it is important to recognize that performance will not be as good at altitude as at sea level.

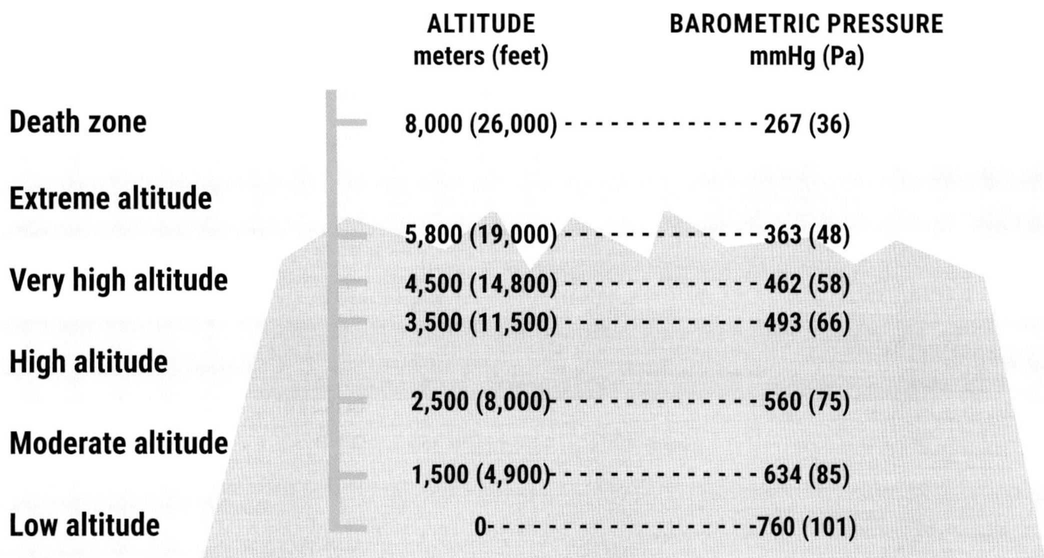

FIGURE 8-14
Exercise at high altitudes

Signs and symptoms of **altitude sickness** include shortness of breath, headache, lightheadedness, and nausea. Generally, altitude sickness can be avoided by properly acclimatizing oneself by gradually increasing exercise and activity levels over the span of several days. The most common everyday experience of altitude sickness is when a person flies into a ski area and tries to ski immediately. Often by the end of the day, they have fairly severe altitude sickness that may take a couple of days to resolve. The higher the destination, the greater the risk, but a good strategy is not to exercise the first night at altitude. This helps many people avoid altitude sickness. A prolonged warm-up and cool-down and frequent exercise breaks at a lower intensity should help most people become accustomed to exercising at higher altitudes.

EXERCISING IN AIR POLLUTION

Some areas have a high degree of airborne pollutants (e.g., smog) that can adversely affect cardiorespiratory exercise performance. These pollutants are the result of the combustion of fossil fuels and primarily include ozone, sulfur dioxide, and carbon monoxide. When these airborne particles are inhaled, they can have a number of deleterious effects on the body, such as irritating the airways and decreasing the O_2-carrying capacity of the blood, both of which hamper cardiorespiratory exercise performance. Inhaled air pollutants have been shown to be associated with the development of both cardiac and pulmonary disease.

One area of risk that is often not well recognized is indoor ice arenas. An ice-preparation machine (or Zamboni) that is powered by propane may leave very high concentrations of pollutants in the air over the ice surface. Thus, while an exerciser is thinking that he or she is safe from the smog outside, he or she may actually be in a very polluted environment.

In individuals with CVD, prolonged exposure to air pollution can even induce ischemia and **angina.** For those with asthma, allergens and irritants (including pollen) can trigger an inflammatory response (see Chapter 13). The overall physiological effects are determined by the degree of exposure (or dose) to pollutants to which an individual is exposed. This dose is related to the amount of pollutants in the air, the length of exposure, and the amount of air breathed. Practical suggestions to minimize the effects of air pollution include exercising early in the morning to avoid the build-up of pollutants associated with increased vehicular traffic and avoiding high-traffic urban areas. Similar to exercising in the heat or at altitude, exercise pace may need to be reduced to keep HR in the desired training range. Under extreme conditions, exercising indoors is probably the best choice.

General Guidelines for Cardiorespiratory Exercise for Health and Fitness

The *2018 Physical Activity Guidelines for Americans* released by the U.S. Department of Health & Human Services (2018) provide comprehensive evidence-based recommendations to reduce the risk of many adverse health outcomes. Many of the recommendations are derived from the knowledge that most health benefits occur with at least 150 minutes a week of moderate-intensity cardiorespiratory activity and that the benefits of physical activity far outweigh the possibility of adverse outcomes. Specific guidelines for adults aged 18 to 64 include the following:

- Any amount of physical activity is more desirable when compared to none. Additionally, a concerted effort should be made to sit less throughout the day.
- Perform 150 to 300 minutes per week of moderate-intensity cardiorespiratory physical activity, or 75 to 150 minutes per week of vigorous-intensity cardiorespiratory physical activity, or a combination of both. Additional health benefits are obtained from performing greater amounts of activity than these quantities.
- Participate in muscle-strengthening activities involving all major muscle groups at least two days per week.

With regard to cardiorespiratory programming, however, widely accepted guidelines for physical activity and basic fitness training are presented by ACSM and the American Heart Association (AHA). These guidelines frequently use the FITT-VP acronym to discuss cardiorespiratory programming (ACSM, 2018; Haskell et al., 2007). This acronym represents frequency, intensity, time (duration), type (modality), volume, and pattern/ progression. Additionally, clients should always enjoy the exercise experience, as this influences the thoughts and emotions that can ultimately dictate participation and **adherence** rates. Frequency, intensity, and duration collectively represent the exercise volume, load, or magnitude of training that is likely to provoke the physiological adaptations to the training response. A **dose-response relationship** exists between volume and the health/fitness benefits achieved, implying that greater benefits are achieved with increased volumes.

Personal trainers generally progress and pattern their clients' programs by manipulating these variables (i.e., frequency, intensity, time, and type) (Table 8-4). The rate of program progression depends on each client's individual health status, exercise tolerance, available time, and program goals. Improvement in cardiorespiratory fitness occurs most quickly from progressive increases in exercise intensity, and fades when training intensity is reduced. Changes in fitness are more sensitive to changes in intensity than to changes in the

TABLE 8-4

Aerobic (Cardiovascular Endurance) Exercise Evidence-based Recommendations

FITT-VP	Evidence-based Recommendation
Frequency	≥5 days/week of moderate exercise, or ≥3 days/week of vigorous exercise, or a combination of moderate and vigorous exercise on ≥3–5 days/week is recommended
Intensity	Moderate and/or vigorous intensity is recommended for most adults. Light-to-moderate intensity exercise may be beneficial in deconditioned individuals.
Time	30–60 minutes/day of purposeful moderate exercise, or 20–60 minutes/day of vigorous exercise, or a combination of moderate and vigorous exercise per day is recommended for most adults. <20 minutes of exercise per day can be beneficial, especially in previously sedentary individuals.
Type	Regular, purposeful exercise that involves major muscle groups and is continuous and rhythmic in nature is recommended.
Volume	A target volume of ≥500–1,000 MET-minutes/week is recommended. Increasing pedometer step counts by ≥2,000 steps/day to reach a daily step count ≥7,000 steps/day is beneficial.* Exercising below these volumes may still be beneficial for individuals unable or unwilling to reach this amount of exercise.
Pattern	Exercise may be performed in one continuous session, in one interval session, or in multiple sessions of ≥10 minutes to accumulate the desired duration and volume of exercise per day. Exercise bouts of <10 minutes may yield favorable adaptations in very deconditioned individuals.
Progression	A gradual progression of exercise volume by adjusting exercise duration, frequency, and/or intensity is reasonable until the desired exercise goal (maintenance) is attained. This approach of "start low and go slow" may enhance adherence and reduce risks of musculoskeletal injury and adverse cardiac events.

*While many groups recommend 10,000 steps, the Centers for Disease Control and Prevention (CDC) recommend that adults engage in 150 minutes of moderate-intensity physical activity per week. To meet the CDC's recommendation, the average person needs to walk approximately 7,000 steps per day.

Note: FITT-VP = Frequency, intensity, time, type, volume, and pattern/progression; MET-minutes = The product of metabolic equivalents (METs) and minutes of exercise (e.g., 5 METs x 30 minutes x 5 days = 750 MET-minutes)

Reprinted with permission from American College of Sports Medicine (2018). *ACSM's Guidelines for Exercise Testing and Prescription* (10th ed.). Philadelphia: Wolters Kluwer.

frequency or duration of training. In the following sections of this chapter, each of the FITT variables is discussed in more detail, while volume, pattern, and progression are addressed extensively in Chapter 11.

FREQUENCY

While minimal health benefits can be attained in as little as one to two sessions per week, current guidelines recommend physical activity on most days of the week (U.S. Department of Health & Human Services, 2018). ACSM (2018) recommendations are presented in Table 8-5. For the beginning adult exerciser, the balance should be in the direction of more moderate-intensity exercise, since higher-intensity exercise has been associated with a risk of exercise-related complications, injury, and a poor experience in beginning exercisers (Foster et al., 2008).

TABLE 8-5

Cardiorespiratory Recommendations for Healthy Adults

Exercise Type	Weekly Frequency
Moderate-intensity cardiorespiratory exercise ▸ 40% to 59% $\dot{V}O_2R$ or HRR ▸ Below VT1 ▸ Can speak comfortably	Minimum of 5 days per week
Vigorous-intensity cardiorespiratory exercise ▸ 60% to 89% $\dot{V}O_2R$ or HRR ▸ VT1 to VT2 ▸ Not sure if speech is comfortable to definitely cannot speak	Minimum of 3 days per week
Combination of moderate- and vigorous-intensity cardiorespiratory exercise	3–5 days per week

Note: $\dot{V}O_2R$ = $\dot{V}O_2$ reserve; HRR = Heart-rate reserve; VT1 = First ventilatory threshold; VT2 = Second ventilatory threshold

Source: American College of Sports Medicine (2018). ACSM's *Guidelines for Exercise Testing and Prescription* (10th ed.). Philadelphia: Wolters Kluwer.

INTENSITY

Exercise intensity is arguably the most important element of the exercise program to monitor. At the same time, it is the most difficult element to present quantitatively. There are numerous methods by which the personal trainer can program and monitor exercise intensity:

- HR [%MHR; % **heart-rate reserve (HRR)**]
- **Rating of perceived exertion (RPE)**
- $\dot{V}O_2$ or **metabolic equivalents (METs)**
- Caloric expenditure
- Talk test and HR at VT1
- Blood lactate and HR at the **second ventilatory threshold (VT2)**

Heart Rate

Using percentage of MHR or HRR is probably the most widely used approach for programming and monitoring exercise intensity. While there is a very large body of evidence supporting this approach, accuracy in using these methods requires knowledge of the individual's MHR. Without a maximal-effort exercise assessment, which is generally not considered appropriate or feasible for most individuals, this marker is not definable. Given the risk associated with conducting a maximal-effort assessment, MHR is normally determined via mathematical formulas. While these calculations are usually easy to compute and provide a simple marker from which personal trainers can anchor exercise intensity (e.g., %MHR), estimated MHR is less useful as an exercise anchor for individual exercise programming and should be questioned due to its inherent error. Numerous variables impact MHR, including the following:

- Genetics
- Exercise modality (e.g., MHR varies between running and cycling due to the involvement of upper-body musculature)
- Medications (see Chapter 5)
- Body size: MHR is generally higher in smaller individuals who have smaller hearts, and hence lower stroke volumes.
- Altitude: Altitude can lower the MHR reached due to most individual's inability to train at higher intensities (see "Exercising at Higher Altitudes" on page 275).
- Age: MHR generally decreases by 1-bpm each year starting in a person's early 20s. However, there is considerable inter-individual variability in the age-associated reduction in MHR based on factors such as genetics, medications, and training status.

MHR does not correlate strongly with performance and is generally not influenced by training. In fact, it may even become lowered with training given the training adaptations of expanded blood volume and stroke volume. Most importantly, MHR varies significantly among people of the same age. For example, the popular formula devised by Fox, Naughton, and Haskell (220 – Age), which was never intended for use with the general population, demonstrates a standard deviation (s.d.) of approximately 12 bpm (Fox, Naughton, & Haskell, 1971). This implies that for 68% of a population (or plus or minus one standard deviation assuming a normal distribution of data), the true MHR would differ from the estimated mathematical calculation by 12 beats on either side of that value (Figure 8-15). The remaining 32% would fall even further outside of this range (e.g., for 95%, or plus or minus two standard deviations, of the population, the true MHR would fall within 24 beats on either side of the calculated value).

Another concern with the 220 – Age formula is the fact that it also tends to overestimate MHR in younger adults and underestimate MHR in older adults [e.g., a 25 year old may never reach 195 bpm (i.e., 220 – 25), while a 60 year old may exceed 160 bpm (i.e., 220 – 60) quite comfortably].

Beyond the invalidity of MHR, a significant concern with using a straight percentage of MHR to design and monitor training intensities stems from the fact that discrepancies in individual

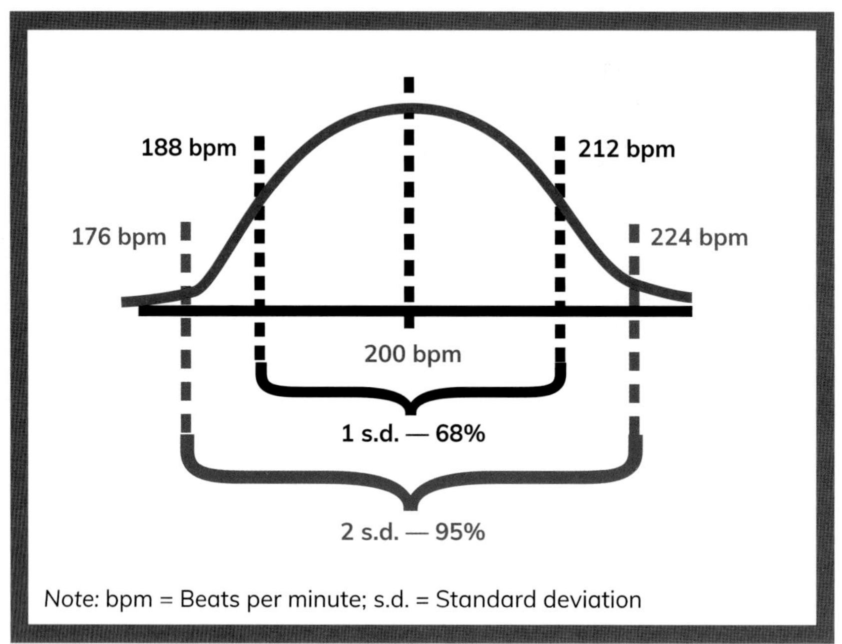

FIGURE 8-15
The standard deviation (i.e., 12 beats per minute) for the 220 – Age maximal heart rate prediction equation for 20 year olds

Resting heart rates (RHRs) are not taken into consideration and may therefore lead the personal trainer to over- or underestimate appropriate exercise intensities.

High-volume training or intensities that are too vigorous for a client increase the risk of injury and creates a potentially negative experience, whereas undertraining can quickly disengage the individual from the exercise experience due to boredom and perhaps insufficient challenge or results. Given that the risk of serious cardiovascular complications during exercise in **previously physically inactive** individuals is associated with inappropriately high exercise intensities (Foster et al., 2008), guiding exercise on the basis of a percentage of estimated age-based MHR is strongly discouraged.

Regardless, ACSM provides guidelines for using %MHR but does make a strong recommendation against using the standardized 220 – Age formula (ACSM, 2018). ACSM suggests formulas with standard deviations closer to 7 bpm (Gellish et al., 2007; Tanaka, Monahan, & Seals, 2001), which still equates to an error of 14 bpm on either side of the calculated HR for 95% of the population, or two standard deviations.

- Gellish et al. formula: MHR = 206.9 – (0.67 × Age)
- Tanaka, Monahan, and Seals formula: MHR = 208 – (0.7 × Age)

Another popular method for monitoring training intensity follows the Karvonen, or HRR, formula. Given the concern with RHR discrepancy, this method is more appropriate, as it does consider potential RHR differences by determining an HRR from which training intensities are calculated. The Karvonen formula reduces discrepancies in training intensities between individuals with different RHRs and accommodates the training adaptation that lowers RHR, therefore expanding HRR (Table 8-6 and Figure 8-16).

TABLE 8-6

Comparing %HRR Estimations in Two 25 Year Olds with Different Resting Heart Rates

	Person A (bpm)	Person B (bpm)
MHR [206.9 – (0.67 x Age)]	190	190
RHR	50	80
HRR (MHR – RHR)	140	110
60% HRR	84	66
Adding RHR	84 + 50	66 + 80
Training HR	134	146
	(12 bpm difference)	

Note: HRR = Heart-rate reserve; MHR = Maximal heart rate; RHR = Resting heart rate; HR = Heart rate; bpm = Beats per minute

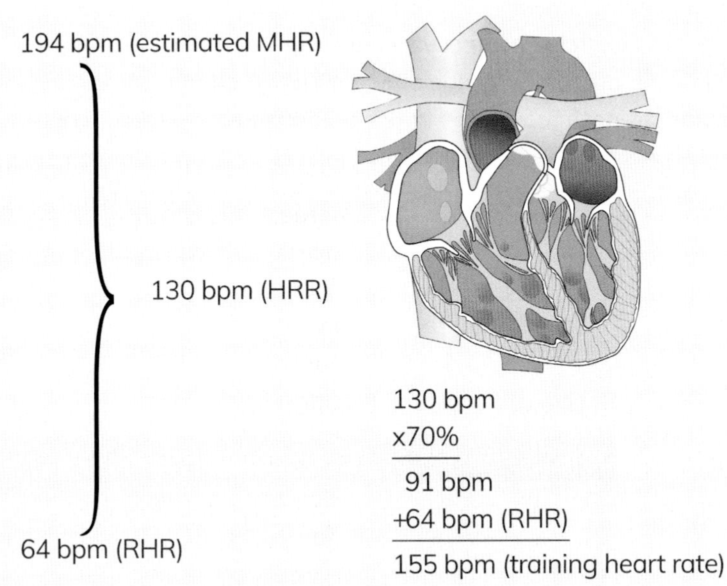

FIGURE 8-16
Use of the Karvonen formula for a 20-year-old man (average shape; resting heart rate = 64 bpm) using the Gellish et al. formula

Note: bpm = Beats per minute; MHR = Maximal heart rate; HRR = Heart-rate reserve; RHR = Resting heart rate

Karvonen Formula
Target HR (THR) = (HRR x % Intensity) + RHR
Where: HRR = MHR – RHR

While the Karvonen formula does reduce the error in estimation, it still has limitations regarding its accuracy and appropriateness:

- As with other exercise-intensity determination techniques, it utilizes a mathematical estimation for MHR. Note: Ideally, the Karvonen formula should be based on measured MHR to yield the most accurate results.

- There is some debate over the body position in which RHR is measured. This formula was created measuring true RHR, taken in the morning in a reclining position. RHR varies by approximately five to 10 beats when a person transitions from lying to standing, thereby reducing the size of the HRR. Given the concern with some inconsistencies with clients measuring their own HR, ACE recommends measuring RHR in the body position in which the client will exercise. This may necessitate the need for two sets of training zones; one for seated/recumbent positions and another for standing activities.

Rating of Perceived Exertion

RPE emerged in the late 1970s and early 1980s as a subjective method of gauging exercise intensity and has since gained wide acceptance. There are two versions of the RPE scale: the classical (6 to 20) scale and the category ratio (0 to 10) scale, which was developed to remedy inconsistencies with the use of the classical RPE scale (Table 8-7) (Borg, 1998). Although fully subjective, the RPE scale (in both forms) has been shown to be capable of defining the ranges of objective exercise intensity associated with effective exercise training programs. The RPE scale works well for most people. Physically inactive individuals often find it difficult to use, as they find any level of exercise fairly hard. However, in previous physically inactive individuals, even a small amount of low-intensity exercise is effective in terms of producing some exercise training benefits and improved health outcomes. At the other end of the continuum, individuals who have high levels of **muscular strength** may under-rate the intensity of exercise if they focus on the muscular tension requirement of exercise rather than on the breathing elements. With practice during cardiorespiratory exercise, these individuals can usually learn to use the RPE scale effectively.

$\dot{V}O_2$ and Metabolic Equivalents

The traditional reference standard for exercise intensity is expressed in terms of percentages of $\dot{V}O_2$max or **$\dot{V}O_2$reserve ($\dot{V}O_2$R).** The great volume of experimental studies conducted in the 1960s and 1970s suggested that there are minimal improvements in $\dot{V}O_2$max if the intensity of training is below a threshold of 40/50% of $\dot{V}O_2$max or $\dot{V}O_2$R (Foster, Porcari, & Lucia, 2008). While acknowledging that lower-intensity exercise can result in improvements in cardiorespiratory fitness in previously physically inactive or unfit individuals, there does seem to be a lower-limit intensity below which exercise is of minimal benefit.

TABLE 8-7

Rating of Perceived Exertion (RPE)

RPE	Category Ratio Scale
6	0 Nothing at all
7 Very, very light	0.5 Very, very weak
8	1 Very weak
9 Very light	2 Weak
10	3 Moderate
11 Fairly light	4 Somewhat strong
12	5 Strong
13 Somewhat hard	6
14	7 Very strong
15 Hard	8
16	9
17 Very hard	10 Very, very strong
18	* Maximal
19 Very, very hard	
20	

Source: Borg, G. (1998). *Borg's Perceived Exertion and Pain Scales.* Champaign, Ill.: Human Kinetics.

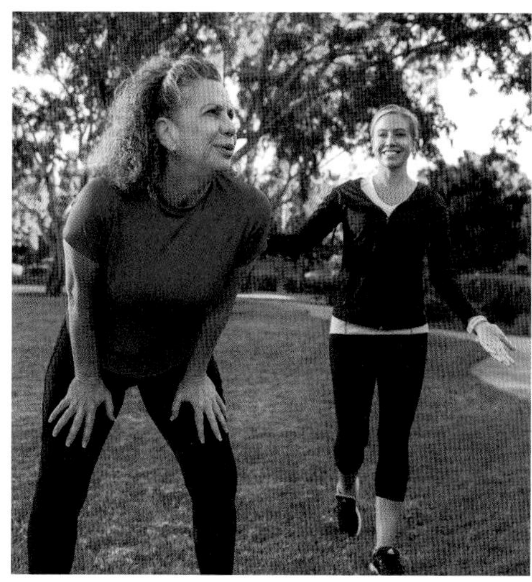

Although the evidence base for percentage of $\dot{V}O_2$max or $\dot{V}O_2$R is extensive, the very large range of acceptable percentages creates the concern that a given percentage is not very specific in terms of recommending exercise. Katch and colleagues (1978) suggested that the "relative percent concept" was essentially flawed and did not take into account the individual metabolic responses to exercise that might more properly represent the lowest effective training stimulus.

Although contemporary guidelines for exercise training are still presented in terms of the relative percent concept, the more than four-decades-old comments of Professor Katch are still remarkably convincing. Although clear experimental evidence is lacking, this lowest effective training intensity at which adaptations might be provoked is probably better defined in terms of VT1. Although training below this threshold may have some benefit, it is highly probable that training very much below this threshold will yield minimal cardiorespiratory fitness benefits (Meyer et al., 2005). It is arguable that very extensive low-intensity training is important in terms of overall health benefits, although there does appear to be a lower limit of exercise intensity that is critical when training for cardiorespiratory fitness. Thus, basing the training program on metabolic or ventilatory responses is much more meaningful than using arbitrary ranges of %$\dot{V}O_2$max or %$\dot{V}O_2$R.

Training programs based on %$\dot{V}O_2$max or %$\dot{V}O_2$R depend on a maximal exercise assessments to be accurate, or on some estimate of $\dot{V}O_2$max derived from a submaximal assessment. Given that maximal assessments are rarely available, and that equations for estimating $\dot{V}O_2$max are not exceedingly accurate, particularly if any handrail support is allowed during treadmill assessment or training (Berling et al., 2006; McConnell et al., 1991), recommending exercise on the basis of this "gold standard" technique probably is much less useful than is widely assumed.

In cases where $\dot{V}O_2$ is not directly measured during either assessment or training, an alternative method for expressing exercise intensity is in terms of METs, which are multiples of an assumed average metabolic rate at rest of 3.5 mL/kg/min. This is very easy and intuitive for many people to understand (e.g., at 5.0 METs, they are working five times harder than resting). It is important to recognize, however, that the resting metabolic rate is not exactly 3.5 mL/kg/min in every individual, or even in the same person at all times. Nevertheless, the utility of using METs rather than directly measured $\dot{V}O_2$ is so substantial that it more than makes up for any imprecision (Table 8-8).

Caloric Expenditure

When the human body burns fuel (e.g., fats and carbohydrates), O_2 is consumed, which yields calories to perform work. While the number of calories produced per liter of O_2 consumed varies according to the fuel utilized (i.e., 4.69 kcal per liter of O_2 for fats and 5.05 kcal per liter of O_2 for glucose), a value of 5 kcal per liter of O_2 is sufficiently accurate considering the fact that people burn a combination of fuels throughout their daily activities.

TABLE 8-8

Metabolic Equivalents (METs) Values of Common Physical Activities Classified as Light, Moderate, or Vigorous Intensity

Light (<3 METs)	Moderate (3–5.9 METs)	Vigorous (≥6 METs)
Walking Walking slowly around home, store, or office = 2.0* **Household and occupation** Standing while performing light work, such as making bed, washing dishes, ironing, preparing food, or store clerk = 2.0–2.5 **Leisure time and sports** Arts and crafts, playing cards = 1.5 Billiards = 2.5 Boating—power = 2.5 Croquet = 2.5 Darts = 2.5 Fishing—sitting = 2.5 Playing most musical instruments = 2.0–2.5	**Walking** Walking 3.0 mph = 3.0* Walking at very brisk pace (4 mph) = 5.0* **Household and occupation** Cleaning, heavy—washing windows, car, clean garage = 3.0 Sweeping floors or carpet, vacuuming, mopping = 3.0–3.5 Carpentry—general = 3.6 Carrying and stacking wood = 5.5 Mowing lawn/walk power mower = 5.5 **Leisure time and sports** Badminton—recreational = 4.5 Basketball—shooting around = 4.5 Dancing—ballroom slow = 3.0; ballroom fast = 4.5 Fishing from riverbank and walking = 4.0 Golf—walking, pulling clubs = 4.3 Sailing boat, wind surfing = 3.0 Swimming leisurely = 6.0† Table tennis = 4.0 Tennis doubles = 5.0 Volleyball—noncompetitive = 3.0–4.0	**Walking, jogging, and running** Walking at very, very brisk pace (4.5 mph) = 6.3* Walking/hiking at moderate pace and grade with no or light pack (<10 lb) = 7.0 Hiking at steep grades and pack 10–42 lb = 7.5–9.0 Jogging at 5 mph = 8.0* Jogging at 6 mph = 10.0* Running at 7 mph = 11.5* **Household and occupation** Shoveling sand, coal, etc. = 7.0 Carrying heavy loads, such as bricks = 7.5 Heavy farming, such as baling hay = 8.0 Shoveling, digging ditches = 8.5 **Leisure time and sports** Bicycling on flat—light effort (10–12 mph) = 6.0 Basketball game = 8.0 Bicycling on flat—moderate effort (12–14 mph) = 8.0; fast (14–16 mph) = 10.0 Skiing cross-country—slow 2.5 mph) = 7.0; fast (5.0–7.9 mph) = 9.0 Soccer—casual = 7.0; competitive = 10.0 Swimming leisurely = 6.0; swimming—moderate/hard = 8.0–11.0† Tennis singles = 8.0 Volleyball—competitive at gym or beach = 8.0

Note: A more complete list of physical activities (and their associated MET values) can be found in the updated version of the "Compendium of Physical Activities" by Ainsworth et al. (2011); MET = Metabolic equivalent; mph = Miles per hour

*On flat, hard surface.

†MET values can vary substantially from person to person during swimming as result of different strokes and skill levels.

Reprinted with permission from American College of Sports Medicine (2018). ACSM's *Guidelines for Exercise Testing and Prescription* (10th ed.). Philadelphia: Wolters Kluwer.

Caloric expenditure is usually calculated in terms of the gross or absolute $\dot{V}O_2$ during an activity by measuring or estimating the total quantity of O_2 consumed per minute and multiplying it by 5 kcal/liter O_2. If the quantity of O_2 consumed is provided or measured in relative terms (i.e., mL/kg/min), this value must first be converted to gross or absolute terms to determine the total amount of O_2 consumed before the caloric value can be calculated. For example, a relative $\dot{V}O_2$ of 40 mL/kg/min for a 220-lb (100-kg) individual is converted to gross or absolute terms as follows:

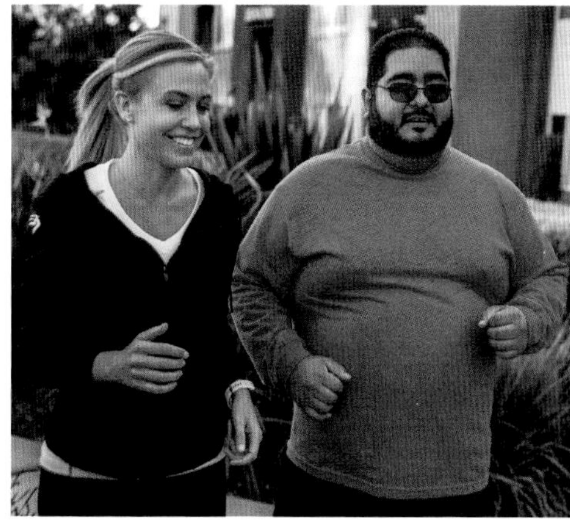

- If this individual consumes 40 mL/kg/min, then it can be represented as 40 mL x 100 kg = 4,000 mL/min, or 4.0 L/min (1,000 mL = 1 L)

Most pieces of commercial cardiorespiratory exercise equipment provide estimates of caloric expenditure in this same manner. While they may not always be 100% accurate, they calculate caloric expenditure by estimating gross or absolute $\dot{V}O_2$ based on the amount of work being performed (i.e., speed, grade, or watts).

If direct measurement of $\dot{V}O_2$ during activity is not available, the personal trainer can use published MET estimates for a variety of activities (see Table 8-8). Caloric-expenditure calculators are available for a variety of physical activities on the ACE website (www.ACEfitness.org/calculators).

VT1 and VT2

Although the increase in HR during exercise is somewhat linear, at least up to fairly high intensities, and although exercise is classically programmed in terms of %MHR, the metabolic response to exercise is generally nonlinear (Foster & Cotter, 2006). Accordingly, it is more reasonable to program exercise in terms of the metabolic response to exercise, which is easily marked by either blood lactate or the ventilatory responses of VT1 and VT2.

At higher intensities, when the buffering mechanism cannot keep up with the extra acid production, and the pH of the blood begins to fall (due to accumulating **hydrogen ions**), the respiratory center is strongly stimulated, and there is yet another increase in breathing (VT2) (see Figure 8-6). This point represents the intensity at which the body can no longer sustain an activity and begins to shut down. In most healthy people, this marker is associated with a flattening of the HR response to increasing intensity, referred to as the **HR turnpoint** (Figure 8-17).

These two metabolic markers—VT1 and VT2—whether based on respiratory responses or blood lactate responses, provide a convenient way to divide intensity into training zones that are determined without any use of, or reference to, MHR (Figure 8-18):

- Zone 1 reflects low-to-moderate intensity exercise with HRs below VT1.
- Zone 2 reflects moderate-to-vigorous intensity exercise with HRs from VT1 to just below VT2.
- Zone 3 reflects vigorous-to-very vigorous intensity exercise with HRs at or above VT2.

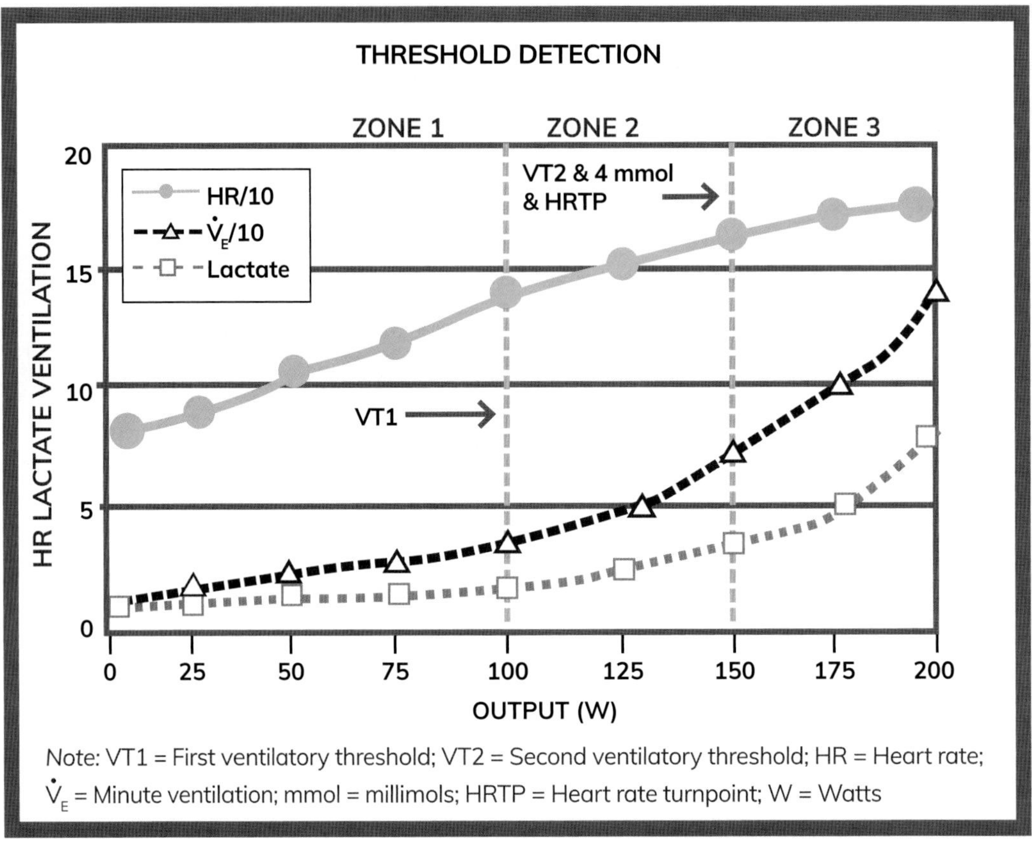

FIGURE 8-17
Schematic of the detection of the first and second thresholds based on increases in ventilation (VT1 and VT2), on lactate (4 mmol/L), and on the non-linearity of the HR increase. This provides for the possibility of three effective training zones based on two thresholds.

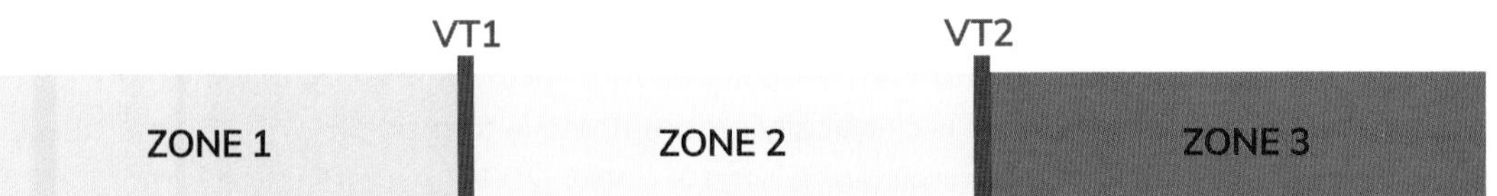

FIGURE 8-18
Three-zone intensity model

Note: VT1 = First ventilatory threshold; VT2 = Second ventilatory threshold

Stated simply, if a client can talk comfortably, he or she is training in zone 1. If the client is not sure if he or she can talk comfortably, he or she is working in zone 2. If the client definitely cannot talk comfortably while training, he or she is working in zone 3.

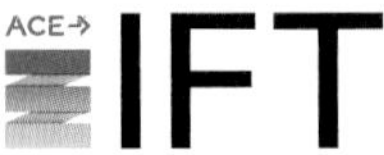

The three phases of the Cardiorespiratory Training component of the ACE IFT Model follow this three-zone system. While this model presents a chronological progression beginning with Base Training, moving through Fitness Training, and culminating with Performance Training (for those with this goal), personal trainers should understand that each client will have a unique point of entry into the ACE IFT Model based on his or her individual needs, goals, and current conditioning level. For example, deconditioned individuals and those seeking to lose weight by building their cardiorespiratory base and ability to efficiently burn more fats (caloric quality) will spend much of their initial training in zone 1, before being introduced to intervals that progress from the higher end of zone 1 to the lower end of zone 2.

DURATION

Exercise duration generally defines the amount of time spent performing a physical activity. ACSM (2018) presents guidelines on recommended durations that reduce the risks for **mortality** and **morbidity,** and improve overall fitness. Personal trainers should consider the following points:

- The quantity of exercise or physical activity may be performed in one continuous bout or be performed intermittently and accumulated in shorter bouts throughout the day.
- While the guidelines provide recommended quantities to improve overall health and fitness, personal trainers should always place the needs and abilities of their clients first.
- Personal trainers should select suitable durations and progressions that fit each client's current conditioning level, tolerance, and availability, and aspire only to attain the recommendations when appropriate.

Benefits gained from exercise and physical activity are dose-related (i.e., greater benefits are derived from greater quantities of activity). For example, physical activity expending ≤1,000 kcal/week generally produces improvements to only health (e.g., lower BP and **cholesterol**). This is considered a minimal recommendation for activity, whereas greater quantities expending ≥2,000 kcal/week promote greater health benefits and significant improvements to overall fitness.

Exercise guidelines related to duration call for the following (U.S. Department of Health & Human Services, 2018):

- Initially, increase the number of minutes per session (duration) and the number of days a week (frequency) of moderate-intensity activity prior to an increase in exercise intensity.
- Be mindful of the magnitude increase in physical activity each week, as this is can be predictive of injury risk. For instance, a 20-minute increase per week is safer for a client who already does 200 minutes a week of jogging (a 10% increase) relative to a client who does 40 minutes a week (a 50% increase).
- High volumes of moderate-to-vigorous physical activity appear to remove the excess risk of all-cause mortality that is associated with high volumes of sitting.
- Decreased sedentary time reduces, but does not eliminate, the risks related to a lack of physical activity throughout the week.

Personal trainers must bear in mind that not all clients will be able to complete a substantial amount of exercise in one bout. For example, beginner exercisers will generally not be able to initially complete 30 minutes of moderate-intensity continuous cardiorespiratory exercise, nor will they be capable of achieving the recommended frequency. For these individuals, brief episodes of moderate-to-vigorous physical activity of any duration of time may be included in the daily accumulated total volume of physical activity. In fact, research now shows that any amount of moderate-to-vigorous physical activity counts toward meeting the daily 30-minute target and will contribute to the overall health benefits associated with the accumulated volume of physical activity (ACSM, 2018; U.S. Department of Health & Human Services, 2018).

The Client with Low Self-efficacy

During the initial consultation with a new client, you determine that due to her current health status and fitness level she should begin her Cardiorespiratory Training with a focus on Base Training to establish a regular exercise habit performing low- to moderate-intensity activities. She knows that exercise is good for her, but she does not believe in her ability to do cardiorespiratory exercise for any amount of time. She admits that she is intimidated by the thought of meeting the recommended guidelines of at least 150 minutes of moderate-intensity cardiorespiratory activity per week. She also does not feel confident that beginning an exercise program is right for her.

ACE ABC APPROACH

The following is an example of how the ACE Mover Method and the ACE ABC Approach can be used when coaching a client with low **self-efficacy.**

Ask: Asking powerful open-ended questions as part of this initial meeting will allow the personal trainer to discover the client's "why" for wanting to work with a personal trainer and keep the conversation moving in a positive direction.

Personal Trainer: You shared with me that you're worried you won't be able to exercise because of your current conditioning level, but you also recognize the value of exercise. In your ideal vision of yourself, what would you like to achieve?

Client: Realistically, I would like to get to a point where I can go for walks without it taking everything out of me and leaving me with no energy. There was a time when I used to walk for fun and felt like I could walk for hours without ever needing a break. I want to travel again and be able to walk around when I visit new places. Right now, I feel like being out of shape is preventing me from doing a lot of things that I would love to do.

Break down barriers: In this step, it is time to further investigate the client's concerns in order to discover what obstacles may prevent her from beginning an exercise program.

Personal Trainer: Right now, you feel limited by your physical conditioning, but in the past you enjoyed walking. You would like to get back to a point where you can walk comfortably and maybe even travel again. What can you start doing to move closer to your goals?

Client: I need to find a starting point that is right for me. I currently have the time to exercise, but I get in my own way with my negative thoughts about how much exercise I need to do.

Personal Trainer: Tell me more about what you feel you need to be doing.

Client: Well, according to the physical-activity guidelines, 150 minutes per week is the minimum amount I should be doing, but the idea of walking for 30 minutes straight seems impossible. I'm frustrated that I'm out of breath after walking to my mailbox.

Personal Trainer: You're right about the physical-activity guidelines, but you might be interested to know that bouts of physical activity of any length contribute to the total accumulation of activity and health benefits that you can achieve. Even the walk you take to get the mail counts!

Collaborate: Working with the client on goals and solutions is the next step now that the client has identified her barrier to getting started and has the information she needs to be in control of where she would like to begin with her exercise program.

Personal Trainer: Based on this idea that even small amounts of activity are beneficial, what steps could you see yourself taking toward including more movement in your day?

Client: I would like to start by meeting with you twice next week. I am not sure where this journey will lead me, but I do enjoy walking and it would be helpful to determine a starting point to know how long I can walk. Knowing that any amount of physical activity is beneficial energizes me to get started—even if it is for less than 30 minutes.

The ACE ABC Approach provides personal trainers with strategies to help clients overcome self-limiting beliefs. By meeting this client where she is, letting her remain in control of the decisions she makes, and providing relevant information, the personal trainer can use his or her expertise of exercise program design to work together with the client to create a safe, effective, and enjoyable exercise experience.

TYPE

Virtually any type of activity that involves a large amount of muscle and can be performed in a rhythmic fashion and sustained for more than a few minutes can be classified as cardiorespiratory exercise. If this type of exercise is performed regularly, there are adaptations in the various organ systems (e.g., circulatory, pulmonary, and musculoskeletal) that improve the ability of the person to move around or otherwise perform sustained exercise (i.e., the cardiorespiratory training effect). Because of the unique muscular requirements of ambulatory exercises (e.g., walking, running, cycling, rowing, and skating), these exercises are usually considered the primary cardiorespiratory exercises. Other related exercises (e.g., stair climbing, elliptical exercise, and arm cranking) can also be classified as cardiorespiratory exercise. Even game-type activities, assuming that they require sustained bodily movement, can be considered cardiorespiratory exercise. In this regard, the cardiorespiratory benefit of game-type exercise is proportional to the amount and intensity of ambulatory activity involved. Thus, golf can be beneficial, as it involves walking for approximately 3 miles (4.8 km) (the average length of a standard 18-hole course) but is less beneficial than a steady walk of the same duration (because of the lower intensity of the intermittent walking during golf). Similarly, singles tennis is probably more valuable from the standpoint of cardiorespiratory exercise than doubles, because of the more extensive running required to cover the entire court. Table 8-9 provides a list of physical activities that promote improvement or maintenance of cardiorespiratory fitness.

Equipment-based Cardiorespiratory Exercise

Exercise equipment designed for cardiorespiratory training is a prominent feature in most fitness facilities, as well as in the home exercise market. This can include treadmills, cycle ergometers,

TABLE 8-9

Physical Activities That Promote Improvement or Maintenance of Cardiorespiratory Fitness

Exercise Description	Recommended Group	Activity Examples
Endurance activities requiring minimal skill or fitness	All adults	Walking, slow-dancing, recreational cycling or swimming
Vigorous-intensity endurance activities requiring minimal skill	Adults participating in regular exercise or having better than average fitness	Jogging, rowing, elliptical training, stepping, indoor cycling, fast-dancing
Endurance activities requiring higher skill levels	Adults with acquired skill and higher fitness levels	Swimming, cross-country skiing
Recreational sports	Adults participating in regular training with acquired fitness and skill levels	Soccer, basketball, racquet sports

elliptical machines, rowing machines, arm ergometers, and a variety of other devices. The cardiorespiratory value of any of these equipment-based approaches is largely based on how the machine is used. Many pieces of higher-end exercise equipment are programed to estimate the MET or caloric cost of exercise. However, the accuracy of estimates for the MET cost of exercising on a particular device is only as good as the research supporting the equation. In many cases, these data are quite good. In other cases, the numbers are much less reliable. Common sense is required when using the MET or caloric values generated by exercise equipment. In many cases, the data are based on university students who are already fairly fit and are exercising without the benefit of handrail support. Thus, in less-fit individuals, and particularly if handrail support is required, the values suggested by the exercise device may overestimate the actual value attained. It is important to understand that the calorie counts on exercise machines (or those obtained from formulas) are simply estimates and will never be 100% accurate. Therefore, it is best to use them as rough benchmarks from workout to workout.

Circuit Training

Because of the **specificity** principle of exercise, muscular-training programs designed to improve muscular strength and endurance are not intrinsically suited to producing cardiorespiratory training effects. As an adaptation of military training exercises, the concept of circuit weight training emerged in the 1950s and 1960s based on the premise that sequential exercises using different muscle groups might allow the exerciser to focus on one muscle group while a previously used group is recovering. The logic behind this practice was that the overall metabolic rate might remain high enough to allow cardiorespiratory training effects, while still focusing the exercises on muscular components. Depending on equipment availability, **circuit training** can be performed either by a single individual or by groups of people rotating in an organized manner through several exercise stations.

Outdoor Exercise

Over the past few decades, a wide variety of outdoor exercises, including **green exercise,** have emerged out of recreational activities, many with the promise of providing cardiorespiratory fitness. Activities that require considerable walking or running are, of course, very likely to provide cardiorespiratory training. Other outdoor activities (e.g., climbing and canoeing) are much more variable in their cardiorespiratory training effects and depend almost entirely on how they are conducted. Additionally, many outdoor activities are very seasonal in their application. For example, cross-country skiing and snowshoeing in the winter months are similar to running and hiking in the warmer months.

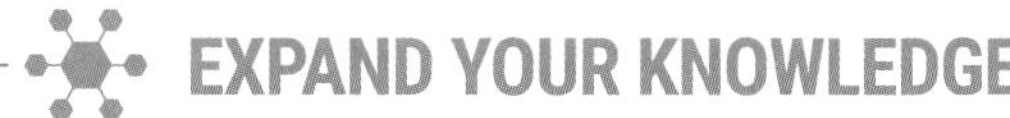

What Is Green Exercise?

The term green exercise refers to exercise performed in natural environments. It is well known that regular exercise training itself confers various health and psychological benefits, including the prevention and management of **hypertension,** obesity, **type 2 diabetes, dyslipidemia**, and CVD. In the past couple of decades, there has been considerable scientific inquiry focused on whether a synergistic effect exists in terms of health benefits when exercise is performed in natural environments. Indeed, there appears to be mounting evidence that green exercise provides an array of beneficial responses ranging from improved cognitive function and enhanced cardiac function to reduced levels of circulating stress hormones (Calogiuri et al., 2015; Grazuleviciene et al., 2015; Barton & Pretty, 2010). Although most people live in a world where much of the required physical work has been eliminated and natural outdoor environments are continuously shrinking, modern humans' intrinsic exercise capacity and requirements are nearly identical to those of our Paleolithic ancestors. Nevertheless, one successful strategy personal trainers can employ is to encourage engagement in green exercise. Here are some practical recommendations:

Strategy #1: Humans were designed to ambulate on grass or dirt. Ideally, the more walking that can be done on natural surfaces, the better. Humans are also genetically adapted to daily, high volumes of low-to-moderate intensity walking. Depending on the individual client and his or her health history, anywhere from 1 to 5 miles/day (1.6 to 8.0 km/day) can be recommended.

Strategy #2: Green exercise can include activities related to the acquisition of food. Indeed, for thousands of years a natural relationship existed between outdoor physical activity and procurement of food and water. Recommended activities include:

- Walking to a restaurant or grocery store
- Fishing
- Gardening
- Hunting

Strategy #3: Encourage clients to select weekly social and/or recreational activities that require a meaningful amount of physical exertion in a green environment. Recommended activities include:

- Golfing
- Group outdoor classes (e.g., boot camp or yoga)
- Tennis or pickleball
- Skiing

Strategy #4: Dose-response relationships between both the intensity and duration of green exercise and health benefits have been established (Barton & Pretty, 2010). Remind clients that they can obtain substantial health benefits from short, light-intensity engagements in green exercise, followed by diminishing, yet still positive improvements, with longer durations and higher intensities.

Strategy #5: It has been shown that increased green space availability and access encourages individuals to spend more time outdoors in green exercise and related activities. However, an unintended health consequence is that increased green exercise has been found to be associated with higher odds of having skin cancer (Astell-Burt et al., 2014). Accordingly, be sure to remind clients to protect themselves from sun exposure by wearing appropriate gear (e.g., hat and UV-protective clothing) and sunscreen when exercising outdoors.

The Outdoorsman

During the cool-down portion of your client's training session, he mentions that he is interested in increasing the amount of physical activity he is doing. He tells you that in addition to his twice-weekly sessions with you, he would like to create a plan to increase his activity level so that he attains even greater health-related benefits. Because of the work you have done establishing rapport with this client, he values your insight and has asked for your help in achieving this new goal.

ACE ABC APPROACH

The following is an example of how the ACE Mover Method and ACE ABC Approach enable the personal trainer to partner with a client in working toward his goals.

Ask: Asking powerful open-ended questions can help the personal trainer uncover what the client is hoping to achieve with his new goal and what types of activity the client enjoys.

Personal Trainer: How will becoming more physically active enhance your life?

Client: I've been feeling great since we began working together six months ago but I know I still have a long way to go. I need to reduce my stress, stay mentally sharp, and keep my heart healthy. I think if I do these things now, I will have the quality of life I want as I get older. Also, I want to be an active participant in the lives of my children and, one day, my grandchildren.

Personal Trainer: You recognize the value in making your health a priority. What types of activities have you enjoyed doing in the past?

Client: I'm starting to, yeah. Unfortunately, the things I enjoy are technically not exercise; they don't involve me going to the gym. I like being outdoors and doing things like hiking, fishing, and riding my bike. These things seem too relaxing to have any real fitness benefit.

Break down barriers: Ask more open-ended questions to uncover beliefs that may be preventing the client from taking action.

Personal Trainer: You want to be more active, and you feel that the activities you enjoy are not strenuous enough to count as physical activity. Interestingly, the type of activities you mentioned fall under a category called green exercise. Are you familiar with this concept?

Client: I can't say that I am, but based on our conversation I am guessing it has something to do with being outside. Is that right?

Personal Trainer: That's correct. Green exercise refers to exercise that takes place in natural environments. Exercising outdoors has been linked to enhanced cardiac function, reduced levels of stress, and improved cognitive function—some of the same things you want to focus on.

Collaborate: Working together with the client on setting more specific goals is the next step now that the client has information about alternative types of physical activity and how they can contribute to long-term goals for overall health improvement.

Client: I had no idea that there were fitness benefits to doing some of the things I already like. I've stopped doing many of these things because they did not seem like a priority.

Personal Trainer: What might you do differently now that you have this new information?

Client: Yesterday, on my way home from work, I noticed that the city made improvements to the park I used to take my kids to when they were younger, which also connects to some hiking trails. I'll start there. My wife has commitments on Tuesday and Thursday evenings, so those would be good days for me to stop and take a hike. Because of the work you and I have been doing, I would like to see if I can hike two days each week for 45 minutes without stopping.

Using the ACE ABC Approach empowered the client to see past barriers and work with the personal trainer to set specific goals for increasing physical activity through sharing relevant information, using open-ended questions, and evoking the client's motivation to improve his quality of life.

Water Exercise

Water exercise can provide a convenient alternative form of exercise that is pleasant, reduces orthopedic loading, and is capable of training different muscle groups than those used during ambulatory activities. While the classical water exercise is swimming, group classes (e.g., water aerobics) and games (e.g., water polo and water volleyball) can be effective methods of exercise as well. Water exercise is particularly valuable for older people, individuals with obesity, or those who may have orthopedic issues, as the buoyancy provided by the water unloads the traditional targets (i.e., weight-bearing joints) of ambulatory exercise. It is important to remember that the energy cost of ambulatory activity in the water is very strongly related to the depth of the water (e.g., walking in thigh-or chest-deep water) and can increase markedly with only very slight increases in the speed of ambulating in the water. Secondly, immersion in water causes the blood to be redistributed to the central circulation, away from the limbs. In people with compromised circulatory function, this can lead to complications (e.g., breathlessness and added cardiac stress). The energy cost of swimming is highly variable and depends not only on swimming velocity, but also on the stroke, technique, and skill of the swimmer.

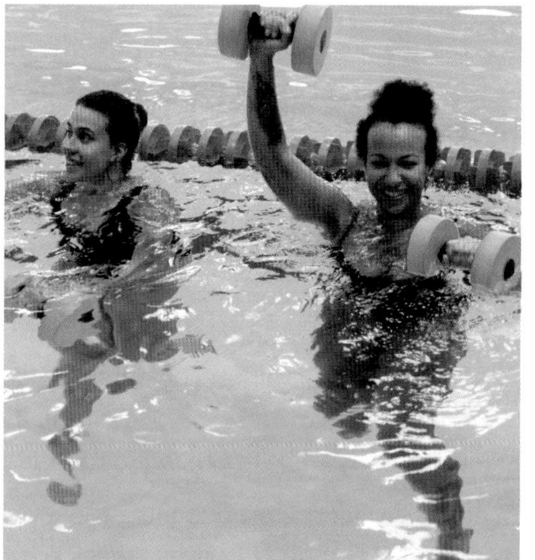

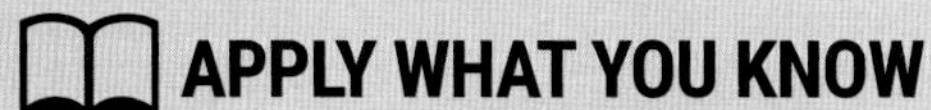

Understanding Exercise Options

Clients tend to adhere to activities that they enjoy and tolerate well. For example, one client may enjoy riding a stationary cycle because she can watch TV while she is working out. Another client might prefer walking outdoors because he enjoys nature and spends the majority of his workweek stuck indoors. As a personal trainer, it is important to discover your clients' activity-mode preferences and design their workout programs accordingly. Consider trying out for yourself all of the modes of activity presented in this chapter so that you will have experience in different types of cardiorespiratory exercise from which to draw when coaching your clients. What specific exercise gear or technology might be helpful to use with different types of activities (e.g., padded bicycle shorts or effective sunscreen for outdoor workouts)? Gaining experience in many different modes of activity will make you a more knowledgeable personal trainer and a more effective resource for your clients.

EXERCISE PROGRESSION

While exercise needs to create an enjoyable and positive experience for clients, the personal trainer will need to determine how to progress each client's program. Progression follows some basic training principles, including the following:

- The principle of **overload** states that when additional stresses are placed on the organs or systems (e.g., cardiorespiratory or muscular) in a timely and appropriate manner, physiological adaptations and improvement will occur. The rate of progression in a program depends on the individual's current conditioning level, program goals, and tolerance for the slight discomfort associated with raising training load or volume.
- The principle of specificity states that the physiological adaptations made within the body are specific to demands placed upon that body—sometimes referred to as the **SAID principle**: specific adaptations to imposed demands. This implies that if a client's goals are consistent with running a half marathon, the training program should progress to mimic the demands of that activity, to provide the specific stimuli that elicit appropriate adaptations within the body. The decision to progress to event- or sport-specific modalities should be made with consideration for the individual's skills and abilities, as well as his or her current conditioning level. Even among cardiorespiratory exercises, the transfer of benefits from one type of exercise to another is far from 100%. Research demonstrates that activities that use similar muscles (e.g., cycling performed by runners) have about 50% of the value of performing specific training (e.g., running) on a minute-by-minute basis. Muscularly non-similar training (e.g., swimming performed by runners) has about 25% of the value of performing specific training on a minute-by-minute basis (Foster et al., 1995; Loy, Holland, & Mutton, 1993).

Exercise duration is probably the most appropriate variable to manipulate initially, building the exercise session by 10% every week or two over the first four to six weeks. Thereafter, and once adherence is developed, personal trainers can implement progressions by increasing exercise frequency and then exercise intensity. Importantly, the progressions should always remain consistent with the client's goals (ACSM, 2018). It may be particularly important to include multiple modalities of exercise (e.g., cross-training, walking, cycling, or elliptical training) and even variations within a modality (e.g., steady-state exercise, interval training, or **Fartlek training**) to limit the risk of boredom, burnout, or orthopedic injury from overuse as the volume of exercise builds. Additional considerations for training program progression are presented in Chapter 11.

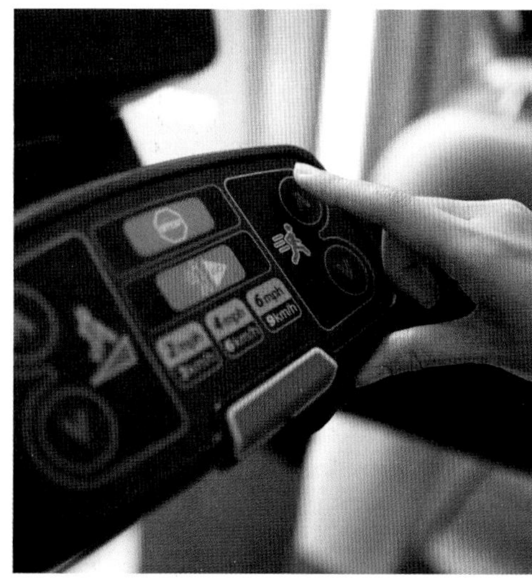

A FITT FOR REDUCING SEDENTARY TIME

The FITT formula can also be applied to designing a program for reducing sedentary time. Table 8-10 outlines evidence-based FITT recommendations that personal trainers can use to assist clients with reducing their sedentary time.

TABLE 8-10

FITT Recommendations for Reducing Sedentary Time

Program Component	Component Recommendation(s)
Frequency	▸ Take breaks from sedentary time every 60 to 120 minutes.
Intensity	▸ Light-intensity activities are recommended for sedentary-break activities. ▸ Light intensity equates to <25 to 50% $\dot{V}O_2$max, >1.5 to <3.0 METs, or below VT1.
Time	▸ Limit overall discretionary sitting time to no more than 2 hours/day. ▸ Each break in sedentary time should last 5 to 10 minutes.
Type	▸ Light-intensity activities include routine household/occupational tasks. ▸ Substitute light-intensity activities for sedentary time whenever possible. ▸ Modify household/occupational environment to limit sitting (e.g., remove chairs from TV area and position computers at a standing height).

Note: $\dot{V}O_2$max = Maximal oxygen uptake; METs = Metabolic equivalents; VT1 = First ventilatory threshold

Source: Dalleck, L.C. & Gibeault, A.N. (2015). *A F.I.T.T. Formula for Sitting? How to Help Your Clients Reduce Sedentary Time and Improve Their Health.* https://www.acefitness.org/education-and-resources/professional/prosource/august-2015/5520/a-f-i-t-t-formula-for-sitting-how-to-help-your-clients-reduce-sedentary-time-and-improve-their

ACE-sponsored research has found that the frequency of breaks from sitting should be every 60 to 120 minutes and that breaks in sedentary time for an average of five to 10 minutes were beneficially associated with decreased metabolic risk (Keeling, Buchanan, & Dalleck, 2018). Additional research by Healy et al. (2008) showed that total sedentary time is linked with obesity, abnormal glucose metabolism, and **metabolic syndrome** and that more frequent breaks in sedentary time lead to favorable metabolic attributes.

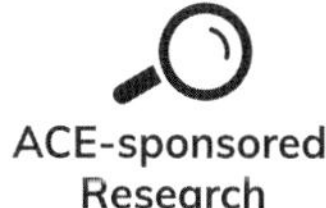

ACE-sponsored Research

Assessments for Cardiorespiratory Fitness

The personal trainer will select and administer cardiorespiratory fitness assessments according to each client's needs and desires using information obtained during the preparticipation health screening. Cardiorespiratory fitness assessments are also determined by a number of other factors, including availability of equipment, client lifestyles, time allotment, and the personal trainer's level of comfort with the assessment procedures. Recommendations for the specific timing of cardiorespiratory fitness assessments should be aligned with client goals and can be found within the "ACE Integrated Fitness Training Model—Cardiorespiratory Training" section on page 304.

During the administration of any exercise assessment involving exertion (e.g., cardiorespiratory or **muscular endurance** and/or muscular strength assessment), personal trainers must always be aware of identifiable signs or symptoms that merit immediate assessment termination and possible referral to a qualified healthcare professional [American College of Sports Medicine (ACSM), 2018]. These signs and symptoms include:

- Onset of angina, chest pain, or angina-like symptoms
- Significant drop (≥10 mmHg) in **systolic blood pressure (SBP)** despite an increase in exercise intensity or a decrease in SBP below the value obtained in the same position prior to assessment
- Excessive rise in BP: SBP reaches >250 mmHg and/or **diastolic blood pressure (DBP)** reaches >115 mmHg
- Shortness of breath, or wheezing (does not include heavy breathing due to intense exercise)
- Signs of poor **perfusion**: lightheadedness, confusion, **ataxia,** pallor (pale skin), **cyanosis** (bluish coloration, especially around the mouth), nausea, or cold and clammy skin
- Failure of HR to increase with increased exercise intensity
- Noticeable change in heart rhythm by **palpation** or **auscultation**
- Subject requests to stop
- Physical or verbal manifestations of severe fatigue
- Failure of assessment equipment

VENTILATORY THRESHOLD ASSESSMENT

Ventilatory threshold assessment is based on the physiological principle of ventilation. During submaximal exercise, ventilation increases linearly with O_2 uptake and CO_2 production. This occurs primarily through an increase in tidal volume. At higher or near-maximal intensities, the frequency of breathing becomes more pronounced and $\dot{V}_E$ rises disproportionately to the increase in O_2 uptake (Figure 8-19).

This disproportionate rise in breathing rate represents a state of ventilation that is no longer directly linked with O_2 demand at the cellular level and is generally termed the ventilatory threshold. The overcompensation in breathing frequency results from an increase in CO_2 production related to the **anaerobic glycolysis** that predominates during near-maximal-

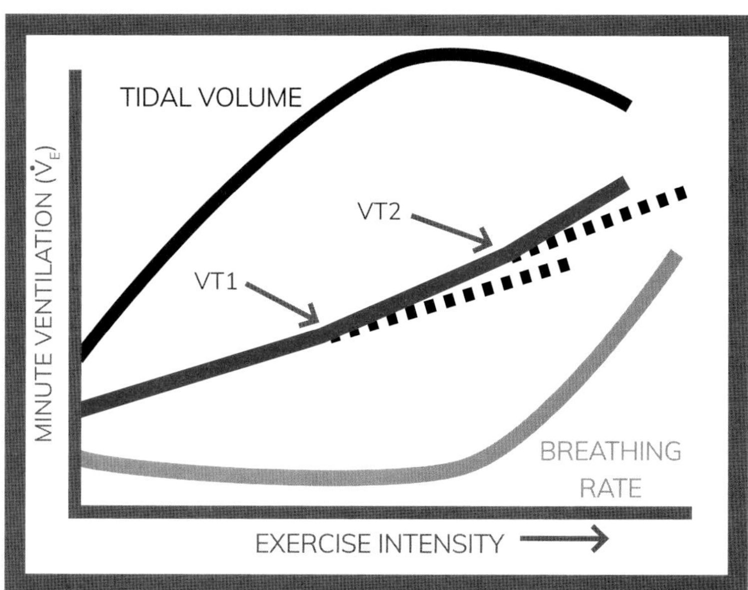

Note: VT1 = First ventilatory threshold; VT2 = Second ventilatory threshold

FIGURE 8-19
Ventilatory effects during aerobic exercise

intensity exercise. During strenuous exercise, breathing frequency may increase from 12 to 15 breaths per minute at rest to 35 to 45 breaths per minute, while tidal volume increases from resting values of 0.4 to 1.0 L up to 3 L or greater (McArdle, Katch, & Katch, 2019).

As exercise intensity increases, ventilation increases in a somewhat linear manner, demonstrating deflection points at certain intensities associated with metabolic changes within the body. One point, called the "crossover" point, or VT1, represents a level of intensity at which blood lactate accumulates faster and must be offset by blood buffers, which are compounds that neutralize acidosis in the blood and muscle fibers. This metabolic change causes the person to alter breathing in an effort to blow off the extra CO_2 produced by the buffering of acid metabolites. The cardiorespiratory challenge to the body at this point lies primarily with inspiration and not with the expiration of additional amounts of CO_2 (associated with buffering lactate in the blood). The need for O_2 is met primarily through an increase in tidal volume and not respiratory rate. As exercise intensity continues to increase past the crossover point, ventilation rates begin to increase exponentially as O_2 demands outpace the O_2-delivery system and lactate begins to accumulate in the blood. Consequently, respiratory rates increase.

The second disproportionate increase in ventilation—VT2, sometimes called the **respiratory compensation threshold**—occurs at the point where lactate is rapidly increasing with intensity and results in hyperventilation even relative to the extra CO_2 that is being produced. This second threshold represents the point at which blowing off the CO_2 is no longer adequate to buffer the increase in acidity that is occurring with progressively intense exercise.

In well-trained individuals, VT1 is approximately the highest intensity that can be sustained for one to two hours of exercise. In elite marathon runners, VT1 is very close to their competitive pace. The VT2 is the highest intensity that can be sustained for 30 to 60 minutes in well-trained individuals.

An important note for assessment purposes is that the exercise intensity associated with the ability to talk comfortably is highly related to VT1. As long as the exerciser can speak comfortably, he or she is almost always below VT1. The first point where it becomes more difficult to speak approximates the intensity of VT1, and the point at which speaking is definitely not comfortable approximates the intensity of VT2.

The majority of personal trainers will not have access to metabolic analyzers for identifying VT1 and VT2 and will need valid field assessments to identify these markers. As such, the most useful and practical approaches for assessing cardiorespiratory fitness are presented here. This section reviews field assessments for measuring HR at VT1 and VT2.

Contraindications

This type of assessment is not recommended for:

- Individuals with certain breathing problems [asthma or **chronic obstructive pulmonary disease (COPD)**]
- Individuals prone to panic/anxiety attacks, as the labored breathing may create discomfort or precipitate an attack
- Those recovering from a recent respiratory infection
- Individuals who are not fit enough to perform or benefit from the assessment

Talk Test

Following up on suggestions from a generation ago, several groups have explored the value of the talk test as a method of monitoring (and controlling) exercise training intensity (Cannon et al., 2004; Persinger et al., 2004; Recalde et al., 2002; Voelker et al., 2002; Porcari et al., 2001; Dehart et al., 2000). The usual experience with the talk test is that if two people are exercising and having a conversation, one of them will eventually turn to the other and say something like, "If we are going to keep talking, you are going to have to slow down." The talk test works on the premise that at about the intensity of VT1, the increase in ventilation is accomplished by an increase in breathing frequency. One of the requirements of comfortable speech is to be able to control breathing frequency. Thus, at the intensity of VT1, it is no longer possible to speak comfortably.

The simple talk test has been shown to work fairly well as an index of the exercise intensity at VT1. Options include asking clients to recite something familiar, such as reciting the alphabet or "A is for apple, B is for boy, etc.," then answer the question, "Can you speak comfortably?" If the answer is yes, the intensity is below the VT1. At the first response that is less than an unequivocal "yes," the intensity is probably right at that of the VT1, and if the answer is "no," the intensity is probably above VT1. When the client can no longer say more than a word or two between breaths, he or she is at or above VT2.

Another option is to compare the number to which an individual can count during the expiration phase of one breath during exercise against the number counted during the expiration phase at rest. Normally, when the number counted to during exercise drops to about 70% of the number that is possible at rest, the intensity is approximately equal to the VT1. For example, if an

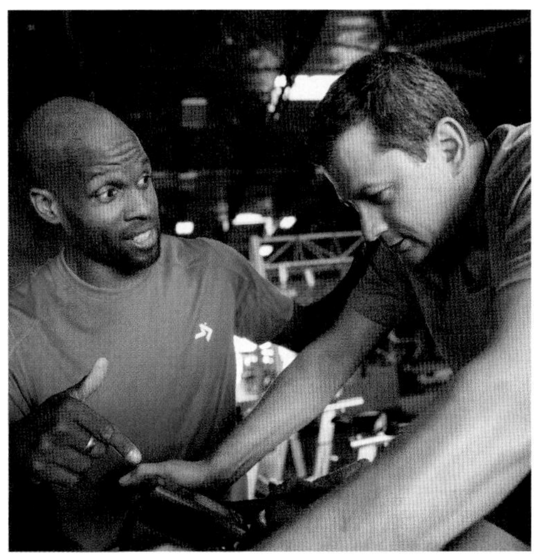

individual can count to 14 during the expiration phase at rest, 70%—the indicator of VT1—represents the exercise intensity at which he or she can no longer count past 10.

The talk test has several advantages as a method of programming and monitoring exercise compared to a given %$\dot{V}O_2$max or %MHR, since it is based off an individual's unique metabolic or ventilatory responses to exercise. Thus, for most people, training at intensities at which the answer to the question, "Can you speak comfortably?" becomes less than an unequivocal "yes" may represent the ideal training intensity marker. Therefore, the talk test is an appropriate marker to use for many individuals, especially for those seeking to lose weight or develop their cardiorespiratory efficiency. Training at or near this intensity (unique to the individual's own metabolism) increases the likelihood of a better exercise experience. Higher-intensity training for those individuals with performance goals can be regulated in terms of VT2.

Submaximal Talk Test for VT1

This test is best performed using HR telemetry (HR strap and watch) for continuous monitoring. To avoid missing VT1, the exercise increments need to be small, increasing steady-state HR by approximately 5 bpm per stage. Consequently, this test will require some preparation to determine the appropriate increments that elicit a 5-bpm increase. Once the increments are determined, the time needed to reach steady-state HR during a stage must also be determined (60 to 120 seconds per stage is usually adequate).

The end-point of the test is not a predetermined HR but is instead based on monitoring changes in breathing rate (technically metabolic changes) that are determined by the client's ability to recite a predetermined combination of phrases. Note: Reading, as opposed to reciting from memory, is not advised, as it compromises balance if testing is being performed on a treadmill.

The objectives of the test are to measure the HR response at VT1 by progressively increasing exercise intensity and achieving steady state at each stage, as well as to identify the HR where the ability to talk continuously becomes compromised. This point represents the intensity where the individual can continue to talk while breathing with minimal discomfort and reflects an associated increase in tidal volume that should not compromise breathing rate or the ability to talk. Progressing beyond this point where breathing rate increases significantly, making continuous talking difficult, is not necessary and will render the test inaccurate.

Equipment:

- Treadmill, cycle ergometer, elliptical trainer, or arm ergometer
- Stopwatch

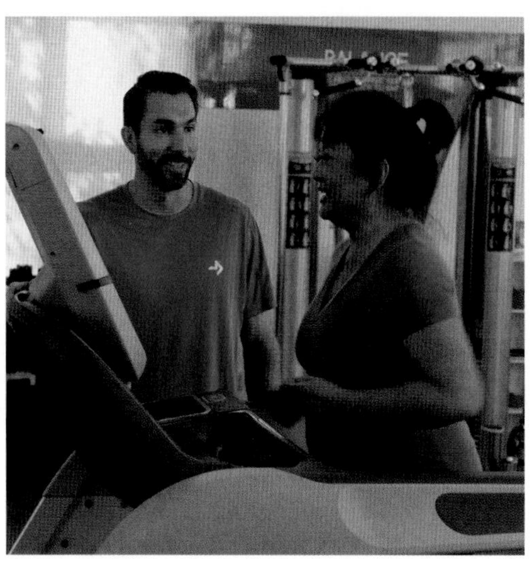

- HR monitor with chest strap (optional)
- Predetermined text that the individual will recite (e.g., alphabet)

Pre-test procedure:

- As this test involves small, incremental increases in intensity specific to each individual, the testing stages need to be predetermined. The goal is to incrementally increase workload in small quantities to determine VT1. Large incremental increases may result in the individual passing through VT1, thereby invalidating the test:
    - Recommended workload increases are approximately 0.5 mph, 1% grade, or 10 to 20 watts.
    - The objective is to increase steady-state HR at each stage by approximately 5 bpm.
    - Plan to complete this test within eight to 16 minutes to ensure that localized muscle fatigue from longer durations of exercise is not an influencing factor.
- Measure pre-exercise HR and BP (if necessary), both sitting and standing, and then record the values on the testing form.
- Describe the purpose of this graded exercise test, review the predetermined protocol, passage to be recited, and allow the client the opportunity to address any questions or concerns. Each stage of the test lasts one to two minutes to achieve steady state HR at each workload.
- Allow the client to walk on the treadmill or use the ergometer to warm up and get used to the apparatus. If using a treadmill, he or she should avoid holding the handrails. If the client is too unstable without holding onto the rails, consider using another testing modality, as this will invalidate the test results.
- Take the client through a light warm-up (RPE of 2 to 3 on the 0 to 10 scale) for three to five minutes, maintaining an intensity comfortably below a moderate level.

Test protocol and administration:

- Once the client has warmed up, adjust the workload intensity so the client is working at a moderate-to-strong intensity level (RPE of 3 to 4 on the 0 to 10 scale).
- Toward the latter part of each stage (i.e., last 20 to 30 seconds), measure/record the HR and then ask the client to recite the predetermined passage. Upon completion of the recital, ask the client to identify whether he or she felt this task was easy or uncomfortable-to-challenging. Note: Conversations with questions and answers are not suggested, as the test needs to evaluate the challenge of talking continuously, not in brief bursts as in conversation. Also, reading as opposed to reciting from memory, is not advised, as it may compromise balance if testing is being performed on a treadmill.
    - The test concludes when the client reports that he or she can speak, but not entirely comfortably.

- If VT1 is not achieved, progress through the successive stages, repeating the protocol at each stage until VT1 is reached.
- Once the HR at VT1 is identified, progress to the cool-down phase (matching the warm-up intensity) for three to five minutes.
- This test should ideally be conducted on two separate occasions with the same exercise modality to determine an average VT1 HR.
    - HR varies between treadmills, bikes, etc., so it is important to conduct the tests with the exercise modality that the client uses most frequently.
    - The VT1 HR will also be noticeably higher if the test is conducted after weight training due to fatigue and increased metabolism. Therefore, clients should be tested before performing muscular-training exercises.

VT2 Threshold Assessment

VT2 is equivalent to another important metabolic marker called the **onset of blood lactate accumulation (OBLA),** the point at which blood lactate accumulates at rates faster than the body can buffer and remove it (blood lactate >4 mmol/L). This marker represents an exponential increase in the concentration of blood lactate, indicating an exercise intensity that can no longer be sustained for long periods, and represents the highest sustainable level of exercise intensity, a strong marker of exercise performance. Continually measuring blood lactate is an accurate method to determine OBLA and the corresponding VT2. However, the cost of lactate analyzers and handling of biohazardous materials make it impractical for most exercise professionals. Consequently, field tests have been created to challenge an individual's ability to sustain high intensities of exercise for a predetermined duration to *estimate* VT2. This method of testing requires an individual to sustain the highest intensity possible during a single bout of steady-state exercise. This obviously mandates high levels of conditioning and experience in pacing. Consequently, VT2 testing is *only* recommended for well-conditioned individuals with fitness and performance goals.

Well-trained individuals can probably estimate their own HR response at VT2 during their training by identifying the highest intensity they can maintain for an extended duration. In cycling, coaches often select a 10-mile time trial or 60 minutes of sustained intensity, whereas in running, a 30-minute run is often used. Given that testing for 30 to 60 minutes is impractical in most fitness facilities, personal trainers can opt to use shorter single-stage tests of highest sustainable intensity to estimate the HR response at VT2.

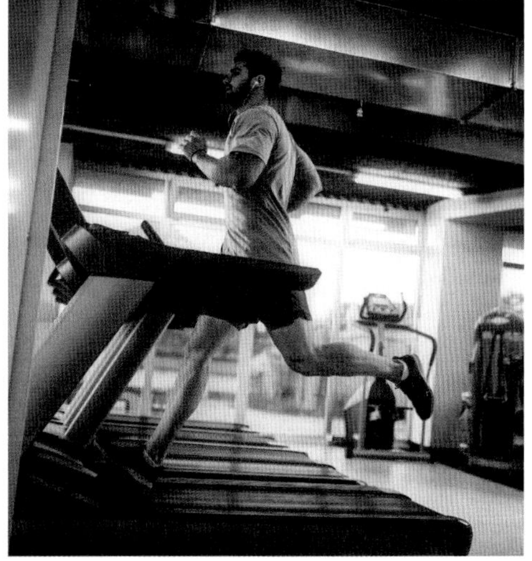

In general, the intensity that can be sustained for 15 to 20 minutes is higher than what could be sustained for 30 to 60 minutes in conditioned individuals. To predict the HR response at VT2 using a 15- to 20-minute test, trainers can estimate that the corrected HR response would be equivalent to approximately 95% of the 15- to 20-minute HR average. For example, if an

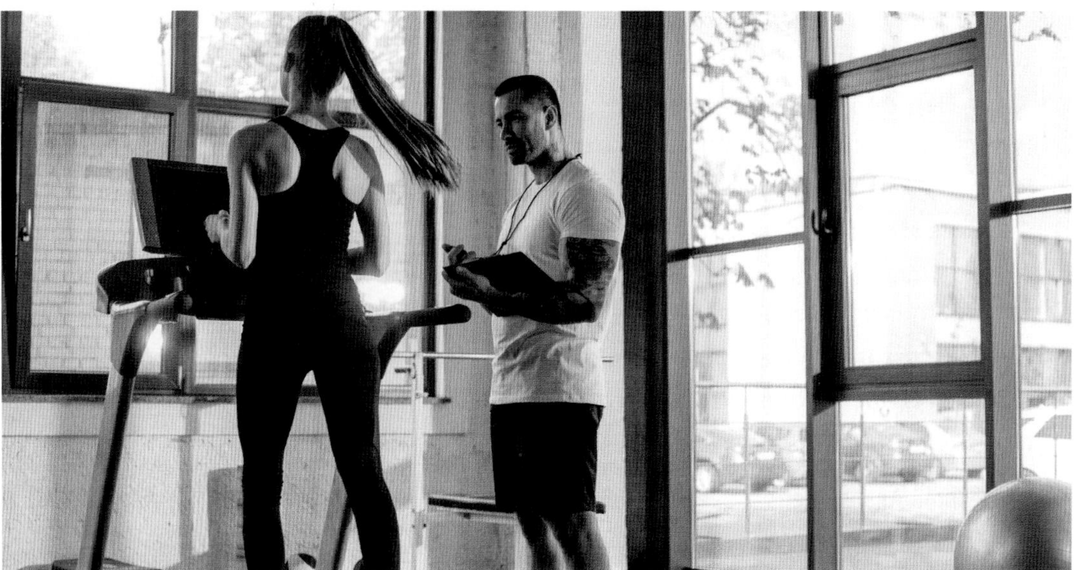

individual's average sustainable HR for a 20-minute bike test is 168 bpm, his or her HR at VT2 would be 160 bpm (168 bpm x 0.95).

This assessment is best performed using HR telemetry (HR strap and watch) for continuous monitoring. Individuals participating in this test need experience with the selected modality to effectively pace themselves at their maximal sustainable intensity for the duration of the bout. In addition, this test should only be performed by clients who are cleared for exercise and ready for Performance Training.

Pre-assessment procedure:

- Briefly explain the purpose of the assessment, review the predetermined protocol, and allow the client the opportunity to address any questions or concerns.
- Take the client through a light warm-up (2- to 3-out-of-10 effort) for three to five minutes, maintaining a heart rate below 120 bpm.

Assessment protocol and administration:

- Begin the assessment by increasing the intensity to the predetermined level.
  - Allow the individual to make changes to the exercise intensity as needed during the first few minutes of the bout. Remember, he or she needs to be able to maintain the selected intensity for 20 minutes.
- During the last five minutes of exercise, record the heart rate at each minute interval.
- Use the average HR collected over the last five minutes to account for any **cardiovascular drift** associated with fatigue, thermoregulation, and changing blood volume.
- Multiply the average HR attained during the 15- to 20-minute high-intensity exercise bout by 0.95 to determine the VT2 estimate.

Components of a Cardiorespiratory Workout Session

There are basically three components of any training session: the warm-up phase, the conditioning phase, and the cool-down phase. In some exercise bouts, the intensity of exercise may be very gradually increased, stabilized, and then decreased, so that the components of the session are almost imperceptibly different. For example, going for a run during which the first and last half miles are slower than the middle portion of the run incorporates all three components of a workout session. In other training sessions, where the conditioning phase may be more challenging, the transitions from warm-up to conditioning to cool-down may be quite distinct.

WARM-UP

The warm-up is a period of lighter exercise preceding the conditioning phase of the exercise bout and should last for five to 10 minutes for most healthy adults. It should begin with low- to moderate-intensity exercise or activity that gradually increases in intensity.

If higher-intensity intervals are planned during the conditioning phase, the latter portion of the warm-up could include some brief higher-intensity exercise to prepare the exerciser for the more intense elements of the stimulus phase. As a general principle, the harder the conditioning phase and/or the older the exerciser, the more extensive the warm-up should be (see Chapters 12 through 15 for specific recommendations for various populations). However, the warm-up should not be so demanding that it creates fatigue that would reduce performance, especially when working with competitive athletes.

CONDITIONING PHASE

The conditioning phase, which must be appropriate for the client's current fitness level and consistent with his or her training goals, should be planned in terms of frequency, duration, intensity (utilizing steady-state or interval-training formats), and modality. The higher-intensity elements of a session should take place fairly early in the conditioning phase, and the session should conclude with more steady-state exercise, even if the intensity is still in the range likely to serve as a stimulus.

Interval training generally involves bouts of steady-state exercise performed at higher intensities for sustained periods, followed by a return to lower cardiorespiratory intensities for the recovery interval. These intervals often utilize exercise-to-recovery ratios between 1:3 and 1:1 (e.g., a one-minute steady-state bout is followed by a two-minute recovery period at a lower intensity when following a 1:2 exercise-to-recovery ratio).

COOL-DOWN

The cool-down should be of approximately the same duration and intensity as the warm-up (i.e., five to 10 minutes of low- to moderate-intensity activity). This phase is directed primarily toward preventing the tendency for blood to pool in the extremities, which may occur when exercise ends. The cessation of significant venous return from the "muscle pump" experienced during exercise can cause blood to accumulate in the lower extremity, reducing blood flow back to the heart and out to vital organs (e.g., the brain, potentially causing symptoms of lightheadedness). An active cool-down also helps remove metabolic waste from the muscles so that it can be metabolized by other tissues. Furthermore, a stretching routine following the cool-down period may improve flexibility.

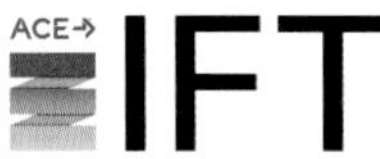

ACE Integrated Fitness Training Model—Cardiorespiratory Training

The basic concept of program design is to create an exercise program with appropriate frequency, intensity, and duration to fit the client's current health and fitness level, with adequate progressions to help the client safely achieve his or her goals. Exercise intensity can be monitored using a variety of methods that have generally been developed through university-based research that included actual measurement of MHR, $\dot{V}O_2$max, blood lactate concentrations and HR at VT1 and VT2, power output (wattage), and other variables. These assessments provide accurate individualized data for use in exercise programming, but they are often not practical or available to most personal trainers. As such, personal trainers generally have to rely on submaximal fitness assessments and prediction equations derived from these studies to predict variables such as MHR and $\dot{V}O_2$max, and then use these predicted values to set appropriate training intensities. Exercise guidelines based upon predictions of MHR or $\dot{V}O_2$max can help clients reach their goals, but they have considerable room for error that must be accounted for when setting and modifying exercise intensities.

The submaximal talk test for VT1 (see page 299) and the VT2 threshold assessment (see page 301) provide personal trainers with submaximal cardiorespiratory fitness assessments that give fairly precise HR data that relates directly to the VT1 and VT2 metabolic markers. The submaximal talk test for VT1 can provide the personal trainer with the client's HR at VT1 to use when designing programs for improving general fitness. The higher-intensity VT2 threshold assessment allows the personal trainer to establish the client's HR at VT2 for use in more advanced programming with clients who have advanced-fitness and endurance sports–performance goals.

The ACE IFT Model has three Cardiorespiratory Training phases (Figure 8-20).

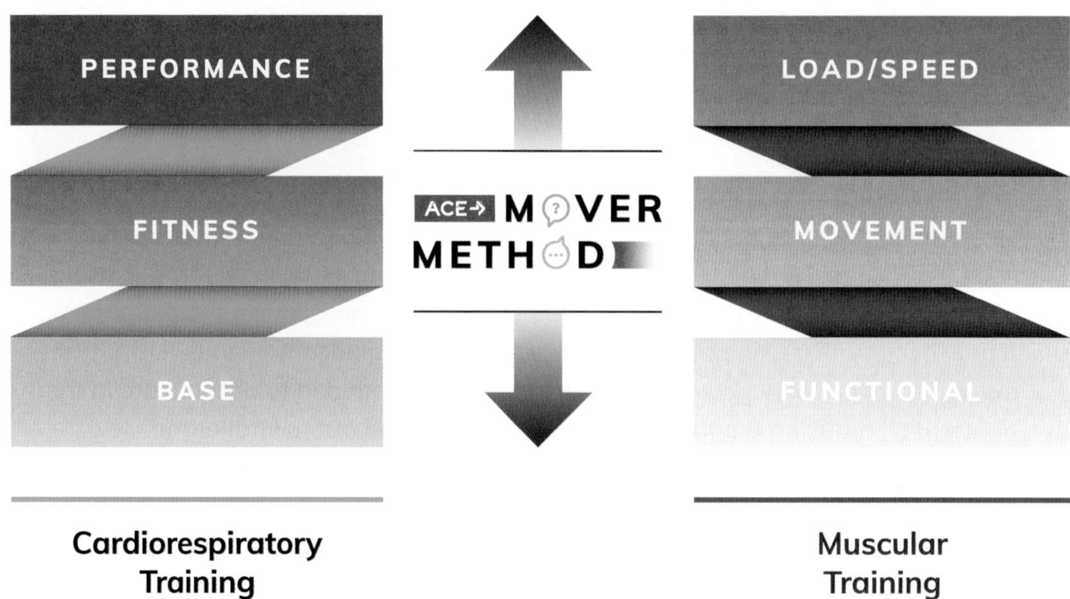

FIGURE 8-20 ACE IFT Model Cardiorespiratory Training phases

Client goals are based on their current health status, fitness levels, and individual preferences. By utilizing the assessment and programming tools for each phase, personal trainers can develop personalized cardiorespiratory programs for clients ranging from physically inactive to endurance athletes. It is important to note that not every client will start in the same phase of training, as many clients will already be regularly participating in cardiorespiratory exercise, and only clients with very specific performance-related objectives will reach the Performance Training phase. Also, clients may have different goals for Cardiorespiratory Training and Muscular Training (see Chapters 9 through 11) based on their current health, fitness, exercise-participation levels, and individual preferences. Programming for each Cardiorespiratory Training phase will be based on the three-zone intensity model shown in Figure 8-18 using HR at VT1 and VT2 to develop personalized programs based on each client's metabolic responses to exercise. It is important to note that training principles in the ACE IFT Model's Cardiorespiratory Training phases can be implemented by personal trainers using various exercise intensity markers, including ones based on predicted values such as %HRR or %MHR, but the exercise intensities will not be as accurate for individual clients as when they utilize measured HR at VT1 and VT2 (Table 8-11).

TABLE 8-11

Three-zone Intensity Model Using Various Intensity Markers

Intensity Markers		Zone 1	Zone 2	Zone 3	Advantages/Limitations
Category terminology for exercise programming	Light	Moderate	Vigorous	Near maximal/ maximal	
Metabolic markers: VT1 and VT2* (HR relative to VT1 and VT2)*		Below VT1 (HR <VT1)	VT1 to just below VT2 (HR ≥VT1 to <VT2)	VT2 and above (HR ≥VT2)	▸ Based on measured VT1 and VT2 ▸ Ideally, VT1 and VT2 are measured in a lab with a metabolic cart and blood lactate ▸ Field assessments are relatively easy to administer, require minimal equipment, and provide accurate corresponding HRs at VT1 and VT2 ▸ Programming with metabolic markers allows for personalized programming
Talk test*		Can talk comfortably Can talk but not sing	Not sure if talking is comfortable Cannot say more than a few words without pausing for a breath	Definitely cannot talk comfortably	▸ Based on actual changes in ventilation due to physiological adaptations to increasing exercise intensities ▸ Very easy for practical measurement ▸ No equipment required ▸ Can easily be taught to clients ▸ Allows for personalized programming
RPE (terminology)*	Very, very weak to light	"Moderate" to "somewhat hard/strong"	"Hard/strong" to "very hard"	"Very strong to very, very hard/strong to maximal"	▸ Good subjective intensity marker ▸ Correlates well with talk test, metabolic markers, and measured %$\dot{V}O_2$max ▸ Easy to teach to clients

Continued on the next page

TABLE 8-11 *(continued)*

Intensity Markers		Zone 1	Zone 2	Zone 3	Advantages/Limitations
RPE (0 to 10 scale)*	0.5 to 2	3 to 4	5 to 6	7 to 10	▸ Good subjective intensity marker ▸ Correlates well with talk test, metabolic markers, and measured %$\dot{V}O_2$max ▸ 0 to 10 scale is easy to teach to clients
RPE (6 to 20 scale)	9 to 11	12 to 13	14 to 17	≥18	▸ Good subjective intensity marker ▸ Correlates well with talk test, metabolic markers, and measured %$\dot{V}O_2$max ▸ 6 to 20 scale is not as easy to teach to clients as the 0 to 10 scale ▸ Note: An RPE of 20 represents maximal effort and cannot be sustained as a training intensity.
%$\dot{V}O_2$R	30 to 39%	40 to 59%	60 to 89%	≥90%	▸ Requires *measured* $\dot{V}O_2$max for most accurate programming ▸ Impractical due to expensive equipment needed for assessment ▸ Increased error with use of *predicted* $\dot{V}O_2$max or *predicted* MHR ▸ Relative percentages for programming are population-based and not individually specific
%HRR	30 to 39%	40 to 59%	60 to 89%	≥90%	▸ Requires *measured* MHR and RHR for most accurate programming ▸ Measured MHR is impractical for the vast majority of trainers and clients ▸ Use of RHR increases individuality of programming vs. strict %MHR ▸ Use of *predicted* MHR introduces potentially large error; the magnitude of the error is dependent on the specific equation used ▸ Relative percentages for programming are population-based and not individually specific
%MHR	57 to 63%	64 to 76%	77 to 95%	≥96%	▸ Requires *measured* MHR for accuracy in programming ▸ Measured MHR is impractical for the vast majority of trainers and clients ▸ Use of *predicted* MHR introduces potentially large error; the magnitude of the error is dependent on the specific equation used ▸ Does not include RHR, as is used in %HRR ▸ Relative percentages for programming are population-based and not individually specific

TABLE 8-11 *(continued)*

Intensity Markers		Zone 1	Zone 2	Zone 3	Advantages/Limitations
METs	2 to 2.9	3 to 5.9	6 to 8.7	≥8.8	▸ Requires measured $\dot{V}O_2$max for most accurate programming ▸ Can use in programming more easily than other intensity markers based off $\dot{V}O_2$max ▸ Limited in programming by knowledge of METs for given activities and/or equipment that gives MET estimates ▸ Relative MET ranges for programming are population-based and not individually specific (e.g., a 5-MET activity might initially be perceived as vigorous by a previously sedentary client)
%$\dot{V}O_2$max	37 to 45%	46 to 63%	64 to 90%	≥91%	▸ Refer to %$\dot{V}O_2$R ▸ Actual measurement is individualized and not based on a prediction

Note: VT1 = First ventilatory threshold; VT2 = Second ventilatory threshold; HR = Heart rate; RPE = Rating of perceived exertion; $\dot{V}O_2$max = Maximal oxygen uptake; $\dot{V}O_2$R = Oxygen uptake reserve; HRR = Heart-rate reserve; MHR = Maximal heart rate; RHR = Resting heart rate; METs = Metabolic equivalents

*These are the preferred intensity markers to use with the three-zone model when designing, implementing, and progressing cardiorespiratory training programs using the ACE Integrated Fitness Training Model.

BASE TRAINING

Training Focus

Base Training has a principal focus of getting clients who are either physically inactive or have little cardiorespiratory fitness to begin engaging in regular cardiorespiratory exercise of a low to moderate intensity with a primary objective of improving health and a secondary objective of building fitness. These clients may have long-term objectives for fitness and possibly even sports performance, but they need to begin in the Base Training phase. The primary emphasis for the personal trainer at this time should be to help the client have positive experiences with cardiorespiratory exercise and to empower him or her to adopt exercise as a regular habit. Base Training helps the client achieve a stable cardiorespiratory base upon which he or she can build further improvements in health, endurance, energy, mood, and caloric expenditure.

The training focus of Base Training is establishing consistent exercise participation, with relatively low- to moderate-intensity exercise of only moderate duration, in order to establish a cardiorespiratory base. Zone 1 training, where the training HR is below the VT1 level, may not be strenuous enough to provoke significant changes in $\dot{V}O_2$max (the classical definition of the cardiorespiratory training effect) but will contribute in a general way to improved health. Once regularity of exercise habits is established, the duration of exercise is extended until the client is able to exercise for 20 to 30 minutes on most days with little residual fatigue. This approach to training ensures the safety of exercise, while at the same time allowing some of the potential physiologic adaptations and most of the health benefits to occur. In clients desiring or requiring higher levels of fitness, higher-intensity training may then be incorporated as they progress to Fitness Training. Within

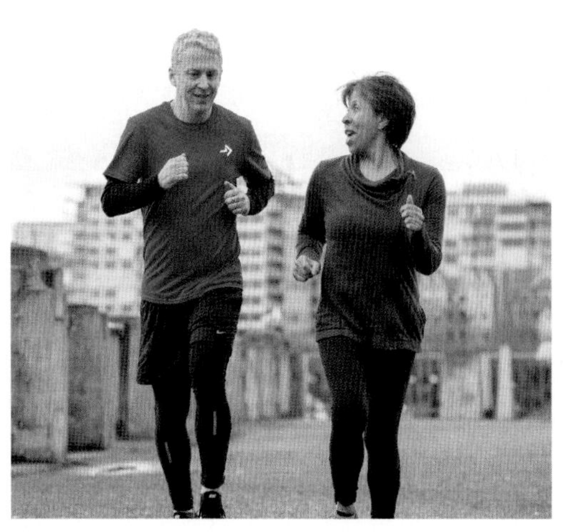

this general design is recognition that the benefit-to-risk ratio of low-intensity zone 1 training is very high for the beginning client, with the possibility for very large gains in health and basic fitness and almost no risk of either cardiovascular or musculoskeletal injury. As the client develops more ambitious exercise training program objectives, more demanding training (either longer or more intense) can be performed.

The underlying foundation of most training programs is the development of cardiorespiratory fitness. The term "training effect" can be thought of as equivalent to the increase in $\dot{V}O_2$max that occurs during the first three to six months of a cardiorespiratory fitness exercise training program.

As long ago as the 1950s, the concept of a minimal-intensity threshold for provoking the training effect was articulated by Karvonen, who made the observation that training at intensities of less than 50% of HRR (approximately 60% of MHR) failed to cause reductions in RHR (Karvonen, Kentala, & Mustala, 1957). This minimal intensity threshold concept was confirmed in randomized training studies throughout the 1970s, 1980s, and 1990s, with $\dot{V}O_2$max as the outcome measure (Swain & Franklin, 2002). A variety of studies have shown that there is a larger increase in $\dot{V}O_2$max with more intense training (Gormley et al., 2008; Swain, 2005). Thus, the cardiorespiratory fitness benefits of training increase markedly with training intensity. However, training is much less comfortable as intensity increases, which means there is an increased risk of clients dropping out during the first few weeks of training. Furthermore, in previously physically inactive adults who might have an underlying risk of CVD, more high-intensity exercise is associated with a greater risk of cardiovascular complications. Thus, an important rule of exercise training for previously physically inactive adults is to start slowly during the beginning weeks of an exercise program. This guideline is sometimes frustrating, as many clients are enthusiastic at the beginning of a program and want rapid gains, and the personal trainer may want to impress clients with challenging, creative workouts. Clearly, restraint, proper education, and careful planning are essential during the early stages of any training program.

Improvements in $\dot{V}O_2$max may continue for six to 12 months after the beginning of a regular exercise program. Lower-intensity exercise programs have been shown to be associated with a variety of beneficial health outcomes, although there may be smaller increases in $\dot{V}O_2$max from training at low exercise intensities than can be achieved with higher-intensity training. Nevertheless, outcomes related to longevity and a reduced incidence of many of the "diseases of civilization" have been achieved with exercise that is not sufficient to cause large increases in $\dot{V}O_2$max (Booth et al., 2002). In any case, with a beginning exerciser, this approach will ensure that not only are there reasonably significant gains in health and functional status, but there will be a minimum of injuries (i.e., a very high benefit/risk ratio).

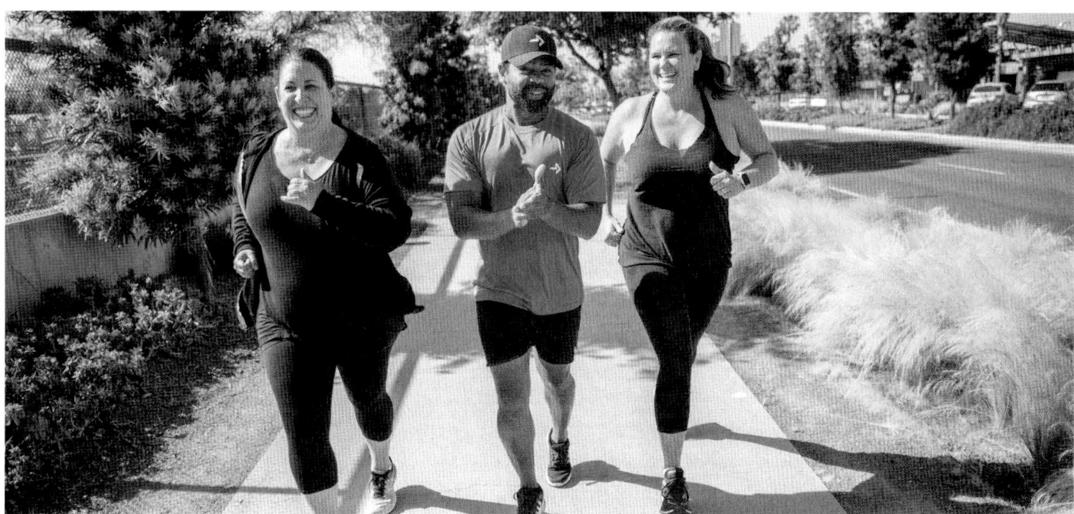

Program Design

The training focus of Base Training is to help clients have positive experiences with exercise to facilitate program adherence and success. Initial cardiorespiratory fitness assessments are not necessary for clients in Base Training, as they will only confirm low levels of fitness and potentially serve as negative reminders about why the physically inactive client with low levels of fitness may not have good self-efficacy regarding exercise. All cardiorespiratory exercise during Base Training falls within zone 1 (sub-VT1), so the personal trainer can use the client's ability to talk comfortably as the upper exercise-intensity limit. The personal trainer can also teach the client to use the 0 to 10 category ratio scale, with the client exercising at an RPE of 3 to 4 (moderate to somewhat hard).

It is not necessary to conduct the submaximal talk test for VT1 assessment to determine HR at VT1 until a client is ready to progress to Fitness Training.

As a general principle, exercise programs designed to improve the cardiorespiratory base begin with zone 1–intensity exercise with HR below VT1 performed for as little as 10 to 15 minutes two to three times each week. However, this should be progressed as rapidly as tolerated to 20 minutes or more at moderate intensity (zone 1 below the talk test threshold), performed three to five times each week. Changes in duration from one week to the next should not exceed a 10% increase versus the week prior. Once this level of exercise can be sustained on a regular basis, the primary adaptation of the cardiorespiratory base will be complete.

For the most part, early training efforts should feature continuous exercise at zone 1 intensity. Depending on how physically inactive a person was prior to beginning the program, this level of exercise may be continued for as little as two weeks or for more than six weeks. The beginning duration of exercise should match what the client is able to perform. For some, this might be 15 continuous minutes, while for others it might be only 5 to 10 continuous minutes. From that point, duration should be increased at a rate of no more than 10% from one week to the next until the client can perform 20 minutes or more of continuous exercise. Once the client is comfortable with assessments and can sustain steady-state cardiorespiratory exercise for at least 20 minutes in zone 1 (RPE of 3 to 4), he or she can move on to Fitness Training.

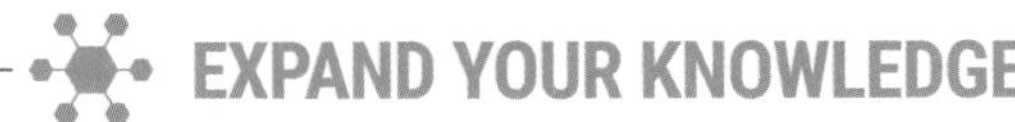

Cardiorespiratory Fitness: The Ultimate Marker for Heart Health

One of the very first studies to explore the connection between cardiorespiratory fitness and heart health was published in 1989. This hallmark paper reported that an inverse relationship existed between $\dot{V}O_2$max values and risk for CVD (Blair et al., 1989); similar findings were reported by Blair and colleagues in 1996. In both studies, these relationships held true for individuals with no other risk factors for CVD, one risk factor for CVD, and two or more CVD risk factors. The question of whether poor cardiorespiratory fitness should be considered a separate risk factor, in addition to lack of physical activity, was addressed in a meta-analysis (a statistical method that combines the results of numerous studies). The author noted that both increased cardiorespiratory fitness and increased physical activity were associated with decreased risk for CVD events (Williams, 2001). Interestingly, it was also found that higher cardiorespiratory fitness levels yielded greater reductions in CVD risk compared to those imparted from increased physical-activity levels. Therefore, it was concluded that being unfit warrants consideration as a separate CVD risk factor—independent of physical inactivity and other traditional CVD risk factors—and merits screening and intervention.

In 2005, researchers reported findings from a study that examined the effect of cardiorespiratory fitness on risk of mortality from CVD in a cohort of men with diabetes within normal weight, overweight, and obese categories (Church et al., 2005). Both diabetes and obesity are associated with increased risk of mortality from CVD. For all weight categories (normal, overweight, and obese), it was shown that the risk of CVD mortality was two- to four-times higher among men with diabetes and low levels of cardiorespiratory fitness compared to those with diabetes and moderate-to-high levels of cardiorespiratory fitness.

Perhaps the strongest case to support cardiorespiratory fitness as the ultimate health outcome was made in a paper published in 2009. The author presented data to show that low cardiorespiratory fitness accounted for more overall deaths, including those from CVD, when compared to deaths that could be attributed to traditional risk factors, such as obesity, smoking, hypertension, high cholesterol, and diabetes (Blair, 2009). Clearly, the personal trainer should recognize that sufficient levels of cardiorespiratory fitness are paramount to overall heart health.

FITNESS TRAINING

Training Focus

This phase has a principal training focus of increasing the time of cardiorespiratory exercise, increasing the frequency of sessions when possible, and introducing intervals to improve fitness and health. Clients who exercise sporadically will progress to this goal only after they have become consistent with their cardiorespiratory exercise and can comfortably perform a minimum of 20 minutes of steady-state cardiorespiratory exercise in zone 1 (RPE of 3 to 4) on three to five days per week. During Fitness Training, the personal trainer will be able to program more variety in terms of exercise frequency and duration. The personal trainer will also be able to challenge the client through the introduction of intervals, first in the lower end of zone 2 and eventually in the upper end of zone 2.

Once the cardiorespiratory base is developed, the client may want to consider the value of additional gains in fitness that will result from increases in exercise intensity, frequency, or duration. However, it is important to understand that after a cardiorespiratory base has been achieved, additional gains in fitness will become progressively smaller, or require disproportionately large increases in training intensity, frequency, or duration. This is the time when the personal trainer needs to carefully evaluate the goals of each client. Do the client's exercise goals center on health and basic fitness benefits? Does he or she have performance-related objectives? Achieving performance-related objectives at the biological limit of the client requires significantly higher training loads, which are addressed in Performance Training. Athletes may have to train at very high loads for only a 1 to 2% increase in performance, with matching increases in the time requirement of training and the risk of injury (Foster et al., 1996).

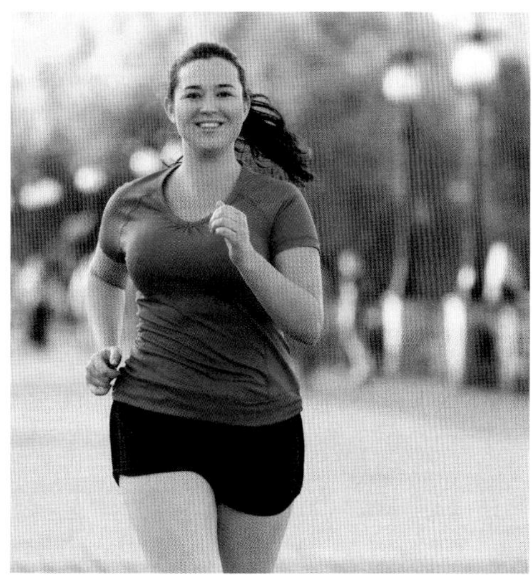

Within the context of cardiorespiratory training, the personal trainer must consider the relative proportion of different intensities of exercise. Early studies suggested that training at about the intensity of VT1 (i.e., zone 1) was the most effective intensity. Subsequent studies have suggested that even very well-trained athletes tend to perform a high proportion of their training (approximately 75 to 80%) at this intensity (Seiler & Kjerland, 2006; Esteve-Lanao et al., 2005). Interestingly, much of this training can be categorized by the verbal anchor "moderate to somewhat hard," or an RPE of 3 to 4 on the 0 to 10 scale. Extensive training at this level requires a motivated individual, so this training goal is reserved for the already motivated and committed client.

Fitness Training is the primary cardiorespiratory training focus for regular clients in a fitness facility who have goals for improving or maintaining fitness and/or health. Fitness Training includes increasing the workload by modifying frequency, duration, and intensity, with intervals introduced that go into zone 2 and eventually approach HR at VT2. The zone 2 intervals for this goal provide a stimulus that will eventually increase the HR at VT1, resulting in the client being able to exercise at a lower HR when at the same level of intensity, and also allowing the client to exercise at higher intensities while at the VT1 HR.

Clients who have a one-time ambition to complete an event, such as a 10K run, can reach their objective of completing the event within the training guidelines of Fitness Training. Once a client begins working toward multiple endurance objectives, trains to improve his or her competitive speed, or simply wants to take on the challenge of training like an athlete, the client should move on to Performance Training.

For the many clients who never develop competitive goals or the desire to train like an endurance athlete, Fitness Training will provide adequate challenges to help them improve and maintain cardiorespiratory fitness for life. The workouts in most nonathletically focused group exercise classes fall into this category. Fitness Training covers the principles for building cardiorespiratory efficiency that are implemented with most personal-training clients and fitness enthusiasts.

Program Design

At the beginning of Fitness Training, the personal trainer should have the client perform the submaximal talk test to determine HR at VT1. This HR will be utilized for programming throughout Fitness Training and will need to be reassessed periodically as fitness improves to see if the HR at VT1 has increased and training intensities need to be adjusted.

The focus of Fitness Training is to enhance the client's cardiorespiratory efficiency by progressing the program through increased duration of sessions, increased frequency of sessions when possible, and the introduction of zone 2 intervals. In Fitness Training, the warm-up, cool-down, recovery intervals, and steady-state cardiorespiratory exercise segments are performed just below VT1 HR (RPE of 3 to 4 on the 0 to 10 scale) to continue advancing the client's cardiorespiratory base. Intervals are introduced at a level that is at or just above VT1 HR, or an RPE of 5 to 6 (0 to 10 scale). The aim of these intervals is to improve cardiorespiratory efficiency by raising the intensity of exercise performed at VT1, improve the client's ability to utilize fat as a fuel source at intensities just below VT1, improve exercise efficiency at VT1, and add variety to the exercise program.

PERFORMANCE TRAINING

Training Focus

Performance Training is designed for clients who have endurance-performance objectives and/or competitive endurance goals such as achieving a personal record, qualifying for a national event, or placing top-five in a championship. The training principles in Performance Training are for clients who have one or more endurance-performance objectives that require specialized training to ensure that adequate training volume and appropriate training intensity and recovery are included to create performance changes that help the client reach his or her objectives. Clients do not need to be highly competitive athletes to participate in Performance Training. They need only to be motivated clients with endurance-performance objectives and the requisite level of fitness achieved from Fitness Training upon which to build.

A variety of studies with different types of athletes, including Nordic skiers, cyclists, and runners, have suggested that 70 to 80% of training by elite endurance athletes is performed at intensities lower than the VT1 (zone 1) (Seiler & Kjerland, 2006; Esteve-Lanao et al., 2005). These same studies suggest that athletes typically perform 5 to 10% of their training at and above the VT2 (zone 3). Thus, even though zone 3 training can be very effective in terms of provoking improvements, only a small amount is tolerable, even for competitive athletes. Surprisingly, very little training is actually performed in the intensity zone between the two thresholds (zone 2). This intensity has been called "the black hole" (where there is a psychological push to do more, but a physiologic pull to do less), since it is the zone where exercise is hard enough to make a person fatigued, but not hard enough to really provoke optimal adaptations (Seiler & Kjerland, 2006).

Most of the studies with training loads have simply observed what athletes spontaneously do during training. In a very well-controlled study of training distribution, researchers randomized cross-country runners into groups, where the total training load was controlled and equalized (Esteve-Lanao et al., 2007). High-intensity (zone 3) training was limited to approximately 10% of total training time in both groups. One group increased the amount of easy (zone 1) training from the spontaneous 70% to about 85% and decreased the amount of moderately hard (zone 2) training from the spontaneous 20% to about 5%. The other group, conversely, decreased zone 1 training from the spontaneous 70% to about 60% and increased zone 2 training from 20% to about 30%. After five months, the improvement in performance signficantly favored those who had performed more zone 1 training. Despite zone 1 being relatively easier training, the results supported the contention that zone 2 training is essentially a "black hole" (Seiler & Kjerland, 2006). It may be that there is an important interaction of the distribution of training with the total volume of training, but the best evidence is that in individuals who are already routinely exercising and who desire to move toward their optimal biological potential, most training (approximately 80%) should be performed at intensities where speech is comfortable (zone 1), and about 10% of training should be performed at intensities at and above VT2 (zone 3), where the physiological provocation to make large gains is present.

It is unclear at this time whether the dominant training intensity within a zone matters. It is easy to speculate that zone 1 training should, for the most part, be performed relatively high in zone 1. Similarly, it would seem to make sense that, except for training designed to augment anaerobic pathways, most zone 3 training should be performed relatively low in zone 3, with progression by duration rather than by intensity. This remains an area in need of controlled studies.

Performance Training also focuses on anaerobic **power.** However, only highly fit and competitive clients with very specific objectives related to high-speed performance during endurance events will require exercise programming focused on anaerobic power. Some examples of athletes who might perform anaerobic-power training include runners and cyclists who compete in events that require repeated accelerations and recovery throughout the race and during the final sprint finish, competitive kayakers who need to paddle vigorously for short periods to navigate through difficult sections of rapids, and athletes in sports such as basketball and soccer where success requires both cardiorespiratory endurance and the ability to sprint repeatedly.

Anaerobic-power training can essentially be thought of as muscular training, although it is specific to the mode of activity (e.g., running or cycling). The intent is to perform very high-intensity training of nearly maximal muscular capacity, but with enough recovery to prevent the rapid accumulation of fatigue, so that the muscular system can be taxed maximally. This is very specialized training intended to be performed by individuals preparing for competition. It is intended to increase the tolerance for the metabolic by-products of high-intensity exercise, including exercise performed at intensities greater than $\dot{V}O_2$max. Since this kind of training is very uncomfortable and, in older individuals, potentially dangerous, it should be performed only after a long period of training.

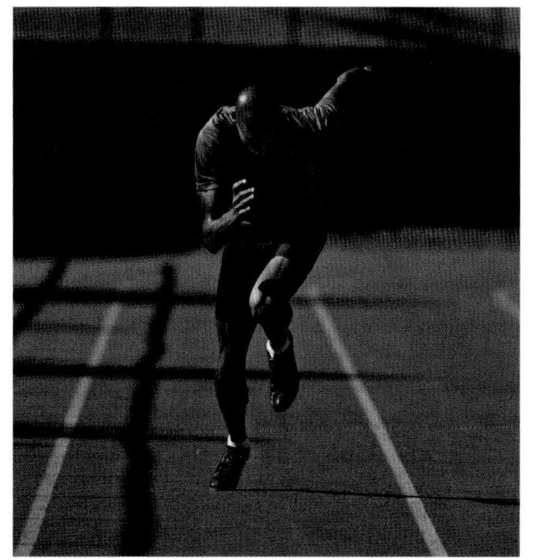

The underlying physiological principle of this type of training is that if there is substantial and sustained depletion of the **phosphagen** stores and accumulation of lactate (and acid metabolites), the body will adapt with a larger phosphagen pool and potentially larger buffer reserves. Studies have suggested that adaptations of this sort can take place but are relatively modest in magnitude (10%) (Tabata et al., 1996). For reasons that are not well understood, men seem able to improve their anaerobic power more than women. Although there are not a lot of well-controlled studies, it appears that interval training with relatively brief (30-second) high-intensity elements is just as effective in terms of producing gains in anaerobic power as longer high-intensity bursts (where phosphagen depletion and lactate accumulation might be larger, and thus be expected to be more provocative of change). Although controlled studies demonstrating the best way to improve anaerobic power are not available, it is generally assumed that high-intensity bouts with relatively short recovery periods that provoke larger disturbances in **homeostasis** are preferred. Thus, a training session of 10 repetitions x 70 seconds at 115% of $\dot{V}O_2$max, with a new repetition beginning every two minutes (after 50 seconds of recovery), might be typical. This kind of training session requires an extended warm-up and cool-down and is tolerable only once or twice weekly.

Program Design

Program design for Performance Training should be focused on helping the client enhance his or her cardiorespiratory efficiency to ensure completion of goal events, while building anaerobic capacity to achieve endurance-performance goals. Improved anaerobic capacity will help the client perform physical work at or near VT2 for an extended period, which will result in improved endurance, speed, and power to meet primary performance objectives.

To program effective intervals for improving anaerobic capacity, the personal trainer should have the client perform the VT2 threshold assessment to determine the client's HR at VT2. Once the personal trainer has current values for the client's HR at VT1 and VT2, the personal trainer can establish a three-zone model that is specific to the client. For example, if a client's HR at VT1 is 143 bpm and HR at VT2 is 162 bpm, the client's HR zones would be as follows:

- Zone 1 = less than 143 bpm
- Zone 2 = 143 to 161 bpm
- Zone 3 = 162 bpm and above

These HR zones can then be used as intensity markers to help the client stay within the correct zone for the desired training outcome of a given workout.

A large volume of zone 1 training time is critical to program success for clients with endurance-performance objectives, as exercise frequency, intensity, and time all add to the total load. Individuals who increase each of these variables too quickly are at risk for burnout and overuse injuries. The personal trainer can help clients avoid the risk for developing **overtraining syndrome** by distributing zone 1 training time across warm-ups, cool-downs, moderate-intensity workouts focused on increasing distance and/or exercise time, recovery intervals following zone 2 and 3 work intervals, and recovery workouts on days following higher-intensity workouts. By completing adequate zone 1 training time, clients will have the mental and physical energy required to perform their zone 2 and 3 intervals as planned. The frequency of zone 2 and 3 interval workouts will be client-specific, based on the client's goals, available training time, available recovery time, and outside stressors. Highly fit competitive clients with adequate recovery time may be able to successfully complete and recover from three to four workouts with zone 2 or 3 intervals during weeks where the aim is to increase the load.

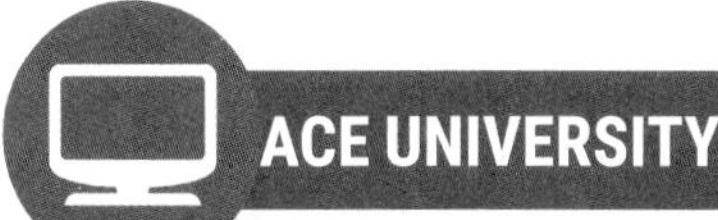

If your study program includes the ACE University, visit www.ACEfitness.org/MyACE and log in to your My ACE Account to take full advantage of the ACE Personal Trainer Study Program and online guided study experience.

A variety of media to support and expand on the material in this text is provided to facilitate learning and best prepare you for the ACE Personal Trainer Certification exam and a career as a personal trainer.

SUMMARY

The ACE IFT Model has three Cardiorespiratory Training phases:

- Base Training
- Fitness Training
- Performance Training

Adequate cardiorespiratory fitness values have been positively linked to heart health. The personal trainer should design Cardiorespiratory Training programs with the explicit goal of improving cardiorespiratory fitness levels in their clients. The basic concept of program design is to incorporate activities that clients enjoy with appropriate frequency, intensity, and duration to match the client's current health status and fitness level, with adequate progressions to help the client safely achieve his or her cardiorespiratory goals. By utilizing the assessment and programming tools for each training phase, personal trainers can develop personalized Cardiorespiratory Training programs for clients ranging from physically inactive individuals to endurance athletes. Programming for each Cardiorespiratory

Training phase will be based on the three-zone intensity model, using HR at VT1 and VT2 to develop personalized programs based on each client's metabolic responses to exercise. This personalized approach to personal training will increase the likelihood of cardiorespiratory fitness training responsiveness.

REFERENCES

Ainsworth, B.E. et al. (2011). 2011 Compendium of Physical Activities: A second update of codes and MET values. *Medicine & Science in Sports & Exercise*, 43, 1575–1581.

American College of Sports Medicine (2018). *ACSM's Guidelines for Exercise Testing and Prescription* (10th ed.). Philadelphia: Wolters Kluwer.

Astell-Burt, T. et al. (2014). Neighbourhood green space and the odds of having skin cancer: Multilevel evidence of survey data from 267072 Australians. *Journal of Epidemiology and Community Health*, 68, 370–374.

Bacon, A.P. et al. (2013). VO_2max trainability and high intensity interval training in humans: A meta-analysis. *PLoS One*, 8, 9, c73182.

Barton, J. & Pretty, J. (2010). What is the best dose of nature and green exercise for improving mental health? A multi-study analysis. *Environmental Science & Technology*, 44, 3947–3955.

Berling, J. et al. (2006). The effect of handrail support on oxygen uptake during steady state treadmill exercise. *Journal of Cardiopulmonary Rehabilitation*, 26, 391–394.

Blair, S.N. (2009). Physical inactivity: The biggest public health problem of the 21st century. *British Journal of Sports Medicine*, 43, 1–2.

Blair, S.N. et al. (1996). Influences of cardiorespiratory fitness and other precursors on cardiovascular disease and all-cause mortality in men and women. *Journal of the American Medical Association*, 276, 205–210.

Blair, S.N. et al. (1989). Physical fitness and all-cause mortality: A prospective study of healthy men and women. *Journal of the American Medical Association*, 262, 2395–2401.

Booth, F.W. et al. (2002). Waging war on physical inactivity: Using modern molecular ammunition against an ancient enemy. *Journal of Applied Physiology*, 93, 3–30.

Borg, G. (1998). *Borg's Perceived Exertion and Pain Scales*. Champaign, Ill.: Human Kinetics.

Brocklebank, L.A. et al. (2015). Accelerometer-measured sedentary time and cardiometabolic biomarkers: A systematic review. *Preventive Medicine*, 76, 92–102.

Calogiuri, G. et al. (2015). Green exercise as a workplace intervention to reduce job stress: Results from a pilot study. *Work*, 53, 99–111.

Cannon, C. et al. (2004). The talk test as a measure of exertional ischemia. *American Journal of Sports Medicine*, 6, 52–57.

Church, T.S. et al. (2005). Cardiorespiratory fitness and body mass index as predictors of cardiovascular disease mortality among men with diabetes. *Archives of Internal Medicine*, 165, 2114–2120.

Dalleck, L.C. & Gibeault, A.N. (2015). *A F.I.T.T. Formula for Sitting? How to Help Your Clients Reduce Sedentary Time and Improve Their Health*. https://www.acefitness.org/education-and-resources/professional/prosource/august-2015/5520/a-f-i-t-tformula-for-sitting-how-to-help-your-clients-reducesedentary-time-and-improve-their

Dehart, M. et al. (2000). Relationship between the talk test and ventilatory threshold. *Clinical Exercise Physiology*, 2, 34–38.

Esteve-Lanao, J. et al. (2007). Impact of training intensity distribution on performance in endurance athletes. *Journal of Strength and Conditioning Research*, 21, 943–949.

Esteve-Lanao, J. et al. (2005). How do endurance runners actually train? Relationship with competition performance. *Medicine & Science in Sports & Exercise*, 37, 496–504.

Foster, C. & Cotter, H.M. (2006). Blood lactate, respiratory and heart rate markers on the capacity for sustained exercise. In: Maud, P.J. & Foster, C. (Eds.) *Physiological Assessment of Human Fitness* (2nd ed.). Champaign, Ill.: Human Kinetics.

Foster, C., Porcari, J.P., & Lucia, A. (2008). Endurance training. In: Durstine, J.L. et al. (Eds.) *Pollock's Textbook of Cardiovascular Disease and Rehabilitation*. Philadelphia: Lippincott Williams & Wilkins.

Foster, C. et al. (2008). The risk of exercise training. *American Journal of Lifestyle Medicine*, 10, 279–284.

Foster, C. et al. (1996). Athletic performance in relation to training load. *Wisconsin Medical Journal*, 95, 370–374.

Foster, C. et al. (1995). Effects of specific vs. cross training on running performance. *European Journal of Applied Physiology*, 70, 367–372.

Fox III, S.M., Naughton, J.P., & Haskell, W.L. (1971). Physical activity and the prevention of coronary heart disease. *Annals of Clinical Research*, 3, 404–432.

Gormley, S.E. et al. (2008). Effect of intensity of aerobic training on VO_2max. *Medicine & Science in Sports & Exercise*, 40, 7, 1336–1343.

Gellish, R.L. et al. (2007). Longitudinal modeling of the relationship between age and maximal heart rate. *Medicine & Science in Sports & Exercise*, 39, 5, 822–829.

Grazuleviciene, R. et al. (2015). The effect of park and urban environments on coronary artery disease patients: A randomized trial. *BioMed Research International*, 2015, 403012.

Haskell, W.L. et al. (2007). Physical activity and public health: Updated recommendations of the American College of Sports Medicine and the American Heart Association. *Medicine & Science in Sports & Exercise*, 39, 1423–1434.

Healy, G.N. et al. (2008). Breaks in sedentary time: Beneficial associations with metabolic risk. *Diabetes Care*, 31, 661–666.

Karvonen, M.J., Kentala, E., & Mustala, O. (1957). The effect of training on heart rate: A longitudinal study. *Annales Medicinae Experimentalis et Biologiae Fenniae*, 35, 307–315.

Katch, V. et al. (1978). Validity of the relative percent concept for equating training intensity. *European Journal of Applied Physiology*, 39, 219–227.

Katzmarzyk, P.T. & Lee, I.M. (2012). Sedentary behaviour and life expectancy in the USA: A cause-deleted life table analysis. *British Medical Journal Open*, 2, e000828.

ACE-sponsored Research

Keeling, S.M., Buchanan, C.A., & Dalleck, L.C. (2018). What is the optimal FIT of sedentary interruption bouts to improve cardiometabolic health? *JEPonline*, 21, 2, 1–18.

Laursen, P.B. et al. (2002). Interval training program optimization in highly trained endurance cyclists. *Medicine & Science in Sports & Exercise*, 34, 1801–1807.

Lightfoot, J.T. (2013). Why control activity? Evolutionary selection pressures affecting the development of physical activity genetic and biological regulation. *Biomedical Research International*, Epub December 24, 2013.

Loy, S.F., Holland, G.J., & Mutton, D.K. (1993). Effects of stair climbing vs. run training on treadmill and track running. *Medicine & Science in Sports & Exercise*, 25, 1275–1278.

McArdle, W., Katch, F., & Katch, V. (2019). *Exercise Physiology: Nutrition, Energy, and Human Performance* (8th ed.). Philadelphia: Lippincott, Williams & Wilkins.

McConnell, T.R. et al. (1991). Prediction of functional capacity during treadmill testing: Effect of handrail support. *Journal of Cardiopulmonary Rehabilitation*, 11, 255–260.

Meyer, T. et al. (2005). A conceptual framework for performance diagnosis and training prescription from submaximal parameters: Theory and application. *International Journal of Sports Medicine*, 26, 1–11.

Owen, N. et al. (2011). Adults' sedentary behavior determinants and interventions. *American Journal of Preventive Medicine*, 41, 189–196.

Persinger, R. et al. (2004). Consistency of the talk test for exercise prescription. *Medicine & Science in Sports & Exercise*, 36, 1632–1636.

Pijl, H. (2011). Obesity: Evolution of a symptom of affluence. *Netherlands Journal of Medicine*, 69, 4, 159–166.

Pontzer, H. et al. (2012). Hunter-gatherer energetics and human obesity. *PLoS ONE*, 7, 7, e40503.

Porcari, J.P., Bryant, C.X., & Comana, F. (2015). *Exercise Physiology*. Philadelphia: F.A. Davis Company.

Porcari, J.P. et al. (2001). Prescribing exercise using the talk test. *Fitness Management*, 17, 9, 46–49.

Rae, D.E. et al. (2008). Heatstroke during endurance exercise: Is there evidence for excessive endothermy? *Medicine & Science in Sports & Exercise*, 40, 1193–1204.

Recalde, P.T. et al. (2002). The talk test as a simple marker of ventilatory threshold. *South African Journal of Sports Medicine*, 9, 5–8.

Seiler, K.S. & Kjerland, G.O. (2006). Quantifying training intensity distribution in elite athletes: Is there evidence for an 'optimal' distribution. *Scandinavian Journal of Medicine & Science in Sports*, 16, 49–56.

Stepto, N.K. et al. (1998). Effect of different interval training programs on cycling time trial performance. *Medicine & Science in Sports & Exercise*, 31, 736–741.

Swain, D.P. (2005). Moderate or vigorous intensity exercise: Which is better for improving aerobic fitness? *Preventive Cardiology*, 8, 1, 55–58.

Swain, D.P. & Franklin, B.A. (2002). $\dot{V}O_2$ reserve and the minimal intensity for improving cardiorespiratory fitness. *Medicine & Science in Sports & Exercise*, 34, 1, 152–157.

Tabata, I. et al. (1996). Effects of moderate-intensity endurance and high-intensity intermittent training on anaerobic capacity and $\dot{V}O_2$ max. *Medicine & Science in Sports & Exercise*, 28, 1327–1330.

Tanaka, H., Monahan, K.D., & Seals, D.R. (2001). Age-predicted maximal heart revisited. *Journal of the American College of Cardiology*, 37, 153–156.

U.S. Department of Health & Human Services (2018). *Physical Activity Guidelines for Americans* (2nd ed.). www.health.gov/paguidelines/

Voelker, S.A. et al. (2002). Relationship between the talk test and ventilatory threshold in cardiac patients. *Clinical Exercise Physiology*, 4, 120–123.

Williams, P.T. (2001). Physical fitness and activity as separate heart disease risk factors: A meta-analysis. *Medicine & Science in Sports & Exercise*, 33, 754–761.

SUGGESTED READINGS

American College of Sports Medicine (2014). *ACSM's Resource Manual for Guidelines for Exercise Testing and Prescription* (7th ed.). Philadelphia: Lippincott Williams & Wilkins.

Daniels, J. (2014). *Daniels' Running Formula* (3rd ed.). Champaign, Ill.: Human Kinetics.

Porcari, J.P., Bryant, C.X., & Comana, F. (2015). *Exercise Physiology*. Philadelphia: F.A. Davis Company.

Powers, S.K. & Howley, E.T. (2017). *Exercise Physiology: Theory and Application to Fitness and Performance* (10th ed.). New York: McGraw-Hill.

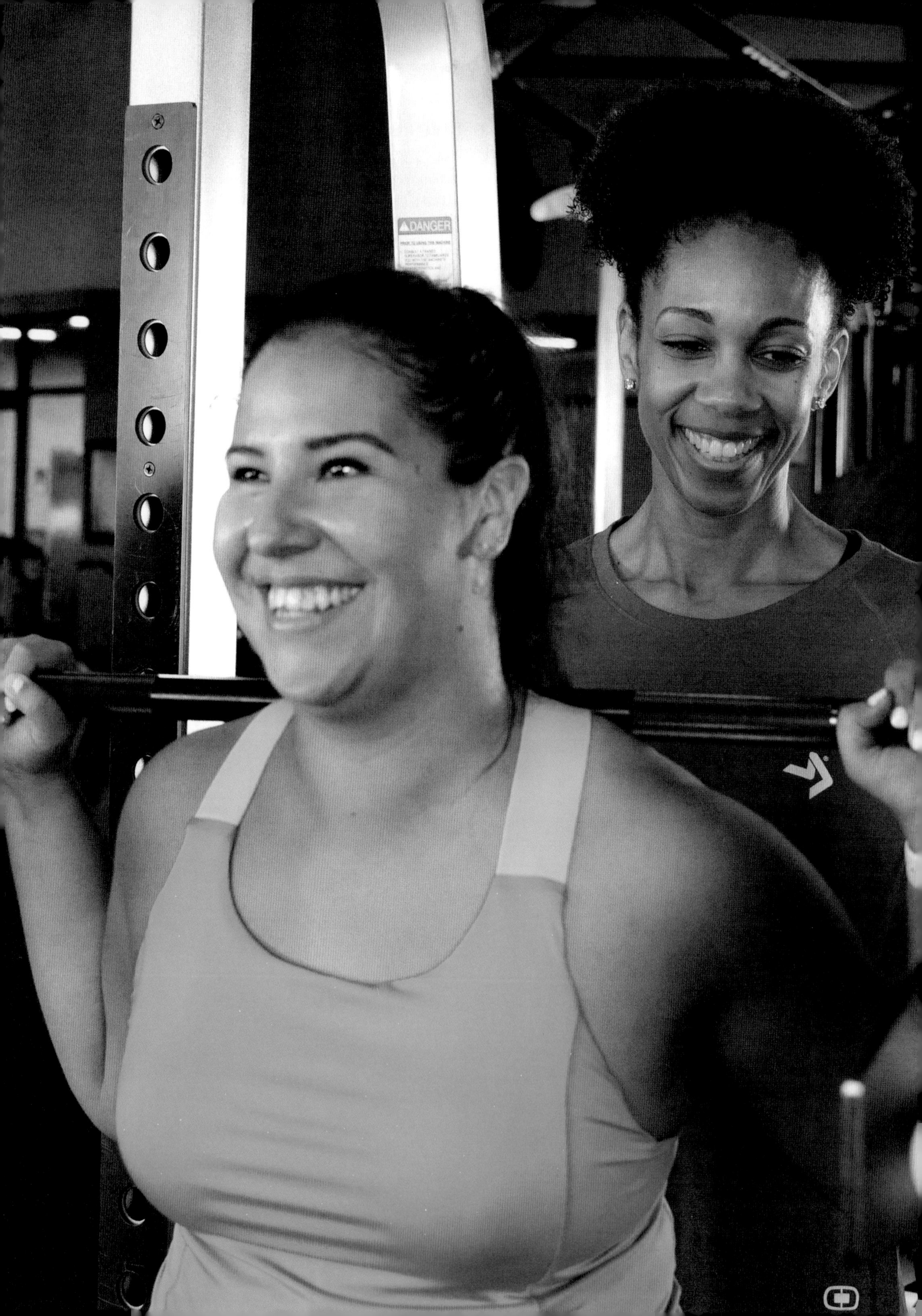
DANGER

CHAPTER 9

Muscular Training: Foundations and Benefits

LANCE C. DALLECK, PhD
Professor of Exercise and Sport Science, Western Colorado University;
Member, ACE Scientific Advisory Panel

IN THIS CHAPTER

LEARNING OBJECTIVES:

Upon completion of this chapter, the reader will be able to:

- Explain the basic anatomy and physiology that underpins muscular training and how this knowledge enhances the design and implementation of safe and effective muscular-training programs
- Recognize the widespread benefits of muscular training
- Understand the acute and chronic physiological adaptations to muscular training
- List the muscular-training principles and recognize how these foundational concepts apply to program design
- Identify key variables for muscular-training program design

ACE UNIVERSITY

If your study program includes the ACE University, visit www.ACEfitness.org/MyACE and log in to your My ACE Account to take full advantage of the ACE Personal Trainer Study Program and online guided study experience.

A variety of media to support and expand on the material in this text is provided to facilitate learning and best prepare you for the ACE Personal Trainer Certification exam and a career as a personal trainer.

Anatomical Systems

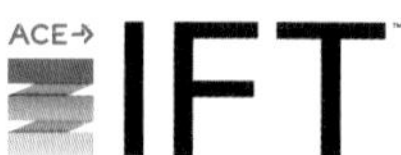

Muscular training, also commonly known as resistance training, strength training, and weight training, is a central feature of the ACE Integrated Fitness Training® (ACE IFT®) Model. Muscular training can positively influence virtually every system of the body and provides widespread benefits, ranging from increased **skeletal muscle** strength to improved **bone mineral density (BMD)** and greater blood **glucose** regulation. It is vital for ACE® Certified Personal Trainers to have an appreciation of the anatomy and physiology that underpins muscular training. This knowledge base will enhance the ability of personal trainers to design and implement safe and effective muscular-training programs for their clients.

SKELETAL SYSTEM

The human skeleton is an active, living tissue that is essential for structural support, movement, organ protection, storage, and formation of blood cells (**hemopoiesis**). The body has a total of 206 bones, most of which are paired (e.g., right and left femurs) (Figure 9-1). The structural functions of bone include giving support to the soft tissues of the body and providing attachment sites for most muscles, which play an important role in movement. Many of the

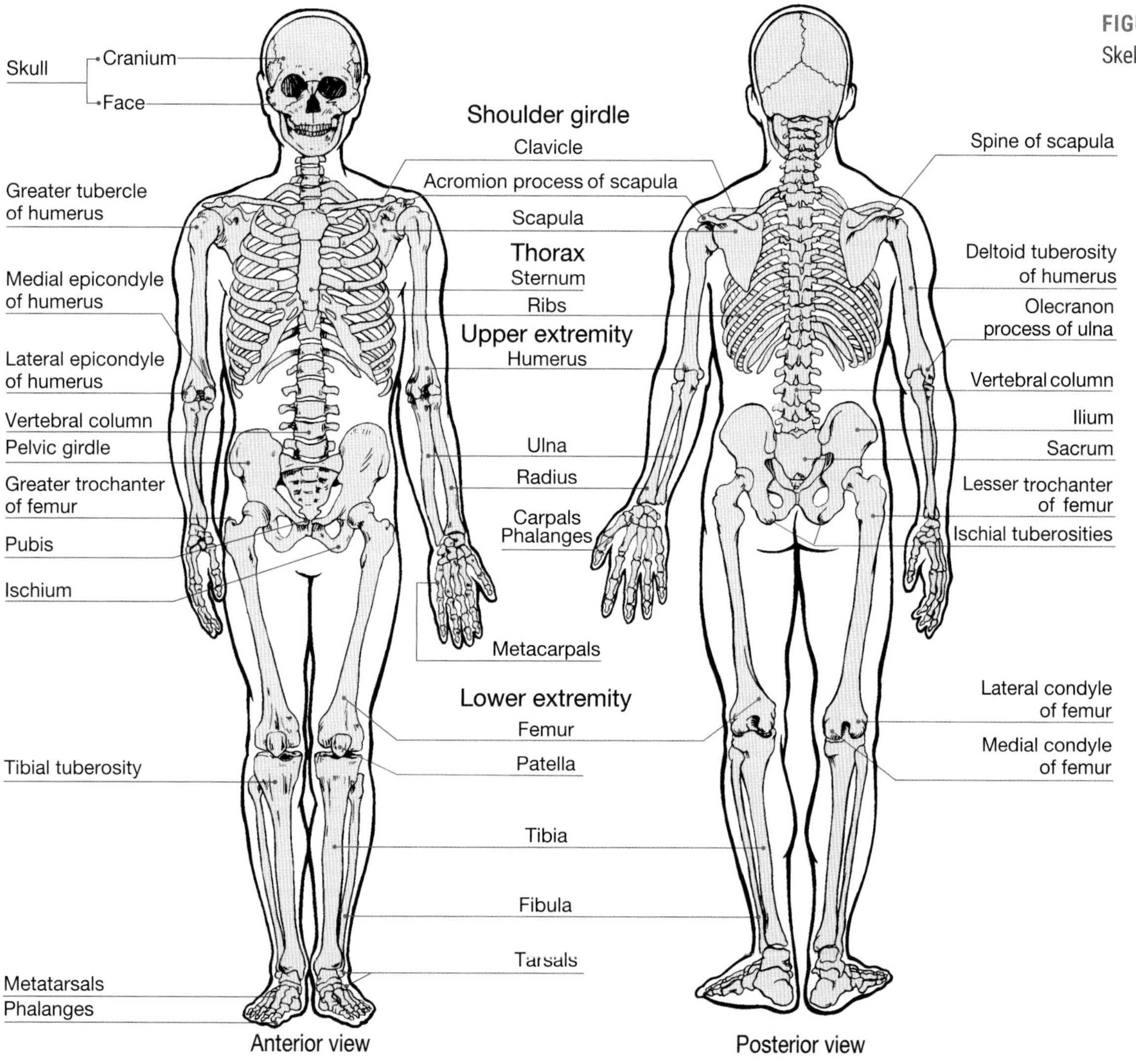

Skull
Cranium
Face
Greater tubercle of humerus
Medial epicondyle of humerus
Lateral epicondyle of humerus
Vertebral column
Pelvic girdle
Greater trochanter of femur
Pubis
Ischium
Tibial tuberosity
Metatarsals
Phalanges
Shoulder girdle
Clavicle
Acromion process of scapula
Scapula
Thorax
Sternum
Ribs
Upper extremity
Humerus
Ulna
Radius
Carpals
Phalanges
Metacarpals
Lower extremity
Femur
Patella
Tibia
Fibula
Tarsals
Spine of scapula
Deltoid tuberosity of humerus
Olecranon process of ulna
Vertebral column
Ilium
Sacrum
Lesser trochanter of femur
Ischial tuberosities
Lateral condyle of femur
Medial condyle of femur
Anterior view
Posterior view

FIGURE 9-1
Skeletal system

body's muscles attach to bone, and when the muscles contract, the bones move at their **articulations** (joints). The skeleton also provides protection for many of the body's organs. For example, the skull encases the brain, the vertebrae form a canal around the spinal cord, the rib cage encases the heart and lungs, and the bony pelvis guards the urinary bladder and internal reproductive organs. The skeleton is also a storehouse for two essential minerals—calcium and phosphorous—that are necessary for the proper functioning of other body systems. In addition, fat, sodium, potassium, and other minerals are stored in the bones. Bones are not static structures. They are constantly breaking down to release minerals and other substances into the blood, while simultaneously rebuilding to provide the body with flexible, yet sturdy, structural support. Following birth, the skeleton is a production site for blood cells found within the circulatory system (e.g., red blood cells, certain white blood cells, and platelets).

The various shapes of bones determine how they are classified (i.e., long, short, flat, or irregular). Long bones are so named because they are longer than they are wide, which means that they have a long axis. Most of the bones of the limbs are classified as long bones (e.g., humerus, radius, ulna, femur, tibia, fibula, and phalanges). Bones that are approximately the same length and width are called short bones (e.g., carpals and tarsals). Flat bones are thin and typically curved (e.g., ribs, sternum, and some bones of the skull). Bones that do not fit into the previous categories are classified as irregular bones because of their diverse shapes (e.g., hip bones, vertebrae, and certain skull bones).

Bones are composed of a dense outer layer, called compact or **cortical bone,** and a honeycomb-like inner structure, called spongy or **trabecular bone.** The cortical shell makes up roughly 75% of the skeleton, whereas the trabecular network makes up the remaining 25%. Cortical bone is essential, because it provides strength, **tendon** attachment sites for muscles, and organ protection without excessive weight. Trabecular bone serves two vital purposes. It provides a large surface area for mineral exchange and helps to maintain skeletal strength and integrity. It is particularly abundant in the vertebrae and at the ends of long bones, sites that are under continuous stress from motion and weight bearing. Areas containing a large percentage of trabecular tissue are most likely to fracture when the bone is weakened due to a disease such as **osteoporosis.**

A closer look at a typical long bone reveals its many structures (Figure 9-2). The shaft, called the **diaphysis,** is located between the two ends, which are named the **proximal** and **distal** epiphyses (singular = **epiphysis**). The hollow space inside the diaphysis is called the medullary cavity, which is used as a storage site for fat and is sometimes called the yellow bone marrow cavity. It is lined by a thin connective tissue layer called the **endosteum.** The diaphysis and outer layers of the epiphyses are made of cortical bone, whereas trabecular bone is concentrated in the central regions of the epiphyses. Certain long bones contain red marrow—which is essential in the manufacture and maturation of red blood cells, most white blood cells, and platelets—in the trabecular tissue of their epiphyses. An **epiphyseal cartilage,** also called a "growth plate," separates the diaphysis and epiphysis in children and young adults, providing a means for the bone to increase in length. In adults, when skeletal growth has been completed, the epiphyseal cartilage is replaced by bone and the area is called the epiphyseal line. A dense connective-tissue layer called the **periosteum** covers the outer surface of bone and is well supplied with blood vessels and nerves, some of which enter the bone.

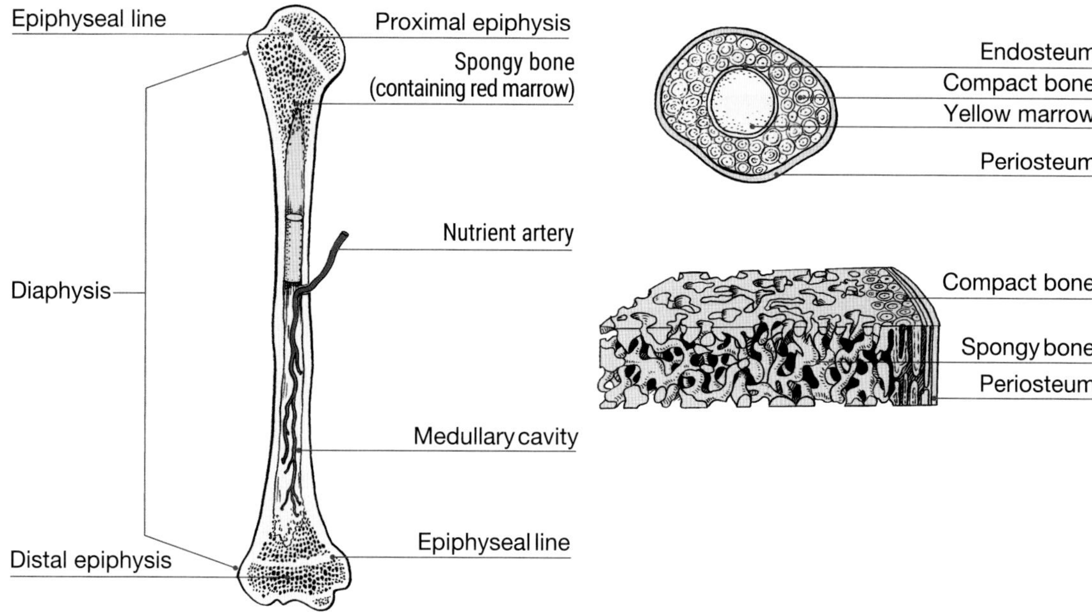

FIGURE 9-2
Long bone gross anatomy

Throughout life, the human skeleton is being continuously broken down while simultaneously being restored. In fact, most of the adult skeleton is replaced approximately every 10 years. In adults, a process called remodeling is responsible for the continual reshaping and rebuilding of the skeleton in response to internal and external signals from specialized bone cells that either build bone (**osteoblasts**) or break it down (**osteoclasts**). Remodeling is vital for bone health for several reasons. First, the remodeling process repairs damage to the skeleton that can result from repeated stresses. It also prevents the accumulation of too much old bone, which can lose its resilience and become brittle. Furthermore, remodeling plays an important role in removing calcium and phosphorous from the bones when these minerals are deficient in the diet or when an increased need exists due to pregnancy or lactation.

Although the size and shape of the skeleton is genetically determined, it can be greatly affected by loading or impact from physical activity. Ultimately, a bone's size and shape fit best with its function. In other words, "form follows function." **Wolff's law** indicates that changes in bone structure coincide with changes in bone function. That is, when the skeleton is subjected to stressful forces, such as those that occur with exercise, it responds by laying down more bone tissue, thereby increasing its density. Conversely, when individuals experience prolonged periods of bed rest due to illness or injury, their bones lose mineral and become less dense. Maintaining adequate bone density is an important issue for all adults.

Axial Skeleton

Of the 206 bones that make up the skeleton, 74 are categorized as the **axial skeleton** (Table 9-1). Consisting of the skull, vertebral column, sternum, and ribs, the axial skeleton's most important functions are to provide the main axial support for the body and protect the **central nervous system (CNS)** and the organs of the thorax. Personal trainers should have a fundamental knowledge of the structure of the vertebral column, since the mechanics of the spine affect exercise performance. The vertebral column consists of 33 vertebrae, which are categorized by regions (Figure 9-3). The upper region (neck area) of the spine contains seven cervical vertebrae, which are the smallest and most delicate. The mid-region, below the cervical

TABLE 9-1

Bones in the Axial and Appendicular Skeletons

Axial Skeleton	Number of Bones
Skull	
Cranium	8
Face	14
Hyoid	1
Vertebral column	26
Thorax	
Sternum	1
Ribs	24
(Auditory ossicles)*	6
Total	80
Appendicular Skeleton	**Number of Bones**
Lower Extremity	
Phalanges	28
Metatarsals	10
Tarsals	14
Patella	2
Tibia	2
Fibula	2
Femur	2
Pelvic Girdle	
Hip or pelvis (os coxae = ilium, ischium, pubis)	2
Shoulder Girdle	
Clavicle	2
Scapula	2
Upper Extremity	
Phalanges	28
Metacarpals	10
Carpals	16
Radius	2
Ulna	2
Humerus	2
Total	126

* The auditory ossicles, three per ear, are not considered part of the axial or appendicular skeletons, but rather a separate group of bones. They were placed in the axial skeleton group for convenience.

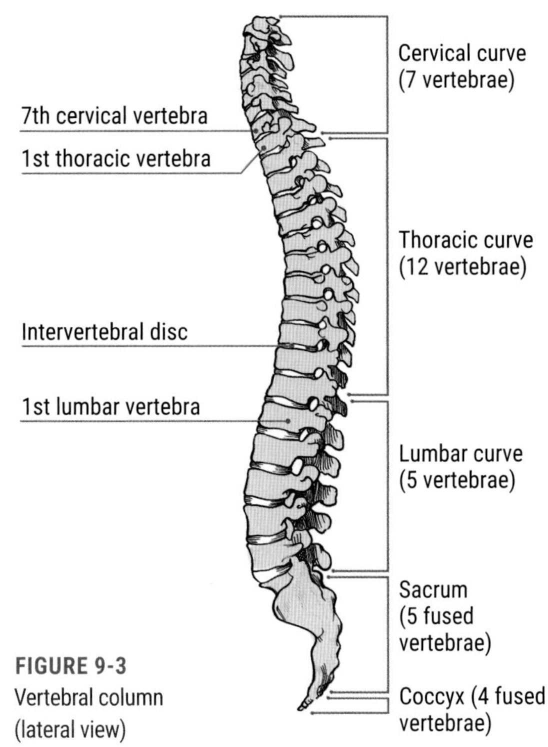

FIGURE 9-3
Vertebral column
(lateral view)

vertebrae, contains 12 thoracic vertebrae that are each attached to a rib. The lower region consists of five lumbar vertebrae, the sacrum (five fused vertebrae), and the coccyx (four fused vertebrae). The lumbar vertebrae are the largest and heaviest vertebrae due to their role in continuously receiving ground reaction forces and axial compression forces.

Appendicular Skeleton

The remaining 126 bones are categorized as the **appendicular skeleton,** which includes the bones of the upper and lower limbs and the shoulder (pectoral) and pelvic (hip) girdles (see Table 9-1). The shoulder and pelvic girdles represent the means by which the appendicular skeleton articulates (joins together) with the axial skeleton. The shoulder girdle (clavicle and scapula) attaches to the axial skeleton only at the sternum, providing little support for the upper-body structures. Still, the support is sufficient, because the upper limbs do not bear the body's weight. This minimal connection with the axial skeleton allows the shoulder girdle to express a wide range of movements at the shoulder. In contrast, the pelvic girdle (ilium, ischium, and pubis—known collectively as the os coxae) does support the body's weight. Therefore, it has more extensive attachments to the axial skeleton through its articulation with the sacrum (see Figure 9-1). Furthermore, each side of the pelvic girdle is united by a strong joint made of cartilage called the pubic symphysis.

Articulations

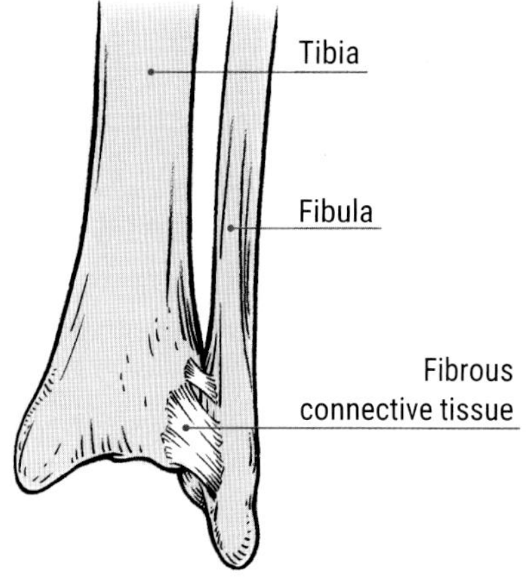

FIGURE 9-4
Example of a fibrous joint

The bones of the skeleton come together at articulations. When two bones meet at a junction, they are said to "articulate" with each other (e.g., the femur articulates inferiorly with the tibia). While most joints allow movement between two bones, some permit little, if any, movement. The three main types of joints are fibrous, cartilaginous, and synovial. Fibrous joints are held tightly together by fibrous connective tissue and allow little or no movement. They are classified as synarthroidal (*syn* = together; *arthro* = joint). In other words, synarthroidal joints are considered immovable joints and include the sutures of the skull and the joint between the distal ends of the tibia and fibula (Figure 9-4). In cartilaginous joints, the bones are connected by cartilage and little or no movement is allowed. A characteristic of one type of cartilaginous joint, a symphysis, is the fibrocartilaginous pad, or disk, that separates two bones. The junction of the two pubic bones (pubic symphysis) and the junctions between the bodies of adjacent vertebrae are examples of symphyses.

The most common type of joint in the body is the synovial joint, which is freely moveable. Because of this freedom, synovial joints are classified as diarthroses (diarthrosis means "through joint"). Synovial joints have four characteristic traits: an articular cartilage, an articular capsule, a synovial membrane, and synovial fluid. Articular cartilage refers to the hyaline cartilage (from the Greek word *hyalos*, meaning glass) that covers the end surfaces of long bones. The articular capsule encloses the joint with a double-layered membrane. The outer layer is composed of a dense fibrous tissue that forms **ligaments** to strengthen the joint. The inner layer is the synovial membrane, which is well supplied with **capillaries** and produces a thick fluid called synovial fluid that nourishes the articular cartilages and lubricates the joint surfaces. Some synovial joints have articular disks made of fibrocartilage, such as the menisci (singular = meniscus) in the knee. The medial and lateral menisci help absorb shock in the knee, increase joint **stability,** direct synovial fluid to aid in nourishment of the knee, and increase joint contact surface area, thereby decreasing overall pressure on the joint.

MOVEMENTS OF SYNOVIAL JOINTS

In order to name various parts of the human body and discuss human movement, anatomists developed a reference position so that the structures and areas of the body could be described in relation to each other. This **anatomical position** refers to a person standing erect with head, eyes, and palms facing forward (**anterior**). The feet are close, with the toes pointing forward and the arms hanging by the sides. A representation of anatomical position is shown in Figure 9-5, along with anatomical **planes of motion.**

Synovial joints move based on the shapes of their bony structures and their articular surfaces. A joint moves around its **axis of rotation,** where the plane of movement is generally perpendicular to the axis (similar to a door moving perpendicular to its axis

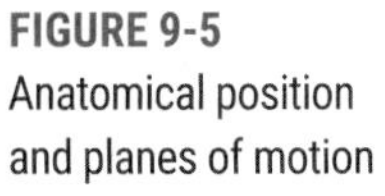

FIGURE 9-5
Anatomical position and planes of motion

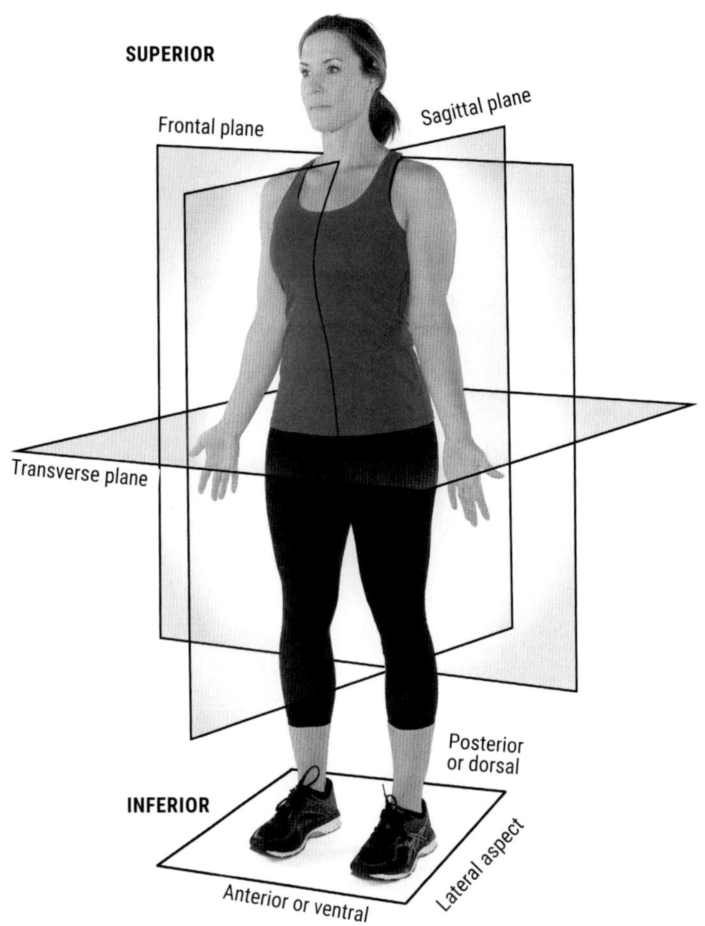

of rotation at the hinges). The axis of rotation is an imaginary line that forms a right angle to the plane of movement about which a joint rotates. For example, the elbow joint allows the forearm to move anteriorly and posteriorly (**sagittal plane**) around an imaginary horizontal line that passes through it from side to side (mediolateral axis of rotation) (Figure 9-6). To review which planes of movement are perpendicular to each other, see Figure 9-5. Some joints have more than one axis of rotation, allowing them to move in multiple planes. Joints that move in one plane only and have one axis of rotation are called uniplanar or uniaxial joints. These joints are also called "hinge" joints, because hinges (like those on a door) allow movement in only one plane. The ankles and elbows are examples of uniaxial joints.

Joints that allow movement in two planes are called biplanar or biaxial joints. Examples of biaxial joints are the foot (calcaneocuboid joint), knee, hand, and wrist. Biaxial joint movement can be observed when the index finger (first phalanx) moves anteriorly and posteriorly (sagittal plane movement around a mediolateral axis) and laterally and medially (**frontal plane** movement around an anteroposterior axis) (see Figure 9-6). Still other joints permit movement in three axes of rotation. These are called multiplanar or triaxial joints and include the hip, thumb, and shoulder. The shoulder, for example, allows the humerus to move anteriorly and posteriorly, laterally and medially, and rotate internally and externally (**transverse plane** movement around a longitudinal

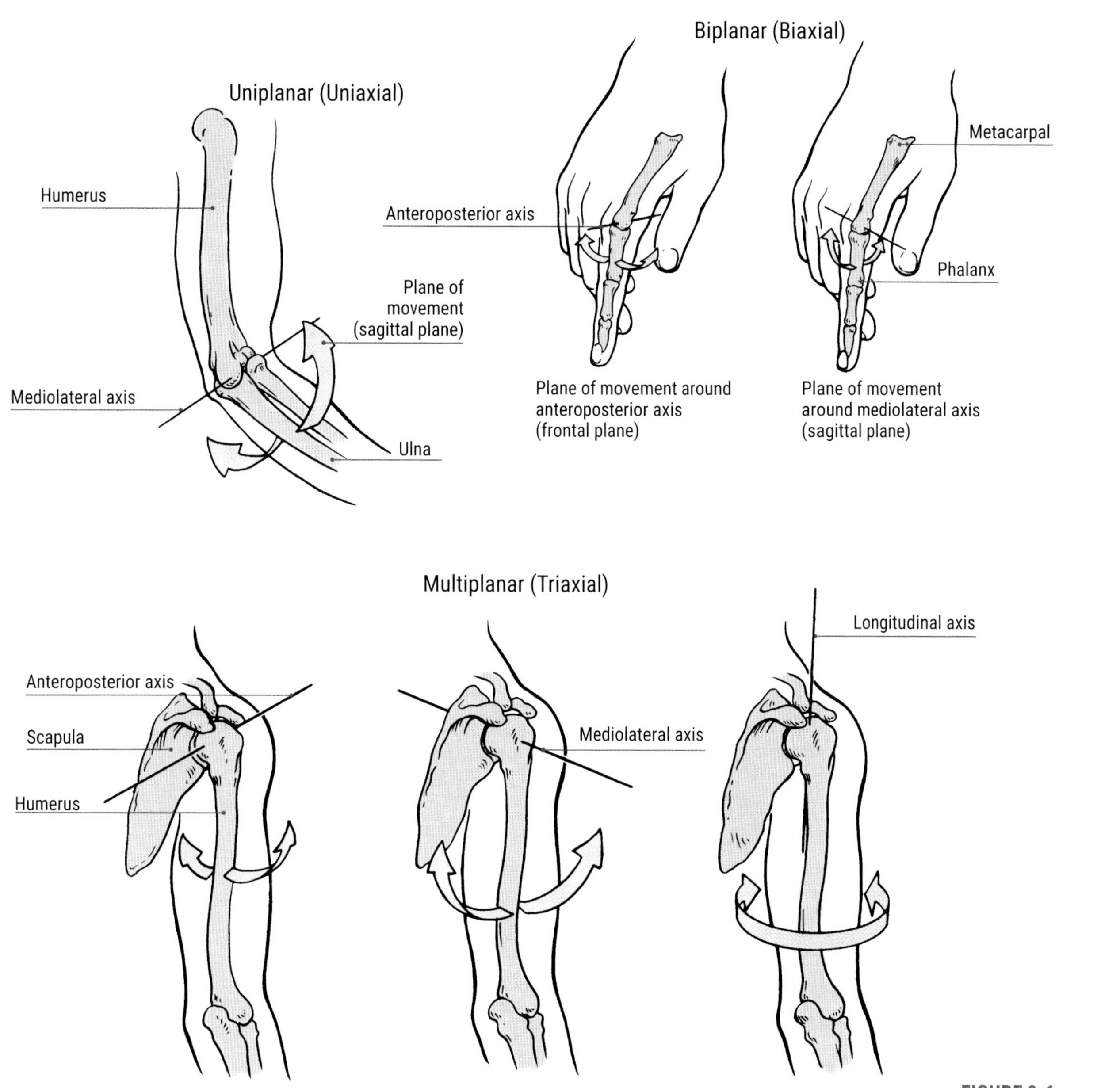

FIGURE 9-6
Movement of synovial (diarthrodial) joints

axis) (see Figure 9-6). A summary of the major joints in the body, with type and possible movements, is presented in Table 9-2.

There are four general groups of movements that occur in synovial joints throughout the body: gliding, angular, circumduction, and rotation. In gliding, the surfaces of two adjoining bones move back and forth upon each other. An example of a gliding joint is the articulation between the head of a rib and the body of its associated vertebra. Angular movement describes an increase or decrease in the angle between two adjoining bones. There are four angular movements defined for synovial joints: **flexion, extension, abduction,** and **adduction.** Flexion describes movement in which the bones comprising

TABLE 9-2
Major Joints in the Body

Region/Joint	Type	Number of Axes of Rotation	Movements Possible
Lower Extremity			
Foot (metatarsophalangeal)	Synovaial (condyloid)	2	Flexion and extension; abduction and adduction; circumduction
Ankle (talocrural)	Synovial (hinge)	1	Plantar flexion and dorsiflexion
Between distal tibia and fibula	Fibrous	0	Slight movement possible
Knee (tibia and femur)	Synovial (modified hinge)	2	Flexion and extension; internal and external rotation
Hip	Synovial (ball and socket)	3	Flexion and extension; abduction and adduction; internal and external rotation
Upper Extremity			
Hand (metacarpophalangeal)	Synovial (condyloid)	2	Flexion and extension; abduction and adduction; circumduction
Thumb	Synovial (saddle)	3	Flexion and extension; abduction and adduction; circumduction; opposition
Wrist (radiocarpal)	Synovial	2	Flexion and extension; abduction and adduction; circumduction
Proximal radioulnar	Synovial (pivot)	1	Pronation and supination
Elbow (ulna and humerus)	Synovial (hinge)	1	Flexion and extension
Shoulder	Synovial (ball and socket)	3	Flexion and extension; abduction and adduction; circumduction; internal and external rotation
Ribs and sternum	Cartilaginous	0	Slight movement possible

a joint move toward each other in the sagittal plane, decreasing the joint angle between them. An example is bringing the forearm upward toward the upper arm, as in elbow flexion. Extension is the opposite of flexion and causes the angle between two adjoining bones to increase in the sagittal plane. An example is starting with the calf upward toward the back of the thigh and moving it downward away from the thigh, as in knee extension (Figure 9-7).

Abduction occurs when a part of the body is moved away from the body, such as lifting an arm or leg away from the midline of the body (Figure 9-8). Adduction is the opposite of abduction and refers to movement of a body part toward the midline of the body, such as lowering an arm or leg from an abducted position toward the side of the body (see Figure 9-8). In the case of the fingers and toes, the reference point for abduction and adduction is the midline of the hand and foot, respectively. For example, abduction of the fingers occurs when they move away from the third digit of the hand (i.e., spreading

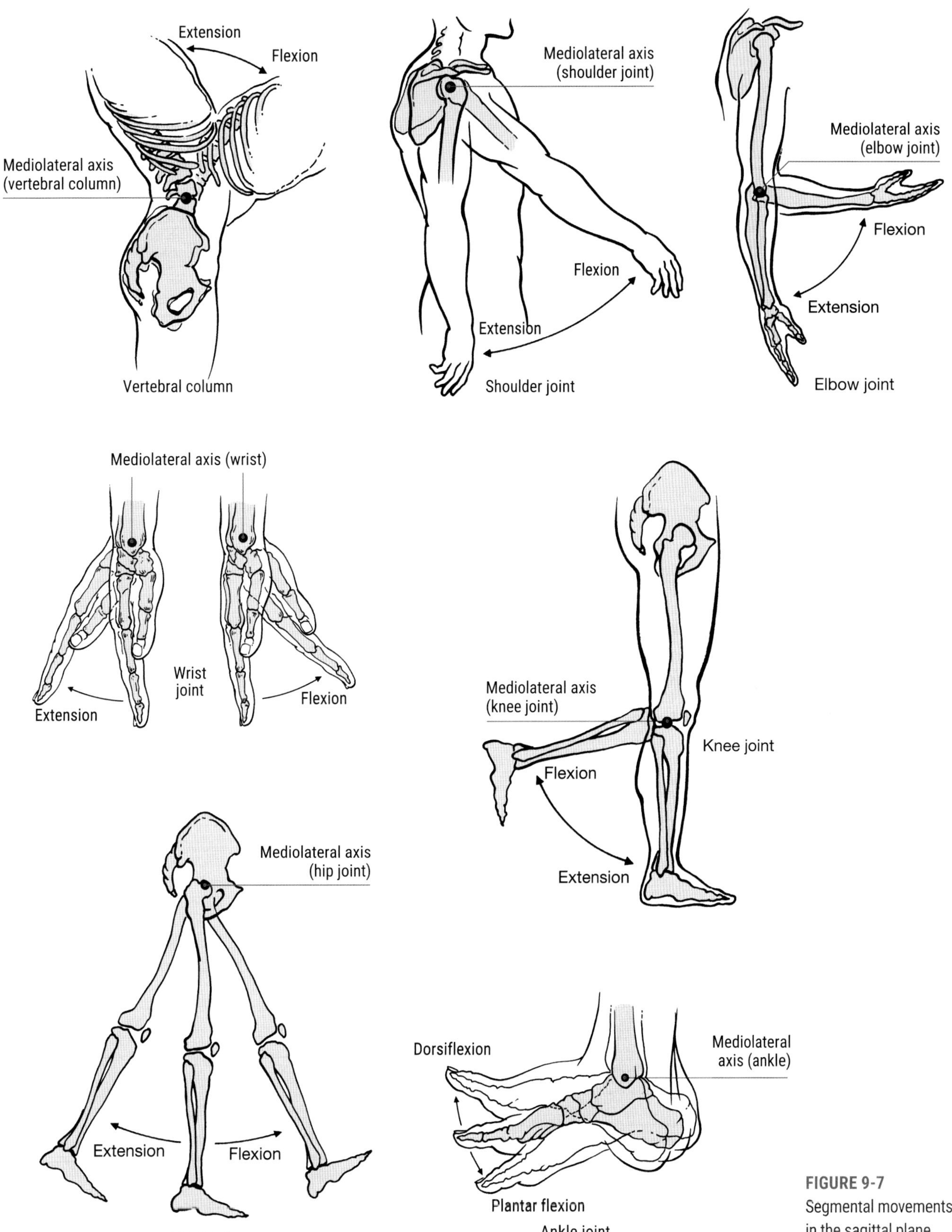

FIGURE 9-7
Segmental movements in the sagittal plane

FIGURE 9-8
Segmental movements in the frontal plane

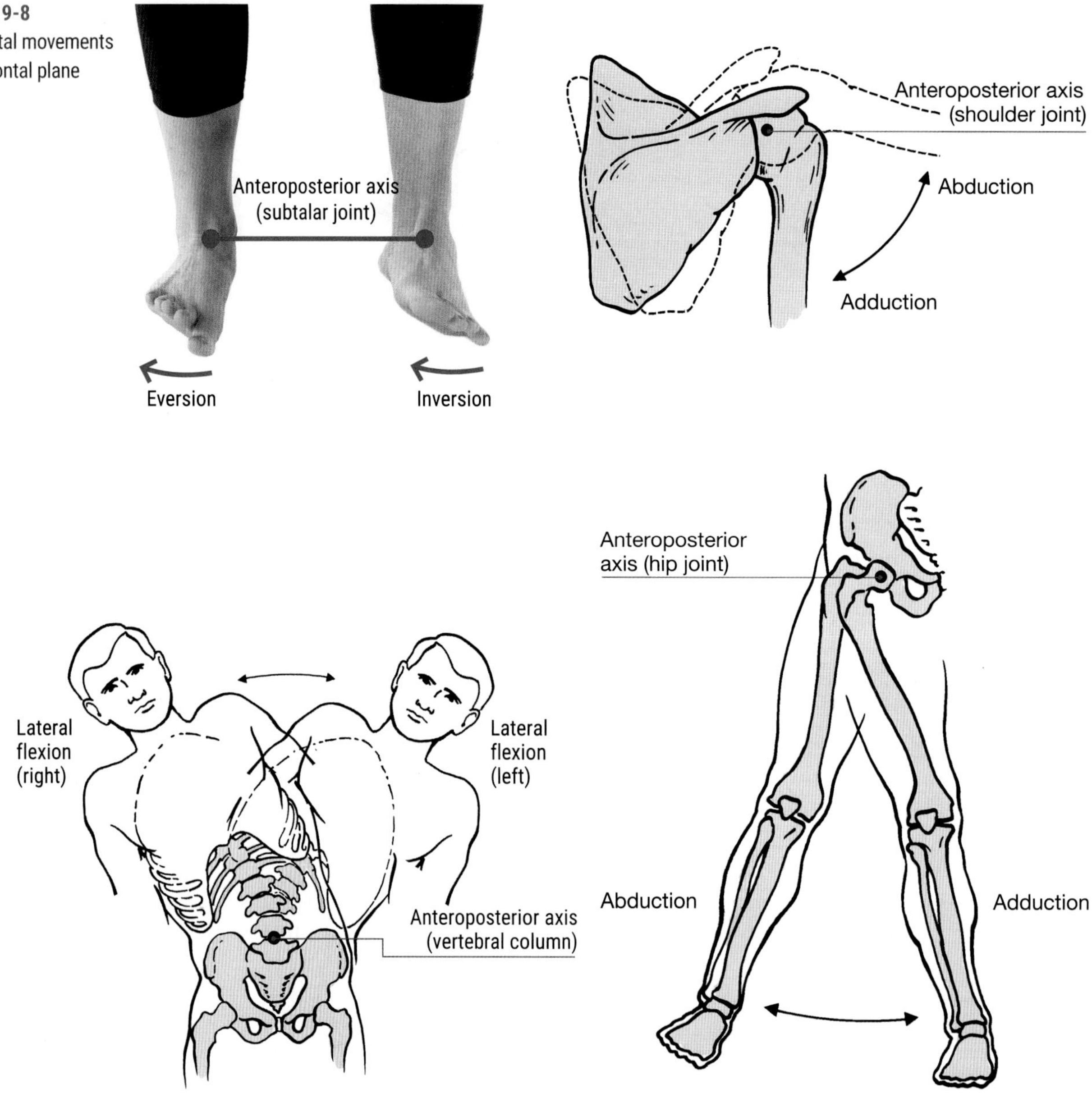

the fingers apart). Conversely, adduction of the fingers refers to the digits moving out of abduction toward the third digit. Abduction of the toes is accomplished by moving them away from the second toe (i.e., spreading the toes apart) and adduction occurs when the toes move out of abduction toward the second toe. All abduction and adduction movements occur in the frontal plane.

Certain joints, such as the shoulder and hip, are capable of incorporating all four angular movements to create one motion called circumduction. That is, the movement is actually a sequential combination of flexion, abduction, extension, and adduction. An easy way to remember circumduction is to picture a swimmer performing arm circles as a warm-up prior to diving in the pool. The circular motion represents circumduction of the shoulder joints.

Rotation describes motion of a bone around a central (longitudinal) axis. From the anatomical position, movement of the anterior surface of the humerus or femur inward is called internal (medial) rotation. Conversely, movement of the anterior surface of the humerus or femur outward is called external (lateral) rotation. A specific type of rotation occurs at the radioulnar joint. Rotating the forearm outward so the palm faces anteriorly with the body in the anatomical position is called **supination,** whereas rotation of the forearm inward so the palm faces posteriorly is called **pronation.** Anatomical position, therefore, requires the forearm to be in a supinated position (see Figure 9-5). Rotation around a longitudinal axis occurs in the transverse plane. This also includes rotation of the spine (Figure 9-9). A summary of the synovial joint fundamental movements by planes of motion is presented in Table 9-3.

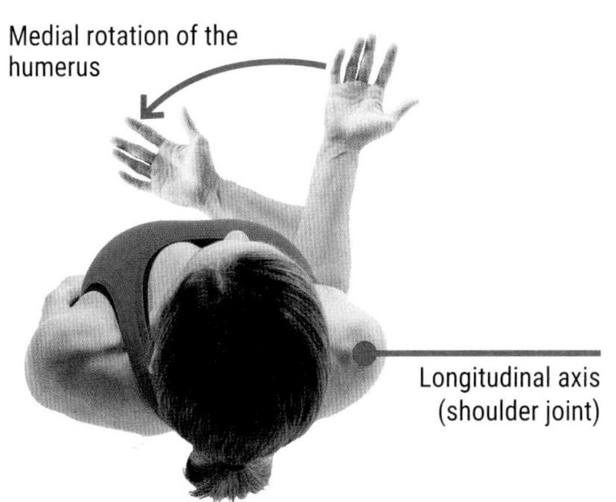

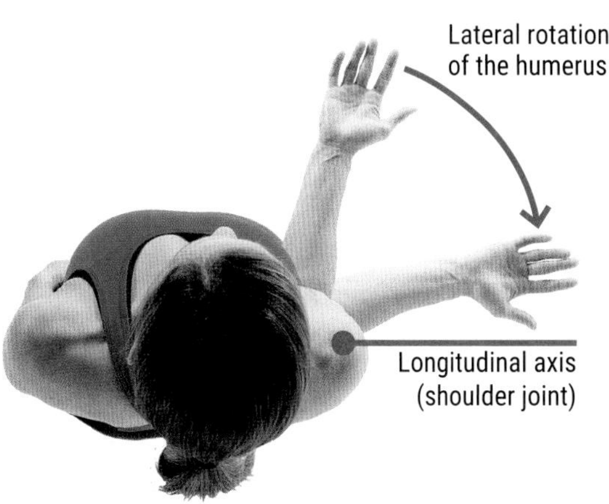

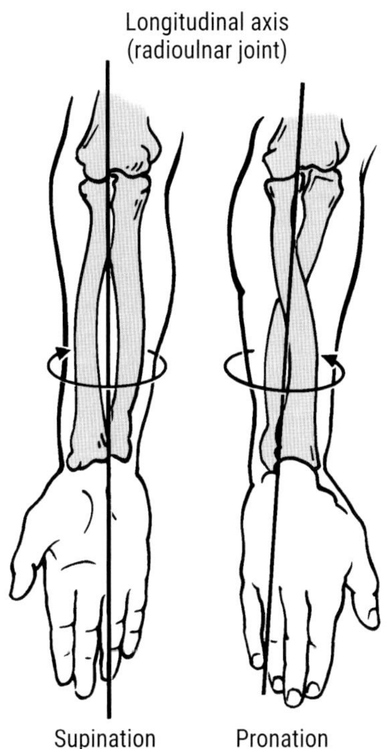

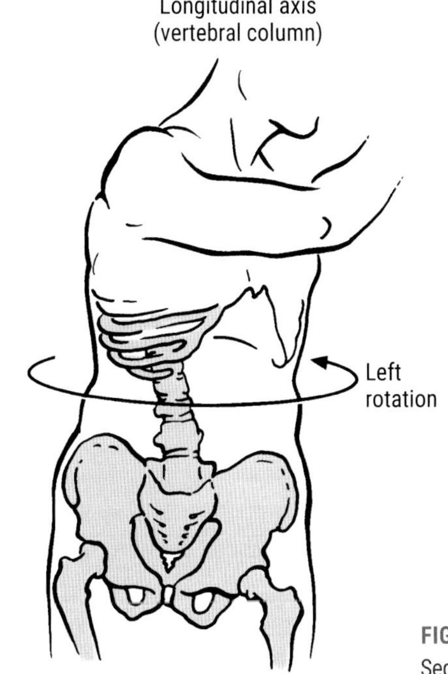

FIGURE 9-9
Segmental movements in the transverse plane

TABLE 9-3

Fundamental Movements (From Anatomical Position)

Plane	Action	Definition
Sagittal	Flexion	Decreasing the angle between two bones
	Extension	Increasing the angle between two bones
	Dorsiflexion	Moving the top of the foot toward the shin (only at the ankle joint)
	Plantar flexion	Moving the sole of the foot downward; "pointing the toes" (only at the ankle)
Frontal	Abduction	Motion away from the midline of the body (or body segment)
	Adduction	Motion toward the midline of the body (or body segment)
	Elevation	Moving to a superior position (only at the scapula)
	Depression	Moving to an inferior position (only at the scapula)
	Inversion	Lifting the medial border of the foot (only at the subtalar joint)
	Eversion	Lifting the lateral border of the foot (only at the subtalar joint)
Transverse	Rotation	Internal (inward) or external (outward) turning about the vertical axis of a bone
	Pronation*	Rotating the hand and wrist medially (palm down position)
	Supination†	Rotating the hand and wrist laterally (palm up position)
	Horizontal flexion (adduction)	From a 90-degree horizontally abducted shoulder or hip position, the humerus or femur, respectively, is flexed (adducted) in toward the midline of the body in the transverse plane
	Horizontal extension (abduction)	From a 90-degree (horizontally) flexed shoulder or hip position, the humerus or femur, respectively, is extended (abducted) out away from the midline of the body in the transverse plane
Multiplanar	Circumduction	Motion that describes a "cone"; combines flexion, abduction, extension, and adduction in sequential order
	Opposition	Thumb movement unique to humans and primates

*Pronation of the foot is a combination of eversion and abduction, raising the lateral edge of the foot.
†Supination of the foot is a combination of inversion and adduction, raising the medial edge of the foot.

APPLY WHAT YOU KNOW

Practicing Movements of the Synovial Joints

Stand up and perform each of the movements depicted in Figures 9-6 through 9-9. What joints are being used in each movement? What type of movement is being performed at each joint?

NERVOUS SYSTEM

A major function of the nervous system is to collect information about conditions in relation to the body's external and internal state, analyze this information, and initialize appropriate responses to fulfill specific needs. In other words, the nervous system gathers information, stores it, and controls various bodily systems in response to this input. The muscular system, which is covered later in this chapter, is composed of more than 600 individual muscles and is responsible for movement of the body. The connection of the muscles to the brain and spinal cord through a network of nerve circuits that direct the ebb and flow of muscular energy is referred to as the neuromuscular system. Connective tissue, which is intricately associated with the neuromuscular system, provides structure, cohesion, and support to the muscles and nerves it surrounds.

Neural Organization

The nervous system is separated into various divisions based on either structural or functional characteristics. Keep in mind that these divisions—which are called nervous systems themselves—are still part of a single, overall nervous system. In terms of structure, the nervous system is divided into two parts: the **central nervous system (CNS)** and the **peripheral nervous system (PNS).** The CNS consists of the brain and spinal cord, which are both encased and protected by bony structures—the skull and the vertebral column, respectively. The CNS is responsible for receiving sensory input from the PNS and formulating responses to this input. This makes the CNS the integrative and control center of the nervous system. The PNS is composed of all the nervous structures located outside of the CNS, namely the nerves and **ganglia** (nerve cell bodies associated with the nerves). In part, the PNS is made up of pairings of nerves that branch out from the brain and spinal cord to innervate organs in different regions. Twelve pairs of cranial nerves, which arise from the brain and brain stem, exit the cranial cavity through **foramina** (small holes) in the skull. Thirty-one pairs of spinal nerves, which arise from the spinal cord, exit the vertebral column through intervertebral foramina. Named for the region of the spine where they originate and the vertebral level from which they emerge, the paired spinal nerves are classified as eight cervical, 12 thoracic, five lumbar, five sacral, and one coccygeal (Figure 9-10).

In terms of function, the PNS is separated into two categories: the afferent (sensory) division and the efferent (motor) division. The afferent division carries nerve impulses to the CNS from receptors located in the skin, **fasciae,** joints, and visceral organs. In other words, afferent sensory data is incoming information. In contrast, the efferent division handles outgoing information and can be divided into the somatic and **autonomic nervous systems.** The **somatic nervous system** is mostly under conscious control and carries nerve impulses from the CNS to the skeletal muscles. In some instances, muscle contractions brought on by the somatic nervous system are not consciously controlled, such as in the case of a reflex response. The autonomic nervous system is made up of nerves that transmit impulses to the **smooth muscles, cardiac muscle,** and glands. These visceral motor impulses generally cannot be consciously controlled. The autonomic nervous system is further divided into the sympathetic and parasympathetic divisions. The **sympathetic nervous system** is activated when there is a stressor or an emergency, such as severe pain, anger, or fear. Called the "fight or flight" response, this activation affects nearly every organ to enable the body to stop storing energy and mobilize all resources to respond to the stressful event or activity. The **parasympathetic nervous system** aids in controlling normal functions when the body is relaxed; it aids in digesting food, storing energy, and promoting growth.

Structures of the Nervous System

The most basic structural and functional component of the nervous system is the **neuron** (nerve cell). The neuron is composed of a cell body (soma) and one or more processes—

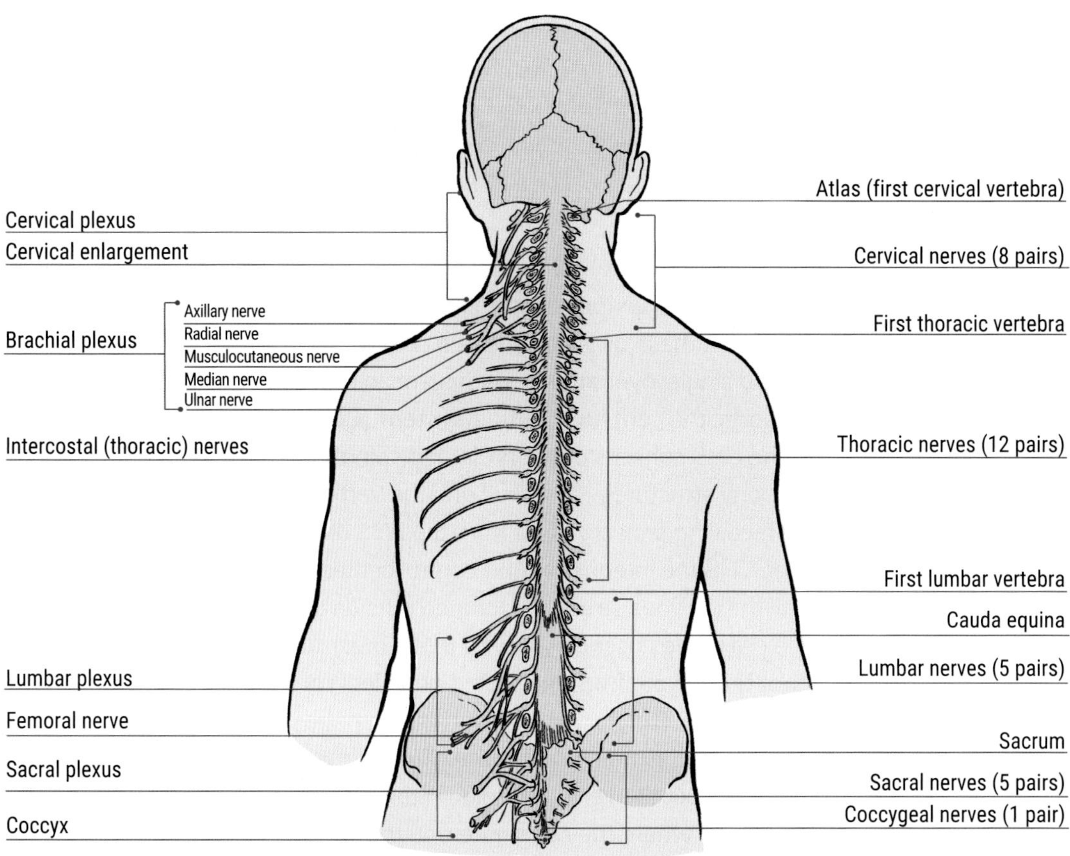

FIGURE 9-10
Spinal cord and spinal nerves (posterior view)

fibrous extensions called **dendrites** and **axons** (Figure 9-11). Dendrites conduct electrical impulses toward the cell body, while axons transmit electrical signals away from the cell body. Neurons may have hundreds of the branching dendrites, depending on the neuron type, but each neuron has only one axon. For an electrical impulse to travel through the nervous system, it must be passed from one neuron to the next. Most neurons do not have direct contact with each other. Instead, neurons remain separated from each other by a small space called a **synapse.** To carry the impulse across the synapse from one neuron to the other, the first neuron releases a chemical transmitter substance that attaches to receptors located on the membrane of the second neuron.

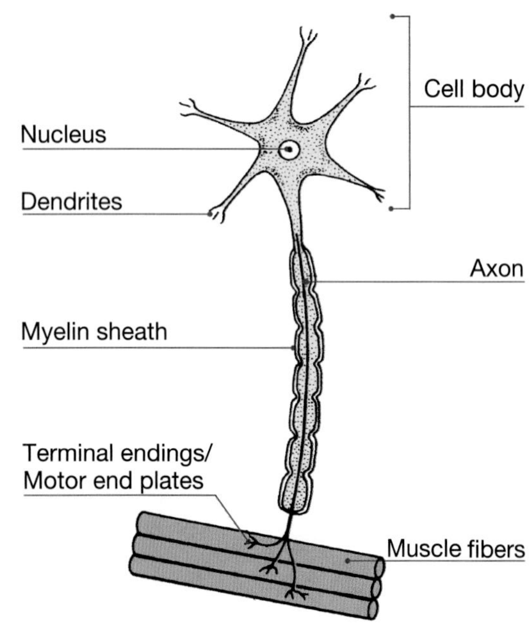

FIGURE 9-11
Basic anatomical structure of a motor neuron (or nerve cell) and motor end plate

Most axons are covered with a fatty substance called **myelin,** which insulates the axon and keeps the electrical current from migrating outside of the neuron. A nerve is made up of the processes of many neurons held together by connective tissue sheaths. Sensory (afferent) nerves carry impulses to the CNS, whereas motor (efferent) nerves carry nerve impulses from the CNS to the PNS. Motor neurons form a **neuromuscular junction** with the skeletal muscles they supply.

Proprioception

The sense of knowing where the body is in relation to its various segments and the external environment is called **proprioception.** The sensory information gathered to achieve this kinesthetic awareness comes from structures called **proprioceptors,** which are receptors located in the skin, in and around the joints and muscles, and in the inner ear. Cutaneous receptors are located in the skin and send sensory information regarding pressure, touch, and movement of the hairs on the skin. Joint receptors are located in the joint capsules and the surrounding ligaments. They transmit sensory information relating to positions, velocities, and accelerations occurring at the joints. In addition, pressure receptors within the joints provide information about pressure changes that is used for important postural adjustments and normal **gait.**

Pacinian corpuscles are receptors located deep within the skin and the joint capsule that are sensitive to pressure. **Meissner's corpuscles** are receptors located in the **superficial** layers of the skin that are responsive to light touch. While most researchers agree that these skin receptors do not play a large part in proprioception, it is believed that injured individuals who have experienced joint and ligament receptor damage benefit from increased reliance on cutaneous receptors for proprioception. **Golgi-Mazzoni corpuscles** are located within the joint capsule and are responsive to joint compression. Thus, any weight-bearing activity stimulates these receptors. Another type of proprioceptor, the musculotendinous receptor, is involved in muscular control and **coordination.** There are two such types of receptors—the **Golgi tendon organ (GTO)** and the **muscle spindle.** Connected to approximately 15 to 20 muscle fibers and located between the muscle belly and its tendon, the GTO senses increased tension within its associated muscle when the muscle contracts or is stretched. One of the GTO's functions when it senses muscle contraction where the tension is too great and may pull the tendon from the bone is to reduce the tension by inhibiting the contraction (**autogenic inhibition**). It has been theorized that this function adjusts muscle output in response to fatigue. That is, when muscle tension is reduced due to fatigue, GTO output is also reduced, which lowers its inhibitory effect in its own muscle and allows the muscle to increase its contractile ability. Furthermore, GTO activation results in an enhanced contraction of the opposing (**antagonist**) muscle group. Both of these properties have important implications in flexibility because a muscle can be stretched more fully and easily when the GTOs are stimulated, resulting in inhibited contraction in the muscle or muscle group being stretched (e.g., hamstrings) and enhanced contraction in the antagonist muscle or muscle group (e.g., hip flexors).

A second type of musculotendinous receptor, the muscle spindle, is located mostly in the muscle belly and lies parallel to the muscle fibers. This arrangement causes the muscle spindle to stretch when the muscle itself experiences a stretch force, thereby exciting the muscle spindle, which causes a reflexive contraction in the muscle known as the stretch reflex. The muscle spindle's reflex contraction of its associated muscle simultaneously causes the antagonist muscle group to relax (**reciprocal inhibition**). For example, if the gastrocnemius (see Figure 9-31, page 362) is stretched rapidly, the muscle spindles within the muscle belly cause it to contract. At the same time, if the opposing muscle group (anterior tibialis) (see Figure 9-32, page 362) is contracting, the muscle spindle reflex causes it to relax. The muscle spindles and the GTOs work together through their reflexive

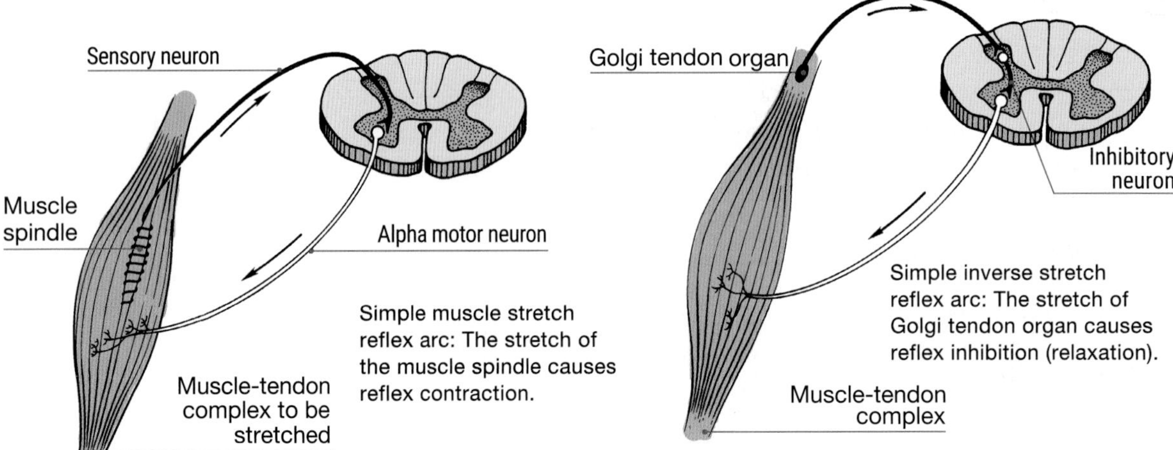

FIGURE 9-12
The stretch reflex and autogenic inhibition

actions to regulate muscle stiffness, and therefore, contribute largely to the body's sense of postural control (Figure 9-12).

Autogenic inhibition and reciprocal inhibition are directly associated with stretching. A practical application of autogenic inhibition is observed during **static stretching.** Low-force, long-duration static stretches evoke a temporary increase in muscle tension due to muscle lengthening. After seven to 10 seconds of a low-force stretch, the increase in muscle tension activates a GTO response. Under GTO activation, muscle spindle activity within the stretched muscle is temporarily inhibited, allowing further muscle stretching. After the removal of the stretch stimulus, however, the muscle spindle quickly reestablishes its stretch threshold.

A practical application of reciprocal inhibition is observed during **proprioceptive neuromuscular facilitation (PNF)** (see Chapter 11). Low-grade muscle contractions (50% of maximal force) of an antagonist muscle for six to 15 seconds inhibit or reduce muscle spindle activity within the agonist muscle. This reduces muscle tonicity, allowing that muscle to be stretched. For example, activation of the hip flexors during a hamstring stretch can temporarily inhibit muscle spindle activity within the hamstrings. For range-of-motion improvement, it is important to initiate a stretch immediately following inhibition of the muscle spindle (as is the case with PNF stretching) due to its rate of recovery.

The body relies on the **vestibular system** for sensory information related to the position of the head in space and to sudden changes in the directional movement of the head. Located in the inner ear, the vestibular system is composed of three fluid-containing semicircular canals that lie at right angles to each other. Each canal contains sensory hair cells that detect the movement of the fluid in the canals. When the angular position of the head changes, fluid rushes over the hair cells and causes them to bend. This response signals to the CNS the direction of the head's rotation and the position of the head during movement. The vestibular system functions to coordinate many motor responses and helps stabilize the eyes to maintain postural stability during stance and locomotion.

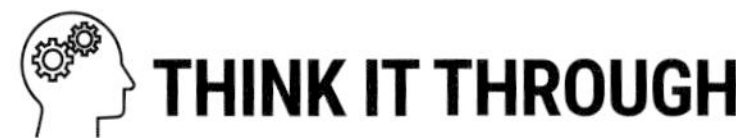

THINK IT THROUGH

The Body's Systems

Before moving on to learn about the muscular system, reflect on the various other systems you read about in Chapter 8 and so far in this chapter and why it is important for a personal trainer to understand their primary functions. How would you explain the role of each system to an interested client?

MUSCULAR SYSTEM

Muscle tissue is categorized into different types based on its function, is controlled both voluntarily and involuntarily, and is able to produce various levels of force based on its size and shape. One property that all muscle tissue has in common is its ability to contract and develop tension. There are three types of muscle tissue—skeletal muscle (Figure 9-13), smooth muscle, and cardiac muscle. Skeletal muscle attaches to the skeleton and, through contraction, exerts force on the bones to move and stabilize them. Skeletal muscle is considered voluntary muscle because it is normally under the conscious control of the individual. When viewed under a microscope, skeletal muscle tissue exhibits alternating light and dark bands, giving it a striped appearance. This characteristic is the reason skeletal muscle is also called striated muscle.

Smooth muscle is found in the walls of hollow organs and tubes, such as the stomach, intestines, and blood vessels, and functions to regulate the movement of materials through the body. It is called smooth muscle because it lacks the striated appearance of skeletal muscle. Because it is not under conscious control, it is considered involuntary.

Cardiac muscle forms the wall of the heart and is a very specialized tissue that functions to maintain the constant pumping action of the heart. Cardiac tissue is involuntary, like smooth muscle, and striated in appearance, like skeletal muscle.

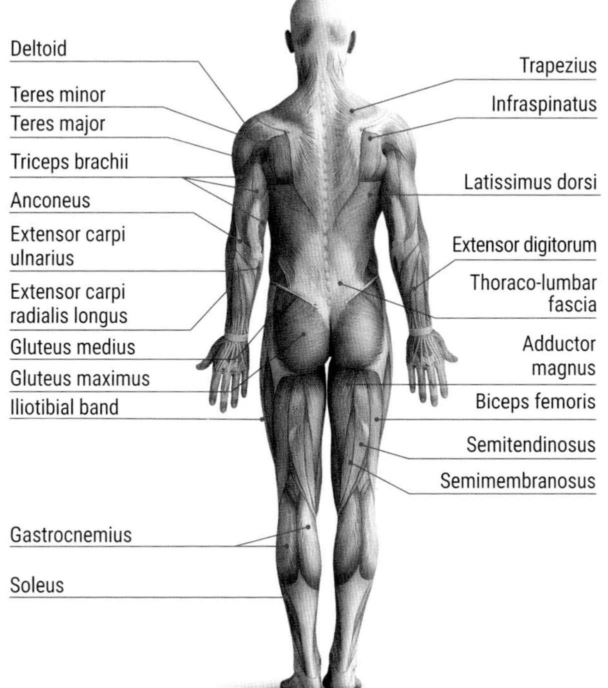

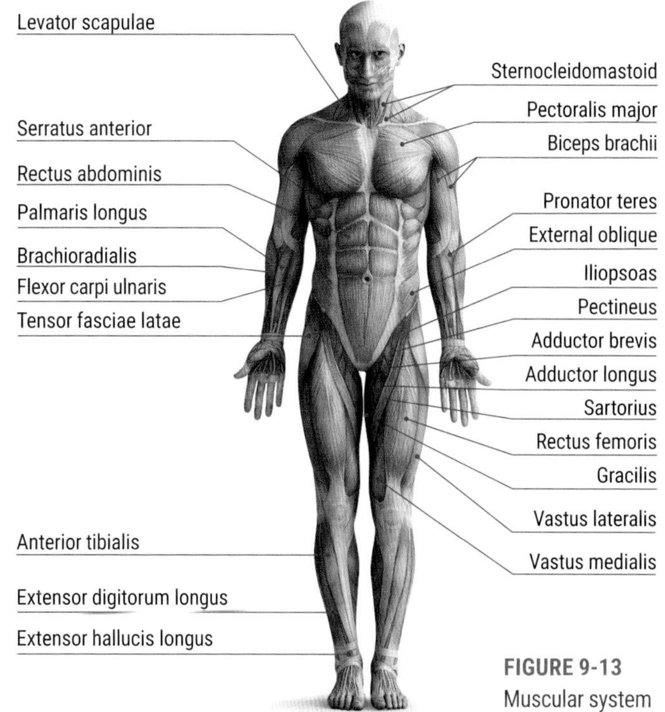

FIGURE 9-13
Muscular system

Muscle Function

Skeletal muscle's role in movement and physical activity is the main focus of this section. At each end of the belly of most skeletal muscles, a specialized form of connective tissue called a tendon attaches the muscle to one or more bones. Fundamentally, skeletal muscles perform their required tasks by pulling on bones to create joint movement. That is, when a muscle contracts, its tendinous attachments move closer together. In contrast, when a muscle is stretched, its tendon attachment points move farther apart. Correct anatomical knowledge of muscle locations and actions is crucial to designing safe and effective exercise programs, but there is more to consider. Each joint movement incorporates all of the supporting structures surrounding it. Pairings of muscles called **agonists** and antagonists help illustrate this point. A muscle that creates a major movement is called a **prime mover,** or agonist. The muscle on the opposite side of the joint is called an opposing muscle, or antagonist. For example, the quadriceps muscle group in the front of the thigh produces knee extension. When the quadriceps contract to extend the knee, it is considered the agonist muscle group, whereas on the opposite side of the joint, the hamstrings (antagonist) are being stretched (Figures 9-14 and 9-15). This type of functional pairing of muscle groups is found throughout the body. Tables 9-4 through 9-11 summarize the major skeletal muscles and their associated primary functions. It is essential that personal trainers understand and are able to apply the content in these tables in practice when working with clients.

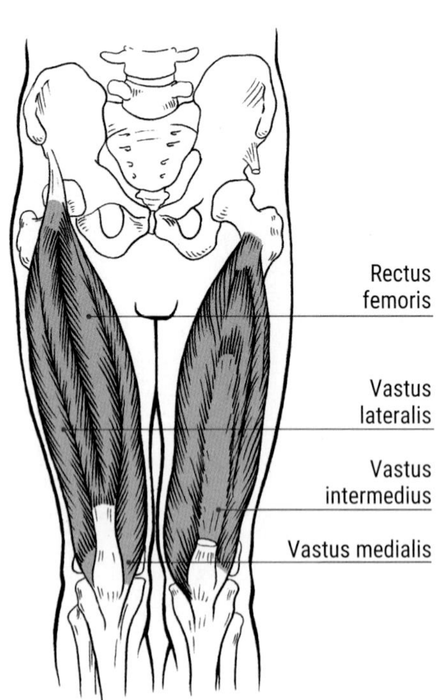

FIGURE 9-14
Quadriceps muscles

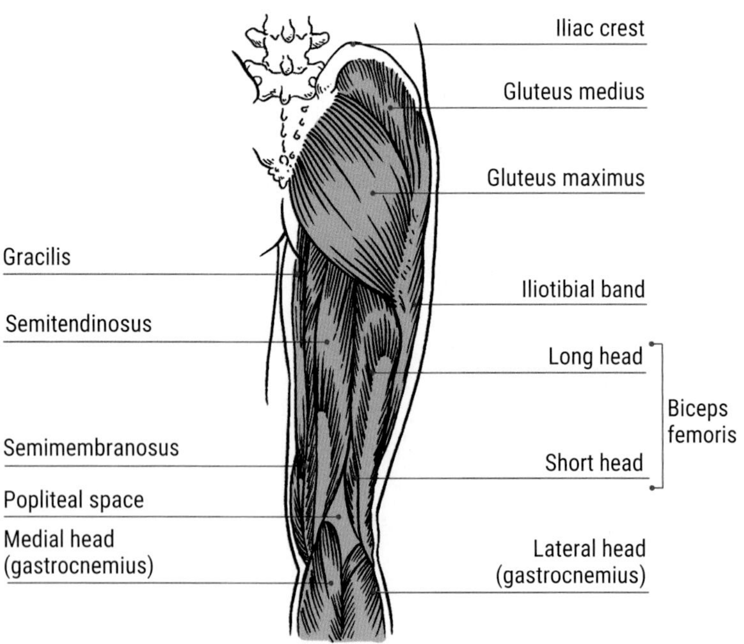

FIGURE 9-15
Posterior musculature of the hip and knee, prime movers for hip extension (gluteus maximus and hamstrings) and knee flexion (hamstrings and gastrocnemius)

TABLE 9-4
Major Muscles That Act at the Ankle and Foot

Muscle	Origin	Insertion	Primary Function(s)	Selected Exercises
Anterior tibialis	Proximal ⅔ of lateral tibia	Medial aspect of 1st cuneiform and base of 1st metatarsal	Dorsiflexion at ankle; inversion at foot	Cycling with toe clips, resisted inversion (with dorsiflexion)
Peroneus longus	Lateral surface of head of tibia, head of fibula, and proximal ⅔ of lateral fibula	Inferior aspects of medial tarsal (1st cuneiform) and base of 1st metatarsal	Plantar flexion at ankle; eversion at foot	Resisted eversion of foot
Peroneus brevis	Distal ⅔ of lateral fibula	Base of the 5th metatarsal	Plantar flexion at ankle; eversion at foot	Resisted eversion of foot
Gastrocnemius	Posterior surfaces of femoral condyles	Posterior surface of calcaneus via Achilles tendon	Plantar flexion at ankle; flexion at knee	Hill running, jumping rope, calf raises, cycling, stair climbing
Soleus	Proximal ⅔ of posterior surfaces of tibia and fibula and popliteal line	Posterior surface of calcaneus via Achilles tendon	Plantar flexion at ankle	Virtually the same as for gastrocnemius; bent-knee toe raises with resistance
Posterior tibialis	Posterior surface of the lateral tibia and medial fibula	Lower medial surfaces of medial tarsals and metatarsals	Plantar flexion at ankle; inversion at foot	Resisted inversion of foot with plantar flexion
Extensor hallucis longus	Anterior middle fibula	Dorsal surface of the distal phalanx of the great toe	Dorsiflexion and inversion of the foot; extension of the great toe	Resisted inversion with dorsiflexion
Extensor digitorum longus	Lateral condyle of tibia, proximal ¾ of the fibula	Dorsal surface of the phalanges of toes 2 through 5	Dorsiflexion and eversion of foot; extension of toes 2 through 5	Resisted eversion with dorsiflexion
Peroneus tertius	Distal ⅓ of the anterior/lateral fibula	Dorsal surface of the base of the 5th metatarsal	Dorsiflexion and eversion of the foot	Resisted eversion with dorsiflexion
Plantaris	Posterior surface of the femur above the lateral condyle	Posterior surface of calcaneus via Achilles tendon	Flexion of the knee; plantar flexion of the ankle	Same as gastrocnemius
Flexor hallucis longus	Distal ⅔ of the fibula	Plantar surface of distal phalanx of great toe	Flexion of the great toe; plantar flexion of the ankle; inversion of the foot	Resisted inversion with plantar flexion
Flexor digitorum longus	Posterior middle ⅓ of tibia	Plantar surfaces of distal phalanges of toes 2 through 5	Flexion of toes 2 through 5; plantar flexion of the ankle; inversion of the foot	Resisted inversion with plantar flexion

TABLE 9-5

Major Muscles That Act at the Knee

Muscle	Origin	Insertion	Primary Function(s)	Selected Exercises
Rectus femoris	Anterior-inferior spine of ilium and upper lip of acetabulum	Superior aspect of patella and patellar tendon	Extension (most effective when the hip is extended)	Cycling, leg press machine, squats, vertical jumping, stair climbing, jumping rope, plyometrics
Vastus lateralis, intermedius, and medialis	Along the surfaces of the lateral, anterior, and medial femur	Patella and tibial tuberosity via the patellar tendon	Extension	Same as for rectus femoris, resisted knee extension
Biceps femoris	Long head: ischial tuberosity; Short head: lower, lateral linea aspera	Lateral condyle of tibia and head of fibula	Flexion and external rotation	Cycling, lunging, hamstring curls
Semitendinosus	Ischial tuberosity	Proximal anterior medial aspect of tibia	Flexion and internal rotation	Same as biceps femoris
Semimembranosus	Ischial tuberosity	Posterior aspect of medial tibial condyle	Flexion and internal rotation	Same as biceps femoris
Gracilis	Pubic symphysis and pubic arch	Medial tibia just below the condyle	Flexion	Side-lying bottom-leg raises, with a flexed knee, resisted adduction with a flexed knee
Sartorius	Anterior superior iliac spine	Proximal anterior medial tibia just below the tuberosity	Flexion and external rotation of the hip; flexion of the knee	Knee lift with hip external rotation, wide stance onto bench
Popliteus	Lateral condyle of the femur	Proximal tibia	Knee flexion; internal rotation of the lower leg to "unlock the knee"	Same as biceps femoris

TABLE 9-6

Major Muscles That Act at the Hip

Muscle	Origin	Insertion	Primary Function(s)	Selected Exercises
Iliopsoas: Iliacus and psoas major and minor	Transverse processes of T12 and L1-L5;* iliac crest and fossa	Lesser trochanter of femur	Flexion and external rotation	Straight-leg sit-ups, running with knees lifted up high, leg raises, hanging knee raises
Rectus femoris	Anterior-inferior spine of ilium and upper lip of acetabulum	Superior aspect of patella and patellar tendon	Flexion	Running, leg press, squat, jumping rope
Gluteus maximus	Posterior ¼ of iliac crest and sacrum	Gluteal line of femur and iliotibial band	Extension and external rotation; Superior fibers: abduction	Cycling, plyometrics, jumping rope, squats, stair-climbing machine

TABLE 9-6 *(continued)*

Muscle	Origin	Insertion	Primary Function(s)	Selected Exercises
Biceps femoris	Long head: ischial tuberosity; Short head: lower, lateral linea aspera	Lateral condyle of tibia and head of fibula	Extension, abduction, and slight external rotation	Cycling, hamstring curls with knee in external rotation
Semitendinosus	Ischial tuberosity	Proximal anterior-medial aspect of tibia	Extension, adduction, and slight internal rotation	Same as biceps femoris
Semimembranosus	Ischial tuberosity	Posterior aspect of medial tibial condyle	Extension, adduction, and slight internal rotation	Same as biceps femoris
Gluteus medius and minimus	Lateral surface of ilium	Greater trochanter of femur	Abduction (all fibers); Anterior fibers: internal rotation; Posterior fibers: external rotation	Side-lying leg raises, walking, running
Adductor magnus	Pubic ramus and ischial tuberosity	Medial aspects of femur	Adduction	Side-lying bottom-leg raises, resisted adduction
Adductor brevis and longus	Pubic ramus and ischial tuberosity	Linea aspera of femur	Adduction	Side-lying bottom-leg raises, resisted adduction
Tensor fasciae latae	Anterior iliac crest and ilium just below crest	Iliotibial band	Flexion, abduction, and internal rotation	Hanging knee raises, side-lying leg raises, running
Sartorius	Anterior superior iliac spine	Proximal anterior medial tibia just below the tuberosity	Flexion and external rotation of the hip; flexion of the knee	Knee lift with hip external rotation, wide stance onto bench
Pectineus	Superior pubic ramus	Lesser trochanter and linea aspera of femur	Flexion, adduction, and external rotation	Hanging knee raises, side-lying bottom-leg raises, resisted external rotation of the thigh
Six deep external (lateral) rotators: Piriformis, obturator internus, obturator externus, superior gemellus, inferior gemellus, and quadratus femoris	Multiple origin points for six muscles on pubis, ischium, sacrum, and obturator foramen	On and just below greater trochanter, and trochanteric fossa of femur	External rotation	Resisted external rotation of the thigh
Gracilis	Pubic symphysis and arch	Medial tibia just below the condyle	Adduction	Side-lying bottom-leg raises, resisted adduction

* T12 = Twelfth thoracic vertebra; L1-L5 = First through fifth lumbar vertebrae

TABLE 9-7

Major Muscles That Act at the Spine

Muscle	Origin	Insertion	Primary Function(s)	Selected Exercises
Rectus abdominis	Pubic crest	Cartilage of 5th through 7th ribs	Flexion and lateral flexion of the trunk	Bent-knee sit-ups, partial curl-ups, pelvic tilts
External oblique	Anterior, lateral borders of lower 8 ribs	Anterior half of ilium, pubic crest, and anterior fascia	Contralateral rotation, lateral flexion, and forward flexion (both sides)	Twisting bent-knee curl-ups (rotation opposite) and curl-ups
Internal oblique	Lumbodorsal fascia, iliac crest, and anterior fascia	Cartilage of last 3 to 4 ribs, linea alba, and superior ramis of pubis	Ipsilateral rotation, lateral flexion, and forward flexion (both sides)	Twisting bent-knee curl-ups (rotation same side) and curl-ups
Transverse abdominis	Iliac crest, lumbar fascia, cartilages of last 6 ribs, and anterior fascia	Xiphoid process of sternum, anterior fascia, and pubis	Compresses abdomen	Prone plank, abdominal bracing
Erector spinae	Posterior iliac crest, sacrum, ribs, and vertebrae	Angles of ribs, transverse processes of all ribs	Extension (both sides) and lateral flexion	Squat, dead lift, prone back extension exercises
Multifidi	Posterior surface of the sacrum, articular processes of the lumbar vertebrae, transverse processes of the thoracic vertebrae, articular processes of C3-7*	The spinous processes spanning 1 to 4 vertebrae above the origin	Contributes to spinal stability during trunk extension, rotation, and side-bending	Bird dog

* C3-7 = Third through seventh thoracic vertebrae

TABLE 9-8

Major Muscles That Act at the Shoulder Girdle

Muscle	Origin	Insertion	Primary Function(s)	Selected Exercises
Trapezius	Occipital bone, spines of 7th cervical and thoracic vertebrae	Lateral third of clavicle, acromion process, and spine of scapula	Upper: upward rotation and elevation of scapula Middle: upward rotation and adduction of scapula Lower: depression of scapula	Upright rows, shoulder shrugs
Levator scapulae	Transverse processes of first four cervical vertebrae	Upper vertebral border of scapula	Elevation of scapula	Shoulder shrugs
Rhomboid major and minor	Spines of 7th cervical through 5th thoracic vertebrae	Middle to lower vertebral border of scapula	Adduction, downward rotation, and elevation of scapula	Chin-ups, supported dumbbell bent-over rows

TABLE 9-8 *(continued)*

Muscle	Origin	Insertion	Primary Function(s)	Selected Exercises
Pectoralis minor	Anterior surface of ribs 3 through 5	Coracoid process of scapula	Stabilization, depression, downward rotation, and abduction of scapula	Push-ups, incline bench press, regular bench press, cable crossover chest flys
Serratus anterior	Lateral, anterior surface of ribs 1 through 9	Ventral surface of vertebral border of scapula	Stabilization, abduction, and upward rotation of scapula	Push-ups, incline bench press, pull-overs

TABLE 9-9

Major Muscles That Act at the Shoulder

Muscle	Origin	Insertion	Primary Function(s)	Selected Exercises
Pectoralis major	Clavicle, sternum, and first six costal cartilages	Greater tubercle of humerus	Flexion, extension, adduction, internal rotation, and horizontal adduction	Push-ups, pull-ups, incline bench press, regular bench press, climbing a rope, all types of throwing, tennis serve
Deltoid	Anterior, lateral clavicle, border of the acromion, and lower edge of spine of the scapula	Deltoid tubercle of humerus on mid-lateral surface	Entire muscle: abduction Anterior fibers: flexion, internal rotation, and horizontal adduction Posterior fibers: external rotation and horizontal abduction	Lateral "butterfly" (abduction) exercises; anterior deltoid has similar functions to the pectoralis major
Latissimus dorsi	Spines of lower six thoracic vertebrae and all lumbar vertebrae, crests of ilium and sacrum, lower four ribs, and inferior angle of scapulae	Medial side of intertubercular groove of humerus	Extension, adduction, horizontal abduction, and internal rotation	Chin-ups, rope climbing, dips on parallel bars, rowing, any exercise that involves pulling the arms downward against resistance (e.g., lat pull-downs on exercise machine)
Rotator cuff	Various aspects of scapula	All insert on greater tubercle of humerus except for the subscapularis, which inserts on the lesser tubercle of the humerus	Infraspinatus and teres minor: external rotation Subscapularis: internal rotation Supraspinatus: abduction All contribute to the stability of the humeral head	Exercises that involve internal and external rotation (e.g., tennis serve, throwing a baseball)
Teres major	Posterior inferior lateral border of scapula, just superior to inferior angle	Intertubercular groove of the humerus	Extension, adduction, and internal rotation	Chin-ups, seated rows, lat pull-downs, rope climbing

TABLE 9-10
Major Muscles That Act at the Elbow and Radioulnar Joints

Muscle	Origin	Insertion	Primary Function(s)	Selected Exercises
Biceps brachii	Long head: tubercle above glenoid cavity; Short head: coracoid process of scapula	Radial tuberosity	Flexion at elbow; supination at forearm	Arm curls, chin-ups, rock climbing, upright rowing
Brachialis	Anterior humerus	Ulnar tuberosity and coronoid process of ulna	Flexion at elbow	Same as for biceps brachii
Brachioradialis	Distal ⅔ of lateral condyloid ridge of humerus	Styloid process of radius	Flexion at elbow; supination at forearm	Same as for biceps brachii
Triceps brachii	Long head: lower edge of glenoid cavity of scapula; Lateral head: posterior humerus; Short head: distal ⅔ of posterior humerus	Olecranon process of ulna	Extension at elbow; arm extension (long head)	Push-ups, dips, bench press, overhead press
Pronator teres	Epicondyle of medial humerus	Middle ⅓ of lateral radius	Flexion at elbow and pronation at forearm	Pronation of forearm with dumbbell
Pronator quadratus	Distal anterior surface of ulna	Distal anterior surface of radius	Pronation at forearm	Resisted pronation
Supinator	Lateral, posterior epicondyle of humerus and supinator crest of ulna	Proximal, lateral surface of radius	Supination at forearm	Resisted supination

TABLE 9-11
Major Muscles That Act at the Wrist

Muscle	Origin	Insertion	Primary Function(s)	Selected Exercises
Flexor carpi radialis	Medial epicondyle of humerus	Anterior base of 2nd and 3rd metacarpals	Flexion	Wrist curls; grip-strengthening exercises for racquet sports
Flexor carpi ulnaris	Medial epicondyle of humerus, medial olecranon process, and upper, posterior ulna	5th metacarpal	Flexion	Same as flexor carpi radialis
Extensor carpi radialis longus	Lateral epicondyle of humerus	Posterior base of 2nd metacarpal	Extension	"Reverse" wrist curls; racquet sports, particularly tennis
Extensor carpi ulnaris	Lateral epicondyle of humerus and middle ½ of posterior ulna	Posterior base of 5th metacarpal	Extension	Same as extensor carpi radialis longus
Palmaris longus	Medial epicondyle of humerus	Palmar aponeurosis	Flexion	Wrist curls

When visually comparing the various skeletal muscles, it is evident that they come in different shapes and muscle-fiber arrangements (Figure 9-16). These characteristics vary from muscle to muscle because of functionality. In some muscles, the muscle fibers run parallel to the long axis of the muscle, forming a long, strap-like arrangement. This type of muscle is classified as a longitudinal muscle, and although it is capable of producing considerable movement, it is relatively weak compared to other muscle-fiber arrangements. The sartorius muscle of the thigh is an example of a longitudinal muscle (Figure 9-17). Other muscles have a tendon that runs the entire length of the muscle, with the muscle fibers inserting diagonally into the tendon. In some muscles of this type, all of the muscle fibers insert onto one side of the tendon (unipennate), and in others, the muscle fibers insert obliquely onto each side of the tendon (bipennate). Unipennate

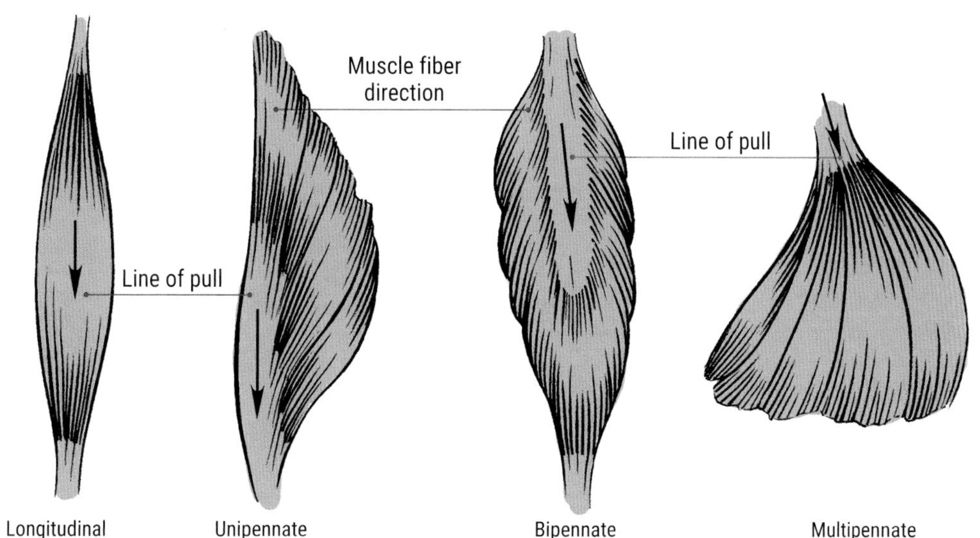

FIGURE 9-16
Muscle fiber arrangements

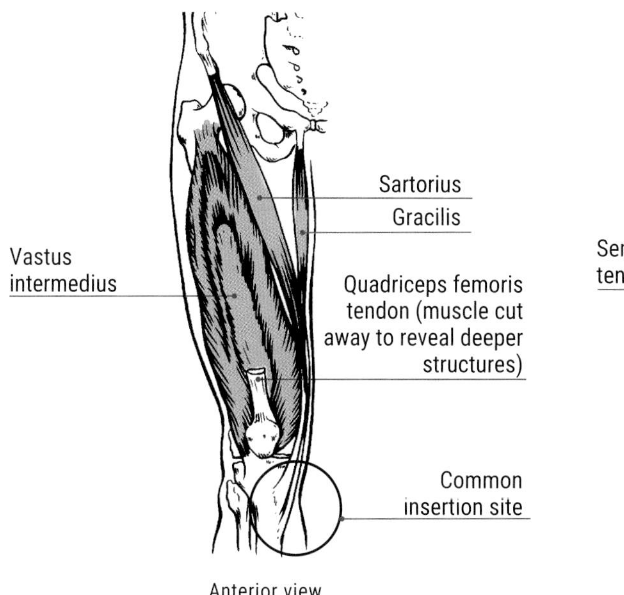

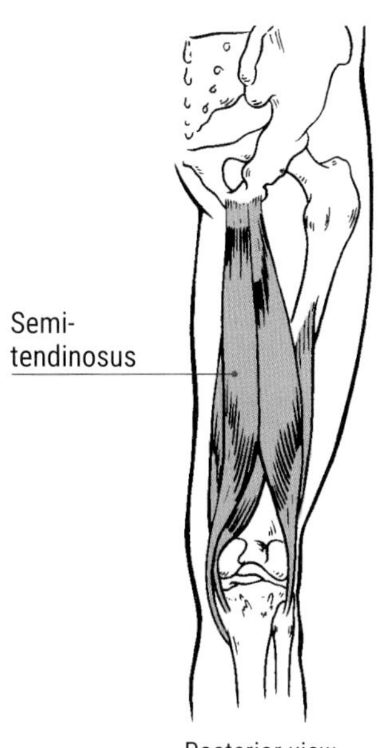

FIGURE 9-17
Pes anserine muscles: sartorius, gracilis, and semitendinosus

(e.g., anterior tibialis; see Figure 9-32, page 362) and bipennate (e.g., rectus femoris; see Figure 9-14) muscles typically produce less movement than longitudinal muscles but are capable of creating greater force during contraction. In multipennate muscles, the muscle fibers have a complex arrangement that involves the convergence of several tendons. The deltoid muscle of the shoulder is a multipennate muscle (Figure 9-18).

Muscle Contraction

Skeletal muscle is composed of tiny, individual muscle cells, called muscle fibers. Muscle fibers are held in place by thin sheets of connective tissue membranes called fasciae (singular = **fascia**). The fascia that encases the entire muscle is known as the **epimysium.** Within the epimysium are bundles of muscle fibers grouped together in a fibrous sheath of fascia known as the **perimysium.** Within the perimysium are individual muscle fibers wrapped in a fascia called **endomysium** (Figure 9-19).

FIGURE 9-18
Superficial musculature of the anterior chest, shoulder, and arm

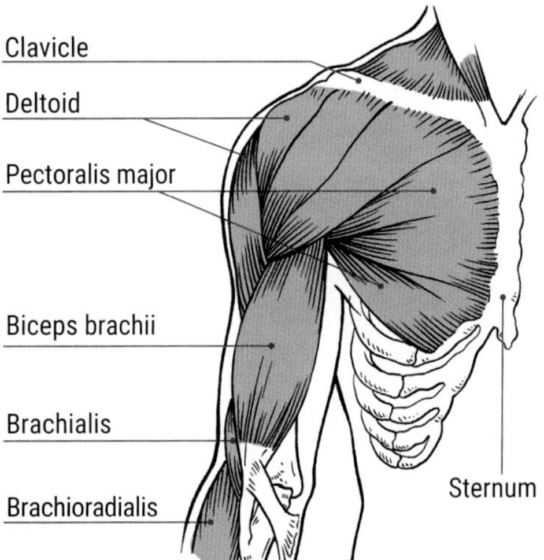

FIGURE 9-19
Organization of muscle

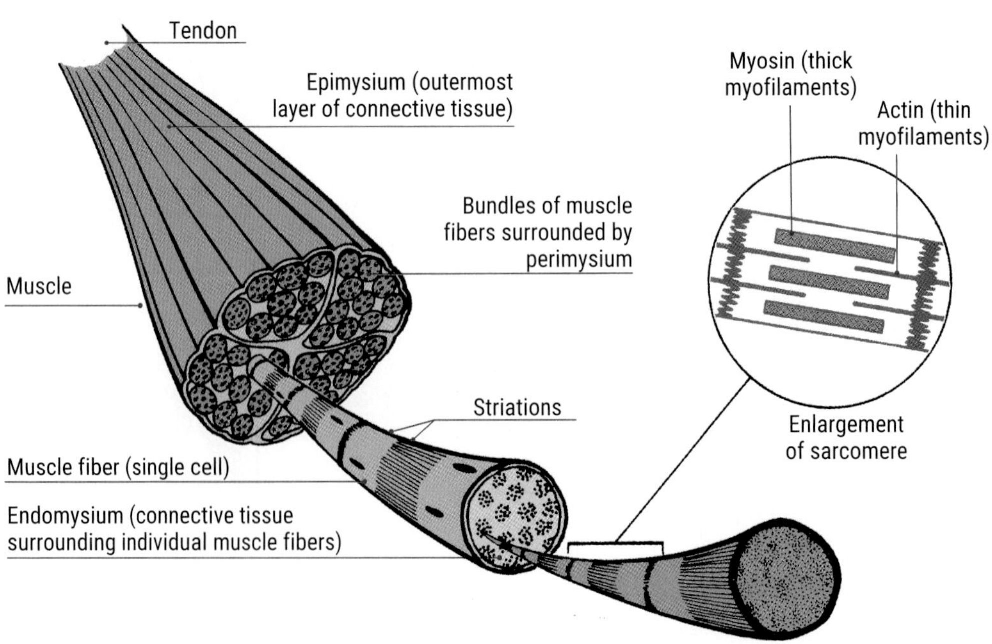

Muscle-fiber Types

Skeletal muscle fibers can be divided into two general categories based on how quickly they contract: **fast-twitch muscle fiber** and **slow-twitch muscle fiber.** Slow-twitch fibers (also called slow-oxidative or **type I muscle fibers**) contain relatively large amounts of **mitochondria** and are surrounded by more capillaries than are fast-twitch fibers. Additionally, slow-twitch fibers contain higher concentrations of **myoglobin** than do fast-twitch fibers (also called **type II muscle fibers**). The high concentration of myoglobin, the large number of capillaries, and the high mitochondrial content make slow-twitch fibers resistant to fatigue and capable of sustaining aerobic metabolism. As the name implies, slow-twitch fibers contract more slowly than fast-twitch fibers. Furthermore, slow-twitch fibers create lower force outputs and are more efficient than fast-twitch fibers.

It is generally agreed that there are two subtypes of fast-twitch fibers—identified as type IIx and IIa. Traditionally, the fastest type of skeletal muscle fiber in humans has been called the type IIb fiber. However, research has led to the discovery of new properties in the skeletal fast-twitch muscle fibers of both rodents and humans, which has prompted scientists to relabel these fibers as type IIx (Gundersen, 2011; Pette, 2001). Type IIx muscle fibers (sometimes called fast-glycolytic fibers) contain a relatively small amount of mitochondria, have a limited capacity for aerobic metabolism, and fatigue more easily than slow-twitch fibers. In fact, these fibers cannot sustain their effort for more than a few seconds. However, they possess a high number of glycolytic **enzymes,** which provide them with a considerable **anaerobic** capacity. Type IIx fibers are the largest and fastest and are capable of producing the most force of all the skeletal muscle fibers but are notably less efficient than slow-twitch fibers, as they also fatigue easily (Sieck et al., 2013; Shoepe et al., 2003). A second subtype of fast-twitch muscle fibers is the type IIa fiber (also called intermediate or fast-oxidative glycolytic fibers). These fibers possess speed, fatigue resistance, and force-production capabilities somewhere between slow-twitch and type IIx fibers. They are also used for strength and **power** activities and can sustain an effort for longer than the type IIx fibers—up to three minutes in highly trained athletes. Type IIa fibers are unique in that they are highly adaptable. That is, with endurance training, they can increase their oxidative capacity to levels similar to those observed in slow-twitch fibers, and with muscular training they become more like type IIx fibers.

A muscle's fiber-type composition is typically a mixture of both fast- and slow-twitch fibers, though some muscle groups are known to be made up of primarily fast-twitch (e.g., soleus) or slow-twitch (e.g., gastrocnemius) fibers (see Figure 9-31, page 362). The percentage of specific fiber types contained in skeletal muscle may be influenced by genetics, **hormones,** and the activity and exercise habits of the individual. Fiber composition of skeletal muscles is thought to play an important role in sport and exercise performance. It is commonly believed that successful power athletes possess a relatively large percentage of fast-twitch fibers, whereas endurance athletes generally possess a large percentage of slow-twitch fibers. However, it should be noted that muscle-fiber composition is only one variable that determines success in overall physical performance.

Muscle-fiber Microanatomy

As noted earlier, when highly magnified with a microscope, skeletal muscle fibers have a cross-striated appearance with alternating light and dark bands (Figure 9-20). Each

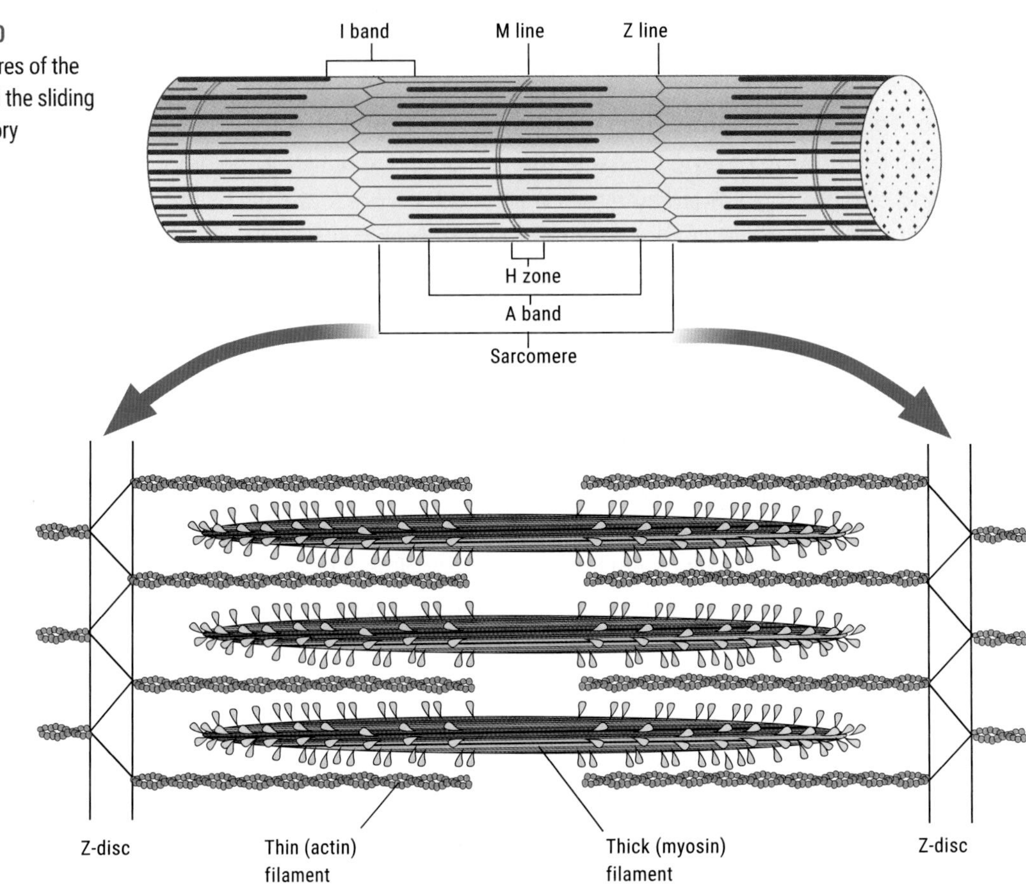

FIGURE 9-20
Microstructures of the myofiber and the sliding filament theory

muscle fiber contains several hundred to several thousand threadlike **myofibrils** (protein filaments) that run parallel to each other and extend lengthwise throughout the cell. The dark bands, called A bands, contain the protein filament **myosin.** The light bands, or I bands, are where the protein filament **actin** is located. Actin filaments also extend into the A bands, where they overlap with the myosin filaments. Crossing the center of each I band is a dense Z line that divides the myofibrils into a series of repeating segments called **sarcomeres.** The sarcomere is considered the functional contracting unit of skeletal muscle and is the portion of a myofibril that is found between two Z lines. In the center of a sarcomere is a lighter, somewhat less dense area called the H zone. This region is lighter in color, because actin does not extend into this area and the myosin filament becomes thinner in this middle region. A thin, darker M line crosses the center of the H zone. The H zone contains only myosin filaments. Actin filaments are found in the I band and in the part of the A band, up to the H zone. Actin filaments attach directly to the Z lines. The myosin filaments have tiny projections called cross-bridges that reach out at an angle toward the actin filaments.

SLIDING FILAMENT MODEL

When a muscle fiber contracts, the energy used to drive the contraction comes primarily from a substance within the cell called **adenosine triphosphate (ATP).** Muscle contraction occurs when the brain and spinal cord direct motor neurons to release a **neurotransmitter** called **acetylcholine** at the neuromuscular junction. Once the acetylcholine is detected, calcium is released into the area surrounding the fiber. The calcium exposes binding sites along the actin filament for the myosin filament. As long as there is sufficient ATP, the myosin filaments bind with receptor sites on the actin filaments and cross-bridges are formed. The myosin pulls the actin toward the center and the sarcomere shortens (i.e., the Z lines are pulled closer together) (see Figure 9-20). Because all of the sarcomeres shorten simultaneously, the overall length of the muscle fiber is shortened. If multiple muscle fibers are stimulated to contract at the same time, the entire muscle will contract.

Connective Tissue

Connective tissue is the material between the cells of the body that gives tissues form and strength. This "cellular glue" is also involved in delivering nutrients to the tissue. Connective tissue is made up of dozens of proteins, including **collagen,** the most abundant protein in the body. The two major physical properties of collagen fibers are their **tensile strength** and relative **inextensibility.** In other words, structures containing large amounts of collagen tend to limit motion and resist stretch. Thus, collagen fibers are the main constituents of tissues such as ligaments and tendons that are subjected to a pulling force.

One of the mechanisms behind collagen's great tensile strength and relative inextensibility is its banded, or striated, structure (much like the pattern observed in muscle tissue). When viewed under a microscope, the collagen of a tendon is arranged in wavy bundles called **fascicles.** Each fascicle is composed of fibrils, which in turn consist of bundles of subfibrils. Each subfibril is composed of bundles of collagen filaments. In addition to a striated pattern, connective tissues contain wavelike folds of collagen fibers known as **crimp.** The mechanical properties of collagen fibers are such that each fibril behaves as a mechanical spring. Thus, each fiber is a collection of springs. When a fiber is pulled, its crimp straightens and its length increases. As in a mechanical spring, energy is stored within the fiber, and it is the release of this energy that returns the fiber to its resting state when the stretch force is removed.

Like collagen, structures called elastic fibers are made up of amino acids. The term **elastin** has been used to describe the structural make-up of these extensible fibers. Unlike collagen, elastic fibers are responsible for determining the possible range of extensibility of muscle cells. There is a large amount of elastic tissue in the connective tissue that surrounds the sarcomere. Elastic fibers also are found in numerous other organs and structures, where their roles include disseminating mechanical stress, enhancing coordination, maintaining tone during muscular relaxation, defending against excessive forces, and assisting organs in returning to their undeformed state once all forces have been removed. As their name implies, elastic fibers succumb readily to stretching, and when released they return to their former length.

Similar to other soft-tissue structures, elastic fibers deteriorate with age. Elastic fibers are subject to fragmentation, fraying, and calcification due to the aging process. These alterations may be in part responsible for the loss of resiliency and increased joint rigidity experienced by older individuals.

Elastic fibers are almost always found together with collagen fibers. These two connective tissues work together to support and facilitate joint movement. Elastic fibers are responsible for reverse elasticity (i.e., the ability of a stretched material to return to its original resting state). Collagen, on the other hand, provides the rigidity that limits the deformations of the elastic elements and gives tissues their tensile strength and relative inextensibility. In tissues containing large amounts of collagen, rigidity, stability, tensile strength, and restricted **range of motion (ROM)** are observed.

While various forms of connective tissue are found throughout the body, the structures related most to the practical applications are tendons, ligaments, and fasciae. Tendons are tough, cord-like tissues that connect muscles to bones. Their primary function is to transmit force from muscle to bone, thereby producing motion. Tendons consist of fibrils that are usually oriented toward the direction of normal physiological stress. The amount of deformation that occurs in a tendon when a stretch load is applied is called a load-deformation curve. The wavy bundles of collagen in tendons straighten when a low level of stretch force is applied. Further stretch results in deformation of the tendon that is linearly related to the amount of tension applied. When stretched within a certain range, tendons will return to their original lengths when unloaded. Stretching the tendon beyond its "yield point" results in permanent length changes and microtrauma to the tendon's structural integrity.

Ligaments function primarily to support a joint by attaching bone to bone. Unlike tendons, ligaments take on various shapes, such as cords, bands, or sheets, depending on their location. Ligaments possess a greater mixture of elastic and fine collagenous fibers woven together than their tendinous counterparts. This results in a tissue that is pliant and flexible that allows freedom of movement, but is also strong, tough, and inextensible so as not to yield easily to **applied forces.**

In gross anatomy, fascia is a term typically used to designate all fibrous connective tissue not otherwise specifically named. There are three general categories of fascia. Superficial fascia lies directly below the skin and usually contains a collection of fat. **Deep** fascia lies directly beneath the superficial fascia and is tougher, tighter, and more compact than the superficial fascia. It encases muscles, bones, nerves, blood vessels, and organs. Finally, subserous fascia forms the fibrous layer of serous membranes that cover and support the innermost body cavities. Examples include the pleura around the lungs, the pericardium around the heart, and the peritoneum around the abdominal cavity and organs.

Intramuscular fascia (deep fascia) is directly related to flexibility and ROM. Its three main functions are:

- To provide a framework that ensures proper alignment of muscle fibers, blood vessels, and nerves
- To enable the safe and effective transmission of forces throughout the whole muscle
- To provide the necessary lubricated surfaces between muscle fibers that allow muscles to change shape during contraction and elongation

Human Motion Terminology

Several terms are important to know when discussing human motion. They are usually one-word descriptions of movements, directions, relationships, and positions, so that discussions can be concise. There also are terms for muscle functions and the roles muscles play during movement.

Synergist muscles assist the agonist in causing a desired action. They may act as joint **stabilizers** or may neutralize rotation or be activated when the external resistance increases or the agonist becomes fatigued. The term **co-contraction** describes when the agonist and antagonist contract together to foster joint stability. For example, the torso muscles must be able to stabilize the spine to safely move external resistance, as is the case when the muscles surrounding the vertebrae co-contract to provide this type of stability. When muscles co-contract to protect a joint and maintain alignment, they are called stabilizers.

TYPES OF MUSCULAR ACTION

When a muscle contracts, it develops tension or force as cross-bridges within muscle fibers are formed. There are several types of muscle actions, each of which is named after the muscle's apparent length during the action. A muscle may actually shorten (come together), lengthen (away from the middle), or remain the same length.

Static (Isometric) Action

In an **isometric** action, no visible movement occurs and the resistance matches the muscular tension. The resistance may come from the opposing muscle group (co-contraction) or from another force such as gravity, an immovable object, or weight-training equipment. Bodybuilders use isometric action when striking a pose to show their muscle development, and physical therapists use isometrics in rehabilitation following an injury when limited joint movement is desired. Isometric action also is used in PNF stretching techniques (see Chapter 11). Isometric muscle action can be used in **balance** and stabilization training and may be included in muscular-training programs. Holding the torso upright in neutral position during a modified V-sit exercise (Figure 9-21) and a brief hold at the top of a push-up (see Figure 11-81, page 545) are good examples. If isometric contractions are used, the person must be able to take deep, fluid breaths throughout the individual muscle action.

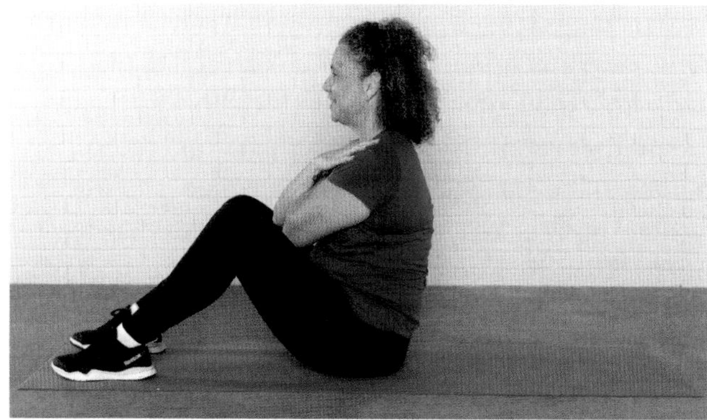

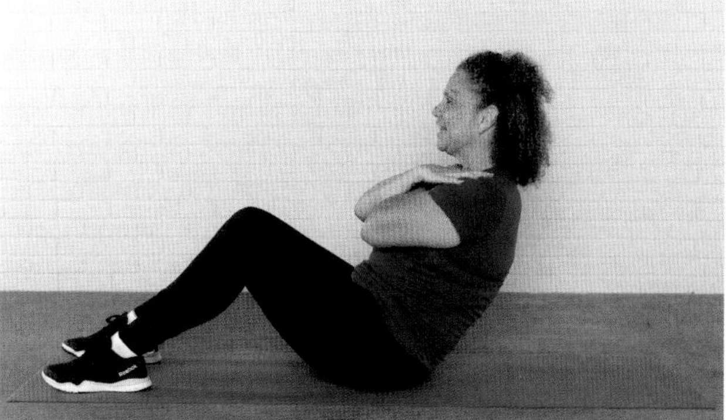

FIGURE 9-21
Modified V-sit exercise

Concentric (Shortening) Action

In a **concentric** action, the muscle shortens and overcomes the resistive force. For example, the biceps brachii act concentrically in the lifting phase of a biceps curl with a dumbbell (Figure 9-22).

Eccentric (Lengthening) Action

In an **eccentric** action, the muscle is producing force and is "lengthening," or returning to its resting length from a shortened position. The muscle "gives in" to, or is overwhelmed by, the external force and can be thought of as "putting on the brakes," or slowing the descent of a weight.

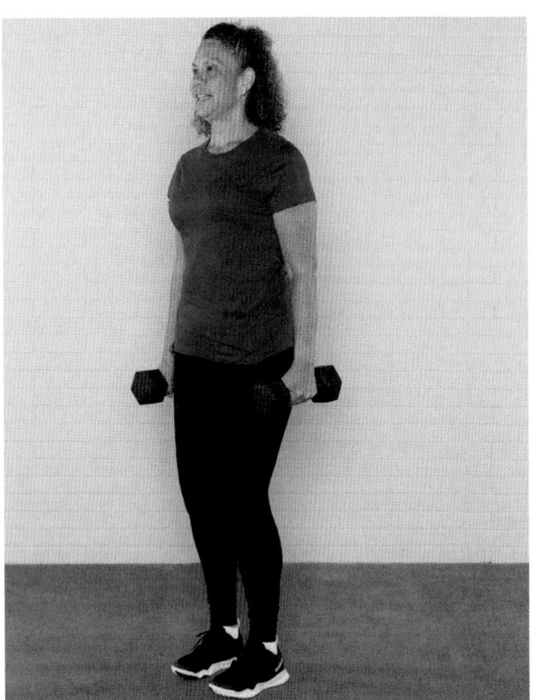
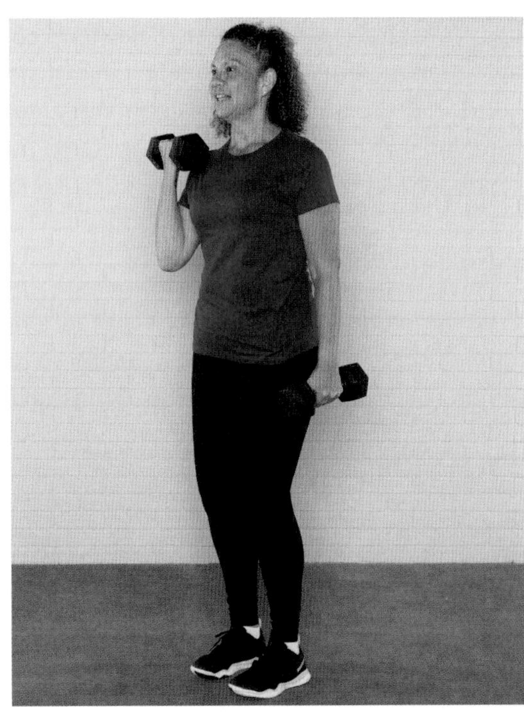

FIGURE 9-22
Biceps curl with a dumbbell

An eccentric action occurs when an external force exceeds the contractile force generated by a muscle. For example, the biceps brachii act eccentrically in the return, or lowering, phase of a biceps curl performed with a dumbbell (see Figure 9-22).

KINETIC CHAIN MOVEMENT

A biomechanical concept that is commonly used in functional training involves the proposition that the body's joints make up a kinetic chain in which each joint represents a link. Drawing on this principle, exercises may be described as either **open-kinetic-chain exercises** or **closed-kinetic-chain exercises.** In a closed-chain movement, the end of the chain farthest from the body is fixed, such as a squat where the feet are fixed on the ground and the rest of the leg chain (i.e., ankles, knees, and hips) moves (Figure 9-23). In an open-chain exercise, the end of the chain farthest from the body is free, such as a seated leg extension (Figure 9-24). Closed-chain exercises tend to emphasize compression of joints, which helps stabilize the joints, whereas open-chain exercises tend to involve more shearing forces at the joints. Furthermore, closed-chain exercises involve more muscles and joints than open-chain exercises, which leads to better neuromuscular coordination and overall stability at the joints.

Optimal performance of movement requires that the body's muscles work together to produce force while simultaneously stabilizing the joints. Typically, people who have weak stabilizer muscles (e.g., deep abdominals, hip stabilizers, and scapular retractors) exhibit problems with performing proper, efficient movement, which may lead to pain and/or injury. Therefore, functional training (or purposeful exercise) that takes advantage of closed-kinetic-chain activity and focuses on the body's stabilizing musculature is often incorporated into rehabilitation and/or post-rehabilitation programs for these individuals.

An example of a program that develops functional strength and ROM is a conditioning routine that incorporates squats, lunges, multidirectional arm reaches, and overhead presses

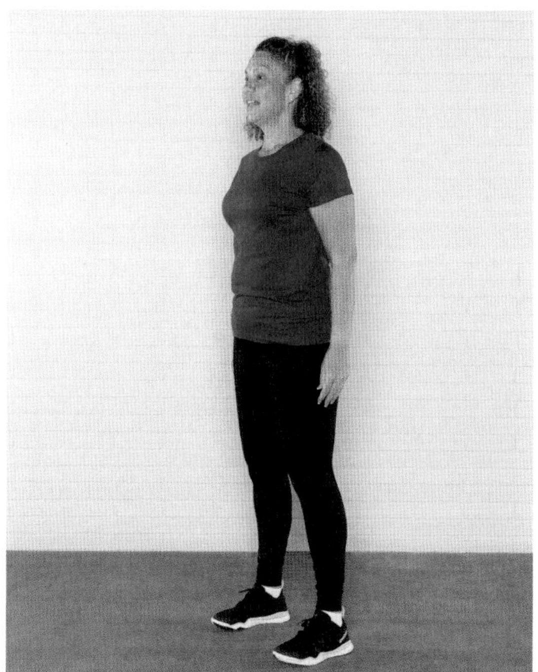
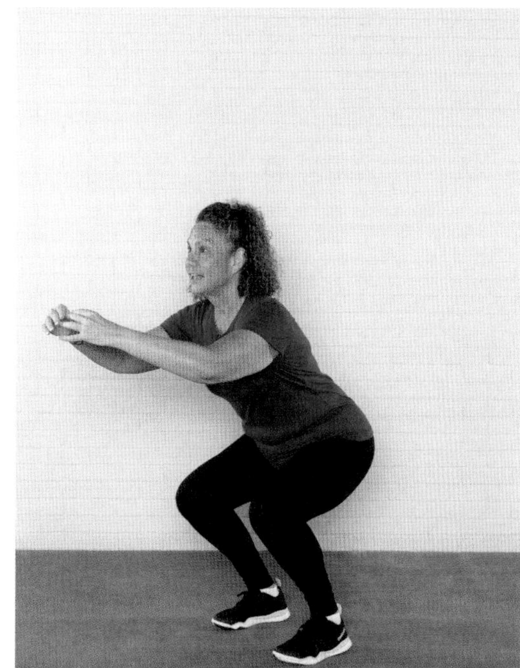

FIGURE 9-23
Closed-chain exercise: Body-weight squat

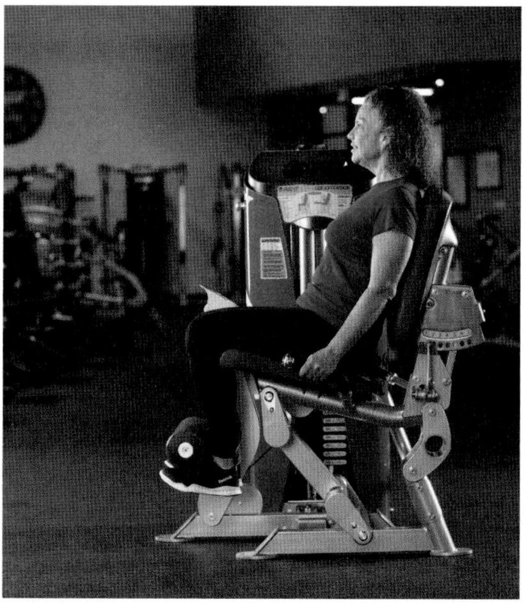
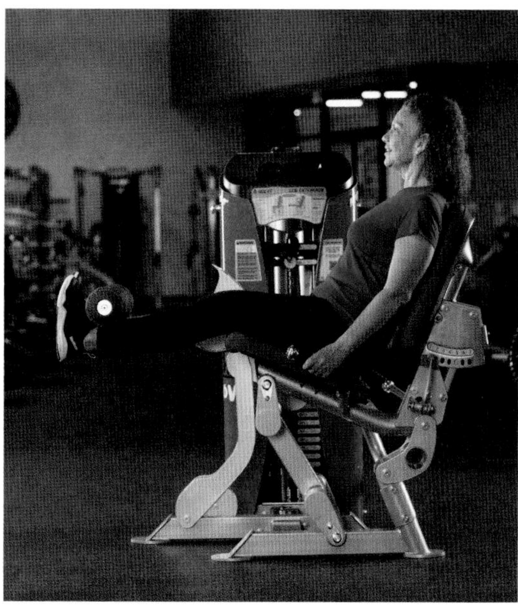

FIGURE 9-24
Open-chain exercise: Seated leg extension

to enhance an older adult's everyday activities. Squatting (see Figure 9-23) and lunging (Figure 9-25) are essential to human movement, as these tasks are required to stand up from a chair or stoop down to pick up a pair of shoes. Multidirectional arm reaches (i.e., reaching one or both arms in front of, to the side of, or behind the body) (Figure 9-26) are important for training balance and postural control during dynamic activities. Balance training is crucial for older adults who find their balance capabilities declining with age. Overhead presses (Figure 9-27) are tied closely to function in older adults because age-associated declines in upper-body strength often make the simplest tasks, such as putting away groceries on a top shelf, a substantial effort.

FIGURE 9-25
Lunge

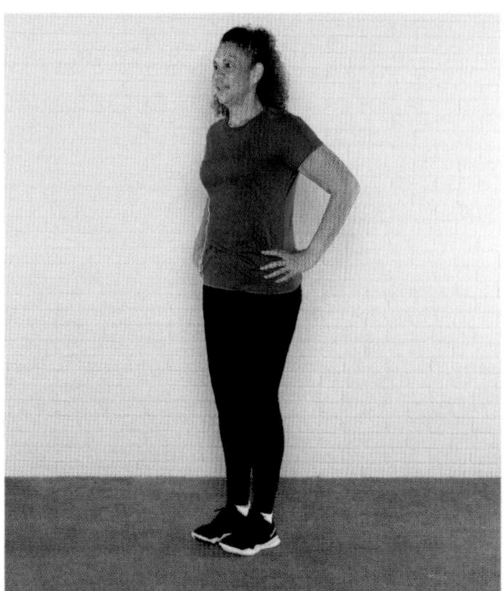
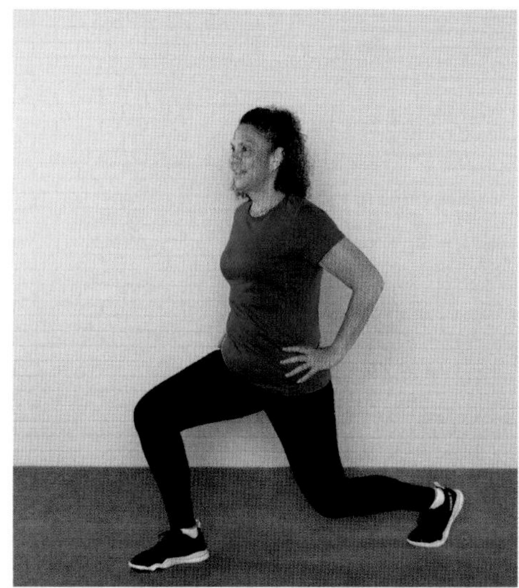

FIGURE 9-26
Multidirectional arm reach

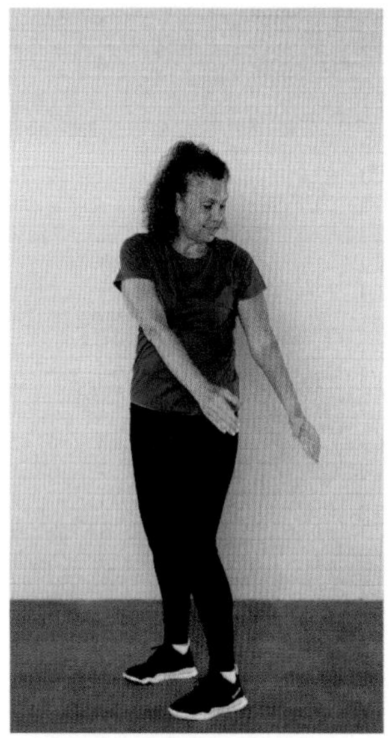
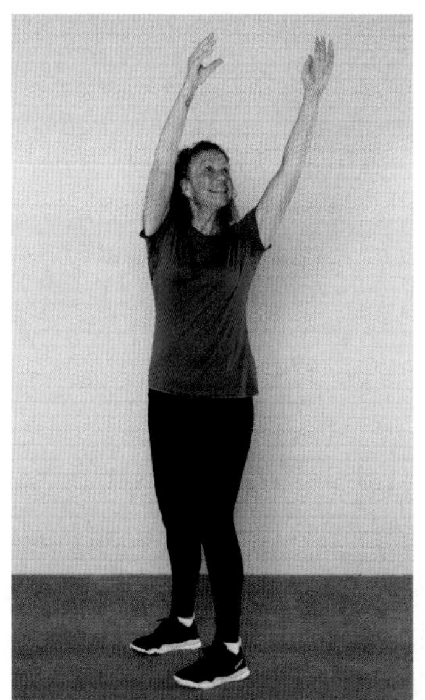
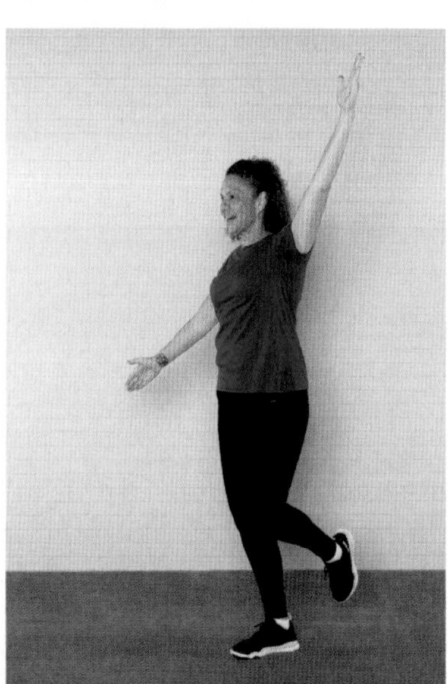

FIGURE 9-27
Overhead press

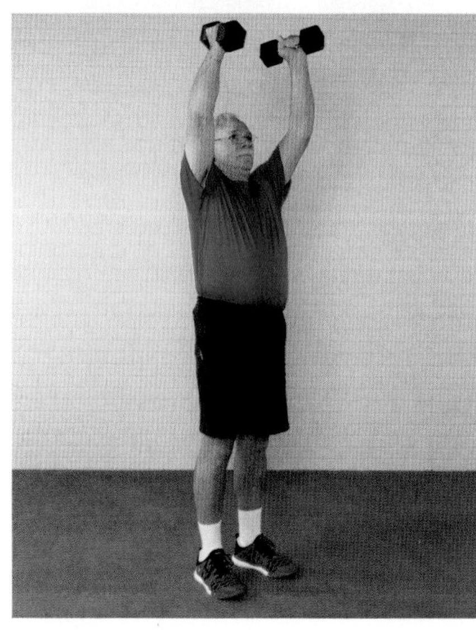

MOBILITY AND STABILITY

Movement involves integrated action along the kinetic chain, where action at one segment affects successive segments within the chain. Joint mobility is the range of uninhibited movement around a joint or body segment. Joint stability is the ability to maintain or control joint movement or position. Both joint mobility and stability are attained by the interaction of all components surrounding the joints and the neuromuscular system. Joint mobility should not be attained by compromising joint stability. Some joints are designed to be more stable than mobile (e.g., foot, knee, lumbar spine, and scapulothoracic), while others are designed to be more mobile than stable (e.g., ankle, hip, thoracic spine, and glenohumeral). Figure 9-28 provides an illustration of the alternating pattern of stable and mobile joints along the kinetic chain, with joints labeled as favoring "stability" or "mobility."

FIGURE 9-28
Mobility and stability of the kinetic chain

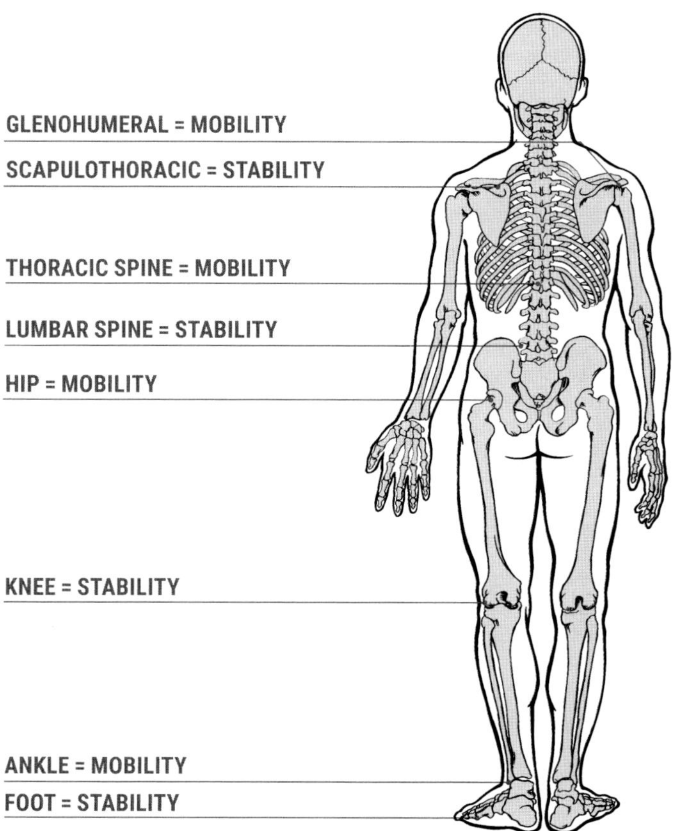

Flawed movement patterns, poor posture, improper exercise technique, and poorly designed exercise equipment may force unnatural joint movements and muscle actions, thereby overtaxing muscles and increasing the potential for muscle imbalance. These types of misalignments and compensated movements due to faulty mechanics may ultimately result in injury. Thus, personal trainers must be especially attuned to each individual's posture and movement patterns to ensure that proper technique is utilized in each exercise session.

BALANCE AND ALIGNMENT

To understand human motion and design appropriate exercise programs, personal trainers must understand several other mechanical principles that relate to the body's balance and alignment: **center of gravity (COG),** the **line of gravity,** and **base of support (BOS).**

Center of Gravity

To track an object's motion, its COG must be identified. In a rigid object of uniform density, like a baseball, this point is at its geometric center. The location of the COG in the human body is more difficult to find. The body's COG is the point at which its mass is considered to concentrate and where it is balanced on either side in all planes (frontal, sagittal, and transverse). Gravity is also exerting its constant downward pull through this point. Thus, a body's center of mass is considered to be its COG.

This point is generally located at the level of the second sacral vertebra, but it changes from person to person, depending on build. It also changes with a person's position in space and depends on whether he or she is supporting external weight. See Figure 9-29 for various locations of a person's COG.

Line of Gravity and Base of Support

Gravity acts on a body in a straight line through its COG toward the center of the earth. This line of gravitational pull is called the line of gravity. To maintain balance without moving, a person's line of gravity must fall within the BOS, the area beneath the body that is encompassed when one continuous line connects all points of the body that are

FIGURE 9-29
Center of gravity

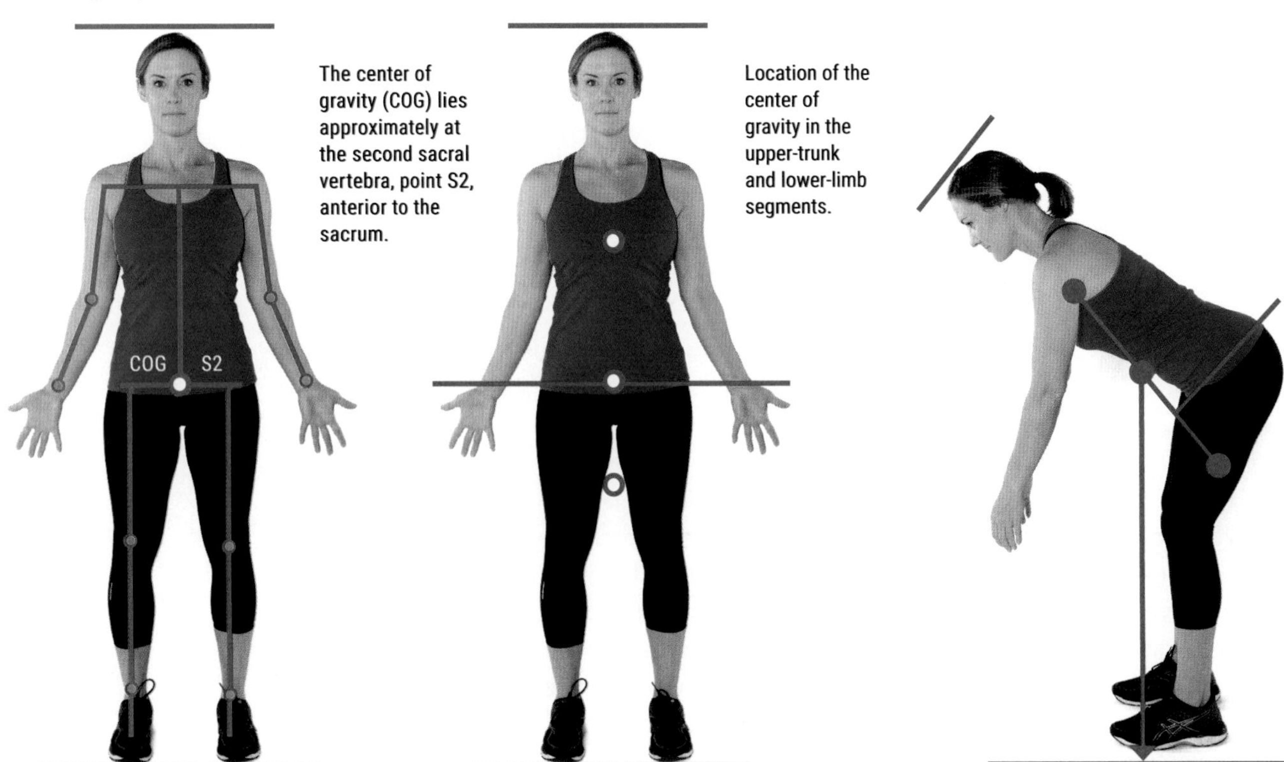

in contact with the ground (e.g., the space between the feet if a person is standing). A large, wide BOS is more stable than a small, narrow one (Figure 9-30). Thus, standing with one's feet apart and toes turned slightly out is more stable than placing them parallel and close together. This is why a person with balance problems will often stand and walk with the feet apart. To work on balance with a client, the personal trainer can make the individual's BOS narrower to stimulate adaptation to the imposed demand.

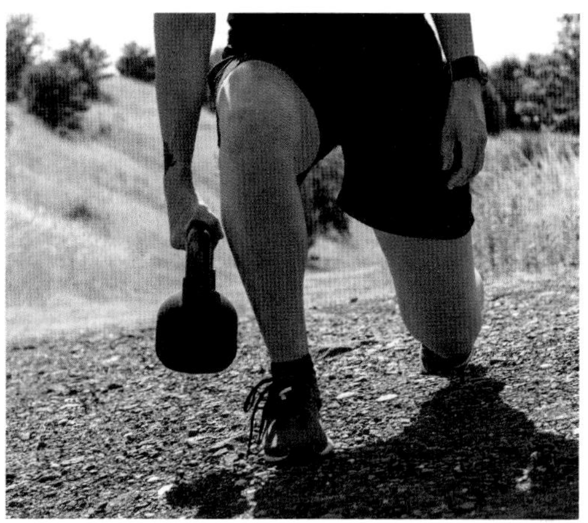

For a person to stand without excessive muscular effort or strain, the body parts must be equally distributed about the line of gravity (within the BOS). Such balanced, neutral alignment prevents excessive stress on muscles and ligaments. An important goal of exercise and training is to stimulate and reinforce neutral, symmetrical alignment about the line of gravity (static balance).

Linear and rotary motion of the whole body (walking, running, or doing a flip or a dive) involve shifting the line of gravity beyond the BOS, then moving to reestablish a new BOS beneath it. The muscles exert forces to rotate and move, then reestablish equilibrium (dynamic balance).

FIGURE 9-29 *(continued)*

The added weight of the suitcase to the shoulder girdle causes the center of gravity to shift up and to the right. The person leans laterally to the left to bring the line of gravity back to the middle of their base of support.

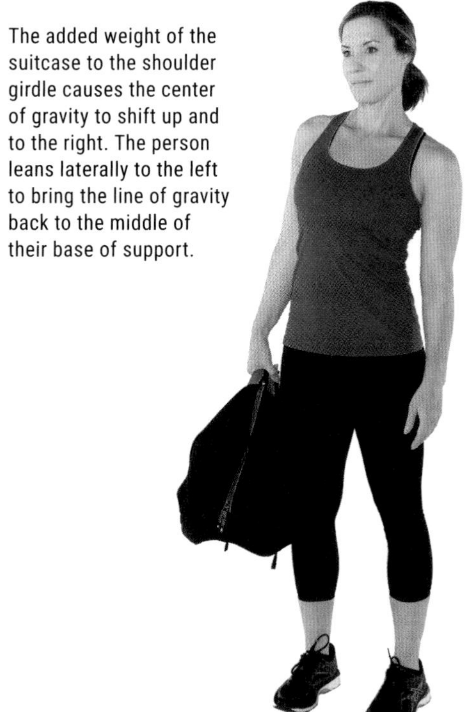

FIGURE 9-30
A wide base of support allows a wide excursion of the line of gravity (LOG) without permitting it to fall outside the base of support.

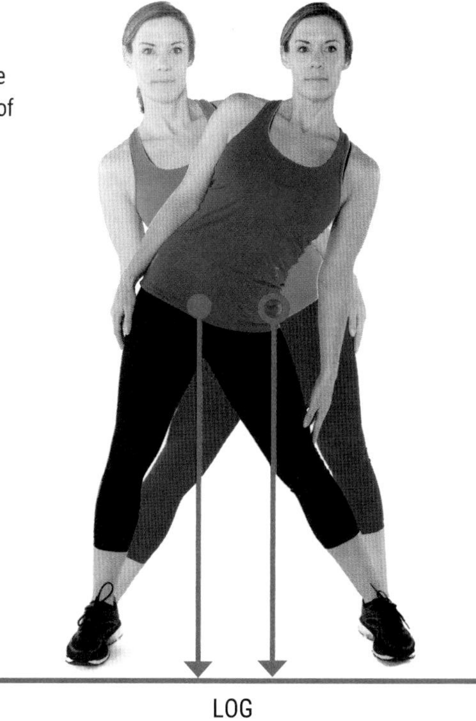

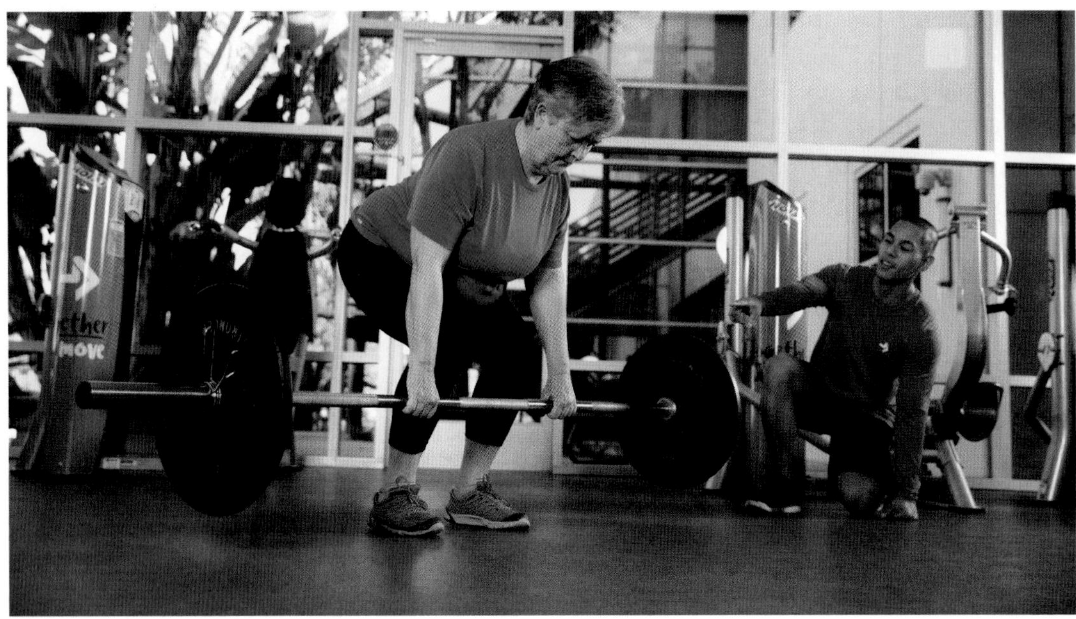

Benefits of Muscular Training

Muscular training is the process of exercising with progressively heavier resistance to stimulate muscle development. The primary outcome of muscular training is an increase in muscle fiber size and contractile strength. Secondary outcomes include increased tensile strength in tendons and ligaments, as well as increased BMD. Properly performed muscular training has a positive impact on the entire musculoskeletal system. While muscular training has obvious implications for improving power production and sports performance, it is equally important from a health and fitness perspective.

INCREASED PHYSICAL CAPACITY

Physical capacity is the ability to perform work or exercise. Muscles utilize energy to produce the forces that enable people to move their body parts and any external resistance, thereby functioning as the engines of the body. Muscular training results in stronger muscles that increase the physical capacity for force production. For example, progressive muscular training enables an individual to perform a single lift with a heavier weightload (**muscular strength**), and to perform more repetitions with a submaximal weightload (**muscular endurance**).

Physical capacity decreases dramatically with age in adults who do not engage in muscular training due to an average 5-pound (2.3-kg) per decade loss of muscle tissue (disuse **atrophy**). Consequently, men and women who want to maintain their physical capacity and performance abilities must make muscular training a regular component of an active lifestyle. Numerous studies have shown that several weeks of traditional muscular training result in about 3.1 pounds (1.4 kg) more muscle, increased **resting metabolic rate (RMR)** of 7%, and 4.0 pounds (1.8 kg) less fat in adults and older adults (Westcott, 2012; Westcott et al., 2009), and these rates of body-composition improvements appear to be maintained for several months (Westcott et al., 2008).

ENHANCED METABOLIC FUNCTION

Muscle tissue is constantly active for purposes of maintenance and remodeling of muscle proteins. Even during sleep, resting skeletal muscles are responsible for more than 25% of the body's calorie use. Logically, the decrease in muscle tissue that results from disuse atrophy is accompanied by a decrease in RMR, and the increase in muscle tissue that results from muscular training is accompanied by an increase in RMR. More specifically, the 5-pound (2.3-kg) per decade muscle loss experienced by adults who do not engage in muscular training leads to a 3 to 8% per decade reduction in RMR (Westcott, 2012). This gradual decrease in metabolism is associated with the gradual increase in body fat that typically accompanies the aging process. When less energy is required for daily metabolic function, calories that were previously used by muscle tissue (that has since atrophied) are stored as fat.

In contrast, muscular training raises RMR and results in more calories burned on a daily basis. Hackney, Engels, and Gretebeck (2008) reported an average 9% increase in resting metabolism for three days after an intense muscular-training workout in untrained individuals, and an average 8% increase in resting metabolism for three days after an intense muscular-training workout in trained individuals. Apparently, the microtrauma-repair and muscle-remodeling processes require increased energy for at least 72 hours following a challenging muscular-training session. As most clients perform muscular training at least every third day, the elevated metabolism would seem to be a continuous physiological response to regular muscular training.

Given a typical RMR of about 1,500 calories per day, an 8% elevation represents 120 additional calories burned at rest on a daily basis. Other things being equal, this would total 3,600 more calories used every 30 days, for a 1-pound (0.5-kg) fat loss per month and a 12-pound (5.5-kg) fat loss per year. While other factors seldom remain the same, it is clear that muscular training can increase muscle mass, decrease fat mass, and raise RMR, effectively countering related degenerative processes of aging. Additionally, the calories used during the muscular-training session and in the post-exercise muscle-remodeling period contribute to fat loss and provide associated health benefits.

REDUCED INJURY RISK AND DISEASE PREVENTION

Muscles serve as shock absorbers and provide stability to the joints. Strong muscles help dissipate the repetitive landing forces experienced in weight-bearing activities such as running and jumping. Balanced muscle development reduces the risk of overuse injuries that result when one muscle group is relatively strong and the opposing muscle group is relatively weak. For example, cycling places greater stress on the hip flexors and quadriceps than the hip extensors and hamstrings, leading to muscle imbalances that may contribute to low-back issues.

To reduce the risk of unbalanced muscle development, personal trainers should include muscular-training exercises for all the major muscle groups, paying special attention to opposing muscles at the joints [e.g., gastrocnemius and anterior tibialis (Figures 9-31 and 9-32), quadriceps and hamstrings (see Figures 9-14 and 9-15), and erector spinae and rectus abdominis (Figures 9-33 and 9-34)]. A comprehensive program of muscular training that addresses all of the major muscle groups may be the most effective means of preventing various musculoskeletal injuries and reducing the risk of many degenerative diseases.

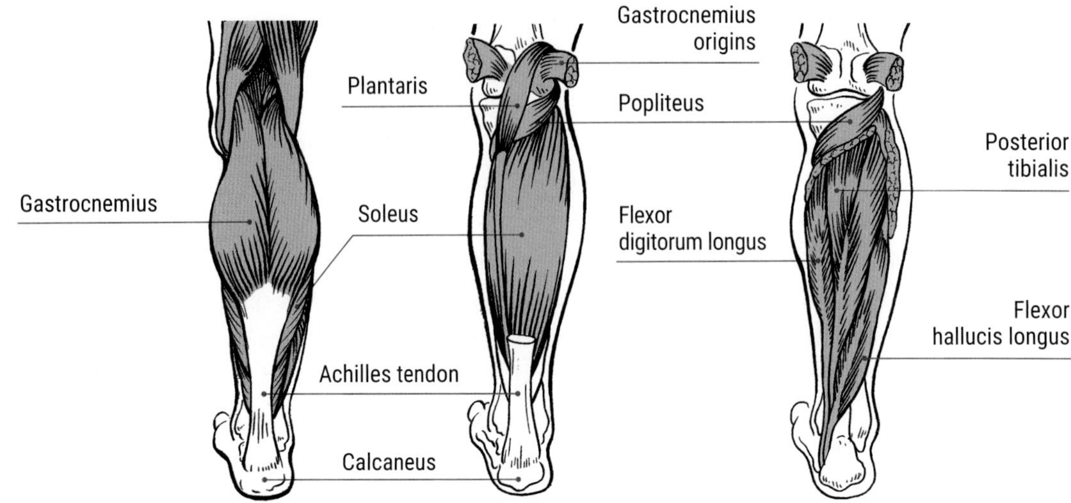

FIGURE 9-31
Triceps surae (i.e., gastrocnemius and soleus) are the posterior tibial compartment muscles primarily responsible for plantar flexion of the ankle.

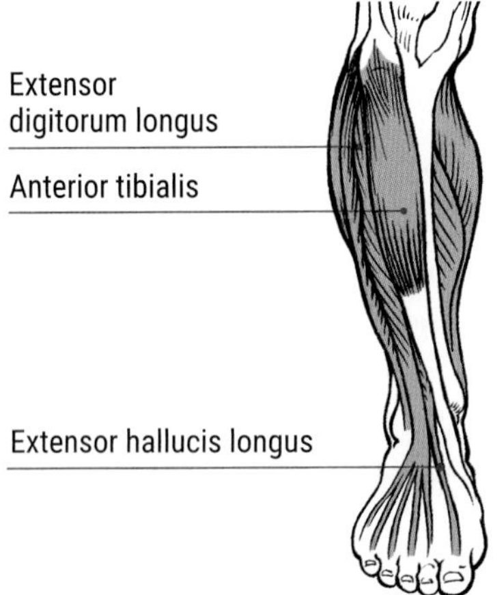

FIGURE 9-32
Anterior tibial compartment muscles—prime movers for dorsiflexion

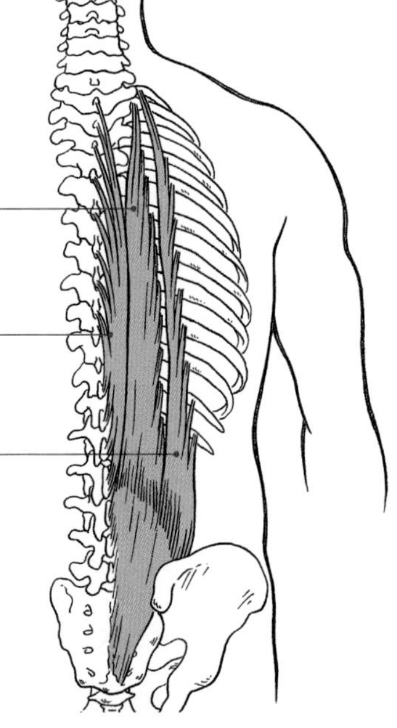

FIGURE 9-33
The erector spinae muscles (posterior view)

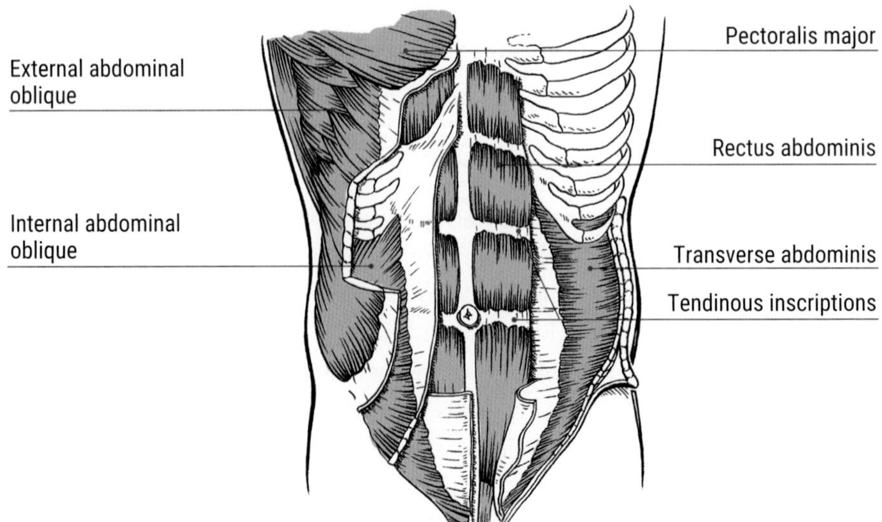

FIGURE 9-34
Muscles of the abdominal wall

One of the most direct benefits of regular muscular training is increased BMD, which may reduce the risk of osteoporosis. Studies have shown a 1 to 3% increase in BMD as a result of a muscular-training program in pre- and postmenopausal women (Westcott, 2016). Other benefits of muscular training include:

- Improved **body composition** (more muscle, less fat), which is associated with a reduced risk of **type 2 diabetes** and **cardiovascular disease (CVD)** (Schwingshackl et al., 2013). With respect to **diabetes,** muscular training has been shown to improve **insulin** response and glucose utilization (Strasser, Siebert, & Schobersberger, 2010). With respect to CVD, muscular training has been demonstrated to lower resting **blood pressure** (Kim & Kim, 2013), improve blood **lipid** profiles (Kelley & Kelley, 2009), enhance vascular function (Kim & Kim, 2013), and improve **metabolic syndrome** risk factors (Normandin et al., 2017).
- Stronger muscles, which appears to be particularly important for low-back health (Smith, Littlewood, & May, 2014)
- Reduced pain of **osteoarthritis** and **rheumatoid arthritis** (Golightly, Allen, & Caine, 2012)
- Decreased prevalence of **depression** in older men and women (Ashdown-Franks et al., 2019)
- Improved functional ability in older adults (Porter Starr, McDonald, & Bales, 2014)

Research has demonstrated numerous health and fitness benefits resulting from regular muscular training. Taken together, these benefits enhance the overall quality of life and lower the risk of premature all-cause **mortality** (Saeidifard et al., 2019).

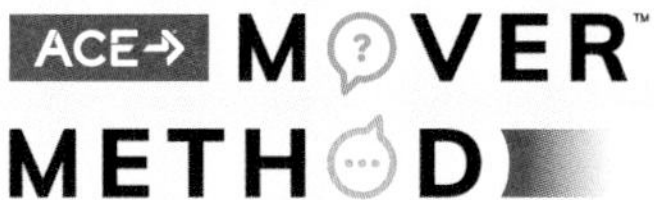

Hesitancy to Add Load

For the past six months, you have been working with a 58-year-old client, Samantha. She currently trains with you three times per week following the ACE IFT Model for Muscular Training. Samantha began her journey with goals to move better, improve balance and posture, and increase mobility in her joints. Samantha has progressed from performing primarily Functional Training movements focusing on core and balance exercises to Movement Training. Here, the emphasis has been on continuing to develop what was accomplished during Functional Training and the development of good control when completing the five primary movement patterns. At this point in her training, Samantha will continue to include exercises specific to the Functional and Movement Training phases of the Muscular Training component of the ACE IFT Model while gradually adding weight to the primary movement patterns. During a training session, you attempt to introduce 5-pound (2.3-kg) hand weights to a bend-and-lift movement pattern and the mood of the exercise session shifts. Samantha's body language and facial expressions change, and it is clear she is not happy about something.

ACE→ABC APPROACH

The following example demonstrates how the ACE ABC Approach™ can be used to explore unique situations that may arise during training sessions.

Ask: Ask open-ended questions to uncover what may have occurred that led to a change in Samantha's demeanor.

Personal Trainer: When I mentioned adding weight to the bend-and-lift pattern exercise, you seemed to hesitate and it looked like you were not too sure about this progression. What caused your hesitation?

Client: I'm happy with the way things are going, and I'm not sure why I need to lift weights when I don't want to be a bodybuilder. The idea of using weights makes me nervous, and I'm not sure I'm ready or that it is even necessary.

Personal Trainer: You enjoy the program as it is, and you don't feel muscular training is important because you don't want to be a bodybuilder.

Client: That's correct. I'm a 58-year-old woman, and I don't want to have big bulky muscles.

Break down barriers: Asking more open-ended questions will enable you to learn about the client's beliefs and hesitations.

Personal Trainer: What do you already know about muscular training and getting bulky?

Client: Well, it seems to me that all the people I see lifting weights get big and muscular, and that is not my goal. Are there other reasons why people lift weights that I am not thinking of? Why do you think it is important for me?

Personal Trainer: Great questions! There are a lot of reasons why people lift weights. One of those reasons may be to get bigger muscles or more defined musculature. Other people might lift weights to increase strength for the activities they do. Some might do it to improve their endurance so they can use their muscles effectively over a long period, or even to maintain or increase muscular power. Weight training is a vital component of slowing the loss of muscle mass that occurs with aging, which can be up to 5 pounds (2.3 kg) of muscle per decade. Other reasons to lift weights would be to increase or maintain BMD to help prevent or combat **osteoporosis.** You could also reduce your risk of injury by becoming stronger through lifting weights. I know this is a lot of information. I don't want to make you feel like it is something you must do. It is up to you to decide if you want to incorporate more resistance into your muscular-training program. Part of my job is to make sure you have all the information you need to make your decision. What else might you want to know about this topic?

Client: I had no idea there was so much to consider. I just thought lifting weights meant you got big. I didn't realize that you lost muscle as you got older! Won't I get bulky if I lift weights?

Personal Trainer: Under natural training conditions, women can enhance muscular strength and size, but they will rarely develop large muscular physiques. Women naturally have lower **anabolic** (muscle building) hormones and less muscle tissue. Even most men have a hard time building big muscles in response to muscular training. Just like in our current program, we would work together, one step at a time, to make sure what we're doing is working. If adding weights to your routine gives you undesired results, we can always just stop.

Client: I'm skeptical, but I'm willing to give it a try, just as long as we can stop at any point if I don't like the way it makes me look or feel.

Collaborate: Work together with the client to determine next steps by partnering with her to decide how she would like to move forward with the introduction of weight to her existing training program.

Personal Trainer: You have my word; you are in control here. I would be doing you a disservice if I didn't give you all the information you need to make the best decision. How would you like to move forward today?

Client: Let's try what you have planned for today and check in at the beginning of our next session to reassess the addition of weight training to my existing program.

Personal Trainer: Great! For your next set of the bend-and-lift movement, we are going to introduce 5-pound (2.3-kg) dumbbells and see how the movement feels and how your body handles the added weight.

Although it may seem like there is not enough time to use the ACE ABC Approach during training sessions, it can be used at any point. Listening to and partnering with your client as soon as a situation arises can add significant value to the experience you are delivering to your client. When you look for coaching moments, you will find them.

Physiological Adaptations to Muscular Training: Acute and Long-term

To perform muscular-training exercises, a number of acute physiological responses must take place. First, nerve impulses must be transmitted from the CNS to activate the appropriate **motor units** and muscle fibers in the prime mover muscles. As the muscle fibers contract to provide the necessary movement force, they use fuel sources such as **creatine phosphate** and **glycogen** for anaerobic energy production. These cellular combustion processes result in metabolic by-products such as hydrogen ions and **lactate.** Acute adaptations to muscular training also occur within the endocrine system. Concentrations of **catabolic** hormones (**cortisol** and **epinephrine**) and anabolic hormones (**growth hormone** and **testosterone**) increase during a muscular training session.

There are two principal long-term physiological adaptations to progressive muscular training: increased muscular strength and increased muscle size (**hypertrophy**). During the first several weeks of training, strength gains are largely the result of neurological factors, which is known as **motor learning.** Repeat performances of a muscular-training exercise result in more efficient activation of the motor units involved in the exercise movement. Motor units that produce the desired movement are facilitated, and motor units that produce the opposing movement are inhibited, thereby resulting in stronger contractions of the prime mover muscles.

Some of the strength gains are the result of muscle hypertrophy. Muscular-training exercise causes varying degrees of muscle tissue microtrauma, depending on the intensity and volume of the training session. During the days following a challenging muscular-training session, muscle tissue remodeling results in growth of muscle fibers coupled with small increases in muscular strength. Satellite cells within the muscle are largely responsible for building larger and stronger muscle fibers. Muscle fibers that have undergone muscular training increase in cross-sectional area as a result of two tissue adaptations. One response to progressive muscular training is an increase in the number of myofibrils (**contractile proteins**) within the muscle fiber. This is referred to as **myofibrillar hypertrophy** and results in greater muscle contraction force.

The second tissue adaptation is an increase in the muscle cell **sarcoplasm** that surrounds the myofibrils but is not directly involved in contractile processes. This is known as **sarcoplasmic hypertrophy** and does not result in greater muscle contraction force, but does increase the cross-sectional area, or size, of the muscle. This form of hypertrophy is related to **transient hypertrophy,** a term denoting the "muscle pump" experienced by many people immediately following muscular training. It is caused by fluid accumulation in the spaces between cells (due to muscle contraction) and it quickly diminishes after exercise as the fluid balance between the various tissues and compartments returns to normal.

FACTORS THAT INFLUENCE MUSCULAR STRENGTH AND HYPERTROPHY

There are several factors that influence the development of muscular strength and size, most of which are genetically determined. These include hormone levels, sex, age, muscle-fiber type, muscle length, limb length, and tendon insertion point.

Hormone Levels

Hormones are produced in the endocrine glands and transported throughout the body by blood circulation. Two hormones associated with tissue growth and development (anabolic processes) are growth hormone and testosterone. Higher levels of these anabolic hormones are advantageous for increasing muscular strength and size. Growth hormone levels are highest during youth and decrease with advancing age. Testosterone is the principal male sex hormone and is largely responsible for the greater size and strength of male muscles compared to female muscles. Testosterone concentrations also decrease with age, which, together with lower growth hormone levels, leads to reduced muscle mass and strength in older adults. Individuals who have higher levels of growth hormone and testosterone typically have enhanced potential for muscle development.

Sex

Male and female muscle tissue is essentially the same with respect to strength production, as each square centimeter (0.4 square inches) of muscle cross-sectional area is capable of

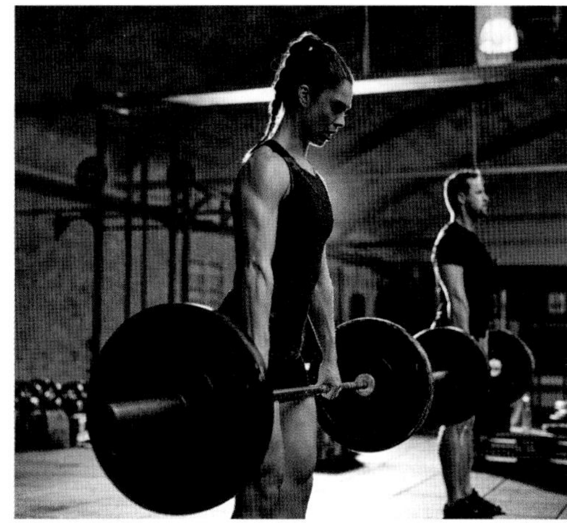

developing 1 to 2 kilograms (2.2 to 4.4 lb) of contractile force. However, while an individual's sex does not affect muscle quality, it does influence muscle quantity. Due to larger body size, higher lean weight percentage, and more anabolic hormones, men typically have greater muscle mass and overall muscular strength than women. For example, in a study of more than 900 men and women, the men were 50% stronger than the women on a standard assessment of quadriceps muscle strength (Westcott, 2016). However, when compared on a pound-for-pound basis of lean (muscle) weight, the average quadriceps muscle force production was almost identical for the male and female subjects.

Age

Advancing age is associated with less muscle mass, leading to a small decrease in RMR, and lower strength levels, at least partly due to lower levels of anabolic hormones. Without muscular training, middle-aged and older adults may experience a loss of 5 to 10% of muscle tissue, a 2 to 3% decrease in RMR, and a 10 to 30% decrease in BMD (Westcott, 2016). Starting at about 30 years of age, strength begins to decline at a rate of about 10 to 15% per decade (Doherty, 2001). Nonetheless, in a study of more than 1,700 men and women, younger adults (20 to 44 years old), middle-aged adults (45 to 64 years old), and older adults (65 to 80 years old) all added statistically similar amounts of lean (muscle) weight after 10 weeks of muscular training (Westcott et al., 2009). It would therefore appear that people of all ages respond favorably to progressive muscular training and gain muscle at approximately the same rate during the initial training period. However, the potential for total-body muscle mass diminishes during the older-adult years.

Muscle-fiber Type

Both type I and type II fibers are involved in muscular training, with the slow-twitch fibers activated at lower force levels and the fast-twitch fibers activated at higher force levels. Likewise, both type I and type II muscle fibers increase in cross-sectional area as a result of muscular training. Because type II muscle fibers experience greater size increases than type I muscle fibers, it would appear that fast-twitch fibers play a larger role than slow-twitch fibers in muscle hypertrophy. This being the case, individuals who are born with higher percentages of type II muscle fibers (e.g., sprinters) may have more potential for muscle hypertrophy than individuals who are born with higher percentages of type I muscle fibers (e.g., marathoner runners). Adaptations to cardiorespiratory and muscular training can create small shifts (<10%) in fiber composition, shifting the number of type IIx fibers to type IIa fibers, while more explosive anaerobic training causes an adaptation where type IIa fibers change to function more like type IIx fibers. Personal trainers should be aware that type I fibers also have the potential for modest hypertrophy. As a result, they should target all muscle fiber types when designing muscular-training programs (Shoepe et al., 2003; Pette, 2001).

Muscle Length

Perhaps the most important factor for attaining large muscle size is muscle length relative to bone length. Muscles typically attach to bones by connective tissues called tendons. Some people have relatively short muscles with long tendon attachments, whereas other people have relatively long muscles with short tendon attachments. Those with relatively long muscles possess greater potential for muscle development than those with relatively short muscles. For example, an individual who has relatively long gastrocnemius muscles with short Achilles tendons possesses more potential to develop large calf muscles than an individual who has relatively short gastrocnemius muscles with long Achilles tendons (see Figure 9-31).

Limb Length

Although limb length does not influence muscle hypertrophy, it definitely affects strength performance. Other things being equal, shorter limbs provide leverage advantages over longer limbs. The relationship between muscle force and resistance force is mediated by leverage factors, as expressed in the following formula:

Motive force (F) x Lever arm of the motive force (Fa) =
Resistance (R) x Lever arm of the resistance (Ra)

The muscle force arm is the distance from the joint axis of rotation to the muscle–tendon insertion point, and the resistance force arm is the distance from the joint axis of rotation to the resistance application point (Figure 9-35). Longer limbs provide longer resistance force arms and require more muscle force to move a given resistance. Conversely, shorter limbs provide shorter resistance force arms and require less muscle force to move a given resistance. Assuming equal biceps muscle strength and tendon insertion points, a person with a shorter forearm can curl a heavier dumbbell than a person with a longer forearm.

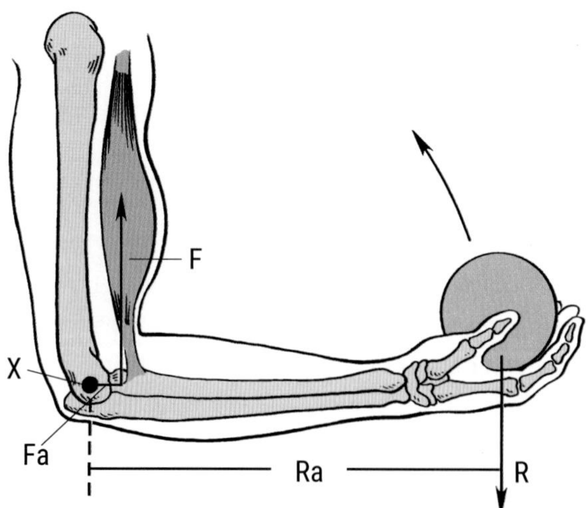

FIGURE 9-35
Example of a lever system in the human body

Note: X = Axis of rotation; F (biceps contraction) = Motive force; R (weight in hand) = Resistance; Fa (biceps force x distance of biceps attachment from axis) = Lever arm of the motive force; Ra (weight x distance from axis) = Lever arm of the resistance

Tendon Insertion Point

Like limb length, the point where the tendon inserts on the bone does not influence muscle hypertrophy, but definitely affects strength performance. Based on the formula presented in the previous section, a longer muscle force arm provides a leverage advantage for moving a heavier resistance. Assuming equal biceps muscle strength and forearm lengths, an individual with a tendon insertion point farther from the elbow joint axis can curl a heavier dumbbell than an individual with a tendon insertion point closer to the elbow joint.

Muscular-training Principles

When muscles are stressed beyond their normal demands, they respond in some way to the imposed stress. If the training stress is much greater than normal, the muscles react negatively to high levels of tissue microtrauma. The resulting (large-scale) cell damage requires several days of muscle repair and rebuilding to regain pretraining strength and functional abilities. Although exceptionally challenging training sessions are typically associated with several days of muscle weakness, fatigue, and discomfort, known as **delayed-onset muscle soreness (DOMS),** they may not lead to larger and stronger muscles. On the other hand, when muscles are systematically stressed in a progressive manner, they gradually increase in size and strength. That is, if the training stress is slightly greater than normal, the muscles respond positively to low levels of tissue microtrauma. The resulting (small-scale) cell damage elicits muscle-remodeling processes that lead to larger and stronger muscles. Research indicates that muscular strength increases significantly above baseline levels 72 to 96 hours after an appropriately stressful session of muscular-training exercise (McLester et al., 2003). However, when the training program no longer produces gains in muscular strength or size, the exercise protocol should be changed in some way to again elicit the desired neuromuscular adaptations.

As mentioned previously, when people with limited muscular-training experience first encounter DOMS, it can create the negative perception that exercise is uncomfortable or painful. It is important to remember to gradually progress exercise intensity and training volume and to not push a new client past his or her current fitness and comfort limits until an ability to adhere to the exercise program has been demonstrated.

PROGRESSION

There are two principal approaches to muscular-training progression. The first and simplest method is to increase the number of repetitions performed with a given resistance (progressive repetitions). This is the standard means for improvement with body-weight exercises. This method works well when a client is working within the repetition ranges specified for each training goal in Table 9-12, page 379, as well as for exercise sets that can be completed using the anaerobic energy system (less than 90 seconds). However, if a client is capable of performing 40 curl-ups (Figure 9-36) in two minutes, increasing the repetitions to 60 in three minutes will have a relatively small effect on abdominal muscle strength.

FIGURE 9-36
Curl-up

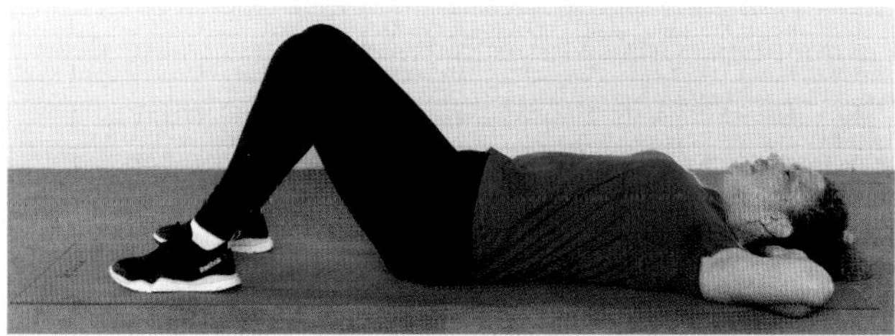

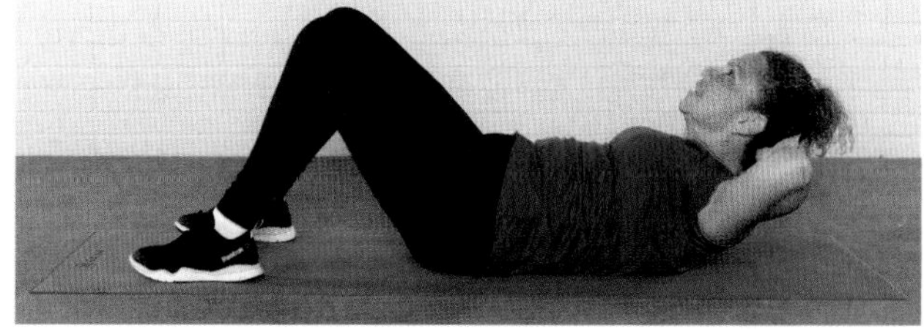

To maximize strength development, the resistance should be heavy enough to fatigue the target muscles within the limits of the anaerobic energy system. This is best achieved by the second method of training progression, which gradually increases the exercise workload (progressive resistance).

By systematically increasing the training resistance, the personal trainer ensures that the exercise set is always completed within the limits of the anaerobic energy system. For example, whenever John can perform incline chest presses for 90 seconds, his weightload is increased by 5%, which reduces his time to muscle fatigue (see Figure 9-44, page 375).

Because it is cumbersome to time each exercise set, repetition ranges provide a more practical means for progressive muscular training. For example, at a movement speed of six seconds per repetition, 10 repetitions would be completed in 60 seconds and 15 repetitions would be completed in 90 seconds. Recommended repetition ranges enable clients to use a **double-progression training protocol** that is effective for strength development and reduces the risk of doing too much too soon.

Assuming a repetition range of 10 to 15 repetitions per set, a double-progression training protocol would be applied in the following manner. Joan can presently perform 10 seated leg presses with 100 pounds (45 kg) (see Figure 11-69, page 537). She continues to train with this weightload until she can complete 15 repetitions with the same weightload. At that point, her exercise resistance is increased by 5% to 105 pounds (48 kg). The heavier weightload reduces the number of leg presses that she can perform to 12 repetitions. She continues to train with 105 pounds (48 kg) until she can again complete 15 repetitions, at which point she increases the weightload another 5% to 110 pounds (50 kg) with an initial goal of 12 repetitions.

The double-progression muscular-training protocol may be used with any repetition range. The first progression is adding repetitions, and the second progression is adding resistance in 5% increments. There is no time limit on double-progression protocol training. Whether it takes one week or one month, the resistance is increased only when the end-range number of repetitions can be completed with proper form.

As a general guideline, a training range of eight to 12 is recommended [American College of Sports Medicine (ACSM), 2018]. Most people can complete eight repetitions with approximately 80% of maximal resistance and 12 repetitions with about 70% of maximal resistance. Progressively training to muscle fatigue with 70 to 80% of maximal resistance represents an anaerobic exercise bout that provides an effective muscle-conditioning stimulus. Another benefit of progression is that a properly organized program allows a client to experience strength gains, which is critical for developing **self-efficacy** and long-term **adherence.**

SPECIFICITY

The principle of training **specificity** has many applications for achieving desired muscular-training objectives. The most obvious aspect of training specificity is to exercise the appropriate muscles. For example, if a client wants to improve his or her rope climbing ability, the prime mover muscles for this activity based on the pulling movement are the latissimus dorsi, teres major, biceps brachii, and forearm flexors (Figures 9-37 and 9-38; see Figure 9-18). Specific muscular-training exercises for strengthening these muscles

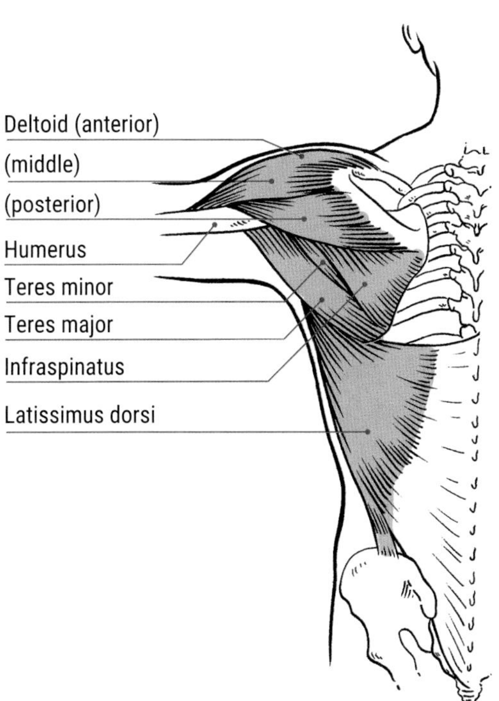

FIGURE 9-37
Superficial musculature of the superior and inferior shoulder joint, prime movers for shoulder abduction (deltoid) and adduction (latissimus dorsi and teres major)

FIGURE 9-38
Muscles of the wrist

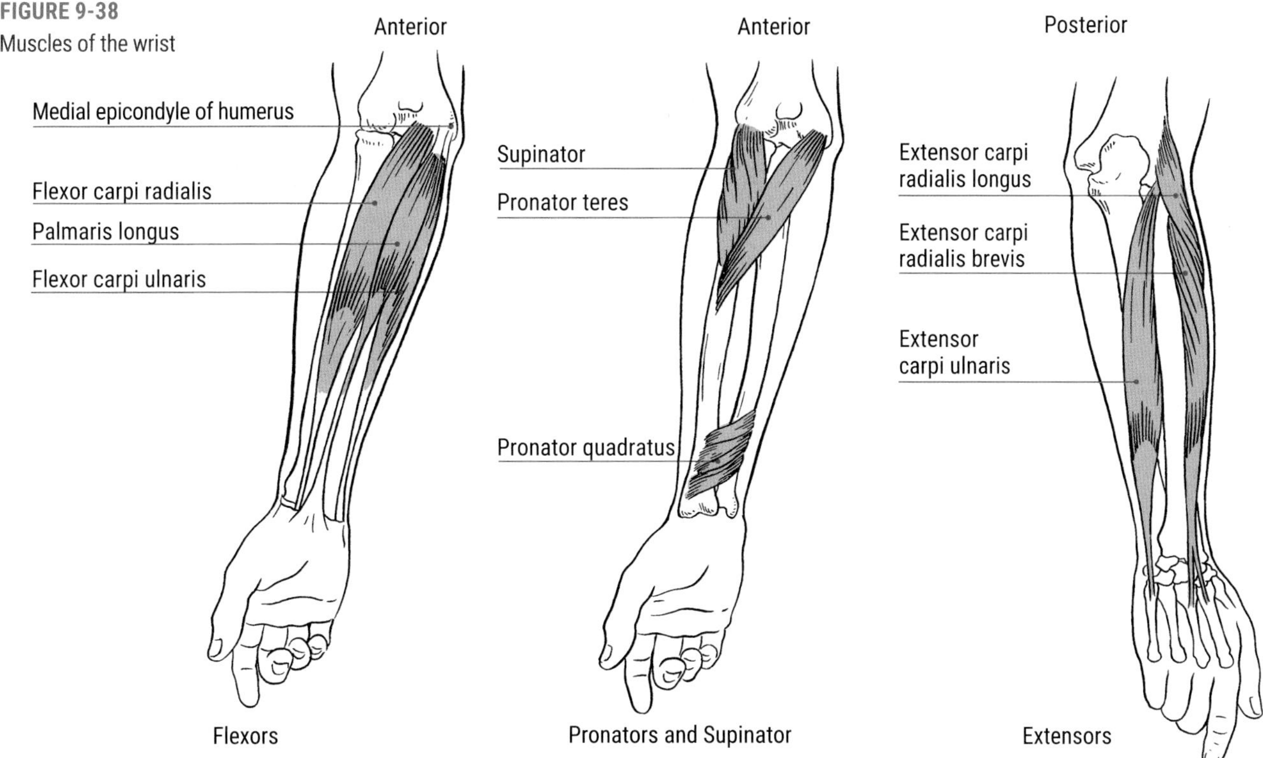

include lat pull-downs, chin-ups, and seated rows (Figures 9-39 through 9-41). Of course, to maintain balanced muscle development, these muscles should not be trained to the exclusion of exercises for the opposing muscle groups responsible for pushing movements (e.g., pectoralis major, deltoids, and triceps brachii; Figure 9-42; see Figures 9-18 and 9-37).

FIGURE 9-39
Lat pull-down

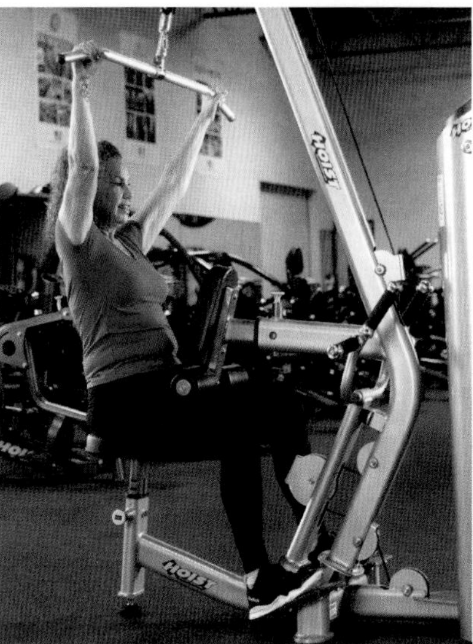

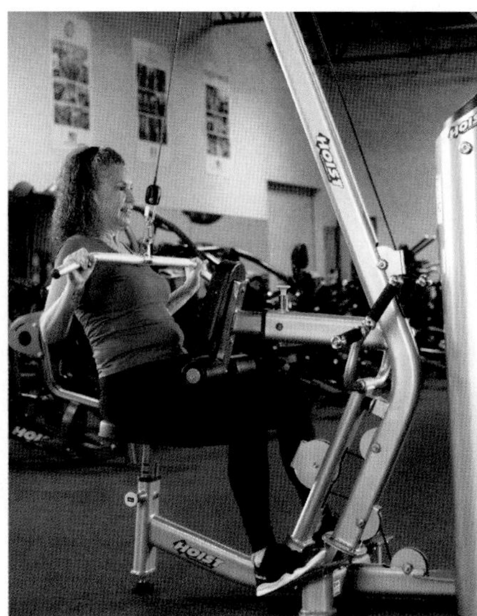

FIGURE 9-40
Chin-up

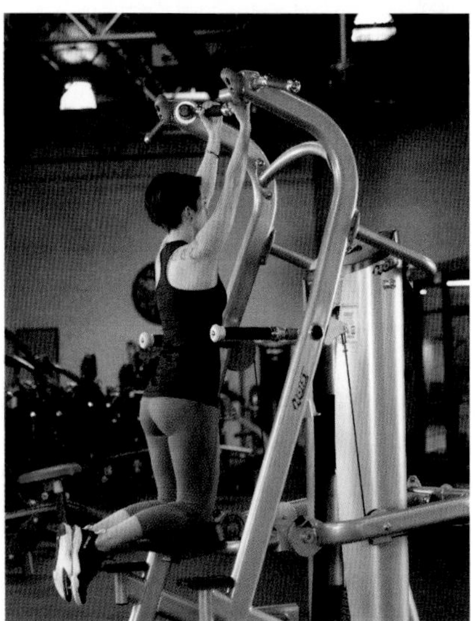

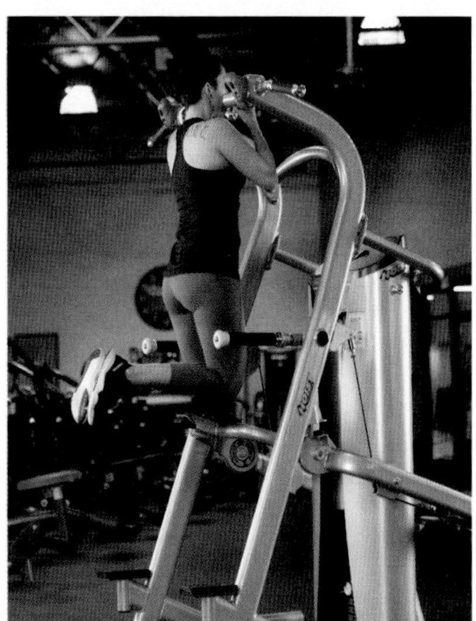

FIGURE 9-41
Seated row

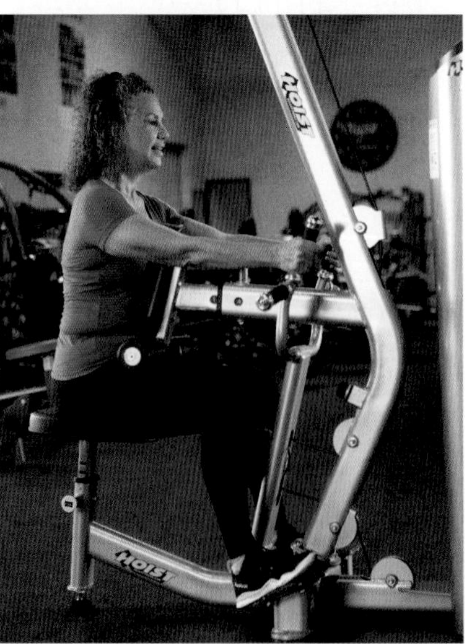

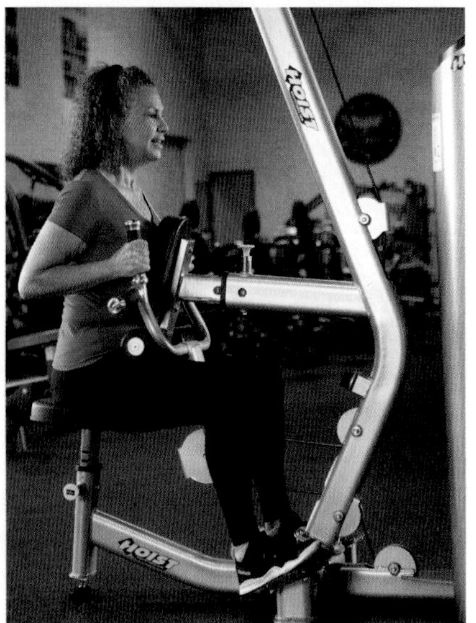

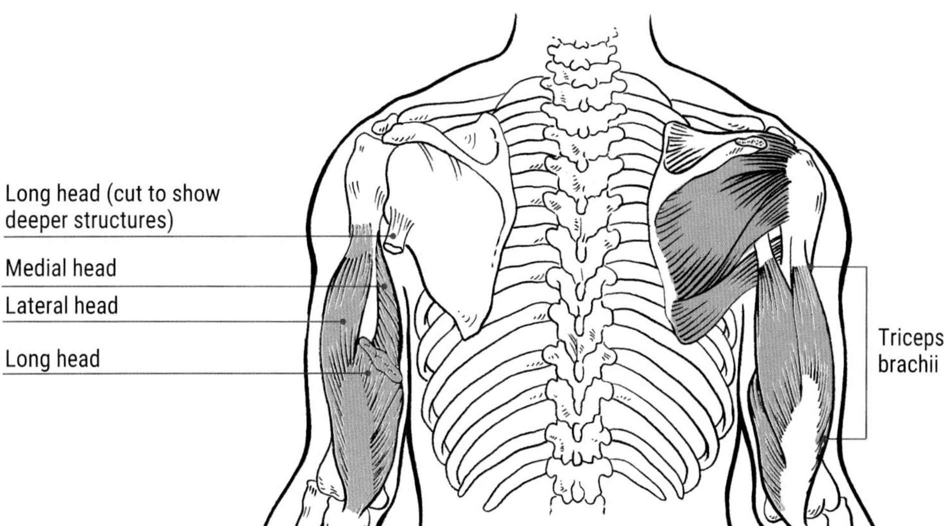

FIGURE 9-42
Triceps: long, medial, and lateral heads

While it is essential to emphasize the specific movements and muscles used in a particular activity, it is equally important to train all of the major muscle groups to reduce the risk of muscle imbalance and overuse injuries.

Another aspect of training specificity is to use appropriate resistance–repetition protocols. For example, a shot putter, whose event requires a one-time maximal effort, should typically train with heavier weightloads and fewer repetitions to emphasize muscular strength development. On the other hand, a rower whose event requires several minutes of strenuous muscular activity should typically train with moderate weightloads and more repetitions to emphasize the development of muscular endurance. Although there is a strong, positive relationship between muscular strength and endurance, specifically designed training protocols are advisable for athletes whose events require greater emphasis on either end of the strength–endurance continuum. The resistance–repetition protocol also affects the energy system that is most prominent during the exercise set. For example, a set of two repetitions performed in 10 seconds primarily uses creatine phosphate for energy, whereas a set of 15 repetitions performed in 75 seconds attains most of the energy from **anaerobic glycolysis.**

OVERLOAD

Muscular endurance can be increased by performing more repetitions with a given resistance, such as by doing more push-ups (see Figure 11-81, page 545). However, to maximize strength development, muscles must be subjected to progressively heavier training loads.

The process of gradually adding more exercise resistance than the muscles have previously encountered is referred to as **overload.** While the degree of overload should be individually determined, a general guideline is to increase the resistance in gradations of about 5%. As presented earlier, a range of eight to 12 repetitions represents approximately 70 to 80% of maximal resistance, which provides an effective training overload, assuming the exercise is continued to the point of muscle fatigue. Once 12 repetitions can be completed, it is advisable to add about 5% more resistance to provide progressive overload and facilitate further strength development. Of course, the overload principle may be applied to other resistance–repetition protocols. Clients training with four to eight repetitions per set should add about 5% more resistance after completing eight repetitions, and those training with 12 to 16 repetitions per set should increase the weightload by 5% after completing 16 repetitions.

REVERSIBILITY

The principle of muscle **reversibility** reinforces the importance of muscular training as a lifestyle component, rather than as a short-term process for attaining a temporary objective. Without muscular training, muscles gradually become smaller and weaker. With progressive muscular-training exercise, regardless of age, muscles increase in size and strength at relatively rapid rates (Westcott et al., 2009). Indeed, an ACE-sponsored research study demonstrated that older individuals experienced similar chest press and leg press five-repetition maximum (5-RM) improvements relative to their younger counterparts following eight weeks of personalized Muscular Training according to the ACE IFT Model (Montano et al., 2018).

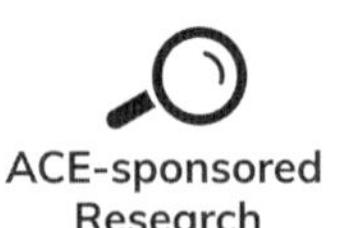

On the other hand, a client who stops performing regular muscular-training exercise will rapidly lose muscle strength. For instance, in an ACE-sponsored study, it was found that muscular strength (as quantified by chest press and leg press 5-RM) decreased significantly with cessation of regular muscular training (Nolan et al., 2018). In fact, with four weeks of detraining, two-thirds of the favorable muscular-strength gains that had been obtained with 13-weeks of Muscular Training according to the ACE IFT Model were abolished (Nolan et al., 2018). Elsewhere, research looking at the effects of detraining on lower-extremity strength in older adults aged 60 to 74 years old suggests that after participating in a high- or moderate-intensity muscular-training program, participants may experience an 18 to 27% decrease in 1-RM strength after 12 weeks of detraining but do not reach pretraining levels, reflecting that some strength improvements are retained (Tokmakidis et al., 2009). Another study looking at upper-body muscular strength in middle-aged adults and detraining also showed that reversibility occurred and 5-RM and local muscular endurance decreased. However, these outcomes did not decrease to pretraining values, again demonstrating that some strength gains were retained (Bezerra et al., 2019).

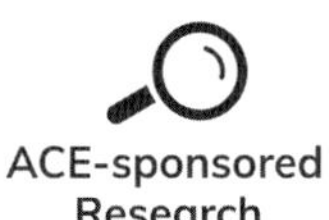

DIMINISHING RETURNS

As clients approach their genetic potential for muscle size and strength, the rate of development decreases accordingly. Regardless of the quality and quantity of training, genetic limitations leave little room for further improvement. The phenomenon of **diminishing returns** can be discouraging to clients who want to attain additional strength gains. One means for addressing this situation, sometimes referred to as a strength plateau, is to change the training exercise. The introduction of a new exercise involves a new neuromuscular stimulus and motor-unit activation pattern that facilitates a period of progressive strength gains. For example, if a client encounters a strength plateau in the chest press exercise (Figure 9-43), it may be helpful to switch to the incline chest press exercise (Figure 9-44). Although both exercises target the pectoralis major, anterior deltoid, and triceps muscles (see Figures 9-18, 9-37, and 9-42), the slight exercise variation offered by the incline chest press can provide a new challenge to stimulate continued improvement.

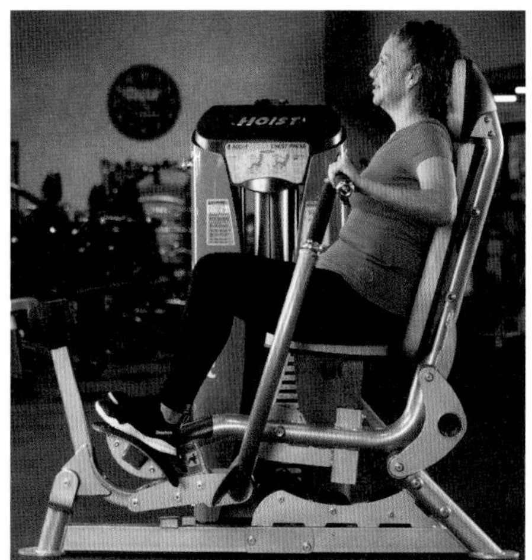
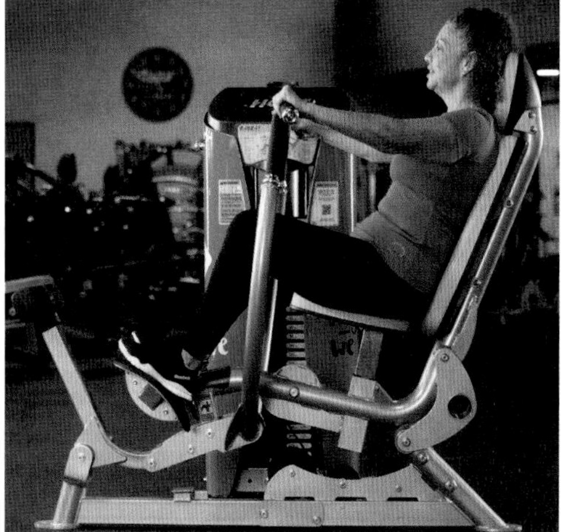

FIGURE 9-43
Chest press

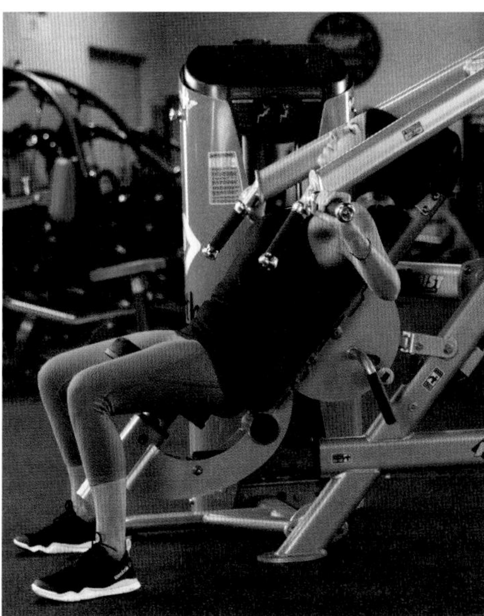
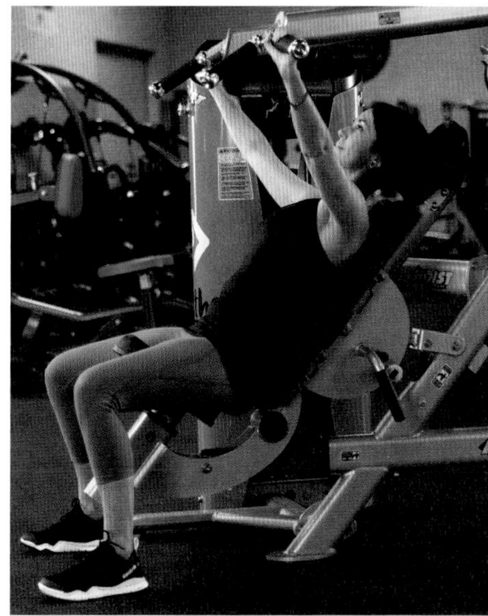

FIGURE 9-44
Incline chest press

Muscular-training Variables Related to Program Design

The design of effective programs requires consideration of several factors and programming variables, including the following:

- A thorough needs assessment on the client
- Appropriate exercise frequency consistent with the client's goals, training experience, current conditioning level, and necessary recovery periods between sessions
- Appropriate exercises and exercise order consistent with program needs and goals, equipment availability, client experience, technique, and conditioning level
- The exercise volume and load—sets, repetitions, and intensity
- The appropriate rest intervals between sets selected according to the client's needs and goals

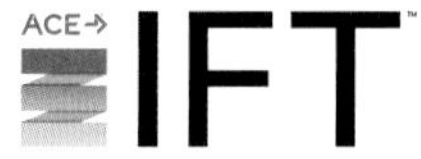

The ACE IFT Model is a comprehensive system for exercise programming that incorporates the multifaceted Muscular Training variables described in this and other chapters that are required to be a successful personal trainer (Figure 9-45). It organizes the latest exercise science

FIGURE 9-45
ACE IFT Model Muscular Training phases

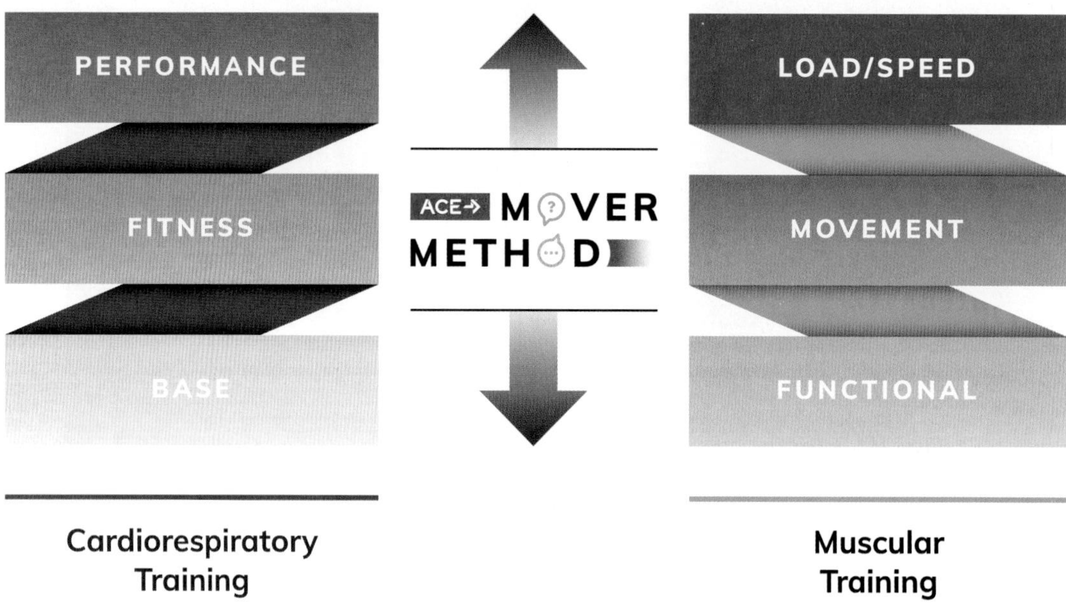

and health-behavior research into a systematic approach to designing, implementing, and modifying exercise programs based on the unique abilities, needs, and goals of each individual. While the general foundational principles of Muscular Training program design are described in the following sections, the ACE IFT Model is expanded upon and detailed further in Chapter 11.

NEEDS ASSESSMENT

Personal trainers can conduct a needs assessment with each client to determine what the appropriate program will entail. The personal trainer should identify what physiological parameters need to be included in the program to achieve success with respect to the client's goals. To complete the needs assessment, the personal trainer should consider the following:

- Evaluation of the goal activity or sport
  - Movement analysis (What movement patterns, speeds, and muscle activation are needed? What mobility, stability, and balance are required? Does it involve job-related movements or activities of daily living?)
  - Physiological analysis (Which energy systems are utilized? Does the activity require muscular endurance, hypertrophy, strength, or power?)
  - Injury analysis (What are prevalent injuries associated with participation in this activity or sport?)
- Individual assessment
  - Current conditioning level
  - Training history and technique
  - History of injury or fear of injury
  - Tolerance for discomfort

Personal trainers who are unfamiliar with a particular activity or sport would be best served to reach out to peer exercise professionals who know the activity, establish communication with some higher-level coaches and athletes, and connect with medical professionals who can provide valuable insight and information into completing the needs assessment.

TRAINING FREQUENCY

Training frequency is inversely related to both training volume and training intensity. Less vigorous exercise sessions produce less muscle microtrauma, require less time for tissue remodeling, and can be performed more frequently. More vigorous exercise sessions produce more muscle microtrauma, require more time for tissue remodeling, and must be performed less frequently for optimal results. Research has revealed that a challenging muscular-training workout elevates RMR by 8 to 9% for three days following the exercise session, presumably due to muscle-building processes (Hackney, Engels, & Gretebeck, 2008). Other studies have shown that standard muscular-training sessions (eight exercises, three sets of 10 repetitions) require at least 72 hours for muscular strength to attain or exceed baseline levels (McLester et al., 2003).

It would therefore appear that advanced exercisers who perform high-volume/high-intensity muscular-training workouts should not train the same muscle groups more frequently than every third day. For example, they could perform workouts that emphasize pushing movements with the chest, shoulders, and triceps on Mondays and Thursdays, workouts that focus on pulling movements with the back, biceps, and trunk on Tuesdays and Fridays, and squatting and lunging movements with the legs on Wednesdays and Saturdays.

On the other hand, a large-scale study on exercise frequency demonstrated similar muscular development for beginning clients who trained two or three days per week. After 10 weeks of basic muscular-training exercise, both training frequencies increased the subjects' lean (muscle) weight by 3.1 pounds (1.4 kg) (Westcott, 2016). Based on these results, two or three weekly muscular-training sessions work equally well for new exercisers, and the choice should be a matter of personal preference. The same study examined the effects of one weekly muscular-training workout on muscle development. Although marginally productive, the one-day-per-week training frequency resulted in significantly less lean (muscle) weight gain than the two-days-per-week and three-days-per-week training frequencies. It is therefore recommended that new exercisers perform resistance training two or three days a week for best results.

EXERCISE SELECTION AND ORDER

Determining exercise selection and order is a complex process that requires consideration of the individual's experience and exercise technique, movement and physiological demands of the activity or sport, equipment availability, and time availability. While hundreds of muscular-training exercises exist, one effective method of exercise selection is to group exercises based on body area (e.g., legs or shoulders) or function (e.g., push versus pull), or by relevance to the activity or sport.

- Primary exercises involve multiple muscles from one or more of the larger muscle areas (e.g., chest or thigh) that span two or more joints (i.e., multijoint exercises) and are generally performed in a linear fashion. Examples include the squat (see Figure 9-23) and overhead press (see Figure 9-27), which involve integrated muscle actions and joint movements working in the same direction.

- Assisted exercises involve smaller muscle groups from more isolated areas that span one joint (i.e., single-joint).

Personal trainers often design programs by grouping specific muscles into a session. While various strategies exist, the muscle grouping should ultimately reflect the specific needs of the client and his or her availability for training. Guidelines from ACSM (2018) recommend targeting each major muscle group two to three days a week, allowing a minimum of 48 hours of recovery between sessions. Therefore, training twice per week may require the use of circuits that target all the major muscle groups within a session, whereas training with greater frequency allows the trainer flexibility to divide sessions into body parts.

Personal trainers can select from a variety of methods to enhance muscle hypertrophy or improve muscular endurance, strength, and power. Some of these options include:

- Performing single-joint exercises followed by accessory exercises within a targeted area
  - This may entail performing single-joint rotary exercises [e.g., movements around one joint—seated leg extension (see Figure 9-24), standing reverse cable fly (see Figure 11-68, page 537), and biceps curl (see Figure 9-22)], followed by multijoint linear exercises [e.g., movement collaboration of several joints moving resistance in one direction—squats (see Figure 9-23), chest press (see Figure 9-43), and overhead press (see Figure 9-27)].
- Alternating upper- and lower-extremity exercises within or between training sessions
- Grouping pushing and pulling muscles within a session (e.g., chest, shoulders, and triceps in a session)
- Alternating pushing and pulling movements or targeting joint agonists and antagonists within a session (e.g., chest muscles and back muscles or biceps and triceps)
- Performing **supersets** or **compound sets** where exercises are done in sequence with little or no rest between them, before an appropriate rest interval is taken (see page 381)
- Performing a muscular-training circuit in which each exercise addresses a different muscle group (see page 290)

TRAINING VOLUME

During each muscular-training session, a certain amount of work is performed. The cumulative work completed is referred to as the training volume. Training volume is calculated in several ways:

- *Repetition-volume calculation:* Volume = Sets x Repetitions (for either the muscle group or the session)
- *Load-volume calculation:* Volume = Exercise weightload x Repetitions x Sets (and then summing the total for each muscle group or the entire session)

Although training volume is an excellent measure of how much work was performed, it may not be an accurate assessment of how hard a person truly worked. For example, Mary can complete four seated leg presses (see Figure 11-69, page 537) with 90 pounds (40.9 kg), eight leg presses with 80 pounds (36.4 kg), and 12 leg presses with 70 pounds (31.8 kg). Although each set requires a high effort and produces similar levels of muscle fatigue (e.g., no additional repetitions can be performed), the training volume varies considerably. Note: Due to rounding error, pound to kilogram values in this example are not exact.

- 1 set x 4 repetitions with 90 pounds (40.9 kg) = 360 pounds (163.6 kg)
- 1 set x 8 repetitions with 80 pounds (36.4 kg) = 640 pounds (290.9 kg)
- 1 set x 12 repetitions with 70 pounds (31.8 kg) = 840 pounds (381.8 kg)

Training volume provides a reasonably good indication of the energy used in a workout, as there is a correlation between the total amount of weight lifted and the total number of calories burned. It is recommended that training volume be changed periodically for physiological and psychological purposes. Training volume is typically lower for competitive powerlifters who perform fewer exercises, repetitions, and sets with heavier weightloads as they focus on improving the muscle's ability to maximally recruit fibers to generate higher amounts of force. Competitive bodybuilders, on the other hand, perform higher-volume workouts with more exercises, repetitions, and sets with moderate weightloads as they focus on increasing the amount of time the muscle spends under tension performing work to stimulate hypertrophy. While each individual's training goals dictate the training volume needed, his or her fitness status provides a good indicator of the appropriate volume. Therefore, personal trainers should consider starting deconditioned or novice clients with manageable volumes prior to progressing their volume to the ranges outlined in Table 9-12.

TABLE 9-12

Training Volume Based on Goal

Training Goal	Sets	Repetitions	Rest Interval	Intensity
General muscular fitness	1–4	8–15	2–3 minutes	20–70% 1-RM
Muscular endurance	2–3	≥12	≤30 seconds	≤67% 1-RM
Muscular hypertrophy	3–6	6–12	30–90 seconds	67–85 1-RM
Muscular strength	2–6	≤6	2–5 minutes	≥85% 1-RM
Power:				
Single-effort events	3–5	1–2	2–5 minutes	80–90% 1-RM
Multiple-effort events	3–5	3–5	2–5 minutes	75–85% 1-RM

Note: 1-RM = One-repetition maximum

The 1-RM load for muscular strength applies to core exercises (e.g., involve large muscle groups and two or more primary joints). Assistance exercises involving small muscle groups and only one primary joint should be limited to loads ≥8-RM.

This table is based on weightlifting-derived movements (e.g., snatch and clean) and the power goal repetitions are not consistent with the %-1RM relationship. In nonexplosive movements, loads of about 80% 1-RM are used in the 2–5 repetitions range.

Sources: American College of Sports Medicine (2018). *ACSM's Guidelines for Exercise Testing and Prescription* (10th ed.). Philadelphia: Wolters Kluwer; Haff, G.G. & Triplett, T.N. (2016). *Essentials of Strength and Conditioning* (4th ed.). Champaign, Ill.: Human Kinetics.

As a client begins a muscular-training program and is in the transition from the **preparation** to the **action** stages of behavioral change (see Chapter 3), the total training volume should be kept relatively low to allow for adaptation and accommodation to the training stress. Another benefit of keeping the training volume low during the initial stages of an exercise program is to allow the client to feel successful after accomplishing the goal of performing a specific volume of training. Training volume can be gradually increased as the client develops adherence to the program, becoming stronger as a result.

TRAINING INTENSITY

Training intensity has two different applications in the area of muscular training. Some experts define training intensity as the percentage of maximal resistance used in an exercise. They would consider four repetitions with 90 pounds (40.1 kg) to be a higher-intensity training bout than eight repetitions with 80 pounds (36.4 kg), even if each exercise set produced similar levels of muscle fatigue (no additional repetitions could be performed), based purely on the amount of weight lifted. Other experts define training intensity as the effort level achieved during an exercise set. They would consider four repetitions with 90 pounds (40.1 kg) and eight repetitions with 80 pounds (36.4 kg) to be equal in training intensity, as long as each exercise bout produced similar levels of muscle fatigue (no additional repetitions could be performed).

Using either definition, training intensity varies inversely with training volume. For most individuals, higher-intensity training sessions require lower exercise volumes, and higher-volume exercise sessions require lower training intensities. Most **periodization** models for muscular-training programs begin with higher-volume/lower-intensity workouts, progress to moderate-volume/moderate-intensity workouts and conclude with lower-volume/higher-intensity workouts. Although both volume and intensity are key components of progressive muscular-training exercise, the more important factor for strength development appears to be the training effort.

When developing an exercise program for a client who is new to muscular training, the initial program should feature exercises with a low level of intensity. A client who is new to muscular training may perceive exercise as painful and uncomfortable. An exercise program with a high level of intensity relative to the client's experience could create significant DOMS and reduce the client's adherence to regular exercise. Intensity can be used to help foster adherence to an exercise program for a client with limited or no muscular-training experience. Designing an exercise program to begin with a low level of intensity in the initial phase, allowing the client to physically and psychologically adapt to the training stress, and gradually progressing the intensity will help the client experience results while developing long-term adherence to exercise. Progressing intensity too quickly could lead to excessive muscle soreness or injury, providing reasons for a client to quit the exercise program.

TRAINING TEMPO

Research has not identified a particular training tempo that is most effective for increasing muscular strength and size. For example, Olympic lifters perform their competitive exercises at fast movement speeds, bodybuilders generally train at moderate movement speeds, and powerlifters do their competitive exercises at slow movement speeds. Controlled movement speeds require a relatively even application of muscle force throughout the entire movement range. Conversely, fast movement speeds require a high level of muscle force to initiate the lift, with momentum becoming increasingly responsible for the remainder of the movement.

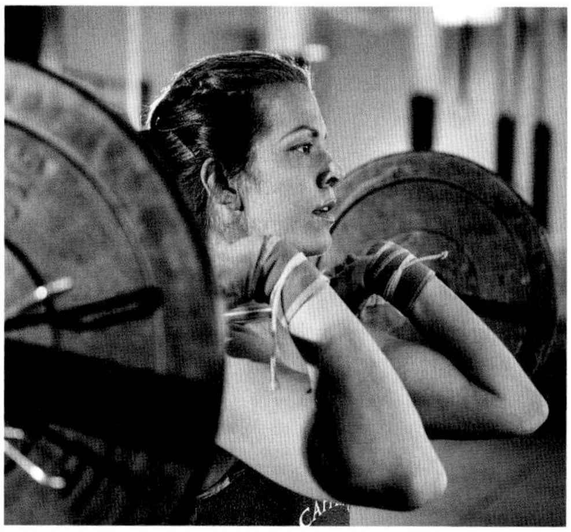

The commonly recommended movement speed of six seconds per repetition is consistent with the repetition speed long recommended for weightstack (or selectorized) machine training (Schoenfeld, 2010). The concentric muscle action should be performed in one to three seconds and the eccentric muscle action should be performed in two to four seconds. Although other controlled movement speeds ranging from four to eight seconds may be equally effective for strength development (Westcott, 2016), six-second repetitions represent an excellent introductory training speed for new exercisers. The personal trainer should emphasize the performance of all exercises through a full ROM. However, as previously discussed, personal trainers may need to consider muscle soreness when planning the duration of the eccentric phase of contraction with new exercisers, as it is this phase that triggers DOMS, which may create a negative experience.

REST INTERVALS

Rest intervals refer to the recovery periods between successive exercises or between successive sets of the same exercise. The length of the rest interval is dependent on the training goal, the client's conditioning status, and the load and amount of work performed. The heavier the load, the longer the rest interval needed for recovery to replenish the muscle's energy pathways. The recommended rest intervals for endurance, hypertrophy, strength, and power are outlined in Table 9-12. A high-effort set of muscular-training exercise reduces the muscle's internal energy stores of creatine phosphate. Replenishment of these local energy substrates is relatively rapid, with 50% renewal within the first 30 seconds, 75% renewal within the first minute, and 95% renewal within the first two minutes. For most practical purposes and general muscular conditioning, one-minute rest intervals between successive exercise sets are sufficient.

Competitive Olympic lifters and powerlifters typically take longer rest intervals between sets to ensure complete muscle recovery and energy replenishment. The longer recovery periods permit the use of relatively heavy weightloads throughout the training session. Exercisers interested in maximizing muscular strength typically take several minutes of rest between sets of the same exercise.

Competitive bodybuilders are less concerned about the exercise resistance and more concerned about "pumping up" their muscles. Therefore, they take relatively short rests

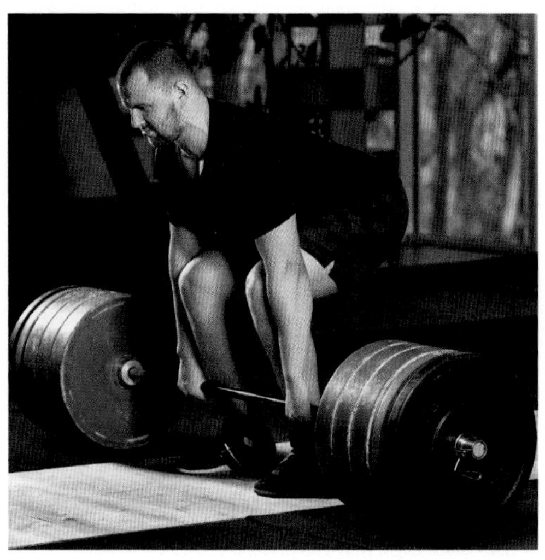

between sets to keep the blood congested in the prime mover muscles. Individuals interested in maximizing muscle size typically rest for 30 to 90 seconds between successive exercise sets.

Rest intervals are an important component of an exercise program because they allow a client to recover after each particular exercise and maintain a consistent level of energy throughout the workout. Clients new to muscular training should have rest intervals long enough to allow them to maintain their comfort levels, but not so long that their **heart rate** and body temperature return to normal resting levels.

When performing a muscular-training circuit in which each exercise addresses a different muscle group, the recovery interval has more impact on the cardiovascular system than on the exercise performance. Shorter rest intervals increase cardiovascular and metabolic responses both during and after the exercise session. This format of muscular training, coupled with higher volumes of resistance work that increase metabolism, is becoming more popular with individuals seeking to lose or manage their weight.

Components of a Muscular-training Session

To safely and effectively provide personalized exercise programming for clients, personal trainers must be mindful of the components of an exercise session, which are described in this section. Regardless of the client's goal, each exercise session should progress from a warm-up to a conditioning portion and conclude with a cool-down.

WARM-UP

Readying the body for a workout is an essential first step of any exercise session. The warm-up is a period of lighter exercise preceding the conditioning portion of the exercise bout and should last for five to 10 minutes for most healthy adults. It should begin with light activity that gradually increases in intensity and takes into account all planes of motion, as well as the various exercises that will be performed in the upcoming training session. By focusing on function and movement at the start of each workout, the proprioceptors are activated (thereby improving balance and coordination), the muscles begin to receive increased blood flow (which carries needed oxygen and nutrients for exertion), and connective tissues benefit from enhanced elasticity. The warm-up sequence should focus on the movement patterns planned for the rest of the workout. In addition, once warmed via light activity, dynamic and static flexibility exercises could be included in the warm-up to further prepare the soft tissues to undergo the necessary ROM required for the upcoming training activity. Further, when a goal of the warm-up is to inhibit an overactive muscle or address postural issues, static stretching may be employed (after a brief bout of light activity). Exercises from the Functional and Movement Training phases of the ACE IFT Model are sensible choices for use in warming up for *both* the Cardiorespiratory and Muscular Training components of the ACE IFT Model.

CONDITIONING

The conditioning portion of an exercise session must be appropriate for the client's current fitness level and consistent with his or her training goals, and should be planned in terms of frequency, duration, intensity, and modality. If high-intensity activities are planned, they should take place fairly early in the conditioning portion of the workout when the client is less likely to be affected by fatigue. In Muscular Training, a variety of areas of focus could comprise the training activities (e.g., endurance, strength, power, **speed, agility,** and/or **quickness**). Accordingly, clients will have unique goals, which are relevant to their skills and abilities. For example, a college-aged client who participates in a recreational volleyball league will have strength and power goals specific to the sport, whereas a retiree who regularly enjoys swimming and hiking may also have goals with a strength and power focus, but the program design would be significantly different compared to the volleyball player. As such, exercises from the Functional, Movement, or Load/Speed phases could be selected for the conditioning portion of a Muscular Training session.

COOL-DOWN

While the warm-up readies a client for activity, the cool-down is the opportunity to focus on stress reduction, returning the heart rate to resting levels and initiating relaxation and the recovery process. The cool-down should be of approximately the same duration and intensity as the warm-up (i.e., five to 10 minutes of light activity). Including static stretching at the conclusion of a Muscular Training session (i.e., in the cool-down period) may inhibit overactive muscles and improve flexibility. Prolonged static stretching is typically performed at the end of a workout, as it may result in neural inhibition and decreased strength, which would be counterproductive if used earlier in an exercise session if strength and power are the intended outcomes. As in the warm-up, exercises from the Functional and Movement Training phases could be good options for the cool-down, with more of a focus on static stretching rather than dynamic flexibility.

The following chapters in this section describe the training and general program-design recommendations for each phase of the Muscular Training component of the ACE IFT Model. In addition, transitions between the phases are further explained. Detailed sample exercise plans, along with the ACE IFT Model Exercise Programming Template, are presented in Chapter 11.

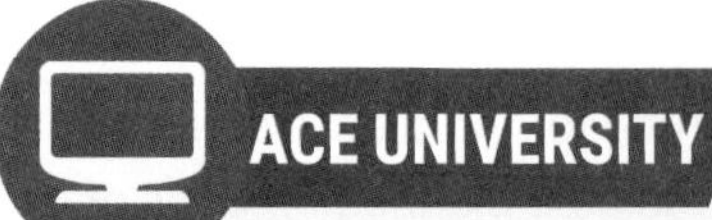

If your study program includes the ACE University, visit www.ACEfitness.org/MyACE and log in to your My ACE Account to take full advantage of the ACE Personal Trainer Study Program and online guided study experience.

A variety of media to support and expand on the material in this text is provided to facilitate learning and best prepare you for the ACE Personal Trainer Certification exam and a career as a personal trainer.

SUMMARY

The first step toward designing and implementing safe and effective exercise programs is gaining an understanding of the anatomy and physiology that serves as the foundation of muscular training. This includes the ability to not only explain the body's anatomical systems and the role that each plays during exercise, but also to utilize scientifically sound terminology to explain human movement to clients. In addition, personal trainers must be able to apply the muscular-training principles to positively influence clients' experiences with exercise as well as their chances for long-term success. Finally, the manipulation of muscular-training variables is a skill that all personal trainers must work to master, as it is the proper relationships among these variables that will ultimately dictate the benefits that clients derive from their muscular-training programs.

REFERENCES

American College of Sports Medicine (2018). *ACSM's Guidelines for Exercise Testing and Prescription* (10th ed.). Philadelphia: Wolters Kluwer.

Ashdown-Franks, G. et al. (2019). Handgrip strength and depression among 34,129 adults aged 50 years and older in six low- and middle-income countries. *Journal of Affective Disorders*, 243, 448–454.

Bezerra, E. et al. (2019). Effects of different strength training volumes and subsequent detraining on strength performance in aging adults. *Journal of Bodywork & Movement Therapies*, https://doi.org/10.1016/j.jbmt.2019.01.010

Doherty, T.J. (2001). The influence of aging and sex on skeletal muscle mass and strength. *Current Opinion in Clinical Nutrition & Metabolic Care*, 4, 6, 503–508.

Golightly, Y.M., Allen, K.D., & Caine, D.J. (2012). A comprehensive review of the effectiveness of different exercise programs for patients with osteoarthritis. *Physician and Sportsmedicine*, 40, 4, 52–65.

Gundersen, K. (2011). Excitation-transcription coupling in skeletal muscle: The molecular pathways of exercise. *Biological Reviews of the Cambridge Philosophical Society*, 86, 3, 564–600.

Hackney, K., Engels, H., & Gretebeck, R. (2008). Resting energy expenditure and delayed-onset muscle soreness after full-body resistance training with an eccentric concentration. *Journal of Strength and Conditioning Research*, 22, 5, 1602–1609.

Haff, G.G. & Triplett, T.N. (2016). *Essentials of Strength Training and Conditioning* (4th ed.). Champaign, Ill.: Human Kinetics.

Kelley, G. & Kelley, K. (2009). Impact of progressive resistance training on lipids and lipoproteins in adults: A meta-analysis of randomized controlled trials. *Preventive Medicine*, 48, 9–19.

Kim, H.S. & Kim, D.G. (2013). Effect of long-term resistance exercise on body composition, blood lipid factors, and vascular compliance in the hypertensive elderly men. *Journal of Exercise Rehabilitation*, 9, 2, 271–277.

McLester, J. et al. (2003). A series of studies: A practical protocol for testing muscle endurance recovery. *Journal of Strength and Conditioning Research*, 17, 2, 259–273.

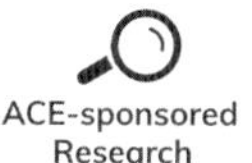

Montano, E. et al. (2018). Do younger and older adults experience similar adaptations to individualized exercise training? *Journal of Exercise Physiology Online*, 21, 2, 41–59.

ACE-sponsored Research

Nolan, P. et al. (2018). The effect of detraining after a period of training on cardiometabolic health in previously sedentary individuals. *International Journal of Environmental Research and Public Health*, 15, 10.

Normandin, E. et al. (2017). Effect of resistance training and caloric restriction on the metabolic syndrome. *Medicine & Science in Sports & Exercise*, 49, 413–419.

Pette, D. (2001). Historical perspectives: Plasticity of mammalian skeletal muscle. *Journal of Applied Physiology*, 90, 3, 1119–1124.

Porter Starr, K.N., McDonald, S.R., & Bales, C.W. (2014). Obesity and physical frailty in older adults: A scoping review of lifestyle intervention trials. *Journal of the American Medical Directors Association*, 15, 4, 240–250.

Saeidifard, F. et al. (2019). The association of resistance training with mortality: A systematic review and meta-analysis. *European Journal of Preventive Cardiology*, May 19:2047487319850718.

Schoenfeld, B.J. (2010). The mechanisms of muscle hypertrophy and their application to resistance training. *Journal of Strength and Conditioning Research*, 24, 10, 2857–2872.

Schwingshackl, L. et al. (2013). Impact of different training modalities on anthropometric and metabolic characteristics in overweight/obese subjects: A systematic review and network meta-analysis. *PLoS One*, 8, 12, e82853.

Shoepe, T. et al. (2003). Functional adaptability of muscle fibers to long-term resistance exercise. *Medicine & Science in Sports & Exercise*, 35, 6, 944–951.

Sieck, G.C. et al. (2013). Mechanical properties of respiratory muscles. *Comprehensive Physiology*, 3, 4, 1553–1567.

Smith, B.E., Littlewood, C., & May, S. (2014). An update of stabilisation exercises for low back pain: A systematic review with meta-analysis. *BMC Musculoskeletal Disorders*, 15, 416.

Strasser, B., Siebert, U., & Schobersberger, W. (2010). Resistance training in the treatment of the metabolic syndrome: A systematic review and meta-analysis of the effect of resistance training on metabolic clustering in patients with abnormal glucose metabolism. *Sports Medicine*, 40, 5, 397–415.

Tokmakidis, S. P. et al. (2009). Effects of detraining on muscle strength and mass after high or moderate intensity of resistance training in older adults. *Scandanavian Society of Clinical Physiology and Nuclear Medicine*, 29, 4, 316–319.

Westcott, W. L. (2016). *Building Strength & Stamina* (3rd ed.). Monterey, Calif.: Healthy Learning.

Westcott, W.L. (2012). Resistance training is medicine: Effects of strength training on health. *Currents Sports Medicine Reports*, 11, 4, 209–216.

Westcott, W. et al. (2009). Prescribing physical activity: Applying the ACSM protocols for exercise type, intensity, and duration across 3 training frequencies. *Physician and Sportsmedicine*, 37, 2, 51–58.

Westcott, W.L. et al. (2008). Protein and body composition. *Fitness Management*, 24, 5, 50–53.

SUGGESTED READINGS

American College of Sports Medicine (2009). Progression models in resistance training for healthy adults. *Medicine & Science in Sports & Exercise*, 41, 3, 687–708.

Haff, G.G. & Triplett, T.N. (2016). *Essentials of Strength Training and Conditioning* (4th ed.). Champaign, Ill.: Human Kinetics.

National Strength and Conditioning Association (2016). *Exercise Techniques Manual for Resistance Training* (3rd ed.). Champaign, Ill.: Human Kinetics.

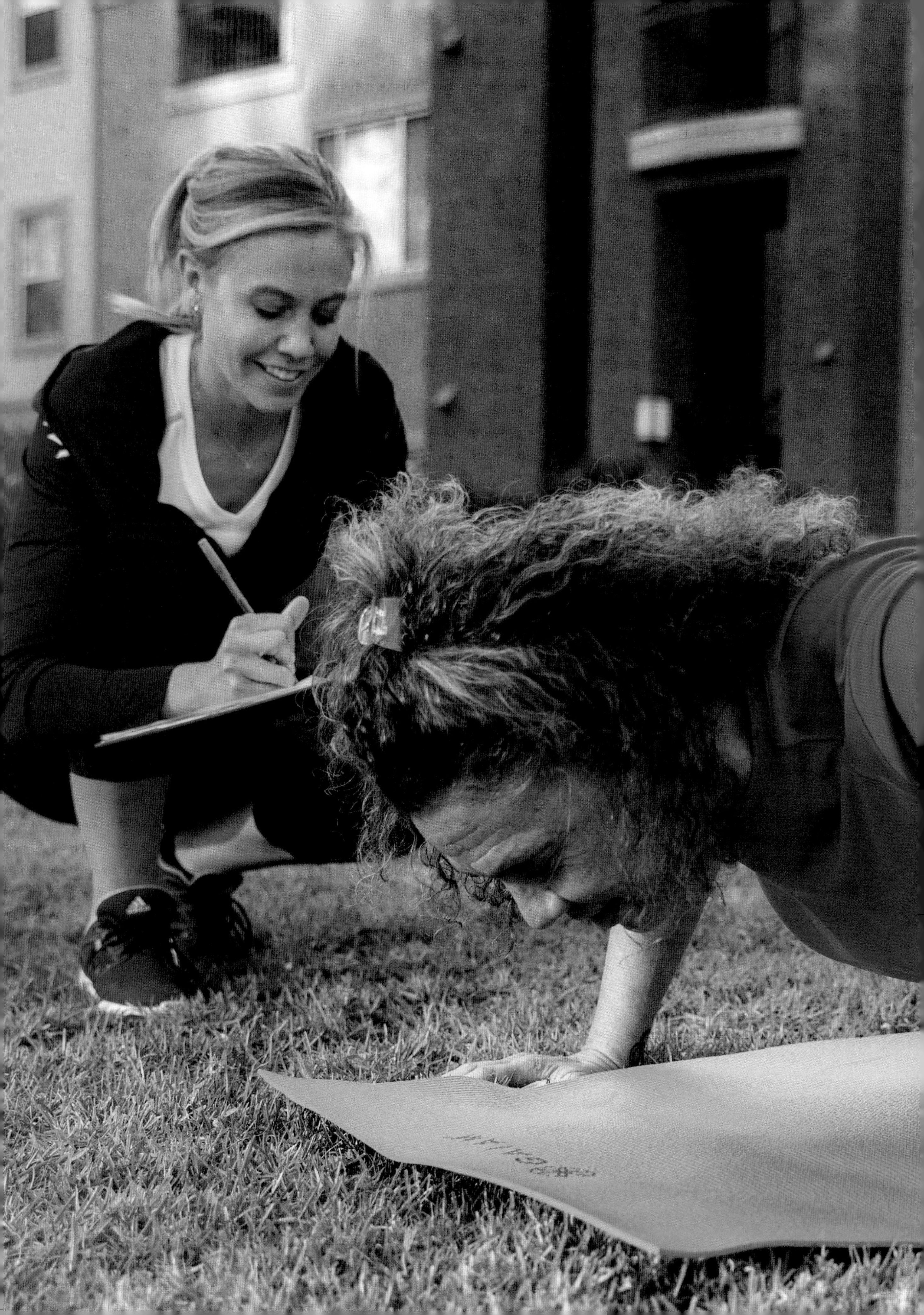

CHAPTER 10

Muscular Training: Assessments

LANCE C. DALLECK, PhD
Professor of Exercise and Sport Science, Western Colorado University;
Member, ACE Scientific Advisory Panel

IN THIS CHAPTER

LEARNING OBJECTIVES:

Upon completion of this chapter, the reader will be able to:

- Select and administer appropriate assessments based on ACE Mover Method™ strategies for client-centered approaches to exercise programming
- Evaluate the results of Functional, Movement, and Load/Speed assessments and apply them to Muscular Training
- Understand when and why Muscular Training assessments should be repeated
- Identify how the results of Muscular Training assessments can be discussed with clients in a personalized and professional manner

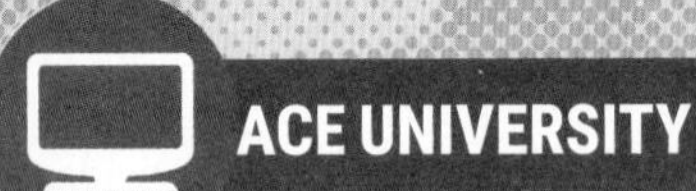

If your study program includes the ACE University, visit www.ACEfitness.org/MyACE and log in to your My ACE Account to take full advantage of the ACE Personal Trainer Study Program and online guided study experience.

A variety of media to support and expand on the material in this text is provided to facilitate learning and best prepare you for the ACE Personal Trainer Certification exam and a career as a personal trainer.

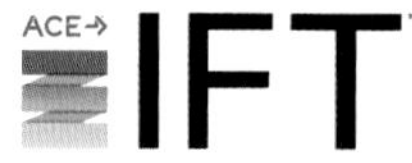

The ACE Integrated Fitness Training® (ACE IFT®) Model provides personal trainers with the option to either conduct evidence-based fitness assessments or lead clients through early sessions that incorporate exercise programming that delivers appropriate movement and fitness challenges while also providing the personal trainer with valuable feedback about a client's current postural **stability,** joint **mobility,** functional movement, **balance, cardiorespiratory fitness,** and **muscular fitness.** Exercises and exercise sequences that can be used for both training sessions and client assessments using the ACE IFT Model are presented in this chapter, along with evidence-based fitness assessments.

APPLY WHAT YOU KNOW

A Client-centered Approach to Integrating Assessments into the Initial Exercise Session

The performance of assessments for Functional, Movement, and Load/Speed Training offers valuable information on joint alignment, muscle balance across joints, and **muscular endurance** and **muscular strength** in clients. In turn, assessment results can be used by personal trainers to design and implement Muscular Training programs according to the ACE IFT Model. However, it is common for many clients to commence an exercise program with very low **self-efficacy** for exercise ability and program success. In fact, this likely holds true for Muscular Training, as many clients may have no previous experience with this exercise modality. It is imperative that personal trainers strike the right balance between integration of Muscular Training assessments within the initial exercise session in order to acquire valuable health- and fitness-related information while simultaneously ensuring clients have a positive exercise experience and are looking forward to subsequent training sessions. The following considerations can assist personal trainers with achieving this critical objective:

- In a client-centered approach to personal training, the client's goals and attributes should dictate all aspects of programming. Accordingly, personal trainers should strategically determine which assessments (if any) are warranted that will best assist with getting clients moving.
- It is unnecessary for the first training session to consist exclusively of assessments. An alternative is to intersperse select assessments with exercise training. Across subsequent training sessions, additional assessments can gradually be performed as clients gain confidence in their exercise abilities.
- It is possible and recommended for personal trainers to perform assessments that are concurrently part of the workout. For instance, the unipedal stance test (see page 410) can be completed as a balance-training exercise for an older adult client. In fact, this strategy can be implemented for the completion of numerous Muscular Training assessments.
- When dealing with a client who opts out of being assessed, a personal trainer may simply move forward with exercise programming, carefully selecting exercises and intensities based on the

client's health history and preferences. In this situation, the personal trainer may have to be creative and collaborate with the client on benchmarks that show improvement due to training (e.g., improved back and shoulder function both at work and during exercise and feeling less daily muscular fatigue).

- Lastly, the personal trainer should be able to observe a client's movement proficiency improving over time. When a personal trainer uses effective communication and coaching skills (see Chapter 4) during training sessions to help the client enhance muscular conditioning, it will inevitably allow him or her to experience improved function. Further, sharing with the client any noticeable improvements in exercise technique, along with advances in volume of exercise, may provide welcomed encouragement.

ACE MOVER METHOD

These strategies align perfectly with the ACE Mover Method philosophy wherein:

- Each professional interaction is client-centered, with a recognition that clients are the foremost experts on themselves. This is especially true for assessments, as personal trainers must select the appropriate assessments to administer (if any) based on the client's willingness to perform them.
- Powerful **open-ended questions** and **active listening** are utilized in every session with clients. To select the appropriate assessments, a personal trainer must be skilled at communicating so that **rapport** is built and clients trust that their needs and preferences are heard and ultimately reflected in their personalized exercise programs.
- Clients are genuinely viewed as resourceful and capable of change. Appropriate assessment selection based on clients' preferences and goals is often the first opportunity for personal trainers to give clients a task about which they can feel successful. Continued encouragement and positively reporting the results of assessments will allow clients to participate in the exercise program feeling confident that what they are doing is a positive step in self-care. When both the client and personal trainer view the client as successful, it empowers the client to succeed in behavior change and promotes client self-efficacy.

The Muscular Training component of the ACE IFT Model provides a systematic approach to training that starts with helping clients to improve poor postural stability and **kinetic chain** mobility, and then incorporates programming and progressions to help people train for general fitness, strength, body building, and athletic performance (as desired). The ACE IFT Model Muscular Training component is divided into three phases, each with a title that defines its training focus (Figure 10-1).

Functional Assessments

Functional Training focuses on establishing or, in many cases, reestablishing postural stability and kinetic chain mobility through the introduction of exercise programs that improve joint function through improved muscular endurance, **flexibility,** core function, **static balance,** and **dynamic balance.** Thus, the functional assessments introduced here are designed to help the personal trainer observe a client's level of postural stabilization, balance, and core function.

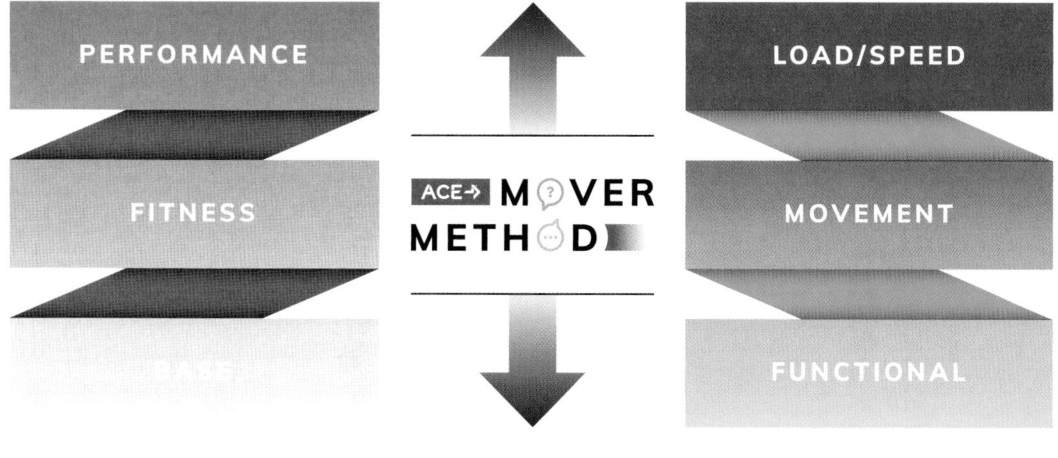

FIGURE 10-1
ACE IFT Model Muscular Training phases

STATIC POSTURAL ASSESSMENT

Movement begins from a position of static posture, which represents the alignment of the body's segments, or how the person holds him- or herself "statically" or "isometrically" in space (Figure 10-2). Therefore, the presence of poor posture is a good indicator that movement may be dysfunctional. Although movement assessments may offer valuable information related to **neuromuscular efficiency,** a static postural assessment may serve as a starting point from which a personal trainer can identify muscle imbalances (Figure 10-3 and Tables 10-1 through 10-4) and potential movement compensations associated with poor posture (Kendall et al., 2005; Sahrmann, 2002). A static postural assessment may offer valuable insight into:

- Muscle imbalance at a joint and the working relationships of muscles around a joint
  - Muscle imbalance often contributes to dysfunctional movement.
- Altered neural action of the muscles moving and controlling the joint
  - For example, tight or shortened muscles are often overactive and dominate movement at the joint, potentially disrupting healthy joint mechanics.

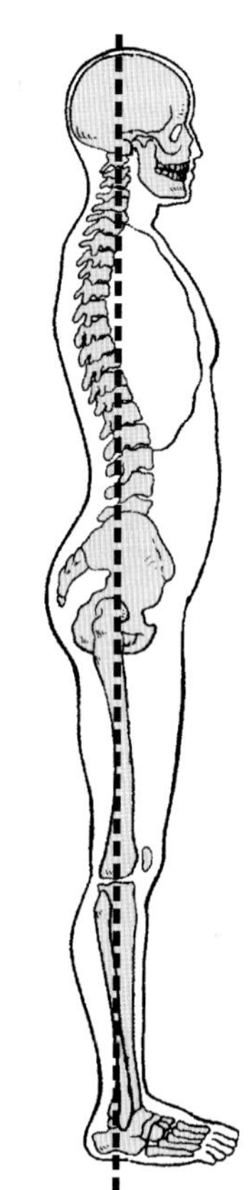

FIGURE 10-2
Neutral spine alignment with slight anterior (lordotic) curves at the neck and low back and a posterior (kyphotic) curve in the thoracic region

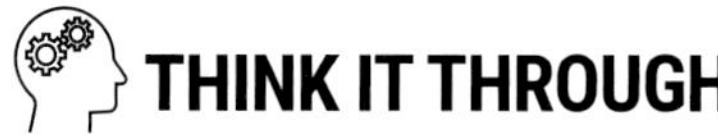

Postural Deviations

Carefully read through the information presented in Tables 10-1 through 10-4. Because the postures depicted are common deviations, you are likely to observe clients with one or more of these variants. Think about methods you would employ as a personal trainer to help clients with these muscle imbalances. Can you come up with at least one stretch for each **hypertonic** or shortened muscle group and one strengthening exercise for each inhibited muscle group?

FIGURE 10-3
Postural deviations

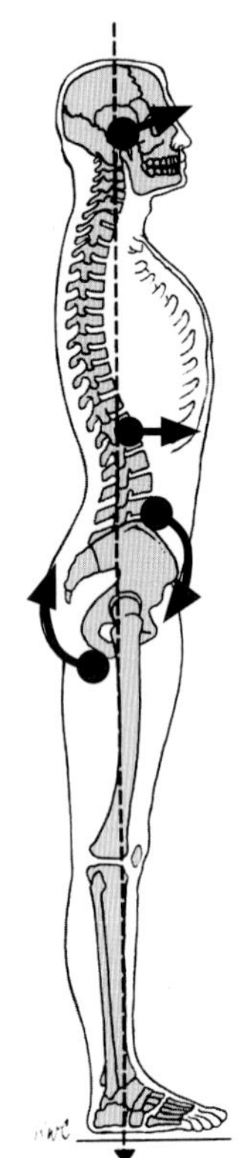
a. Lordosis: increased anterior lumbar curve from neutral

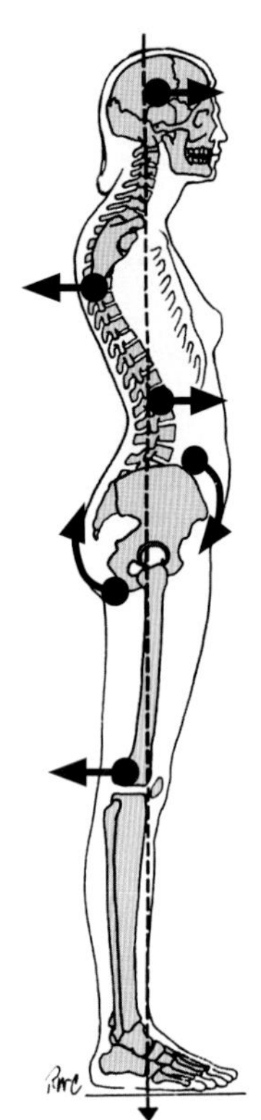
b. Kyphosis: increased posterior thoracic curve from neutral

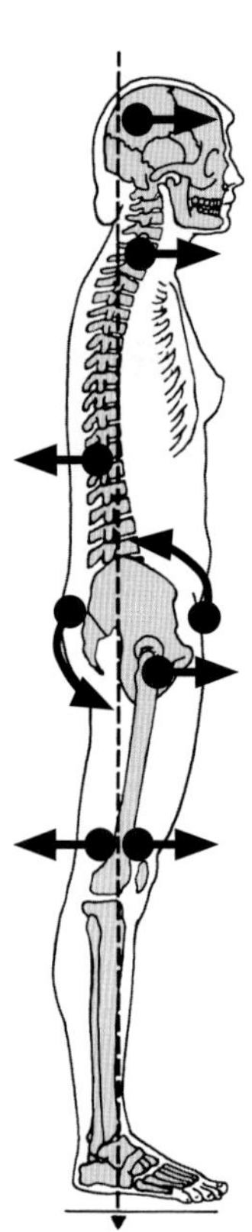
c. Flat back: decreased anterior lumbar curve

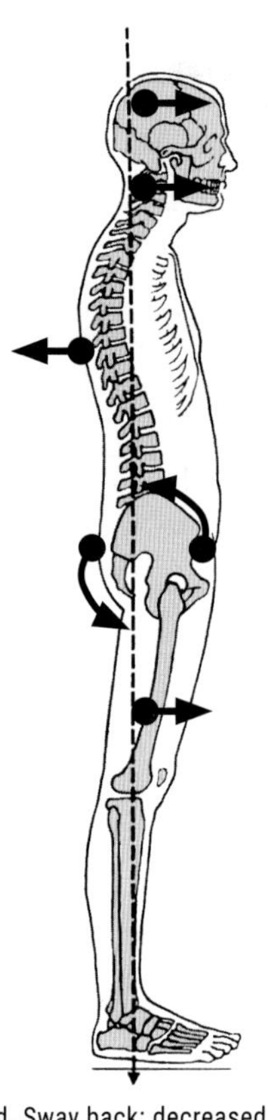
d. Sway back: decreased anterior lumbar curve and increased posterior thoracic curve from neutral

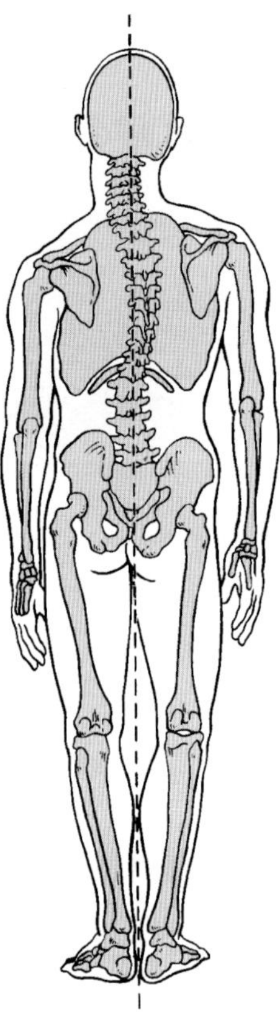
e. Scoliosis: lateral spinal curvature often accompanied by vertebral rotation

TABLE 10-1

Muscle Imbalances Associated with Lordosis Posture

Facilitated/Hypertonic (Shortened)	Inhibited (Lengthened)
Hip flexors	Hip extensors
Lumbar extensors	External obliques
	Rectus abdominis

TABLE 10-2

Muscle Imbalances Associated with Kyphosis Posture

Facilitated/Hypertonic (Shortened)	Inhibited (Lengthened)
Anterior chest/shoulders	Upper-back extensors
Latissimus dorsi	Scapular stabilizers
Neck extensors	Neck flexors

TABLE 10-3

Muscle Imbalances Associated With Flat-back Posture

Facilitated/Hypertonic (Shortened)	Inhibited (Lengthened)
Rectus abdominis	Iliacus/psoas major
Upper-back extensors	Internal obliques
Neck extensors	Lumbar extensors
Ankle plantar flexors	Neck flexors

TABLE 10-4
Muscle Imbalances Associated With Sway-back Posture

Facilitated/Hypertonic (Shortened)	Inhibited (Lengthened)
Hamstrings	Iliacus/psoas major
Upper fibers of posterior obliques	Rectus femoris
Lumbar extensors	External oblique
Neck extensors	Upper-back extensors
	Neck flexors

Muscle imbalance and postural deviations can be attributed to many factors that are both correctible and non-correctible, including the following:

- Correctible factors:
  - Repetitive movements (muscular pattern overload)
  - Awkward positions and movements (habitually poor posture)
  - Side dominance
  - Lack of joint stability
  - Lack of joint mobility
  - Imbalanced strength-training programs
- Non-correctible factors:
  - Congenital conditions (e.g., **scoliosis**)
  - Some pathologies (e.g., **rheumatoid arthritis**)
  - Structural deviations (e.g., tibial or femoral **torsion,** or **femoral anteversion**)
  - Certain types of trauma (e.g., surgery, injury, or amputation)

When joints are correctly aligned, the **length-tension relationships** and **force-couple relationships** function efficiently. This facilitates proper joint mechanics, allowing the body to generate and accept forces throughout the kinetic chain, and promotes joint stability and mobility and movement efficiency.

When assessing posture, a personal trainer can start by observing a client's stance following the right-angle rule of the body (Kendall et al., 2005). This rule describes how the body represents itself in vertical alignment across the major joints—the ankle, knee, hip, shoulder, and spine. Applying the right-angle rule allows the personal trainer to observe postural deviations in all three planes, noting specific "static" asymmetries at the joints (e.g., front to back and left to right). The right-angle rule implies a state in the **frontal plane** wherein the two hemispheres are equally divided, and in the **sagittal plane** wherein the **anterior** and **posterior** surfaces appear in balance. The body is in good postural position when the body parts are symmetrically balanced around the body's **line of gravity** (Figure 10-4), which is the intersection of the mid-frontal and mid-sagittal planes.

While this rule helps personal trainers identify postural compensations and potential muscle imbalances, it is important to recognize that limitations exist in using this rule.

FIGURE 10-4
The right-angle rule (frontal and sagittal plane views)

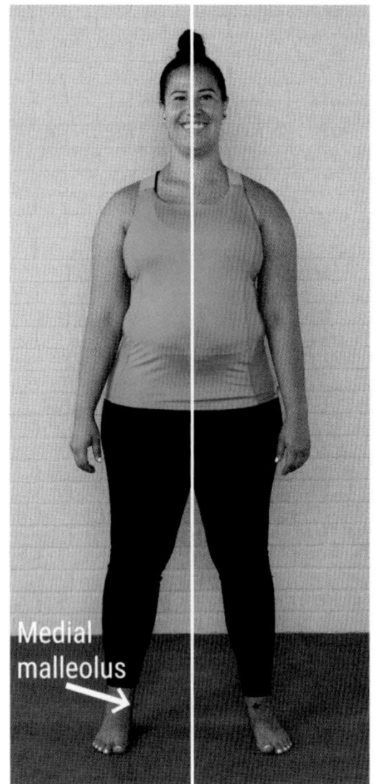

a. Frontal plane view (anterior)

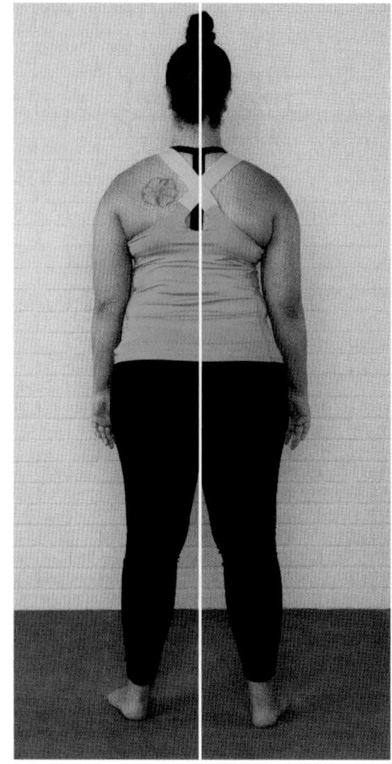
b. Frontal plane view (posterior)

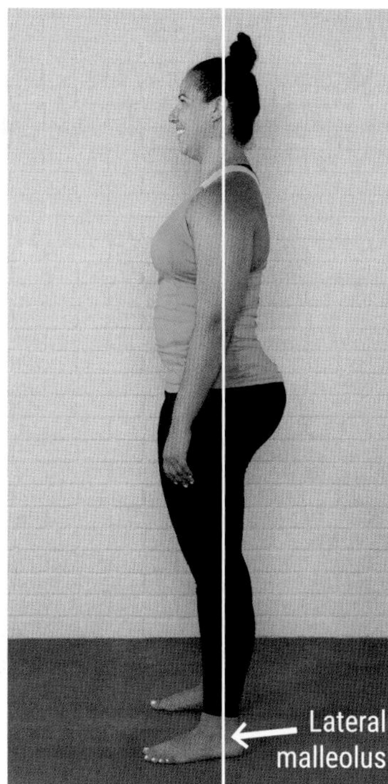

c. Sagittal plane view

Protocol

Select a location that offers a solid, plain backdrop or a grid pattern with vertical and horizontal lines that offer contrast against the client. Encourage the client to wear form-fitting, athletic-style clothing to expose as many joints and bony landmarks as possible, and have the client remove his or her shoes and socks.

The objective of this assessment is to observe the client's symmetry against the right angles that the weight-bearing joints make relative to the line of gravity. Individuals will consciously or subconsciously attempt to correct posture when they are aware they are being observed, so personal trainers should encourage clients to assume a normal, relaxed posture, and utilize distractions such as casual conversation to encourage this relaxed posture.

Personal trainers should focus on the obvious, gross imbalances and avoid getting caught up in minor postural asymmetries. Bear in mind that the body is rarely perfectly symmetrical and that overanalyzing asymmetries is time-consuming, potentially intimidating to clients, and may induce muscle fatigue in the client that can alter his or her posture even further. Therefore, when looking for gross deviations, the personal trainer should select an acceptable margin of asymmetry and focus on larger, more obvious discrepancies. For example, start by focusing on gross deviations that differ by a quarter-inch (0.6 cm) or more between the compartments of the body.

Observations

Frontal Views (Anterior and Posterior)

- For the anterior view, good posture presents as a line of gravity that bisects the right and left sides of the body equally, falling between the feet and ankles, and intersecting the pubis, umbilicus, sternum, mandible (chin), maxilla (face), and frontal bone (forehead) (see Figure 10-4a).

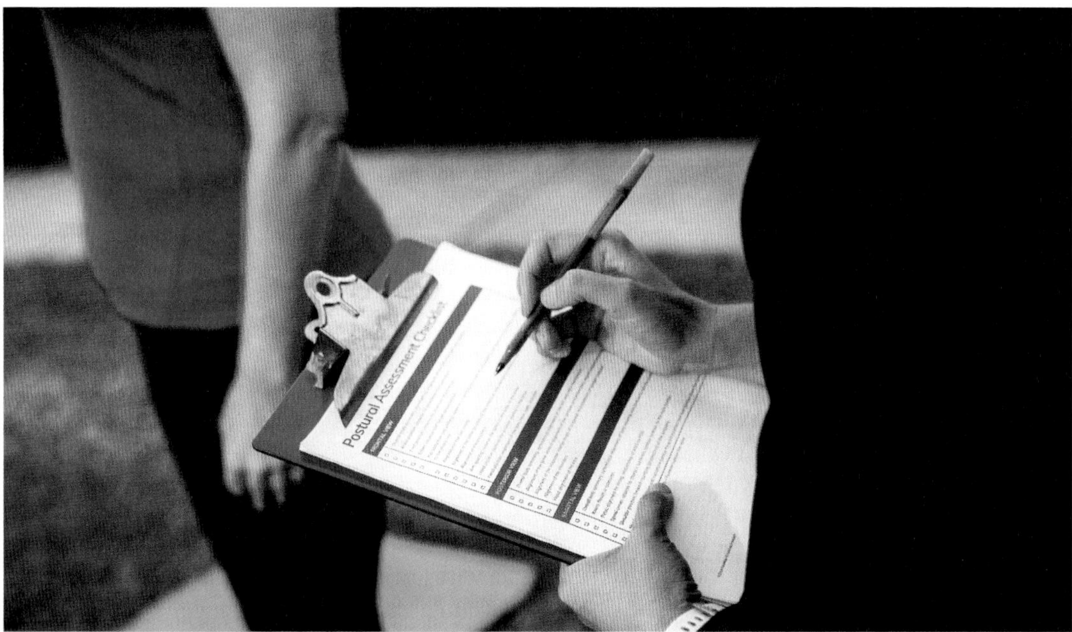

- For the posterior view, good posture is indicated if the line of gravity bisects the sacrum and overlaps the spinous processes of the vertebrae, leaving the right and left sides of the body equally balanced (see Figure 10-4b).

Sagittal View

- Observing the client from the side, good posture presents as a line of gravity that passes through the anterior third of the knee, the greater trochanter of the femur, and the acromioclavicular (AC) joint, and slightly anterior to the mastoid process of the temporal bone of the skull (in line with, or just behind, the ear lobe) (see Figure 10-4c).

Transverse View

- All transverse plane observations of the limbs and torso are performed from the frontal- and sagittal-view positions and include observing rotation, **pronation,** and **supination.**
- For the anterior view, good posture presents as the palms facing the **lateral** aspect of the thighs with the thumbs visible, the patellae pointing straight ahead, and the feet pointing straight ahead or turned slightly outward.
- For the posterior view, good posture is indicated when the calcaneus is oriented perpendicular to the floor and the palms of the hands are not visible (as they are facing the lateral aspect of the thighs with the pinky side of the hand visible).
- For the sagittal view, good posture presents as the feet pointing forward, the knees facing neither outward or inward, and the backs of the hands visible, as the palms are facing the lateral aspect of the thighs.

Common Postural Deviations

The following sections address five key postural deviations that a personal trainer is likely to observe. The content included here is intended to provide a foundational overview of some of the important principles of specific postural deviations and how they might affect joints up and down the kinetic chain.

DEVIATION 1: SUBTALAR PRONATION/SUPINATION AND THE EFFECT ON TIBIAL AND FEMORAL ROTATION

Both feet should face forward in parallel or with slight (12 to 18 degrees) **external rotation** (toes pointing outward from the midline, as the ankle joint lies in an oblique plane with the medial malleolus slightly anterior to the lateral malleolus) (Houglum, 2016) (see Figure 10-4). The toes should be aligned in the same direction as the feet and any excessive pronation (arch flattening) or supination (high arches) at the subtalar joint should be noted.

APPLY WHAT YOU KNOW

Kinetic Chain: Subtalar Position and Tibial and Femoral Rotation

Because the body is one continuous kinetic chain, the position of the subtalar joint will impact the position of the tibia and femur. Barring structural differences in the skeletal system (e.g., tibial torsion or femoral anteversion), a pronated subtalar joint position typically forces internal rotation of the tibia and slightly less internal rotation of the femur (Figure 10-5 and Table 10-5). To demonstrate this point, stand with shoes off and place the hands firmly on the fronts of the thighs. Notice what happens to the orientation of the knees and thighs when moving between pronation and supination. Additionally, notice how the calcaneus everts as the subtalar joint is pronated.

FIGURE 10-5
Foot pronation and supination and the effects up the kinetic chain

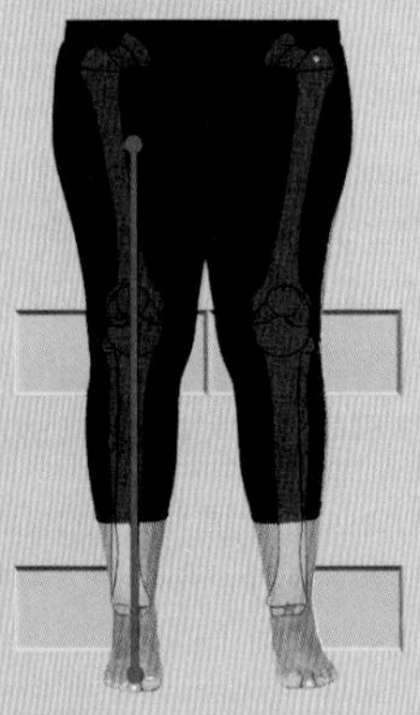

Neutral subtalar joint position with neutral knee alignment

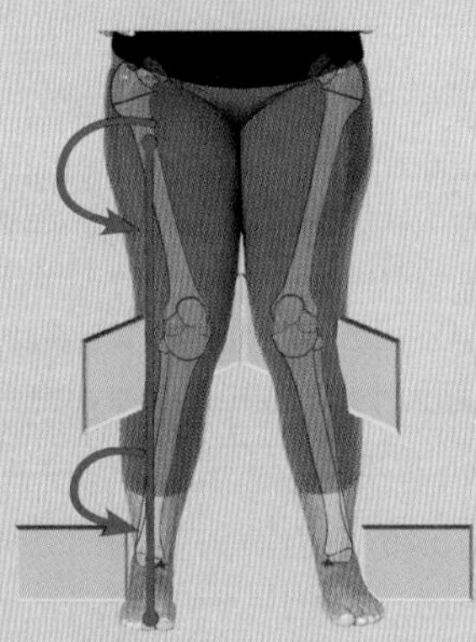

Pronation with internal rotation of the knee

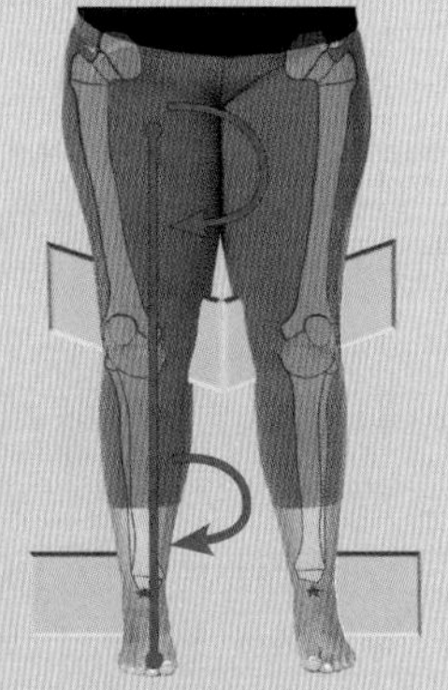

Supination with external rotation of the knee

TABLE 10-5

Subtalar Joint Pronation/Supination and the Effect on the Feet, Tibia, and Femur

Subtalar Joint Movement	Foot Movement	Tibial (Knee) Movement	Femoral Movement	Frontal Plane
Pronation	Eversion	Internal rotation	Internal rotation	Anterior view
Supination	Inversion	External rotation	External rotation	Anterior view

Subtalar joint pronation forces internal rotation at the tibia, flexion at the knee, and hip flexion and internal rotation when weight bearing. Additional stresses on some knee ligaments and the integrity of the joint itself may lead to injury during ambulation if the joint remains in pronation (Houglum, 2016). Additionally, closed-chain pronation tends to move the calcaneus into **eversion,** which may actually lift the outside of the heel slightly off the ground (moving the ankle into **plantar flexion**). In turn, this may tighten the calf muscles and potentially limit ankle **dorsiflexion,** but personal trainers should keep in mind that the opposite is also true: A tight gastrocnemius and soleus complex (triceps surae) (see Figure 9-31, page 362) may force **calcaneal eversion** in an otherwise neutral subtalar joint position (Gray & Tiberio, 2006).

To illustrate this point, stand barefoot facing a wall with the feet 36 inches (0.9 m) away. Extend both arms in front of the body, placing the hands on the wall for support. Slowly lean forward, flexing the elbows and dorsiflexing the ankles while keeping both heels firmly pressed into the floor. Observe for any movement in the feet (e.g., appearance of the arch collapsing with calcaneal eversion). As a tight gastrocnemius and soleus complex reach the limit of their extensibility, the body may need to evert the calcaneus to allow further movement. This scenario may occur repeatedly in **gait** immediately prior to the push-off phase if the gastrocnemius and soleus complex are tight, forcing calcaneal eversion and subtalar joint pronation.

DEVIATION 2: HIP ADDUCTION

In standing and in gait, hip **adduction** is a lateral tilt of the pelvis that elevates one hip higher than the other (also called "hip hiking"), which may be evident in individuals who have a limb-length discrepancy (Sahrmann, 2002). If a person raises the right hip as illustrated in Figure 10-6, the line of gravity following the spine tilts over toward the left, moving the right thigh closer to this line of gravity. Consequently, the right hip is identified as moving into adduction. This position progressively lengthens and weakens the right hip abductors, which are unable to hold the hip level (Table 10-6). Sleeping on one's side can produce a similar effect, as the hip abductors of the upper hip fail to hold the hip level.

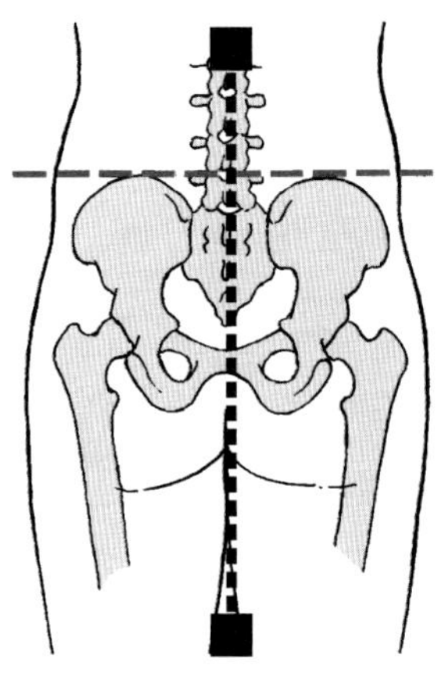

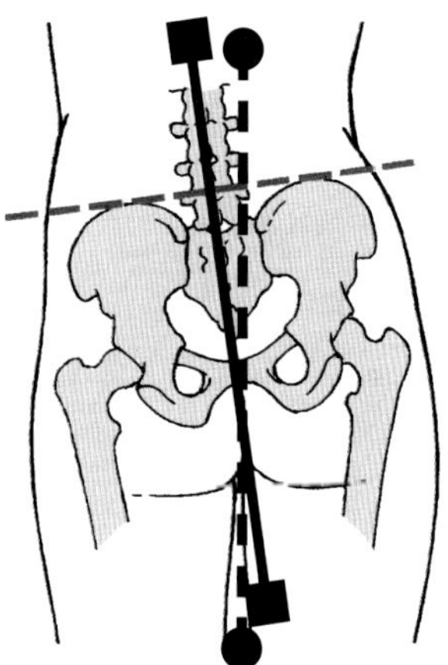

FIGURE 10-6
Normal hip position versus right hip adduction (posterior view)

Source: LifeART image copyright 2008 Wolters Kluwer Health, Inc., Lippincott Williams & Wilkins. All rights reserved.

TABLE 10-6
Hip Adduction

Observation	Position	Alignment	Frontal Plane
Right hip adduction	Elevated (vs. left side)	Hips usually shifted right	Posterior view
Left hip adduction	Elevated (vs. right side)	Hips usually shifted left	Posterior view

DEVIATION 3: PELVIC TILTING (ANTERIOR OR POSTERIOR)

Anterior tilting of the pelvis frequently occurs in individuals with tight hip flexors, which is generally associated with **physically inactive** and **sedentary** lifestyles where individuals spend countless hours in seated (i.e., shortened hip flexor) positions (Kendall et al., 2005) (Figure 10-7). With standing, this shortened hip flexor pulls the pelvis into an anterior tilt (i.e., the superior, anterior portion of the pelvis rotates downward and forward) (Figure 10-8). As illustrated in Figure 10-9, an anterior pelvic tilt rotates the superior, anterior portion of the pelvis forward and downward, spilling water out of the front of the bucket, whereas a posterior tilt rotates the superior, posterior portion of the pelvis backward and downward, spilling water out of the back of the bucket. Figure 10-10 illustrates the alignment of the anterior superior iliac spine and posterior superior iliac spine in neutral alignment, as well in anterior and posterior pelvic tilts.

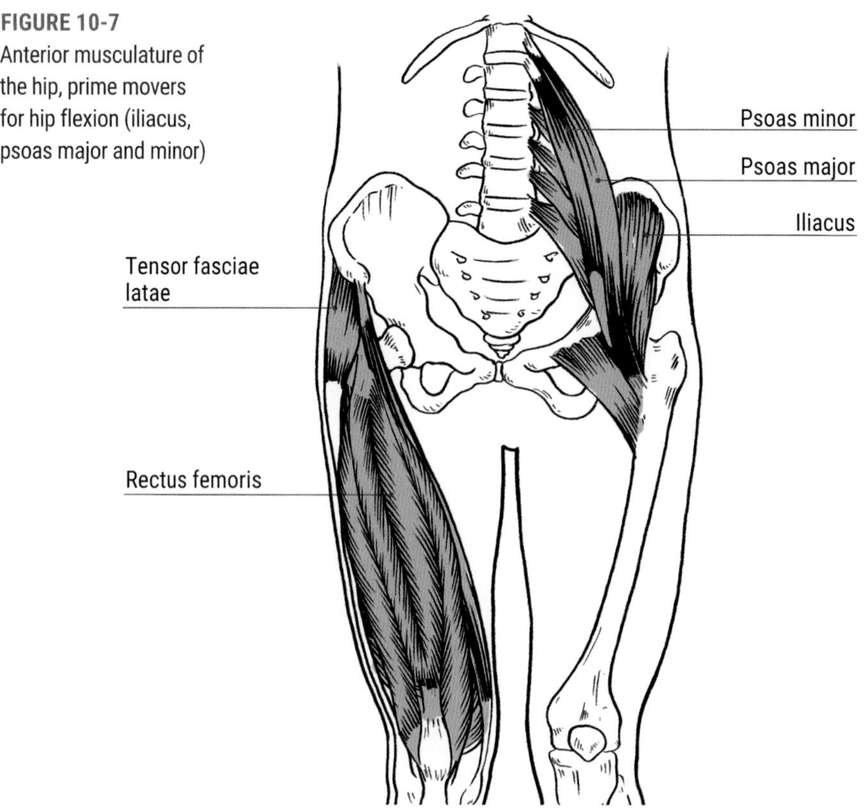

FIGURE 10-7
Anterior musculature of the hip, prime movers for hip flexion (iliacus, psoas major and minor)

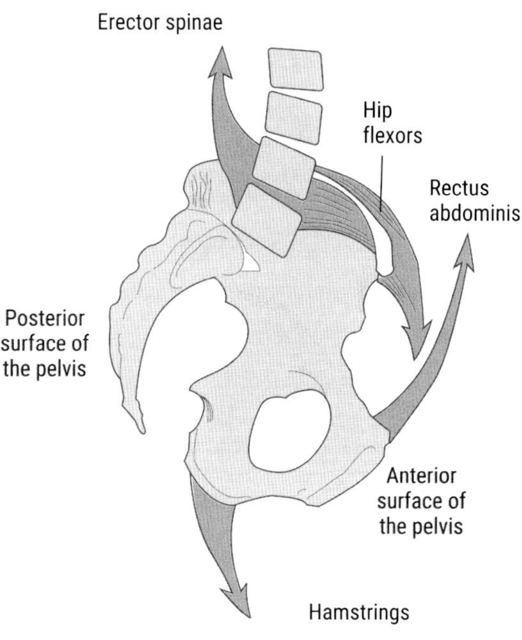

FIGURE 10-8
Muscular control of the pelvis by the abdominals and hip flexors (iliopsoas and rectus femoris) anteriorly and the spinal extensors (erector spinae) and hamstrings posteriorly

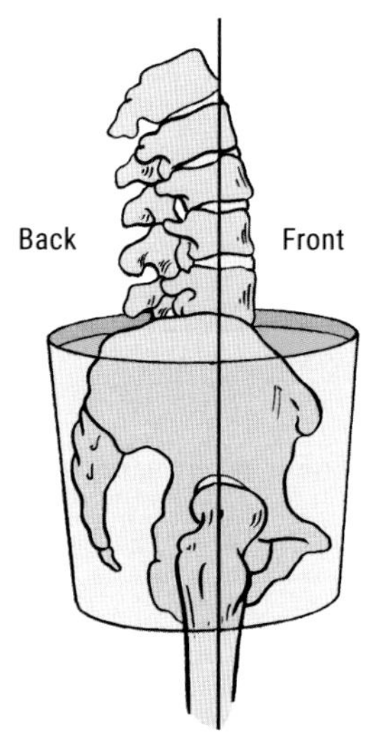

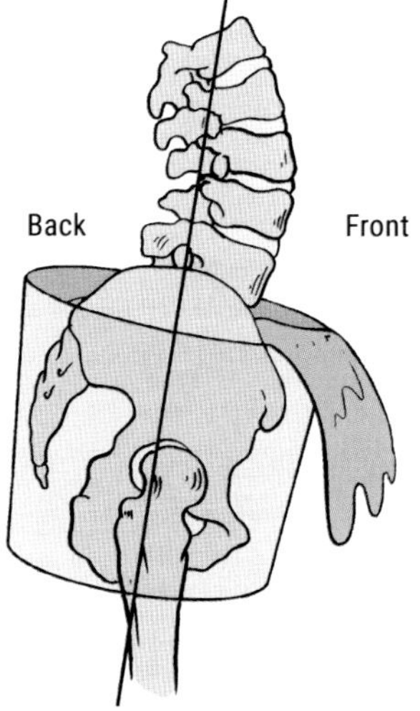

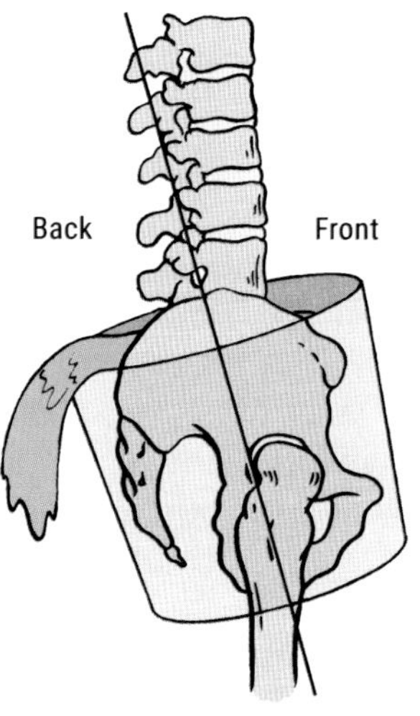

FIGURE 10-9
Anterior and posterior tilting of the pelvis—sagittal (side) view

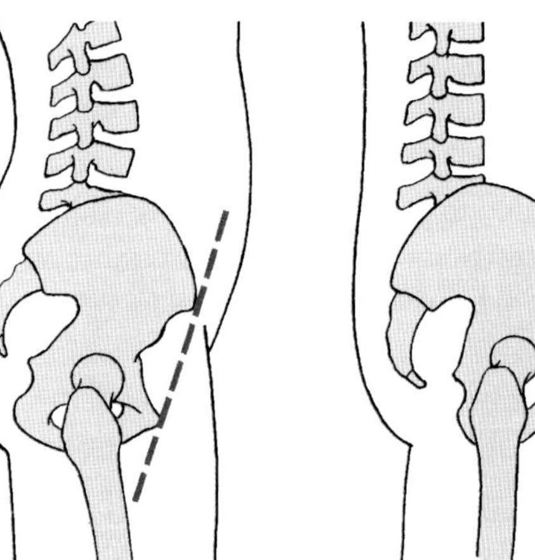

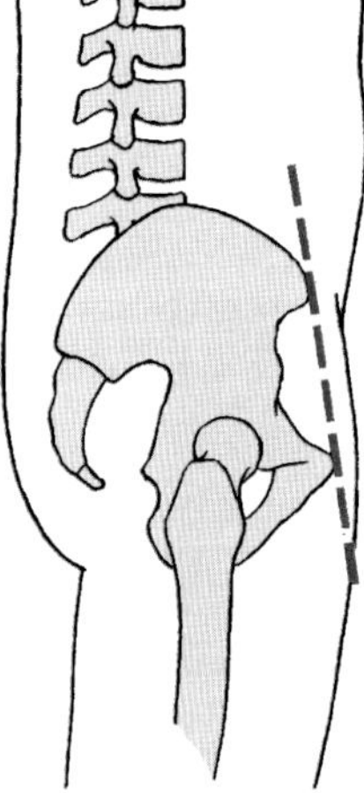

FIGURE 10-10
Alignment of the anterior superior iliac spine (ASIS) and pubic bone

Source: LifeART image copyright 2008 Wolters Kluwer Health, Inc., Lippincott Williams & Wilkins. All rights reserved.

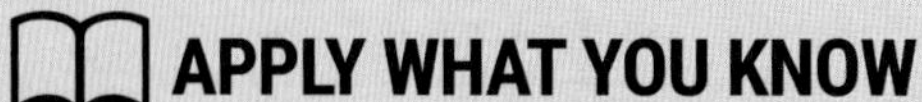

APPLY WHAT YOU KNOW

Pelvic Tilt

An anterior pelvic tilt will increase lordosis in the lumbar spine, whereas a posterior pelvic tilt will reduce the amount of lordosis in the lumbar spine. To demonstrate this point, stand with hands placed on the hips and gently tilt the pelvis anteriorly, noticing the change in position and increase in muscle tension in the lumbar region. Likewise, tilt the pelvis posteriorly and notice how the lumbar spine flattens and reduces tension in the lumbar extensors.

Tight or hypertonic hip flexors may be coupled with tight erector spinae muscles, producing an anterior pelvic tilt, while tight or hypertonic rectus abdominis muscles may be coupled with tight hamstrings, producing a posterior pelvic tilt (Table 10-7). With foot pronation and accompanying internal femoral rotation, the pelvis may tilt anteriorly to better accommodate the head of the femur, demonstrating the point of an integrated kinetic chain whereby foot pronation can increase lumbar lordosis due to an anterior pelvic tilt (Sahrmann, 2002).

TABLE 10-7
Pelvic Tilt

	Anterior Tilt	Posterior Tilt
Rotation	ASIS tilts downward and forward	ASIS tilts upward and backward
Muscles suspected to be tight	Hip flexors, erector spinae	Rectus abdominis, hamstrings
Muscles suspected to be lengthened	Hamstrings, rectus abdominis	Hip flexors, erector spinae
Plane of view	Sagittal	Sagittal

Note: ASIS = Anterior superior iliac spine

DEVIATION 4: SHOULDER POSITION AND THE THORACIC SPINE

Limitations and compensations to movement at the shoulder occur frequently due to the complex nature of the shoulder girdle design and the varied movements performed at the shoulder. While the glenohumeral joint is highly mobile and perhaps a less stable joint, the scapulothoracic joint is designed to offer greater stability with less mobility (Figure 10-11). However, it is important to remember that it still contributes approximately 60 degrees of movement in raising the arms overhead, with the glenohumeral joint contributing the remaining 120 degrees (Figure 10-12). This relationship is referred to as **scapulohumeral rhythm** and approximates that for every 2 degrees of humeral motion, 1 degree of scapular motion takes places throughout the available **range of motion (ROM)** for flexion/extension and abduction/adduction. The scapulothoracic joint also promotes many important movements of the scapulae (Figure 10-13). Collectively, however, they allow for a diverse range of movements in the shoulder complex. Observation of the position of the scapulae in all three planes provides good insight into a client's quality of movement at the shoulders.

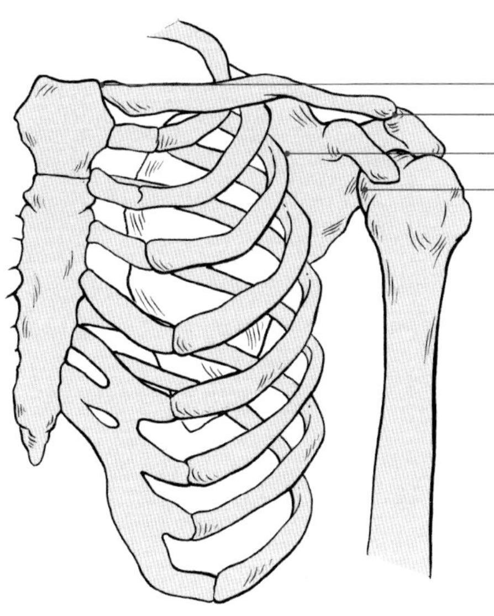

FIGURE 10-11
The four articulations of the shoulder-joint complex

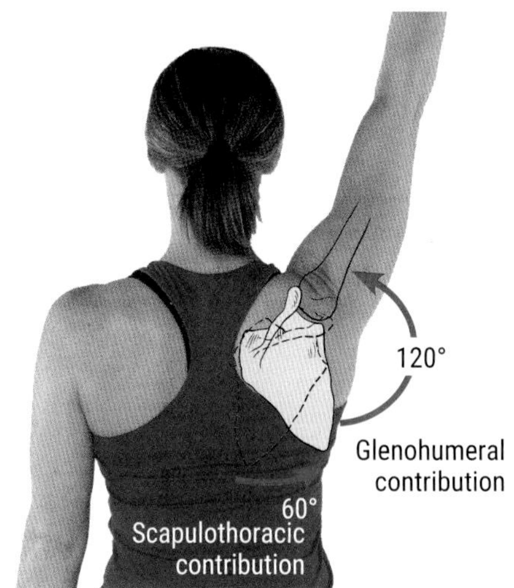

FIGURE 10-12
Scapulohumeral rhythm

The movement of the arm is accompanied by movement of the scapula—a ratio of approximately 2° of arm movement for every 1° of scapular movement occurs during shoulder abduction and flexion.

FIGURE 10-13
Scapular movements

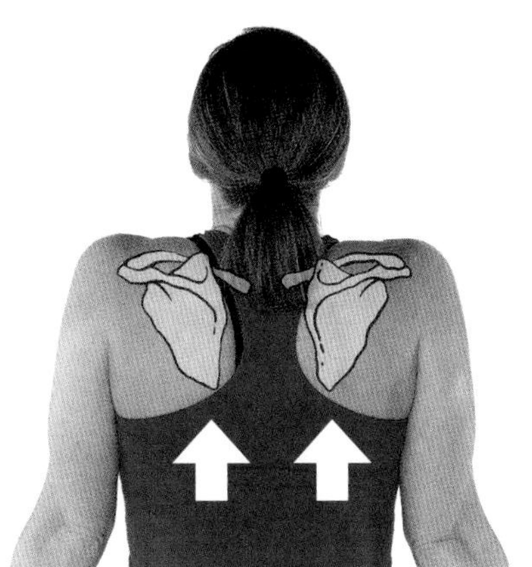
Elevation

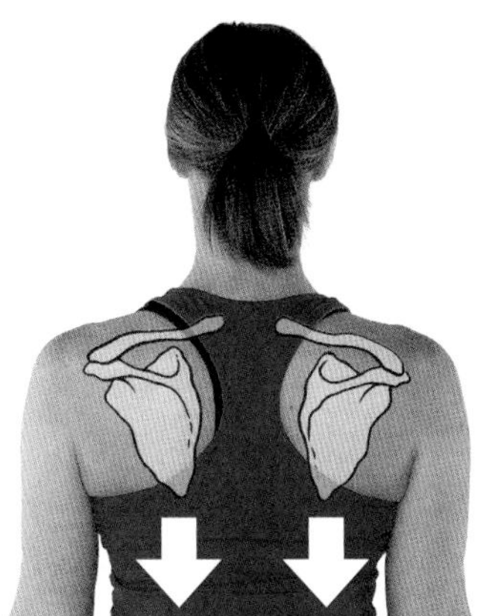
Depression

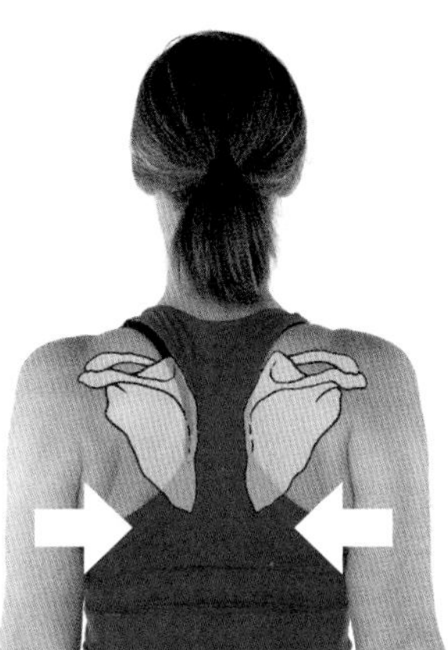
Adduction (retraction)

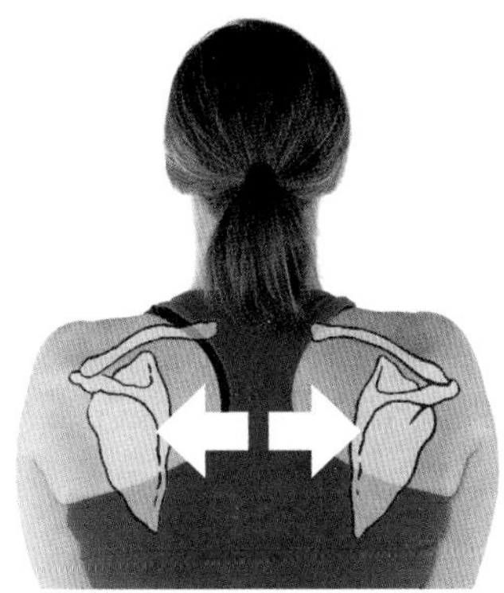
Abduction (protraction)

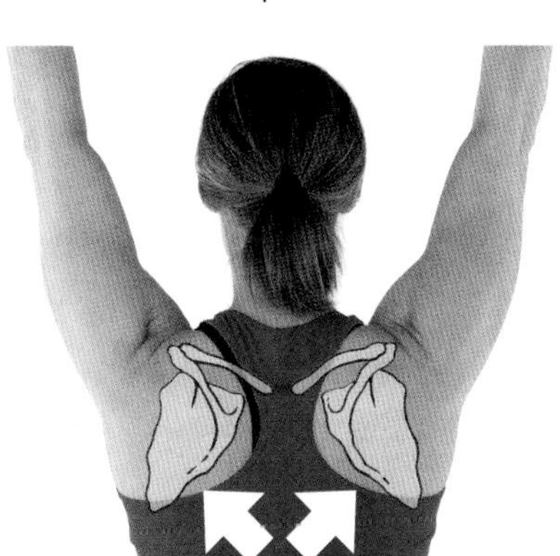
Upward rotation

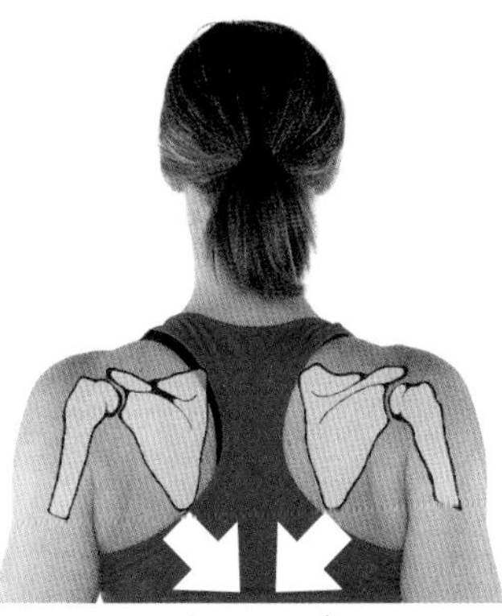
Downward rotation (return to anatomical position)

Figure 10-14 illustrates the "resting" position of the scapulae, which can vary considerably from person to person. The scapulae are typically positioned against the rib cage between the second and seventh ribs about 2 inches (5.1 cm) from the spinous processes (Houglum, 2016; Kendall et al., 2005). While the glenoid fossa is tilted upward 5 degrees and anteriorly 30 degrees to optimally articulate with the head of the humerus, the scapulae usually lie flat against the rib cage (Kendall et al., 2005). While the scapulae should appear flat against the rib cage, their orientation depends on the size and shape of the person and the rib cage.

FIGURE 10-14
The normal position of the scapulae

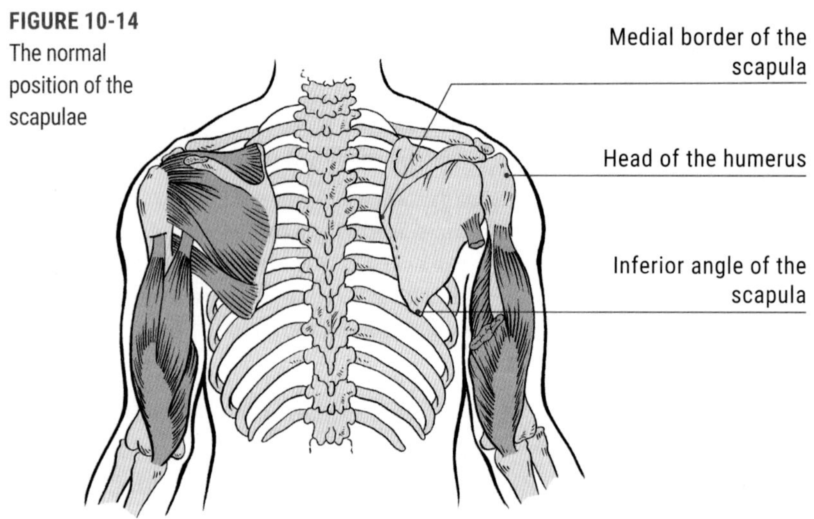

APPLY WHAT YOU KNOW

Scapular Winging and Scapular Protraction

Personal trainers can perform a quick observational assessment to identify scapular winging and scapular protraction. While looking at the client from the posterior view, if the vertebral (medial) and/or inferior angle of the scapulae protrude outward, this indicates an inability of the scapular stabilizers (primarily the rhomboids and serratus anterior) to hold the scapulae in place. Noticeable protrusion of the vertebral (medial) border outward is termed "scapular protraction" (Figure 10-15a), while protrusion of the inferior angle and vertebral (medial) border outward is termed "winged scapulae" (Figure 10-15b).

Scapular protraction can also be identified from the anterior view (Figure 10-16). If the palms face backward instead of to the sides, this generally indicates internal (medial) rotation of the humerus and/or scapular protraction.

Table 10-8 lists key deviations of the thoracic spine and shoulders in various planes of view.

Note: There is often a natural amount of "shrugging" inward with scapular protraction.

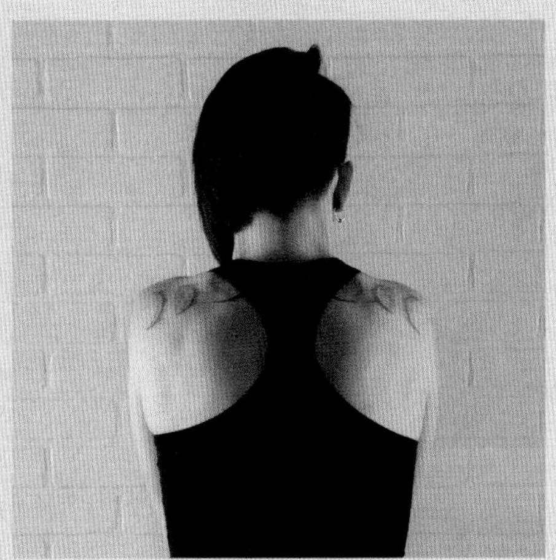
a. Scapular protraction

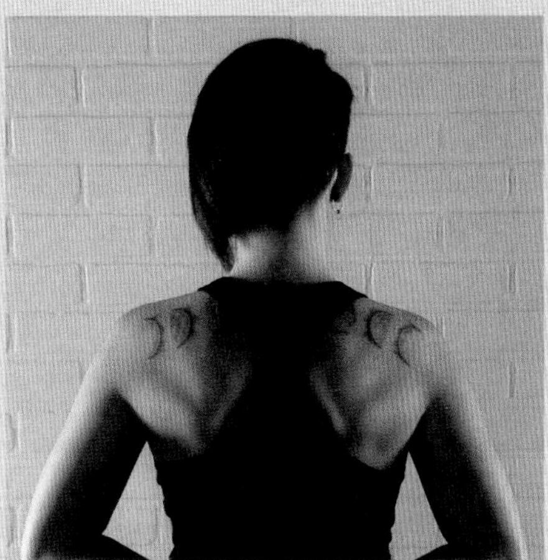
b. Scapular winging

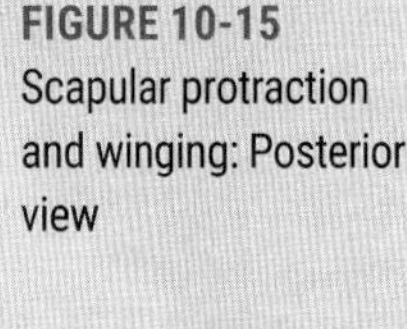
FIGURE 10-15
Scapular protraction and winging: Posterior view

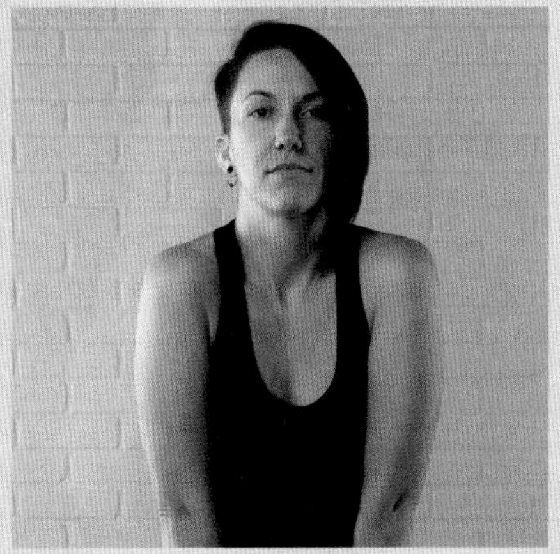
FIGURE 10-16
Scapular protraction: Anterior view

TABLE 10-8
Shoulder Position

Observation	Muscles Suspected to Be Tight	Plane of View
Shoulders not level	Upper trapezius, levator scapula, rhomboids on the elevated side	Frontal
Asymmetry to midline	Lateral trunk flexors (flexed side)	Frontal
Protracted (forward, rounded)	Serratus anterior*, anterior scapulo-humeral muscles†, upper trapezius	Sagittal
Medially rotated humerus	Pectoralis major and latissimus dorsi (shoulder adductors), subscapularis	Frontal
Kyphosis and depressed chest	Shoulder adductors, pectoralis minor, rectus abdominis, internal oblique	Sagittal

*Serratus anterior is usually tight with scapular protraction and is usually lengthened with scapular winging.

†A group of seven muscles (coracobrachialis, deltoids, four rotator cuff muscles, and teres major) that connect the humerus to the scapula and function to stabilize the glenohumeral joint.

DEVIATION 5: HEAD POSITION

With good posture, the earlobe should align approximately over the acromion process in the sagittal view, but given the many awkward postures and repetitive motions of daily life, a forward-head position is very common (Table 10-9) (Kendall et al., 2005). This altered position does not tilt the head downward, but simply shifts it forward so that the earlobe appears significantly forward of the AC joint (Figure 10-17). A forward-head position may represent tightness in the cervical extensors and lengthening of the cervical flexors.

TABLE 10-9
Head Position

Observation	Muscles Suspected to Be Tight	Plane of View
Forward-head position	Cervical spine extensors, upper trapezius, levator scapulae	Sagittal

FIGURE 10-17
Alignment of the acromioclavicular joint with the ear

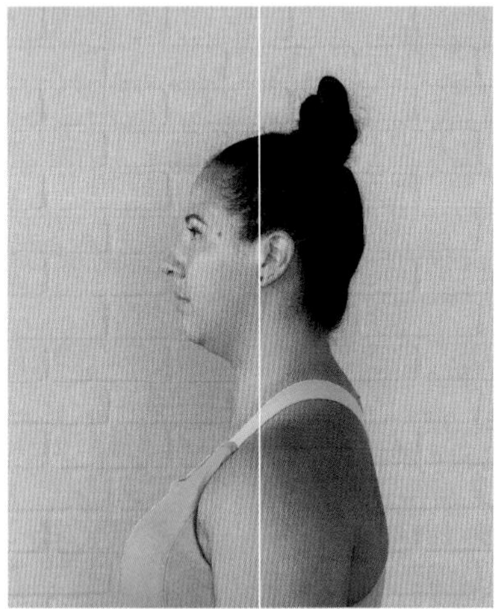

Postural alignment

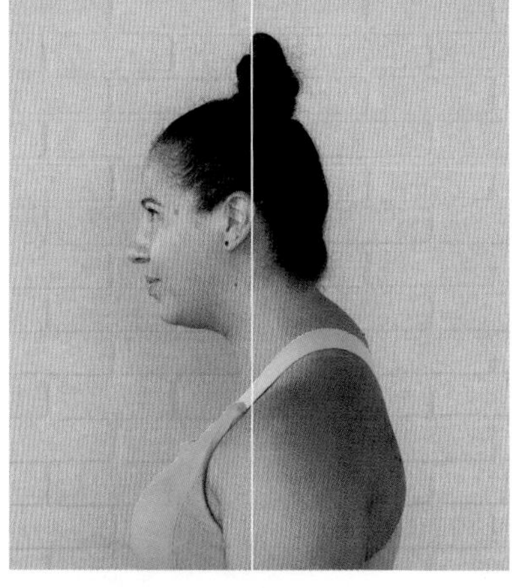

Forward-head position

Postural Assessment Checklist and Worksheets

When performing basic postural assessments, personal trainers can use the checklist provided in Figure 10-18 to guide themselves through their observations, and complete the worksheets provided in Figures 10-19 and 10-20 to mark any postural compensations they identify.

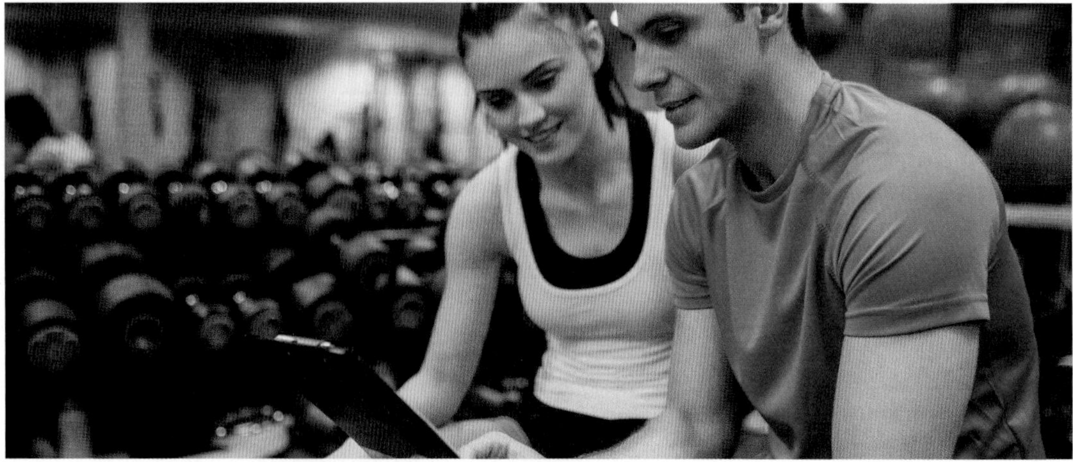

FIGURE 10-18
Postural assessment checklist

	ANTERIOR VIEW
☐	Overall body symmetry: symmetrical alignment of the left and right hemispheres
☐	Ankle position: observe for pronation and supination
☐	Foot position: observe for inversion and eversion
☐	Knees: rotation and height discrepancies
☐	Hip adduction and shifting: observe for shifting to a side as witnessed by the position of the pubis in relation to the line of gravity
☐	Alignment of the iliac crests
☐	Alignment of the torso: position of the umbilicus and sternum in relation to the line of gravity
☐	Alignment of the shoulders
☐	Arm spacing: observe the space to the sides of the torso
☐	Hand position: observe the position relative to the torso
☐	Head position: alignment of the ears, nose, eyes, and chin
	POSTERIOR VIEW
☐	Overall body symmetry: symmetrical alignment of the left and right hemispheres
☐	Alignment of the spine: vertical alignment of the spinous processes (may require forward bending)
☐	Alignment of the scapulae: inferior angle of scapulae and presence of winged scapulae
☐	Alignment of the shoulders
☐	Head: alignment of the ears
	SIDE VIEW
☐	Overall body symmetry: symmetrical alignment of load-bearing joint landmarks with the line of gravity
☐	Knees: flexion or extension
☐	Pelvic alignment for tilting: relationship of ASIS to PSIS
☐	Spinal curves: observe for thoracic kyphosis, lumbar lordosis, or flat-back position
☐	Shoulder position: forward rounding (protraction) of the scapulae
☐	Head position: neutral cervical curvature (versus forward position) and level (position above the clavicle)

Note: ASIS = Anterior superior iliac spine; PSIS = Posterior superior iliac spine

ANTERIOR VIEW:			POSTERIOR VIEW:		
L	R	OBSERVATION	L	R	OBSERVATION
☐	☐	1.	☐	☐	1.
☐	☐	2.	☐	☐	2.
☐	☐	3.	☐	☐	3.
☐	☐	4.	☐	☐	4.
☐	☐	5.	☐	☐	5.
☐	☐	6.	☐	☐	6.
☐	☐	7.	☐	☐	7.
CIRCLE OR MARK OBSERVATIONS			CIRCLE OR MARK OBSERVATIONS		

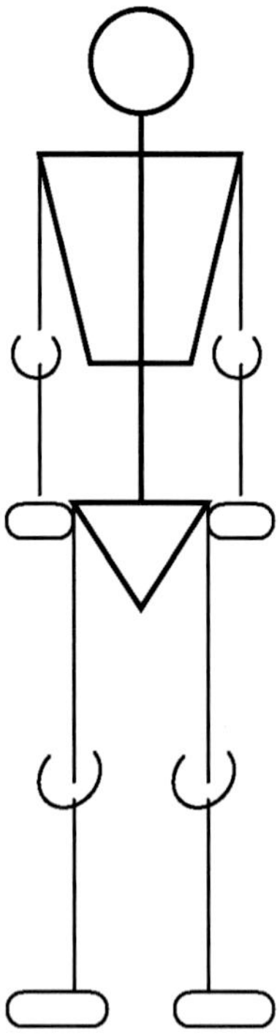

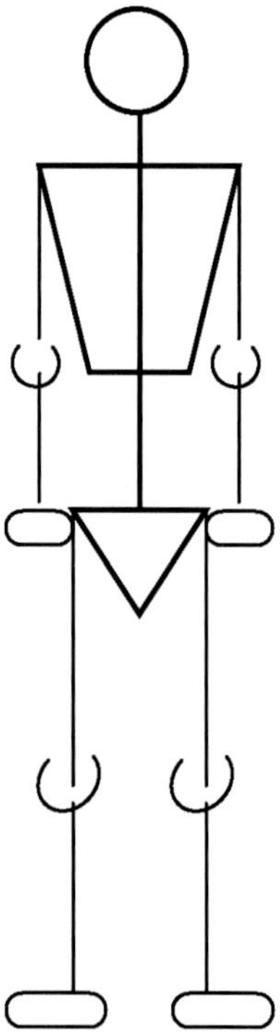

FIGURE 10-19
Anterior/posterior worksheet

LEFT SIDE VIEW:		RIGHT SIDE VIEW:	
L	OBSERVATION	R	OBSERVATION
☐	1.	☐	1.
☐	2.	☐	2.
☐	3.	☐	3.
☐	4.	☐	4.
☐	5.	☐	5.
☐	6.	☐	6.
☐	7.	☐	7.
CIRCLE OR MARK OBSERVATIONS		CIRCLE OR MARK OBSERVATIONS	

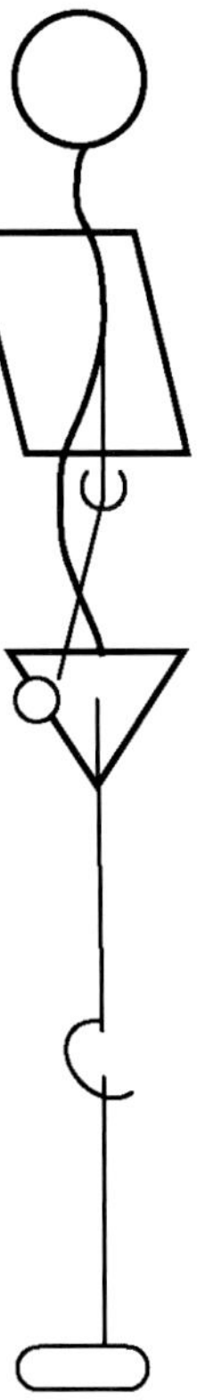

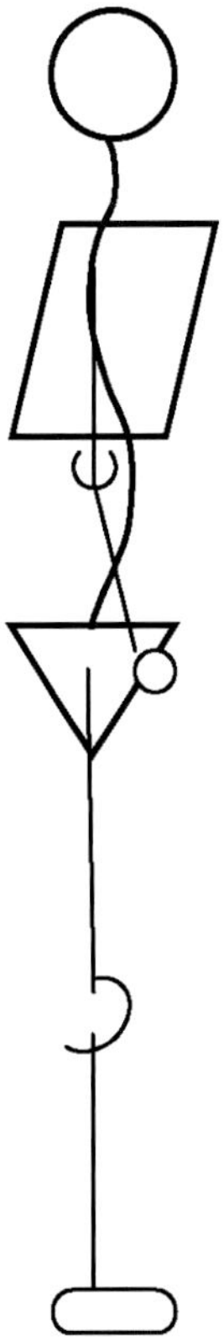

FIGURE 10-20
Sagittal worksheet

STATIC BALANCE: UNIPEDAL STANCE TEST

Fall incidence rates currently pose a serious health problem for older adults. Among those who are 65 or older, it has been estimated that more than one in four older adults fall at least once a year (Centers for Disease Control and Prevention, 2018). The unipedal stance test (also sometimes referred to as the timed one-leg stance test) provides personal trainers with a simple, yet valid and reliable option to assess the static balance of their clients. Outcome measures from the unipedal stance test provide personal trainers with valuable information regarding their client's risk for falls, abilities to perform **activities of daily living (ADL),** and risk of low-back pain (Gibson, Wagner, & Heyward, 2019).

Equipment:

- Stop watch or wrist watch
- 10-feet x 10-feet clear space with firm flooring

Pre-test procedure:

- Explain the purpose of the test and that the client will be spotted for safety.
- Have the client kick a ball to identify the dominant leg.
- Model body position and demonstrate test procedures (with and without eyes closed) for the client.

Test protocol and administration:

- Instruct the client to stand barefooted with arms folded across the chest.
- Instruct the client to focus his or her eyesight on an eye-level point on the wall directly in front. The test can be performed with eyes either open or closed. If performing the test with eyes closed, instruct the client to close his or her eyes after focusing on the point on the wall.

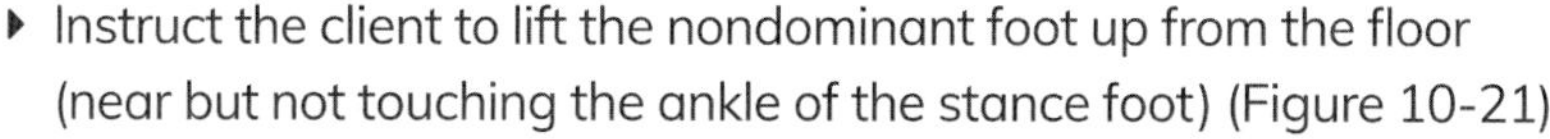

- Instruct the client to lift the nondominant foot up from the floor (near but not touching the ankle of the stance foot) (Figure 10-21).
- The test commences when the client lifts the nondominant foot from the floor.
- The test progresses until any of the following termination criteria occurs:
    - Client opens eyes during an eyes-closed trial
    - Dominant weight-bearing foot moves in order to maintain balance
    - Nondominant foot touches the floor or moves away from the dominant weight-bearing limb
    - Client achieves the maximum 45-second duration of the test
- Administer three trials and record the best performance.

FIGURE 10-21
Unipedal stance test

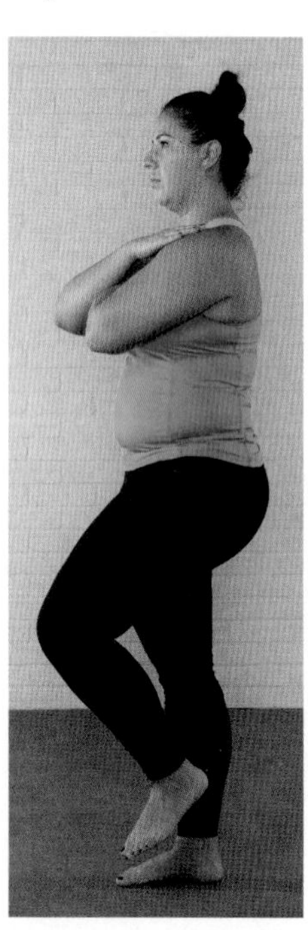

Interpretation:

Table 10-10 can be used to interpret the unipedal stance test compared to normative data including men and women of various age groups.

TABLE 10-10
Normative Data for the Unipedal Stance Test

	Eyes Open (seconds)		Eyes Closed (seconds)	
Age Category (years)	**Female**	**Male**	**Female**	**Male**
18–39	45.1	44.4	13.1	16.9
40–49	42.1	41.6	13.5	12.0
50–59	40.9	41.5	7.9	8.6
60–69	30.4	33.8	3.6	5.1
70–79	16.7	25.9	3.7	2.6
80–99	10.6	8.7	2.1	1.8

Reprinted with permission from Gibson, A.L., Wagner, D.R., & Heyward, V.H. (2019). *Advanced Fitness Assessment and Exercise Prescription* (8th ed.). Champaign, Ill.: Human Kinetics, page 354.

DYNAMIC BALANCE: Y BALANCE TEST

The Y balance test can be used to assess dynamic balance (Chimera, Smith, & Warren, 2015). Asymmetries between legs during the Y balance test are related to injury risk and may indicate the need for guided injury-prevention strategies (e.g., a focused balance-training program) in athletes (Lisman et al., 2018). The Y balance test is appropriate for athletic populations and clients with sport-related goals (Chimera, Smith, & Warren, 2015). This assessment is not recommended for older adult clients and/or those with balance impairments.

The Y balance test requires clients to balance on one leg and concurrently reach as far as possible with the other leg in three directions (Figure 10-22): anterior, posteromedial, and posterolateral. The naming of the three reaches is based on the directional terms of the stance foot (e.g., anterior, posterior, and lateral). For example, using the left foot as the stance foot, a reach to the right corresponds to the medial side of the left foot (i.e., posteromedial reach; see Figure 10-22b) and a reach to the left (with the

FIGURE 10-22
The three directions of the Y balance test

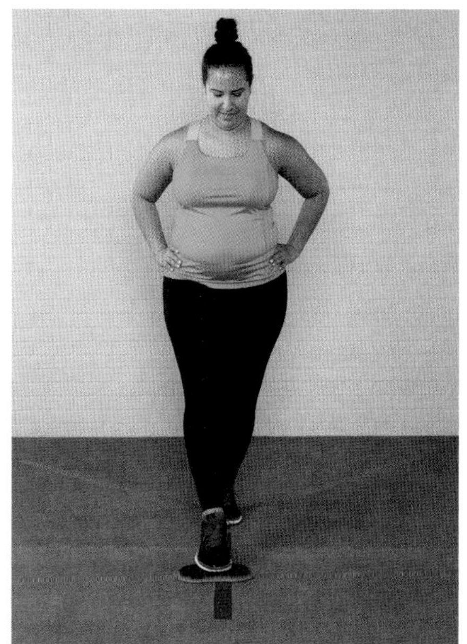
a. Anterior reach

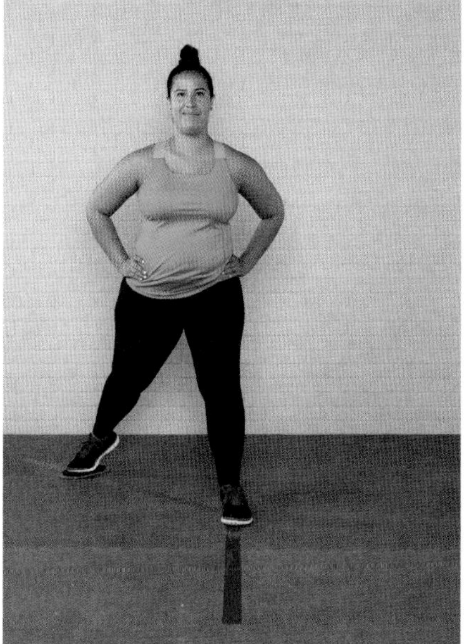
b. Posteromedial reach

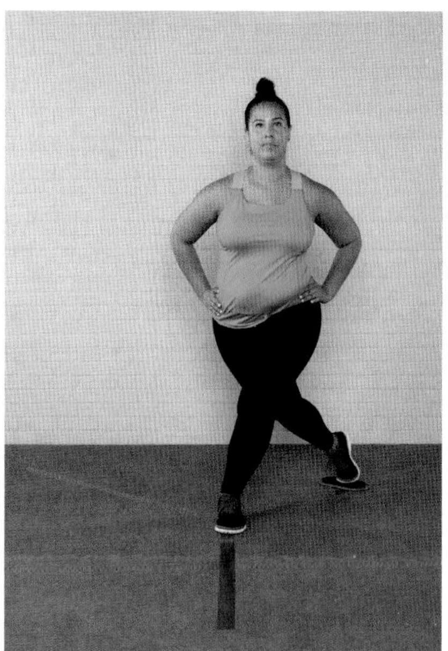
c. Posterolateral reach

right foot) corresponds to the lateral side of the left foot (i.e., posterolateral reach; see Figure 10-22c). Essentially, if the client is reaching away from the medial side of the stance foot, the directional term is posteromedial, and if the client is reaching toward the lateral aspect of the stance foot, the directional term is posterolateral.

Equipment:

- Adequate space of 6 feet x 6 feet
- Tape measure, adhesive tape, protractor, and 3- x 5-inch furniture or exercise sliders
- Data collection sheet

Pre-assessment procedures:

- Set up the assessment area according to dimensions presented in Figure 10-23.
- The client should perform a five-minute warm-up of light cardiorespiratory exercise followed by five minutes of gentle **static stretching** of the major lower-extremity muscle groups.

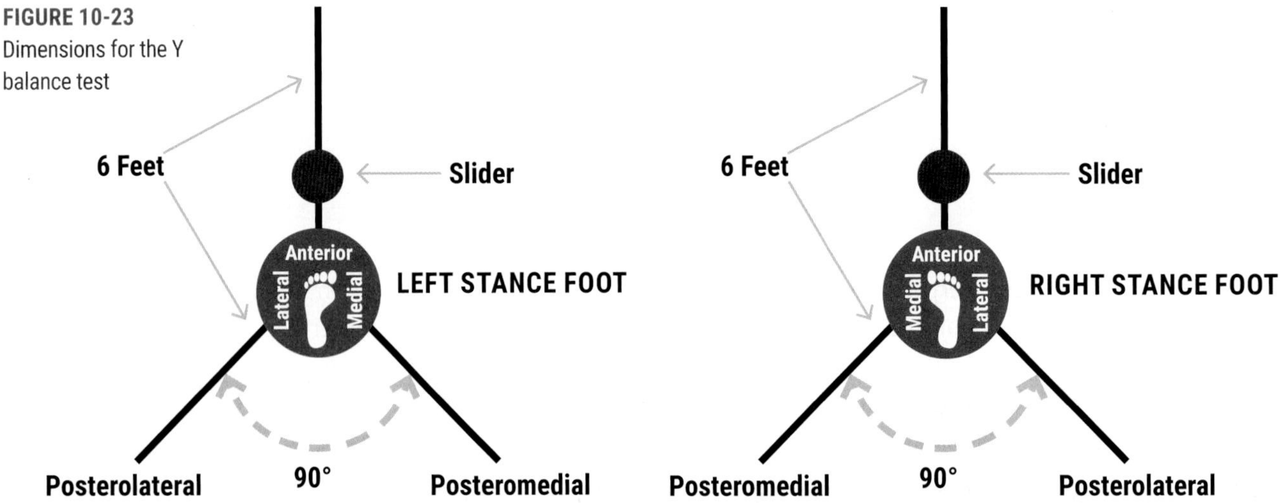

FIGURE 10-23
Dimensions for the Y balance test

Assessment protocol and administration:

- Testing is completed in the following leg/direction order: (1) right leg anterior, (2) left leg anterior, (3) right leg posteromedial, (4) left leg posteromedial, (5) right leg posterolateral, and (6) left leg posterolateral.
- While balancing on the left leg, clients should place hands on hips and slide the furniture slider forward (i.e., anterior) as far as possible, and then return to a two-feet standing position.
- Sliding forward with the right foot should be performed three consecutive times, followed by sliding forward three consecutive times with the left foot.
- The Y balance test progresses in the order described above after three consecutive slides with each foot in each direction.
- The following scenarios constitute failed attempts:
    - The client cannot touch the reach foot to the ground prior to returning to the starting position.

- The client is unable to maintain contact between the reach foot and slider throughout the reach.
- The client kicks the slider forward to achieve a better score.

Interpretation:

- The personal trainer records the best slide for each leg/direction combination to the nearest 0.25 inch (0.6 cm) using the scoring sheet provided in Table 10-11.
- A greater than 1.6-inch (4-cm) difference in anterior symmetry has been demonstrated to increase risk of lower-extremity injury (Chimera, Smith, & Warren, 2015).
- Upon periodic reassessment of dynamic balance, personal trainers can compare follow-up Y balance test measures to baseline values to quantify improvements and training program effectiveness.

TABLE 10-11
Scoring Sheet for Y Balance Test

Direction	Right Foot Stance (Left Foot Reach)	Left Foot Stance (Right Foot Reach)	Difference
Anterior			
Posteromedial			
Posterolateral			

MCGILL'S TORSO MUSCULAR ENDURANCE TEST BATTERY

Optimally functioning core muscles help clients perform ADL like lifting a heavy laundry basket or recreational activities like swinging a golf club. Further, back dysfunction may be reversed by having a conditioned core. To evaluate balanced core endurance and stability, it is important to assess all sides of the torso. Each of the following assessments is performed individually, then evaluated collectively. Poor endurance capacity of the torso muscles or an imbalance among these three muscle groups is believed to contribute to low-back dysfunction and core instability.

Trunk Flexor Endurance Test

The trunk flexor endurance test is the first in the battery of three tests that assesses muscular endurance of the trunk flexors (i.e., rectus abdominis, external and internal obliques, and transverse abdominis) (Figure 10-24; see Figure 9-34, page 362). It is a timed test involving a static, **isometric** contraction of the anterior muscles, stabilizing the spine until the individual exhibits fatigue and can no longer hold the assumed position. This test may not be suitable for individuals who suffer from low-back pain, have had recent back surgery, and/or are in the midst of an acute low-back flare-up.

Equipment:

- Stopwatch
- Board (or step)
- Strap (optional)

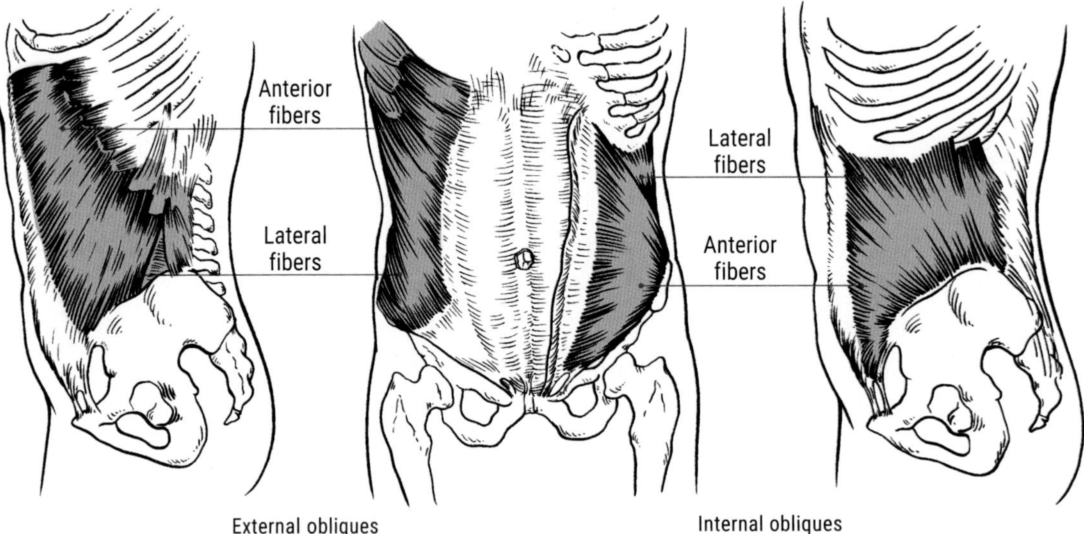

FIGURE 10-24
External and internal obliques

Pre-assessment procedure:

- After explaining the purpose of the flexor endurance test, describe the proper body position.
  - The starting position requires the client to be seated, with the hips and knees bent to 90 degrees, aligning the hips, knees, and second toe.
  - Instruct the client to fold his or her arms across the chest, touching each hand to the opposite shoulder, lean against a board positioned at a 50- to 60-degree incline, and keep the head in a neutral position (Figure 10-25).
  - It is important to ask the client to press the shoulders into the board and maintain this "open" position throughout the test after the board is removed.
  - Instruct the client to engage the abdominals to maintain a flat-to-neutral spine. The back should never be allowed to arch during the test.
  - The personal trainer can anchor the toes under a strap or manually stabilize the feet if necessary.
- The goal of the test is to hold this 50- to 60-degree position for as long as possible without the benefit of the back support.
- Encourage the client to practice this position prior to attempting the test.

Assessment protocol and administration:

- The personal trainer starts the stopwatch as he or she moves the board about 4 inches (10 cm) back, while the client maintains the 50- to 60-degree, suspended position.
- Terminate the test when there is a noticeable change in the trunk position:
  - Watch for a deviation from the neutral spine (i.e., the shoulders rounding forward) or an increase in the low-back arch.
  - No part of the back should touch the back rest.
- Record the client's time on the testing form.

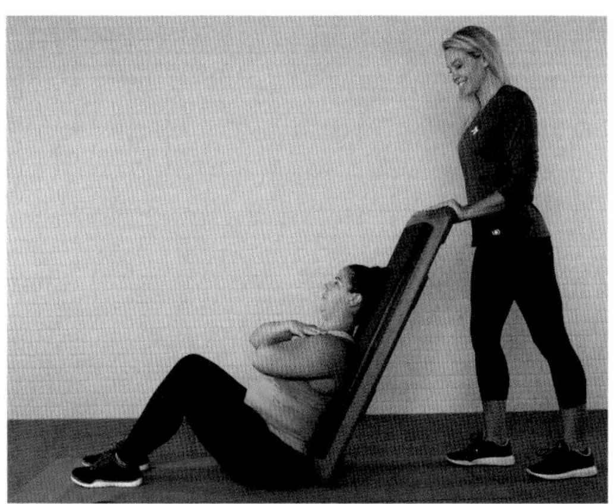
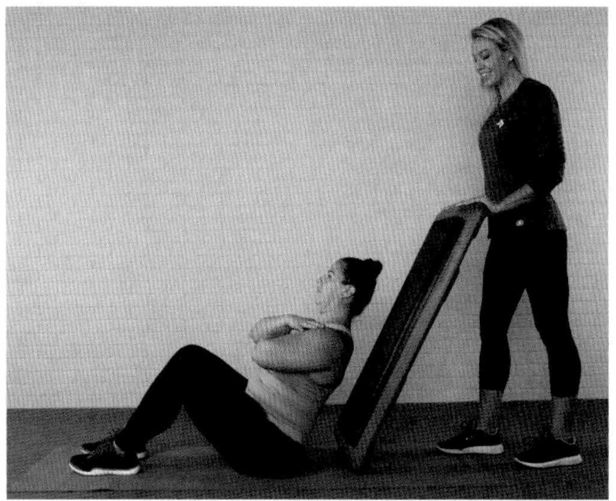

FIGURE 10-25
Trunk flexor endurance test

Trunk Lateral Endurance Test

The trunk lateral endurance test, also called the side-bridge test, assesses muscular endurance of the lateral core muscles (i.e., transverse abdominis, obliques, quadratus lumborum, and erector spinae) [Figure 10-26; see Figures 9-34 (page 362) and 10-24]. This timed test involves static, isometric contractions of the lateral muscles on each side of the trunk that stabilize the spine. This test may not be suitable for individuals with shoulder pain or weakness and who suffer from low-back pain, have had recent back surgery, and/or are in the midst of an acute low-back flare-up.

Equipment:

- Stopwatch
- Mat (optional)

Pre-assessment procedure:

- After explaining the purpose of this test, describe the proper body position.
  - The starting position requires the client to be on his or her side with extended legs, aligning the feet on top of each other or in a tandem position (heel-to-toe).
  - Have the client place the lower arm under the body and the upper arm on the side of the body.
  - When the client is ready, instruct him or her to assume a full side-bridge position, keeping both legs extended and the sides of the feet on the floor. The elbow of the lower arm should be positioned directly under the shoulder with the forearm facing out (the forearm can be placed palm down for balance and support) and the upper arm should be resting along the side of the body or across the chest to the opposite shoulder.
  - The hips should be elevated off the mat and the body should be in straight alignment (i.e., head, neck, torso, hips, and legs). The torso should only be supported by the client's foot/feet and the elbow/forearm of the lower arm (Figure 10-27).
    - *Modification*: If a client is unable to support his or her body weight while balancing on the feet, an alternative is for the client to rest on the side of the lower leg with both knees bent in the hook-lying position (Figure 10-28), thereby

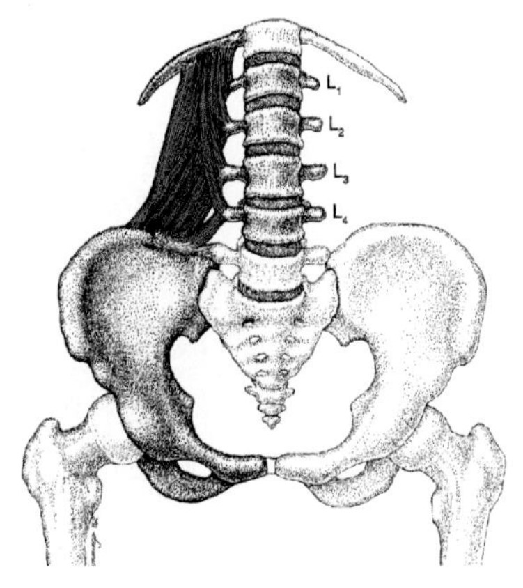

FIGURE 10-26
Quadratus lumborum

Source: LifeART image copyright 2008 Wolters Kluwer Health, Inc., Lippincott Williams & Wilkins.

shortening the lever of the legs and increasing the surface area on which to balance. If this modification is used, be sure to perform subsequent assessments in the modified position so that the results are comparable. Because the original test battery was not performed using this modification, the scoring and reliability of results will vary.

- The goal of the test is to hold this position for as long as possible. Once the client breaks the position, the test is terminated.
- Encourage the client to practice this position prior to attempting the test.

Assessment protocol and administration:

- The personal trainer starts the stopwatch as the client moves into the side-bridge position.
- Terminate the test when there is a noticeable change in the trunk position
  - A deviation from the neutral spine (i.e., the hips dropping downward)
  - The hips shifting forward or backward in an effort to maintain balance and stability
- Record the client's time on the testing form.
- Repeat the test on the opposite side and record this value on the testing form.

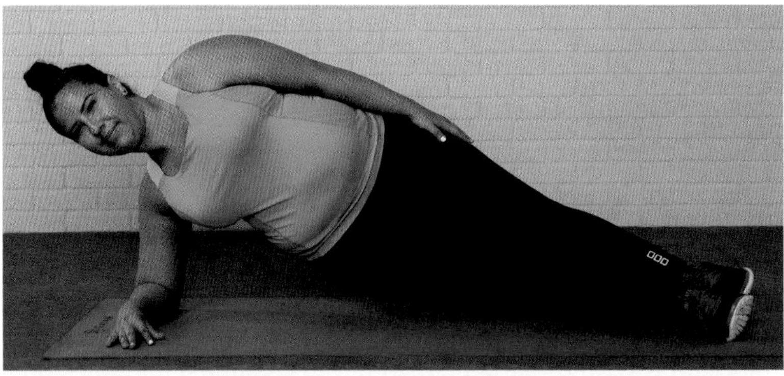

FIGURE 10-27
Trunk lateral endurance test

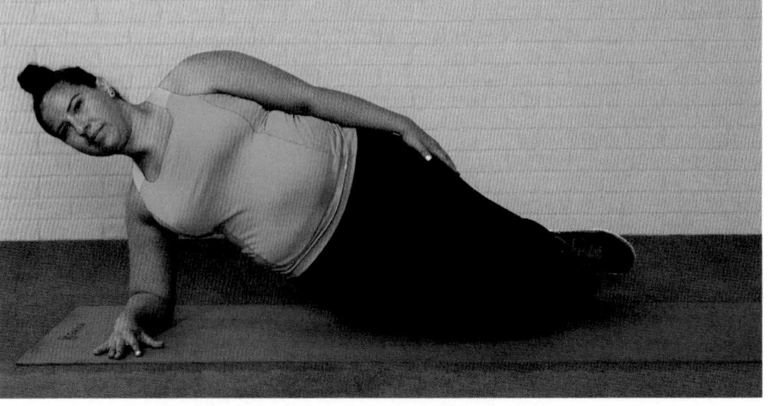

FIGURE 10-28
Trunk lateral endurance test: Modified hook-lying position

Trunk Extensor Endurance Test

The trunk extensor endurance test is generally used to assess muscular endurance of the torso extensor muscles (i.e., erector spinae and multifidi) (see Figure 9-33, page 362; Figure 10-29). This is a timed test involving a static, isometric contraction of the trunk extensor muscles that stabilize the spine. This test may not be suitable for a client with major strength deficiencies, where the individual cannot even lift the torso from a forward flexed position to a neutral position, a client with a high body mass, in which case it would be difficult for the personal trainer to support the client's suspended upper-body weight, and individuals who suffer from low-back pain, have had recent back surgery, and/ or are in the midst of an acute low-back flare-up.

FIGURE 10-29
Multifidi

Source: LifeART image copyright 2008 Wolters Kluwer Health, Inc., Lippincott Williams & Wilkins. All rights reserved.

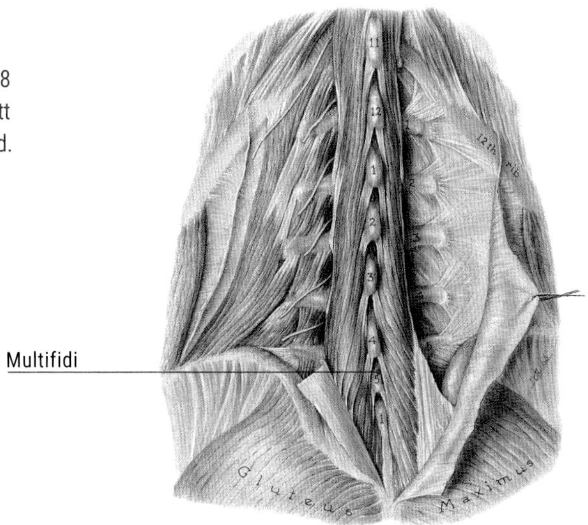

Equipment:

- Elevated, sturdy exam table
- Nylon strap
- Stopwatch

Pre-assessment procedure:

- After explaining the purpose of the test, explain the proper body position.
  - The starting position requires the client to be prone, positioning the iliac crests at the table edge while supporting the upper extremity on the arms, which are placed on the floor or on a riser.
  - While the client is supporting the weight of his or her upper body, anchor the client's lower legs to the table using a strap. If a strap is not used, the personal trainer will have to use his or her own body weight to stabilize the client's legs (Figure 10-30a).
- The goal of the test is to hold a horizontal, prone position for as long as possible. Once the client falls below horizontal, the test is terminated.
- Encourage the client to practice this position prior to attempting the test.

Assessment protocol and administration:

- When ready, the client lifts/extends the torso until it is parallel to the floor with his or her arms crossed over the chest (Figure 10-30b).
  - *Modification:* If a client is unable to support his or her body weight while hanging off the edge of a table, an alternative is for the client to lie prone on the floor and come into spinal extension (Figure 10-31), thereby eliminating the need for a table and strap (or for the personal trainer to hold the client's legs). The client should be instructed to keep the thighs in contact with the floor throughout the duration of the assessment. If this modification is used, be sure to perform subsequent assessments in the modified position so that the results are comparable. Because the original test battery was not performed using this modification, the scoring and reliability of results will vary.
- Start the stopwatch as soon as the client assumes this position.
- Terminate the test when the client can no longer maintain the position.
- Record the client's time on the testing form.

FIGURE 10-30
Trunk extensor endurance test

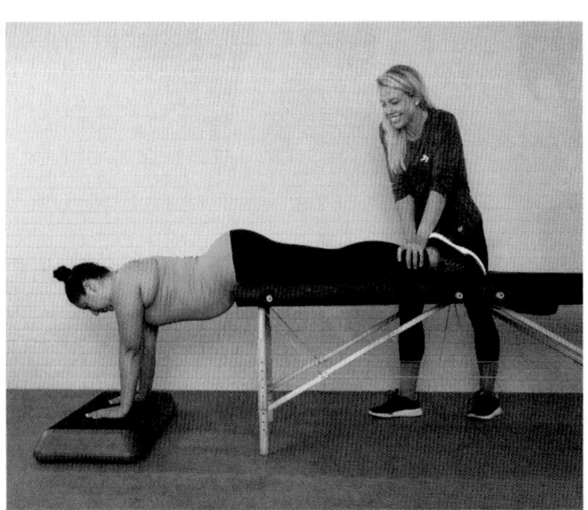

a. Starting position

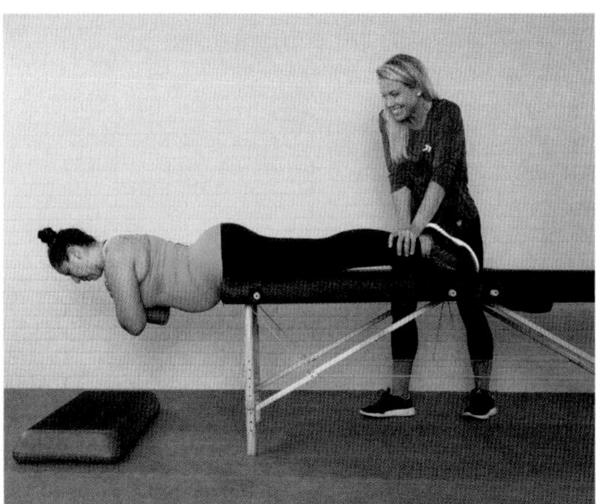

b. Test position

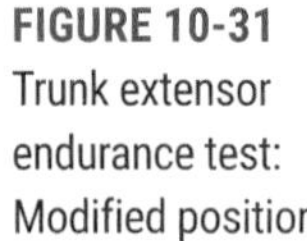

FIGURE 10-31
Trunk extensor endurance test: Modified position

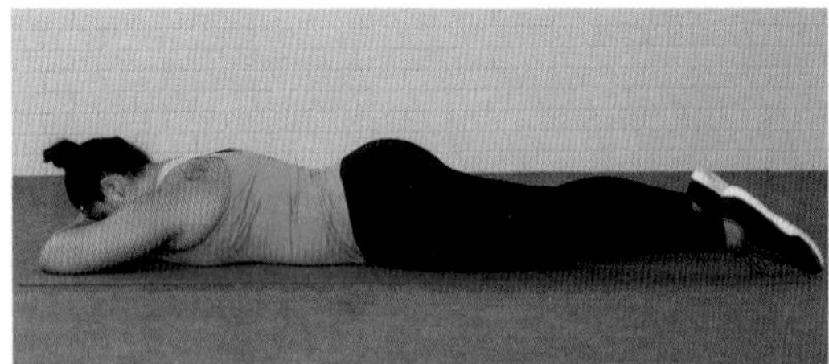

a. Starting position

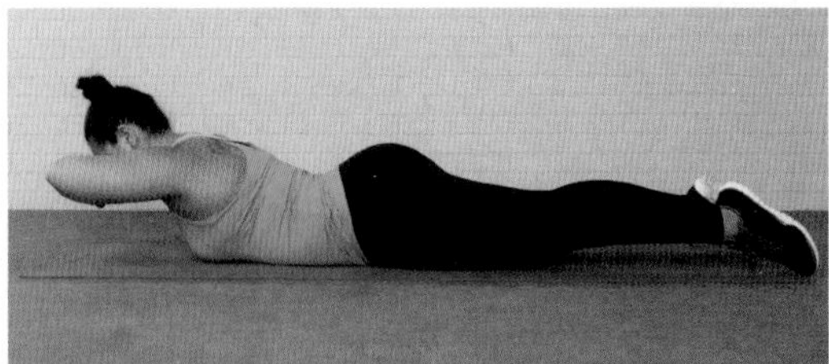

b. Test position

Total Test Battery Interpretation

Each individual test in this testing battery is not a primary indicator of current or future back problems. McGill (2016) has shown that the relationships among the tests are more important indicators of muscle imbalances that can lead to back pain compared to looking at the individual results of each test because the torso extensors, flexors, and lateral musculature are involved in virtually all tasks. In fact, even in a person with little or no back pain, the ratios can still be off, suggesting that low-back pain may eventually occur without diligent attention to a solid core-conditioning program. McGill (2016) suggests the following ratios indicate balanced endurance among the muscle groups:

- Flexion:extension ratio should be less than 1.0
  - For example, a flexion score of 120 seconds and extension score of 150 seconds generates a ratio score of 0.80
- Right-side bridge (RSB):left-side bridge (LSB) scores should be no greater than 0.05 from a balanced score of 1.0 (i.e., 0.95 to 1.05)
  - For example, a RSB score of 88 seconds and an LSB score of 92 seconds generates a ratio score of 0.96, which is within the 0.05 range from 1.0
- Side bridge (either side):extension ratio should be less than 0.75
  - For example, a RSB score of 88 seconds and an extension score of 150 seconds generates a ratio score of 0.59

Demonstrated deficiencies in these core functional assessments should be addressed during exercise programming as part of the foundational exercises for a client. The goal is to create ratios consistent with McGill's recommendations. Muscular endurance, more so than muscular strength or even ROM, has been shown to be an accurate predictor of back health (McGill, 2016). Low-back stabilization exercises have the most benefit when performed daily (see pages 710–712). When working with clients with low-back dysfunction, it is prudent to include daily stabilization exercises in their home exercise plans. After completing all elements of McGill's torso muscular endurance test battery, personal trainers can use Figure 10-32 to record the client's data.

Trunk flexor endurance test

Time to completion: ____________

Trunk lateral endurance test

Right side time to completion: _________ Left side time to completion:_________

Trunk extensor endurance test

Time to completion: ____________

Ratio of Comparison	Criteria for Good Relationship Between Muscles
Flexion:extension	Ratio less than 1.0
Right-side bridge:left-side bridge	Scores should be no greater than 0.05 from a balanced score of 1.0
Side bridge (each side):extension	Ratio less than 0.75

Flexion:extension ratio: ________________ Rating: ❑ Good ❑ Poor

Right-side bridge:left-side bridge ratio: ______ Rating: ❑ Good ❑ Poor

Side-bridge (each side):extension ratio: ______ Rating: ❑ Good ❑ Poor

FIGURE 10-32 McGill's torso muscular endurance test battery—record sheet

FLEXIBILITY ASSESSMENTS

A client and personal trainer may collaborate on whether to assess the flexibility of specific muscle groups. The results of initial flexibility assessments could provide information on progress achieved due to a training program if compared against data from follow-up assessments. Or, if a client comments that he or she experiences tightness or stiffness in an area, it could be valuable to assess the associated joint ROM to evaluate if there are notable differences between right and left sides of the body or if the client's ROM is remarkably different than average. While Figures 10-33 through 10-35 illustrate normal ROMs for healthy adults at each major joint, only a select few muscle groups that commonly appear tight are discussed in this section. In addition, Table 10-12 presents the average ROM at various joints for healthy adults. Figure 10-36 can be used to keep records when conducting the flexibility assessments presented in this section.

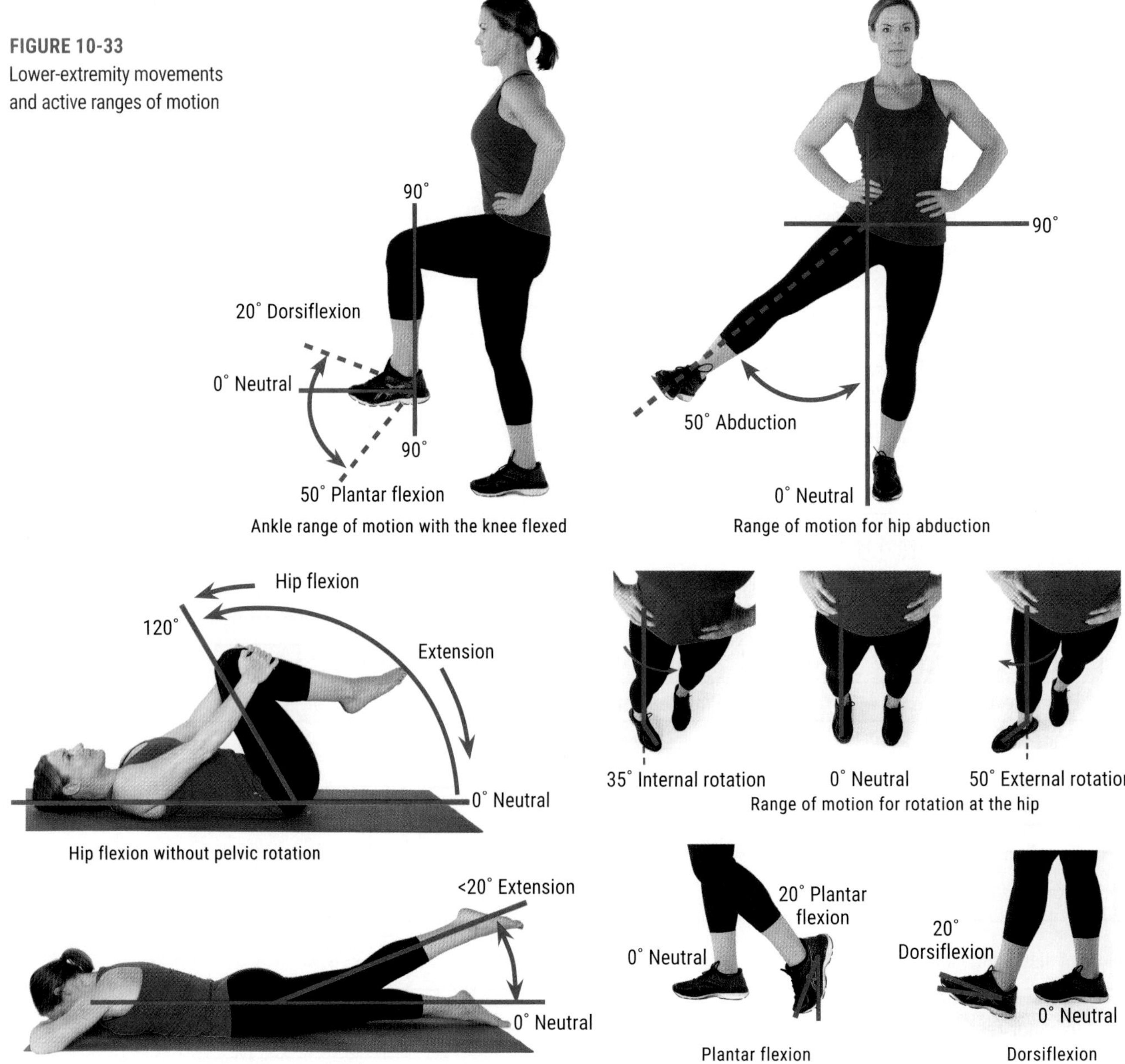

FIGURE 10-33
Lower-extremity movements and active ranges of motion

FIGURE 10-34
Shoulder joint range of motion

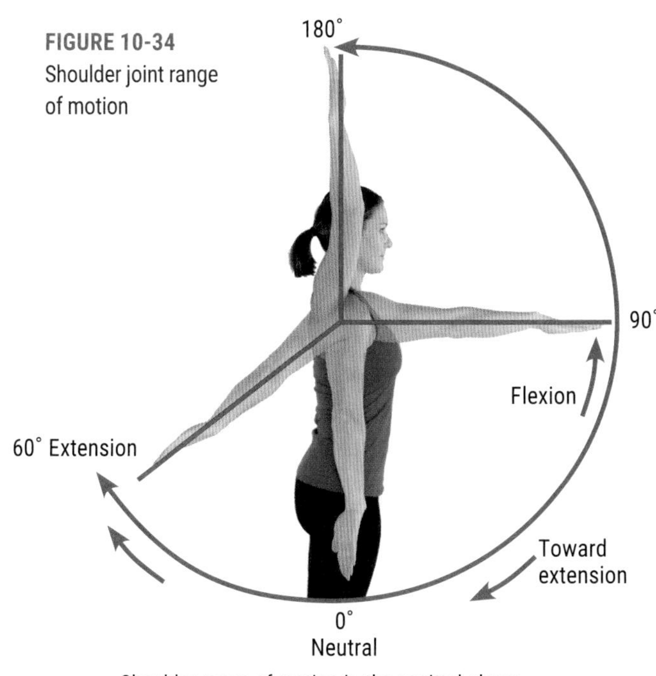

Shoulder range of motion in the sagittal plane: Flexion 180°, extension to 0°, hyperextension 60°

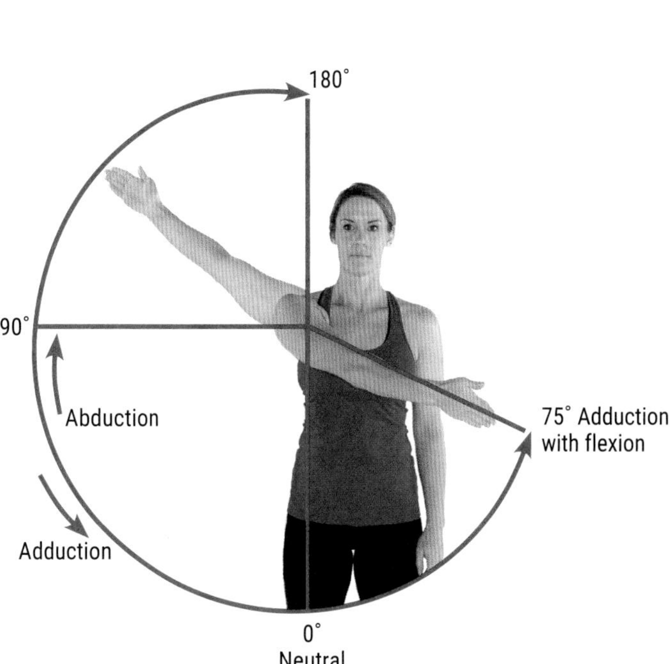

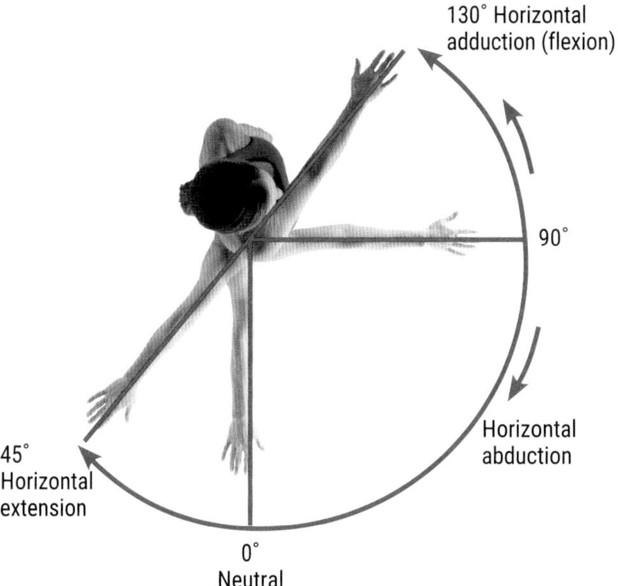

Shoulder range of motion in the transverse plane: Horizontal adduction (flexion) 130°, horizontal abduction to 0°, horizontal extension 45° past neutral

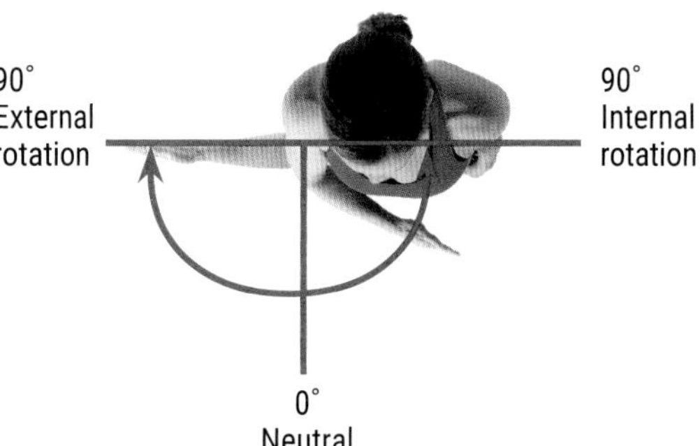

Shoulder rotation range of motion in the transverse plane (shoulder is adducted to 0°): External rotation 90°, internal rotation 90°

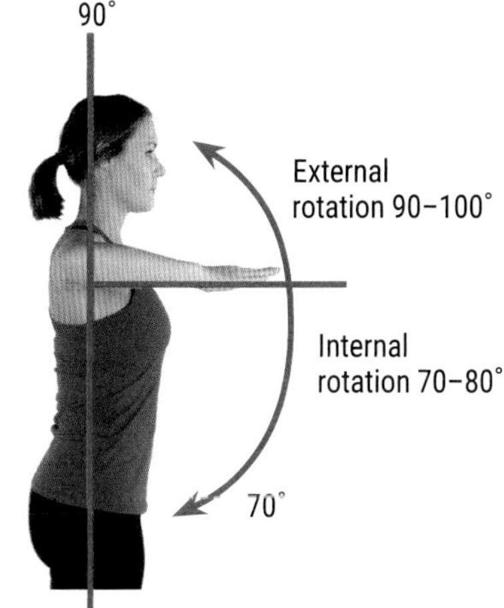

Shoulder rotation range of motion in the sagittal plane: External rotation 90–100°, internal rotation 70–80°

FIGURE 10-35
Active range of motion of the thoracic and lumbar spine

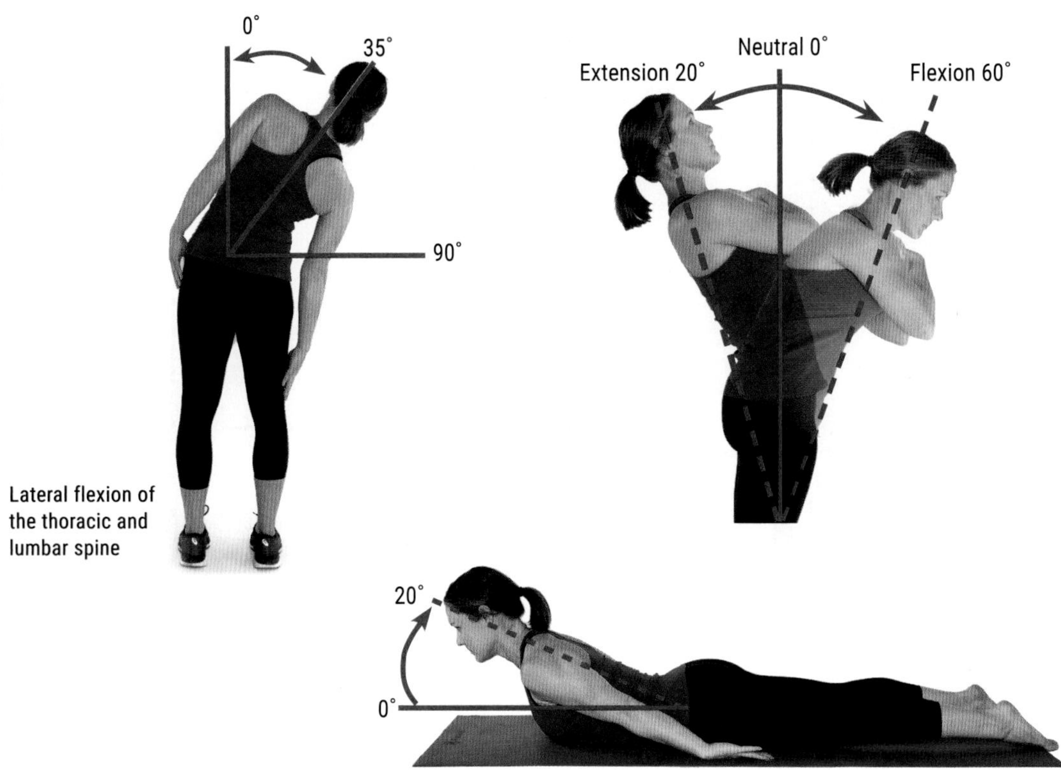

Spinal extension (thoracic and lumbar spine)

TABLE 10-12
Average Range of Motion for Healthy Adults

Joint and Movement	ROM (°)	Joint and Movement	ROM (°)
Shoulder/Scapulae		*Thoraco-lumbar Spine*	
Flexion	150–180	Lumbar flexion	40–45
Extension	50–60	Thoracic flexion	30–40
Abduction	180	Lumbar extension	30–40
Internal/medial rotation	70–80	Thoracic extension	20–30
External/lateral rotation	90	Lumbar rotation	10–15
Shoulder horizontal adduction	90*	Thoracic rotation	35
Shoulder horizontal abduction	30–40*	Lumbar lateral flexion	20
		Thoracic lateral flexion	20–25
Elbow		*Hip*	
Flexion	145	Flexion	100–120
Extension	0	Extension	10–30
		Abduction	40–45
		Adduction	20–30
		Internal/medial rotation	35–45
		External/lateral rotation	45–60

TABLE 10-12 *(continued)*

Joint and Movement	ROM (°)	Joint and Movement	ROM (°)
Radio-ulnar		Knee	
Pronation	90	Flexion	125–145
Supination	90	Extension	0–10
Wrist		*Ankle*	
Flexion	80	Dorsiflexion	20
Extension	70	Plantar flexion	45–50
Radial deviation	20		
Ulnar deviation	45		
Cervical Spine		*Subtalar*	
Flexion	45–50	Inversion	30–35
Extension	45–75	Eversion	15–20
Lateral flexion	45		
Rotation	65–75		

*Zero point (0 degrees) is with the arms positioned in frontal-plane abduction at shoulder height.

Source: Kendall, F.P. et al. (2005). *Muscles Testing and Function with Posture and Pain* (5th ed.). Baltimore, Md.: Lippincott Williams & Wilkins.

THOMAS TEST

Left hip: Normal ❑ Tight ❑ Right hip: Normal ❑ Tight ❑

Additional notes:_______________ Additional notes:_______________

PASSIVE STRAIGHT-LEG RAISE

Left Hamstrings: Normal ❑ Tight ❑ Right Hamstrings: Normal ❑ Tight ❑

Additional notes:_______________ Additional notes:_______________

SHOULDER FLEXION

Left shoulder: Normal ❑ Tight ❑ Right shoulder: Normal ❑ Tight ❑

Additional notes:_______________ Additional notes:_______________

SHOULDER EXTENSION

Left shoulder: Normal ❑ Tight ❑ Right shoulder: Normal ❑ Tight ❑

Additional notes:_______________ Additional notes:_______________

FIGURE 10-36
Worksheet for conducting flexibility assessments

Thomas Test for Hip Flexor Length

Objective: To evaluate the length of the muscles involved in hip flexion (i.e., hip flexors and rectus femoris). This test assesses the length of the primary hip flexors. It should not be conducted on clients suffering from low-back pain, unless cleared by their physician.

Equipment:

- Stable table

Instructions:

- Given the nature of the movement associated with this test, personal trainers may want to consider draping a towel over the client's groin area.
- Explain the objective of the test and allow a warm-up.
- Instruct the client to sit at the end of a table with the mid-thigh aligned with the table edge (Figure 10-37a).
- While supporting the client, instruct him or her to flex one thigh toward the chest and gradually assist as he or she rolls to the table top with back and shoulders flat.
- Instruct the client to continue to pull one knee toward the chest only until the low back is flat (Figure 10-37b).

FIGURE 10-37
Thomas test for hip flexor length

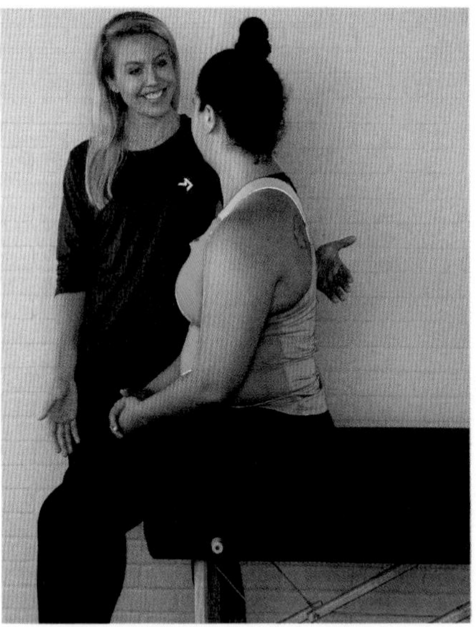

a. Starting position

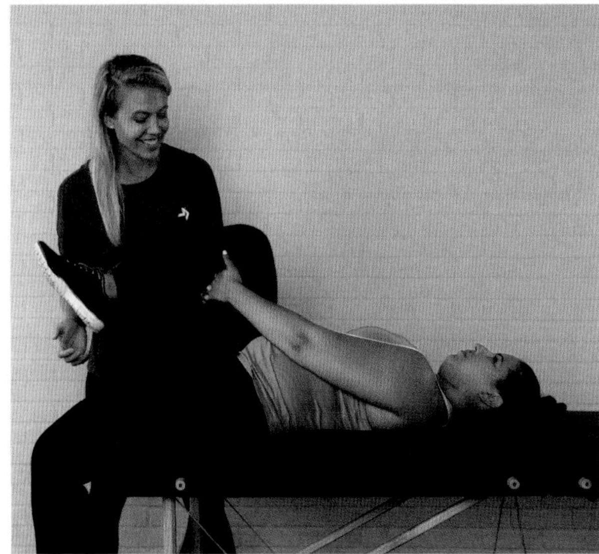

b. Test position

Observations:

- Observe whether the back of the lowered thigh touches the table (hips positioned in 10 degrees of extension).
- Observe whether the knee of the lowered leg achieves 80 degrees of flexion.
- Observe whether the knee remains aligned straight or falls into internal or external rotation.

Interpretation:

- Use the information provided in Table 10-13 to determine the location and identity of the tight or limiting muscles.

TABLE 10-13
Interpretation of the Thomas Test

Movement/Limitation	Suspected Muscle Tightness
With the back and sacrum flat: ▸ The back of the lowered thigh *does not* touch the table ▸ The knee *does not* flex to 80 degrees	Primary hip flexor muscles
With the back and sacrum flat: ▸ The back of the lowered thigh *does not* touch the table ▸ The knee *does* flex to 80 degrees	The iliopsoas, which is preventing the hip from rotating posteriorly and inhibiting the thigh from being able to touch the table
With the back and sacrum flat: ▸ The back of the lowered thigh *does* touch the table ▸ The knee *does not* flex to 80 degrees	The rectus femoris, which does not allow the knee to bend

Source: Kendall, F.P. et al. (2005). *Muscles Testing and Function with Posture and Pain* (5th ed.). Baltimore, Md.: Lippincott Williams & Wilkins.

Passive Straight-leg Raise

Objective: To assess the length of the hamstrings

Equipment:

- Stable table or exercise mat

Instructions:

- Explain the objective of the assessment and allow a warm-up.
- Instruct the client to lie supine on a mat or table with the legs extended and the low back and sacrum flat against the surface.
- Place one hand under the calf of the leg that will be raised while instructing the client to keep the opposite leg extended on the mat or table. Restrain that leg from moving or rising during the assessment.
- Slide the other hand under the lumbar spine into the space between the client's back and the mat or table (Figure 10-38).
- Advise the client to gently plantar flex his or her ankles to point the toes away from the body. This position avoids an assessment limitation due to a tight gastrocnemius muscle (which would limit knee extension with the ankle in dorsiflexion). Additionally, a straight-leg raise with dorsiflexion may increase tension within the sciatic nerve and create some discomfort.
- Slowly raise the one leg, asking the client to keep that knee loosely extended throughout the movement.
- Continue to raise the leg until firm pressure can be felt from the low back pressing down against the hand (Figure 10-39).

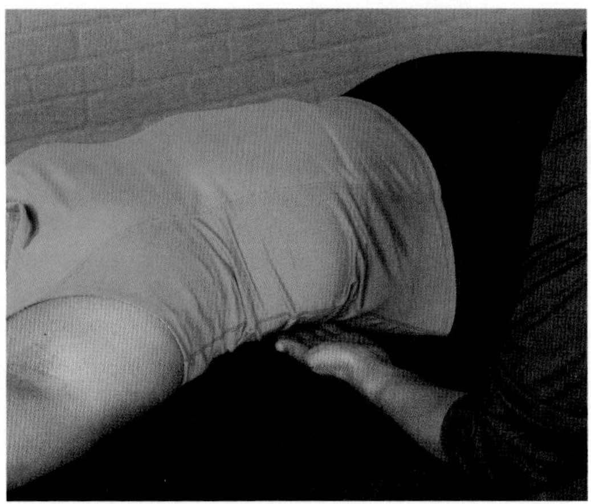

FIGURE 10-38
Passive straight-leg raise: Personal trainer's hand position

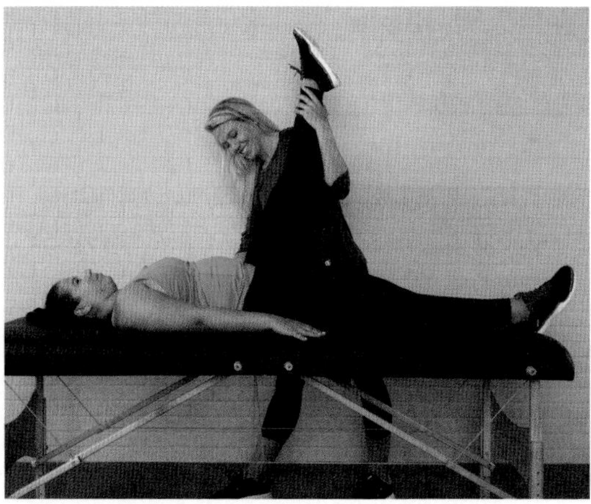

FIGURE 10-39
Passive straight-leg raise: Assessment position

- This indicates an end-ROM of the hamstrings, with movement now occurring as the pelvis rotates posteriorly.
- Throughout the movement, the client needs to maintain extension in the opposite leg and keep the sacrum and low back flat against the mat or table.
    - If the assessment is performed with the opposite hip in slight flexion, this allows the pelvis more freedom to move into a posterior tilt, allowing a greater ROM and falsely increasing the length of the hamstrings.

Observation:

- Note the degree of movement attained from the table or mat that is achieved before the spine compresses the hand under the low back or the opposite leg begins to show visible signs of lifting off the table or mat.
    - The mat or table represents 0 degrees.
    - The leg perpendicular to the mat or table represents 90 degrees.

Interpretation:

- Use the information provided in Table 10-14 to determine the limitation(s).

TABLE 10-14
Interpretation of the Passive Straight-leg Raise

Movement/Limitation	Hamstrings Length
The raised leg achieves ≥80 degrees of movement before the pelvis rotates posteriorly.	Normal hamstrings length
The raised leg achieves <80 degrees of movement before the pelvis rotates posteriorly or there are any visible signs in the opposite leg lifting off the mat or table.	Tight hamstrings

Source: Kendall, F.P. et al. (2005). *Muscles Testing and Function with Posture and Pain* (5th ed.). Baltimore, Md.: Lippincott Williams & Wilkins.

Shoulder Flexion and Extension

Objective: To assess the degree of shoulder flexion and extension

Equipment:

- Exercise mat
- Pillow (optional)

Instructions:

- Explain the purpose of the assessment.
- Shoulder flexion:
  - Instruct the client to lie supine on a mat, with the back flat and a bent-knee position (knees and second toe aligned with the hips), and with the arms at the sides.
  - Have the client engage the abdominal muscles to hold a neutral spine without raising the hips from the mat.
  - Instruct the client to raise both arms simultaneously into shoulder flexion, moving them overhead, keeping them close to the sides of the head, and bringing them down to touch the floor or as close to the floor as possible (Figure 10-40).
    - The client must maintain extended elbows and neutral wrist position (the arms will naturally rotate internally during this movement).
    - Have the client avoid any arching in the low back during the movement.
    - Have the client avoid any depression of the rib cage, which may pull the shoulders off the mat.
- Shoulder extension:
  - Instruct the client to lie prone, extending both legs, with arms at the sides, and resting the forehead gently on a pillow or the mat.
  - Ask the client to slowly raise both arms simultaneously into extension, lifting them off the mat while keeping the arms close to the sides (Figure 10-41) (the arms will naturally rotate internally during this movement).
    - A small amount of extension in the thoracic spine is acceptable during the movement.
    - The client should avoid any arching in the low back or any rotation of the torso during the movement.
    - The client should avoid any attempts to lift the chest or head off the mat during the movement.

Observations:

- Measure the degree of movement in each direction.
- Note any bilateral differences between the left and right arms in performing both movements.

Interpretation:

- Use the information provided in Table 10-15 to determine the limitation(s) in these shoulder flexibility assessments.

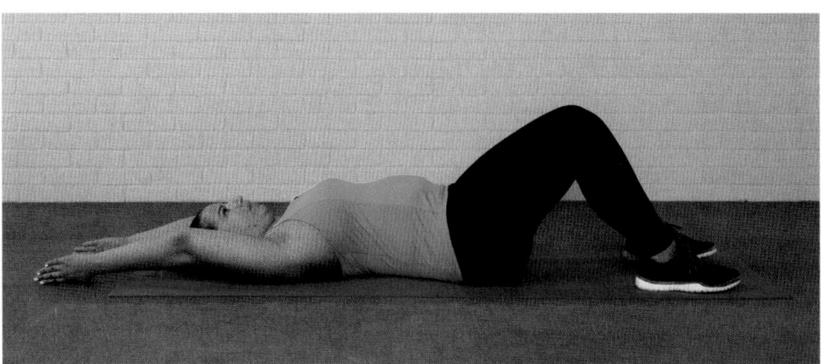

FIGURE 10-40
Shoulder flexion assessment

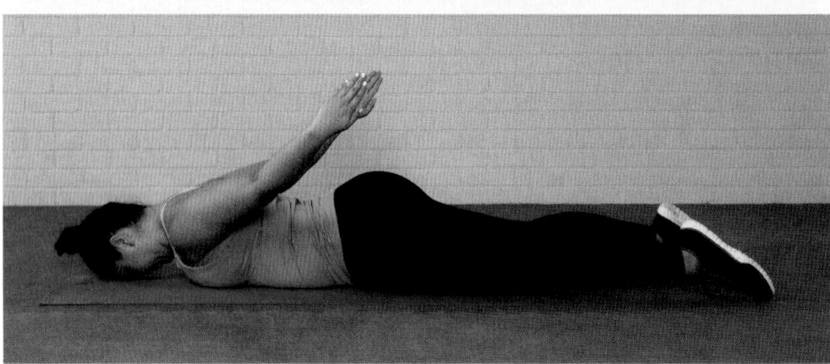

FIGURE 10-41
Shoulder extension assessment

TABLE 10-15
Interpretation of the Shoulder Flexion and Extension Assessments

Movement/Limitation—Flexion	Shoulder Mobility
Ability to flex the shoulders to 170–180 degrees (hands touching/nearly touching floor)	Good shoulder mobility
Inability to flex the shoulders to 170 degrees or discrepancies between the limbs	Potential tightness in the pectoralis major and minor, latissimus dorsi, teres major, rhomboids, and subscapularis ▸ Tightness in the latissimus dorsi will force the low back to arch. ▸ Tightness of the pectoralis minor may tilt the scapulae forward (anterior tilt) and prevent the arms from touching the floor. ▸ Tight abdominals may depress the rib cage, tilting the scapulae forward (anterior tilt), and prevent the arms from touching the floor. ▸ Thoracic kyphosis may round the thoracic spine and prevent the arms from touching the floor.
Movement/Limitation—Extension	**Shoulder Mobility**
Ability to extend the shoulders to 50–60 degrees off the floor	Good shoulder mobility
Inability to extend the shoulders to 50 degrees or discrepancies between the limbs	Potential tightness in pectoralis major, abdominals, subscapularis, certain shoulder flexors (anterior deltoid), coracobrachialis, and biceps brachii ▸ Tightness in the abdominals may prevent normal extension of the thoracic spine and rib cage. ▸ Tightness in the biceps brachii may prevent adequate shoulder extension with an extended elbow (but may permit extension with a bent elbow).

Source: Houglum, P.A. (2016). *Therapeutic Exercise for Musculoskeletal Injuries* (4th ed). Champaign, Ill.: Human Kinetics.

Movement Assessments

Movement Training focuses on establishing efficient movement through healthy ROMs specific to each client, essentially teaching clients to perform the five primary movements effectively in all three **planes of motion** without compromising postural or joint stability. Thus, the movement assessments introduced here are designed to help the personal trainer observe a client's ability to control mobility as he or she performs the five primary movements:

- *Bend-and-lift:* Hip-hinging and squatting movements performed throughout the day (e.g., sitting on or standing up from a chair or squatting down to lift up an object off the floor)
- *Single-leg:* Movements done while balancing on one leg, including lunging [e.g., alternate foot stance during walking (gait cycle), stepping forward to reach down with one hand to pick up something off the floor, or walking down/up a flight of stairs)]
- *Pushing:* Movements performed in a forward direction (e.g., during a push-up exercise or when pushing open a door), in an overhead direction (e.g., during an overhead press or when putting an item on a high shelf), or in a lateral direction (e.g., pushing open double sliding doors or lifting one's torso when getting up from a side-lying position)
- *Pulling:* Movements performed during an exercise such as a bent-over row or pull-up or during a movement like pulling open a car door
- *Rotation:* Movements, such as the rotation of the thoracic spine during gait or reaching across the body to pick up an object on one's left side and placing it on the right side (e.g., when putting on a seatbelt in a car)

BEND-AND-LIFT ASSESSMENT: SQUAT PATTERN

Objective: To assess symmetrical lower-extremity mobility and stability and trunk mobility and stability during a bend-and-lift movement

Equipment:

- None

Instructions:

- Briefly discuss the protocol so the client understands what is required.
- Ask the client to stand with the feet shoulder-width apart with the arms hanging freely to the sides.
- Ask the client to perform five to 10 bend-and-lift movements (i.e., squats), lowering as deep as is comfortable. It is important not to cue the client to use good technique, but instead observe his or her natural movement.

Observations (Table 10-16):

- Anterior view (Figure 10-42):
  - Feet: Is there evidence of pronation, supination, eversion, or **inversion**?
  - Knees: Do they move inward or outward?
  - Torso: How is the overall symmetry of the entire body over the **base of support**? Is there evidence of a lateral shift or rotation?

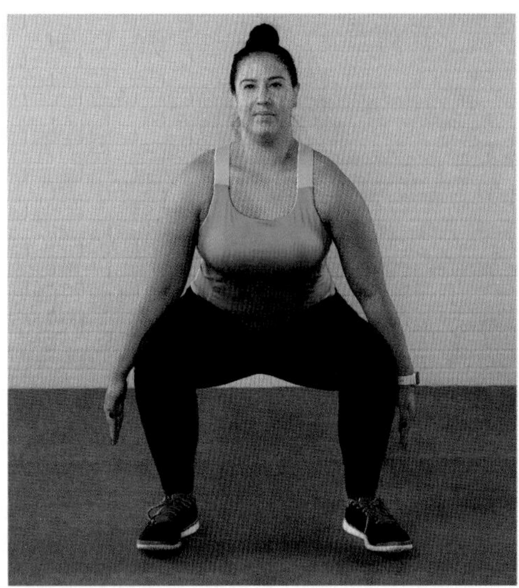

FIGURE 10-42
Bend-and-lift assessment (squat pattern): Anterior view

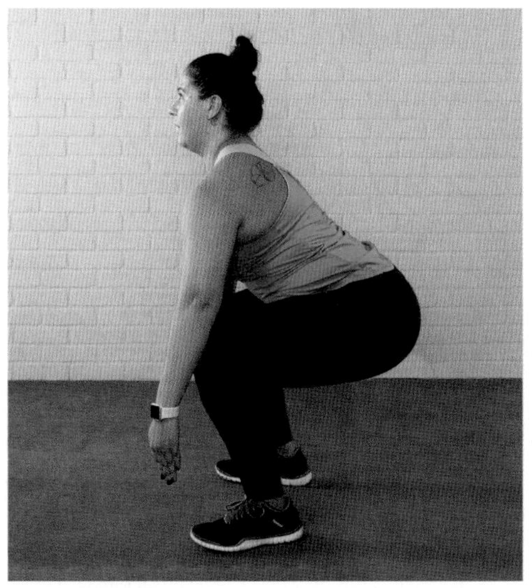

FIGURE 10-43
Bend-and-lift assessment (squat pattern): Side view

- Side view (Figure 10-43):
  - Feet: Do the heels remain in contact with the floor throughout the movement?
  - Hip and knee: Does the client exhibit "glute" or "quadriceps dominance" (i.e., is the descent initiated by driving the knees forward or by pushing the hips backward)?
  - Hip and knee: Does the client achieve a parallel position between the top of the thighs and the floor?
  - Knee: Does the client control the descent to avoid resting the hamstrings against the calves at the bottom of the squat?
  - Lumbar and thoracic spine: Does the client exhibit an exaggerated curve in the lumbar (i.e., "lumbar dominance") or thoracic spine during the descent?
  - Head: Are any changes in the position of the head observed during the movement?

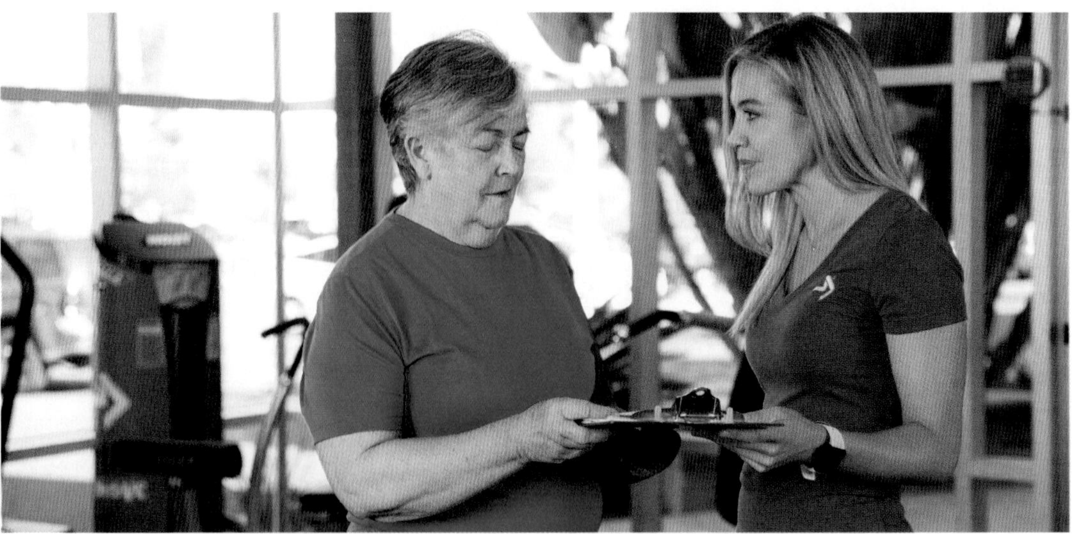

Interpretation:

- Identify origin(s) of movement limitation or compensation.
- Evaluate the impact on the entire kinetic chain.

TABLE 10-16
Bend-and-Lift Assessment: Squat Pattern

View		Location	Compensation	Key Suspected Compensations: Overactive (Tight)	Key Suspected Compensations: Underactive (Lengthened)
☐	Anterior	Feet	Lack of foot stability: Ankles collapse inward/feet turn outward	Soleus, lateral gastrocnemius, peroneals	Medial gastrocnemius, gracilis, sartorius, tibialis group
☐	Anterior	Knees	Move inward	Hip adductors, tensor fascia latae	Gluteus medius and maximus
☐	Anterior	Torso	Lateral shift to a side	Side dominance and muscle imbalance due to potential lack of stability in the lower extremity during joint loading	
☐	Side	Feet	Unable to keep heels in contact with the floor	Plantar flexors	None
☐	Side	Hip and knee	Initiation of movement	Movement initiated at knees may indicate quadriceps and hip flexor dominance, as well as insufficient activation of the gluteus group	
☐	Side	Hip and knee	Unable to achieve tops of thighs parallel to the floor	Poor mechanics, lack of dorsiflexion due to tight plantar flexors (which normally allow the tibia to move forward)	
		Contact behind knee	Hamstrings contact back of calves	Muscle weakness and poor mechanics, resulting in an inability to stabilize and control the lowering phase	
☐	Side	Lumbar and thoracic spine	Back excessively arches (i.e., lumbar dominance)	Hip flexors, back extensors, latissimus dorsi	Core, rectus abdominis, gluteal group, hamstrings
			Back rounds forward	Latissimus dorsi, teres major, pectoralis major and minor	Upper back extensors
☐	Side	Head	Downward	Increased hip and trunk flexion	
			Upward	Compression and tightness in the cervical extensor region	

Sources: Kendall, F.P. et al. (2005). *Muscles Testing and Function with Posture and Pain* (5th ed.). Baltimore, Md.: Lippincott Williams & Wilkins; Cook, G. (2003). *Athletic Body in Balance*. Champaign, Ill.: Human Kinetics; Donnelly, D.V. et al. (2006). The effect of directional gaze on kinematics during the squat exercise. *Journal of Strength and Conditioning Research*, 20, 145–150; Fry, A.C., Smith J.C., & Schilling, B.K. (2003). Effect of knee position on hip and knees torques during the barbell squat. *Journal of Strength and Conditioning Research*, 17, 629–633; Abelbeck, K.G. (2002). Biomechanical model and evaluation of a linear motion squat type exercise. *Journal of Strength and Conditioning Research*, 16, 516–524; Sahrmann, S.A. (2002). *Diagnosis and Treatment of Movement Impairment Syndromes*. St. Louis, Mo.: Mosby.

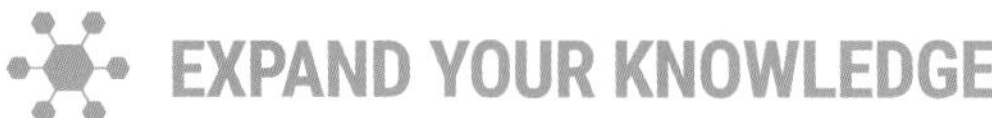

Movement Patterns during a Squat

The gluteals and core musculature play an important role in the squat movement, during which individuals can exhibit "lumbar dominance," "quadriceps dominance," or "glute dominance."

- *Lumbar dominance:* This implies a lack of core and gluteal muscle strength to counteract the force of the hip flexors and erector spinae as they pull the pelvis forward during a squat movement. In this scenario, the individual experiences excessive loads within the lumbar spine as it moves into extension during the squat. The muscles of the abdominal wall and gluteal complex do not contribute enough in this situation to spare the back and foster proper execution of the squat (McGill, 2017). Chronically tight hip flexors, such as those experienced by individuals who sit for prolonged periods throughout the day, may also contribute to the problem.
- *Quadriceps dominance:* This implies reliance on loading the quadriceps group during a squat movement. The first 10 to 15 degrees of the downward phase are initiated by driving the tibia forward, creating shearing forces across the knee as the femur slides over the tibia. In this lowered position, the gluteus maximus does not eccentrically load and cannot generate much force during the upward phase. Quadriceps-dominant squatting transfers more pressure into the knees, placing greater loads on the **anterior cruciate ligament (ACL)** (Wilthrow et al., 2005).
- *Glute dominance:* This implies reliance on eccentrically loading the gluteus maximus during a squat movement. The first 10 to 15 degrees of the downward phase are initiated by pushing the hips backward, creating a hip-hinge (Figure 10-44). In the lowered position, this maximizes the eccentric loading on the gluteus maximus to generate significant force during the upward, concentric phase. The glute-dominant squat pattern is the preferred method of squatting, as it spares the lumbar spine and relieves undue stress on the knees. Glute dominance also helps activate the hamstrings, which pull on the posterior surface of the tibia and help unload the ACL to protect it from potential injury (Hauschildt, 2008).

FIGURE 10-44
Hip hinge

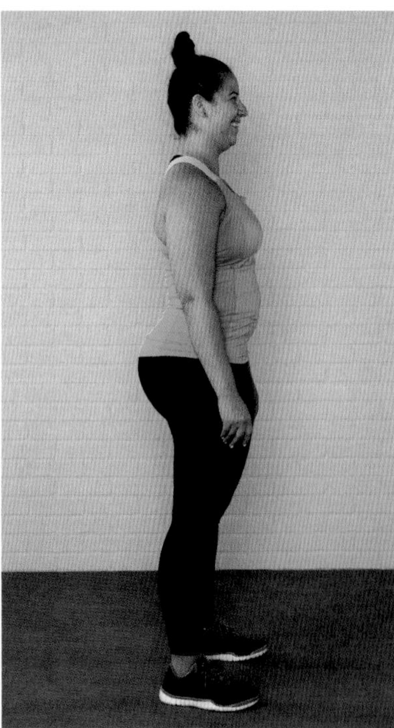

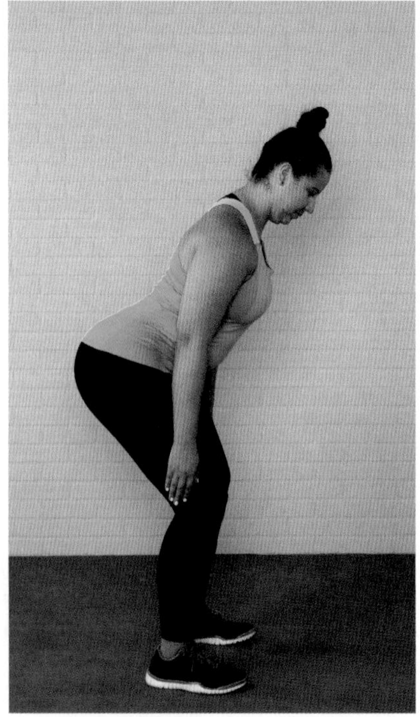

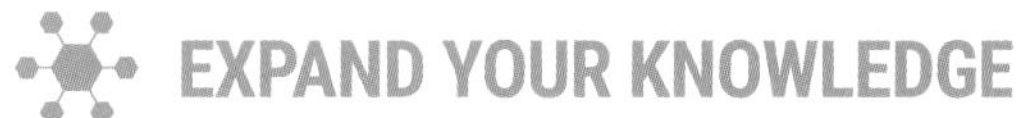

Squat and Lunges: Is "Never Let the Knees Go Past the Toes" an Appropriate Movement Cue?

While it is appropriate to avoid excessive forward movement of the knee during squatting and lunging movements, it is a myth that exercisers should "never let the knees go past the toes" while doing a squat or lunge. This common movement cue originated from a 1978 study that found that keeping the lower leg as vertical as possible reduced shearing forces on the knees during a squat (McLaughlin, Lardner, & Dillman, 1978). In truth, leaning the trunk too far forward is more likely the cause of any injury.

In 2003, researchers confirmed that knee stress increased by 28% when the knees were allowed to move past the toes while performing a squat (Fry, Smith, & Schilling, 2003). However, hip stress increased by nearly 1,000% when forward movement of the knee was restricted. In addition, in group exercise, the cue "don't let your knees go over your toes" has long been an effective general rule when trying to teach an exercise to a room full of people with different skill levels, abilities, and goals. When a class has a large number of participants, it is difficult to help each individual participant with his or her specific ROM, so providing this general cue is an effective way of erring on the side of caution for the group fitness instructor.

The general pointer while performing a lunge is to try to keep the knees aligned over the second toe so that the knee is moving in the same direction as the ankle joint. However, in reality, clients often find the knee translating forward to the toes or beyond in a squat or lunge movement, so there are other things that must be considered, specifically limb length.

During lunge or squat movements, personal trainers should always emphasize beginning the movement by pushing the hips backward before lowering toward the floor (an action referred to as "hip hinging"; see Figure 10-44). This technique prevents premature forward movement of the knee by shifting the hips backward. As the exerciser continues to lower his or her body downward, this creates a healthy hinge effect at the knee, but there comes a time where the knee (tibia) will begin to move forward in order to maintain balance (keeping the **center of mass** within the base of support). If an exerciser happens to have long limbs, then it is realistic to expect the knees to move forward over or beyond the toes. Any attempt to prevent this motion will result in either the client falling backward or bad squat or lunge technique that places increased loads on the low back. As long as personal trainers teach the lunge/squat movement correctly by first initiating the movement at the hips and avoid premature forward movement of the knees, then the fact that the knees are moving forward is quite safe.

SINGLE-LEG ASSESSMENT: STEP-UP

Objective: To assess symmetrical lower-extremity mobility and stability and trunk mobility and stability during a single-leg (step-up) movement

Equipment:

- Bench; select a bench height that allows the client to start with the hip and knee at approximately a 90-degree angle.

Instructions:

- Briefly discuss the protocol so the client understands what is required.
- Ask the client to stand with the feet shoulder-width apart with the arms hanging freely to the sides.
- Instruct the client to place one leg up squarely on the bench while maintaining an upright posture.

- Instruct the client to push off with the heel of the foot on the bench while simultaneously bringing the opposite leg up to a 90-degree angle.
- Instruct the client to return slowly to the starting position in a one-two-three rhythm.
- Ask the client to perform five to 10 single-leg (step-up) movements.
- Switch the leg positioned on the bench and repeat the above steps.
- It is important not to cue the client to use good technique, but instead observe his or her natural movement.

Observations (Table 10-17):

- Anterior view (Figure 10-45):
    - First repetition: Observe the stability of the foot (i.e., evidence of pronation, supination, eversion, or inversion).
    - Second repetition: Observe the alignment of the stance-leg knee over the foot (i.e., evidence of knee movement in any plane).
    - Third repetition: Watch for excessive hip adduction greater than 2 inches (5.1 cm) as measured by excessive stance-leg adduction or downward hip-tilting toward the opposite side.
    - Fourth repetition: Observe the stability of the torso.
    - Fifth repetition: Observe the alignment of the moving leg (i.e., lack of dorsiflexion at the ankle, deviation from the sagittal plane at the knee or ankle, or hiking of the moving hip).

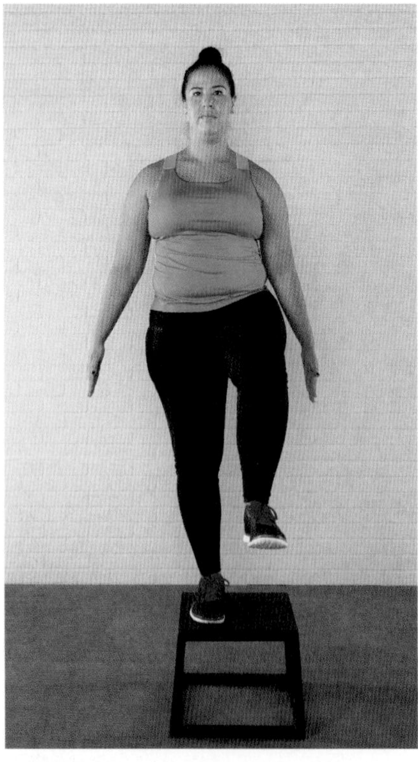

FIGURE 10-45
Step-up: Anterior view

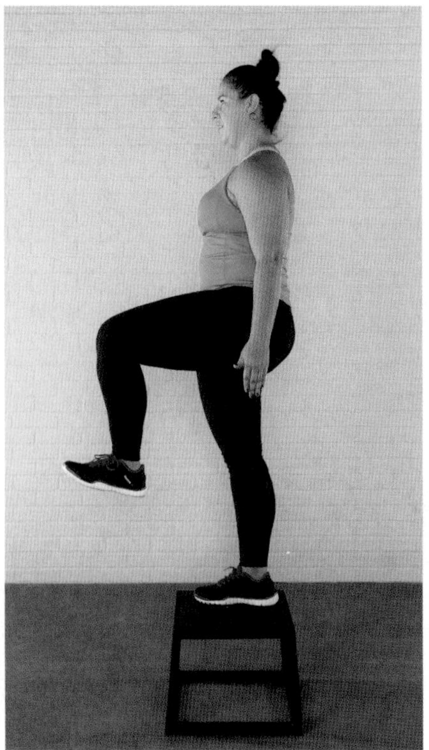

FIGURE 10-46
Step-up: Side view

- Side view (Figure 10-46):
  - First repetition: Observe the stability of the torso and stance leg.
  - Second repetition: Observe the mobility of the hip (i.e., allowing 70 degrees of hip flexion without compensation—anterior tilting) of the moving leg.

Interpretation:

- Identify origin(s) of movement limitation or compensation.
- Evaluate the impact on the entire kinetic chain.

TABLE 10-17

Single-leg Assessment: Step-up

View	Location	Compensation	Key Suspected Compensations: Overactive (Tight)	Key Suspected Compensations: Underactive (Lengthened)
☐ Anterior	Feet	Lack of foot stability: Ankles collapse inward/feet turn outward	Soleus, lateral gastrocnemius, peroneals	Medial gastrocnemius, gracilis, sartorius, tibialis group, gluteus medius and maximus—inability to control internal rotation
☐ Anterior	Knees	Move inward	Hip adductors, tensor fascia latae	Gluteus medius and maximus
☐ Anterior	Hips	Hip adduction* >2 inches (5.1 cm)	Hip adductors, tensor fascia latae	Gluteus medius and maximus
		Stance-leg hip rotation (inward)	Stance-leg or raised-leg internal rotators	Stance-leg or raised-leg external rotators
☐ Anterior	Torso	Lateral tilt, forward lean, rotation	Lack of core stability	
☐ Anterior	Raised-leg	Limb deviates from sagittal plane	Ankle plantar flexors	Ankle dorsiflexors
		Hiking the raised hip	Raised-leg hip extensors	Raised-leg hip flexors
			Stance-leg hip flexors—limiting posterior hip rotation during raise	
☐ Side	Pelvis and low back	Lack of ankle dorsiflexion	Stance-leg hip flexors	Rectus abdominis and hip extensors
		Anterior tilt with forward torso lean	Rectus abdominis and hip extensors	Stance-leg hip flexors
		Posterior tilt with hunched-over torso		

*Hip adduction involves weight transference over the stance leg while preserving hip, knee, and foot alignment. This weight transference requires a 1- to 2-inch (2.5- to 5-cm) lateral shift over the stance-leg, with a small hike in the stance-hip of 4 to 5 degrees or less.

Sources: Kendall, F.P. et al. (2005). *Muscles Testing and Function with Posture and Pain* (5th ed.). Baltimore, Md.: Lippincott Williams & Wilkins; Cook, G. (2003). *Athletic Body in Balance*. Champaign, Ill.: Human Kinetics; Sahrmann, S.A. (2002). *Diagnosis and Treatment of Movement Impairment Syndromes*. St. Louis, Mo.: Mosby.

PUSH ASSESSMENT: SHOULDER PUSH STABILIZATION

Objective: To assess stabilization of the scapulothoracic joint and core control during closed-kinetic-chain pushing movements

Instructions:

- Briefly discuss the protocol so the client understands what is required.
  - The client presses his or her body off the ground as the personal trainer evaluates the ability to stabilize the scapulae against the thorax (rib cage) during pushing-type movements (Figure 10-47).
- Instruct the client to lie prone on the floor with arms abducted in the push-up position or bent-knee push-up position.
- Ask the client to perform several push-ups to full arm extension.
  - Subjects should perform full push-ups; modify to bent-knee push-ups if necessary (see Figures 10-52 and 10-53, page 444).
  - It is important to remember not to cue the client to use good technique, but instead observe his or her natural movement.
  - Repetitions need to be performed slowly and with control.

Observations (Table 10-18):

- Observe any notable changes in the position of the scapulae relative to the rib cage at both end-ranges of motion (i.e., the appearance of scapular "winging") (see Figure 10-15b).
- Observe for lumbar hyperextension in the press position.

General interpretations:

- Identify the origin(s) of movement limitation or compensation.
- Evaluate the impact on the entire kinetic chain.

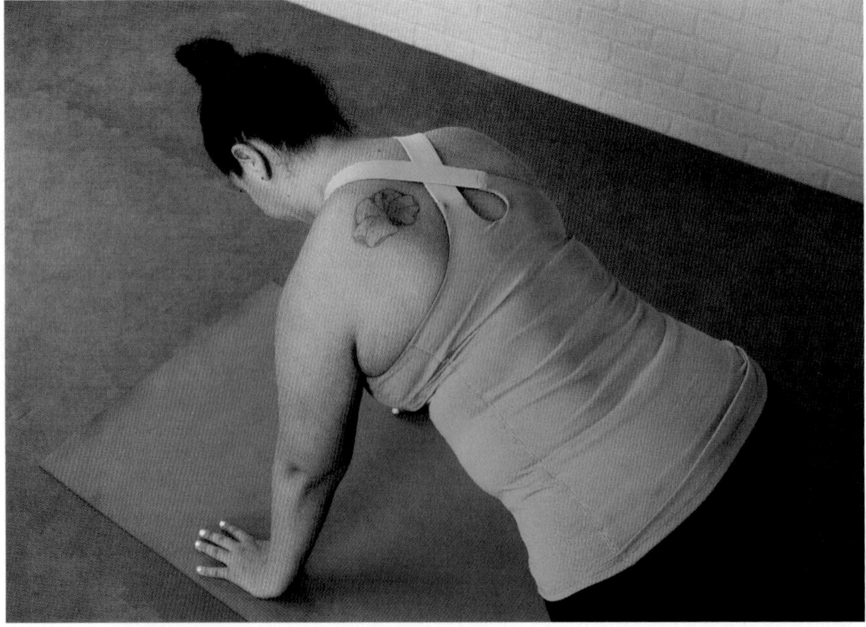

FIGURE 10-47
Push assessment: Shoulder push stabilization

TABLE 10-18

Push Assessment: Shoulder Push Stabilization

View	Joint Location	Compensation	Key Suspected Compensations
☐ Side	Scapulothoracic	Exhibits "winging" during the push-up movement	Inability of the parascapular muscles (i.e., serratus anterior, trapezius, levator scapula, rhomboids) to stabilize the scapulae against the rib cage. Can also be due to a flat thoracic spine.
☐ Side	Trunk	Hyperextension or "collapsing" of the low back	Lack of core, abdominal, and low-back strength, resulting in instability

Sources: Kendall, F.P. et al. (2005). *Muscles Testing and Function with Posture and Pain* (5th ed.). Baltimore, Md.: Lippincott Williams & Wilkins; Sahrmann, S.A. (2002). *Diagnosis and Treatment of Movement Impairment Syndromes.* St. Louis, Mo.: Mosby.

PULL ASSESSMENT: STANDING ROW

Objective: To assess movement efficiency and potential muscle imbalances during pulling movements

Equipment:

- Selectorized cable machine with handle attachments or resistance band with handles

Instructions:

- Briefly discuss the protocol so the client understands what is required.
- A light resistance appropriate for the client should be selected.
- Ask the client to stand with feet shoulder-width apart and knees slightly bent.
- Position the anchor point at a height that aligns with the client's xiphoid process.
- Instruct the client to grab the handles.
- Instruct the client to pull the bar or handle toward his or her pectoral muscles/torso while keeping the chest forward and back straight (Figure 10-48). The client should briefly pause and then return to the starting position.
- Ask the client to perform several repetitions slowly and with control.
- It is important to remember not to cue the client to use good technique, but instead observe his or her natural movement.

Observations (Table 10-19):

- Observe for shoulder elevation or head migrating forward.
- Observe for lumbar hyperextension in the pull position.

General interpretations:

- Identify the origin(s) of movement limitation or compensation.
- Evaluate the impact on the entire kinetic chain.

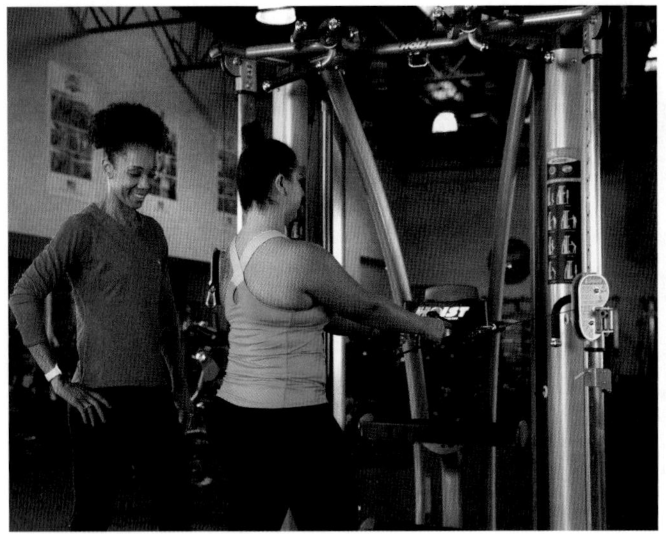
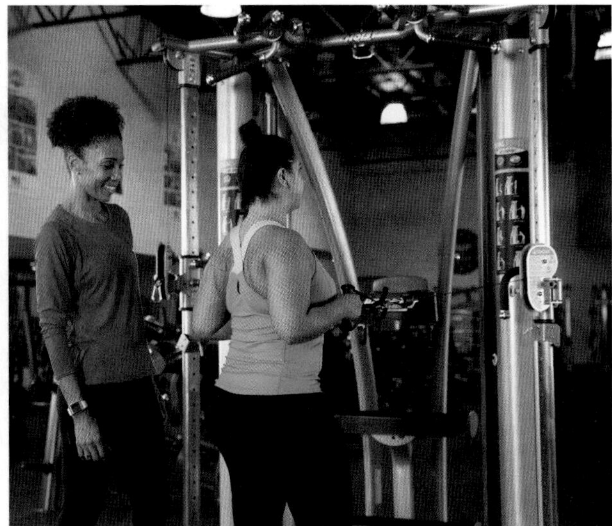

FIGURE 10-48
Pull assessment: Standing row

TABLE 10-19
Pull Assessment: Standing Row

View	Location	Compensation	Key Suspected Compensations: Overactive (Tight)	Key Suspected Compensations: Underactive (Lengthened)
Side	Lumbar spine	Hyperextension	Hip flexors, back extensors	Core, rectus abdominis, gluteal group, hamstrings
Posterior	Scapulothoracic	Elevation	Upper trapezius, levator scapulae, rhomboid major and minor	Mid and lower trapezius
Side	Head	Migrates forward (protraction)	Cervical spine extensors, upper trapezius, levator scapulae	Cervical spine flexors
Posterior	Scapulothoracic	Abduction (protraction)	Serratus anterior, anterior scapulohumeral muscles, upper trapezius	Rhomboid major and minor, middle trapezius

ROTATION ASSESSMENT: THORACIC SPINE MOBILITY

Objective: To assess bilateral mobility of the thoracic spine. Lumbar spine rotation is considered insignificant, as it only offers approximately 15 degrees of rotation.

Equipment:

- Chair
- Squeezable ball or block
- 48-inch (1.2-m) dowel

Instructions:

- Briefly discuss the protocol so the client understands what is required.

- Instruct the client to sit upright toward the front edge of the seat with the feet together and firmly placed on the floor. The client's back should not touch the backrest.
- Place a squeezable ball or block between the knees and a dowel across the front of the shoulders, instructing the client to hold the bar in the hands (i.e., front barbell squat grip) (Figure 10-49a).
- While maintaining an upright and straight posture, the client squeezes the block to immobilize the hips and gently rotates left and right to an end-ROM without any bouncing (Figure 10-49b).
  - It is important to remember not to cue the client to use good technique, but instead observe his or her natural movement.
  - Ask the client to perform a few repetitions in each direction, slowly and with control.

Observation (Table 10-20):

- Observe any bilateral discrepancies between the rotations in each direction.

General interpretations:

- Identify the origin(s) of movement limitation or compensation. As an individual rotates, the facet joints of each vertebra experience shearing forces against each other. One way to reduce this force and promote greater movement is to laterally flex the trunk during the movement or at the end-range of movement. This assessment evaluates trunk rotation in the transverse plane. Therefore, any lateral flexion of the trunk (dowel tilting up or down) must be avoided.
- Evaluate the impact on the entire kinetic chain. Remember that the lumbar spine generally exhibits limited rotation of approximately 15 degrees (Sahrmann, 2002), with the balance of trunk rotation occurring through the thoracic spine. If thoracic spine mobility is limited, the body strives to gain movement in alternative planes within the lumbar spine (e.g., increase in lordosis to promote greater rotation).

FIGURE 10-49
Rotation assessment: Thoracic spine mobility

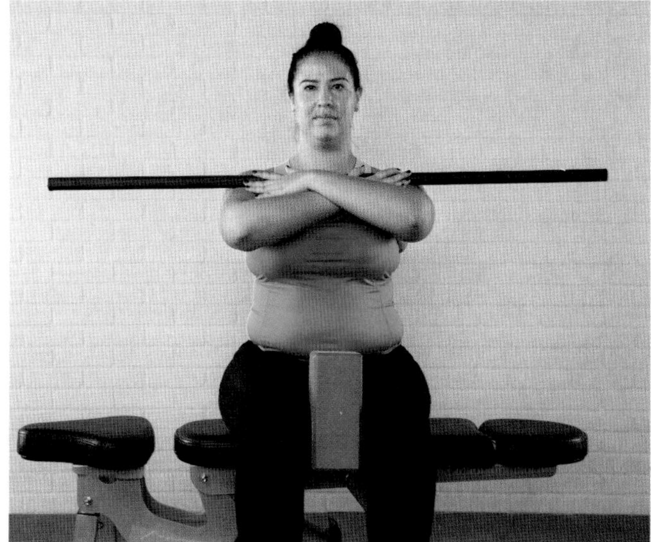

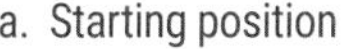
a. Starting position

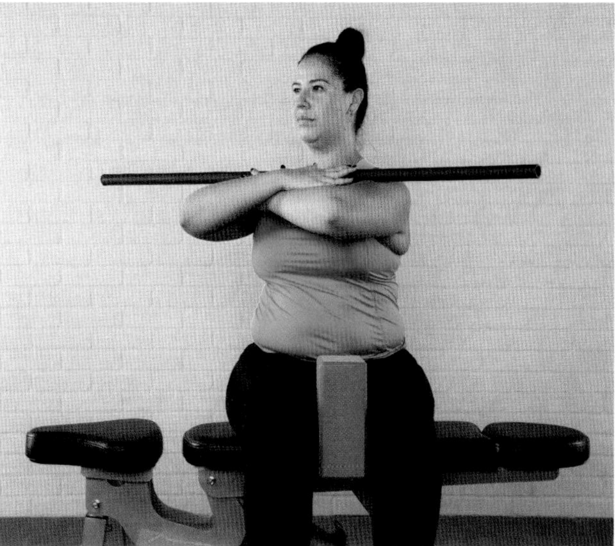

b. Assessment position

TABLE 10-20

Rotation Assessment: Thoracic Spine Mobility

View		Location	Compensation	Possible Biomechanical Problems
☐	Anterior or posterior	Trunk	None if trunk rotation achieves 45 degrees in each direction	
☐	Anterior or posterior	Trunk	Bilateral discrepancy (assuming no existing congenital issues in the spine)	Side-dominance Differences in paraspinal development Torso rotation, perhaps associated with some hip rotation Note: Lack of thoracic mobility will negatively impact glenohumeral mobility

Source: Sahrmann, S.A. (2002). *Diagnosis and Treatment of Movement Impairment Syndromes.* St. Louis, Mo.: Mosby.

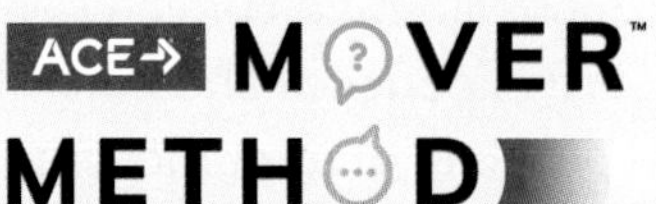

Assessing a Client Who Is Uncomfortable Being "Judged"

For the past five months, you have been working with a client focusing on reestablishing postural stability and kinetic chain mobility. Initial programming consisted of improving joint function, muscular endurance, flexibility, core function, and balance. In addition to working in the Functional Training phase of the Muscular Training component of the ACE IFT Model, this client has been working to reestablish a cardiorespiratory base. The client is now ready to progress to the Movement Training phase of the ACE IFT Model. The following assessments will be used to observe postural and joint stability in the five primary movement patterns and will be incorporated into the client's upcoming session: the squat pattern, step-up, shoulder push stabilization, standing row, and thoracic spine mobility.

The client begins with a 10-minute warm-up, incorporating exercises that she is familiar with from her Functional Training program. You explain to the client that today's workout will include new and challenging exercises that will provide the opportunity to observe her natural movement patterns. The results will help direct the focus of her next training phase.

While performing her first set of the standing row exercise, you notice that she seems uneasy. Following is an example of how to address an uncomfortable situation while using the principles of the ACE Mover Method and the skills of the ACE ABC Approach™.

ACE ABC APPROACH™

Ask: Asking powerful open-ended questions will enable you to discover the root of the client's concerns and keep the workout on track.

Personal Trainer: Today is about starting a new phase of your training program and learning more about the way you move. During your row exercise, you seemed unsure of me assessing your movements. What is the most challenging part of this for you?

Client: Today feels different than the other sessions we've had in the past five months. I know you mentioned that it would be an opportunity to make observations about the way I move, and I understand that. But the way you're watching me from multiple angles is making me nervous. I feel uncomfortable.

Break down barriers: Asking more open-ended questions will allow you to learn more about the client's concerns.

Personal Trainer: Thank you for sharing your concerns with me. Are you able to tell me what exactly has made you nervous?

Client: It feels awkward, the way you're moving around me while I exercise. I feel like I'm on display and like you're judging me. I think the most uncomfortable part is the silence.

Collaborate: Work together with the client to find solutions to barriers to ensure the client feels understood and respected while also keeping on track with the focus of the exercise session.

Personal Trainer: You feel like I'm silently judging you while I am making my observations and that is making you self-conscious. What can I do to alleviate that feeling?

Client: I know I'm getting a good workout and I want to finish. Is it possible for you to walk me through what is going on in your mind as you are making observations and share with me what you're seeing? I think that will help me to have a better understanding of what we are accomplishing today.

Personal Trainer: Yes, of course. I would be happy to do that. Beginning with our next exercise, I can walk you through each step and let you know what I am seeing. You can ask me questions at any point, and you will be able to see how we go from observing how you move into creating an exercise program. My only ask of you is that you do not change how you move because you know I am watching you. It's vital that you continue to move as you usually would so that I can make an honest assessment.

Client: I am curious to learn more about how my body moves so I will do my best to move normally. Thank you for hearing me out. It helps me to feel like you understand what I'm feeling.

In this scenario, the personal trainer observed the client's body language and acted on it at an appropriate time. The use of open-ended questions and reflective listening allowed the personal trainer to gather the information necessary to put the client at ease. By valuing and respecting the client's feelings, the personal trainer can enhance the working relationship that will keep the client experience focused and productive.

Load/Speed Assessments

The Load/Speed Training phase emphasizes muscular endurance and strength, and/or improved skill performance in activities that rely on **power, speed, agility,** and **quickness.** Thus, the load/speed assessments introduced here are designed to help the personal trainer observe a client's performance in these areas.

As noted earlier in this chapter, deciding which assessments to include must be a collaborative process between the client and personal trainer. If a client has muscular conditioning goals that include improving muscular endurance, strength, or athletic performance, conducting assessments included in this section could offer valuable information for designing a personalized training program, as well as comparative data for checking progress against follow-up assessments as the program advances. However, because these assessments are designed to push clients beyond that to which they are ordinarily accustomed (e.g., perform as many push-ups as possible or squat as much load as is tolerable), great care and consideration should be given to which ones are selected and the appropriateness of the assessments for the individual client.

MUSCULAR-ENDURANCE ASSESSMENTS

Muscular-endurance assessments evaluate the ability of a specific muscle group, or groups, to perform repeated or sustained contractions to sufficiently invoke muscular fatigue. The following are important considerations prior to any muscular-endurance assessment:

- Always check for low-back pain and other orthopedic issues before conducting any of these assessments.
- As with any assessment, any indication of pain during an assessment merits immediate termination of the assessment and referral to a more qualified professional.
- If a client has a history of orthopedic issues, such as diagnosed low-back pain or is currently experiencing pain and/or discomfort, these assessments should not be performed until he or she has consulted with a doctor.

Push-up Assessment

The push-up assessment measures upper-body endurance, specifically of the pectoralis muscles, triceps, and anterior deltoids (Figures 10-50 and 10-51; see Figures 9-18, page 348, and 9-42, page 373). Due to common variations in upper-body strength between men and women, women are assessed while performing a modified push-up. The push-up is useful not only as an evaluation tool for measuring upper-body strength and endurance, but is also a prime activity for developing and maintaining upper-body muscular fitness. This assessment may not be appropriate for clients with shoulder, elbow, or wrist problems. A major problem associated with assessments that require performance to

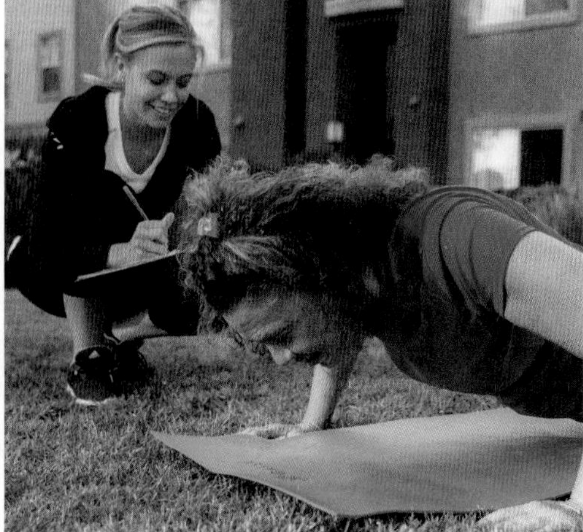

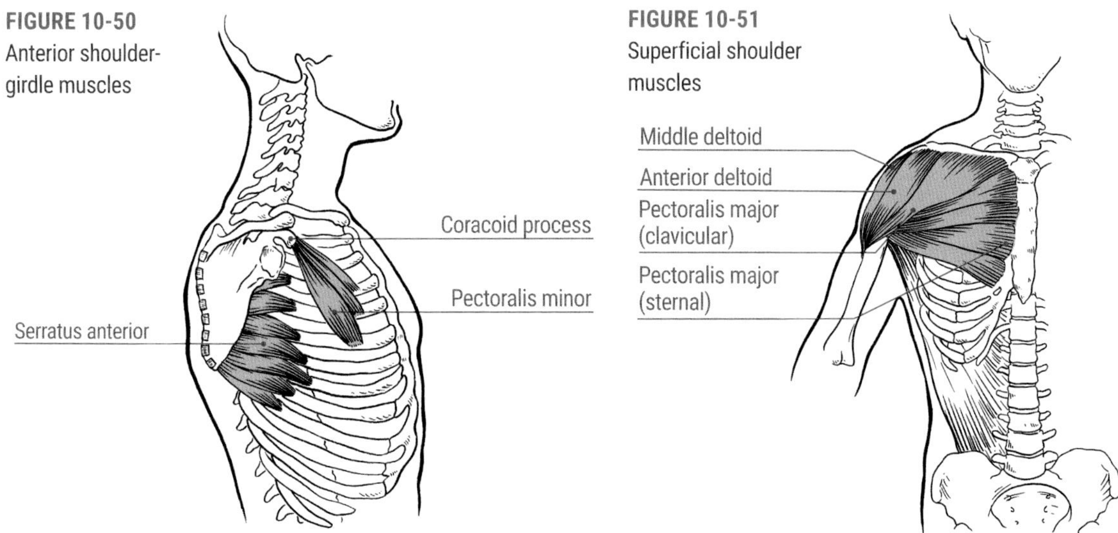

FIGURE 10-50 Anterior shoulder-girdle muscles

FIGURE 10-51 Superficial shoulder muscles

fatigue is that the point of "exhaustion" or fatigue is highly influenced by an individual's level of motivation. Novice exercisers may not push themselves to the maximal point of exertion.

Objective: To measure upper-body endurance

Equipment:

- Mat (optional)
- Towel or foam block

Pre-assessment procedure:

- After explaining the purpose of the assessment, explain and demonstrate the correct push-up version (standard or modified).
- The hands should point forward and be positioned shoulder-width apart, directly under the shoulders. The hips and shoulders should be aligned (i.e., rigid trunk) and the head should remain in a neutral to slightly extended position.
- The goal of the assessment is to perform as many consecutive and complete push-ups as possible before reaching a point of fatigue. The push-ups must be steady, without any rest in between the repetitions. Explain that only correctly performed push-ups are counted.
- Encourage the client to perform a few practice trials before the assessment begins.

Assessment protocol and administration:

- The assessment starts in the "down" position and the client can begin the assessment whenever he or she is ready (Figure 10-52).
- Count each *complete* push-up until the client reaches fatigue. A complete push-up requires:
  - Full elbow extension with a straight back and rigid torso in the "up" position (Figure 10-53)
  - The chest touching the personal trainer's fist, a rolled towel, or a foam block, without resting the stomach or body on the mat in the "down" position

- The assessment is terminated when the client is unable to complete a repetition or fails to maintain proper technique for two consecutive repetitions.
- Record the score on the assessment form.
- Classify the client's score using Table 10-21. Note that categories are based on the performance of standard push-ups for men and modified push-ups for women.

Clients who are physically inactive or unaccustomed to working the upper body are likely lacking in upper-body strength and endurance. If the muscles of the upper body are weak, this can lead to poor posture and a variety of musculoskeletal problems.

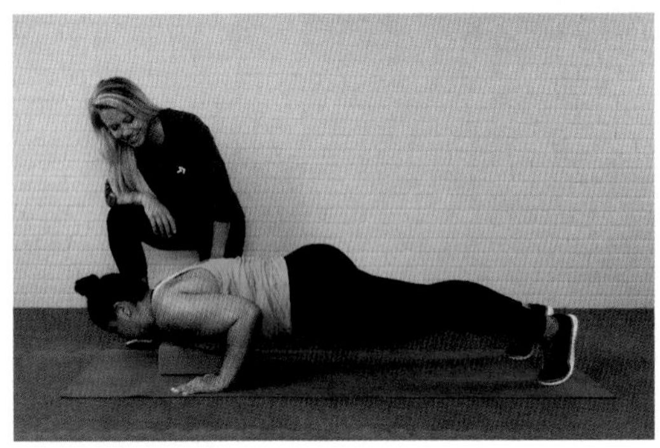

a. Standard push-up starting position

b. Modified push-up starting position

FIGURE 10-52
Push-up assessment: Starting position

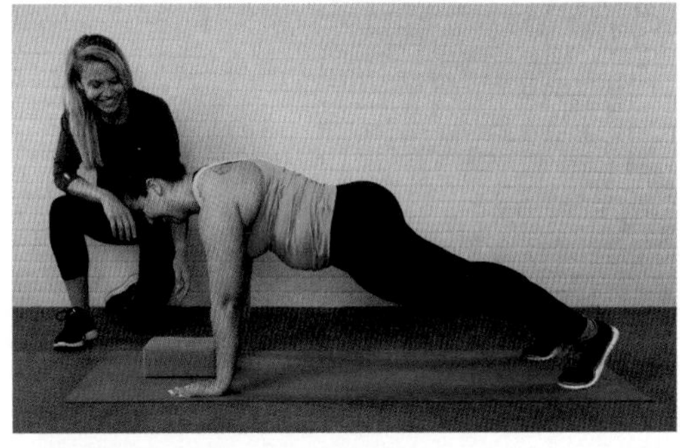

a. Standard push-up “up” position

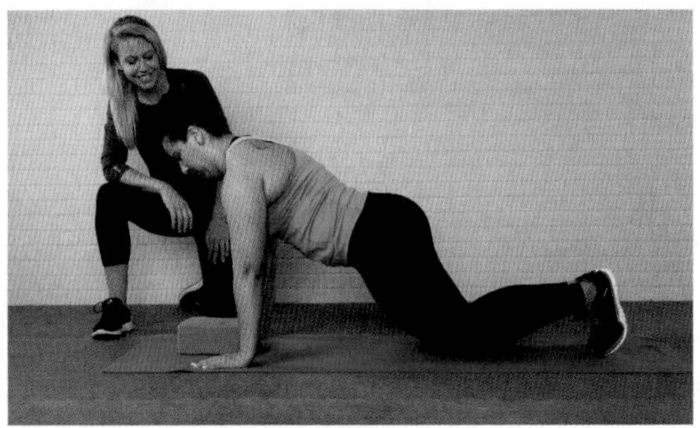

b. Modified push-up “up” position

FIGURE 10-53
Push-up assessment: "Up" position

TABLE 10-21

Converting the Push-up Score (Number) to a Health Benefit Rating

	Age (years)											
Category	15–19		20–29		30–39		40–49		50–59		60–69	
Sex	M	W	M	W	M	W	M	W	M	W	M	W
Excellent	≥39	≥33	≥36	≥30	≥30	≥27	≥25	≥24	≥21	≥21	≥18	≥17
Very good	29–38	25–32	29–35	21–29	22–29	20–26	17–24	15–23	13–20	11–20	11–17	12–16
Good	23–28	18–24	22–28	15–20	17–21	13–19	13–16	11–14	10–12	7–10	8–10	5–11
Fair	18–22	12–17	17–21	10–14	12–16	8–12	10–12	5–10	7–9	2–6	5–7	2–4
Needs improvement	≤17	≤11	≤16	≤9	≤11	≤7	≤9	≤4	≤6	≤1	≤4	≤1

Note: M = Men; W = Women

Reprinted with permission from Canadian Society for Exercise Physiology (2019). *CSEP Physical Activity Training for Health (CSEP-PATH) Resource Manual* (2nd ed.). Ottawa: Canadian Society for Exercise Physiology.

Body-weight Squat Assessment

This assessment evaluates muscular endurance of the lower extremity when performing repetitions of a squat-to-stand movement. This assessment is suitable *only* for individuals who demonstrate proper form when performing a squat. It can be used to effectively gauge relative improvements in a client's lower-extremity muscular endurance. While this assessment mimics a primary movement that most individuals perform daily, it may not be suitable for clients who are deconditioned or who are frail with lower-extremity weakness, or clients with balance concerns and orthopedic issues (especially in the knees).

Objective: To evaluate muscular endurance of the lower extremity

Pre-assessment procedure:

- After explaining the purpose of the body-weight squat assessment, explain and demonstrate the proper technique (Figure 10-54). See page 429 for proper squat technique.
- Allow for adequate warm-up and stretching if needed.
- Evaluate the depth of the squat using the following criterion:
    - The thighs reach parallel to the floor
- To enhance balance and stability, the client may extend his or her arms to the sides or front for balance.
- The goal of the assessment is to complete as many controlled and proper repetitions as possible. Once the client exhibits fatigue where he or she can no longer complete a full repetition, terminate the assessment. This includes an inability to fully lower into the down position, pausing to rest, or faltering as he or she stands.
- Encourage the client to practice this movement prior to attempting the assessment.

Assessment protocol and administration:

- When ready, the client begins performing squat repetitions.
- Count only complete repetitions until any assessment-termination criteria is reached.

Interpretation:

- Use the information presented in Table 10-22 to categorize the client's performance.

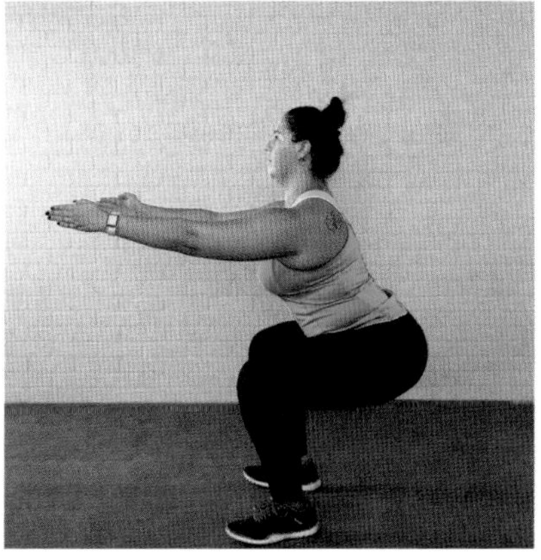

FIGURE 10-54
Body-weight squat assessment

TABLE 10-22

Norms for Body-weight Squats

Males	18–25	26–35	36–45	46–55	56–65	65+
Excellent	>49	>45	>41	>35	>31	>28
Good	44–49	40–45	35–41	29–35	25–31	22–28
Above average	39–43	35–39	30–34	25–38	21–24	19–21
Average	35–38	31–34	27–29	22–24	17–20	15–18
Below average	31–34	29–30	23–26	18–21	13–16	11–14
Poor	25–30	22–28	17–22	13–17	9–12	7–10
Very poor	<25	<22	<17	<9	<9	<7
Females	**18–25**	**26–35**	**36–45**	**46–55**	**56–65**	**65+**
Excellent	>43	>39	>33	>27	>24	>23
Good	37–43	33–39	27–33	22–27	18–24	17–23
Above average	33–36	29–32	23–26	18–21	13–17	14–16
Average	29–32	25–28	19–22	14–17	10–12	11–13
Below average	25–28	21–24	15–18	10–13	7–9	5–10
Poor	18–24	13–20	7–14	5–9	3–6	2–4
Very Poor	<18	<13	<7	<5	<3	<2

Reprinted with permission from Mackenzie, B. (2005). *101 Performance Evaluation Tests.* London: Green Star Media. Reused by permission of Peak Performance. www.peakendurancesport.com

MUSCULAR-STRENGTH ASSESSMENTS

Muscular strength is an important component of physical fitness. Strength is dependent on variables such as muscle size (diameter), limb length, and neurological adaptations. Maintaining muscular strength is important for everything from performance of ADL to sports performance. Strength can be expressed as either **absolute strength** or **relative strength.** Absolute strength is defined as the greatest amount of weight that can be lifted one time and can be defined as a **one-repetition maximum (1-RM).** On the other hand, relative strength takes the person's body weight into consideration and is used primarily when comparing individuals.

Relative strength is the maximal force a person is able to exert in relation to his or her body weight and is calculated using the following formula:

Relative strength = Absolute strength/Body weight

Note: Absolute strength equals the amount of weight lifted

Just as in previous assessments, it is important to understand the goals of the client being assessed and then choose assessments that are associated with those goals.

- Does the client want to improve overall function or is he or she interested in precise performance gains?
- Is the client interested in total-body fitness or is he or she interested in specific muscle fitness (e.g., to rehabilitate an injury)?
- Does the client need to enhance muscular power, strength, and/or endurance? For example, 1-RM training is not well-correlated to muscular endurance.

When a personal trainer is deciding on an appropriate strength assessment, any 1-RM assessment should be chosen with thoughtful consideration. 1-RM assessments should only be performed during the Load/Speed Training phase of the ACE IFT Model, as appropriate. A certain amount of injury risk is associated with maximal exertion. Submaximal strength assessments can be used with a high amount of accuracy to determine a client's likely 1-RM.

There is no single assessment that evaluates total-body muscular strength. Therefore, a variety of assessments would be appropriate to determine strength in different muscle groups. Strength assessments are important to determine muscular fitness, identify areas of weakness or imbalances, monitor rehabilitation progress, and assess training effectiveness. The following strength assessments are described in this section:

- 1-RM bench-press assessment
- 1-RM squat assessment

Strength assessments will likely be incorporated into a comprehensive assessment session. A client should warm up prior to strength assessments to reduce the likelihood of injury and enhance overall strength. Prolonged static stretching prior to strength assessments should be discouraged, as it may decrease performance.

Normative data are not available for all forms of 1-RM assessments and, in most cases, this form of assessment is most valuable as a source of baseline data against which the personal trainer can measure a client's future performance. Improvements in 1-RM can be very motivating for many clients, as they are a clear indication of strength development. Many strength assessments are performed using free weights, so proper form and control are necessary elements. Novice exercisers may not have the familiarity or skill to handle the heavier free weights. Additionally, beginning exercisers are often unsure of their abilities and tend to quit before their true maximum. Proper breathing patterns are necessary. Clients should avoid the **Valsalva maneuver** or any other form of breath-holding. Individuals with **hypertension** and/or a history of **vascular disease** should avoid 1-RM assessments.

Conducting maximal exertion assessments, such as the 1-RM bench-press and squat assessments, is not necessary for most clients as a starting point (or baseline) for training. Personal trainers may have success showing their clients how their strength improves over time by simply keeping a record of training sessions that documents increases in clients' abilities to lift heavier loads. Clients may find this approach more appealing and, as a result, more motivating than being asked to perform 1-RM assessments.

1-RM Bench-press Assessment

This assessment is suitable *only* for individuals who demonstrate proper form in performing a bench press and are free from a history of shoulder problems.

Objective: To evaluate upper-body strength using a fundamental upper-extremity movement: the bench press

Equipment:

- Barbell and bench
- Weights, ranging from 2.5-lb to 45-lb plates (1-kg to 20-kg plates)
- Collars
- Spotter (in addition to the personal trainer is preferred)

Pre-assessment procedure:

- After explaining the purpose of the assessment, explain and demonstrate the proper technique for the bench press.
  - The client is supine with eyes below the racked bar and both feet planted firmly on the floor or on a riser to accommodate a neutral or flat back. The head, shoulders, and buttocks should be placed firmly and evenly on a bench. The back and neck should be relaxed and the body should maintain all points of contact throughout the movement to maintain stability and support the spine.
  - The hands should be in closed pronated grip and positioned slightly wider than shoulder-width apart, so that the elbows are at a 90-degree angle (or slightly less) at the bottom of the movement range.
  - Proper ROM during the bench press is from arms fully extended (bar positioned above the chest) to the bar lightly touching the chest (bar located over the lower part of the sternum).
  - The client should inhale while slowly lowering the bar and exhale while raising the bar. Breath-holding (or the Valsalva maneuver) should be avoided.
  - It is important for the client to communicate with the spotter if he or she cannot complete the repetition.
  - Instruct the client not to lock the elbows and not to bounce the bar off the chest. Poor technique can cause injuries, so the client should not contort his or her body in an effort to display strength beyond his or her capabilities.
- Encourage the client to perform a few practice trials to ensure proper technique.
- The responsibilities of the spotter include providing assistance in racking and unracking the barbell and raising the bar during an incomplete attempt.
  - *Single spotting:* The spotter stands behind the client in a split-stance position with a dead-lift or closed, alternated grip (i.e., a mix of an overhand grip and an underhand grip) on the bar with the hands placed in the area between the client's hands (Figure 10-55).
  - *Double spotting:* The two spotters grasp either end of the barbell (Figure 10-56).
- The goal of the assessment is to determine the maximal amount of weight that can be lifted one time (i.e., the 1-RM). It is important to avoid fatiguing the client by having him or her perform too many "unnecessary" repetitions. Finding a suitable starting weight is important for an accurate assessment of the client's strength.

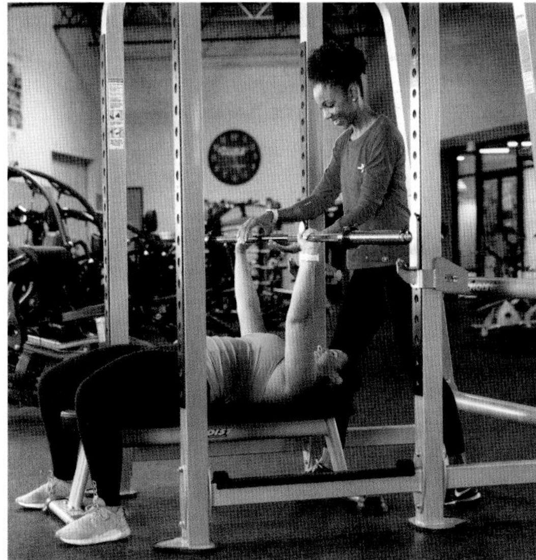
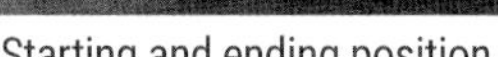
Starting and ending position

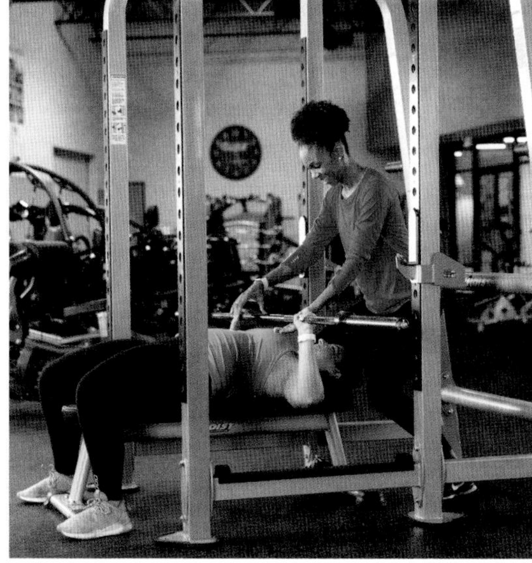
Mid-range position

FIGURE 10-55
Bench press assessment

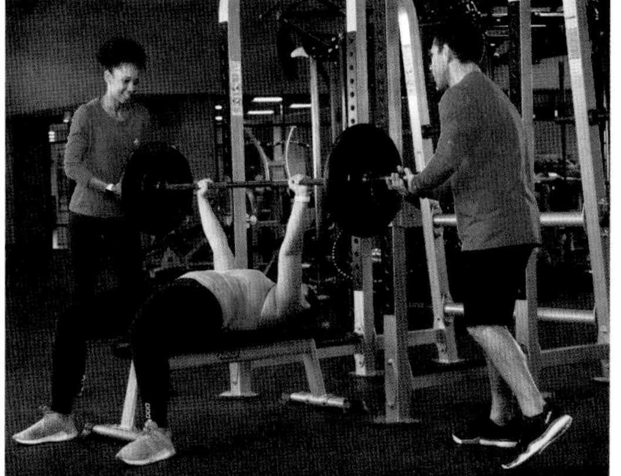
Starting and ending position

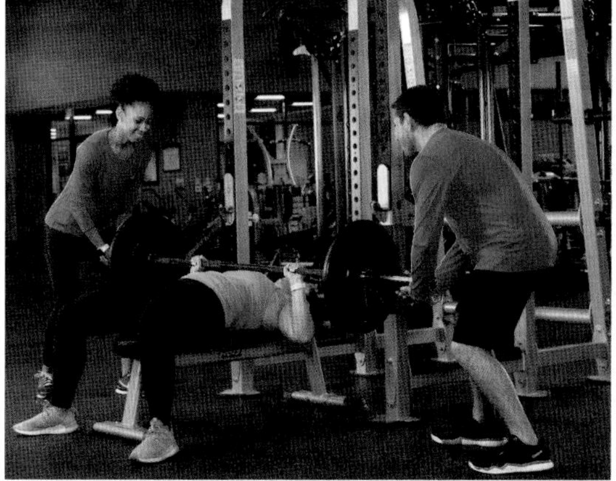
Mid-range position

FIGURE 10-56
Bench press assessment with two spotters

Assessment protocol and administration:

- Administer the assessment protocol for a 1-RM bench press.
  - The client should warm up with one set of light resistance that allows five to 10 repetitions, and then rest for one minute.
  - Based on the client's warm-up effort, determine a suitable starting workload for the second set that allows for three to five repetitions, and then allow the client to rest for two minutes. Use the following guideline for determining workload increases throughout this assessment:
    - In general, increase by approximately 5 to 10%.
- Next, have the client perform one heavy set of two to three repetitions and rest for two to four minutes.
- Based on the client's third set, determine the next workload to find the client's 1-RM effort. The 1-RM chart provided in Table 10-25 on page 455 can be used to make these calculations.
- Allow the client to attempt this set. If the client is successful, he or she should rest for two to four minutes and repeat the 1-RM effort with a heavier load.

- If the attempt was unsuccessful, decrease the load accordingly (by 2.5 to 5%) and have the client try again after resting for two to four minutes.
- Continue to adjust the resistance level until a true 1-RM is achieved. *Ideally, the client should achieve his or her 1-RM in three to five sets.*
- Use the assessment form to record the weight, progression, sets, repetitions, and any comments on the client's progress. The final weight/load is recorded as the absolute strength.
- Calculate relative strength and record that value as well.
  - For example, if Jose's actual 1-RM was measured at 205 lb (93.2 kg) and he weighs 175 lb (79.5 kg), then his strength-to-weight ratio, or relative strength, would be 1.17 (205/175 or 93.2/79.5).

Interpretation:

Use Table 10-23 or 10-24 to rank the client's ability, which should be recorded on the assessment form as well.

TABLE 10-23
Upper-body Strength (Men)

One-repetition Maximum Bench Press (Bench Press Weight Ratio = Weight Pushed / Body Weight)							
		Age					
	%	<20	20–29	30–39	40–49	50–59	60+
Superior	95	1.76	1.63	1.35	1.20	1.05	0.94
Excellent	80	1.34	1.32	1.12	1.00	0.90	0.82
Good	60	1.19	1.14	0.98	0.88	0.79	0.72
Fair	40	1.06	0.99	0.88	0.80	0.71	0.66
Poor	20	0.89	0.88	0.78	0.72	0.63	0.57
Very Poor	5	0.76	0.72	0.65	0.59	0.53	0.49

Reprinted with permission from The Cooper Institute, Dallas, Texas from *Physical Fitness Assessments and Norms for Adults and Law Enforcement*. Available online at www.cooperinstitute.org.

TABLE 10-24
Upper-body Strength (Women)

One-repetition Maximum Bench Press (Bench Press Weight Ratio = Weight Pushed / Body Weight)							
		Age					
	%	<20	20–29	30–39	40–49	50–59	60+
Superior	95	0.88	1.01	0.82	0.77	0.68	0.72
Excellent	80	0.77	0.80	0.70	0.62	0.55	0.54
Good	60	0.65	0.70	0.60	0.54	0.48	0.47
Fair	40	0.58	0.59	0.53	0.50	0.44	0.43
Poor	20	0.53	0.51	0.47	0.43	0.39	0.38
Very Poor	5	0.41	0.44	0.39	0.35	0.31	0.26

Reprinted with permission from The Cooper Institute, Dallas, Texas from *Physical Fitness Assessments and Norms for Adults and Law Enforcement*. Available online at www.cooperinstitute.org.

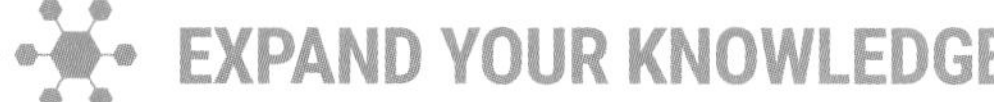

EXPAND YOUR KNOWLEDGE

Considerations for Spotting

Personal trainers must be prepared to properly spot clients as needed throughout their muscular-training workouts. Consider the following recommendations (Gibson, Wagner, & Heyward, 2019):

- Personal trainers can help prevent client injuries with proper spotting techniques.
- Personal trainers who are spotting during 1-RM assessments should have the leverage and strength needed to safely do so.
- It is suggested that personal trainers provide clients with spotting for all free weight exercise performed with barbells or dumbbells moving over the head (Figure 10-57), in front of the shoulders (Figure 10-58), on the back (see Figure 10-59, page 453), or moving over the face (see Figures 10-55 and 10-56) (with the exception of power exercises).
- Personal trainers should establish a stable base of support and maintain good posture via a neutral spine when spotting heavier weights.
- Personal trainers will generally assist clients with positioning the barbell or dumbbells in the correct starting position (e.g., the liftoff phase).
- Personal trainers should spot as close to the dumbbell as possible for dumbbell exercises.
- Over-the-face exercises (e.g., bench press) should be spotted by personal trainers with an alternated grip narrower than that of the client when gripping the bar to lift or lower it. A supinated grip should be used to spot the bar during the exercise itself (see Figure 10-55).
- Exercises should be performed within a power rack when lifting overhead or loading a movement with a bar placed in back or in front of the shoulders.
- Personal trainers will generally need to provide modest assistance to clients in order to finish a repetition. However, during 1-RM assessments, the personal trainer should anticipate the need to take the bar immediately if a client is unable to perform the 1-RM.

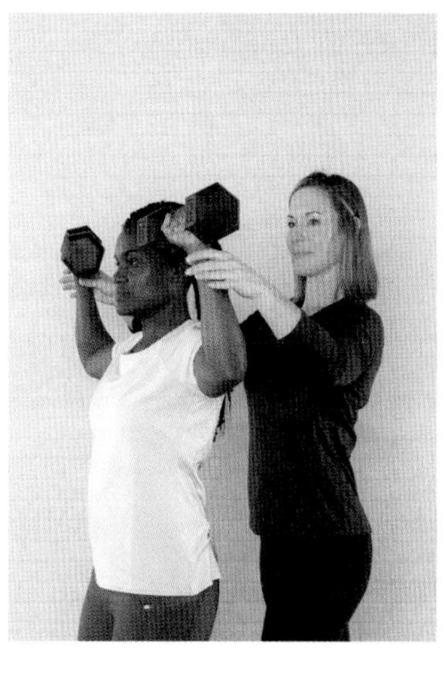

FIGURE 10-57 Proper spotting of an overhead press

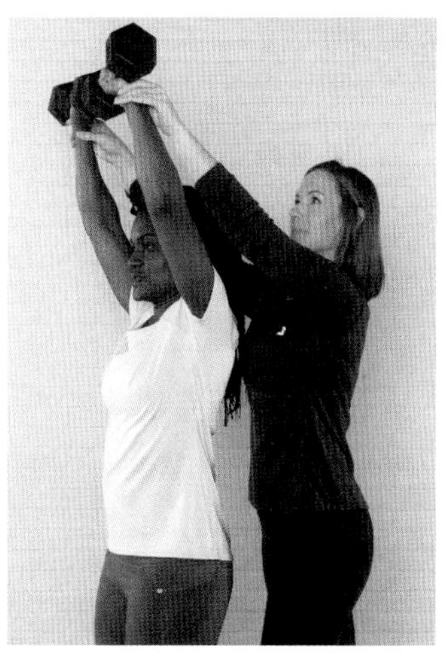

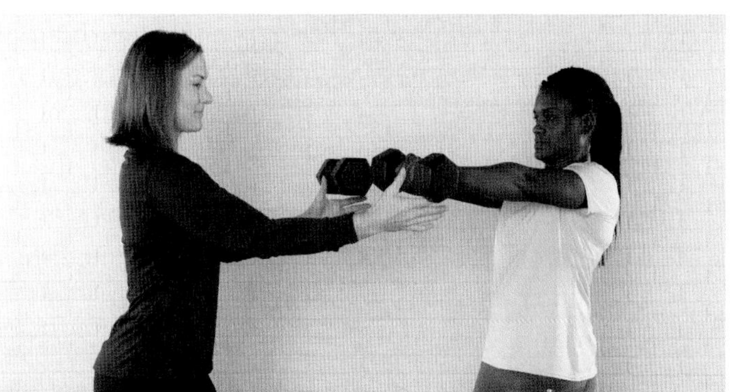

FIGURE 10-58 Proper spotting of a front arm raise

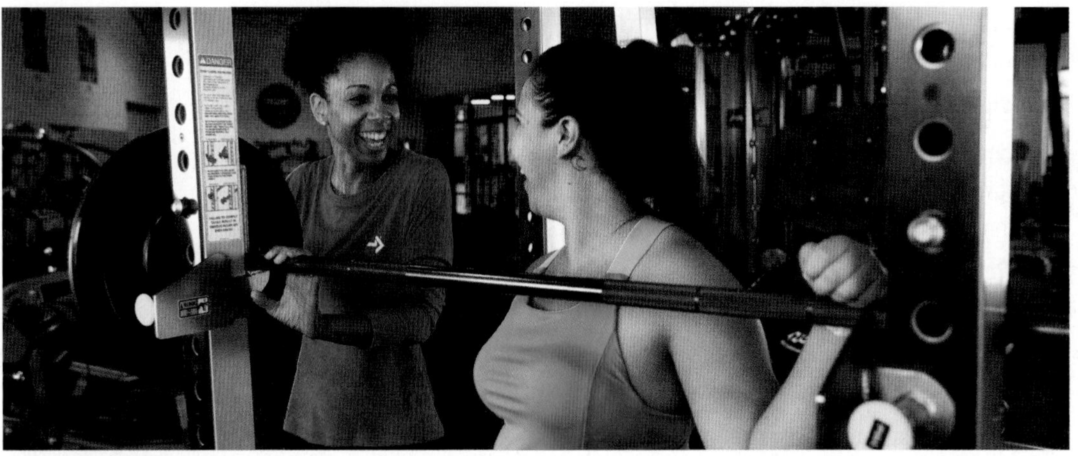

1-RM Squat Assessment

This assessment is suitable *only* for individuals who demonstrate proper form when performing a squat and are free of low-back or knee pain.

Objective: To evaluate lower-extremity strength using an unsupported, functional movement: the squat

Equipment:

- Barbell and squat rack
- Weights, ranging from 2.5-pound plates to 45-pound plates (1-kg to 20-kg plates)
- Collars
- Spotter (in addition to the personal trainer is preferred)

Pre-assessment procedure:

- After explaining the purpose of the assessment, explain and demonstrate the proper technique for the squat (Figure 10-59).
    - The client should stand behind a racked bar that is positioned below the shoulders, but above the nipple line.
    - He or she should grasp the bar with a closed, pronated (overhead) grip (hand placement depends on bar position) and step under the bar with the feet parallel to unrack the bar.
    - Position the barbell in the high-bar position (i.e., the bar is placed above the posterior deltoids, resting on the upper trapezius at the base of the neck with the hands slightly wider than shoulder-width apart), or the low-bar position, where the bar is placed across the posterior deltoids along the spine of the scapulae using a wider hand position.
    - The client engages the core and abdominal muscles to brace the trunk, then uses the lower extremity to unrack the bar and move into the starting position.
    - The client stands with the feet shoulder-width apart, back neutral, feet flat, chest up and out, and the head neutral or positioned facing slightly upward.
    - The lowering phase is initiated with flexion at the hips first, pushing the buttocks backward prior to bending the knees. This hip-hinge movement reduces the stress across the knee joint.

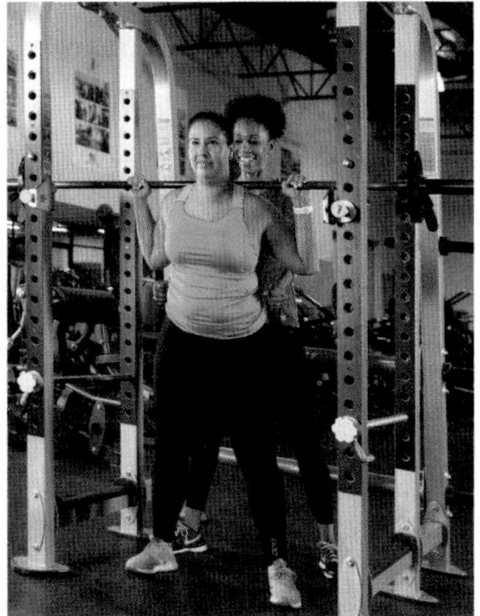
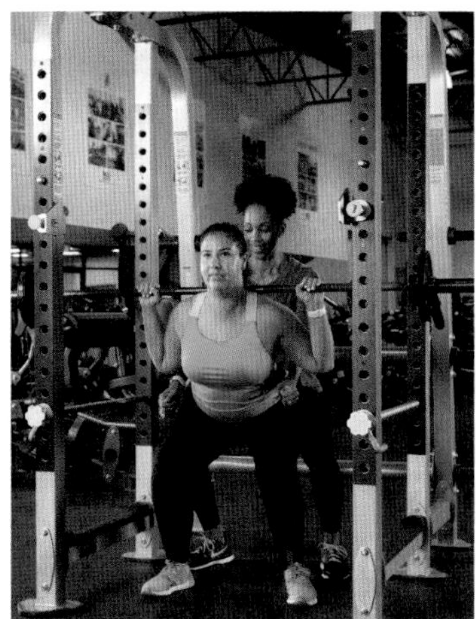
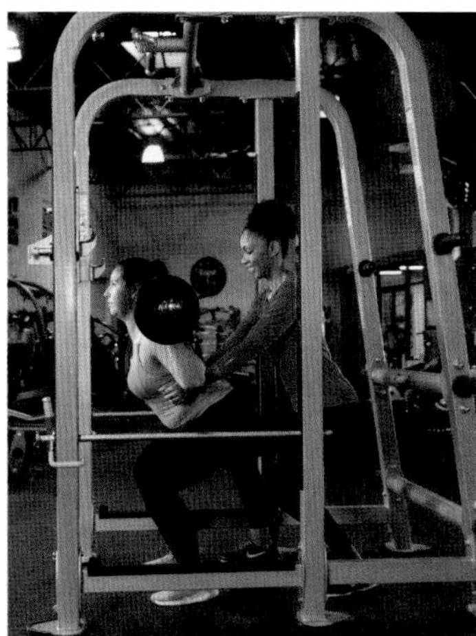

FIGURE 10-59
Squat assessment

- ROM during the squat is from standing with legs straight to a squatting position with the knees bent slightly more than 90 degrees, or until the thighs are parallel to the floor.
- The client inhales during the lowering phase and exhales during the lifting phase. Breath-holding (i.e., Valsalva maneuver) should be avoided.
- Throughout the movement, the heels must remain in contact with the floor, and the upward phase is performed by pushing through the heels.
- It is important for the client to communicate with the spotter if he or she cannot complete the repetition.
- Instruct the client to avoid locking the knees and not to exceed a parallel-with-the-floor position with the thighs.

- Encourage the client to perform a few practice trials to ensure proper technique.
- The goal of this assessment is to determine the client's 1-RM. It is important not to fatigue the client by having him or her perform too many "unnecessary" repetitions. Finding a suitable starting weight is important.

Assessment protocol and administration:

- Explain the assessment protocol for a 1-RM squat.
  - The client should warm up with one set of light resistance that allows five to 10 repetitions, and then rest for one minute.
  - Based on the client's warm-up effort, determine a suitable workload for the second set that allows for three to five repetitions by increasing the weight by 30 to 40 pounds (13.7 to 18.2 kg) or 10 to 20%, after which the client will rest for two minutes. Use the following guideline for determining workload increases throughout this assessment:
    - Increase the weight by 10 to 20%.
  - Next, have the client perform one heavy set of two to three repetitions and rest for two to four minutes.
- Based on the client's third set, determine the next workload to find the client's 1-RM effort.

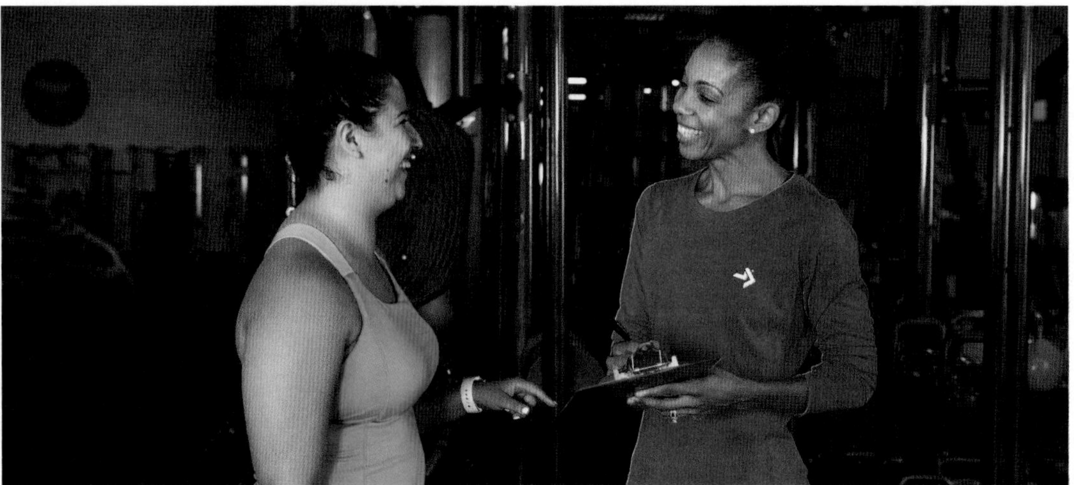

- Allow the client to attempt this set. If the client is successful, he or she should rest for two to four minutes and repeat the 1-RM effort with a heavier load.
- If the attempt was unsuccessful, decrease the load accordingly [by 15 to 20 pounds (6.8 to 9.1 kg) or 5 to 10%] and have the client try again after resting for two to four minutes.
- Continue to adjust the resistance level until a true 1-RM is achieved. *Ideally, the client should achieve his or her 1-RM in three to five testing sets.*
- The final successful load is recorded as the absolute strength.
- Record the weight, progression, sets, repetitions, and any comments on the client's progress on the assessment form.
- Calculate relative strength and record that value as well.
    - For example, if Jose's actual 1-RM was measured at 230 lb (104.5 kg) and he weighs 175 lb (79.5 kg), then his strength-to-weight ratio, or relative strength, would be 1.31 (230/175 or 104.5/79.5).

Interpretation:

- Record the client's performance and use the results as a baseline against which to measure future progress.

Submaximal Strength Assessments

When working with inexperienced exercisers or individuals with health considerations that would preclude them from performing a 1-RM assessment, it is appropriate to assess strength during various exercises using submaximal efforts that do not exceed 10 repetitions. Submaximal assessments that exceed 10 repetitions are moving toward the muscular endurance end of the strength–endurance continuum.

Objective: To evaluate upper- and lower-extremity strength using submaximal loads

Assessment protocol:

- Determine the number of repetitions that are appropriate for the client based upon his or her current training regimen or experience [e.g., Mary usually performs three sets of eight repetitions at 60 pounds (27 kg)].

- Sets:
  - Have the client perform one or two warm-up sets at a lower intensity than the target weight and allow one to two minutes of recovery between the sets.
  - Instruct the client to perform the first attempt at a personal best, completing the targeted number of repetitions consistent with his or her current training [e.g., Mary completes one set of eight repetitions at 60 pounds (27 kg)].
  - If the client is successful, he or she should rest for approximately two minutes and repeat the personal-best effort with a heavier load.
  - If the client is unsuccessful at achieving the goal repetitions, simply use the actual number completed in the calculation (see Table 10-27) [e.g., If Mary completes five squat repetitions with an increased load of 70 lb (32 kg), her predicted 1-RM would equal 84 lb (38 kg), as 70 lb x 1.2 = 84 lb].

The 1-RM chart provided in Table 10-25 can be used to make these calculations.

TABLE 10-25
1-RM—Repetition Table

Repetitions	% 1-RM
1	100
2	95
3	93
4	90
5	87
6	85
7	83
8	80
9	77
10	75
11	70
12	67
15	65

Note: 1-RM = One-repetition maximum

Reprinted with permission from Sheppard, J.M & Triplett, N.T. (2016). Program design for resistance training. In: Haff, G.G. & Triplett, N.T. (Eds.) *Essentials of Strength Training and Conditioning* (4th ed.). Champaign, Ill.: Human Kinetics, 452. Data from Chapman et al., 1998; Lander, 1984; Mayhew, Whitehead, & Binkert, 1992; and Morales & Sobonya, 1996.

Assessments can also be performed to determine left-to-right muscle balance or appropriate ratios of **agonist** to **antagonist** muscle strength. Muscle imbalances occur from improper training, overuse of one side of the body (e.g., tennis serves or golf swings), or from structural imbalances caused by injury or poor posture or body mechanics. Muscle balance is essential to prevent injury, enhance sports performance, and avoid chronic conditions later in life. Table 10-26 presents the recommended strength ratios between opposing muscle groups.

TABLE 10-26
Appropriate Strength Ratios

Joint	Movements	Muscles	Ratio
Shoulder	Flexion:Extension	Anterior deltoids:Trapezius, posterior deltoids	2:3
Shoulder	Internal rotation: External rotation	Subscapularis:Supraspinatus, infraspinatus, teres minor	3:2
Elbow	Flexion:Extension	Biceps:Triceps	1:1
Lumbar spine	Flexion:Extension	Iliopsoas, abdominals:Erector spinae	1:1
Hip	Flexion:Extension	Iliopsoas, rectus abdominis, tensor fascia latae:Erector spinae, gluteus maximus, hamstrings	1:1
Knee	Flexion:Extension	Hamstrings:Quadriceps	2:3
Ankle	Plantar flexion:Dorsiflexion	Gastrocnemius:Tibialis anterior	3:1
Ankle	Inversion:Eversion	Tibialis anterior:Peroneals	1:1

Source: Gibson, A.L., Wagner, D.L., & Heyward, V.H. (2019). *Advanced Fitness Assessments and Exercise Prescription* (8th ed.). Champaign, Ill.: Human Kinetics.

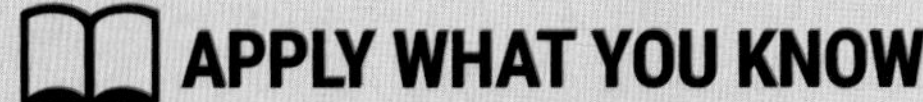

APPLY WHAT YOU KNOW

Estimating 1-RM

Table 10-27 offers personal trainers a way to estimate a client's 1-RM without requiring the client to perform an exercise with maximal effort. In fact, the client's 1-RM can be estimated by simply observing a workout and making the appropriate calculation. For example:

- A client is performing bench presses during his or her workout and the personal trainer observes that he or she consistently completes eight repetitions with 160 pounds (73 kg). Using the coefficient of 1.255, the client's estimated 1-RM is calculated as follows:
  - 1-RM = 160 pounds x 1.255 = 201 pounds (91 kg)

TABLE 10-27

One-repetition Maximum (1-RM) Prediction Coefficients

Number of repetitions completed	Squat or leg press coefficient	Bench or chest press coefficient
1	1.000	1.000
2	1.0475	1.035
3	1.13	1.08
4	1.1575	1.115
5	1.2	1.15
6	1.242	1.18
7	1.284	1.22
8	1.326	1.255
9	1.368	1.29
10	1.41	1.325

Source: Brzycki, M. (1993). Strength testing: Predicting a one-rep max from reps-to-fatigue. *Journal of Physical Education, Recreation, and Dance*, 64, 1, 88–90.

POWER ASSESSMENT

Human power is defined as the rate at which mechanical work is performed under a defined set of conditions. Power correlates to the immediate energy available through the phosphagen energy system. **Anaerobic** power involves a single repetition or event and represents the maximal amount of power the body can generate, whereas anaerobic capacity represents the sustainability of power output for brief periods of time.

Strength and power are closely related, but for assessment purposes, they should be evaluated independently. Power is also sport- or activity-specific. Evaluation and subsequent correction of athletic performance is closely related to body mechanics and movement. Evaluation of fluid movements like a golf swing or a swimming stroke may require digital movement analysis or other technology. The power assessments covered in this section are also related to skills and performance in a variety of sports and have been observed to have a correlation to sports success.

Field assessments that assess power measure how fast the body can move in a short time period. The vertical jump assessment is used to assess anaerobic power.

Power Equations
Power = Force x Velocity
or
Power = Work/Time
Where:
Force = Mass x Acceleration
Velocity = Distance/Time
Work = Force x Distance

Personal trainers must keep in mind that power assessments are designed for clients interested in Load/Speed Training. Therefore, the majority of normative data presented with these assessments has been obtained from studies involving college and professional athletes. Little, if any, data exists for middle-aged or older adults. The results of these assessments are perhaps best utilized as baseline data against which to measure a client's future performance.

Contraindications for Field Assessments of Power, Speed, Agility, and Quickness

Because these assessments are intended for athletes and those interested in advanced forms of training, individuals in "special populations" are not likely candidates. When working with a client who has an orthopedic limitation or is still recovering from an injury, it is wise to omit these assessments.

Vertical Jump Assessment

The vertical jump assessment is very simple and quick to administer. It is especially valuable when assessing the vertical jump height in athletes who participate in sports that require skill and power in jumping (e.g., basketball, volleyball, or football).

Objective: To evaluate standing vertical jump height

Equipment:

- A smooth wall with a relatively high ceiling
- A flat, stable floor that provides good traction
- Chalk (different color than the wall)
- Measuring tape or stick
- Stepstool or small ladder

Assessment protocol and administration:

- After explaining the purpose of the vertical jump assessment, describe and demonstrate the procedure. Allow the client to perform a few practice trials before administering the assessment.

- Instruct the client to stand adjacent to a wall, with the inside shoulder of the dominant arm approximately 6 inches (15 cm) from the wall. Measure the client's standing height by marking the fingers with chalk, extending the inside arm overhead, and marking the wall (Figure 10-60). This mark will then be compared to the maximal height achieved on a vertical jump.

FIGURE 10-60
Vertical jump assessment

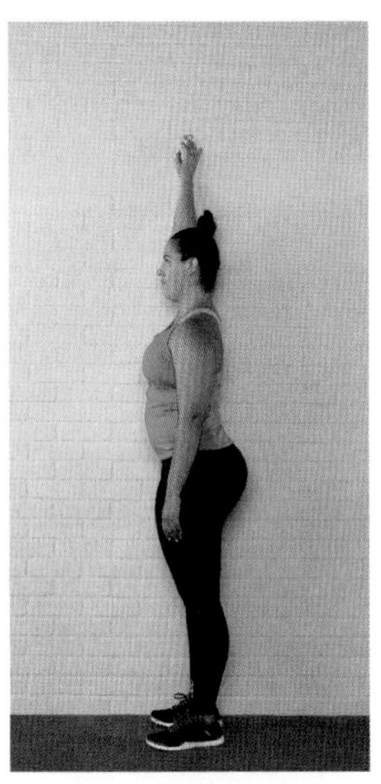
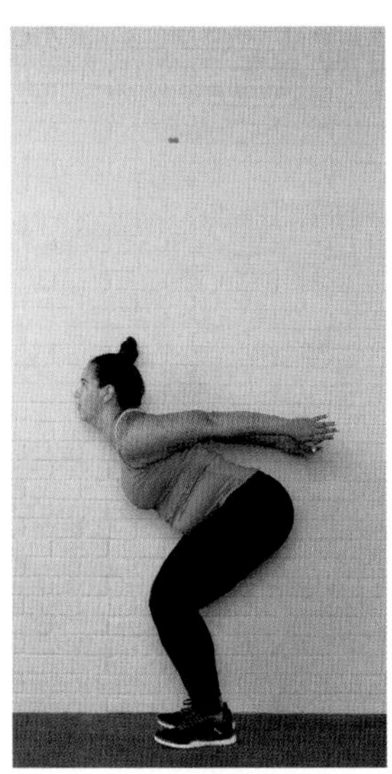
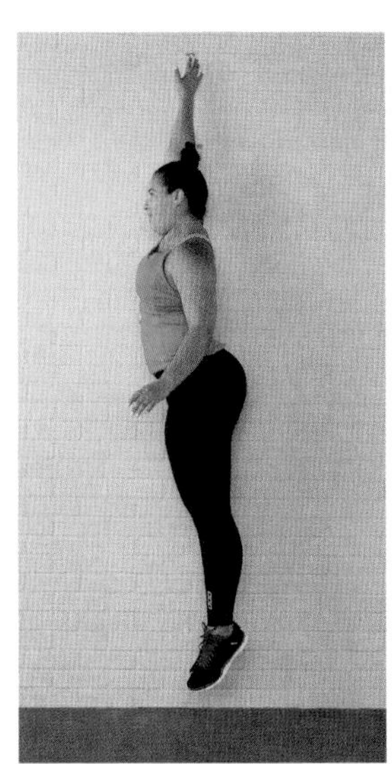

- The client then lowers the arms and, without any pause or step, drops into a squat movement before exploding upward into a vertical jump.
- The goal of this assessment is to jump as high as possible from a standing position.
- Since proper technique plays a role in achieving maximal jump height, encourage the client to use the arms and legs for propulsion.
- At the highest point, the athlete touches the wall, marking it with chalk.
- The vertical jump measurement is determined by the vertical distance between the new chalk mark and the starting height.
- Allow three repetitions and record the maximal height achieved on the assessment form.
- Use Table 10-28 to categorize the client's performance.

TABLE 10-28

Norms for the Vertical Jump Assessment (cm)

Men						
Age (years)	15–19	20–29	30–39	40–49	50–59	60–69
Excellent	≥56	≥58	≥52	≥43	≥41	≥33
Very good	51–55	54–57	46–51	36–42	34–40	29–32
Good	46–50	48–53	40–45	32–35	28–33	25–28
Fair	42–45	42–47	31–39	26–31	18–27	18–24
Needs Improvement	≤41	≤41	≤30	≤25	≤17	≤17

TABLE 10-28 (continued)

Women						
Age (years)	15-19	20-29	30-39	40-49	50-59	60-69
Excellent	≥40	≥38	≥36	≥31	≥25	≥19
Very good	36–39	34–37	32–35	27–30	21–24	15–18
Good	32–35	29–33	28–31	23–26	16–20	11–14
Fair	28–31	25–28	24–27	18–22	10–15	7–10
Needs improvement	≤27	≤24	≤23	≤17	≤9	≤6

Reprinted with permission from Gibson, A.L., Wagner, D.R., & Heyward, V.H. (2019). Advanced Fitness Assessment and Exercise Prescription (8th ed.). Champaign, Ill.: Human Kinetics, 175.

SPEED, AGILITY, AND QUICKNESS ASSESSMENT

Speed and agility assessments require maximal effort and swift limb movement. To perform well and avoid injury, it is imperative that the client warms up adequately. A sample warm-up includes a five- to 10-minute jog or light cardiorespiratory activity combined with some short sprints. Light, dynamic stretching should be included for the involved muscle groups (i.e., quadriceps, hamstrings, calves, and hip flexors).

T-Test

Objective: To assess multidirectional movement ability (Kainoa et al., 2000)

Equipment:

- A marked football field, but the assessment can be conducted on any hard, flat surface that offers good traction
- Measuring tape
- Four cones
- Stopwatch
- Timing gates (optional)

Pre-assessment procedure:

- Set up the cones as depicted in Figure 10-61.
- After explaining the purpose of the assessment, describe and demonstrate the proper route and technique. Allow the client to warm up and perform a few practice trials before administering the assessment.
- The goal of the assessment is to complete the course as quickly as possible.
- The client must keep his or her body facing forward at all times and must physically

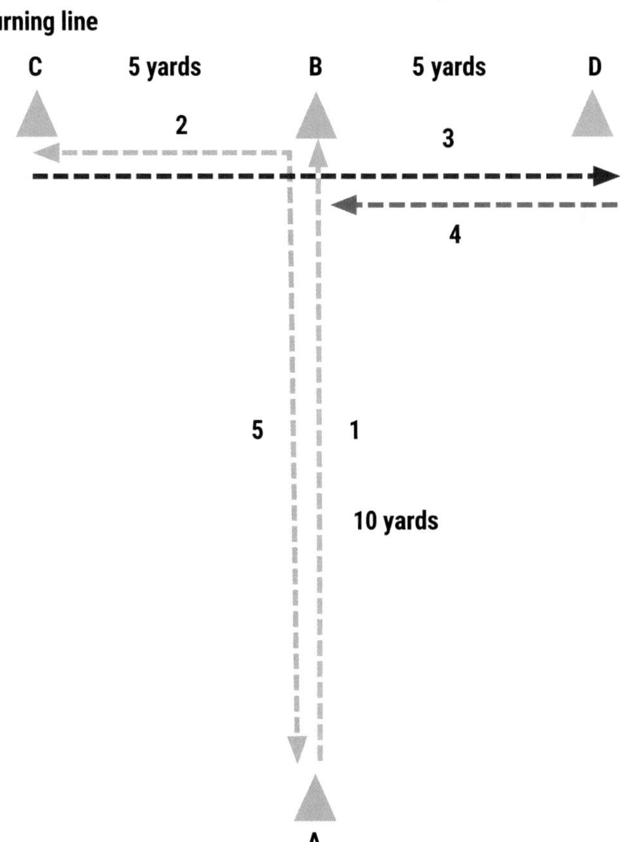

FIGURE 10-61
Layout for the T-test

touch each cone with the correct hand. The client shuffles through the course and cannot allow the feet to crossover at any time. Proper technique must be followed, or the run will not count.

Assessment protocol and administration:

- The client starts at cone A. On the personal trainer's command, the client sprints to cone B and touches the base of the cone with the right hand.
- Client shuffles left to cone C and touches the base of the cone with the left hand.
- Client shuffles right to cone D and touches the base of the cone with the right hand.
- Client then shuffles back to cone B and touches the base with the left hand before running backward to the start (cone A).
- Stop the stopwatch as the client passes cone A.
- The T-test is performed two times with a few minutes of recovery between each assessment.

Interpretation:

- Record the fastest time on an assessment form and use it as a baseline against which to compare future performance.

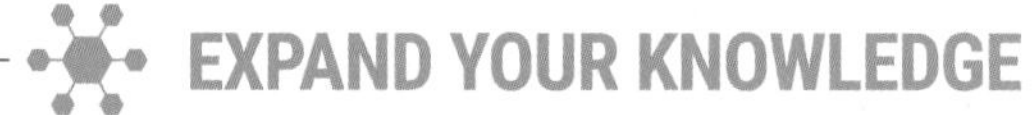

When and Why Should Assessments Be Repeated?

Assessments are not exclusively relegated to the initial phase of training. The performance of follow-up assessments is valuable for numerous reasons. For example, repeated assessments may be warranted to account for favorable training adaptations that have occurred in order to make the necessary adjustments to various Muscular Training variables. Moreover, as highlighted in Chapter 4, effective goal setting should include **SMART goals,** as this strategy can be effective for promoting positive behavior change, including initiation and maintenance of regular physical activity. Accordingly, measurable and time-bound goals that have been established can be evaluated with follow-up assessments that have been mutually agreed upon by the client and personal trainer.

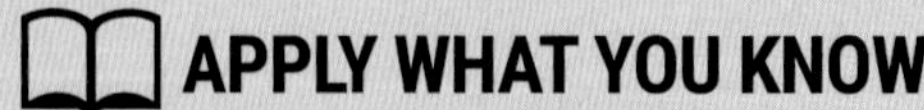

Discussing Muscular-training Assessment Results with Clients

Collecting assessment information through conducting physical fitness assessments can be an important step in exercise program development for clients. The baseline data, as well as follow-up data, can be invaluable in guiding clients through the journey of improving health and fitness that ultimately helps them achieve their goals. For this information to be meaningful and motivating to the client, the personal trainer must present assessment results in a way that is easily understood and relevant to the client's goals. The following example illustrates how personal trainers can effectively communicate a client's physical-fitness assessment data in a clear manner that teaches the client how the results apply to his or her personal situation.

Jennifer, a busy personal trainer who works in a fitness facility, has just retained Ben as a client. Ben is a 65-year-old retiree who is interested in improving lower-body strength because he has noticed that rising up out of a chair is becoming more challenging the older he gets. Ben has just completed the body-weight squat assessment (see page 445) and reports that he felt the work mainly in the "tops of his thighs." Additionally, Jennifer observed the following characteristics during Ben's assessment:

- Completed 20 repetitions at a depth of 30 degrees of knee flexion
- Both knees dropped in an inward direction during the movement

To help Ben understand the assessment results and make them relevant to his personal goals, Jennifer explained the data in the following way:

"Ben, you did very well and completed 20 repetitions, which is above average for your age. This indicates that your muscular endurance—or the ability to sustain exercise without becoming too fatigued—is at the right level. I also noticed that the depth of your squat was less than 90 degrees and that your knees had a tendency to drop inward during the movement. This lets me know that you could benefit from working on improving muscular strength in your legs as well as on increasing your ability to maintain proper knee alignment during squat-type movements. Working on alignment is important so that as you gain strength you also move properly, protecting the joints from unnecessary wear and tear. I have some very effective exercises and stretches in mind to address these issues, which will also help you with your goal of standing up from a seated position more easily."

While the scenario described above portrays just one component of a client's overall conditioning program, it gives an example of how technical assessment data can be delivered in a meaningful way. The personal trainer can take this approach with all assessment-result information to facilitate the client's understanding of why the assessments were performed and how they apply directly to the client. For clients who have a good understanding of physiology and kinesiology, it may be more appropriate to communicate assessment results using more technical language. In these situations, it is up to the personal trainer to gauge the knowledge level and interest of the client in using exercise science–related terminology. If, through the initial interview process and the course of conversation, it is discovered that a client possesses advanced knowledge of anatomical and health-related topics, it would be prudent to speak to the level of understanding of the client. Communicating in such a manner adds to the perceived professionalism of the personal trainer and lets the client know that the trainer is not attempting to "speak down" to him or her.

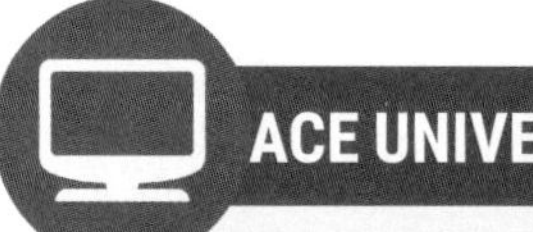

If your study program includes the ACE University, visit www.ACEfitness.org/MyACE and log in to your My ACE Account to take full advantage of the ACE Personal Trainer Study Program and online guided study experience.

A variety of media to support and expand on the material in this text is provided to facilitate learning and best prepare you for the ACE Personal Trainer Certification exam and a career as a personal trainer.

SUMMARY

The performance of assessments for Functional and Movement Training will offer valuable information on joint alignment and muscle balance across joints in clients. The ACE IFT Model provides a comprehensive and integrated muscular-training approach that spans from initial programming for a previously physically inactive client who has to build a foundation of health before moving on to working on fitness, all the way to a highly skilled client striving to enhance performance. Good joint alignment facilitates effective muscle action and joint movement, serving as the platform upon which good exercise technique is built.

REFERENCES

Abelbeck, K.G. (2002). Biomechanical model and evaluation of a linear motion squat type exercise. *Journal of Strength and Conditioning Research*, 16, 516–524.

Brzycki, M. (1993). Strength testing: Predicting a one-rep max from reps-to-fatigue. *Journal of Physical Education, Recreation, and Dance*, 64, 1, 88–90.

Canadian Society for Exercise Physiology (2019). *CSEP Physical Activity Training for Health (CSEP-PATH) Resource Manual* (2nd ed.). Ottawa: Canadian Society for Exercise Physiology.

Centers for Disease Control and Prevention (2018). *Older Adults Falls*. https://www.cdc.gov/features/falls-older-adults/index.html.

Chapman, P.P., Whitehead, J.R., & Binkert, R.H. (1998). The 225-lb reps-to fatigue test as a submaximal estimate of 1RM bench press performance in college football players. *Journal of Strength & Conditioning Research*, 12, 4, 258–261.

Chimera, N.J., Smith, C.A., & Warren, M. (2015). Injury history, sex, and performance on the functional movement screen and Y balance test. *Journal of Athletic Training*, 50, 475–485.

Cook, G. (2003). *Athletic Body in Balance*. Champaign, Ill.: Human Kinetics.

Donnelly, D.V. et al. (2006). The effect of directional gaze on kinematics during the squat exercise. *Journal of Strength and Conditioning Research*, 20, 145–150.

Fry, A.C., Smith J.C., & Schilling, B.K. (2003). Effect of knee position on hip and knees torques during the barbell squat. *Journal of Strength and Conditioning Research*, 17, 629–633.

Gibson, A.L., Wagner, D.L., & Heyward, V.H. (2019). *Advanced Fitness Assessments and Exercise Prescription* (8th ed.). Champaign, Ill.: Human Kinetics.

Gray, G. & Tiberio, D. (2006). *Chain Reaction Function*. Adrian, Mich.: The Gray Institute.

Hauschildt, M. (2008). Landing mechanics: What, why and when? *NSCA's Performance Training Journal*, 7, 1, 13–16.

Houglum, P.A. (2016). *Therapeutic Exercise for Musculoskeletal Injuries* (4th ed). Champaign, Ill.: Human Kinetics.

Kainoa, P. et al. (2000) Reliability and validity of the T-test as a measure of agility, leg power, and leg speed in college-aged men and women. *The Journal of Strength and Conditioning Research*, 14, 443–450.

Kendall, F.P. et al. (2005). *Muscles: Testing and Function with Posture and Pain* (5th ed.). Baltimore, Md.: Lippincott Williams & Wilkins.

Lander, J. (1984). Maximum based on reps. *NSCA Journal*, 6, 6, 60–61.

Lisman, P. et al. (2018). Functional movement screen and Y-Balance test scores across levels of American football players. *Biology of Sport*, 35, 253–260.

Mackenzie, B. (2005). *101 Performance Evaluation Tests*. London: Electric Word.

Mayhew, J.L. et al. (1992). Relative muscular endurance performance as a predictor of bench press strength in college men and women. *Journal of Applied Sport Science Research*, 6, 4, 200–206.

McGill, S.M. (2017). *Ultimate Back Fitness and Performance* (6th ed.). Waterloo, Canada: www.Backfitpro.com

McGill, S.M. (2016). *Low Back Disorders: Evidence-Based Prevention and Rehabilitation* (3rd ed.). Champaign, Ill.: Human Kinetics.

McLaughlin, T., Lardner, T., & Dillman, C. (1978). Kinetics of the parallel squat. *Research Quarterly*, 49, 2, 175–189.

Morales, J. & Sobonya, S. (1996). Use of submaximal repetition tests for predicting 1-RM strength in class athletes. *Journal of Strength & Conditioning Research*, 10, 3, 186–189.

Sahrmann, S.A. (2002). *Diagnosis and Treatment of Movement Impairment Syndromes*. St. Louis, Mo.: Mosby.

Sheppard, J.M. & Triplett, N.T. (2016). Program design for resistance training. In: Haff, G.G. & Triplett (Eds.) *Essentials of Strength Training and Conditioning* (4th ed.). Champaign, Ill.: Human Kinetics.

Wilthrow, T.J. et al. (2005). The relationship between quadriceps muscle force, knee flexion and anterior cruciate ligament strain in an in vitro simulated jump landing. *American Journal of Sports Medicine*, 34, 2, 269–274.

SUGGESTED READING

Gibson, A.L., Wagner, D.L., & Heyward, V.H. (2019). *Advanced Fitness Assessments and Exercise Prescription* (8th ed.). Champaign, Ill.: Human Kinetics.

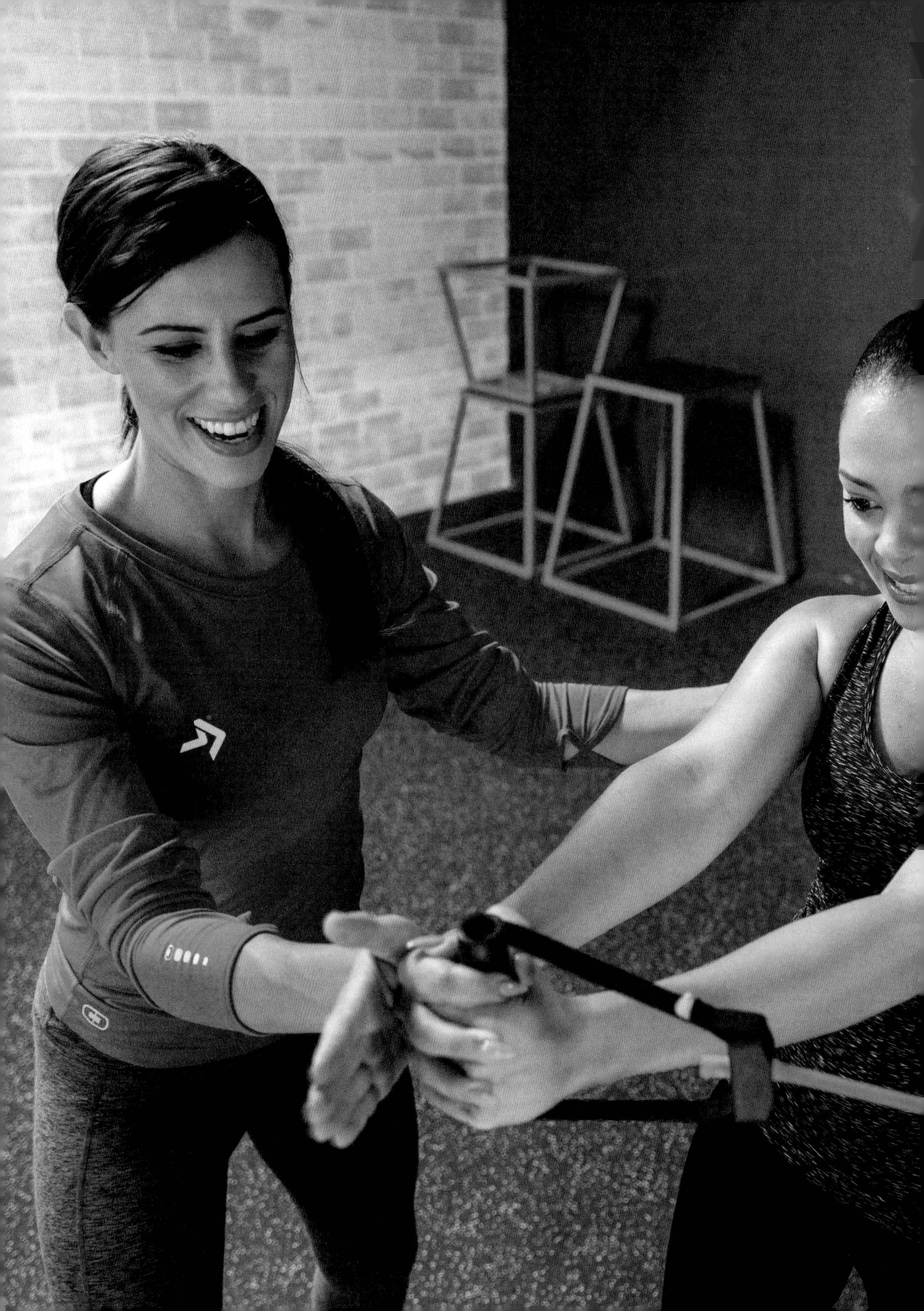

CHAPTER 11

Integrated Exercise Programming: From Evidence to Practice

LANCE C. DALLECK, PhD
Professor of Exercise and Sport Science, Western Colorado University;
Member, ACE Scientific Advisory Panel

IN THIS CHAPTER

LEARNING OBJECTIVES:

Upon completion of this chapter, the reader will be able to:

- Define and list the steps of evidence-based practice
- Apply the concept of evidence-based practice to exercise programming
- Discuss personalized implementation and progression strategies for exercise programming for clients
- List key considerations for program maintenance
- Identify programming considerations for training recovery
- Design personalized, evidence-based Cardiorespiratory and Muscular Training programs for clients ranging from physically inactive to highly active individuals using research and programming tools from each phase of the ACE Integrated Fitness Training® Model

ACE UNIVERSITY

If your study program includes the ACE University, visit www.ACEfitness.org/MyACE and log in to your My ACE Account to take full advantage of the ACE Personal Trainer Study Program and online guided study experience.

A variety of media to support and expand on the material in this text is provided to facilitate learning and best prepare you for the ACE Personal Trainer Certification exam and a career as a personal trainer.

All aspects of personalized exercise programming should be based on a combination of three factors: (1) client attributes, goals, and preferences, (2) personal trainer experience and expertise, and (3) the latest research findings in health and fitness (Amonette, English, & Kraemer, 2016). This multifaceted approach to personalized exercise programming is known as **evidence-based practice** (Figure 11-1). Evidence-based practice aligned with specific goals is a client-centered approach to optimal decision making with respect to exercise program design, implementation, supervision, and evaluation. Accordingly, evidence-based practice is a valuable skill for personal trainers to acquire and subsequently apply with current and future clients.

FIGURE 11-1
An exercise program underpinned by evidence-based practice (EBP) equally considers the client, personal trainer expertise and experience, and research findings in health and fitness

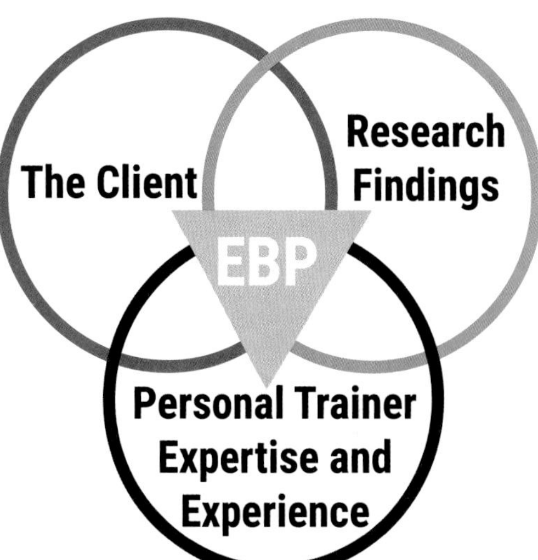

Evidence-based Practice

The first series of client–personal trainer interactions are focused on the personal trainer learning more about his or her client. For instance, personal trainers gather personal attribute–related data about their clients, including age, health history, chronic-disease status, and exercise training goals. Baseline assessments also provide important preliminary information about the client. Moreover, personal trainers identify client preferences regarding physical activity, including factors such as exercise equipment/program likes and dislikes, weekly availability for training, and potential barriers to regular physical activity. Evaluation of the client is a vital preliminary step in evidence-based practice. The formal process of evidence-based practice consists of five steps (Figure 11-2): (1) formulating a question, (2) searching for health and fitness research evidence that best answers the formulated question, (3) scrutinizing the quality of the research evidence, (4) incorporating the research evidence into exercise program design and implementation, and (5) evaluating exercise program outcomes and periodically reevaluating the research evidence (Amonette, English, & Ottenbacher, 2010). Keeping current with exercise science research helps personal trainers build the knowledge required for steps 2 and 3.

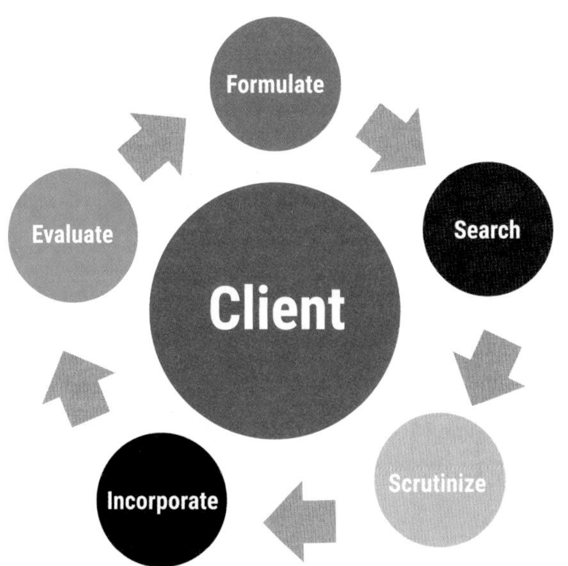

FIGURE 11-2
The five-step process of evidence-based practice

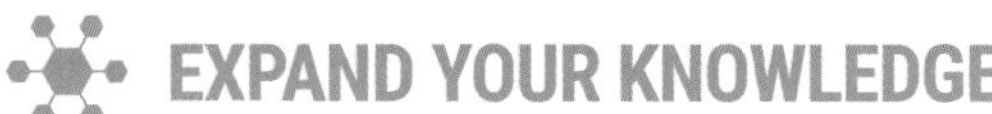

Basic Concepts for Interpreting Scientific Research

As practitioners in a science-based field, ACE® Certified Personal Trainers must carefully choose which information they will utilize when making decisions about training their clients. As such, personal trainers should be aware of factors that either support or detract from reported evidence. Figure 11-3 provides some basic guidance on how to recognize evidence-based science.

FIGURE 11-3
Steps to recognizing evidence-based science

Search for bias

Ask yourself, "Does the claimant have anything to gain by promoting this point of view or product?"

Read the research

If research is cited, review the full research paper to get an idea of sample size, study design, conclusions, study limitations, and validity and reliability. This information will shed light on potential logical fallacies. If no research is cited, the claim is likely not an example of evidence-based science.

Evaluate for truth

Signs that something is not true include overstating or overgeneralizing research results, misinterpreting correlations, reliance on anecdotal experience, and selective reporting.

Look for consensus

For topics with a public health impact, respected organizations (e.g., the American Heart Association, Centers for Disease Control and Prevention, and World Health Organization) often offer a consensus opinion. These are widely available at no cost.

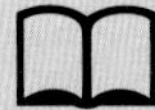

APPLY WHAT YOU KNOW

Six Steps for Client-centered Exercise Programming

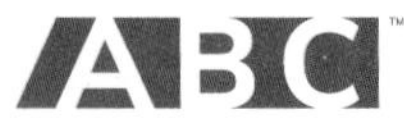

The better you are able to combine the foundational exercise science content with the evidence-based practical application principles and behavior-change strategies presented in this textbook, the better you will be at providing the best possible experience for your clients. The following list will help you implement a process for training clients, organized in a way that incorporates the important concepts of the ACE ABC Approach™, SMART goal setting, and exercise program design based on the ACE Integrated Fitness Training (ACE IFT®) Model guidelines. The steps outlined may be used with any client at any point on his or her path toward improved health and/or fitness.

Step 1—Establish rapport and identify client goals (see Chapter 4).

Ask **open-ended questions,** such as:

- "What do you want to achieve through working with a personal trainer?"
- "How would you describe your current level of physical activity?"
- "Which activities have you found enjoyable in the past?"

Step 2—Administer an exercise preparticipation health screening (see Chapter 5).

- Is medical clearance necessary?

Step 3—Identify barriers and collaborate on next steps (see Chapter 4).

Break down barriers by asking more open-ended questions, such as:

- "What do you need to start doing now to move closer to your goals?"
- "What obstacles might get in the way of your goals?"

Collaborate on ways to set and then achieve **SMART goals** based on the client's input by asking more open-ended questions, such as:

- "How would you describe successful achievement of your goals (e.g., in what ways will your life be different when your goals have been accomplished)?"
- "What do you think you will do?"
- "How will you move forward today?"

Step 4—Determine if physiological or movement assessments are necessary (see Chapters 8 and 10).

Step 5—Determine in which phase(s) of the ACE IFT Model to begin (see Chapter 2).

Step 6—Prioritize program design and select exercise order (see subsequent sections of this chapter).

ACE IFT Model Cardiorespiratory Training Programming

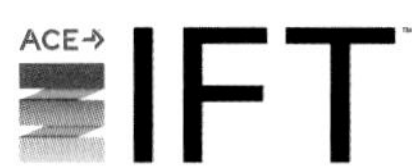

In Chapter 8, the foundations of exercise science, assessments, and initial programming recommendations for cardiorespiratory fitness were presented. In this section, the programming concepts are expanded to include progressions for each phase of the Cardiorespiratory Training component of the ACE IFT Model. Recall that the ACE IFT Model provides a systematic approach to cardiorespiratory training that can take a client all the way from being **physically inactive** to training for a performance goal such as running a competitive race. A summary of these basic programming guidelines is shown in Table 11-1. The Cardiorespiratory Training component is divided into three phases, each with a title that defines its training focus (Figure 11-4).

TABLE 11-1

Cardiorespiratory Training

Base Training	▸ Focus on moderate-intensity cardiorespiratory exercise (RPE = 3 to 4), while keeping an emphasis on enjoyment. ▸ Keep intensities below the talk-test threshold (below VT1). ▸ Increase duration and frequency of exercise bouts. ▸ Progress to Fitness Training when the client can complete at least 20 minutes of cardiorespiratory exercise below the talk test threshold.
Fitness Training	▸ Progress cardiorespiratory exercise duration and frequency based on the client's goals and available time. ▸ Integrate vigorous-intensity (RPE = 5 to 6) cardiorespiratory exercise intervals with segments performed at intensities below, at, and above VT1 to just below VT2.
Performance Training	▸ Progress moderate- and vigorous-intensity cardiorespiratory exercise. ▸ Program sufficient volume for the client to achieve goals. ▸ Integrate near-maximal and maximal intensity (RPE = 7 to 10) intervals performed at and above VT2 to increase aerobic capacity, speed, and performance. ▸ Periodized training plans can be used to incorporate adequate training time below VT1, from VT1 to just below VT2, and at or above VT2.

Note: RPE = Rating of perceived exertion (0 to 10 scale); VT1 = First ventilatory threshold; VT2 = Second ventilatory threshold

FIGURE 11-4
ACE IFT Model Cardiorespiratory Training phases

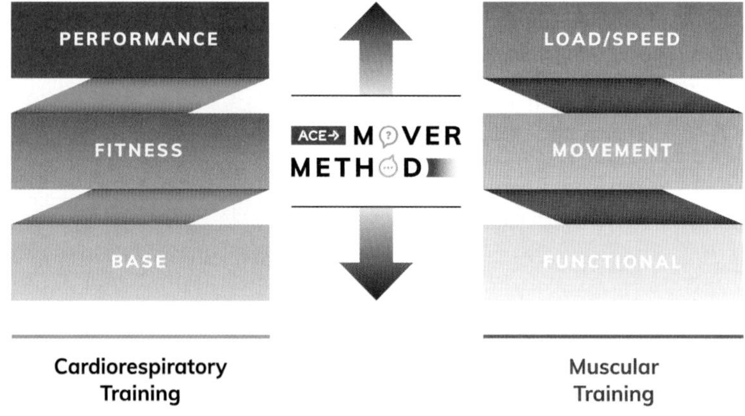

BASE TRAINING

The exercise programming in the Base Training phase is intended to help people move more consistently to establish basic cardiorespiratory endurance. This, in turn, will lead to improved overall health, energy, and mood, and increased caloric expenditure. Encouragement and exercise activities that can be successfully completed in each workout are crucial for building client **self-efficacy** in this phase.

Training Focus

Any client who is not already consistently performing moderate-intensity cardiorespiratory exercise should begin with Base Training. As such, the goal for all clients in Base Training is to gradually increase exercise duration and frequency until the client is performing cardiorespiratory exercise three to five days per week for a duration of 20 minutes or more. No cardiorespiratory assessments are recommended during the Base Training phase, as many of the clients who start in this phase will be unfit and may have difficulty completing an assessment of this nature. Personal trainers can learn about their clients' current cardiorespiratory exercise participation during the investigation stage of the client–personal trainer relationship (see Chapter 5).

The easiest method for monitoring intensity with clients during Base Training is to use the informal **talk test.** If the client can perform the exercise and talk comfortably, he or she is likely below the **first ventilatory threshold (VT1).** By exercising below VT1, clients should be exercising at a moderate intensity classified by a **rating of perceived exertion (RPE)** of 3 to 4 (Note: All RPEs presented in this chapter are based on the 0 to 10 scale) (see Chapter 8).

Program Design

For the most part, early training efforts should feature continuous exercise at zone 1 intensity (see Chapter 8). Depending on how **physically active** a person was prior to beginning the program, this level of exercise may be continued for as little as two weeks or for more than six weeks. The beginning duration of exercise should match what the client is able to perform. For some, this might be 15 continuous minutes, while for others it might be only five to 10 continuous minutes. From that point, duration should be increased at a rate of no more than 10% from one week to the next until the client can perform 20 minutes or more of continuous exercise. Once the client is comfortable with assessments and can sustain **steady state** cardiorespiratory exercise for 20 minutes in zone 1 (RPE of 3 to 4), he or she can move on from Base Training to Fitness Training.

A sample Cardiorespiratory Training progression for a client exercising four days per week in zone 1 is illustrated in Table 11-2. This sample shows appropriate progressions for weekly duration, with different options for session duration during most weeks to add variety and accommodate other program objectives. The client in this sample could be ready to move to Fitness Training after week 4 or 5 if he or she is comfortable progressing.

TABLE 11-2
Sample Base Training Progression

Training Parameter	Week 1	Week 2	Week 3	Week 4	Week 5
Frequency	4 times/week	4 times/week	4 times/week	4 times/week	4 times/week
Total Weekly Duration (increase by ~10% each week)	60 minutes 4 x 15 min	66 minutes 4 x 16.5 min Or 2 x 15min 2 x 18 min	72 minutes 4 x 18 min Or 2 x 17 min 2 x 19 min	80 minutes 4 x 20 min Or 2 x 18 min 2 x 22 min	88 minutes 4 x 22 min Or 2 x 20 min 2 x 24 min
Intensity	<VT1 HR	<VT1 HR	<VT1 HR	<VT1 HR	<VT1 HR
Intervals: Work-to-Recovery Intervals	None	None	None	None	None

Note: VT1 = First ventilatory threshold; HR = Heart rate

FITNESS TRAINING

It is likely that clients in the Fitness Training phase will have a wide variety of goals. Those looking to improve fitness and overall health can benefit from increased exercise frequency, duration, and the introduction of intervals.

Training Focus

Both new and existing clients who can consistently perform moderate-intensity cardiorespiratory exercise for bouts of 20 minutes or more on at least three days per week can perform cardiorespiratory Fitness Training. This phase is focused on enhancing the client's aerobic efficiency by progressing the program through increased duration of sessions, increased frequency of sessions when possible, and the integration of exercise performed at and above VT1 to just below VT2 (see Chapter 8).

The more formal submaximal talk test for VT1 may be administered during this phase, and the results may be used to personalize the clients' exercise recommendations for Fitness Training. The inclusion of zone 2 cardiorespiratory exercise performed at and above VT1 to just below VT2 allows personal trainers to blend moderate-intensity exercise (below VT1) with vigorous-intensity exercise (at or above VT1 to just below VT2; RPE = 5 to 6) in a client's program to add variety to individual sessions and to introduce more intense training stimuli to elicit desired physiological adaptations to exercise. By providing clients with intervals that offer increased yet achievable challenges, personal trainers can help their clients simultaneously increase fitness and self-efficacy.

Program Design

As a general principle, intervals should start out relatively brief (initially about 30 seconds), with an approximate hard-to-easy ratio of 1:3 (e.g., a 60-second work interval followed by a 180-second recovery interval), eventually progressing to a ratio of 1:2 and then 1:1. The duration of these intervals can be increased in regular increments, depending on client objectives, but should be increased cautiously over several weeks depending on the client's fitness level. Typically, the exercise load should be increased by no more than 10% per week. Early in Fitness Training, exercise bouts wherein the client reports an RPE greater than 5 (e.g., hard exercise) should be performed infrequently. As the client's fitness increases, steady-state exercise bouts with efforts just above VT1 (RPE of 5) can be introduced.

Low zone 2 intervals should first be progressed by increasing the time of each interval and then moving to a 1:1 work-to-recovery (hard-to-easy) interval ratio. As the client progresses, intervals can progress into the upper end of zone 2 (RPE of 6) at a 1:3 work-to-recovery ratio, progressing first to longer intervals and then eventually moving to intervals with a 1:1 work-to-recovery ratio. Well-trained and motivated nonathletes can progress to where they are performing as much as 50% of their cardiorespiratory training in zone 2, while endurance athletes will typically follow a Performance Training program.

Programming variables and variety during Fitness Training are diverse enough for clients who do not have competitive objectives to train for many years. A sample cardiorespiratory training progression for a client in Fitness Training is presented in Table 11-3. This sample shows appropriate progressions during a five-week period.

TABLE 11-3
Sample Fitness Training Progression

Training Parameter	Week 1	Week 2	Week 3	Week 4	Week 5
Frequency	3 times/week	3 times/week	3 times/week	3 times/week	3 times/week
Session Duration (increase by ~10% each week)	30 minutes	33 minutes	36 minutes	40 minutes	44 minutes
Intensity	Zone 1 (HR <VT1): Warm-up, cool-down, and recovery intervals Zone 2 (HR ≥VT1 to <VT2): Work intervals	Zone 1 (HR <VT1): Warm-up, cool-down, and recovery intervals Zone 2 (HR ≥VT1 to <VT2): Work intervals	Zone 1 (HR <VT1): Warm-up, cool-down, and recovery intervals Zone 2 (HR ≥VT1 to <VT2): Work intervals	Zone 1 (HR <VT1): Warm-up, cool-down, and recovery intervals Zone 2 (HR ≥VT1 to <VT2): Work intervals	Zone 1 (HR <VT1): Warm-up, cool-down, and recovery intervals Zone 2 (HR ≥VT1 to <VT2): Work intervals
Intervals: Work-to-Recovery Intervals	1:3 30 seconds work: 90 seconds recovery	1:3 45 seconds work: 135 seconds recovery	1:3 60 seconds work: 180 seconds recovery	1:2 60 seconds work: 120 seconds recovery	1:1½ 60 seconds work: 90 seconds recovery

Note: HR = Heart rate; VT1 = First ventilatory threshold; VT2 = Second ventilatory threshold

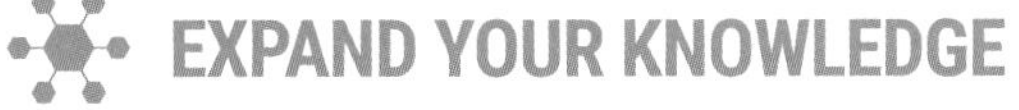

Is High-intensity Interval Training (HIIT) a Time Saver?

Despite its widespread benefits, regular engagement in physical activity or exercise remains scarce, primarily due to a reported "lack of time" (Trost et al., 2002). Over the past decade, the concept of HIIT has captivated the attention of the scientific community due to its superior ability to improve cardiorespiratory fitness and cardiometabolic health for a lesser weekly time commitment relative to the current exercise guidelines [American College of Sports Medicine (ACSM), 2018] for **moderate-intensity continuous training (MICT).** HIIT involves multiple (~four to 10 repetitions) brief bouts (20 seconds to five minutes) of high-intensity exercise [80 to 100% of **maximal heart rate (MHR)**], interspersed with either rest or low-intensity workloads throughout an exercise session. Another prominent form of interval training is known as **sprint interval training (SIT),** which is characterized by repeated (six to 10 bouts) 20- to 30-second all-out supramaximal sprints [>100% of **maximal oxygen uptake ($\dot{V}O_2$max)**]. This strategy enables relatively unfit individuals to accumulate periods of vigorous or high-intensity exercise that would otherwise not be possible if executed continuously. However, one drawback to the protocols employed in the majority of previous SIT/HIIT studies is that they were not actually time-efficient, with most SIT/HIIT protocols requiring a time commitment (~120 minutes/week) that is similar to the current recommended exercise guideline of 150 minutes per week of MICT (Vollaard & Metcalfe, 2017). Moreover, it has also been suggested that the potential for a negative perceptual response to high-intensity exercise heightens with increasing repetition (Vollaard & Metcalfe, 2017). Thus, for HIIT or SIT to be a feasible option to improve public health and a viable option for personal trainers, it must be made time-efficient by specifically reducing the number of bouts (intervals) performed at vigorous to high intensity. This type of HIIT is known as **reduced-exertion high-intensity interval training (REHIT).** ACE-sponsored research has reported cardiorespiratory REHIT to be an effective, time-efficient, and safe strategy for achieving meaningful health and fitness benefits (Cuddy, Ramos, & Dalleck, 2019).

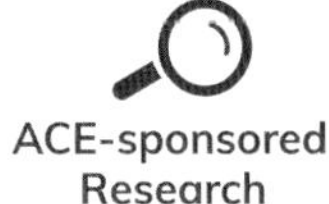
ACE-sponsored Research

PERFORMANCE TRAINING

Individuals who progress to Performance Training will have goals that are focused on success in endurance sports and events. The training programs will progress beyond the outcomes of fitness to focus on performance through increased **speed, power,** and endurance.

Training Focus

Performance Training requires adequate training volume to prepare clients to comfortably complete their events. To help clients achieve higher-level performance goals, personal trainers should design programs that continue to build on moderate- and vigorous-intensity exercise, while integrating zone 3 intervals that push clients up to and beyond VT2, where efforts are of very high intensity (RPE = 7 to 10) and short duration (see Chapter 8). To program effective intervals, the personal trainer should administer the VT2 threshold assessment to determine the client's **heart rate (HR)** at VT2 (see Chapter 8).

Program Design

Training intensity should be varied, with 70 to 80% of training in zone 1, approximately 10 to 20% of training in zone 3, and only brief periods (~10%) in zone 2. This large volume of zone 1 training time is critical to program success for clients with endurance-performance goals, as exercise frequency, intensity, and time all add to the total load. Individuals who increase each of these variables too quickly are at risk for burnout and overuse injuries. The volume of training should be progressively increased (≤10% per week) until the total weekly volume reaches a maximum of three times the anticipated duration of the target event for which the client is training. This "rule of threes" is a classic concept from marathon running. Although there is a lack of direct experimental evidence, the concept is generally well-supported.

Intervals should be programmed to meet the unique aspects of a client's goal event. Using running events as a model, the volume of intervals performed on hard days will vary with the duration of the event. Thus, a person preparing for a 1-mile (1.6-km) race might do about 2.5 times the racing distance (e.g., performing 10 x 400 m intervals is a very reasonable training load), whereas someone preparing for a 10K race might do approximately equal to the race distance in his or her higher-intensity intervals (6 x 1-mile intervals might be appropriate). Someone preparing for a marathon might have a multiplier of approximately 0.25 (6 x 1-mile intervals might be appropriate) (Figure 11-5). Obviously, these kinds of volume multipliers are highly empirical and probably best fit serious competitive athletes. Scaled-down versions, based more on common sense and time available rather than on experimentally derived data, are appropriate for more recreational competitors.

Intervals performed in zone 2 will generally be of longer duration than intervals performed in zone 3. This is due to the inability to sustain long intervals at zone 3 intensities where HR equals or exceeds HR at VT2 (RPE ≥7), as compared to zone 2 intervals where HR will range from HR at VT1 to just below VT2 (RPE of 5 or 6). Higher-intensity zone 3 work will also require greater recovery intervals relative to work intervals when compared to those used in zone 2. Table 11-4 illustrates the work in zones 1, 2, and 3 that might be performed by a client training for a marathon during a four-week training period.

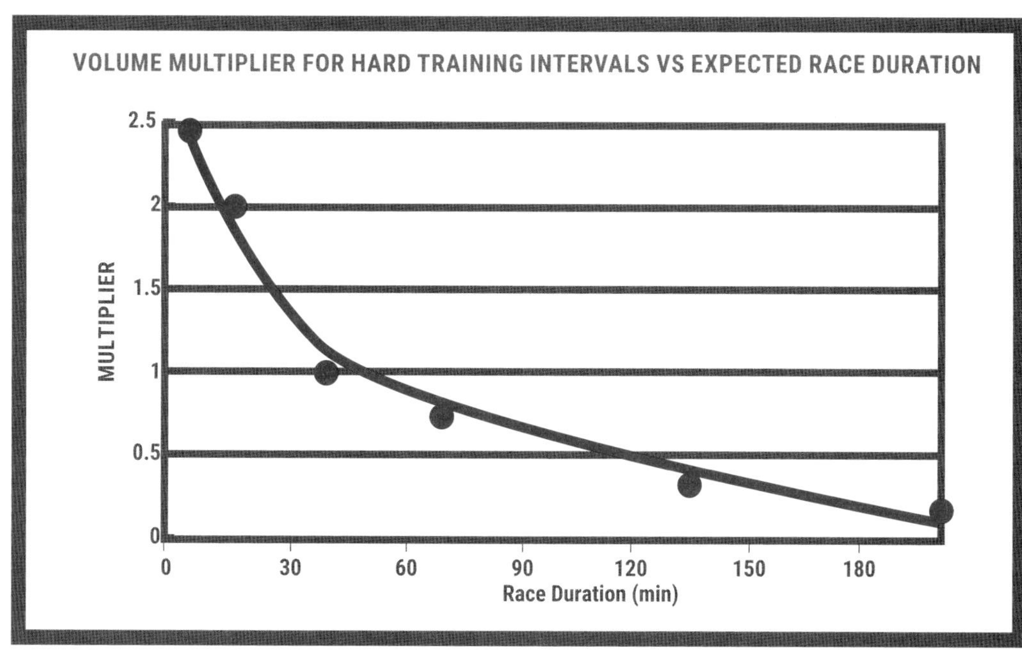

FIGURE 11-5
Schematic volume multiplier for the amount of high-intensity training within a "hard day" in relation to the expected duration of a competitive event. When preparing for a short event (e.g., running 1 mile), it might be appropriate to perform 2.5 times the race distance or duration (with appropriate recovery interval) (e.g., 10 x 400 m/ 400 m jog). For a longer event, such as a marathon (for a three-hour competitor), the multiplier might be quite low (0.25) (e.g., 6 x 1 mile). Although experimental evidence for such a multiplier is absent, it does represent a consensus of opinion.

TABLE 11-4

Sample Performance Training Program: Four-week Mesocycle for Marathon Training

Training Parameter	Week 1	Week 2—Increase Intensity	Week 3—Increase Intensity	Week 4—Recovery Week
Frequency	5 sessions/week	5 sessions/week	5 sessions/week	5 sessions/week
Zone 1 sessions (3 per week) **Intensity for zone 1 sessions:** <VT1 (RPE = 3–4)	1 session/week Long run = 2 hours 30 min 1 session/week 90-min run 1 session/week 60-min run	1 session/week Long run = 2 hours 45 min 1 session/week 90-min run 1 session/week 60-min run	1 session/week Long run = 3 hours 1 session/week 90-min run 1 session/week 60-min run	1 session/week Long run = 2 hours 1 session/week 60-min run 1 session/week 45-min run
Zone 2 sessions (1 per week) **Intensity for zone 2 sessions:** Warm-up, cool-down, and recovery intervals at zone 1: <VT1 (RPE = 3–4) Work intervals at zone 2: ≥VT1 but <VT2 (RPE = 5–6)	3 x 4-min intervals 1:1½ ratio (4-min work:6-min recovery) 60-min workout with warm-up and cool-down	4 x 4-min intervals 1:1½ ratio (4-min work:6-min recovery) 70-min workout with warm-up and cool-down	5 x 4-min intervals 1:1½ ratio (4-min work:6-min recovery) 75-min workout with warm-up and cool-down	2 x 6-min intervals 1:2 ratio (6-min work:12-min recovery) 60-min workout with warm-up and cool-down

Continued on the next page

TABLE 11-4 *(continued)*

Training Parameter	Week 1	Week 2—Increase Intensity	Week 3—Increase Intensity	Week 4—Recovery Week
Zone 3 sessions (1 per week)	2 sets: 3 x 60-sec intervals	3 sets: 3 x 45-sec intervals	3 sets: 3 x 60-sec intervals	2 sets: 3 x 30-sec intervals
Intensity for zone 3 sessions: Warm-up, cool-down, and recovery intervals at zone 1: <VT1 (RPE = 3–4)	1:3 ratio 60-sec work:180-sec recovery 10-min recovery between sets	1:3 ratio 45-sec work:135-sec recovery 10-min recovery between sets	1:3 ratio 60-sec work:180-sec recovery 10-min recovery between sets	1:3 ratio 30-sec work:90-sec recovery 10-min recovery between sets
Work intervals at zone 3: ≥VT2 (RPE ≥7)	60-min workout with warm-up and cool-down	70-min workout with warm-up and cool-down	75-min workout with warm-up and cool-down	45-min workout with warm-up and cool-down

Note: RPE = Rating of perceived exertion (0 to 10 scale); VT1 = First ventilatory threshold; VT2 = Second ventilatory threshold

If the client begins showing signs of **overtraining syndrome** [e.g., increased **resting heart rate (RHR),** disturbed sleep, or decreased hunger on multiple days], the personal trainer should decrease the frequency and/or intensity of the client's intervals and provide more time for recovery. Also, if the client cannot reach the desired intensity during an interval or is unable to reach the desired recovery intensity or HR during the recovery interval, the interval session should be stopped and the client should recover with cardiorespiratory exercise at an RPE of 3, and no more than 4.

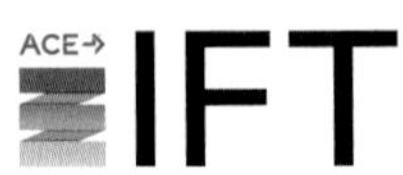

ACE IFT Model Muscular Training Programming

In Chapters 9 and 10, the foundations of exercise science, assessments, and basic programming recommendations for muscular fitness were presented. In this section, the programming concepts are expanded to include progressions for each phase of the Muscular Training component of the ACE IFT Model. Recall that the Muscular Training component provides a systematic approach to training that starts with helping clients improve poor postural **stability** and **kinetic chain** mobility, and then incorporates programming and progressions to help people train for general fitness, strength, and athletic performance. A summary of these basic programming guidelines is shown in Table 11-5. Exercises that target improving postural stability and kinetic chain **mobility** are associated with **neuromotor** and **flexibility** elements, respectively, whereas muscular conditioning exercises mainly target fitness, strength, and performance outcomes. The ACE IFT Model Muscular Training component is divided into three phases, each with a title that defines its training focus (Figure 11-6).

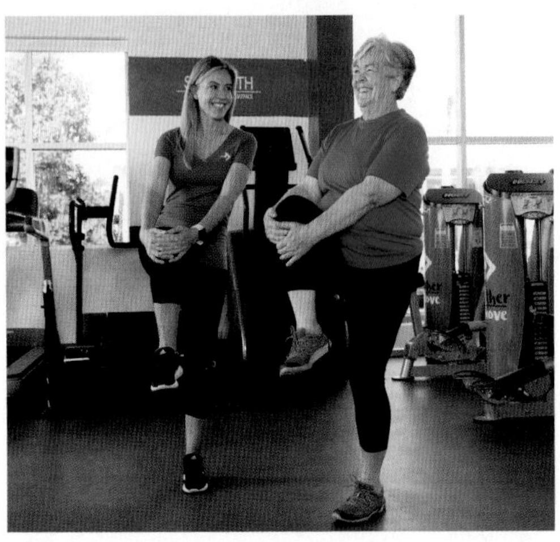

TABLE 11-5

Muscular Training

Functional Training	▸ Focus on establishing/reestablishing postural stability and kinetic chain mobility. ▸ Exercise programs should improve muscular endurance, flexibility, core function, and static and dynamic balance. ▸ Progress exercise volume and challenge as function improves.
Movement Training	▸ Focus on developing good movement patterns without compromising postural or joint stability. ▸ Programs should include exercises for all five primary movement patterns in varied planes of motion. ▸ Integrate Functional Training exercises to help clients maintain and improve postural stability and kinetic chain mobility.
Load/Speed Training	▸ Focus on application of external loads to movements to create increased force production to meet desired goals. ▸ Integrate the five primary movement patterns through exercises that load them in different planes of motion and combinations. ▸ Integrate Functional Training exercises to enhance postural stability and kinetic chain mobility to support increased workloads. ▸ Programs should focus on adequate resistance training loads to help clients reach muscular strength, endurance, and hypertrophy goals. ▸ Clients with goals for athletic performance will integrate exercises and drills to build speed, agility, quickness, and power.

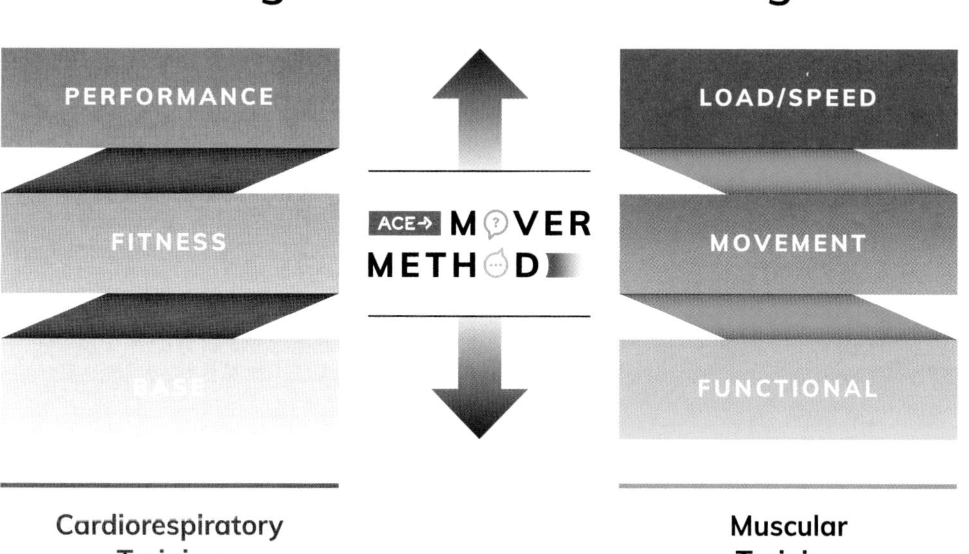

FIGURE 11-6
ACE IFT Model Muscular Training phases

FUNCTIONAL TRAINING

Functional Training focuses on establishing, or in many cases reestablishing, postural stability and kinetic chain mobility (i.e., neuromotor and flexibility outcomes) through the introduction of exercise programs that improve joint function through improved **muscular endurance,** flexibility, core function, **static balance,** and **dynamic balance.**

Training Focus

Exercise selection for Functional Training will focus on core and **balance** exercises that improve the strength and function of the muscles responsible for stabilizing the spine during static positions and dynamic movements. As clients progress to Movement Training and Load/Speed Training, it is important to still include Functional Training exercises in their workouts. These can be included as part of either the warm-up or cool-down, or by incorporating progressions that increase the challenge of the Functional Training exercises by increasing the resistance or balance challenge.

Program Design

Exercises for Functional Training will initially use primarily body weight or body-segment weight resistance, with a targeted focus on the muscles that support the spine. If functional assessments were administered, any noted deviations in **posture,** decrements in flexibility, or problems with balance are addressed with exercises in this phase.

Programming should begin by first promoting stability of the lumbar region through the action and function of the core. Once an individual demonstrates the ability to stabilize this region, the program should then progress to the more **distal** segments. An example of an exercise progression that addresses **proximal** stability first and then advances the challenge with upper and lower extremity movement is shown in Figure 11-7 and Table 11-6.

Adjacent to the lumbar spine are the hips and thoracic spine, both of which are primarily mobile (see Figure 9-28, page 357). As thoracic spine mobility is restored, the program can target stability of the scapulothoracic region. An example of an exercise that promotes thoracic spine mobility is the cat-cow (Figure 11-8) and an exercise for scapulothoracic stability is the rocking quadruped (Figure 11-9). Finally, once stability and mobility of the lumbo-pelvic, thoracic, and shoulder regions have been established, the program can then shift to enhancing mobility and stability of the distal extremities. Attempting to improve mobility within distal joints without developing more proximal stability only serves to compromise any

FIGURE 11-7
Adopt a quadruped position with the knees under the hips and the hands beneath the shoulders. Maintain a neutral spine throughout all movements.

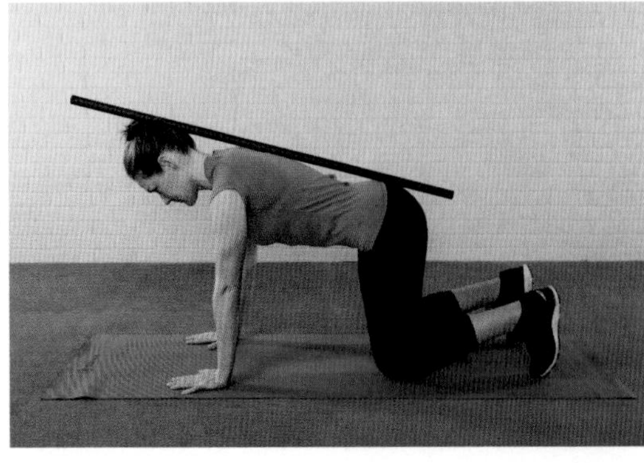

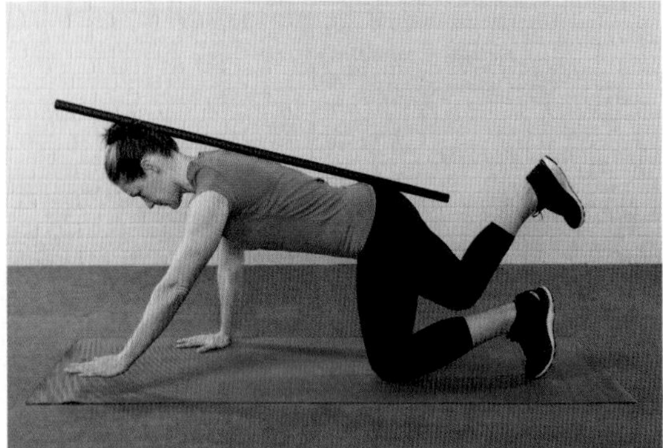

TABLE 11-6
Exercise Progression for Core Stabilization

1. Raise one arm 0.5 to 1 inch (1.25 to 2.5 cm) off the floor and perform the sequence of controlled shoulder movements: ▸ 6–12 inch (15–30 cm) sagittal plane shoulder movements (flexion/extension) ▸ 6–12 inch (15–30 cm) frontal plane shoulder movements (abduction/adduction) ▸ 6–12 inch (15–30 cm) multiplanar shoulder movements (circles or circumduction)	Perform 1–2 sets x 10 repetitions with a 2-second tempo, use 10–15 second rest intervals between sets
2. Raise one knee 0.5 to 1 inch (1.25 to 2.5 cm) off the floor and perform the sequence of controlled hip movements: ▸ 6–12 inch (15–30 cm) sagittal plane hip movements (flexion/extension) ▸ 6–12 inch (15–30 cm) frontal plane hip movements (abduction/adduction) ▸ 6–12 inch (15–30 cm) multiplanar hip movements (circles)	Perform 1–2 sets x 10 repetitions with a 2-second tempo, use 10–15 second rest intervals between sets
3. Raise contralateral limbs (i.e., one arm and the opposite knee) 0.5 to 1 inch (1.25 to 2.5 cm) off the floor and perform the sequence of movements: ▸ Repeat the above movements in matching planes (i.e., simultaneous movement in the same plane with both limbs) or alternating planes (i.e., mixing the planes between the two limbs). ▸ This contralateral movement pattern mimics the muscle-activation patterns used during the push-off phase portion of walking and is an effective exercise to train this pattern.	Perform 1–2 sets x 10 repetitions with a 2-second tempo, use 10–15 second rest intervals between sets

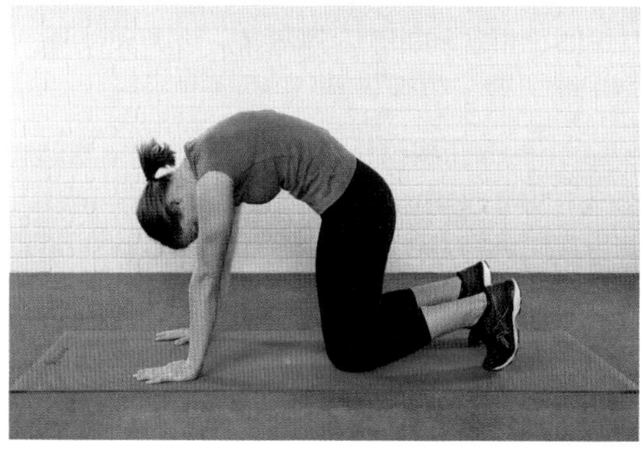
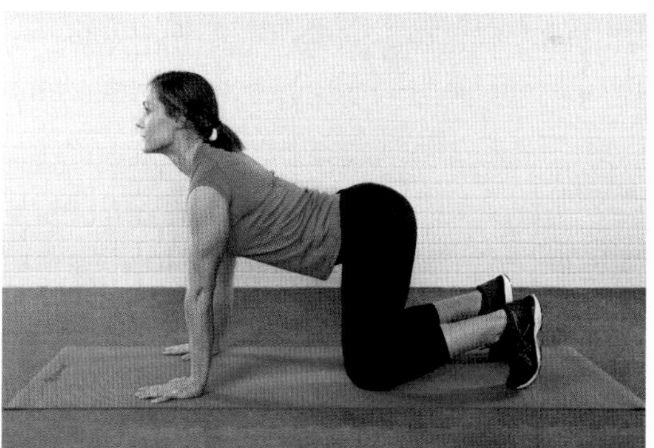

FIGURE 11-8
Cat-cow

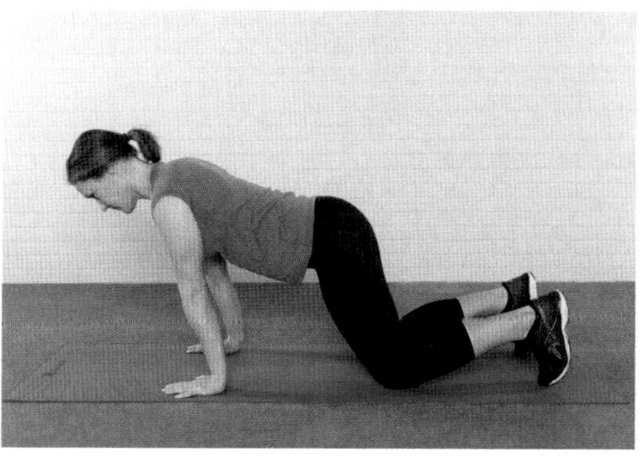
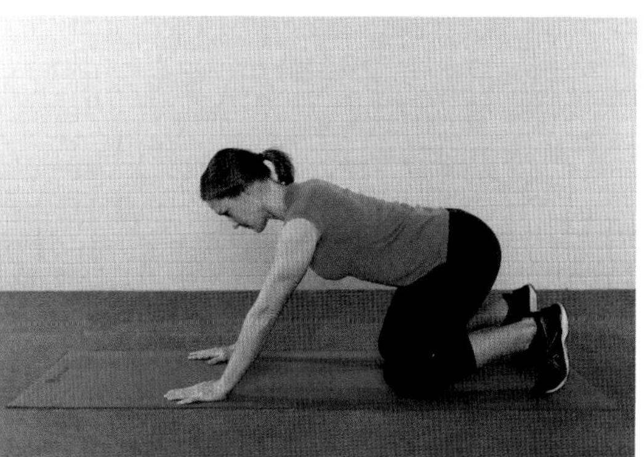

FIGURE 11-9
Rocking quadruped

existing stability within these segments. When a joint lacks stability, many of the muscles that normally mobilize that joint may need to alter their true functions to assist in providing stability. For example, if an individual lacks stability in the scapulothoracic joint, the deltoids, which are normally responsible for many glenohumeral movements, may need to compromise some of their force-generating capacity and assist in stabilizing scapulothoracic movement. This altered deltoid function decreases force output and may increase the potential for dysfunctional movement and injury.

FLEXIBILITY EXERCISE

Flexibility is an essential component of fitness and decreases with age and physical inactivity. Poor flexibility, coupled with decreased musculoskeletal strength, has been associated with a diminished ability to perform **activities of daily living (ADL)** (ACSM, 2018). Consequently, the beneficial effect of stretching on the achievement and maintenance of flexibility should not be overlooked. Flexibility exercise will promote increases in joint **range of motion (ROM),** which is why a focus on flexibility is included in the Functional Training phase. For example, stretching techniques are important for balancing muscle groups on all sides of a joint, which could result in improved postural alignment, better static and dynamic balance abilities, and more efficient movement patterns. Various types of flexibility exercise, which are described here, are effective at improving ROM around a joint.

There are three key properties of tissue that personal trainers should understand: **elasticity, plasticity,** and **viscoelasticity.** Elasticity is the mechanical property that allows a tissue to return to its original shape or size when an applied force is removed (often defined as "temporary deformation") (Figure 11-10). **Ballistic stretching** and **dynamic stretching** are examples of this principle. While they offer no permanent improvement to tissue extensibility, these stretching modalities activate neuromuscular patterns in preparation for activity.

A critical region called the "elastic limit" is reached when a tissue is stretched beyond the point where it can return to its normal length after the tensile force is removed (Figure 11-11). The difference (or deformity) between the original resting length of the tissue and the new resting length, after being stretched beyond its elastic limit, is termed permanent set, permanent deformation, or strain. This new state of permanent elongation is also called plastic stretch. This transition is called the yield point. **Static stretching,** which illustrates this principle, improves tissue extensibility, as the tissue deformation remains after the tension is removed. If further tensile force is applied to a tissue beyond its yield point, gradual tissue failure occurs.

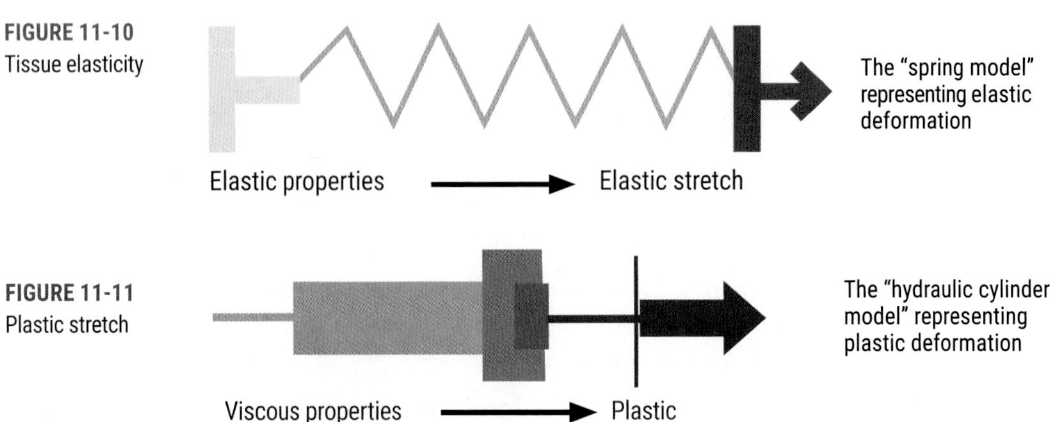

FIGURE 11-10
Tissue elasticity

The "spring model" representing elastic deformation

FIGURE 11-11
Plastic stretch

The "hydraulic cylinder model" representing plastic deformation

The mechanical property known as plasticity allows a tissue to deform when it is loaded past its elastic limit. Once a tissue is set past its yield point, it may succumb to considerable amounts of additional deformation due to relatively small increases in force. Plasticity of tissues can be observed with long-term, repetitive microtrauma. This type of chronic stress leads to tissues that are less stable and less efficient. An unmistakable example of long-term microtrauma is the deformation that occurs in postural muscles as a result of poor posture when sitting in a chair. Over time, the body may adapt to a faulty sitting posture by increased deformation of the back tissues and shortening of the **anterior** trunk tissues. Hence, an exercise program to improve posture could take the approach of promoting plasticity of the anterior trunk muscles through stretching and developing strength in the back muscles through resistance training.

Viscosity is the property of tissues that allows them to resist loads and, unlike elasticity and plasticity, is dependent on time and temperature. Tissue viscosity is an important principle for exercisers and athletes. Properly warming up the body's tissues and fluids reduces viscosity and allows adequate extensibility.

As the name implies, viscoelasticity is the property that allows tissues to exhibit both plastic and elastic behaviors. Most structures in the body are neither completely elastic nor completely plastic. Instead, they exhibit a combination of both properties. When subjected to low loads, most tissues exhibit elastic behavior. Conversely, when subjected to higher loads, tissues exhibit a plastic response. Furthermore, when loads are repeated over time, tissues exhibit viscous deformation.

Although the evidence is unclear, many fitness and sports professionals engage in regular flexibility training in an attempt to improve performance and reduce the risk of musculoskeletal injuries. This section presents commonly used stretching techniques and the acute improvements and chronic adaptations to flexibility training. First, it is important for personal trainers to understand two neurological properties of stretching: **autogenic inhibition** and **reciprocal inhibition.**

Autogenic inhibition is a principle stating that activation of a **Golgi tendon organ (GTO)** inhibits a **muscle spindle** response.

- When a static stretch is initially performed (low-force, longer-duration), the small change in muscle length stimulates low-grade muscle spindle activity and a temporary increase in muscle tension.
- This low-grade muscle response progressively decreases due to a gradual desensitization of the muscle spindle activity as the duration of the stretch progresses. This response is referred to as stress-relaxation.
- After seven to 10 seconds of a low-force stretch, the increase in muscle tension activates a GTO response.
- Under GTO activation, muscle spindle activity and any tension in the muscle are temporarily inhibited, allowing further muscle stretching.
- Now that the muscle tension is removed, holding the stretch beyond 10 seconds places stresses along the **collagen** fibers, remodeling them as they pull apart (plastic deformation) and lengthening the tissue. The lengthening that occurs when a stretch force is applied is called **creep.** Reductions in tension (stress-relaxation response) and

creep are possible explanations for the increases in ROM observed after an acute static-stretching session.

- After terminating the stretch, the muscle spindle quickly reestablishes its stretch threshold again (approximately a 70% recovery of the muscle spindle within the first five seconds).
- Repeating the static stretch a finite number of times produces a gradual increase in muscle extensibility.
- As an example, holding a hamstrings stretch for seven to 10 seconds will inhibit the muscle and allow greater stretching.

Reciprocal inhibition is the principle stating that activation of a muscle on one side of a joint (i.e., the **agonist**) coincides with neural inhibition of the opposing muscle on the other side of the joint (i.e., the **antagonist**) to facilitate movement. When a contraction or active movement in an agonist is performed (<50% of maximal force is suggested) for more than six seconds, the antagonist muscle becomes inhibited (reduced muscle spindle activity), allowing it to be stretched. For example, firing the gluteus maximus for six to 15 seconds reciprocally inhibits the hip flexors temporarily, thereby allowing the hip flexors to then be stretched.

Commonly used stretching techniques include the following:

- **Static stretching:** A static stretch is performed by moving the joints to place the targeted muscle group in an end-range position and holding that position for up to 30 seconds. Static stretching is one of the most commonly practiced forms of flexibility training because it is easily performed without the requirement of a partner and it does not elicit the **stretch reflex** (i.e., a reflexive muscle contraction that occurs in response to rapid stretching of the muscle), reducing the likelihood of injury. As long as the stretch is not too intense (i.e., does not provoke pain), there are no disadvantages to static stretching if proper technique is used.

  Static stretching can be performed actively or passively. An active stretch occurs when the individual applies added force to increase the intensity of the stretch. For example, leaning further to the side during a side bend stretch increases the intensity of the stretch to the **lateral** flexors on the opposite side of the torso. Since the side-bending action is performed by the person stretching, he or she is "actively" involved in the exercise. In contrast, a passive stretch occurs when a partner or assistive device provides added force for the stretch. An example of a passive stretch is an individual performing a lying hamstrings stretch with the leg propped against a sturdy structure, such as a vertical equipment stanchion or a door jamb (Figure 11-12). Another example is when a personal trainer applies a slight force to the back of the person's leg to allow the client to reach the point of resistance in his or her ROM.

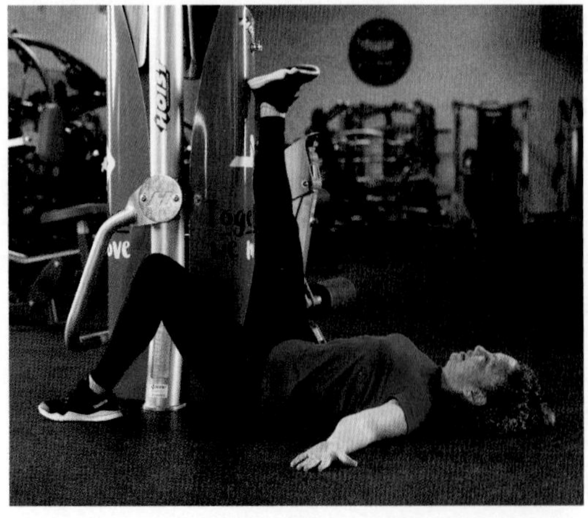

FIGURE 11-12
Passive static stretch of the hamstrings

- **Proprioceptive neuromuscular facilitation:** Originally developed and used to treat increased tissue tonicity in the rehabilitation setting, **proprioceptive**

neuromuscular facilitation (PNF) capitalizes on the principles of autogenic inhibition and reciprocal inhibition. There are three basic types of PNF stretching techniques: hold-relax, contract-relax, and hold-relax with agonist contraction. For each of the three techniques, a partner provides a passive pre-stretch of 10 seconds as the initial step. The actions that follow the passive pre-stretch are different for each technique. These unique differences give each technique its name.

- Hold-relax: After the passive 10-second pre-stretch, the hold-relax technique requires the individual to hold and resist the force provided by the personal trainer so that an **isometric** muscle action occurs for six seconds in the muscle group targeted for the stretch. Then, the individual relaxes the muscle group and allows a passive stretch force from the personal trainer (held for 30 seconds) to increase the ROM in the target muscle group. This final stretch should be of greater magnitude due to autogenic inhibition. Figure 11-13 illustrates proper hand placement for PNF stretching of the hamstrings.
- Contract-relax: After a passive 10-second pre-stretch, the contract-relax technique requires the individual to push against the force provided by the personal trainer so that a **concentric** muscle action occurs throughout the full ROM of the muscle group targeted for the stretch. In other words, the personal trainer provides enough resistance to slightly counteract the individual's force of contraction, but not so much that he or she cannot move the joint through its ROM. Then, similar to the hold-relax method, the individual relaxes the muscle group and allows a passive stretch force from the personal trainer (held for 30 seconds) to increase the ROM in the muscle group that was previously concentrically active. This final stretch should be of greater magnitude due to autogenic inhibition.
- Hold-relax with agonist contraction: The hold-relax with agonist contraction technique is identical to the hold-relax technique, except a concentric action of the opposing muscle group is added during the final passive stretch to add to the stretch force. With this technique, the final stretch should be of greater magnitude primarily due to reciprocal inhibition and, secondarily, to autogenic inhibition. This PNF technique is considered the most effective since it utilizes both reciprocal and autogenic inhibition.

- **Dynamic stretching:** A dynamic stretch mimics a movement pattern to be used in the upcoming workout or sporting event. It is commonly used to help athletes prepare for competition by allowing them to increase sport-specific flexibility. An example of an athlete preparing for an event using dynamic stretches would be a track sprinter performing long walking strides that emphasize hip **extension** while maintaining a **posterior** pelvic tilt. This type of activity-specific movement enhances the flexibility of the hip joints and prepares the tissues for the upcoming physical exertion.

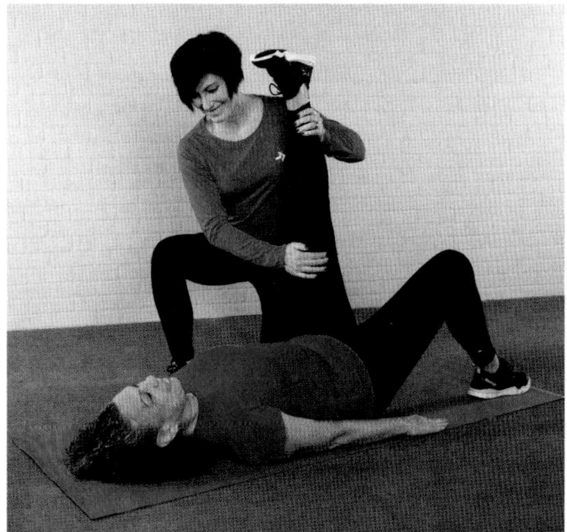

FIGURE 11-13 Hand placement for proprioceptive neuromuscular facilitation of the hamstrings

- **Ballistic stretching:** A stretch that incorporates bouncing-type movements is a ballistic stretch. Ballistic stretching has been used in athletic drills and in pre-training warm-ups. The bouncing movements associated with ballistic stretching usually trigger the stretch reflex and thus may be associated with an increased risk for injury. As a result, the use of ballistic stretching has not been widely advocated (Page, 2012). However, the absolute exclusion of ballistic stretching from flexibility programs has been questioned, particularly in the case of athletes whose functional demands include ballistic-type movements.

Programming for flexibility exercise should focus on the major **tendon** units, including ankles, anterior and posterior legs, chest, hips, lower back, neck, shoulder girdle, and trunk (ACSM, 2018). A summary of evidence-based recommendations for flexibility exercise are presented in Table 11-7.

Much scientific inquiry has examined the topic of stretching and performance/risk of injury. Collectively, present research findings suggest that there are no **ergogenic** benefits, and potentially detrimental effects (decreased **muscular strength** and muscular endurance, impaired balance, and diminished **reaction time**), resulting from the incorporation of static stretching exercises into the warm-up routine (ACSM, 2018). These findings are consistent among different populations and research designs, including untrained and trained individuals, recreational and competitive athletes, males and females, and those with or without a general warm-up (ACSM, 2018). Personal trainers should be mindful of this evidence when designing programs for clients and consider sequencing the workout so that flexibility follows the cardiorespiratory and muscular training components.

TABLE 11-7

Flexibility Exercise Evidence-based Recommendations

FITT-VP	Evidence-based Recommendation
Frequency	≥2–3 days/week with daily being most effective
Intensity	Stretch to the point of feeling tightness or slight discomfort.
Time	Holding a static stretch for 10–30 seconds is recommended for most adults. In older individuals, holding a stretch for 30–60 seconds may confer greater benefit For proprioceptive neuromuscular facilitation (PNF) stretching, a 3–6 second light-to-moderate contraction (e.g., 20–75% of maximum voluntary contraction) followed by a 10- to 30-second assisted stretch is desirable.
Type	A series of flexibility exercises for each of the major muscle-tendon units is recommended. Static flexibility (i.e., active or passive), dynamic flexibility, ballistic flexibility, and PNF are each effective.
Volume	A reasonable target is to perform 60 seconds of total stretching time for each flexibility exercise.
Pattern	Repetition of each flexibility exercise 2–4 times is recommended. Flexibility exercise is most effective when the muscle is warmed through light-to-moderate aerobic activity or passively through external methods such as moist heat packs or hot baths.
Progression	Methods for optimal progression are not known.

Reprinted with permission from American College of Sports Medicine (2018). ACSM's *Guidelines for Exercise Testing and Prescription* (10th ed.). Philadelphia: Wolters Kluwer.

EXPAND YOUR KNOWLEDGE

Understanding Self-myofascial Release

Understanding the concept behind self-myofascial release requires an understanding of the fascial system itself. **Fascia** is a densely woven, specialized system of connective tissue that covers and unites all of the body's compartments. The result is a system where each part is connected to the other parts through this web of tissue. Essentially, the purpose of the fascia is to surround and support the bodily structures, which provides stability as well as a cohesive direction for the line of pull of muscle groups. For example, the fascia surrounding the quadriceps keeps this muscle group contained in the anterior compartment of the thigh (stability) and orients the muscle fibers in a vertical direction so that the line of pull is more effective at extending the knee. In a normal healthy state, fascia has a relaxed and wavy configuration. It has the ability to stretch and move without restriction. However, with physical trauma, scarring, or inflammation, fascia may lose its pliability.

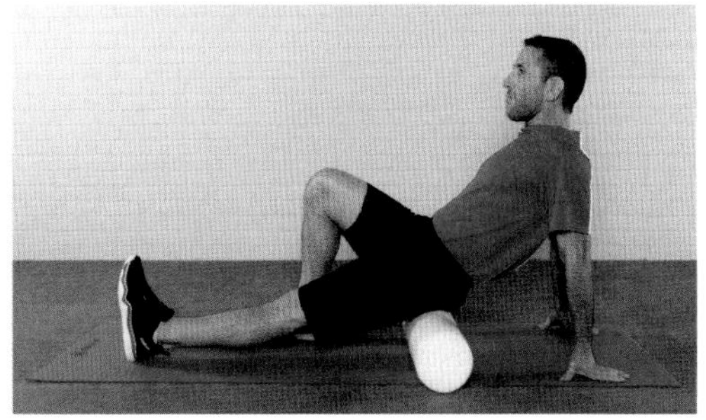

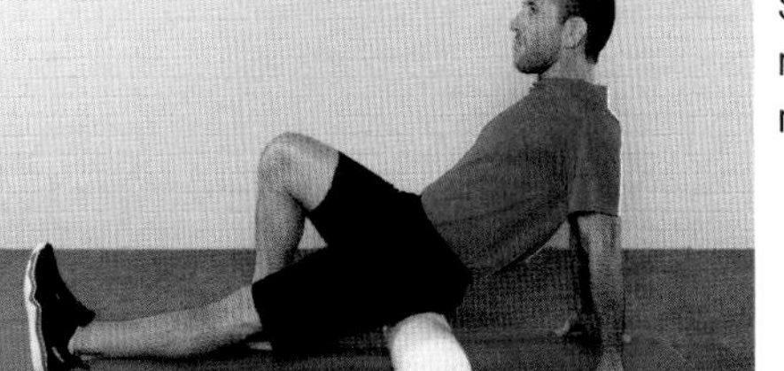

a. Gluteals

b. Quadriceps

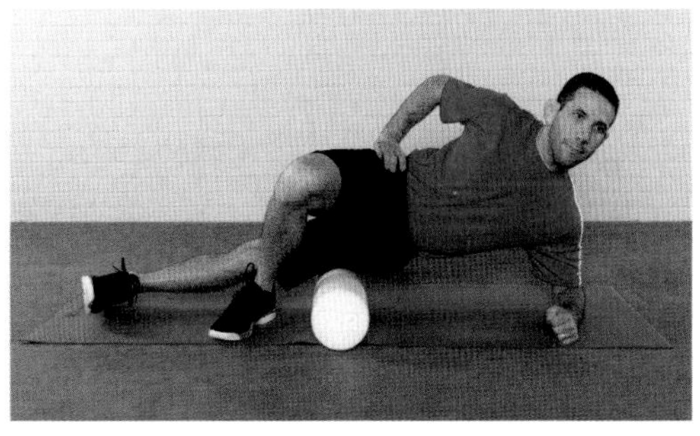

c. Iliotibial band

FIGURE 11-14
Self-myofascial release using a foam roller

Self-myofascial release is a technique that applies pressure to tight, restricted areas of fascia and underlying muscle in an attempt to relieve tension and improve flexibility. It is thought that applying direct sustained pressure to a tight area can inhibit the tension in a muscle. Tightness in soft tissue may be diminished through the application of pressure (e.g., self-myofascial release) followed by static stretching.

The practical application of myofascial release in the fitness setting is commonly done through the use of a foam roller, where the client controls his or her own intensity and duration of pressure. A common technique is to instruct clients to perform small, continuous, back-and-forth movements on a foam roller, covering an area of 2 to 6 inches (5 to 15 cm) over the tender region for 30 to 60 seconds (Figure 11-14). Because exerting pressure on an already tender area requires a certain level of pain tolerance, the intensity of the application of pressure determines the duration for which the client can withstand the discomfort. Personal trainers should always be cognizant of the pain tolerance for rolling of their clients. For some individuals, using a foam roller will simply feel too painful. In these cases, a softer foam roller or a soft, small ball can be used in place of the traditional, denser foam roller.

Evidence is lacking on the mechanisms and benefits of performing self-myofascial release, with some experts disparaging the use of the word "release" as an accurate depiction of what actually occurs. Personal trainers who encourage the use of this technique to improve flexibility with clients should make every effort to stay current with research as it becomes available in this area.

BALANCE EXERCISE

Lastly, exercises that promote static and dynamic balance (e.g., neuromotor exercise) may be included in the Functional Training phase, as these aspects of fitness rely heavily on proper kinetic chain stability and joint mobility. The same programming recommendations as those found in Table 11-8 apply for program design in this phase.

Fall incidence rates currently pose a serious health problem for older adults. In persons 65 years and older, it has been estimated that 35 to 45% of otherwise healthy, community-dwelling adults fall at least once a year (American Geriatrics Society, British Geriatrics Society, and American Academy of Orthopedic Surgeon Panel on Falls Prevention, 2001). Decreased balance is attributable to an age-related decline in multiple physiological systems that contribute to decreased muscle flexibility and strength, reduced central processing of sensory information, and slowed motor responses (American Geriatrics Society, British Geriatrics Society, and American Academy of Orthopedic Surgeon Panel on Falls Prevention, 2001). In addition to an increased risk of falls, diminished balance and mobility may limit performance of ADL or participation in leisure-time activities. Accordingly, personal trainers must include balance exercises in exercise programming for adults, particularly for older adults. Although research has yet to identify the optimal frequency, duration, and type of balance exercises, it has been recommended that balance exercises be performed three days per week for 10 to 15 minutes each session (Nelson et al., 2007). Balance training can be integrated into the various components of an exercise session, including the warm-up, main conditioning component, or cool-down.

Clients with no previous balance-training experience should initially perform basic sitting and standing exercises as a means to improve balance performance. As these initial exercises become easier, an increase in difficulty can be accomplished in numerous ways (ACSM, 2018):

- **Arm progressions:** Vary the use and position of the arms in numerous ways to make a given balance exercise more difficult. Hands may at first need to be grasping or touching another object, such as a wall or back of chair, to facilitate balance. Progressively, exercises can be performed with arms spread out and raised to shoulder height in order to assist with stability. Ultimately, clients can move arms in from sides to a folded position across the chest.
- **Surface progressions:** Alter the surface or apparatus on which clients perform balance exercises, progressively increasing the difficulty. For instance, foam pads and balance disks can be substituted for a hard, flat surface while performing multiple standing balance exercises. Similarly, stability balls can be exchanged for regular chairs when performing seated exercises.
- **Visual progressions:** Mitigate the visual sensory cues provided to the client during nearly all balance exercises. For example, lighting of the room can be gradually dimmed, sunglasses may be worn inside, or eyes may be shut completely.
- **Tasking progressions:** Require clients to initially master each balance exercise performed as a singular task. When this level of achievement is attained, additional tasks should be incorporated into the routine. Cognitive tasks or added physical tasks are a few of the readily available options.

Sample balance exercises and training progressions (from simple to complex) are presented in Table 11-9 and Figure 11-15.

TABLE 11-8

Neuromotor Exercise Evidence-based Recommendations

FITT-VP	Evidence-based Recommendation
Frequency	≥2-3 days/week is recommended.
Intensity	An effective intensity of neuromotor exercise has not been determined.
Time	≥20–30 minutes/day may be needed.
Type	Exercises involving motor skills (e.g., balance, agility, coordination, and gait), proprioceptive exercise training, and multifaceted activities (e.g., tai chi and yoga) are recommended for older individuals to improve and maintain physical function and reduce falls in those at risk for falling. The effectiveness of neuromotor exercise training in younger and middle-aged individuals has not been established, but there is probable benefit.
Volume	The optimal volume (e.g., number of repetitions, intensity) is not known.
Pattern	The optimal pattern of performing neuromotor exercise is not known.
Progression	Methods for optimal progression are not known.

Reprinted with permission from American College of Sports Medicine (2018). ACSM's *Guidelines for Exercise Testing and Prescription* (10th ed.). Philadelphia: Wolters Kluwer.

TABLE 11-9

Balance Exercises and Training Progressions

Position	Balance Exercise
Seated	▸ Sit upright and complete progressions listed below. ▸ Perform leg activities while seated (heel raises, toe raises, or single-leg raises; marching).
Standing	▸ Clock: Balance on one leg (non-support leg knee flexed at 45 or 90° angle); the personal trainer calls out a time and the client moves the non-support leg to the time called (e.g., 5 o'clock or 9 o'clock); alternate legs ▸ Perform various leg activities while standing [heel raises, toe raises, or single-leg raises (non-support leg knee flexed at 45 or 90° angle); marching] ▸ Spelling: Balance on one leg (non-support leg knee flexed at 45 or 90° angle); the personal trainer asks the client to spell a word using the non-support leg (e.g., the client's name, day of the week, or a favorite food); alternate legs
In Motion	▸ Heel-to-toe walking along a 15-foot line on the floor (first with and then without a partner) ▸ Excursion: Alternating legs, lunge over a space separated by two lines of tape; progress t o hopping or jumping (using single-leg or double-leg actions) back and forth across the space ▸ Dribble a basketball around cones that require the client to change direction multiple times
Training Progressions	▸ Arm progressions: Use a surface for support, hands on thighs, hands folded across the chest ▸ Surface progressions: Chair, balance disks, foam pad, stability ball ▸ Visual progressions: Open eyes, sunglasses or dim room lighting, closed eyes ▸ Tasking progressions: Single tasking, multitasking (e.g., balance exercise plus pass/catch a ball)

Note: Number of repetitions per exercise and rest intervals will be dependent on client conditioning and functional status.

FIGURE 11-15
Sample progressions of balance exercises

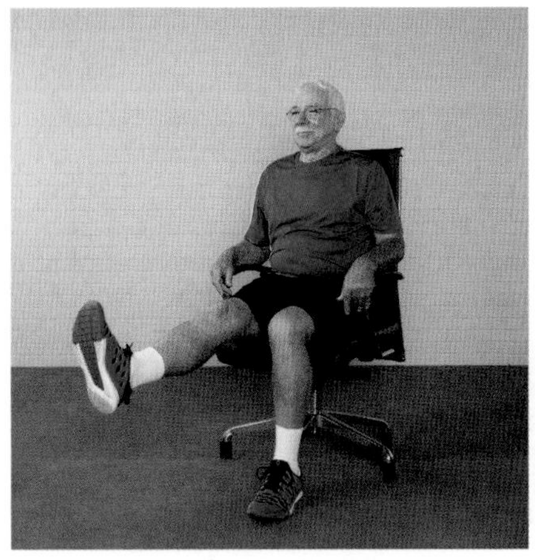
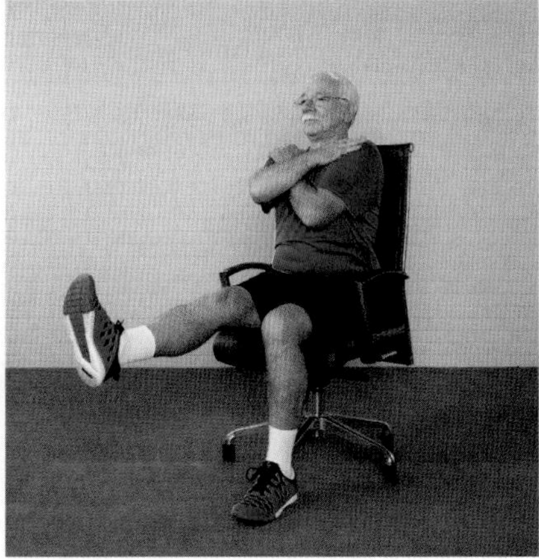
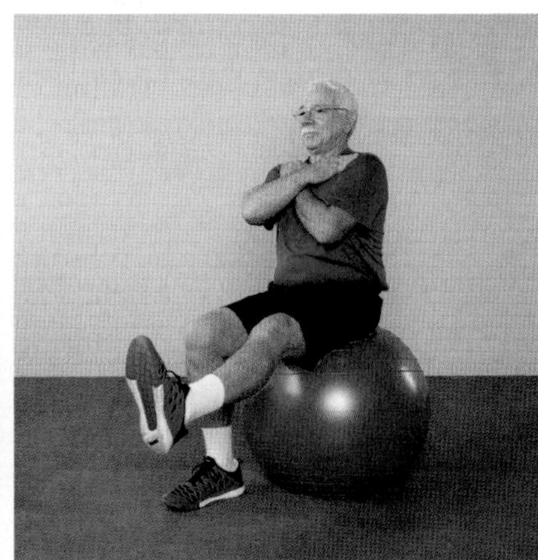

Sample progression of seated balance exercises (closed eyes, arms crossed, stability ball)

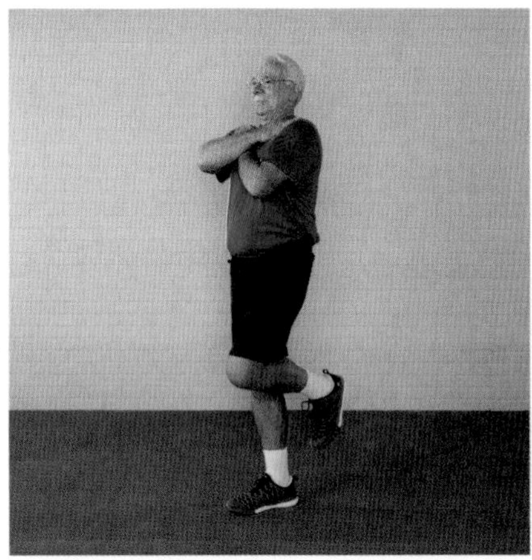
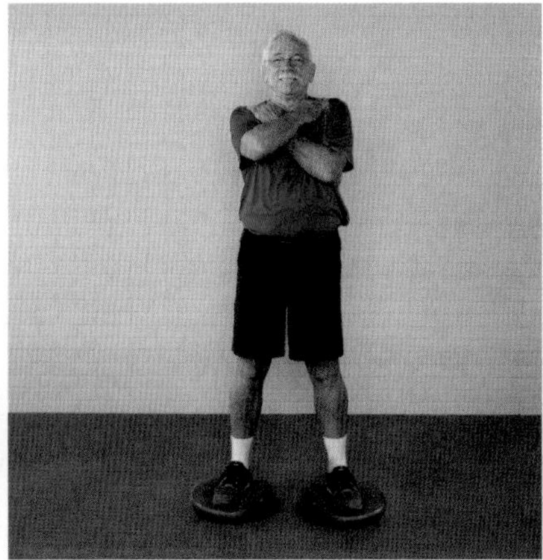
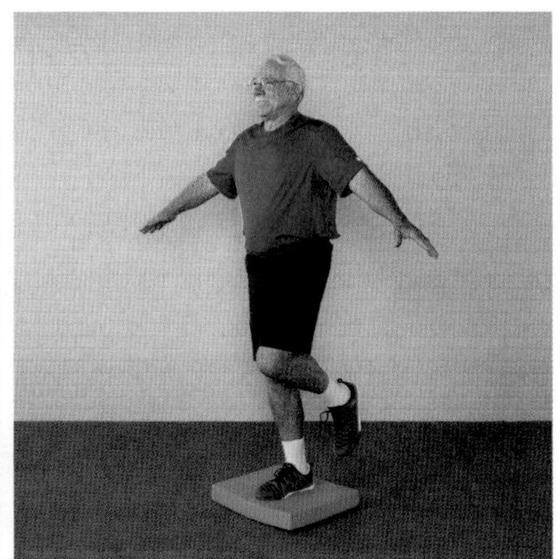

Sample progression of standing balance exercises (arms crossed, balance disks, foam pad)

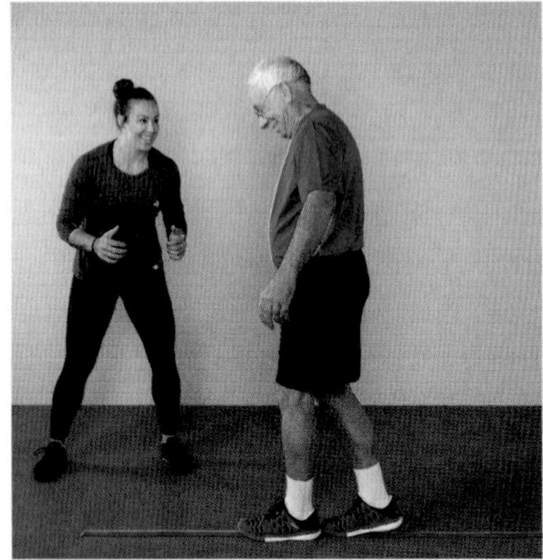
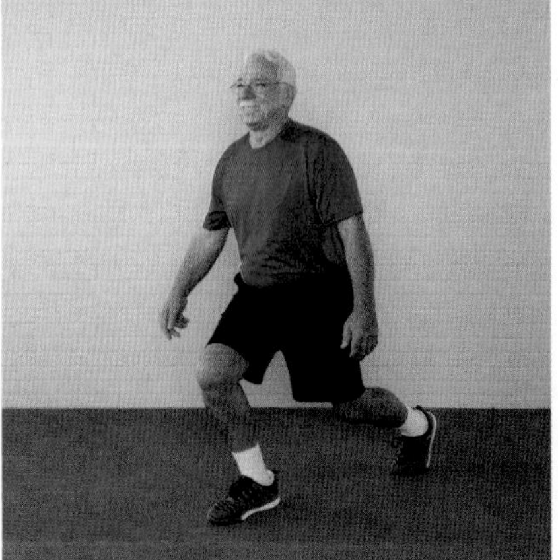
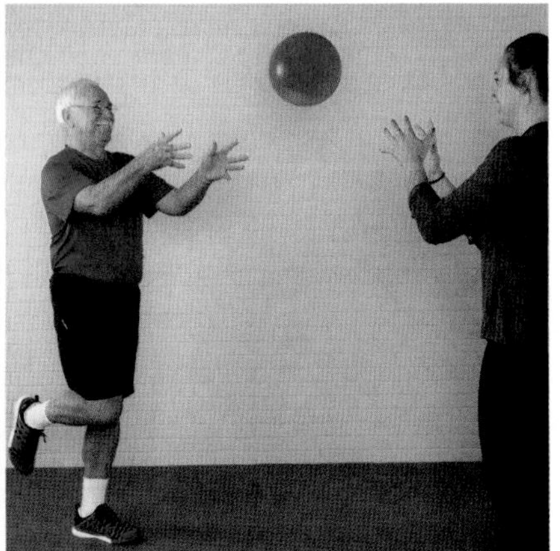

Sample progression of in-motion balance exercises (heel-to-toe, excursion, multitasking)

MOVEMENT TRAINING

The next phase in the Muscular Training component of the ACE IFT Model is Movement Training, which includes exercises that are categorized based on the five primary movement patterns (i.e., bend-and-lift single-leg, push, pull, and rotation).

Training Focus

A blend of neuromotor, flexibility, and muscular conditioning occur in the Movement Training phase, as the focus is on developing movement efficiency, essentially teaching clients to perform the five primary movements effectively in all three planes. Training these movements will improve the client's ability to perform his or her daily activities. During the Movement Training phase, motor learning plays a major role in the desired physical development and movement patterns. Consequently, during this training period, exercise repetition should be emphasized over exercise intensity.

Program Design

If movement assessments were conducted, any noted problems with form or technique may be addressed in the Movement Training phase. Further, any dynamic balance work that was initiated in the Functional Training phase may be progressed in this phase. Most pushing, pulling, and squatting motions can be performed either unilaterally or bilaterally, while lunges require combined acyclical unilateral movements of the legs. Most everyday pushing, pulling, and squatting movements also have a rotational component that requires either motion or stabilization to prevent motion in the **transverse plane,** yet traditional exercise selection often emphasizes linear movements that do not require individuals to produce or control torque (i.e., rotational force). A client who learns how to perform the basic movement patterns with control and without compensation will address asymmetries of limb strength and muscle imbalance, reducing the risk of injury as the intensity of the exercise program is eventually progressed through repetition and the addition of external loads.

Once the five primary movements can be performed with proper form and controlled speed, external resistance may be applied for progressive muscle conditioning. Adding light external load [e.g., up to 50–60% of **one-repetition maximum (1-RM)**] to exercises that comprise the primary movement patterns is a safe and effective way to challenge clients' muscular capabilities after they have demonstrated they can perform the five primary movement patterns well and before they progress to even heavier resistances or more rapid movements in the Load/Speed Training phase. It is essential that the external loads are increased gradually so that correct movement patterns are not altered during the performance of the exercises. The timeframe for Movement Training may be two weeks to two months, depending on each client's initial level of movement ability and his or her rate of progression. The same programming

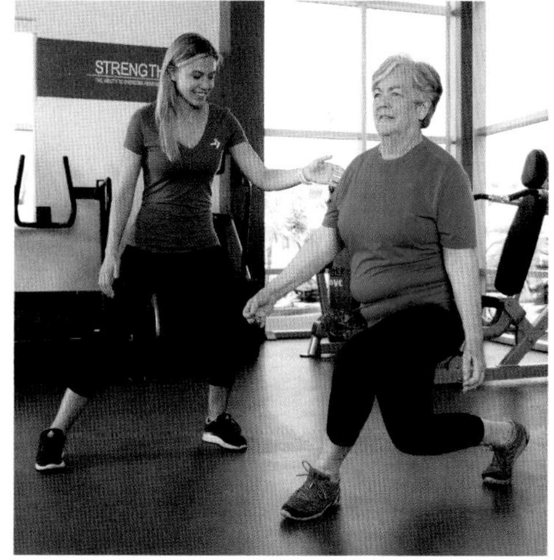

recommendations as those found in Table 11-10 apply for designing programs in this phase, with a specific focus on very light to moderate intensities. The transition from Movement Training to Load/Speed Training often occurs naturally as clients gain experience and become more efficient at controlling the body's **center of gravity** throughout the normal ROM with both body weight and light external loads.

TABLE 11-10

Resistance Exercise Evidence-based Recommendations

FITT-VP	Evidence-based Recommendation
Frequency	Each major muscle group should be trained on 2–3 days/week.
Intensity	60–70% 1-RM (moderate-to-vigorous intensity) for novice to intermediate exercisers to improve strength Experienced strength trainers can gradually increase to ≥80% 1-RM (vigorous-to-very vigorous intensity) to improve strength. 40–50% 1-RM (very light-to-light intensity) for older individuals beginning exercise to improve strength 40–50% 1-RM (very light-to-light intensity) may be beneficial for improving strength in sedentary individuals beginning a resistance-training program <50% 1-RM (light-to-moderate intensity) to improve muscular endurance 20–50% 1-RM in older adults to improve power
Time	No specific duration of training has been identified for effectiveness.
Type	Resistance exercises involving each major muscle group are recommended. Multijoint exercises affecting more than one muscle group and targeting agonist and antagonist muscle groups are recommended for all adults. Single-joint exercises targeting major muscle groups may also be included in a resistance-training program, typically after performing multijoint exercise(s) for that particular muscle group. A variety of exercise equipment and/or body weight can be used to perform these exercises.
Repetitions	8–12 repetitions are recommended to improve strength and power in most adults. 10–15 repetitions are effective in improving strength in middle-aged and older individuals starting exercise. 15–25 repetitions are recommended to improve muscular endurance.
Sets	2–4 sets are recommended for most adults to improve strength and power. A single set of resistance exercise can be effective, especially among older and novice exercisers. ≤2 sets are effective in improving muscular endurance.
Pattern	Rest intervals of 2–3 minutes between each set of repetitions are effective. A rest of ≥48 hours between sessions for any single muscle group is recommended.
Progression	A gradual progression of greater resistance, and/or more repetitions per set, and/or increasing frequency is recommended.

Note: FITT-VP = Frequency, intensity, time, type, volume, and pattern/progressions; 1-RM = One-repetition maximum

Reprinted with permission from American College of Sports Medicine (2018). *ACSM's Guidelines for Exercise Testing and Prescription* (10th ed.). Philadelphia: Wolters Kluwer.

APPLY WHAT YOU KNOW

Adding Load to Movement Training

The following list describes examples of how to add light loads to the five primary movement patterns to prepare clients as they transition from the Movement Training phase to the Load/ Speed phase.

- **Bend-and-lift (squat):** External loading may be applied with various types of resistance equipment. A client may begin by holding a medicine ball while doing squats. Another resistance option is placing an elastic band under the feet and holding each end of the band while performing squats. A third resistance option is free weights, beginning with dumbbells and progressing to a light barbell. An alternative exercise to the barbell squat is the leg press, which trains the same pattern of movement without the influence of gravity, while strengthening the quadriceps, hamstrings, and gluteus maximus muscles.
- **Single-leg (lunge):** Lunge movements (in any direction) may be performed with external loads by holding a medicine ball or dumbbells.
- **Pushing movements:** Pushing movements may be performed with added resistance by using resistance bands or cables in a standing position, by performing machine chest presses from a seated position, or by lifting free weights (dumbbells or a light barbell) from a lying (**supine**) position.
- **Pulling movements:** Pulling movements may be performed with external loads by using resistance bands or cables in a standing position, by performing machine rows and pull-downs from a seated position, and by lifting dumbbells from a bent-over standing position with the torso parallel to the floor and supported by one arm (bent-over row exercise).
- **Rotational movements:** External resistance may be applied to rotational movements by using resistance bands or cables in a standing position, by using machines from a seated position, or by lifting medicine balls from a variety of positions (standing, seated, and lying). Dumbbells can be used in movements that directly oppose gravity's line of pull.

LOAD/SPEED TRAINING

Applying external loads to movements that create a need for increased force and/or speed production that results in muscular adaptations is a primary focus of in the Load/Speed Training phase.

Training Focus

In the Load/Speed Training phase, neuromotor, flexibility, and muscle conditioning are taken to the next level, as the training emphasis may progress to muscle force production and speed, which can be addressed in different ways to attain specific developmental objectives.

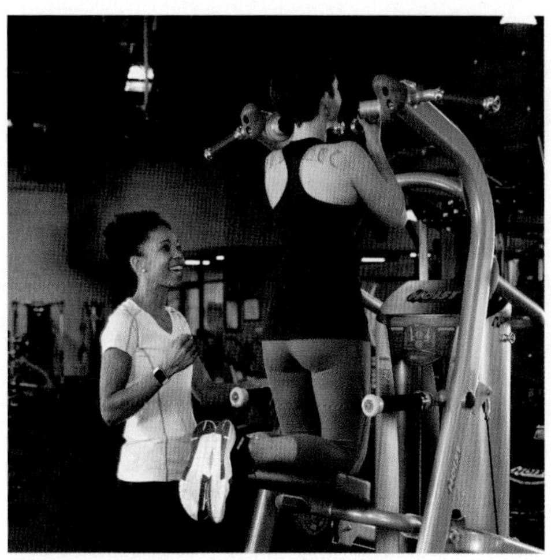

The training objectives may include increased muscular endurance, increased muscular strength, and increased muscle **hypertrophy,** in addition to improved **body composition,** movement, function, health, and performance. Regardless of the specific objective of the Load/Speed Training phase for a particular client, it is recommended that Functional and Movement Training exercises continue to be included in the warm-up and cool-down activities.

Load/Speed Training incorporates specific load/speed training (i.e., power) related to performance enhancement. Power training during this phase is an important component of sports-conditioning programs that prepare athletes for the rigors of their specific sport. Typically, this type of program is not appropriate for the average client who is interested in improving general health and fitness. However, there are individuals who could benefit from adding power training to their fitness programs, such as middle-aged clients who have been exercising for months and are looking to improve their performance in competitive or recreational sport activities. Older-adult clients may also benefit from this type of Load/Speed Training that emphasizes power and quickness to help avoid falls. Furthermore, if designed and progressed appropriately, power training can add interest and fun to an existing exercise program. Personal trainers can program this form of conditioning for their clients, as long as the clients have demonstrated appropriate postural stability and movement abilities, as well as progressed accordingly through Functional and Movement Training.

Program Design

If assessments were administered to determine a client's abilities in muscular strength, power, speed, quickness, or **agility,** any noted unfavorable outcomes may be addressed with exercises in the Load/Speed Training phase. Alternatively, it could be the case that clients perform well on the load/speed assessments and have goals of bettering their performance on those outcomes based on athletic goals. Clients who have athletic performance goals can benefit from training that builds speed, agility, quickness, and power. Before advancing to training for athletic performance goals, clients should consistently exhibit good postural stability, kinetic chain mobility, and movement patterns. They should also have a good foundation of muscular strength to produce and control the force generated during athletic performance–focused exercises and drills. Exercise selection for clients with athletic performance goals can include Olympic lifting, power lifting, **plyometrics,** speed work, and drills for agility, coordination, and quickness. The same programming recommendations as those found in Table 11-10 apply for program design in this phase, with a specific focus on moderate to vigorous intensities.

During the Load/Speed Training phase, muscular, flexibility and neuromotor components should be periodically assessed to facilitate program design and to quantify training effectiveness. If, for some reason, the client has a significant period without exercise, it may be prudent to conduct postural, movement, and flexibility assessments to determine if any postural deviations, muscle imbalances, or movement issues have reappeared due to lack of training. If so, these should be addressed before reintroducing the Load/Speed Training phase.

Client Prerequisites and Preparation for Sport-related Load/Speed Training

Effective sports conditioning in Load/Speed Training requires that clients demonstrate movement proficiency and control during loading and against reactive forces. Specifically, clients must be proficient at acceleration, deceleration, and stabilization during the powerful movements required for performance training. To ensure program safety and success, clients should have the following prerequisites:

- A foundation of strength and joint integrity (joint mobility and stability)
- Adequate static balance and dynamic balance
- Effective core function
- **Anaerobic efficiency** (training of the anaerobic pathways)
- Athleticism (sufficient skills to perform advanced movements)
- No **contraindications** for load-bearing, dynamic movements
- No medical concerns that affect balance and motor skills

Speed is the ability to achieve high velocity and incorporates reaction time and speed of travel over a given distance. Agility is the ability to decelerate an explosive movement and reactively couple it with acceleration and/or a change in direction. For example, a basketball player who sprints down the court at a high velocity (speed), quickly brakes (decelerates), and cuts to the left and jumps (accelerates) to make a shot is a perfect example of an athlete using speed and agility to his or her advantage.

Fast movement speeds require a high level of muscle force to initiate the movement, with momentum mostly responsible for the remainder of the movement. Given the element of momentum in high-velocity movements, a personal trainer must be certain that his or her clients have the postural stability and muscular strength to safely and effectively execute these types of sports-conditioning activities. Once a client achieves an appropriate level of conditioning and expresses a desire to improve athletic skills, techniques to improve power, speed, agility, and reaction time can help the client reach his or her performance goals.

Prior to starting each sports-conditioning session, a personal trainer should plan on having the client perform a specific low-intensity warm-up that incorporates movements that are similar to the high-intensity exercises that are planned during the training session. For example, exaggerated marching (with high knees and pumping arms) mimics running and emphasizes the posture and movement techniques involved in running. This type of pattern-specific warm-up readies the client's **neuromuscular system** for a more intense version of the movement, while simultaneously preparing the client mentally for the challenge ahead. Similarly, adding low-intensity activity-specific movements to a client's cool-down is a good practice because it can contribute to the recovery and relaxation process. The more power necessary for a given sport or activity, the more important the warm-up and cool-down.

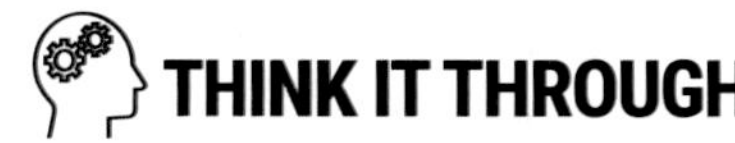

Sport-specific Considerations

If a client meets all of the prerequisites for Load/Speed Training and expresses an interest in amplifying his or her training regimen through high-intensity sports conditioning, the next step is to determine the purpose of the program. That is, the personal trainer must learn which fitness parameters or sports skills the client hopes to improve and then set out to design a safe and effective program to meet the client's goals.

- Which movement patterns and activities (aerobic vs. anaerobic) are required for the client to be successful in reaching his or her performance goals?
- What are the athletic skills and abilities the client currently lacks?
- What are the common injuries associated with the activity? For example, lateral ankle sprains are common in soccer, especially if the athlete has high arches, so incorporating drills designed to enhance a client's ankle reactivity, and thus stability, would be appropriate.

Considerations for Improving Power

To improve the production of muscular force and power, plyometric exercise can be implemented. Plyometric exercise incorporates quick, powerful movements and involves the **stretch-shortening cycle** [an active stretch (**eccentric** action) of a muscle followed by an immediate shortening (concentric action) of that same muscle].

Muscles and tendons experience an increase in their elastic energy when they are rapidly stretched (eccentric action). When immediately followed by a concentric muscle action, this stored energy is released, resulting in an increased total force production. The period of time between the eccentric and concentric actions is called the **amortization phase** and should be kept to a minimum to produce the greatest amount of muscular force. The production of muscular power can also be explained in terms of the stretch reflex (the body's reflexive response to concentrically act after it has been rapidly stretched). Muscle spindles sense differences in the rate and magnitude of stretching imposed on a muscle. When a quick stretch is detected (such as the pre-stretch performed in plyometric exercise), the muscle spindles respond by invoking an involuntary concentric muscle action (stretch reflex), thus increasing the activity in the agonist muscle and increasing muscular force production.

Timing is another important factor in the stretch-shortening cycle, such that if the concentric muscle action does not occur immediately following the pre-stretch (a prolonged amortization phase), or if the eccentric phase is too long, the stored musculotendinous energy dissipates and is lost as heat, and the reflexive potential is negated. Thus, an individual's ability to quickly perform dynamic activity is a strong determinant of his or her potential for power output. This phenomenon explains the increase in vertical jump height experienced by an athlete who squats down (incorporating a pre-stretch) immediately prior to jumping, versus an athlete who jumps up after holding a static squat position for several seconds.

PLYOMETRICS FOR THE LOWER AND UPPER BODY

Plyometric training can be programmed specifically for either the lower body or upper body. Lower-body plyometrics are appropriate for clients who play virtually any sport, as well as for those who want to enhance their reaction and balance abilities. Lower-body plyometric exercises include jumps, hops, and bounds (involving one leg or both legs) (Table 11-11). Upper-body plyometrics, which are covered later in this chapter, are appropriate for individuals interested in improving upper-body power for sports such as softball, tennis, or golf that require rapid force production with an implement like a bat, racquet, or club. Other sports requiring upper-body power include crew, volleyball, American football, lacrosse, and rugby. Upper-body plyometric exercises include medicine-ball throws and catches and various types of push-ups.

TABLE 11-11

Plyometric Jumps, Hops, and Bounds

Type of Jump	Description
Jumps in place	Jumps require taking off and landing with both feet simultaneously. Jumps in place emphasize the vertical component of jumping and are performed repeatedly with no rest between jumps.
Single linear jumps or hops	These exercises emphasize the vertical and horizontal components of jumping and are performed at maximal effort with rest between actions.
Multiple linear jumps or hops	These exercises move the client in a single linear direction, emphasize the vertical and horizontal components of jumping or hopping, and are performed repeatedly with no rest between actions.
Multidirectional jumps or hops	These exercises move the client in a variety of directions, emphasize the vertical and horizontal components of jumping, and are performed repeatedly with no rest between actions.
Hops and bounds	Hops involve taking off and landing with the same foot, while bounds involve the process of alternating feet during the take-off and landing (e.g., taking off with the right foot and landing with the left foot). Hops and bounds emphasize horizontal speed and are performed repeatedly with no rest between actions.
Depth jumps or hops	These exercises involve jumping or hopping off of a box, landing on the floor, and immediately jumping or hopping vertically, horizontally, or onto another box.

Movement-pattern progression is another consideration of programming plyometric exercise. Patterns should begin with linear-forward movements and then progress to lateral, then backward, then rotational, and then crossover, cutting, or curving movements (Figure 11-16).

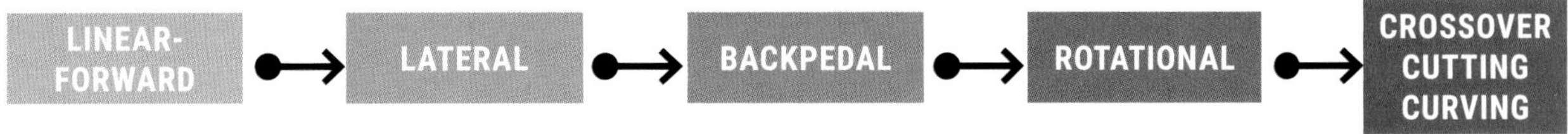

FIGURE 11-16 Movement-pattern progressions for velocity training

PRECAUTIONARY GUIDELINES

Given the ballistic nature of plyometric-training drills, appropriate strength, flexibility, and postural mechanics are required to avoid injury. The following recommendations are provided to reduce the potential for injury and increase the likelihood of performance-related goal achievement for clients.

- Plyometric drills should be performed at the beginning of a training session after the completion of a dynamic warm-up (while clients are not fatigued) to reduce the risk of injury.

- Proper technique is crucial. Clients should not jump unless they know how to land. Ensure that clients are capable of landing correctly by initially teaching small, low-intensity jumps and using appropriate landing techniques.

APPLY WHAT YOU KNOW

Jumping and Hopping Tips to Ensure Safety and Effectiveness

- Clients should land softly on the midfoot, and then roll forward to push off the ball of the foot. Landing on the heel or ball of the foot must be avoided, as these errors increase impact forces. Landing on the midfoot also shortens the time between the eccentric and concentric actions (i.e., the amortization phase), thus increasing the potential for power development if another jump follows.
- Ensure alignment of the hips, knees, and toes due to the potential for injury, especially in women.
- Encourage clients to drop the hips to absorb the impact forces and develop gluteal dominance (see page 432).
- Clients must avoid locking out the knees upon landing, which leads to the development of quadriceps dominance (see page 432). Poor landing technique can increase the risk of knee injuries. Proper hip mechanics during **flexion** and extension, along with the requisite muscular strength, is extremely important for developing lower-body power, which is why it is recommended that clients go through both the Functional and Movement Training phases before progressing to Load/Speed Training exercises.
- Instruct clients to engage the core musculature, which stiffens the torso, protects the spine during landing, and allows for increased force transfer during the subsequent concentric muscle action (or jump).
- Clients should land with the trunk inclined slightly forward, the head up, and the torso rigid. Personal trainers can cue clients to keep their "chests over their knees" and their "nose over their toes" during the landing phase of jumps.

FREQUENCY

The number of plyometric-training workouts per week should range from one to three. The relatively low frequency underscores the importance of recovery time between plyometric exercise sessions. The recommended recovery period between high-intensity plyometric workout sessions is 48 to 72 hours.

INTENSITY

The most important aspect of determining plyometric exercise intensity is to understand the amount of stress placed on the muscles, connective tissues, and joints. Factors such as points of contact (e.g., one foot or both feet), speed, vertical height of the movement, the client's body weight, and the complexity of the movement all contribute to the forces experienced by the body, thus affecting intensity (Table 11-12). Intensity of plyometric drills should be progressed from light, to moderate, to high intensity as indicated in Figure 11-17.

REPETITIONS AND SETS

Volume in plyometric training is expressed as the number of repetitions and sets performed in a given workout. Repetitions for lower-body plyometric training are normally counted as the number of foot contacts (i.e., each time one foot or both feet together make contact with the training surface) per session. For example, four sets of 10 repetitions of knee-tuck jumps equal 40 foot contacts. Upper-body plyometric-training repetitions are counted as the number

TABLE 11-12
Intensity Factors Related to Lower-body Plyometric Drills

Points of contact	The feet are the points of contact for lower-body drills. Single-leg drills impart more stress on the body than double-leg drills.
Speed	Faster movements increase intensity more than slower movements.
Vertical height	The higher the body's center of gravity, the greater the forces of impact upon landing.
Body weight	The greater the client's weight, the more intense the drill. Additional external weight (e.g., medicine ball or weighted vest) can be added to increase the drill's intensity.
Complexity of the exercise	Increasing the complexity, such as adding more body segments or increasing the balance challenge, increases the intensity of the drill.

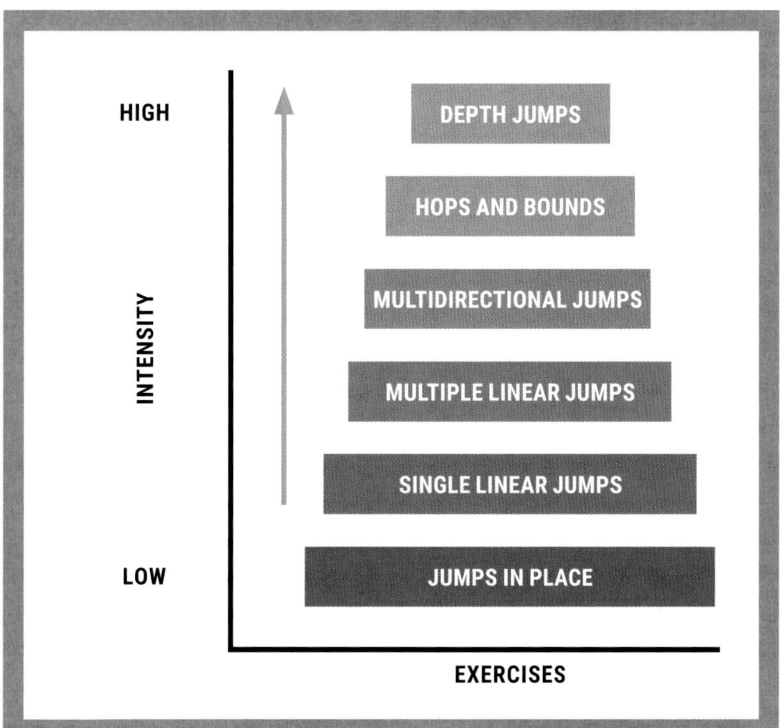

FIGURE 11-17
Plyometric drill classification model

TABLE 11-13

Plyometric Volume Guidelines (Given in Contacts per Session)

Plyometric Experience	Beginning Volume
Beginner (no experience)	80–100
Intermediate (some experience)	100–120
Advanced (considerable experience)	120–140

Reprinted with permission from Potach, D.H. & Chu, D.A. (2016). Program design and technique for plyometric training. In: Haff, G.G. & Triplett, N.T. (Eds.) *Essentials of Strength Training and Conditioning* (4th ed.). Champaign, Il.: Human Kinetics, 477.

of hand contacts (push-up exercises), as well as the number of throws or catches per workout. A progressive-volume format should be followed when programming plyometric workouts for clients (Table 11-13). Generally, as intensity increases, volume should decrease.

TYPE

Plyometric exercises consist of quick, powerful movements for the lower and upper body. Tables 11-14 and 11-15 list common plyometric drills.

TABLE 11-14

Lower-body Plyometric Drills

Drill	Description
Jump in place	Jumps require taking off and landing on both feet simultaneously. Jumps in place require multiple explosive jumps with no rest between repetitions.
Jumping jacks	Jumping jacks involve simultaneous lower- and upper-body movements. The traditional jumping jack involves both the arms and legs moving in the frontal plane. However, arm and leg actions can take place in all three planes and could occur either in-synch (where the arms and legs move the same direction at the same time), or out-of-synch (where the arm and leg actions occur during opposing movements).
Alternating push-off [<12-inch (30-cm) box]	Clients begin with the right foot on the top of a step or small box and the left foot placed behind on the floor. The client explosively pushes off with the right leg and switches feet in the air to land with the left foot on the box and the right foot on the floor.
Single linear jump	These exercises emphasize the vertical and horizontal components of jumping and are performed at maximal effort with rest between jumps.
Standing long/vertical jump	These exercises emphasize an explosive action in either the horizontal (long jumps) or vertical direction and are performed with little to no rest between repetitions.
Single front/lateral box jump	These exercises require an explosive action to move either forward or laterally to land on top of a stable box or platform. The client should explosively jump to the top of the box, and then step back down to perform the next repetition.
Multiple linear jumps	These exercises move the client in a single linear direction, emphasize the vertical and horizontal components of jumping, and are performed repeatedly with no rest between jumps.
Tuck jump	These exercises challenge the client to pull the knees up to the chest during the flight time in the air. They can be performed one at a time, or repeatedly with no rest between jumps.
Front/lateral cone jump	These exercises require jumping over cones in either a forward or lateral direction. The height of the cones can vary to change the intensity of the jumps.
Multidirectional jump	These exercises move in a variety of directions, emphasize the vertical and horizontal components of jumping, and are performed repeatedly with no rest between jumps.
Hexagon drill	The personal trainer marks off a hexagon on the ground using 18-inch (46-cm) lines. The drill involves jumping in and out of the hexagon and moving from one line to the next to complete two full revolutions around the hexagon.
Diagonal cone jump	These exercises require jumping over cones in a diagonal direction. The height of the cones can vary to change the intensity of the jumps.

TABLE 11-15
Upper-body Plyometric Drills

Drill	Description
Push-ups	
Power push-up (Figure 11-18)	▸ Adopt a push-up position with the hands slightly wider than shoulder-width apart. ▸ Flex the elbows to approximately 90 degrees and then explosively extend the elbows so that the hands lift off the floor slightly. ▸ Land with the elbows slightly flexed.
FIGURE 11-18 Power push-up	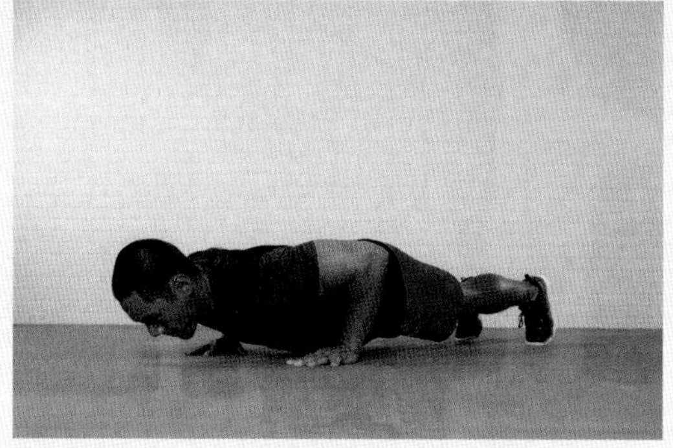 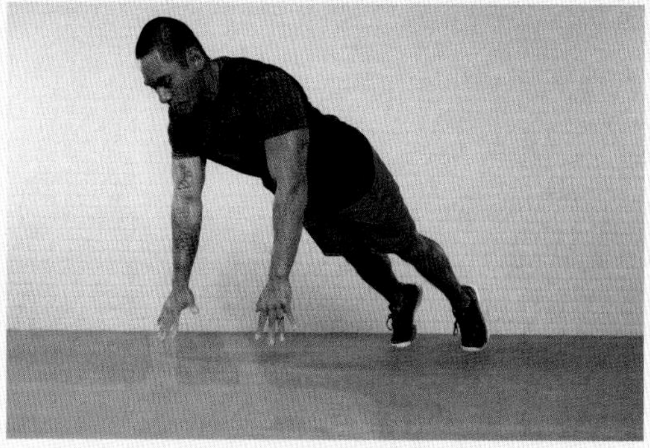
Medicine ball power push-up (Figure 11-19)	▸ Adopt a push-up position with both hands on top of a 5- to 8-lb (~2- to 3.5-kg) medicine ball. ▸ Quickly remove the hands and drop them to the floor slightly wider than shoulder-width apart. ▸ Make sure to land with the elbows slightly flexed. ▸ Continue to flex the elbows and drop the chest to almost touch the medicine ball. ▸ Explosively extend the elbows and push up so that the hands return to the top of the ball. **Note: This exercise is appropriate for elite-level clients only.**
FIGURE 11-19 Medicine ball power push-up	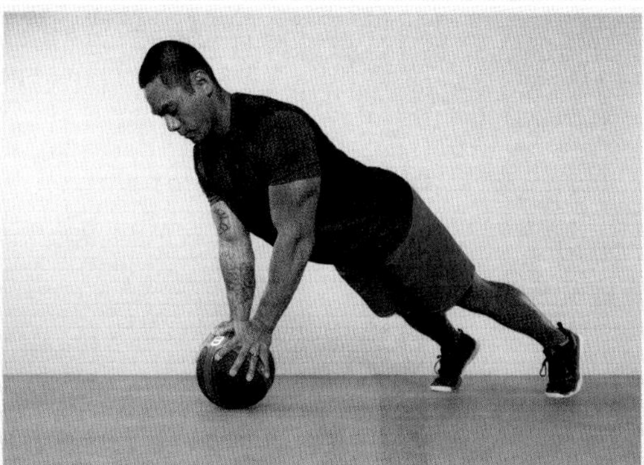 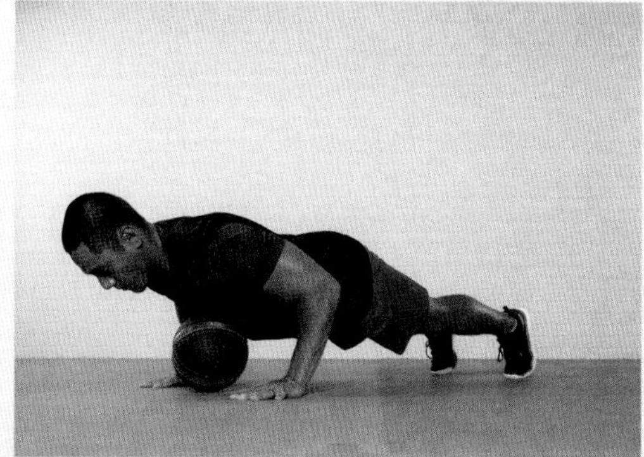 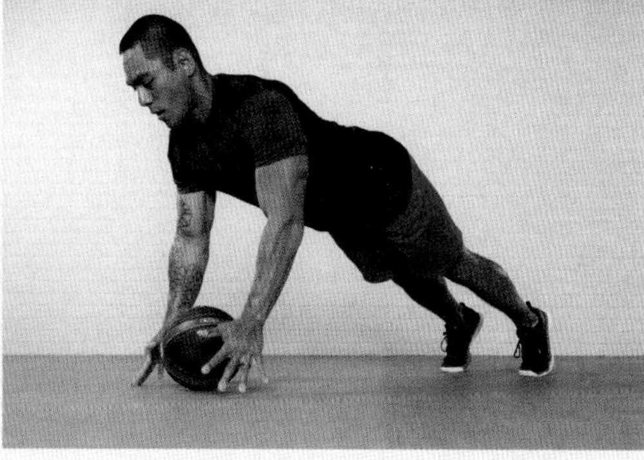

Continued on the next page

TABLE 11-15 *(continued)*

Drill	Description
Throws and catches	
Horizontal chest pass* (Figure 11-20)	▸ Hold a 2- to 8-lb (~1- to 3.5-kg) medicine ball with both hands directly in front of the chest with the elbows flexed. ▸ Throw the ball to a partner or a rebounder by extending the elbows and releasing the ball through the fingertips. ▸ Upon return, catch the ball at chest level and immediately repeat the pass.
FIGURE 11-20 Horizontal chest pass	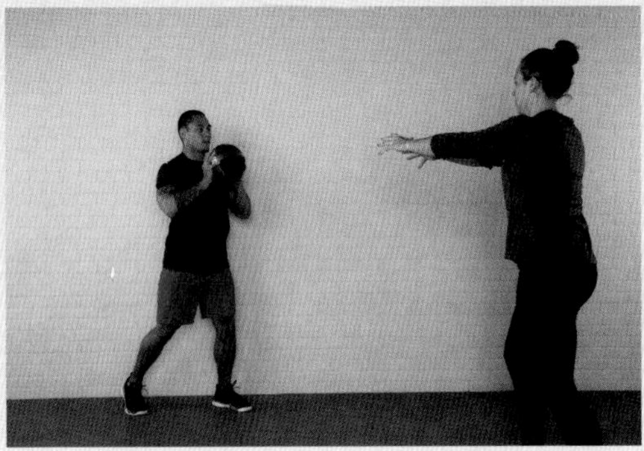 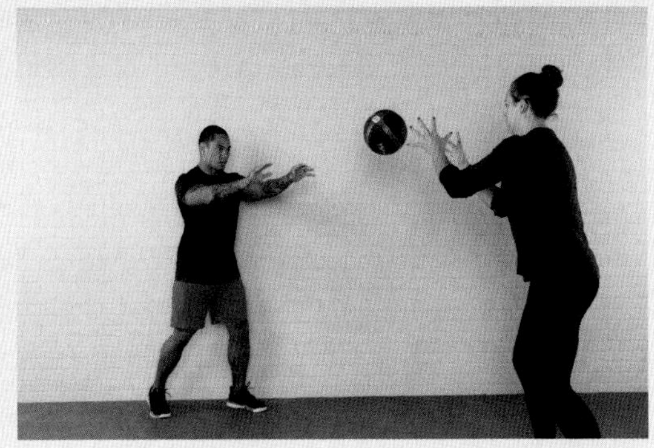
Supine vertical chest toss (Figure 11-21)	▸ Lie supine with the arms extended upward (shoulders at approximately 90 degrees of flexion). ▸ A partner stands on top of a box and holds a 2- to 8-lb (~1- to 3.5-kg) medicine ball above the exerciser's arms. ▸ When the partner drops the ball, catch the ball using both arms and immediately toss the ball back up to the partner.
FIGURE 11-21 Supine vertical chest toss	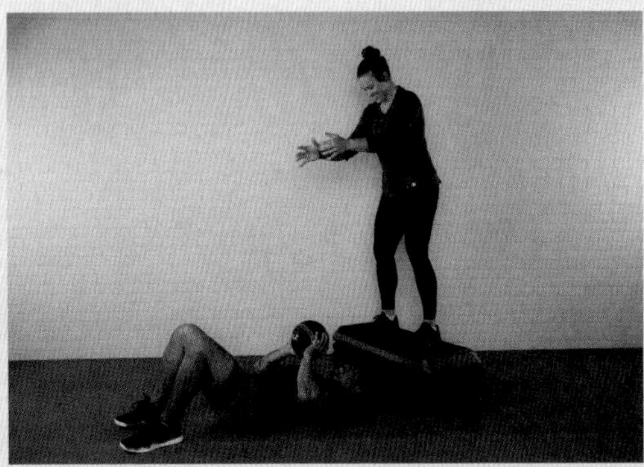 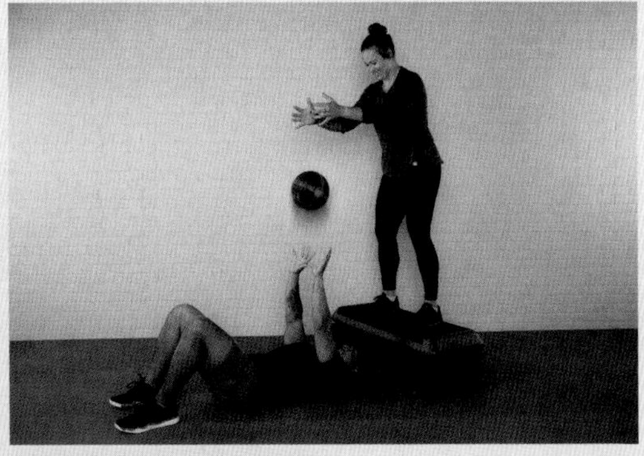 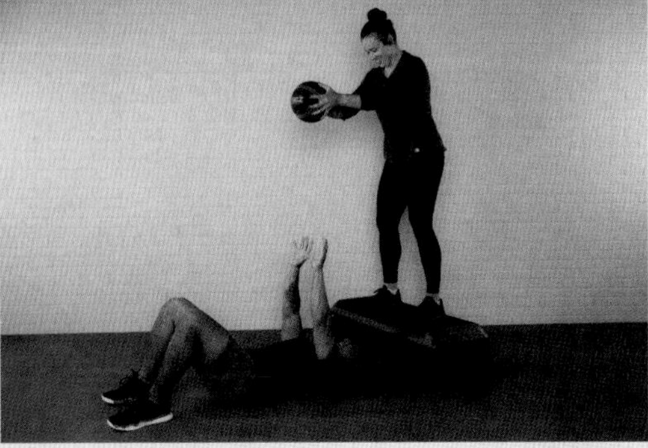

*Can be performed seated, kneeling, or standing

Considerations for Improving Speed, Agility, and Reactivity

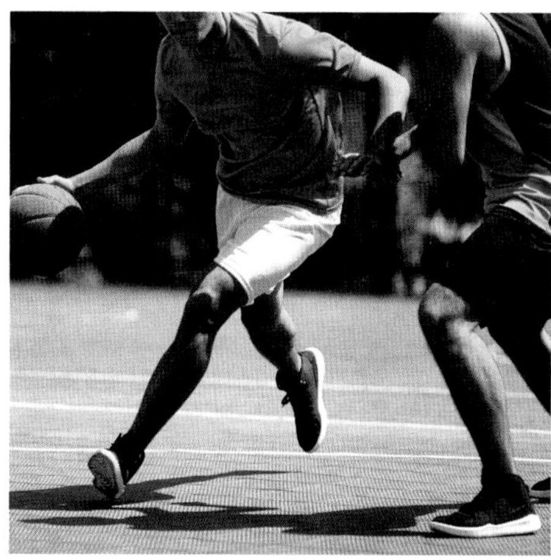

Terms used to describe functional-movement speed include quickness, reactivity, and explosive strength. An individual's ability to move quickly while simultaneously overcoming the forces imposed by his or her own body weight or an external load is determined by the rate of muscle shortening (or concentric action). **Speed-strength** is the ability to develop force at high velocities and relies on a person's reactive ability. **Speed-endurance** refers to the ability of an individual to maintain maximal velocity over an extended time period, such as a sprinter running at all-out velocity for 20 seconds. Both speed-strength and speed-endurance are important components of agility training. A client's reactive ability can be improved through training that applies explosive force to specific movements, such as the movements performed in speed and agility drills.

Agility training involves the components of acceleration, deceleration, and balance, and requires the client to control the **center of mass (COM)** over the **base of support (BOS)** while rapidly changing body position. Speed training incorporates moving rapidly from one point to another in the shortest timeframe possible. Speed and agility drills should be preceded by practice drills that are initially performed at submaximal speed to ensure proper technique.

APPLY WHAT YOU KNOW

Training Tips for Speed and Agility Drills

Speed Drills

- Body position or lean
  - Maintain a slight forward lean during the acceleration phase.
  - Transition to a more vertical position with top speed to facilitate hip and knee extension for stride length.
- Head position
  - Assume a relaxed, neutral position.
- Arm action
  - Drive from the shoulders, not the elbows.
  - Short strokes (or pumping actions) are utilized during the acceleration and deceleration phases.
  - Long strokes are utilized during top speed and sustained speed phases.
  - Relax the hands and maintain an open hand position.

- Leg action
  - At toe-off, kick upward explosively and directly under the buttocks while simultaneously driving the knee forward and upward until the thigh is parallel to the ground.
  - The foot then swings below the knee, moving to a fully extended knee position while maintaining a dorsiflexed ankle position.

Agility Drills

- Progress drills by increasing the speed of movement, complexity of tasks, and direction of movement, and by introducing resistance (e.g., bands and ankle weights).
- Drills can be predetermined (i.e., the client is informed of the expected task) or reactive (i.e., the client reacts to unexpected verbal or visual cues).
- Aim to progressively narrow the BOS to improve agility.

FREQUENCY

The same guidelines for safe and effective plyometric training can be used for programming speed and agility training. The number of speed and agility training workouts should range from one to three non-consecutive days per week.

INTENSITY

The high-intensity, explosive nature of speed and agility drills requires that these activities be performed early in a training session, after an appropriate warm-up but before other fatiguing exercises. Intensity is determined by the energy system that predominates during a drill, which is influenced by the duration of a drill. Table 11-16 lists the energy systems associated with specific durations during speed and agility drills, along with the appropriateness of each for different participant skill levels.

TABLE 11-16

Duration, Energy System, and Associated Participant Skill Level for Speed and Agility Drills

	Duration	Energy System
Beginner	15–30 seconds	Glycolytic system
Intermediate	<10 seconds	Phosphagen system
Advanced	10–60 seconds	Glycolytic and phosphagen systems

REPETITIONS AND SETS

Volume for speed and agility training is determined by the duration of time spent working in each of the energy systems (see Table 11-16). Stationary drills can be performed for one to three sets for 10 to 15 seconds per repetition, eventually progressing to 20 to 30 seconds. Dynamic drills can be performed for one to three sets for 20 to 30 yards per repetition, eventually progressing to 100 yards. Training sessions should be planned to include a minimum duration of two- to three-minute rest periods between repetitions to allow the exerciser to recover and produce maximal power for successive repetitions.

TYPE

Various speed and agility drills are presented in Tables 11-17 through 11-19.

TABLE 11-17
Speed Drills

Basic Arm Drills*	Description
Arm squeeze and rear arm drive (Figure 11-22)	▸ Position one arm in rear-cocked position, forming a triangle with 90 degrees of elbow flexion (place the hand "in a side pocket"). ▸ Squeeze the arm to the side of the body moving only in the sagittal plane. ▸ Allow the upper arm to move slowly forward to align with the torso, then pop back explosively. ▸ Minimal torso rotation is allowable. ▸ Perform 1–2 sets x 10–15 repetitions per arm.
FIGURE 11-22 Arm squeeze and rear arm drive	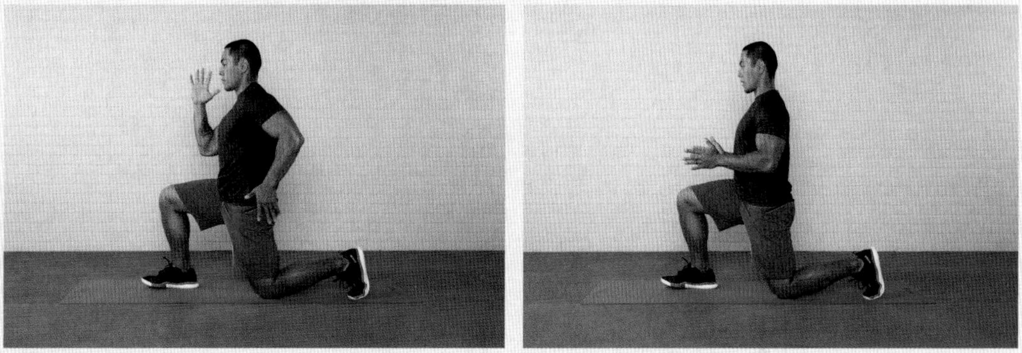
Arm squeeze and forward arm drive (Figure 11-23)	▸ Position one arm at the side of the body, forming 90 degrees of elbow flexion. ▸ Squeeze the arm to the side of the body moving only in the sagittal plane. ▸ Short strokes drive the arm to align the fingertips with the clavicle/chin level. ▸ Long strokes drive the arm to align the fingertips with the nose level or higher. ▸ Minimal torso rotation is allowable. ▸ Perform 1–2 sets x 10–15 repetitions per arm.
FIGURE 11-23 Arms squeeze and forward arm drive	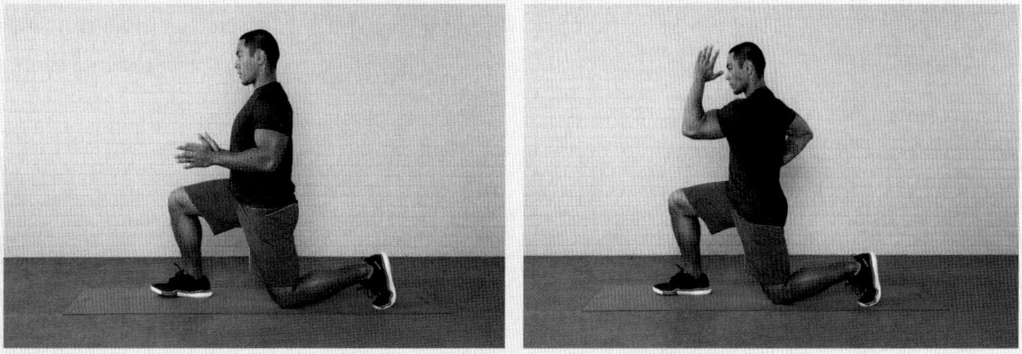
Arm squeeze and full cycles	▸ Integrate the previous two drills into full cycles. ▸ Minimal torso rotation is allowable.

*Can be performed seated, kneeling, or standing

Continued on the next page

TABLE 11-17 *(continued)*

Basic Leg Drills	Description
ABC drills	▸ These drills improve leg mechanics for stride length and leg turnover. Perform 1–2 sets x 20–30 yards of each drill. ▸ During each of these drills, assume a slight forward lean (5°), maintaining a rigid torso, but a relaxed head position.
A: High knees (Figure 11-24)	▸ While incorporating arm cycles, march in place, driving each knee high while maintaining dorsiflexed ankles. ▸ Progress to walking, skipping, and then slow running, attempting to explode off the stance leg (extension of the ankle, knees, and hips) with each step.
	FIGURE 11-24 High knees
B: High marches (Figure 11-25)	▸ While incorporating arm cycles, march in place, driving each knee high while maintaining dorsiflexed ankles. ▸ Once the knee reaches peak height, quickly kick the knee out (knee extension) before returning to the ground. Hip flexion must precede knee extension. Avoid the "soccer kick" movement (i.e., swinging the entire leg forward from the ground). ▸ Progress to walking, skipping, and then slow running, attempting to explode off the stance leg (extension of the ankle, knees, and hips) with each step.
C: Butt kicks (Figure 11-26)	▸ Drive the stance leg positioned under the hips directly upward to strike the heel of the foot under the butt. ▸ Return the leg to the ground slightly in front of the body, attempting to "paw" the ground with the mid-foot, cycling the leg backward under the hip, before driving the knee upward again. Avoid the "mule kick" movement (i.e., swinging the leg behind the body); performing this exercise while standing against a wall will help clients avoid this movement. ▸ Start with single leg cycles before progressing to walking, slow running, and then incorporating the arm cycles.

FIGURE 11-25
High marches

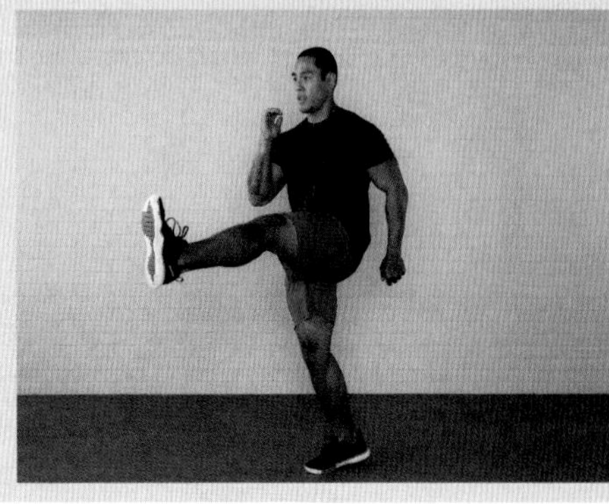

FIGURE 11-26
Butt kicks

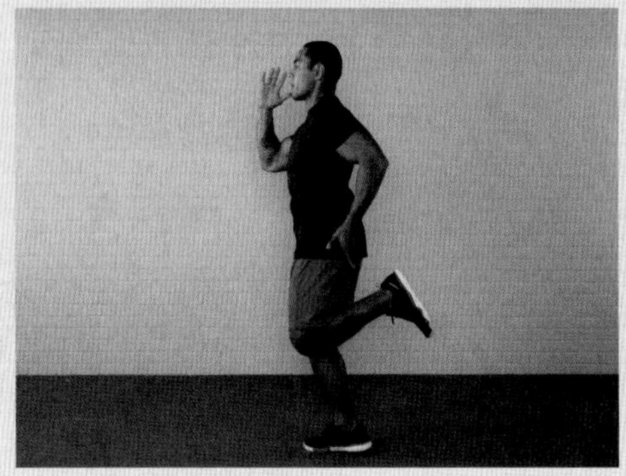

TABLE 11-18
Agility—Ladder/Hurdle Drills

Agility Ladder/Hurdle Drills	Examples (Complete 30 feet per drill/leg)
Forward (Figure 11-27a)	▸ Single step-in ▪ One foot in each rung ▸ Double step-in ▪ Two feet in each rung
Forward jumps/hops	▸ Double foot (jumps) ▸ Jumping jacks (side-straddle jumps) ▪ Both feet inside one rung, then on either side of the following rung ▸ Hopscotch ▸ Single foot (hops)
Lateral (Figure 11-27b)	▸ Basic shuffle ▪ Both feet in each rung ▸ Carioca
Lateral jumps/hops	▸ Double foot (jumps) ▸ Single foot (hops) ▸ Crossovers ▪ Moving left-to-right, start with one foot in each rung (left in 1st rung, right in 2nd rung) ▪ Jump laterally, moving the left foot into the 3rd rung, keeping the right foot in the 2nd rung ▪ Jump, moving the right foot into the 4th rung, while the left foot remains in the 3rd rung ▪ Repeat the sequence
Backpedal	▸ Steps ▸ Jumps and hops

FIGURE 11-27
Agility ladder/hurdle drills

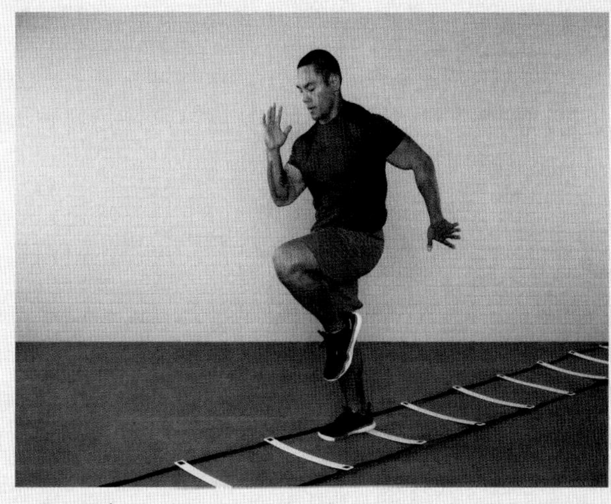
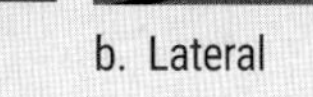
a. Forward

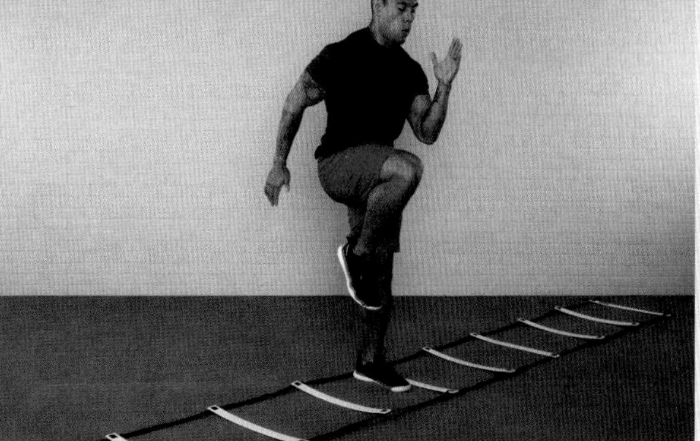
b. Lateral

Continued on the next page

TABLE 11-18 *(continued)*

Agility Ladder/Hurdle Drills	Examples (Complete 30 feet per drill/leg)
Multidirectional (Figure 11-27c)	▸ Single side-ins (zigzags or slalom) ▪ One foot contacts outside the rung on each side ▸ Double slalom ▪ Two-feet contact outside the rung on each side ▸ W's ▪ Lateral-diagonal movements forming the letter "W" ▪ Moving left-to-right, step back into the rung with the right, follow with the left ▪ Step forward out of the rung with the right, follow with the left ▪ Repeat ▸ M's ▪ Opposite movement to form the letter "M" (i.e., start moving forward) ▸ James Bonds ▪ Alternating push-jumps—moving left-to-right, start with the right foot in the rung and the left foot out ▪ Perform alternating push-jumps, switching foot positions, moving down the ladder ▸ Machine gunners ▪ Rapid fire, forward-backward stepping (>2x/foot) in each rung, moving down the ladder

FIGURE 11-27 *(continued)*

c. Multidirectional

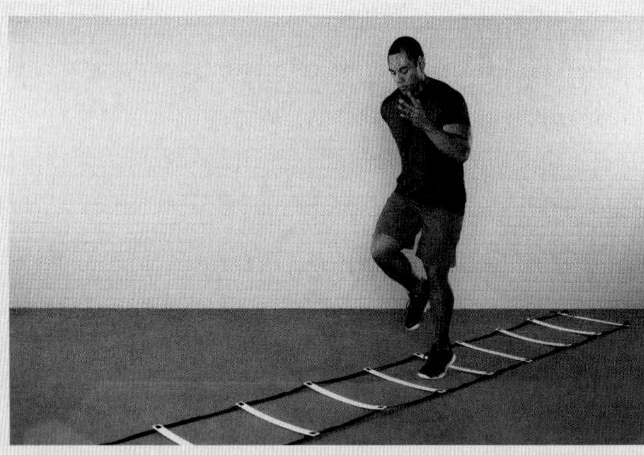

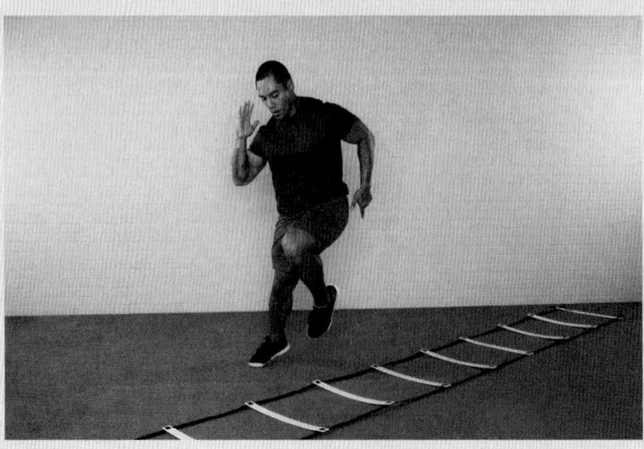

TABLE 11-19

Agility—Cone/Marker Drills

Cone/Marker Drills	Description (1–2 sets x 5–15 seconds)
Lateral shuffles	▸ Set two cones 5–10 yards apart ▪ Shuffle back and forth, touching each cone with the outside hand ▪ Do not cross feet over
Pro agility drill	▸ Set three cones in a line, 5 yards apart ▪ Start by straddling the center cone ▪ On a cue, turn and run right (5 yards) to touch the right cone with the outside hand ▪ Turn and run left to the far left cone (10 yards), touching it with the outside hand ▪ Turn again and run through the middle cone (5 yards)
Multidirectional drill	▸ Hexagon drill ▪ Predetermined—where directions are structured in advance ▪ Reactive—the individual moves to the cone markers identified by the trainer ▸ T-drill (see Figure 10-61, page 459) ▪ Set three cones in a line, 5 yards apart, and one cone 10 yards from the middle cone to form the letter "T" ▪ Start on the baseline, run to the middle cone, touch it with the left hand, then shuffle right to the right cone, touching it with the outside hand ▪ Proceed to shuffle to the left cone, touching it with the outside hand ▪ Shuffle back to the middle cone, touching it with the right hand, then run backward through the line ▪ Run the course in both directions
Curved or cutting drills	▸ Figure 8s ▪ Use the same cone configuration as the T-drill ▪ Individual starts on the baseline and completes the course outline ▪ Run the course in both directions

Periodization

Periodization refers to planned progression of exercise that intentionally varies the training stimuli, especially with respect to intensity and volume. Systematically changing the exercise variables (e.g., resistance, repetition, and sets) appears to be more effective for attaining both strength development and peak performance than standardized muscular-training protocols (Kraemer et al., 2000; Fleck, 1999). The advantage of periodized over non-periodized exercise programs is the frequently changing demands on the neuromuscular system that require progressively higher levels of stress adaptation.

Periodized training is divided into time segments referred to as **macrocycles, mesocycles,** and **microcycles** (Figure 11-28). The overall time frame for a specific periodization program is called the macrocycle, which may cover a training period of six to 12 months. The long-range

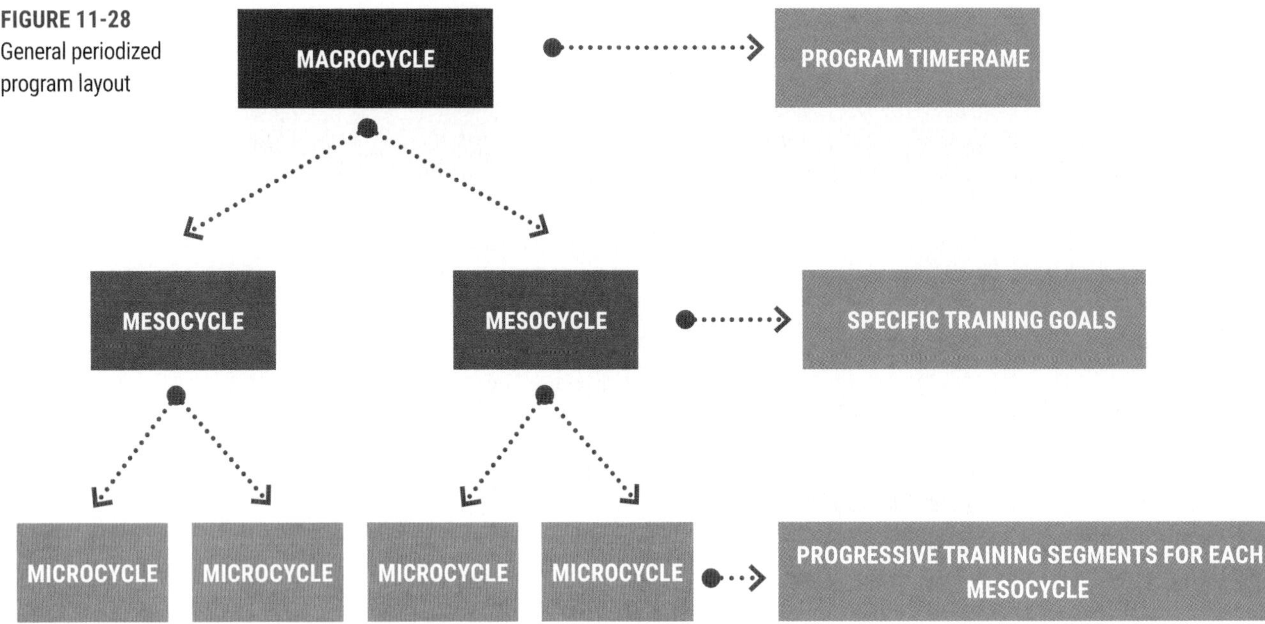

FIGURE 11-28
General periodized program layout

goal to be attained by the end of the macrocycle is divided into shorter-term goals that are addressed in time segments of less duration. For example, a six-month macrocycle may consist of two three-month mesocycles. Each mesocycle would provide sequential goals leading to the ultimate goal of the six-month macrocycle. Because even three-month mesocycles represent a relatively long period for goal attainment, these are divided into more manageable microcycles, which are typically two to four weeks in length and provide regular reinforcement for making small steps toward the larger goals.

Periodized programs may be performed in either a linear manner or an undulating approach (Figure 11-29). Basically, **linear periodization** provides a consistent training protocol *within* each microcycle and changes the training variables *after* each microcycle. On the other hand, **undulating periodization** provides different training protocols *during* the microcycles in addition to changing the training variables *after* each microcycle.

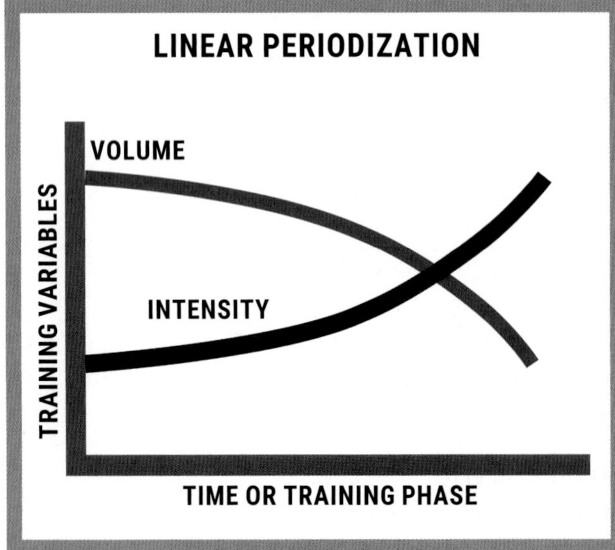

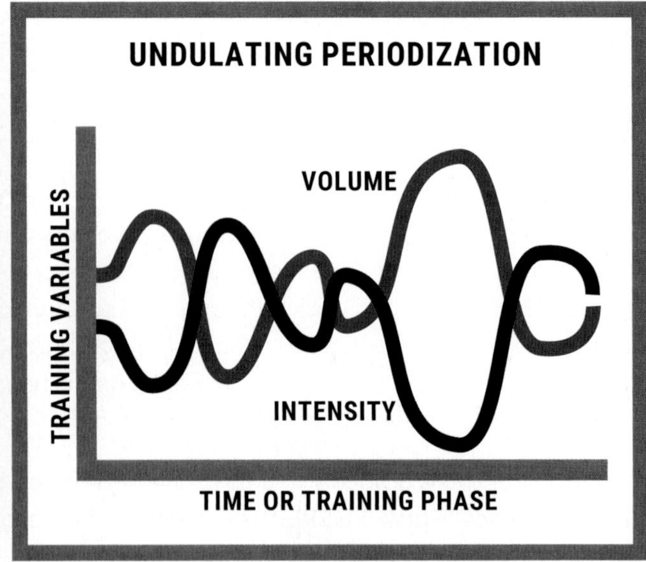

FIGURE 11-29
Linear vs. undulating periodization

APPLY WHAT YOU KNOW

Periodization Program—Sample Protocols

Abraham has a goal of bench pressing 250 pounds (114 kg). He can presently perform a maximal bench press of 200 pounds (91 kg). The following sample bench press training programs use the linear and undulating periodization models.

- One macrocycle with a six-month goal of bench pressing 250 pounds (114 kg)
- Two mesocycles of three months each: The goal of the first mesocycle is to bench press 230 pounds (105 kg). The goal of the second mesocycle is to bench press 250 pounds (114 kg).
- 12 microcycles of two weeks each: A linear periodization model is presented in Table 11-20, while an undulating periodization model is presented in Table 11-21.

Although the overall muscular-training program includes exercises for all of the major muscle groups, only the bench press protocols are presented here. The training weightload progressions are consistent with research data, but the recommended number of repetitions may not apply to all individuals.

Abraham should perform as many repetitions as possible with each exercise set, even if this is slightly lower or higher than the target number. Abraham is advised to perform two progressive bench press warm-up sets, followed by two sets with the training weightload.

TABLE 11-20
Linear Periodization Model—Six-month Macrocycle

Mesocycle 1 (3 months)	Monday	Wednesday	Friday
Microcycle 1 (2 weeks)	140 lb (64 kg) x 12 repetitions	140 lb (64 kg) x 12 repetitions	140 lb (64 kg) x 12 repetitions
Microcycle 2 (2 weeks)	160 lb (73 kg) x 8 repetitions	160 lb (73 kg) x 8 repetitions	160 lb (73 kg) x 8 repetitions
Microcycle 3 (2 weeks)	180 lb (82 kg) x 4 repetitions	180 lb (82 kg) x 4 repetitions	180 lb (82 kg) x 4 repetitions
Microcycle 4 (2 weeks)	155 lb (70 kg) x 12 repetitions	155 lb (70 kg) x 12 repetitions	155 lb (70 kg) x 12 repetitions
Microcycle 5 (2 weeks)	175 lb (79 kg) x 8 repetitions	175 lb (79 kg) x 8 repetitions	175 lb (79 kg) x 8 repetitions
Microcycle 6 (2 weeks)	195 lb (89 kg) x 4 repetitions	195 lb (89 kg) x 4 repetitions	195 lb (89 kg) x 4 repetitions
Interim Week	230 lb (104 kg) x 1 repetition (goal assessment)	Rest	Rest

Continued on the next page

TABLE 11-20 *(continued)*

Mesocycle 2 (3 months)	Monday	Wednesday	Friday
Microcycle 1 (2 weeks)	170 lb (77 kg) x 12 repetitions	170 lb (77 kg) x 12 repetitions	170 lb (77 kg) x 12 repetitions
Microcycle 2 (2 weeks)	190 lb (86 kg) x 8 repetitions	190 lb (86 kg) x 8 repetitions	190 lb (86 kg) x 8 repetitions
Microcycle 3 (2 weeks)	210 lb (95 kg) x 4 repetitions	210 lb (95 kg) x 4 repetitions	210 lb (95 kg) x 4 repetitions
Microcycle 4 (2 weeks)	180 lb (82 kg) x 12 repetitions	180 lb (82 kg) x 12 repetitions	180 lb (82 kg) x 12 repetitions
Microcycle 5 (2 weeks)	200 lb (91 kg) x 8 repetitions	200 lb (91 kg) x 8 repetitions	200 lb (91 kg) x 8 repetitions
Microcycle 6 (2 weeks)	220 lb (100 kg) x 4 repetitions	220 lb (100 kg) x 4 repetitions	220 lb (100 kg) x 4 repetitions
Interim Week	250 lb (114 kg) x 1 repetition (goal assessment)	Rest	Rest

TABLE 11-21
Undulating Periodization Model—Six-month Macrocycle

Mesocycle 1 (3 months)	Monday	Wednesday	Friday
Microcycle 1 (2 weeks)	140 lb (64 kg) x 12 repetitions	160 lb (73 kg) x 8 repetitions	180 lb (82 kg) x 4 repetitions
Microcycle 2 (2 weeks)	140 lb (64 kg) x 12 repetitions	160 lb (73 kg) x 8 repetitions	180 lb (82 kg) x 4 repetitions
Microcycle 3 (2 weeks)	140 lb (64 kg) x 12 repetitions	160 lb (73 kg) x 8 repetitions	180 lb (82 kg) x 4 repetitions
Microcycle 4 (2 weeks)	155 lb (70 kg) x 12 repetitions	175 lb (79 kg) x 8 repetitions	195 lb (89 kg) x 4 repetitions
Microcycle 5 (2 weeks)	155 lb (70 kg) x 12 repetitions	175 lb (79 kg) x 8 repetitions	195 lb (89 kg) x 4 repetitions
Microcycle 6 (2 weeks)	155 lb (70 kg) x 12 repetitions	175 lb (79 kg) x 8 repetitions	195 lb (89 kg) x 4 repetitions
Interim Week	230 lb (104 kg) x 1 repetition (goal assessment)	Rest	Rest
Mesocycle 2 (3 months)	**Monday**	**Wednesday**	**Friday**
Microcycle 1 (2 weeks)	170 lb (77 kg) x 12 repetitions	190 lb (86 kg) x 8 repetitions	210 lb (95 kg) x 4 repetitions
Microcycle 2 (2 weeks)	170 lb (77 kg) x 12 repetitions	190 lb (86 kg) x 8 repetitions	210 lb (95 kg) x 4 repetitions
Microcycle 3 (2 weeks)	170 lb (77 kg) x 12 repetitions	190 lb (86 kg) x 8 repetitions	210 lb (95 kg) x 4 repetitions

TABLE 11-21 *(continued)*

Mesocycle 2 (3 months)	Monday	Wednesday	Friday
Microcycle 4 (2 weeks)	180 lb (82 kg) x 12 repetitions	200 lb (91 kg) x 8 repetitions	220 lb (100 kg) x 4 repetitions
Microcycle 5 (2 weeks)	180 lb (82 kg) x 12 repetitions	200 lb (91 kg) x 8 repetitions	220 lb (100 kg) x 4 repetitions
Microcycle 6 (2 weeks)	180 lb (82 kg) x 12 repetitions	200 lb (91 kg) x 8 repetitions	220 lb (100 kg) x 4 repetitions
Interim Week	250 lb (114 kg) x 1 repetition (goal assessment)	Rest	Rest

Program Maintenance

An underappreciated aspect of exercise training is that continuous progression and improvement are unrealistic training outcomes. For a variety of reasons, including work travel, family vacations, illness, and the busy holiday seasons, clients may experience interruptions to their regular exercise routines, which can make maintaining fitness a daunting task. In fact, research shows that as little as a one- or two-week interruption to regular exercise can quickly result in lost fitness and declines in cardiometabolic health (Nolan et al., 2018). Fortunately, there are research-substantiated solutions that personal trainers can offer clients to avoid **detraining** and maintain cardiometabolic health and fitness throughout challenges to regular training.

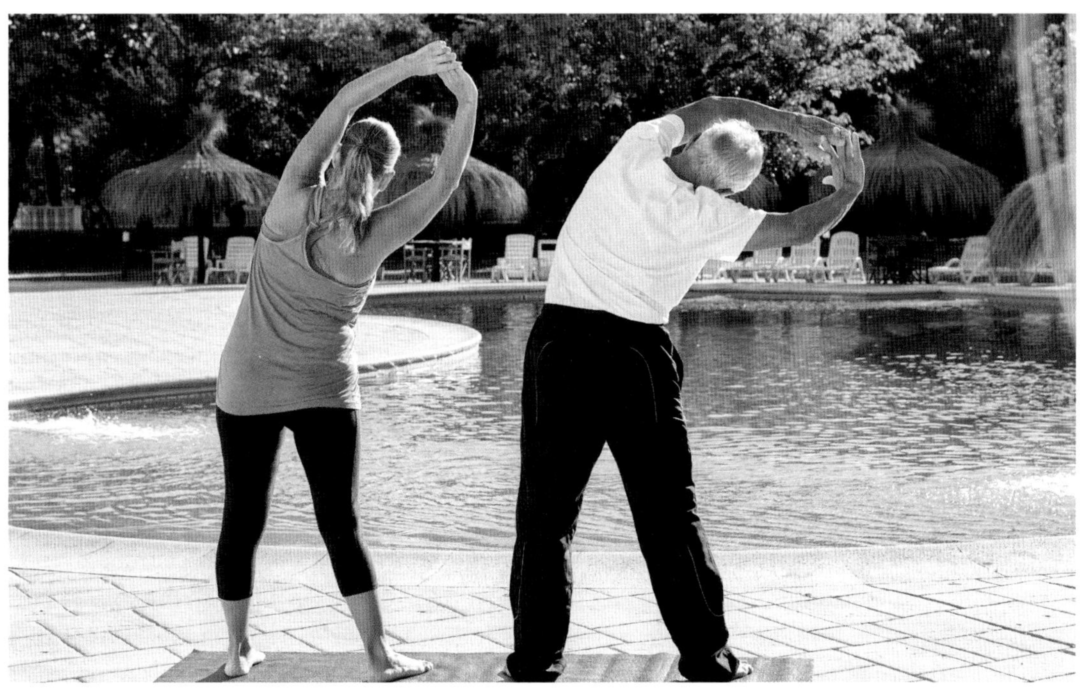

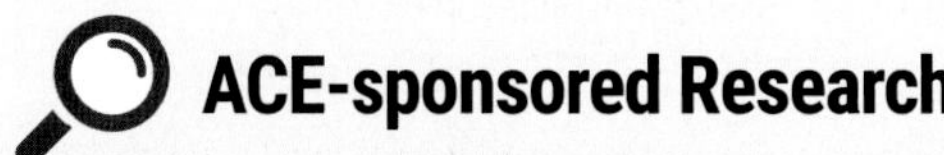

How Fast Does Fitness Fade?

In a randomized controlled trial, researchers (Nolan et al., 2018) examined the physiological implications when one hits the "pause button" on a regular exercise training program. The goal was to quantify the timing and magnitude of changes in physical fitness and cardiometabolic health outcomes that occur with the cessation of regular exercise training. Initially, all participants completed a personalized 13-week exercise program based on the ACE IFT Model. Upon completion of the 13-week program and post-program testing (repeating the baseline measures), participants were randomly placed into two groups. The "train" group continued the personalized exercise program for an additional four weeks. The "detrain" group discontinued regular exercise and did not perform any structured exercise for four weeks, though they were permitted to maintain other lifestyle habits.

Conclusions

- A personalized exercise program elicits significant improvements in all areas of physical fitness and key cardiometabolic risk factors over 13 weeks of exercise training that continue to be further enhanced with an additional month of training.
- Cessation of regular exercise rapidly abolishes all training adaptations within a one-month timeframe, with **systolic blood pressure, high-density lipoprotein (HDL)** cholesterol, and **triglyceride** improvements all completely lost after a one-week interruption to training.

- **Training Strategy #1: The minimum dose of activity to maintain weight and cardiometabolic health equates to 1 mile per day:** Researchers have demonstrated that a minimal level of physical activity is required to maintain body weight and cardiometabolic health (Slentz, Houmard, & Kraus, 2007). Indeed, it has been reported that the minimal physical-activity level for weight maintenance occurred at approximately 8 miles (12.9 km) of walking per week (or an equivalent energy expenditure). This equates to a little more than 1 mile (1.6 km) each day. Additionally, the researchers highlighted that body-weight changes are a good proxy of the dose of physical-activity levels required to maintain cardiometabolic health. An increase in body weight can be interpreted to mean that additional physical activity is required to maintain weight and cardiometabolic health.
- **Training Strategy #2: Low-dose HIIT (12 minutes/week) improves cardiometabolic health:** HIIT involves alternating brief bouts (30 seconds to 5 minutes) of higher-intensity exercise with either rest or lower-intensity workloads throughout an exercise routine. Different forms of HIIT have captivated the attention of both researchers and exercise professionals alike due to its reported ability to improve health outcomes for a lesser weekly time commitment relative to the current exercise guidelines for moderate-intensity continuous training. Researchers have demonstrated that a very

low dose of HIIT, consisting of a single four-minute interval bout at 85 to 95% of MHR performed three times per week, was sufficient to significantly improve $\dot{V}O_2$max and lower **blood pressure (BP)** in a group of individuals with **metabolic syndrome (MetS)** (Ramos et al., 2016). Each HIIT session was preceded by a 10-minute warm-up and concluded with a three-minute cool-down. Both the warm-up and cool-down were performed at an intensity of 60 to 70% of MHR.

- Training Strategy #3: Integrate a single long training session into the biweekly training routine: More than one-third (37.6%) of U.S. adults have **prediabetes** (Benjamin et al., 2019). People with prediabetes have a two- to sixfold increased risk of developing **type 2 diabetes** in their lifetimes. Moreover, individuals with type 2 diabetes have a life expectancy, on average, that is 10 years shorter than their counterparts without type 2 diabetes. Prediabetes is underpinned by impaired blood **glucose** and poor **insulin sensitivity.** Both of these physiological markers worsen considerably with even brief periods of inactivity (i.e., less than one week). Arguably, the single best workout to augment insulin sensitivity and improve blood glucose control is a prolonged bout of exercise that decreases muscle **glycogen** stores. For example, Schenk and Horowitz (2007) saw an impressive 25% improvement in insulin sensitivity among study participants following a single 90-minute moderate-intensity (65 to 75% of MHR) exercise session.
- Training Strategy #4: Combined cardiorespiratory and muscular training is an antidote to detraining: While the best option is to consistently avoid inactivity and **sedentary** behaviors altogether, some degree of physical inactivity and sedentary behavior is inevitable. With this in mind, try to design clients' exercise training programs in advance of interruptions to regular activity in a manner that attenuates the rate of detraining. Combined cardiorespiratory and muscular training results in numerous favorable effects (e.g., body composition, muscular strength, and **lipid** profile) that persisted for longer following training cessation when compared with either cardiorespiratory or muscular training alone (Theodorou et al., 2016).

Recovery

Post-exercise recovery is a vital component of the overall exercise training paradigm, and essential for high-level performance and continued improvement. If the rate of recovery is appropriate, higher training volumes and intensities are possible without the detrimental effects of overuse. Personal trainers play a critical role in helping clients identify the most appropriate training recovery program, a process that requires purposeful trial and error. Frequency, intensity, time, and type of recovery between each bout of exercise must also be considered to optimize recovery.

EXERCISE PROGRAM FITT FOR ACCELERATING RECOVERY

Training recovery can be optimized by correctly managing the various components surrounding the exercise program (ACSM, 2018). To accomplish this endeavor, personal trainers are encouraged to plan an appropriate FITT (frequency, intensity, time, and type) for training recovery itself (Figure 11-30). In the following sections, different features of the training recovery aspect of the exercise program are described in more detail.

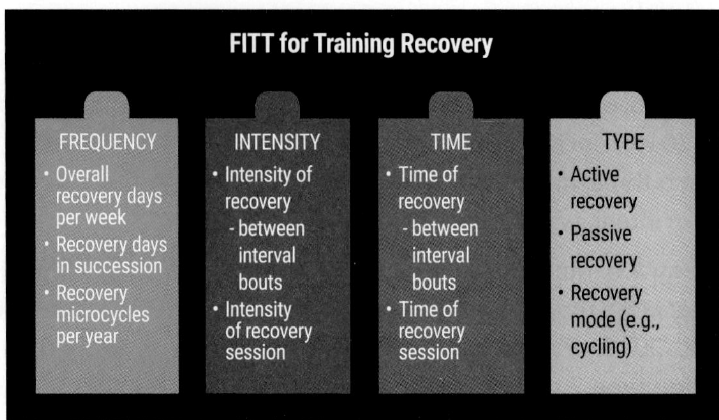

FIGURE 11-30
FITT for training recovery

Frequency of Recovery

This component of training recovery refers to the number of days per week (i.e., frequency) specifically devoted to recovery. For instance, if a client is simply recovering from a somewhat hard training session, the frequency of recovery may be a single day. Conversely, a client recovering from a 10K run may require several days of recovery.

Intensity of Recovery

For a client performing an interval session that consists of four repetitions of four minutes at 60 to 89% of HRR (HR ≥VT1 to <VT2) interspersed with two minutes of **active recovery** bouts, personal trainers need to program a specific intensity (e.g., 40 to 59% of HRR, or HR <VT1) to be performed for the active recovery bouts. The intensity of recovery may also extend to the overall intensity of a daily session of exercise dedicated to recovery (e.g., a moderate-intensity, 60-minute bicycle ride at 40 to 59% of HRR or HR <VT1).

Time (Duration) of Recovery

This component can refer to either the recovery time between interval bouts or the duration of an entire recovery session.

Type of Recovery between Bouts

This component refers to the type of recovery and may refer to either active recovery or **passive recovery.** Active recovery involves continued exercise at a substantially lower intensity or workload, while passive recovery consists of resting completely. The type of recovery to be performed is a consideration for both the time between interval bouts and daily recovery sessions. In terms of an active recovery, the mode of exercise to be performed is an additional variable to be contemplated. It is common for clients who normally run to cross-train; for example, an active recovery day for a runner may consist of swimming or exercising on an elliptical trainer.

PRACTICAL APPLICATIONS FOR THE PERSONAL TRAINER

Personal trainers should recognize that current and future clients will spend more time throughout the week in training recovery compared to actual exercise training. This fact necessitates a purposeful approach to the overall training recovery paradigm. This section provides personal trainers with practical applications supported by the scientific literature and ACE-sponsored research aimed at augmenting post-exercise recovery.

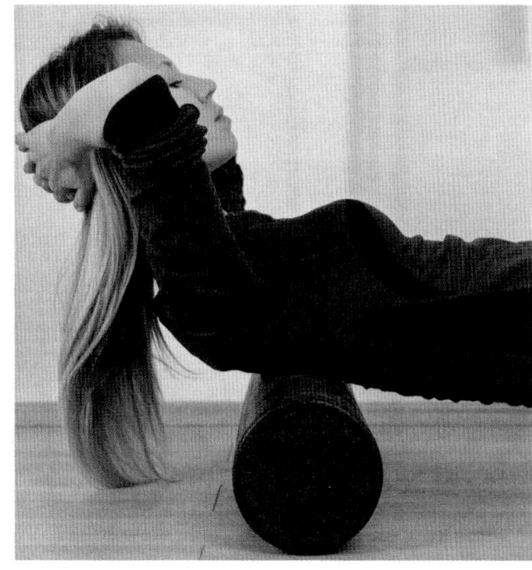

Program Active Recovery

Whether it is between interval bouts, immediately after an interval session, or the day following strenuous exercise, there is compelling evidence that an active recovery is superior to passive recovery (Del Coso et al., 2010). Logically, from a physiological perspective, this practice should make sense. Continued blood flow to the skeletal muscle best promotes the resynthesis of **creatine phosphate** and glycogen stores; it also facilitates the removal of **protons.** Collectively, these factors aid in recovery.

Program Specific Recovery Intensities

Regrettably, it is common for many clients and athletes to exercise too hard during periods of recovery, be it between interval bouts, following an interval workout, or the day after competition. Personal trainers can help clients to avoid or minimize this error by establishing specific target intensities for recovery scenarios. Research has reported that active recovery bouts of very light intensity (<50 % of MHR) are optimal for decreasing **lactate** and proton levels (Del Coso et al., 2010). In terms of coupling the very light recovery intensity with a proper cool-down, research has identified approximately 10 minutes as an ideal duration. In terms of an exercise intensity for recovery sessions, research has generally reported moderate-intensity (65 to 75% of MHR) exercise to be sufficient (Powers & Howley, 2017).

Program High-intensity Interval Training

Research shows HIIT elicits several physiological adaptations that aid in recovery, including improved $\dot{V}O_2$max, increased **buffering capacity** and a greater concentration of **monocarboxylate transport (MCT) proteins** (Thomas et al., 2012; Bishop et al., 2008). MCT proteins are found on cell membranes and help transport lactate and proton molecules from inside the cell out into the bloodstream. Exercise training leads to an increased MCT concentration, which results in a greater capacity for removal of excessive lactate and protons from the cell. However, to elicit these improvements, there are several important considerations for the exercise program. The intensity of intervals should be high (~90 to 95% of MHR), but not maximal. The duration of interval bouts should equate to two minutes with a shorter recovery period (e.g., one minute). The number of interval bouts can range from three to 12 per session, and the number of HIIT sessions per week can range from one to three, with at least 48 hours between sessions.

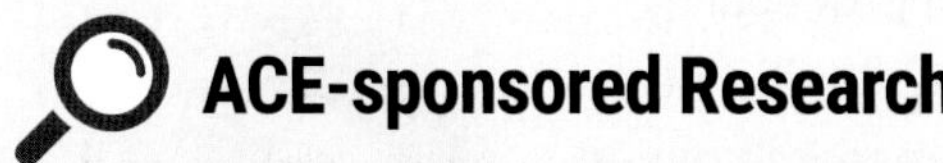

Active vs. Passive Recovery and Exercise Performance: Which Strategy Is Best?

Researchers examined the effect of active vs. passive recovery on exercise performance (St. Pierre et al., 2018). The purpose of this study was threefold: (1) to compare the effect of active vs. passive recovery on endurance-related performance, (2) to compare the effect of active vs. passive recovery on power-related performance, and (3) to compare the effect of different intensities of active recovery on exercise performance.

Conclusions

- Active recovery is more effective than passive recovery at maintaining endurance performance.
- Active recovery is superior to passive recovery for sustaining power output.
- Active recovery should be performed at a moderate intensity [i.e., 80 to 90% of VT2, which is approximately 55 to 60% of **heart-rate reserve (HRR)**] in order to sustain endurance performance and promote greater blood lactate removal. In contrast, when active recovery is performed at a vigorous intensity (i.e., at VT2, which corresponds to 75 to 85% of HRR), there is delayed blood lactate removal and a resultant decrease in endurance performance.

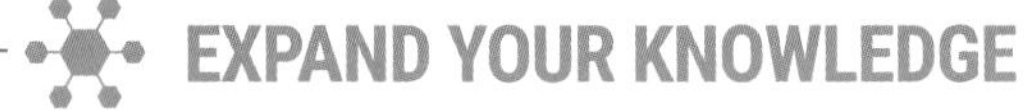

Small-group Training

In addition to one-on-one training sessions with clients, many personal trainers are getting into the practice of seeing clients in a small-group setting. A small-group workout can be thought of as two or more clients sharing the same training session. A personal trainer who has experience teaching group fitness classes may be comfortable instructing 10 to 15 clients at once, provided the clients all do the same exercises simultaneously, have similar fitness abilities, and do not require extra individual attention during exercise. However, groups consisting of more than four or five people could potentially be too large for one personal-trainer to effectively instruct and supervise, especially considering that most clients will need individual attention at some point during the training session. Thus, in general, the size of a small-group training session should be limited to the number of clients that the personal trainer can safely and effectively manage.

Benefits

There are many benefits of small-group training that extend to both the personal trainer and the client. From the personal trainer's perspective, semiprivate training provides advantages in the areas of finance, time management, and referrals. For the client, benefits include a lower cost per session, enhanced camaraderie among workout partners, and an opportunity to receive instruction in a small-group setting from a qualified exercise professional.

Group Homogeneity

When selecting a group of clients to work together in a group session, a personal trainer should ensure that the individuals are somewhat homogenous in characteristics such as level of physical conditioning, fitness goals, training experience, and even physique. From a leadership perspective, personal trainers benefit from working with groups of clients who are as similar as possible with regard to health history and physical ability. For example, one client who requires more attention than the others can make the other clients sharing the session feel that they are not getting the instruction and supervision that they deserve. When dealing with clients who require extra focus, it is best to direct them to participate in a personalized program, at least until they are capable of performing the exercises autonomously without the undivided attention of a personal trainer. Clients with similar fitness goals also work better together in a group. For example, an athlete who is interested in increasing his or her vertical jump height through plyometric training would not be a good match if paired with a middle-aged client concerned with lowering BP and losing weight. From a psychological perspective, clients can experience a certain level of social physique anxiety, which has a negative correlation with exercise adherence, if they perceive that they are being compared to more fit members of their group. Thus, a client who is intimidated by physical activity and anxious about his or her appearance should be placed in a group with others who have similar concerns. That way, the clients can support and encourage each other while simultaneously enhancing self-efficacy.

Personal Attention

For clients who are used to the traditional personal-training approach where individual-focused attention and personal interaction are standard, small-group training can seem less than ideal. The best way to deal with this issue is to have an upfront, honest conversation with clients about the level of personal interaction they can expect during a semiprivate training session. Group size ultimately determines what clients can expect. A group with fewer participants obviously allows the personal trainer to devote more individual attention to each client and provide more hands-on instruction, if necessary. Larger groups can provide an atmosphere of robust energy and excitement, but they also can spread the personal trainer a little thin as he or she tries to manage the clients and various pieces of equipment. As long as each client is aware that there is limited personal attention from the personal trainer in a group setting, small-group training can be an enjoyable social and physical experience for all participants.

Case Studies

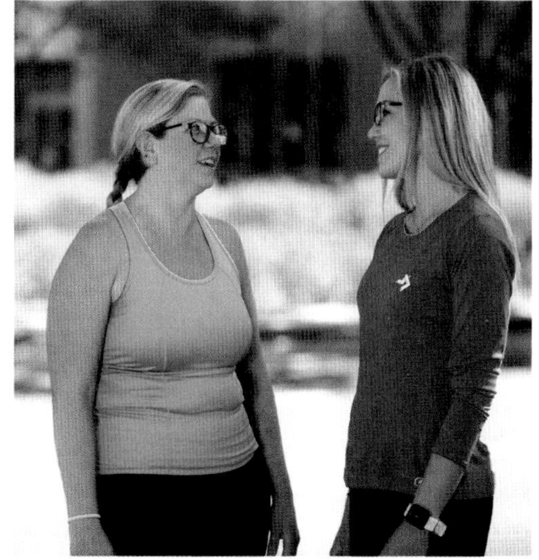

This section offers examples of how to put into practice the content described thus far on supporting clients through their behavior-change efforts in increasing physical activity. Aligning with the ACE Mover™ Method philosophy, the personal trainer in the following scenarios makes each interaction a client-centered experience, while drawing upon skills used in the ACE ABC Approach to learn more about the client and then design the most appropriate exercise program possible. Figure 11-31 provides a blank ACE IFT Model Exercise Programming Template, while the case studies that follow provide examples of how a personal trainer can use this tool when working with a variety of clients.

FIGURE 11-31
ACE IFT Model Exercise Programming Template

Client Name: ____________________

Client Goals: ____________________

Client-centered Considerations: ____________________

Frequency (active and rest days): ____________________

Cardiorespiratory Training Phase:

☐ **Base Training**
Focus on moderate-intensity exercise below the talk test threshold

☐ **Fitness Training**
Build on Base Training through the introduction of zone 2 intervals performed from VT1 to just below VT2

☐ **Performance Training**
Build on Fitness Training and introduce zone 3 intervals performed at and above VT2

Muscular Training Phase:

☐ **Functional Training**
Focus on establishing postural stability and kinetic chain mobility

☐ **Movement Training**
Focus on training the five primary movement patterns while incorporating Functional Training exercises in the warm-up and cool-down

☐ **Load/Speed Training**
Focus on load and speed goals while including Functional Training exercises in the warm-up and cool-down and loading primary movement patterns

Exercise Goal*	Exercise/Exercise Mode	Intensity†	Volume‡
Warm-up:			
Conditioning:			

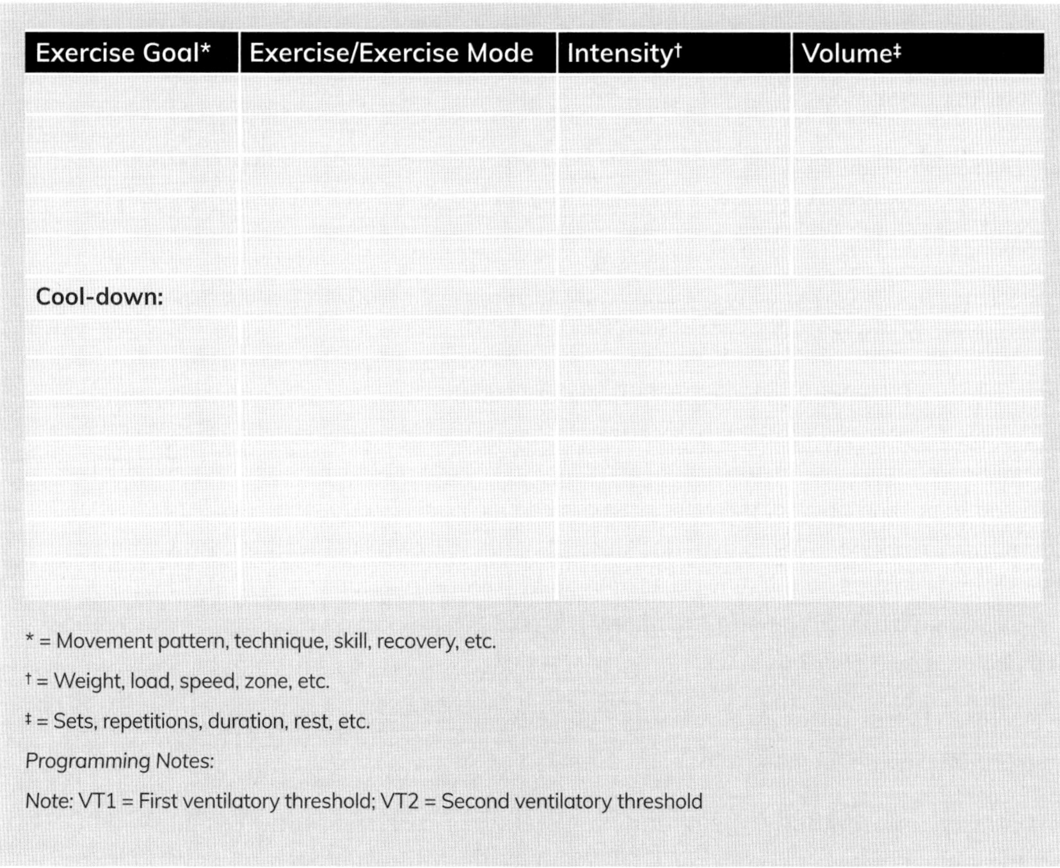

Exercise Goal*	Exercise/Exercise Mode	Intensity†	Volume‡
Cool-down:			

* = Movement pattern, technique, skill, recovery, etc.

† = Weight, load, speed, zone, etc.

‡ = Sets, repetitions, duration, rest, etc.

Programming Notes:

Note: VT1 = First ventilatory threshold; VT2 = Second ventilatory threshold

FIGURE 11-31
(continued)

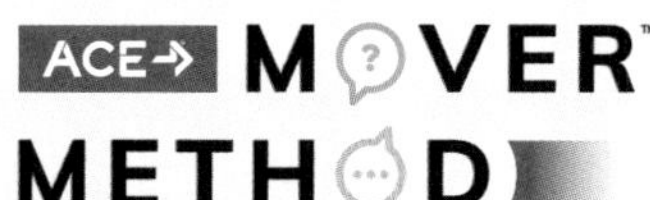

Busy Mom Who Wants to Run a 5K Race

Valerie, a 39-year-old mother of three children, has scheduled an introductory session with an ACE Certified Personal Trainer at the gym she recently joined. Valerie is looking forward to working with a personal trainer to prepare for her goal of running a 5K race, her first in more than 12 years. Valerie was highly active for most of her life, competing in youth sports and participating in 5K and 10K races as an adult and gradually became physically inactive during her first pregnancy. Valerie has been cleared for exercise by her doctor and recently began running again. To stay motivated, she registered for a 5K race.

ACE ABC APPROACH

Following is an example that demonstrates how the ACE Mover Method philosophy is embraced by using the ACE ABC Approach for gathering the necessary information to create and implement an exercise program. This method can help guide Valerie toward reaching her fitness-related goals.

Ask: Asking powerful, open-ended questions during this initial session will help to spark discussion about client expectations and identify what Valerie is hoping to accomplish by working with a personal trainer.

Personal Trainer: Thank you for taking the time to meet with me for this initial session. How do you envision me helping to support your goals?

Client: I think working with a personal trainer can help me be more accountable and efficient with my training program. I haven't done any structured physical activity for nearly 12 years. Six months ago, I decided I need to get back in shape, so I started running again.

Personal Trainer: Efficiency and accountability are important to you as you work on getting back in shape. What does being "in shape" mean to you?

Client: Being in shape means being able to keep up with all my children's activities but also being able to run 5Ks again. Before my 12-year-old son was born, I used to run all the time and raced in multiple 5K and 10K events each year. Sometimes I would participate in as many as eight events per year. When I think about how active I used to be, and how for the past 12 years I haven't been exercising, I get frustrated with myself! So, six months ago I decided to join a gym and dedicate time to exercising. I started slowly by just walking on a treadmill, and I've worked my way up to running at a moderate pace for 30 minutes, three days per week. I'm averaging a 12-minute mile. I'm happy with the progress, even though I am not yet back to running like I was before having my kids.

Personal Trainer: Over the past six months, you've made some significant improvements to your physical conditioning. When do you plan on running in your first event?

Client: That's part of why I'm here today. I've already registered for a 5K run that takes place in 18 weeks. It's during the week of my 40th birthday. I'm hoping to get some guidance and a structured plan from you to help me to prepare for this event. My 5K record is 24 minutes and 48 seconds. For my comeback race, I'd like to maintain a pace just under a 10-minute mile and finish the run in under 31 minutes.

Break down barriers: Ask open-ended questions to discover potential obstacles that may get in the way of Valerie reaching her goal of running in a 5K race in 18 weeks and finishing the event in under 31 minutes.

Personal Trainer: What do you need to start doing now to move closer to this goal?

Client: I need a schedule that allows me to train four days per week. I want to meet with you once a week to make sure I'm on track with my goals and train three days per week on my own. Before having my children, I could run whenever I wanted, and as often as my body could handle. Now, I need to be efficient with my training if I'm going to reach my goal since I don't always have a set schedule or know when I will have time to train.

Personal Trainer: Creating an efficient schedule, as well as taking care of your physical health, is crucial to your success. Not having enough structure to your plan may be a barrier to reaching this goal.

Client: That's right! I haven't had any structure with my current training program. I need a "master calendar" for my entire family, where I can track my training schedule. If I make it just as important as the other events we have going on, it will be easier to stay on track.

Collaborate: Working together with the client on solutions to barriers is the next step, along with setting SMART goals for implementing a strategic training program for preparing for a 5K run in 18 weeks.

Personal Trainer: What can you do within the next week to get started?

Client: I want to get started working with you as soon as possible. This week I'll work with my family to get all our events for the next few months written on one calendar, including my exercise time. Then, next week, I will meet with you twice per week, and I will run on my own two days per week from now until my race while following the exercise plan that you create for me.

Personal Trainer: Creating an exercise plan based on the goals and information you shared with me will be our next step. For our first training session, we will perform an initial assessment to help determine the best training intensities and program for you. Next week, once you have your master family schedule created, we can work together to define which specific days you will train each week and how you would like to be held accountable for adhering to your plan.

Because Valerie is already completing 30-minute runs at a moderate intensity three days per week, it is determined that she is currently performing in the Base Training phase of the ACE IFT Model and is ready to progress to Fitness Training, where the frequency of her runs will increase and interval training will be added at HRs at and above VT1. In order to utilize effective intervals, Valerie's HR at VT1 must be determined. During her initial training session, Valerie completed the VT1 talk test and it revealed that her HR at VT1 is 138 beats per minute (bpm). Also, during this first session Valerie was assessed as she performed body-weight exercises in the five primary movement patterns during her warm-up. Because of how she performed during the movement assessments (i.e., displaying adequate postural stability and kinetic chain mobility), she will begin her program in the Movement Training phase of the Muscular Training component of the ACE IFT Model. Based on observations, assessment results, and the timeline Valerie established, the exercise plan in Figure 11-32 was created.

FIGURE 11-32
ACE IFT Model Exercise Programming Template—Busy Mom Who Wants to Run a 5K Race

Client Name: Valerie, a busy 39-year-old mother of three who wants to run a 5K race

Client Goals: In 18 weeks, run a 5K in under 31 minutes and improve the strength of the arms, legs, and core muscles

Client-centered Considerations: Needs programming that fits within a busy family schedule; include workouts in family calendar

Frequency (active and rest days): ***Muscular training + running*** (2 days/week): Focus on movement training, with a 30-minute run below VT1. ***Interval running*** (2 days/week): 35-minute interval run with work intervals performed at and above VT1 to just below VT2 and a 1:3 work-to-recovery ratio

Cardiorespiratory Training Phase:

[ ] **Base Training**
Focus on moderate-intensity exercise below the talk test threshold

[X] **Fitness Training**
Build on Base Training through the introduction of zone 2 intervals performed from VT1 to just below VT2

Muscular Training Phase:

[ ] **Functional Training**
Focus on establishing postural stability and kinetic chain mobility

[X] **Movement Training**
Focus on training the five primary movement patterns while incorporating Functional Training exercises in the warm-up and cool-down

Continued on the next page

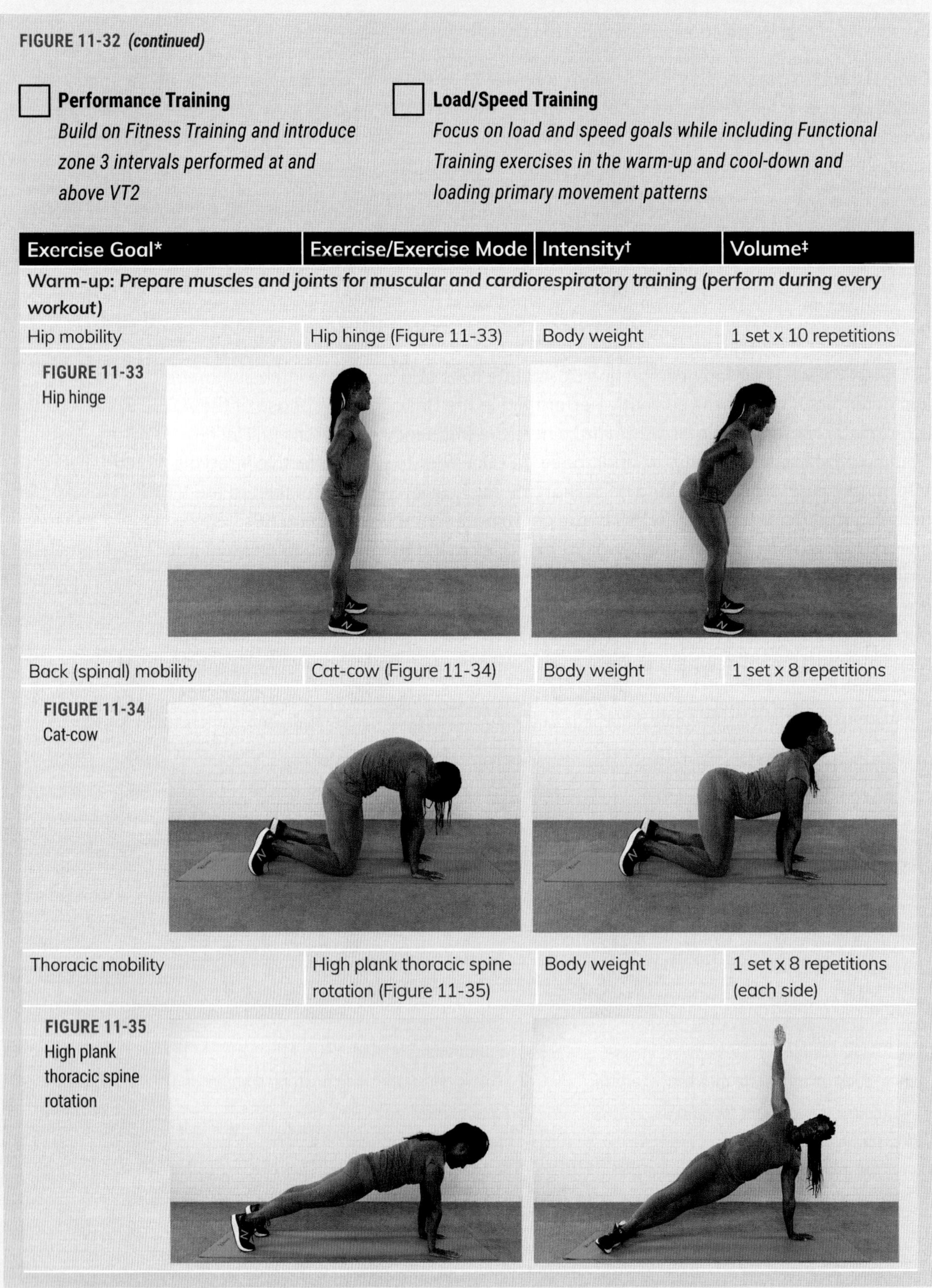

FIGURE 11-32 *(continued)*

☐ **Performance Training**
Build on Fitness Training and introduce zone 3 intervals performed at and above VT2

☐ **Load/Speed Training**
Focus on load and speed goals while including Functional Training exercises in the warm-up and cool-down and loading primary movement patterns

Exercise Goal*	Exercise/Exercise Mode	Intensity†	Volume‡
Warm-up: Prepare muscles and joints for muscular and cardiorespiratory training (perform during every workout)			
Hip mobility	Hip hinge (Figure 11-33)	Body weight	1 set x 10 repetitions
Back (spinal) mobility	Cat-cow (Figure 11-34)	Body weight	1 set x 8 repetitions
Thoracic mobility	High plank thoracic spine rotation (Figure 11-35)	Body weight	1 set x 8 repetitions (each side)

FIGURE 11-33
Hip hinge

FIGURE 11-34
Cat-cow

FIGURE 11-35
High plank thoracic spine rotation

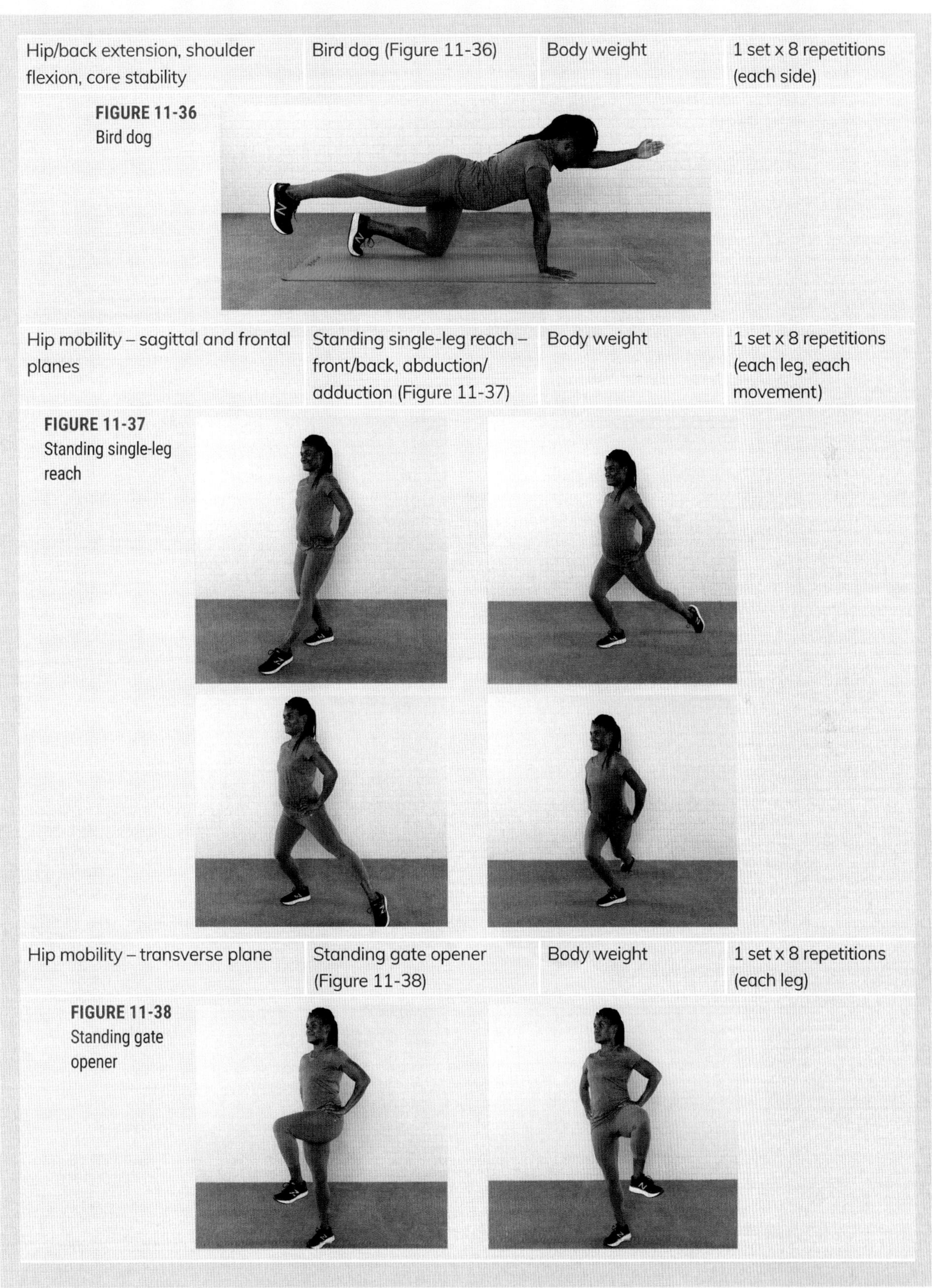

Hip/back extension, shoulder flexion, core stability	Bird dog (Figure 11-36)	Body weight	1 set x 8 repetitions (each side)

FIGURE 11-36
Bird dog

Hip mobility – sagittal and frontal planes	Standing single-leg reach – front/back, abduction/adduction (Figure 11-37)	Body weight	1 set x 8 repetitions (each leg, each movement)

FIGURE 11-37
Standing single-leg reach

Hip mobility – transverse plane	Standing gate opener (Figure 11-38)	Body weight	1 set x 8 repetitions (each leg)

FIGURE 11-38
Standing gate opener

Continued on the next page

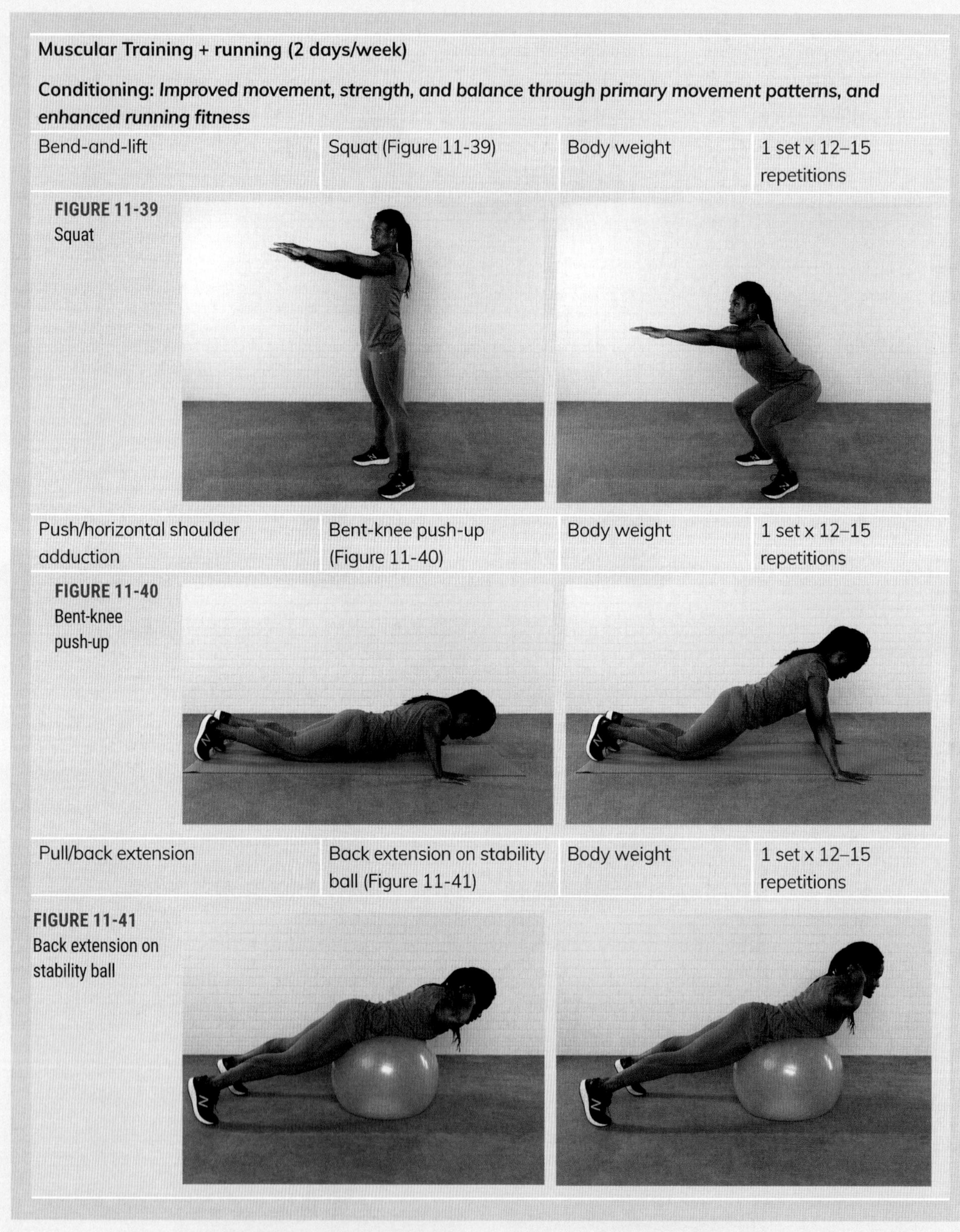

Muscular Training + running (2 days/week)

Conditioning: *Improved movement, strength, and balance through primary movement patterns, and enhanced running fitness*

Movement pattern	Exercise	Resistance	Sets/repetitions
Bend-and-lift	Squat (Figure 11-39)	Body weight	1 set x 12–15 repetitions

FIGURE 11-39
Squat

Movement pattern	Exercise	Resistance	Sets/repetitions
Push/horizontal shoulder adduction	Bent-knee push-up (Figure 11-40)	Body weight	1 set x 12–15 repetitions

FIGURE 11-40
Bent-knee push-up

Movement pattern	Exercise	Resistance	Sets/repetitions
Pull/back extension	Back extension on stability ball (Figure 11-41)	Body weight	1 set x 12–15 repetitions

FIGURE 11-41
Back extension on stability ball

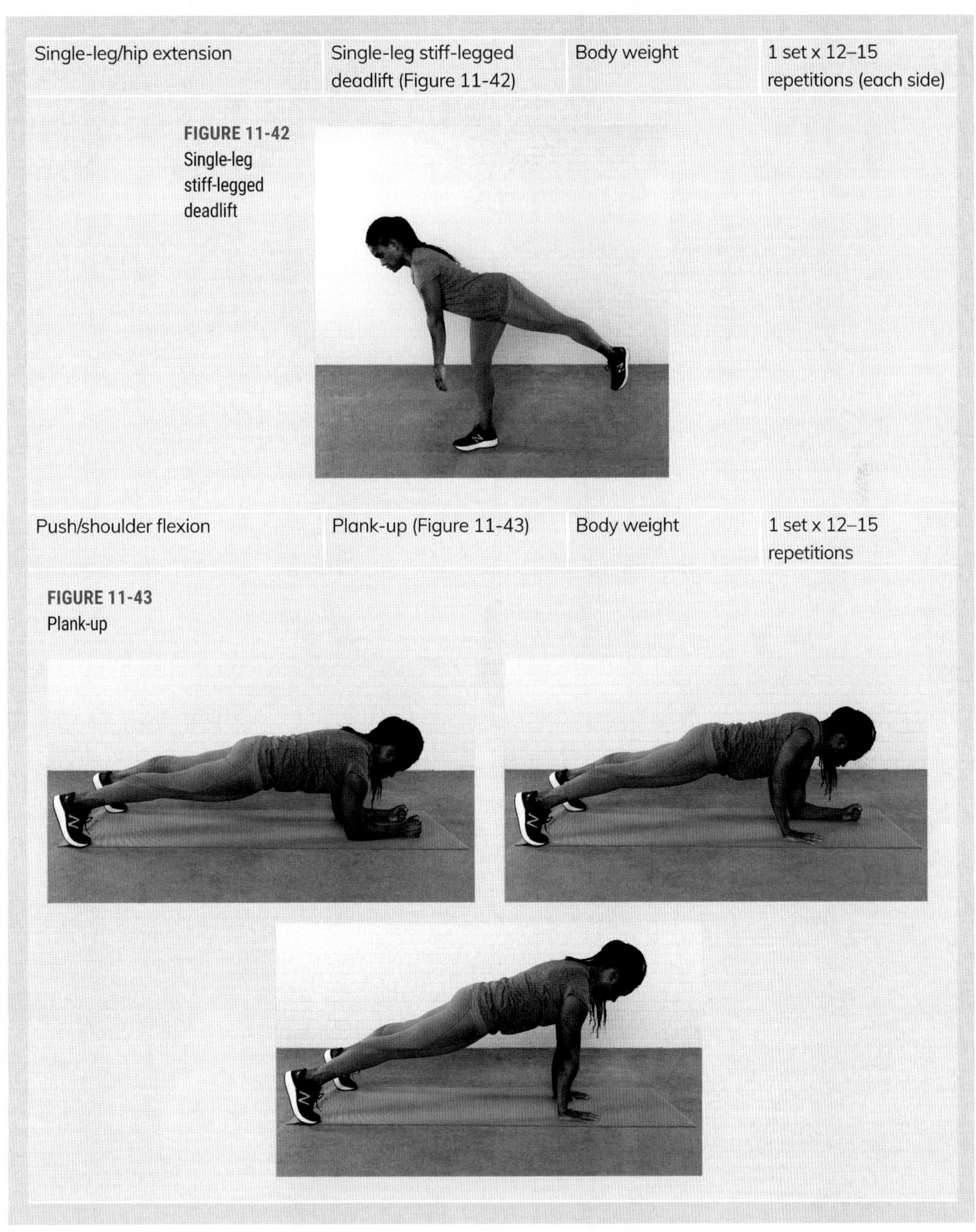

Single-leg/hip extension	Single-leg stiff-legged deadlift (Figure 11-42)	Body weight	1 set x 12–15 repetitions (each side)

FIGURE 11-42
Single-leg stiff-legged deadlift

Push/shoulder flexion	Plank-up (Figure 11-43)	Body weight	1 set x 12–15 repetitions

FIGURE 11-43
Plank-up

Continued on the next page

Pull/scapular retraction/shoulder flexion and horizontal abduction	Stability ball shoulder stabilization – I, Y, T, W (Figure 11-44)	Body weight	1 set x 5 repetitions (I, Y, T, W)

FIGURE 11-44
Stability ball shoulder stabilization – I, Y, T, W

I

Y

T

W

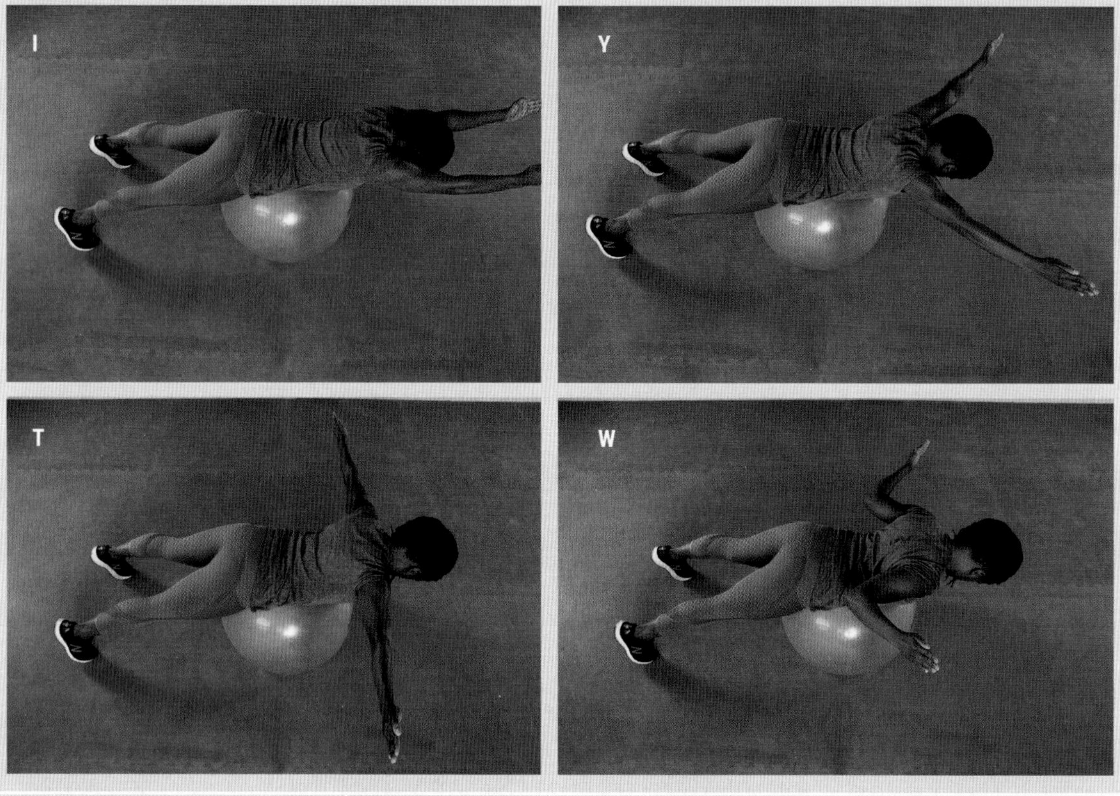

Single-leg in frontal plane	Side lunge (Figure 11-45)	Body weight	1 set x 12–15 repetitions (each side)

FIGURE 11-45
Side lunge

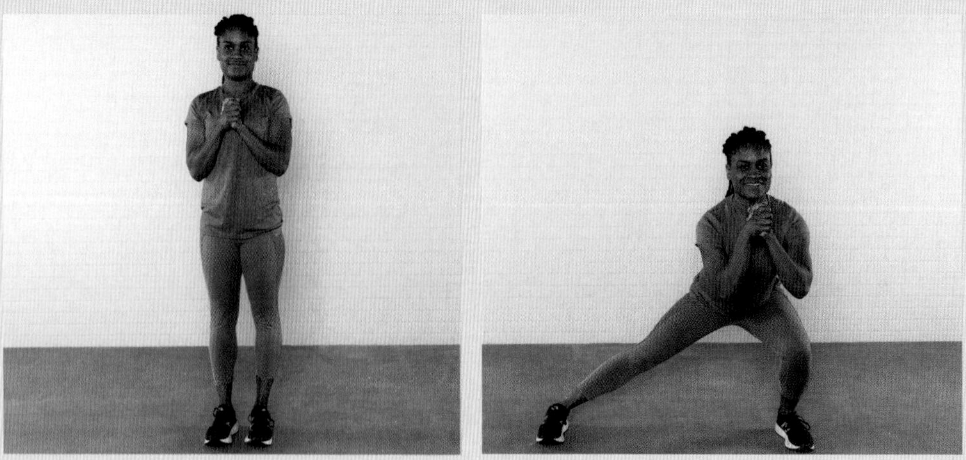

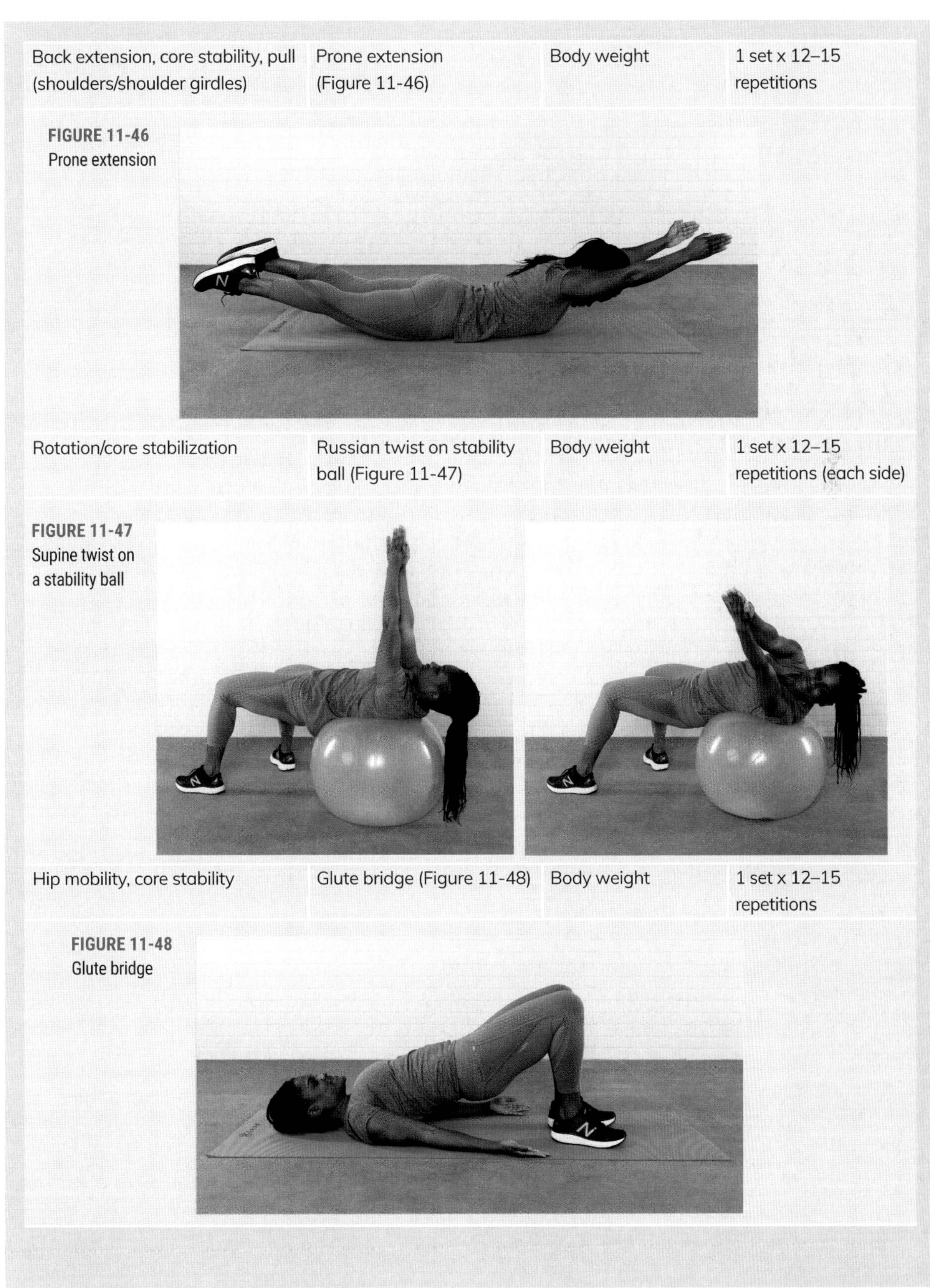

Back extension, core stability, pull (shoulders/shoulder girdles)	Prone extension (Figure 11-46)	Body weight	1 set x 12–15 repetitions
FIGURE 11-46 Prone extension			
Rotation/core stabilization	Russian twist on stability ball (Figure 11-47)	Body weight	1 set x 12–15 repetitions (each side)
FIGURE 11-47 Supine twist on a stability ball			
Hip mobility, core stability	Glute bridge (Figure 11-48)	Body weight	1 set x 12–15 repetitions
FIGURE 11-48 Glute bridge			

Continued on the next page

Core stability	Side bridge (Figure 11-49)	Body weight	1 set x 5 repetitions (10 seconds each)
FIGURE 11-49 Side bridge			
Cardiorespiratory fitness training	Running	Zone 1 – Pacing just below VT1 (HR = 130–137 bpm)	30 minutes
Interval Running Days (2 days/week)			
Conditioning: *Increased running pace for sustained efforts*			
Warm-up segment of run	Jogging	Zone 1 – HR below 138 bpm	10 minutes
Work intervals	Running interval	Zone 2 – HR ≥VT1 to just below VT2 (138–145 bpm)	1 minute x 5 repetitions
Recovery intervals	Jogging recovery interval	Zone 1 – HR below 138 bpm	3 minutes x 5 repetitions (following each work interval)
Cool-down segment of run	Jogging	Zone 1 – HR below 138 bpm	5 minutes
Cool-down: *Active recovery to reduce HR and core temperature while working on flexibility (perform during every workout)*			
Hip and shoulder mobility/ROM	Downward-facing dog (Figure 11-50)	Body weight	1 x 15–30 seconds
FIGURE 11-50 Downward-facing dog			

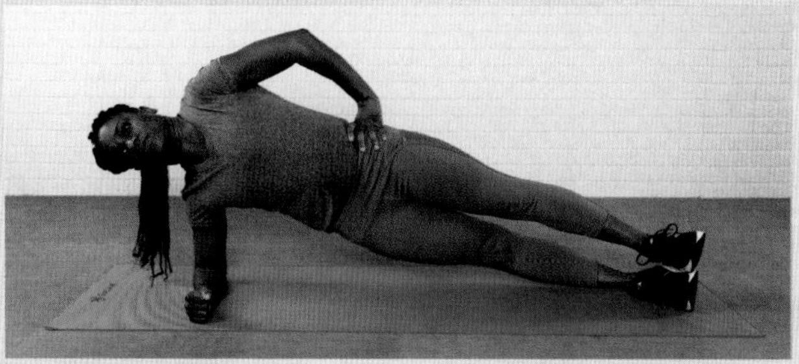

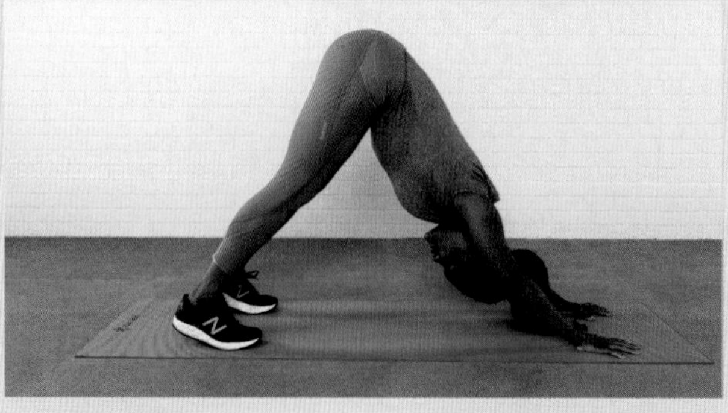

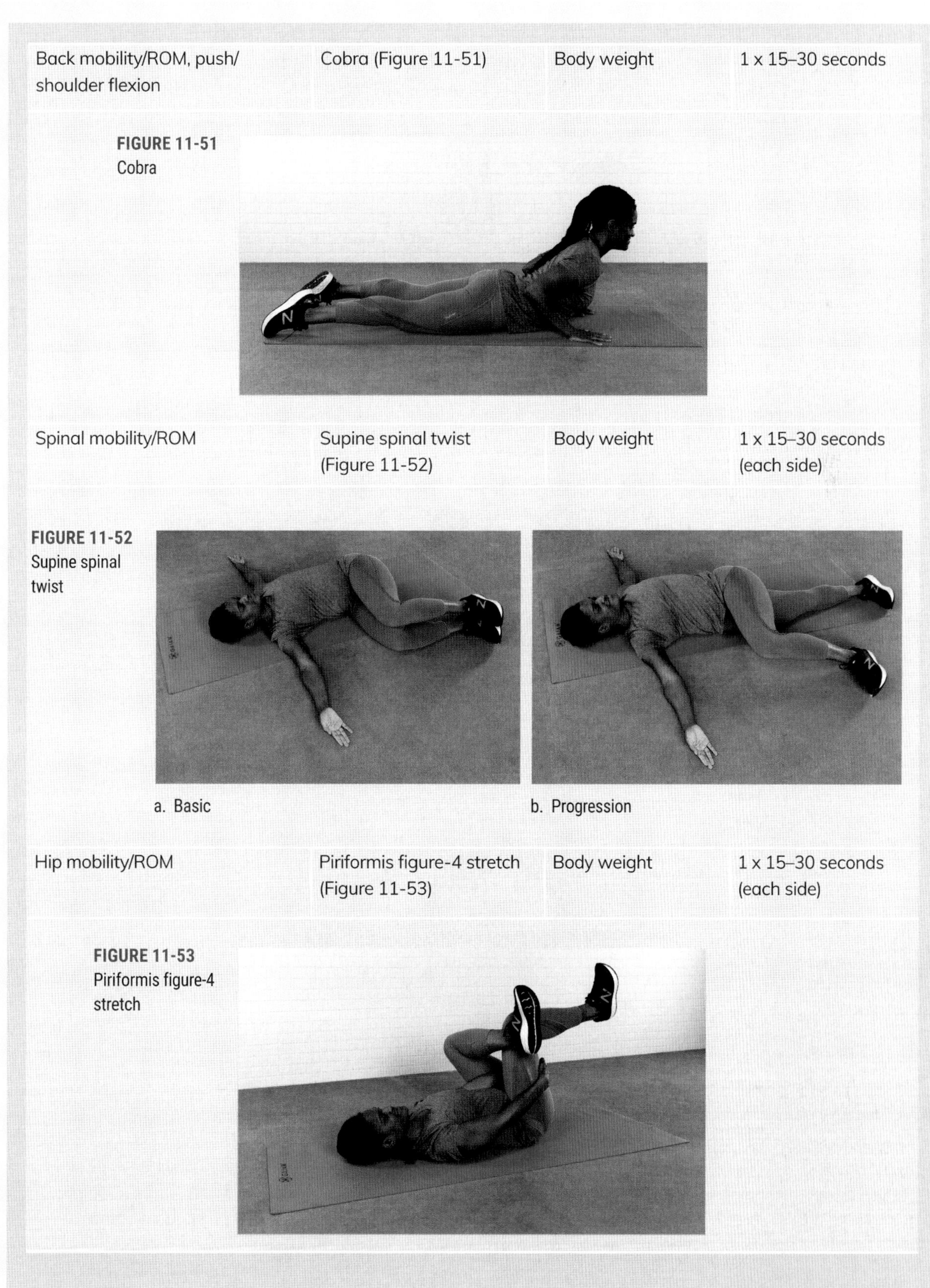

Back mobility/ROM, push/shoulder flexion	Cobra (Figure 11-51)	Body weight	1 x 15–30 seconds

FIGURE 11-51
Cobra

Spinal mobility/ROM	Supine spinal twist (Figure 11-52)	Body weight	1 x 15–30 seconds (each side)

FIGURE 11-52
Supine spinal twist

a. Basic

b. Progression

Hip mobility/ROM	Piriformis figure-4 stretch (Figure 11-53)	Body weight	1 x 15–30 seconds (each side)

FIGURE 11-53
Piriformis figure-4 stretch

Continued on the next page

Hip mobility/ROM	Kneeling hip flexor stretch (Figure 11-54)	Body weight	1 x 15–30 seconds (each side)

FIGURE 11-54
Kneeling hip flexor stretch

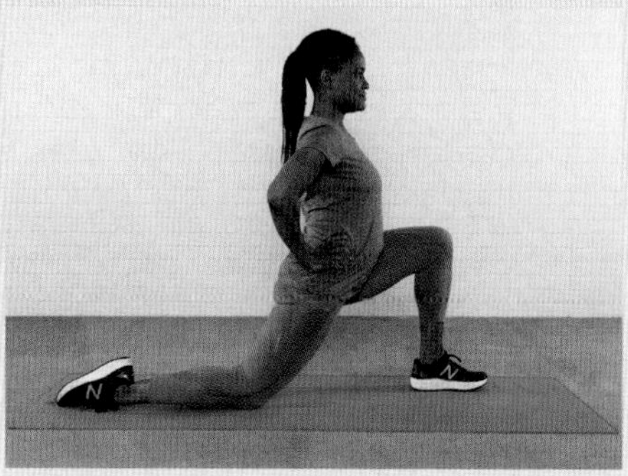

Hip mobility/ROM	Modified hurdler stretch (Figure 11-55)	Body weight	1 x 15–30 seconds (each side)

FIGURE 11-55
Modified hurdler stretch

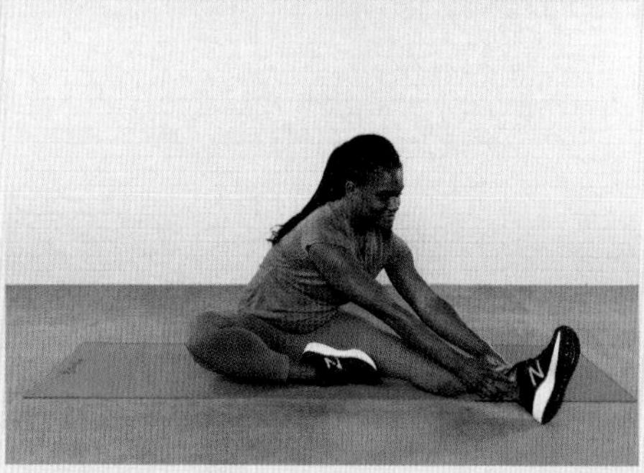

Hip mobility/ROM	Seated butterfly stretch (Figure 11-56)	Body weight	1 x 15–30 seconds

FIGURE 11-56
Seated butterfly stretch

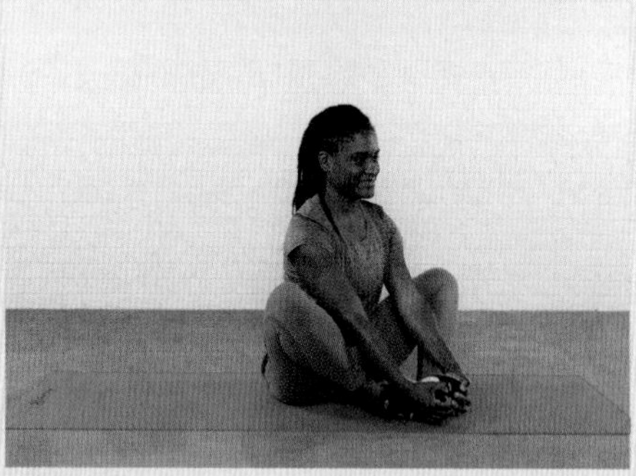

* = Movement pattern, technique, skill, recovery, etc.

† = Weight, load, speed, zone, etc.

‡ = Sets, repetitions, duration, rest, etc.

Programming Notes: Progress Muscular Training by increasing to 15 repetitions and two sets, and then introduce new multiplanar exercises and advance to Load/Speed Training, when appropriate. Initial Cardiorespiratory Training program focus is Fitness Training, with intervals introduced at and just above VT1, progressing work intervals up to 90 seconds and the work-to-rest interval to a ratio of 1:2 (e.g., 90 seconds:180 seconds). As Valerie moves closer to her goal event, introduce intervals at or above VT2 through Performance Training, based on her progress.

Note: HR = Heart rate; VT1 = First ventilatory threshold; VT2 = Second ventilatory threshold; ROM = Range of motion

Using the ACE ABC Approach allowed the personal trainer to not only build rapport with Valerie, but also gather relevant information to collaborate on designing an effective exercise program. This approach will continue to be used throughout the client–personal trainer relationship as Valerie progresses from this initial exercise program and moves closer to her goal event in 18 weeks.

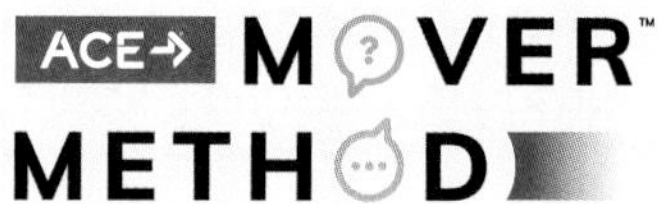

Warehouse Worker with a History of Shoulder Problems

Phillip is 35 years old and has spent the past 15 years working as a warehouse operator at a large distribution center. His daily functions include driving a forklift and manually lifting and placing heavy objects onto overhead shelving units. Phillip has a history of work-related shoulder pain from lifting boxes overhead. He completed six weeks of physical therapy per his doctor's recommendation for the treatment of shoulder impingement and was under the care of his physician during that time. Phillip has been cleared for exercise as tolerated by his doctor and has been pain-free for over a year. He would like to maintain the improvements he made in physical therapy and improve his overall physical health to reduce the risk of recurring shoulder issues.

ACE→ ABC APPROACH™

The following scenario is an example of how the ACE ABC Approach can be used to work with Phillip. This conversation style is used to discover the information needed to create and implement an enjoyable exercise program that supports his goals and promotes adherence.

Ask: Asking powerful open-ended questions will help to identify what Phillip would like to accomplish by working with a personal trainer.

Personal Trainer: Hi, Phillip. It's nice to meet you. Thank you for taking the time to meet with me today. What would you like to achieve by working with a personal trainer?

Client: I work in a warehouse, and my job is labor-intensive. I'm always moving, lifting boxes, and squatting down to pick up things. Over the years, I've had a variety of aches and pains. About two years ago, I started having shoulder pain that got progressively worse, and it began to affect my job. I went to the doctor and was diagnosed with shoulder impingement in both shoulders. I completed six weeks of physical therapy that focused on fixing my shoulders and have been pain-free for about one year. Now I want to work with you to maintain the strength and flexibility I gained in physical therapy so I can be productive at work and enjoy my personal life. Also, even though I am active at work, I would like to become healthier and exercise more.

Personal Trainer: Maintaining the integrity of your shoulders is important to you, as well as improving your overall physical health.

Client: Keeping my shoulders healthy is my top priority, yes. I learned a lot in physical therapy, and it made me aware of the reasons to take better care of myself. I want to include some cardio in my routine, but during my sessions working with you, I want to improve my shoulder flexibility and strength. I would also like to make sure that the rest of my body stays healthy and feeling good.

Break down barriers: Asking more open-ended questions will help the personal trainer discover if any potential obstacles may get in the way of Phillip reaching his goals.

Personal Trainer: What have your past experiences with adopting healthier habits been like?

Client: Over the years, I've tried making exercise a regular part of my routine but usually feel too tired to do anything after work. I've tried some diets in the past, but not for long because they required too much work and I had to stop eating the foods I like. I've always thought about exercising more but finding the time to do it is another story. However, I have surprised myself, and I've recently made some healthy changes that are now a part of my routine.

Personal Trainer: Restrictive diets and finding a time to exercise that works for you has been a challenge. You are feeling motivated now because you have been able to make some healthy changes. How are you able to be successful with the healthy behaviors you do now?

Client: The good things I am doing now are part of my daily routine, and I can stick with these changes because of how important they are to me. I was eating a lot of junk food while at work and knew that it was not good for me. I replaced the junk food with healthy snacks on most days. I never thought I could make this change, but it is important to me, and it doesn't require that much work.

Personal Trainer: What do you need to do more of to continue moving closer to your goals?

Client: I've already made up my mind that my health is a priority. Working with a personal trainer to maintain my shoulder health is crucial to my success at work. My biggest concern is that I won't have the time to exercise and that I'll be too tired after work. With physical therapy, I was approved by my employer to go to the appointments while on the clock. Now that I have completed therapy, exercise needs to happen on my own time.

Collaborate: Working together with the client on goals and solutions is the next step and allows the client to work toward what he would like to accomplish. Even though the personal trainer is the expert in exercise program design, Phillip will play a contributory role in the development of the program.

Personal Trainer: Being tired after work and finding the time to exercise are concerns, but your health is important and a priority right now. How do you see your program unfolding over the next few months?

Client: I can see myself working with you three times per week, every week. I want to try working out in the mornings before I have a long, tiring day at work. I also would like to have a structured plan for exercise I can do on my own. A key to the success of my program will be to find the right amount of exercise to do so that I reach my goals and still have the energy to do my job.

Personal Trainer: You want to concentrate on your health by working with me three times per week, with a focus on shoulder health. You would like to exercise in the mornings before work and having a structured plan will help keep you on track. It is also essential that the intensity of your workouts does not impact your job performance. How will you move forward today?

Client: I'd like to start working with you next week, and for the rest of this week, I'll get up earlier at the time I would need to for the gym and see how challenging that is for me. I'll also leave for work early and drive past the gym to see what traffic is like at that time of day. What do you think our next steps should be?

Personal Trainer: We know what you would like to achieve and what you need to be successful, and we can schedule a day and time to begin working together next week. I'll create an exercise program that we implement together, being mindful of intensity and duration so as not to affect your job performance.

Because Phillip is not consistently performing regular cardiorespiratory exercise, he will begin in the Base Training phase of the ACE IFT Model. This means that no initial cardiorespiratory assessments are needed and intensity will be based on the talk test. He will work at a tolerable intensity and duration while moving toward being able to perform bouts of at least 20 minutes at a moderate intensity on at least three days per week. During the first scheduled session, Phillip demonstrated that he can perform exercises across the five primary movement patterns without compromising postural or joint stability, so he will begin in the Load/Speed Training phase of the ACE IFT Model, where the focus will be on applying external loads to movement that create a need for increased force production. Elements of Functional and Movement Training will be included throughout all exercise sessions, while working to find a balance between the work done in the gym and the physical demands of Philip's job.

This interaction between Phillip and his personal trainer is an example of how the ACE ABC Approach is used to uncover client information to design and implement the appropriate exercise program. Based on the information provided by Phillip, the personal trainer's experience, and completed assessments, the initial program in Figure 11-57 was created.

FIGURE 11-57
ACE IFT Model Exercise Programming Template—Warehouse Worker with a History of Shoulder Problems

Client Name: Phillip, a 35-year-old warehouse worker with a history of shoulder impingement issues

Client Goals: Improve overall strength, improve shoulder mobility and strength to reduce the risk of future impingement, and establish a cardiorespiratory base to improve upon as he works toward increased cardiorespiratory fitness

Client-centered Considerations: Completed six weeks of physical therapy; pain-free for one year; performs daily labor-intensive work

Frequency (active and rest days): Total-body Muscular and Cardiorespiratory Training 3 days/week with one rest day between workouts

Cardiorespiratory Training Phase:

[X] **Base Training**
Focus on moderate-intensity exercise below the talk test threshold

[ ] **Fitness Training**
Build on Base Training through the introduction of zone 2 intervals performed from VT1 to just below VT2

[ ] **Performance Training**
Build on Fitness Training and introduce zone 3 intervals performed at and above VT2

Muscular Training Phase:

[ ] **Functional Training**
Focus on establishing postural stability and kinetic chain mobility

[ ] **Movement Training**
Focus on training the five primary movement patterns while incorporating Functional Training exercises in the warm-up and cool-down

[X] **Load/Speed Training**
Focus on load and speed goals while including Functional Training exercises in the warm-up and cool-down and loading primary movement patterns

Continued on the next page

Exercise Goal*	Exercise/Exercise Mode	Intensity†	Volume‡
Warm-up: Prepare the muscles and joints for muscular and cardiorespiratory training			
Warm-up muscles and joints	Walk on treadmill	Zone 1 – below talk test threshold	5 minutes
Scapular stabilization	Scapular retraction and depression (shoulder packing) (Figure 11-58)	Body weight	1 set x 8 repetitions

FIGURE 11-58 Scapular retraction and depression (shoulder packing)

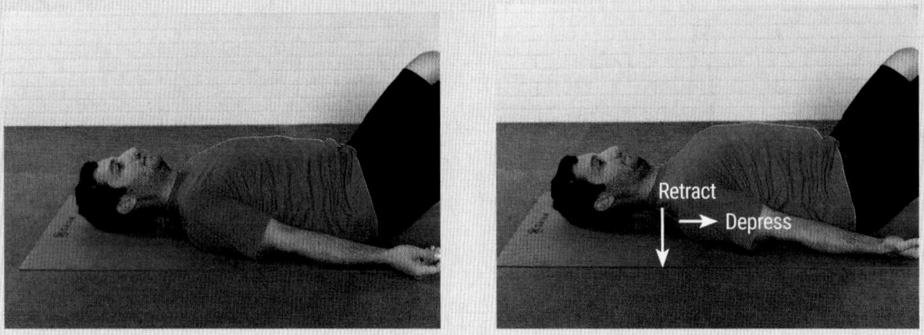

Exercise Goal*	Exercise/Exercise Mode	Intensity†	Volume‡
Shoulder mobility	Supine shoulder flexion (Figure 11-59)	Body weight	1 set x 8 repetitions

FIGURE 11-59 Supine shoulder flexion

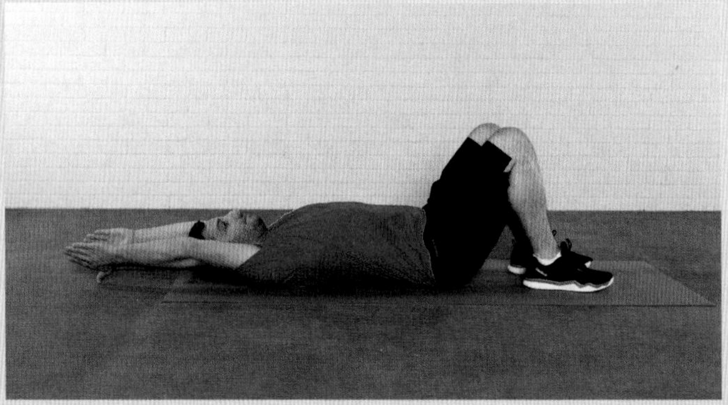

Exercise Goal*	Exercise/Exercise Mode	Intensity†	Volume‡
Shoulder mobility	Supine internal and external shoulder rotation (Figure 11-60)	Body weight	1 set x 8 repetitions

FIGURE 11-60 Supine internal and external shoulder rotation

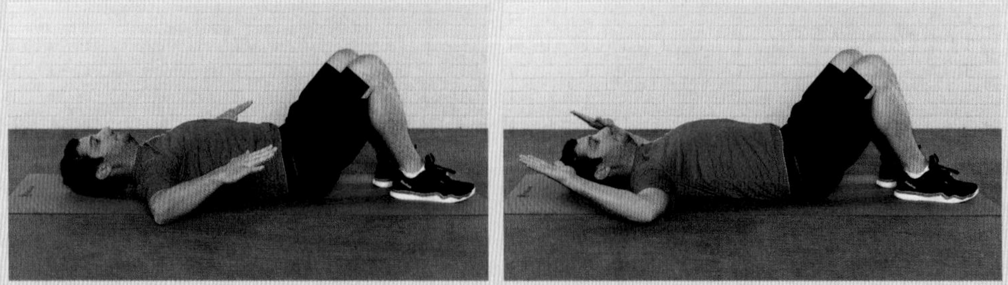

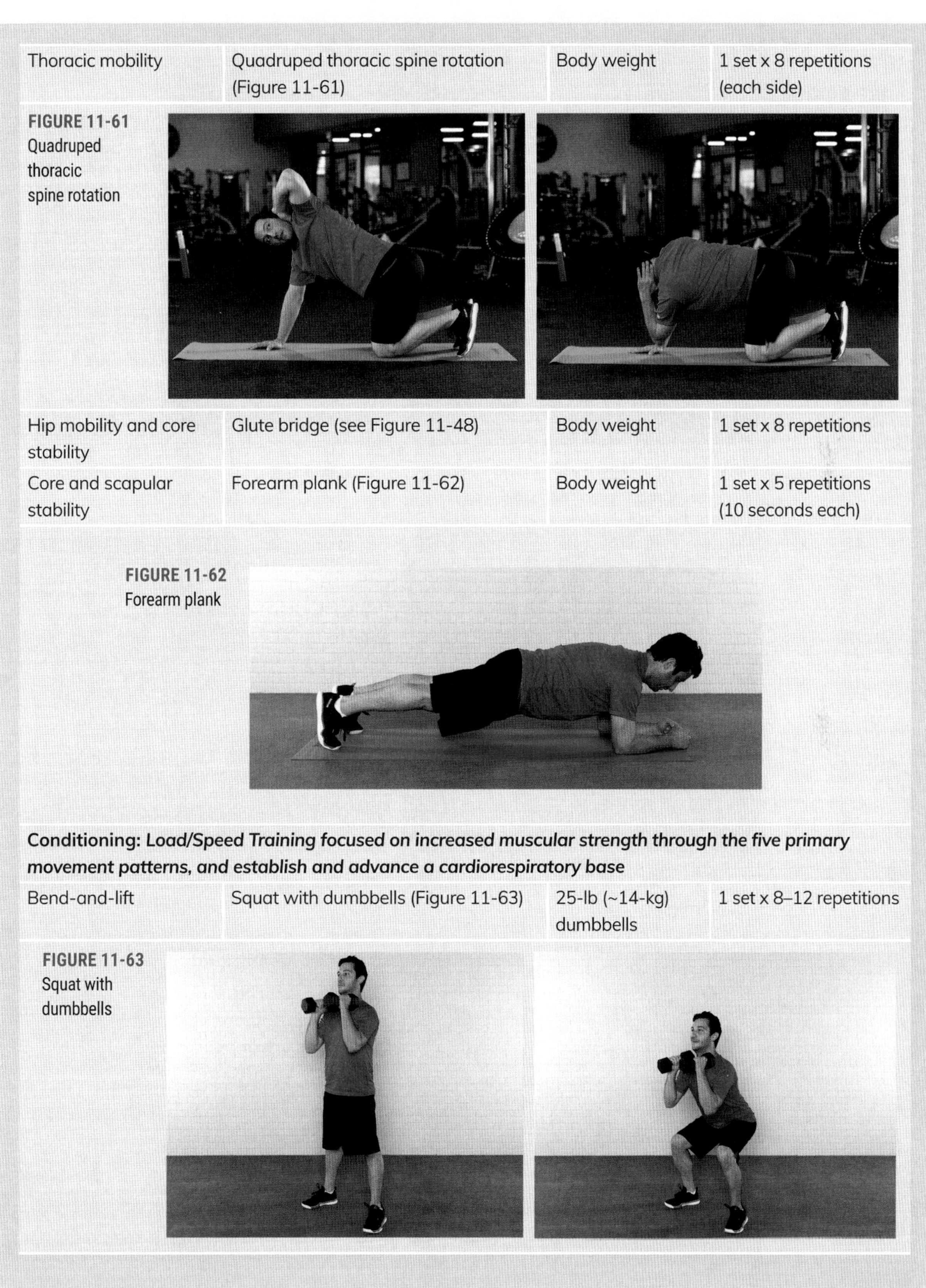

Thoracic mobility	Quadruped thoracic spine rotation (Figure 11-61)	Body weight	1 set x 8 repetitions (each side)

FIGURE 11-61
Quadruped thoracic spine rotation

Hip mobility and core stability	Glute bridge (see Figure 11-48)	Body weight	1 set x 8 repetitions
Core and scapular stability	Forearm plank (Figure 11-62)	Body weight	1 set x 5 repetitions (10 seconds each)

FIGURE 11-62
Forearm plank

Conditioning: *Load/Speed Training focused on increased muscular strength through the five primary movement patterns, and establish and advance a cardiorespiratory base*			
Bend-and-lift	Squat with dumbbells (Figure 11-63)	25-lb (~14-kg) dumbbells	1 set x 8–12 repetitions

FIGURE 11-63
Squat with dumbbells

Continued on the next page

Push/horizontal shoulder adduction	Seated cable chest press (Figure 11-64)	40-lb (~18-kg)	1 set x 8–12 repetitions (each side)

FIGURE 11-64
Seated cable chest press

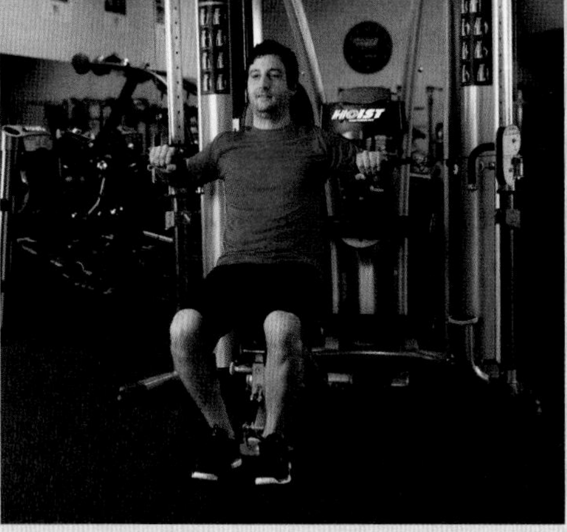

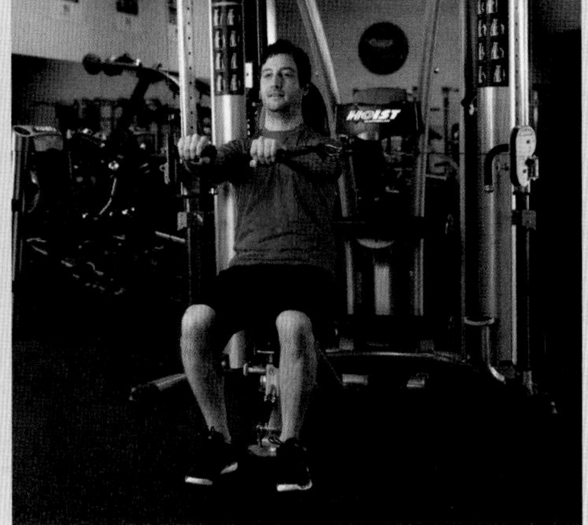

Pull/shoulder extension	Standing single-arm cable row (Figure 11-65)	40 lb (~18-kg)	1 set x 8–12 repetitions (each side)

FIGURE 11-65
Standing single-arm cable row

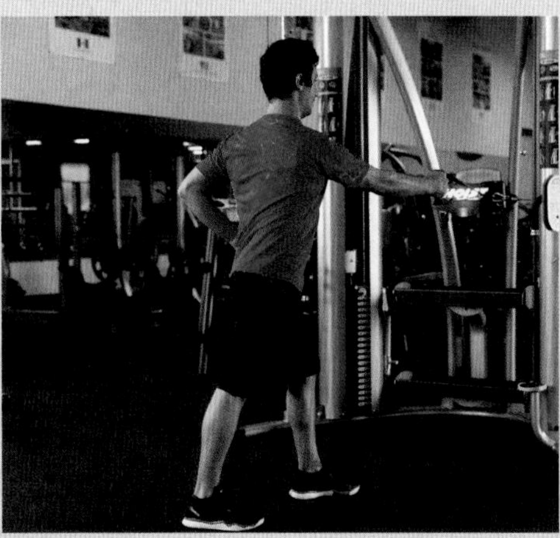

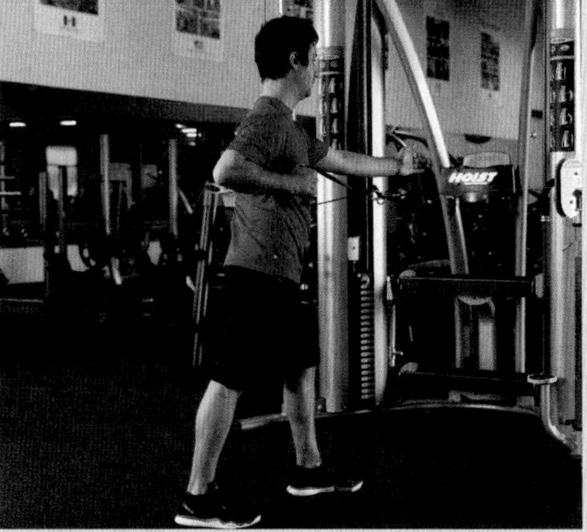

Single-leg in sagittal plane	Step-up with dumbbells (Figure 11-66)	15-lb (~7-kg) dumbbells	1 set x 8–12 repetitions (each side)

FIGURE 11-66
Step-up with dumbbells

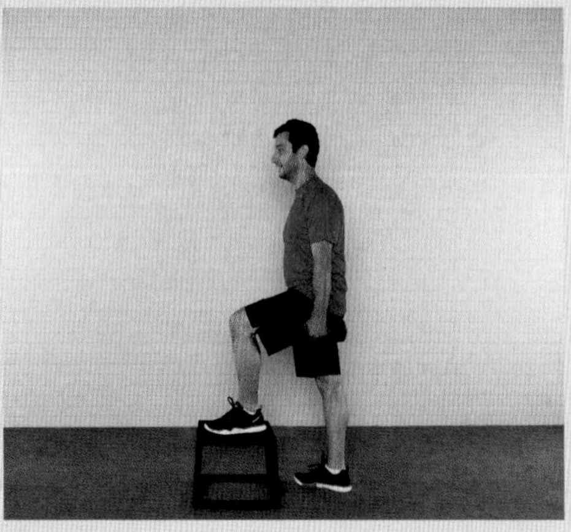

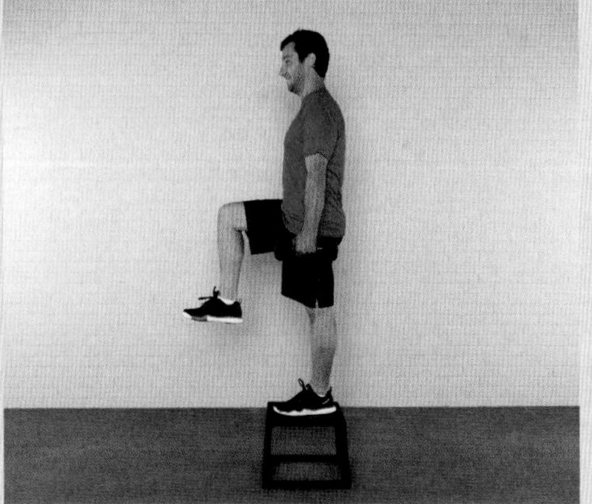

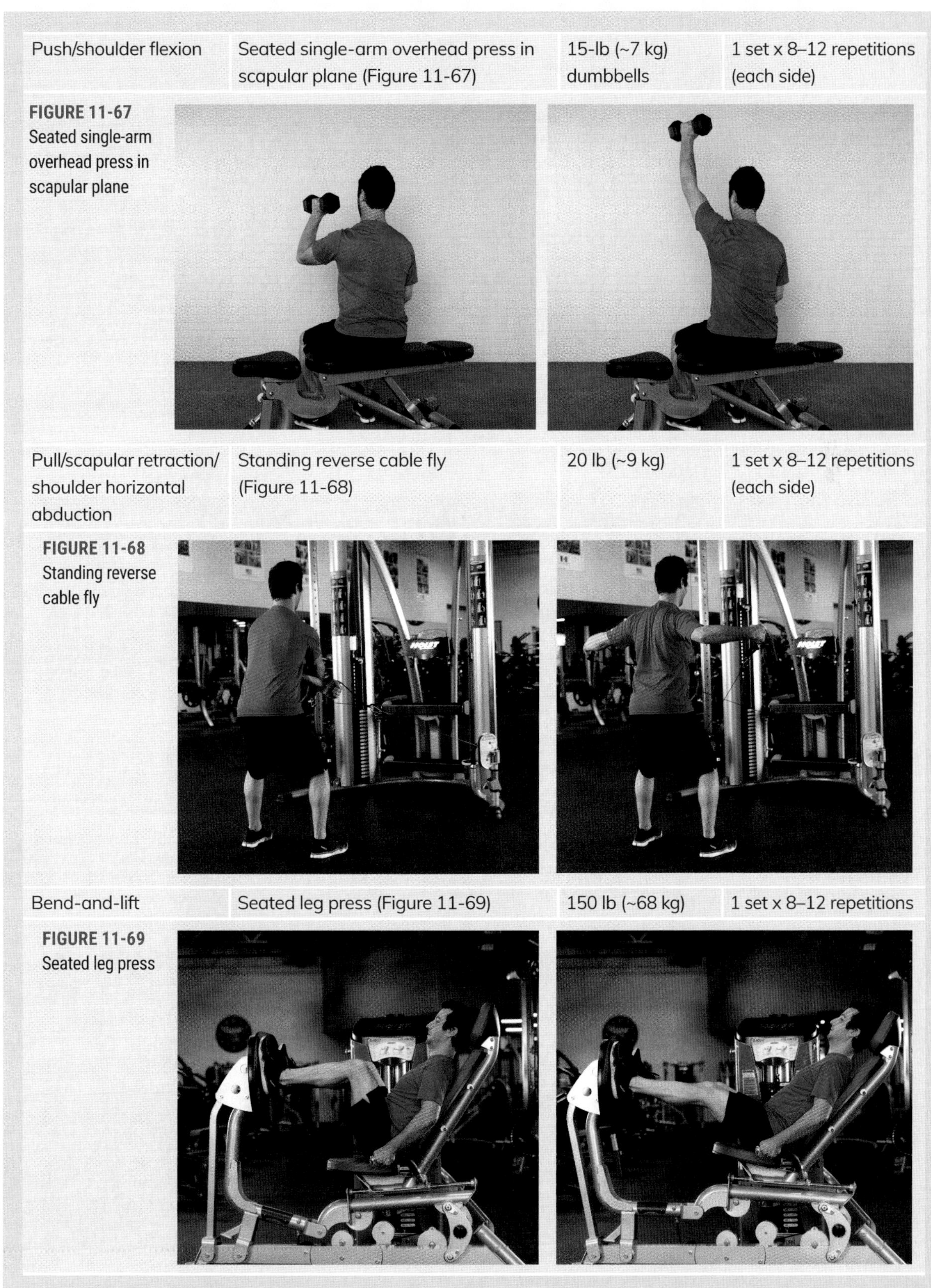

Push/shoulder flexion	Seated single-arm overhead press in scapular plane (Figure 11-67)	15-lb (~7 kg) dumbbells	1 set x 8–12 repetitions (each side)

FIGURE 11-67
Seated single-arm overhead press in scapular plane

Pull/scapular retraction/ shoulder horizontal abduction	Standing reverse cable fly (Figure 11-68)	20 lb (~9 kg)	1 set x 8–12 repetitions (each side)

FIGURE 11-68
Standing reverse cable fly

Bend-and-lift	Seated leg press (Figure 11-69)	150 lb (~68 kg)	1 set x 8–12 repetitions

FIGURE 11-69
Seated leg press

Continued on the next page

Core rotation/shoulder pull	Standing cable wood chop (Figure 11-70)	30 lb (~14 kg)	1 set x 8–12 repetitions (each side)
FIGURE 11-70 Standing cable wood chop			
Core rotation/shoulder push	Standing cable hay baler (Figure 11-71)	30 lb (~14 kg)	1 set x 8–12 repetitions (each side)
FIGURE 11-71 Standing cable hay baler			
Single-leg lateral movement	Side lunge (see Figure 11-45)	Body weight	1 set x 8–12 repetitions (each side)
Shoulder rotation	Standing cable shoulder internal rotation (Figure 11-72)	10 lb (~5 kg)	1 set x 8 repetitions (each side)
FIGURE 11-72 Standing cable shoulder internal rotation			

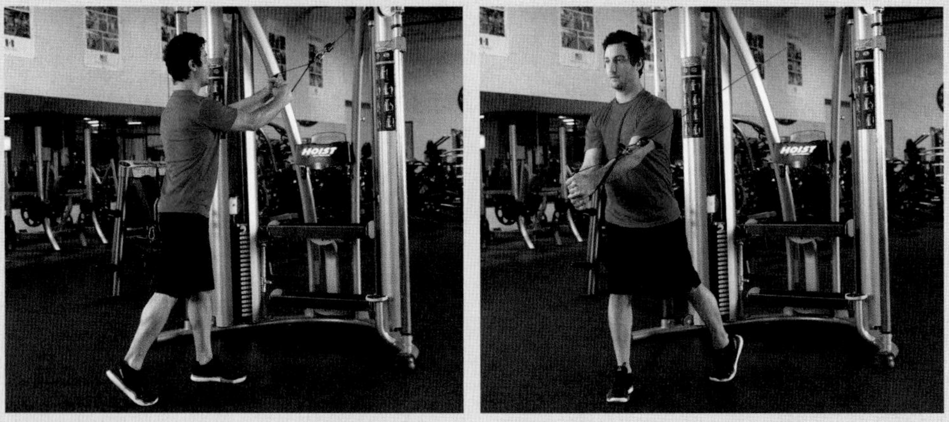

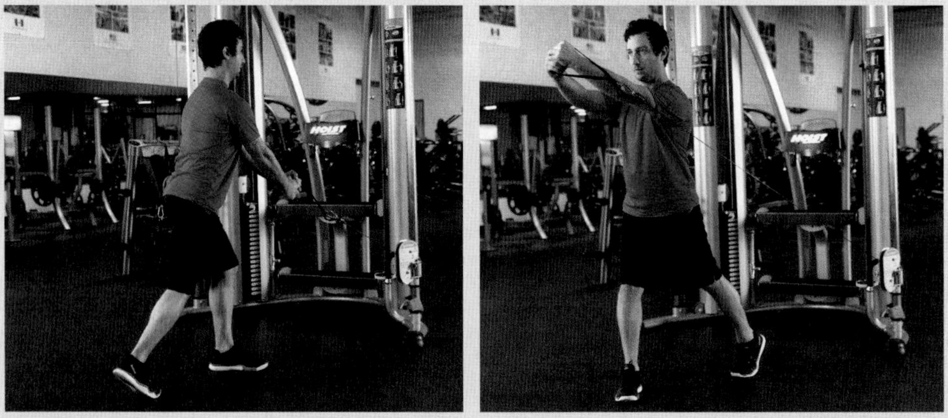

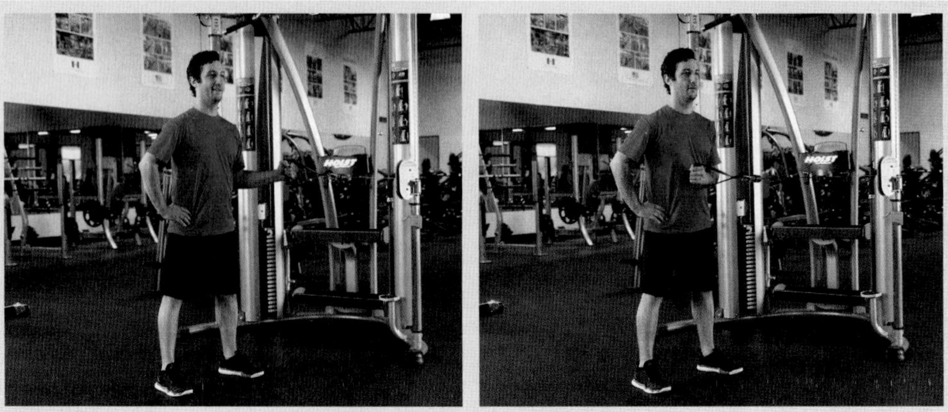

Shoulder rotation	Standing cable shoulder external rotation (Figure 11-73)	10 lb (~5 kg)	1 set x 8 repetitions (each side)

FIGURE 11-73
Standing cable shoulder external rotation

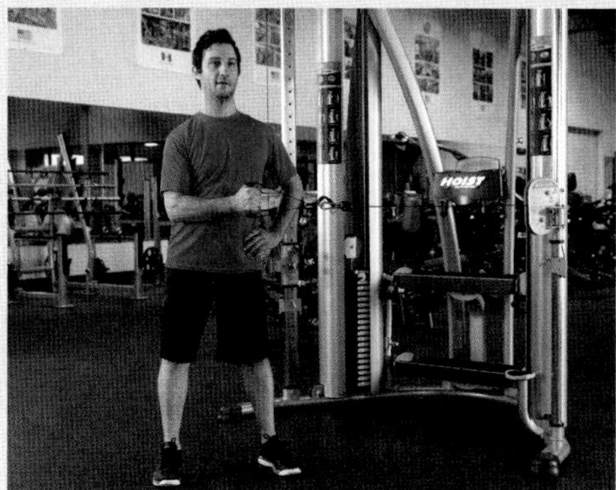

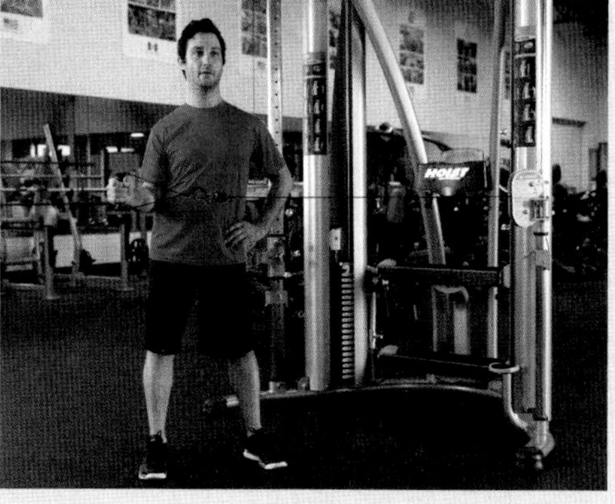

Cardiorespiratory base training	Stationary bike or elliptical trainer	Zone 1 – below talk test threshold	15 minutes
Cool-down: ***Active recovery allowing for reduced HR and core temperature while working work on flexibility***			
Shoulder mobility/ROM	Anterior shoulder and chest wall stretch (Figure 11-74)	Body weight	1 x 15–30 seconds (each side)

FIGURE 11-74
Anterior shoulder and chest wall stretch

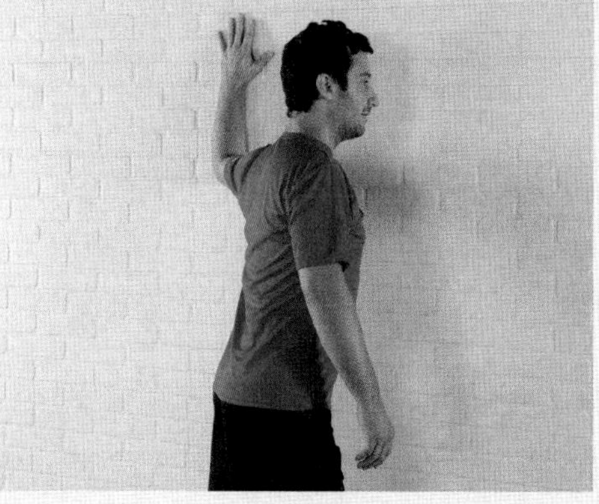

Shoulder mobility/ROM	Overhead triceps stretch (Figure 11-75)	Body weight	1 x 15–30 seconds (each side)

FIGURE 11-75
Overhead triceps stretch

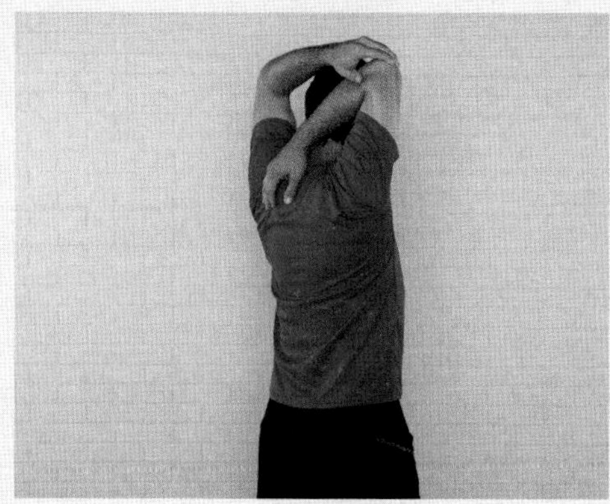

Continued on the next page

Hip mobility/ROM	Kneeling hip flexor stretch (see Figure 11-54)	Body weight	1 x 15–30 seconds (each side)
Spinal mobility/ROM	Supine spinal twist (see Figure 11-52)	Body weight	1 x 15–30 seconds (each side)
Hip mobility/ROM	Piriformis figure-4 stretch (see Figure 11-53)	Body weight	1 x 15–30 seconds (each side)
Hip mobility/ROM	Supine hamstrings stretch (Figure 11-76)	Body weight	1 x 15–30 seconds (each side)

FIGURE 11-76
Supine hamstrings stretch

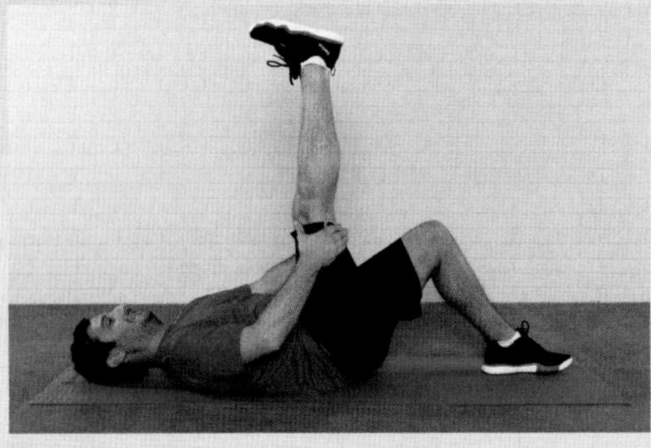

Spinal mobility	Child's pose (Figure 11-77)	Body weight	1 x 30 seconds

FIGURE 11-77
Child's pose

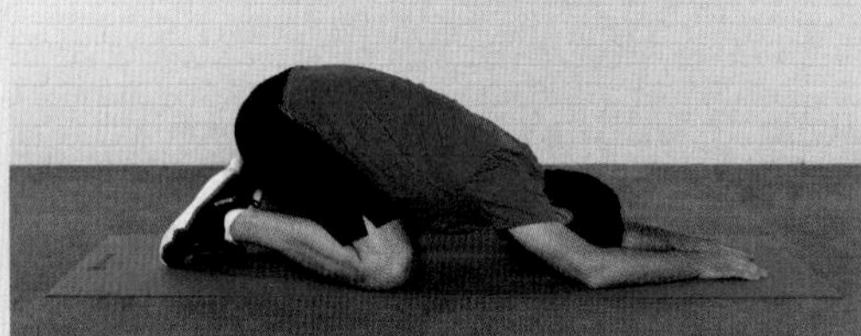

* = Movement pattern, technique, skill, recovery, etc.
† = Weight, load, speed, zone, etc.
‡ = Sets, repetitions, duration, rest, etc.
Programming Notes: Include exercises for scapular stability, shoulder mobility, strength of the rotator cuff and muscles acting on the scapula, and postural mobility and stability to help prevent future shoulder impingement issues. Progress Muscular Training over time by increasing resistance, adding a second set, and introducing new exercises. Progress Cardiorespiratory Training from Base to Fitness Training by extending duration gradually to at least 20 minutes (no more than 10% at a time), and then moving to cardiorespiratory Fitness Training by first completing the VT1 talk test and adding short intervals at and above the HR at VT1.
Note: ROM = Range of motion; HR = Heart rate

In this scenario, you can see how the ACE Mover Method philosophy helps build the client–personal trainer relationship. Further, the communication skills used in the ACE ABC Approach were called upon to help design an effective exercise program following the ACE IFT Model that takes the client's goals, concerns, and values into consideration. The ACE ABC Approach will continue to be used as the relationship unfolds and as the client progresses through the phases of the ACE IFT Model.

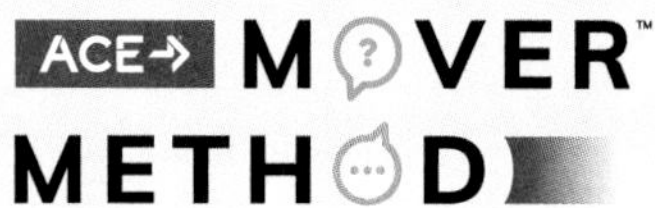

Physically Inactive Office Worker with a Weight-loss Goal

Clare is a 60-year-old office worker who spends eight hours per day seated at a desk and does not currently perform any moderate- or vigorous-intensity physical activity. She has been contemplating becoming more physically active for the past six months and has yet to act. Clare intends to move forward with her plan for becoming more active and has support from her doctor, who encouraged working toward a 20-pound (9.1-kg) weight loss goal. Clare is apparently healthy and has been cleared by her physician for exercise as tolerated without any limitations. Clare has signed up for an initial session with a personal trainer. She is eager to get started so that she is in better shape and can fully enjoy her impending retirement.

ACE→ ABC APPROACH

The following scenario is an example of how the ACE ABC Approach can be used when partnering with Clare to design and implement a structured exercise program to promote enjoyment and adherence.

Ask: Asking powerful open-ended questions during the initial session allows the personal trainer to identify what Clare wants to achieve by working with a personal trainer and what activities she enjoys.

Personal Trainer: Clare, it's nice to meet you, and thank you for taking the time to schedule this session with me. Tell me more about what you would like to achieve by working with a personal trainer.

Client: I made up my mind that I need to start exercising. I'm hoping that working with you will help me stay focused, structured, and safe, while having fun. I used to be very active when I was younger and I enjoyed walking, playing sports, hiking, and spending as much time outdoors as possible. I'm a little embarrassed to admit it, but for the past 25 years, I have not done much physical activity at all.

Personal Trainer: You've decided that now is the time to focus on improving your physical fitness. A fun, safe, and structured exercise program is important to you. What value does fun bring to an exercise program for you?

Client: If I'm going to stick with an exercise program, it needs to have activities that I enjoy. For the past six months, I've been trying to exercise, but I keep coming up with excuses for not doing it. At this point in my life, it seems like a chore instead of something fun. I think if I'm having fun and enjoying what I'm doing, it will be easier to think of reasons to exercise instead of reasons to skip it.

Personal Trainer: Any exercise program you do must be fun so that you look forward to it. You mentioned being active when you were younger. What types of activities have you done in the past that you enjoyed?

Client: When I was younger, I liked playing soccer, hiking, and swimming. It never felt like exercise because I was having fun. What I want right now is to feel stronger and be able to walk longer distances without getting tired. I know that it's possible if I can stay consistent.

Break down barriers: Follow up with more open-ended questions to keep the conversation moving forward in a positive direction. The focus of these questions will be to uncover any potential barriers that Clare may face that could stand in the way of her reaching her goals.

Personal Trainer: Consistency will be the key to achieving this goal. Tell me about your current level of physical activity and what, if anything, might prevent you from being consistent?

Client: Currently, my life is filled with the same routine every day. I wake up, have coffee, go to work, sit for eight hours, come home, eat dinner, watch tv, and go to bed. It's my lack of physical activity that concerns me the most. One thing that may get in the way, besides not having fun, would be feeling discouraged. I still remember what it felt like to be young, strong, and athletic. I tend to be hard on myself when I don't feel that way anymore. I know I can make the time to exercise. I just need to stay motivated and consistent.

Personal Trainer: You are very aware of the barriers you could encounter—inconsistency, lack of motivation, and being discouraged. But if exercise is fun, safe, and enjoyable, you believe you'll be able to maintain consistency. What will help you to feel encouraged about your progress?

Client: Being able to see progress toward my goals would be encouraging. For instance, if we could gauge my level of enjoyment with different exercises and track if I'm getting stronger and fitter, that will help. I know with weight loss we would expect to see changes on the scale, and that motivates me.

Collaborate: Now that the personal trainer knows more about Clare, her barriers, and what she would like to achieve, it is time to move forward with setting specific goals and establishing next steps.

Personal Trainer: Being as specific as possible, how will you know when you have achieved success?

Client: Once exercise becomes part of my weekly routine, and I start looking forward to being active, I will know that the right activities are in place. Losing the 20 pounds (9.1 kg) that my doctor suggested will be a success and being able to walk without getting tired will tell me I'm on the right track. Seeing improvements in strength and cardio will also be a success for me.

Personal Trainer: There are many ways to build on your success in this program, and we can collaborate on a plan for tracking your progress. How will you move forward today?

Client: I'd like to get started working with you as soon as possible. Today, I plan on getting appropriate exercise shoes and clothing. To start, I'd like to meet with you three days per week for an hour, and perhaps discuss some suggestions for being active throughout my workday as the program unfolds.

Personal Trainer: Yes, that is all very doable! I appreciate you sharing so much with me today and I look forward to working with you. Based on our discussion, I will develop a program that includes ways to track your progress and emphasizes activities you might find to be fun. This initial program will be a work in progress that enables us to make sure you're enjoying what we are doing and that we are monitoring the right information. Please feel free to let me know at any time if something I've included isn't working for you. I can't stress enough that you are steering the ship on this journey.

Because Clare is currently inactive and not doing any physical activity beyond basic movements of daily living, she will begin in the Base Training phase of the Cardiorespiratory Training component of the ACE IFT Model at an intensity below the talk test threshold. During Clare's initial exercise session, the personal trainer had her perform a variety of warm-up exercises covering the five primary movement patterns and determined that her initial Muscular Training programming will begin in the Functional Training phase. No muscular or cardiorespiratory assessments are needed at this point and early programming will focus on enjoyment, building a cardiorespiratory base, establishing postural stability, improving kinetic chain mobility, and making physical activity a regular part of her life.

Using the ACE ABC Approach, Clare and her personal trainer have partnered to uncover what Clare would like to achieve and what she needs to be successful. Clare plays a critical role in the client–personal trainer relationship and will continue to do so as the relationship develops. Based on the initial information gathered, Clare's personal trainer developed the program shown in Figure 11-78.

FIGURE 11-78
ACE IFT Model Exercise Programming Template—Physically Inactive Office Worker with a Weight-loss Goal

Client Name: Clare, a 60-year-old, physically inactive office worker with overweight

Client Goals: Begin exercise program to improve health, lose 20 pounds (9.1 kg), walk for longer distances, and feel stronger like when she was young

Client-centered Considerations: Activity as tolerated; eager to get started; previously enjoyed soccer, hiking, and swimming

Frequency (active and rest days): Total-body Muscular and Cardiorespiratory Training 3 days/week, with at least one rest day in between

Cardiorespiratory Training Phase:

- [X] **Base Training**
  Focus on moderate-intensity exercise below the talk test threshold
- [ ] **Fitness Training**
  Build on Base Training through the introduction of zone 2 intervals performed from VT1 to just below VT2
- [ ] **Performance Training**
  Build on Fitness Training and introduce zone 3 intervals performed at and above VT2

Muscular Training Phase:

- [X] **Functional Training**
  Focus on establishing postural stability and kinetic chain mobility
- [ ] **Movement Training**
  Focus on training the five primary movement patterns while incorporating Functional Training exercises in the warm-up and cool-down
- [ ] **Load/Speed Training**
  Focus on load and speed goals while including Functional Training exercises in the warm-up and cool-down and loading primary movement patterns

Continued on the next page

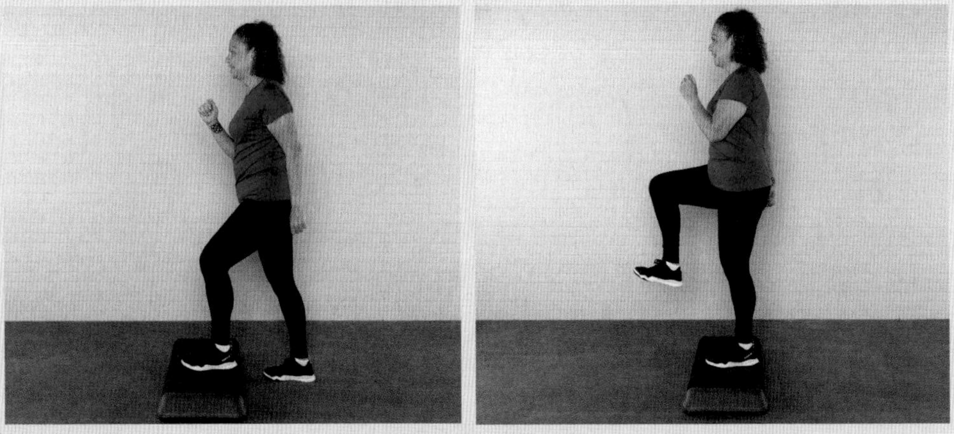

Exercise Goal*	Exercise/Exercise Mode	Intensity†	Volume‡
Warm-up: *Prepare the muscles and joints for Muscular and Cardiorespiratory Training*			
Warm-up muscles and joints	Walk on treadmill	Zone 1 – below talk test threshold	35 minutes
Scapular stabilization	Scapular retraction and depression (shoulder packing) (see Figure 11-58)	Body weight	1 set x 8 repetitions
Hip mobility	Hip hinge (see Figure 11-33)	Body weight	1 set x 8 repetitions
Spinal mobility	Cat-cow (see Figure 11-34)	Body weight	1 set x 5 repetitions
Thoracic mobility	Quadruped thoracic spine rotation (see Figure 11-61)	Body weight	1 set x 5 repetitions (each side)
Conditioning: *Functional Training focused on improved postural stability, kinetic-chain mobility, and building a cardiorespiratory base*			
Single-leg stability and balance	Step-up (4-inch step) (Figure 11-79)	Body weight	1 set x 10–15 repetitions (each side)
Scapular stability/ shoulder mobility	Stability ball shoulder stabilization – I, Y, T, W (see Figure 11-44)	Body weight	1 set x 10–15 repetitions
Double-leg stability	Quarter squat – with external support if needed (Figure 11-80)	Body weight	1 set x 10–15 repetitions

FIGURE 11-79
Step-up

FIGURE 11-80
Quarter squat

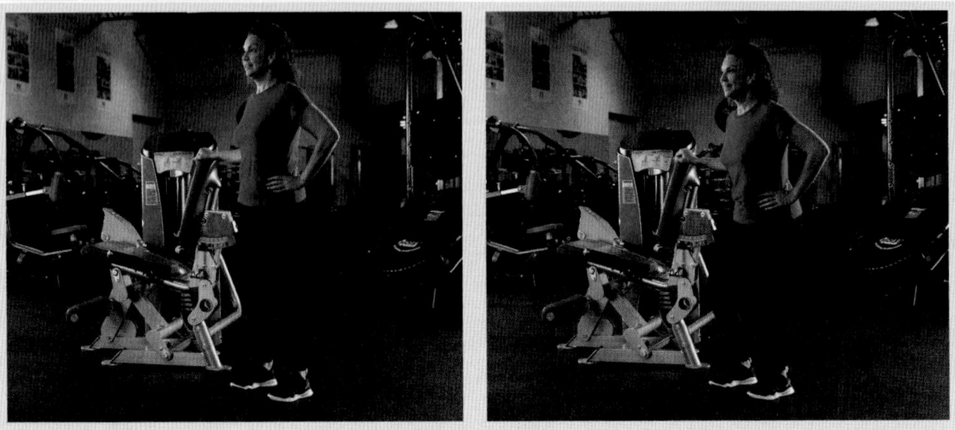

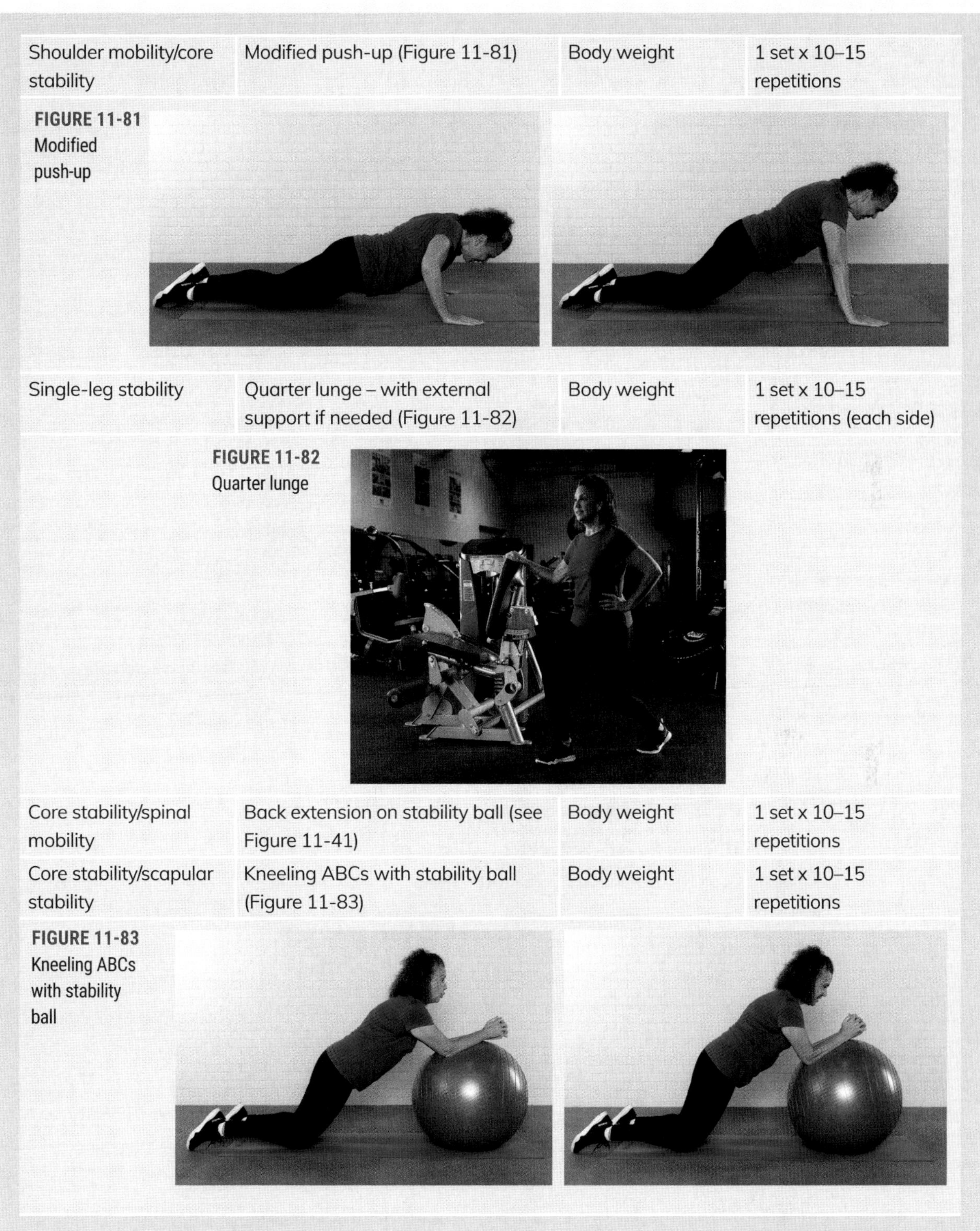

Shoulder mobility/core stability	Modified push-up (Figure 11-81)	Body weight	1 set x 10–15 repetitions

FIGURE 11-81
Modified push-up

Single-leg stability	Quarter lunge – with external support if needed (Figure 11-82)	Body weight	1 set x 10–15 repetitions (each side)

FIGURE 11-82
Quarter lunge

Core stability/spinal mobility	Back extension on stability ball (see Figure 11-41)	Body weight	1 set x 10–15 repetitions
Core stability/scapular stability	Kneeling ABCs with stability ball (Figure 11-83)	Body weight	1 set x 10–15 repetitions

FIGURE 11-83
Kneeling ABCs with stability ball

Continued on the next page

Spinal mobility/core stability	Modified curl-up with one leg straight, one leg bent (Figure 11-84)	Body weight	1 set x 10–15 repetitions

FIGURE 11-84
Modified curl-up

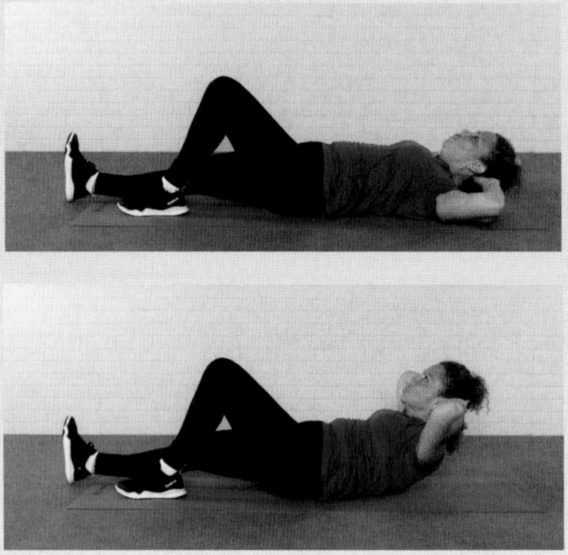

Core stability/shoulder and hip mobility	Bird dog (see Figure 11-36)	Body weight	1 set x 5 repetitions (each side)
Core stability	Side bridge – bent knee (Figure 11-85)	Body weight	1 set x 5 repetitions (5 seconds each) (each side)

FIGURE 11-85
Side bridge – bent knee

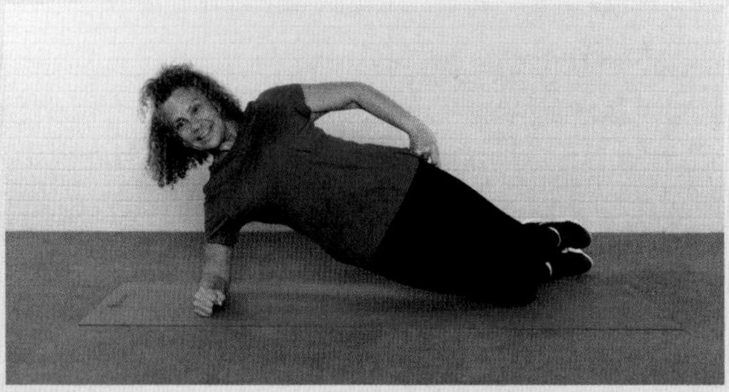

Cardiorespiratory base training	Walking on treadmill	Zone 1 – below talk test threshold	10 minutes
Cool-down: Active recovery allowing for reduced HR and core temperature while working on flexibility			
Shoulder mobility/ROM	Anterior shoulder and chest wall stretch (see Figure 11-74)	Body weight	1 x 15–30 seconds (each side)
Shoulder mobility/ROM	Overhead triceps stretch (see Figure 11-75)	Body weight	1 x 15–30 seconds (each side)

Ankle mobility/ROM	Standing calf stretch (Figure 11-86)	Body weight	1 x 15–30 seconds (each side)

FIGURE 11-86
Standing calf stretch

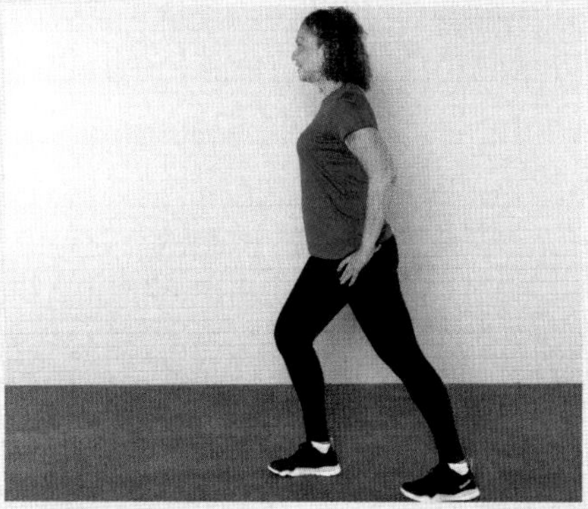

Hip mobility/ROM	Side-lying hip flexor stretch (Figure 11-87)	Body weight	1 x 15–30 seconds (each side)

FIGURE 11-87
Side-lying hip flexor stretch

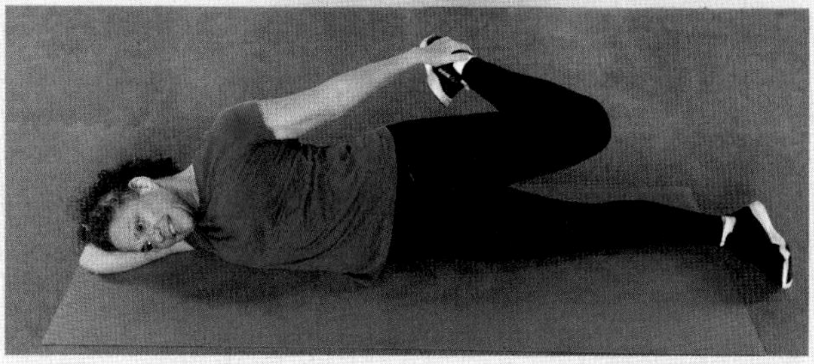

Hip mobility/ROM	Supine hamstrings stretch (see Figure 11-76)	Body weight	1 x 15–30 seconds (each side)

* = Movement pattern, technique, skill, recovery, etc.

† = Weight, load, speed, zone, etc.

‡ = Sets, repetitions, duration, rest, etc.

Programming Notes: Initial program is focused on Functional Training to improve postural stability and joint mobility. Progress Muscular Training to 15 repetitions per set, then transition to Movement Training with body-weight exercises once good postural stability and kinetic-chain mobility is established. Progress Cardiorespiratory Training by extending duration by 5 to 10% per week with a goal of walking up to 20 to 30 minutes per session. Add 2% incline to treadmill walking for short (1 to 2 minute) segments with 3- to 6-minute recovery at 0% incline, once client can consistently walk 25 or more minutes comfortably. Add sport-like exercises based on preferences noted in initial interview once good postural stability, kinetic-chain mobility, and movement patterns are established.

Note: HR = Heart rate; ROM = Range of motion

In this scenario, the client–personal trainer relationship develops during the initial meeting and leads to a point where an introductory exercise program can be implemented. Collaboration allows the client to take an active role in her program. As the client becomes more physically active, the ACE ABC Approach will be used as often as possible to identify and plan for obstacles as they arise and ensure the client remains an active partner in progressing a plan to assist her in reaching her health-related goals.

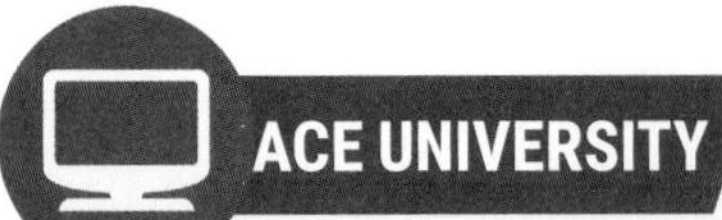

If your study program includes the ACE University, visit www.ACEfitness.org/MyACE and log in to your My ACE Account to take full advantage of the ACE Personal Trainer Study Program and online guided study experience.

A variety of media to support and expand on the material in this text is provided to facilitate learning and best prepare you for the ACE Personal Trainer Certification exam and a career as a personal trainer.

SUMMARY

Evidence-based practice is a client-centered approach to optimal decision making with regard to all aspects of exercise programming. Accordingly, evidence-based practice is a valuable skill for personal trainers to acquire and subsequently apply with current and future clients. Personal trainers can design, implement, supervise, and evaluate personalized Cardiorespiratory and Muscular Training programs by considering client attributes and preferences, ACE-sponsored research evidence statements, and other scientific-based guidelines, combined with their own expertise and experience.

REFERENCES

American College of Sports Medicine (2018). ACSM's *Guidelines for Exercise Testing and Prescription* (10th ed.). Philadelphia: Wolters Kluwer.

American Geriatrics Society, British Geriatrics Society, and American Academy of Orthopedic Surgeon Panel on Falls Prevention (2001). Guideline for the prevention of falls. *Journal of the American Geriatrics Society*, 49, 5, 664–672.

Amonette, W.E., English, K.L., & Ottenbacher, K.J. (2010). Nullius in verba: A call for the incorporation of evidence-based practice into the discipline of exercise science. *Sports Medicine*, 40, 449–457.

Amonette, W.E., English, K.L., & Kraemer, W.J. (2016). *Evidence-Based Practice in Exercise Science.* Champaign, Ill: Human Kinetics.

Benjamin, E.J., et al. (2019). Heart Disease and Stroke Statistics-2019 Update: A Report from the American Heart Association. *Circulation*, 39, 10, e56–e528.

Bishop, D. et al. (2008). Effects of high-intensity training on muscle lactate transporters and postexercise recovery of muscle lactate hydrogen ions in women. *American Journal of Physiology. Regulatory, Integrative and Comparative Physiology*, 295, R1991–R1998.

Cuddy, T.F., Ramos, J.S., & Dalleck, L.C. (2019). Reduced exertion high-intensity interval training is more effective at improving cardiorespiratory fitness and cardiometabolic health than traditional moderate-intensity continuous training. *International Journal of Environmental Research and Public Health*, 16, 3.

Del Coso, J. et al. (2010). Restoration of blood pH between repeated bouts of high-intensity exercise: Effects of various active-recovery protocols. *European Journal of Applied Physiology*, 108, 523–532.

Fleck, S.J. (1999). Periodized strength training: A critical review. *Journal of Strength and Conditioning Research*, 13, 1, 82–89.

Kraemer, W.J. et al. (2000). Influence of resistance training volume and periodization on physiological and performance adaptations in collegiate women tennis players. *The American Journal of Sports Medicine*, 28, 5, 626–633.

Nelson, M.E., et al. (2007). Physical activity and public health in older adults: Recommendation for adults from the American College of Sports Medicine and the American Heart Association. *Medicine & Science in Sports & Exercise*, 39, 8, 1435–1445.

Nolan, P.B. et al. (2018). The effect of detraining after a period of training on cardiometabolic health in previously sedentary individuals. *International Journal of Environmental Research and Public Health*, 15, 10.

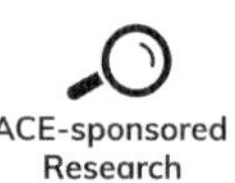

Page, P. (2012). Current concepts in muscle stretching for exercise and rehabilitation. *International Journal of Sports and Physical Therapy*, 7, 1, 109–119.

Potach, D.H. & Chu, D.A. (2016). Program design and technique for plyometric training. In: Haff, N.T. & Triplett, N.T. (Eds.) *Essentials of Strength Training and Conditioning* (4th ed.). Champaign, Ill.: Human Kinetics.

Powers, S.K. & Howley, E.T. (2017). *Exercise Physiology: Theory and Application to Fitness and Performance* (10th ed.). New York: McGraw-Hill.

Ramos, J.S. et al. (2016). 12 min/week of high-intensity interval training reduces aortic reservoir pressure in individuals with metabolic syndrome: A randomized trial. *Journal of Hypertension*, 34, 1977–1987.

Schenk, S. & Horowitz, J.F. (2007). Acute exercise increases triglyceride synthesis in skeletal muscle and prevents fatty acid-induced insulin resistance. *The Journal of Clinical Investigation*, 117, 1690–1698.

Slentz, C.A., Houmard, J.A., & Kraus, W.E. (2007). Modest exercise prevents the progressive disease associated with physical inactivity. *Exercise & Sport Sciences Reviews*, 35, 18–23.

St. Pierre, I.A. et al. (2018). ACE-sponsored Research: *Active vs. Passive Recovery and Exercise Performance: Which Strategy Is Best?* https://www.acefitness.org/education-and-resources/professional/certified/march-2018/6919/ace-sponsored-research-active-vs-passive-recovery-and-exercise-performance-which-strategy-is-best

Theodorou, A.A. et al. (2016). Aerobic, resistance and combined training and detraining on body composition, muscle strength, lipid profile and inflammation in coronary artery disease patients. *Research in Sports Medicine*, 24, 171–184.

Thomas, C. et al. (2012). Effects of acute and chronic exercise on sarcolemmal MCT1 and MCT4 contents in human skeletal muscles: Current status. *American Journal of Physiology. Regulatory, Integrative and Comparative Physiology*, 302, R1–R14.

Trost, S.G. et al. (2002). Correlates of adults' participation in physical activity: Review and update. *Medicine & Science in Sports & Exercise*, 34, 1996–2001.

Vollaard, N.B.J. & Metcalfe, R.S. (2017). Research into the health benefits of sprint interval training should focus on protocols with fewer and shorter sprints. *Sports Medicine*, 47, 2443–2451.

SUGGESTED READINGS

Amonette, W.E., English, K.L., & Kraemer, W.J. (2016). *Evidence-Based Practice in Exercise Science*. Champaign, Ill: Human Kinetics.

Amonette, W.E., English, K.L., & Ottenbacher, K.J. (2010). Nullius in verba: A call for the incorporation of evidence-based practice into the discipline of exercise science. *Sports Medicine*, 40, 449–457.

Dalleck, L.C. (2017). *ACE Scientific Advisory Panel Reports: The Science of Post-Exercise Recovery*. https://acewebcontent.azureedge.net/SAP-Reports/Post-Exercise_Recovery_SAP_Reports.pdf

Jo, S. (2019). *ACE Scientific Advisory Panel Reports: Integrating Science with Practice*. https://acewebcontent.azureedge.net/SAP-Reports/Integrated_Science_SAP_Reports.pdf

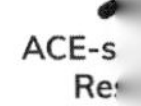

SECTION IV

Program Modifications for Clients with Special Considerations

CHAPTER 12
Considerations for Clients with Obesity

CHAPTER 13
Considerations for Clients with Chronic Disease

CHAPTER 14
Exercise Considerations across the Lifespan

CHAPTER 15
Considerations for Clients with Musculoskeletal Issues

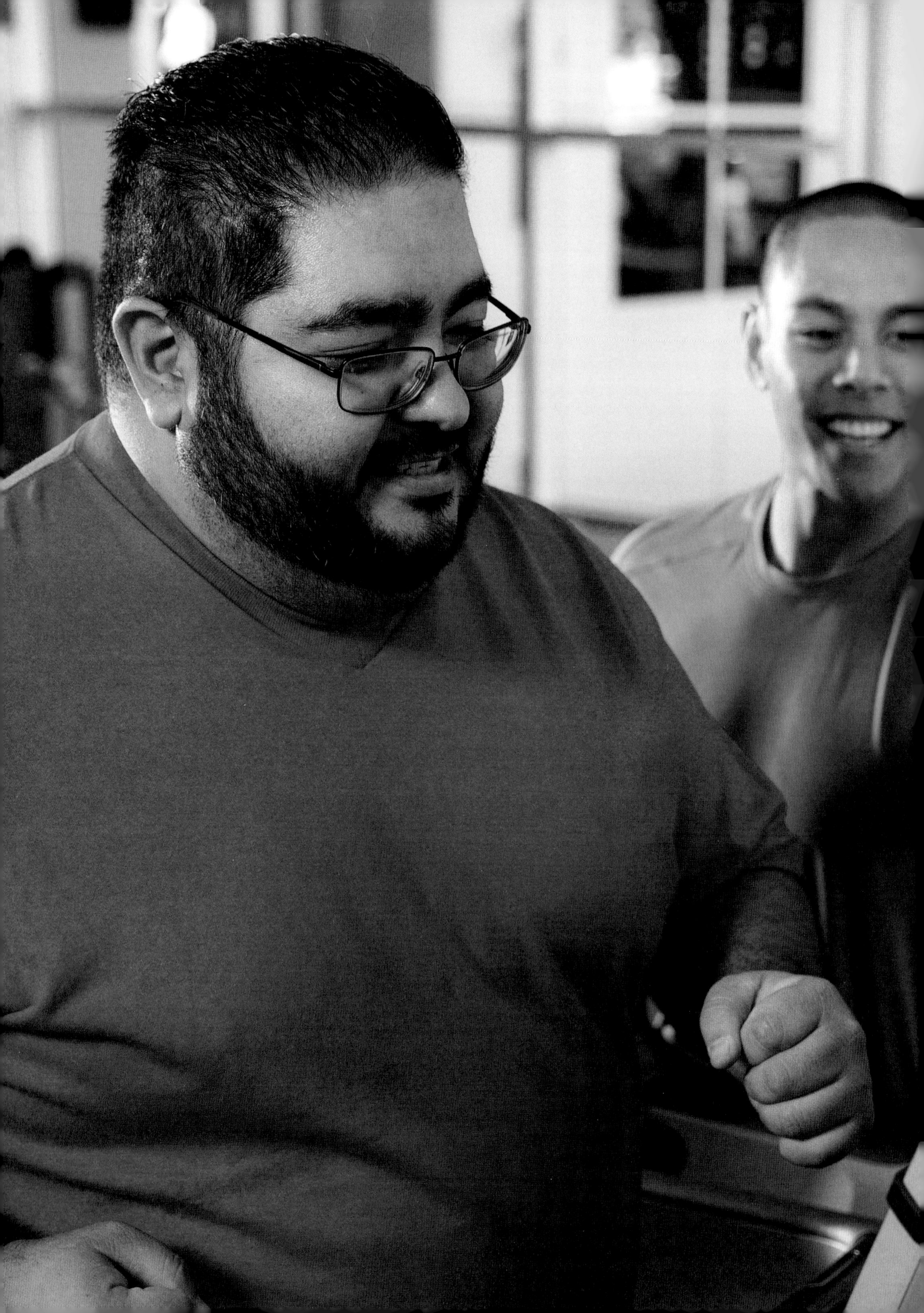

CHAPTER 12

Considerations for Clients with Obesity

JAMES S. SKINNER, PhD
Senior Advisor for Exercise Science, American Council on Exercise; Professor Emeritus, Indiana University; Former President, American College of Sports Medicine

IN THIS CHAPTER

LEARNING OBJECTIVES:

Upon completion of this chapter, the reader will be able to:

- Describe the major factors that contribute to obesity
- Explain the chief components of a behavioral weight-loss plan
- Outline key dietary strategies for weight loss and weight maintenance
- Discuss the role of physical activity and exercise in the prevention and treatment of overweight and obesity

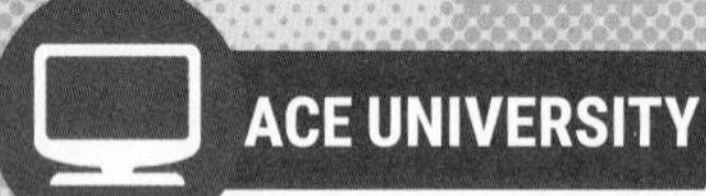

If your study program includes the ACE University, visit www.ACEfitness.org/MyACE and log in to your My ACE Account to take full advantage of the ACE Personal Trainer Study Program and online guided study experience.

A variety of media to support and expand on the material in this text is provided to facilitate learning and best prepare you for the ACE Personal Trainer Certification exam and a career as a personal trainer.

Often, **overweight** and **obesity** are described simplistically as the result of an imbalance between calories consumed [energy intake (EI)] and calories expended [energy expenditure (EE)]. An increased EI, without an equal increase in EE, leads to an increase in weight. Similarly, decreased EE with no change in EI will also result in an energy imbalance and lead to weight gain. While these are contributing variables, obesity is a multifactorial disease involving a complex interplay among environmental, behavioral, genetic, and hormonal factors. With a multidimensional view of health and **wellness,** ACE® Certified Personal Trainers are in a unique position to offer much-needed support as key allies in the fight against obesity.

Once associated with high-income countries, obesity is now also prevalent in low- and middle-income countries. Worldwide projections by the World Health Organization (WHO, 2018) indicate that 1.9 billion people age 18 years or older have overweight, with approximately 650 million of them having obesity. Some contributing factors to this epidemic can be attributed largely to the progression from a rural lifestyle to a highly technological urban existence, and the tempting capacity of the modern environment to encourage individuals to eat more and move less. Almost all countries are experiencing this dramatic increase in overweight and obesity.

Excess body weight is associated with an increased likelihood to develop heart disease, **hypertension, type 2 diabetes,** sleep disorders, gallstones, breathing problems, musculoskeletal disabilities, and certain forms of cancer (endometrial, breast, and colon) [National Institutes of Health (NIH), 2012]. It is also associated with reduced life expectancy and early **mortality** [American College of Sports Medicine (ACSM), 2018]. In addition, obesity has a deleterious effect on the economy of all countries, as it increases the associated costs for treating the related diseases.

Possible Causes of Obesity

While it is clear that obesity develops when EI is greater than EE, the relative contribution of each is not well understood. According to Nguyen and El-Serag (2010), obesity is caused by "a complex interaction between the environment, genetic predisposition, and human behavior," but environmental factors are probably the major factor contributing to the obesity epidemic. Other factors include stress (Sominsky & Spencer, 2014), greater use of medicines that cause weight gain (Heymsfield & Wadden, 2017), and inadequate sleep (Kahan, 2017).

ENVIRONMENTAL FACTORS

Environmental factors include the availability, quantity, and energy density of foods consumed (EI), as well as the availability of labor-saving devices, more time spent sitting, and less availability of facilities where one can be active in the built environment (EE).

STRESS

Stress causes or contributes to many diseases and disorders, including obesity and other eating-related disorders. Immediately after a stressful event, food intake is suppressed. However, with chronic psychological stress, hunger is stimulated, particularly the consumption

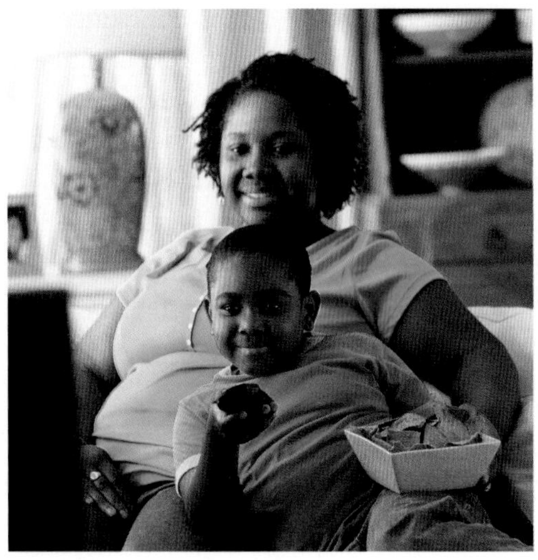

of high-calorie "palatable" food (Sominsky & Spencer, 2014). Research suggests that psychological benefits from exercise can be observed in a single acute exercise session, which may play a role in supporting long-term participation in exercise (Elkington et al., 2017). As such, personal trainers should inform clients that participation in regular exercise may empower them to reduce their stress levels.

GENETICS

There has been a rapid increase in the prevalence of overweight and obesity in the United States over the past 60 years. The magnitude of the change in prevalence has been too sudden to be caused solely by genetic factors and is more likely to be caused by behavioral and environmental factors.

Estimates from twin, family, and adoption studies show that the rate of heritability of **body mass index (BMI)** ranges from 40 to 70% (Bray et al., 2016). Nevertheless, specific genes associated with BMI and **body fat** account for less than 5% of the total variation (Pigeyre et al., 2016). In other words, genes are a factor, but are not as important as lifestyle. Li et al. (2010) studied the effect of different genes associated with body weight. The more **obesogenic** genes a person had, the higher his or her body weight. Interestingly, the average increase in weight was greater in **physically inactive** persons (1.3 lb; 0.6 kg) compared to that of active persons (0.8 lb; 0.36 kg). Thus, the genetic predisposition to obesity can be reduced by about 40% by being physically active.

Genetic factors can also influence how much weight is gained or lost. Bouchard et al. (1988) overfed identical twins by 1,000 calories each day for 100 days in a very controlled environment. Although there was a large variation in how much weight was gained (9 to 29 lb; 4.1 to 13.2 kg), the amount gained by each set of twins was more similar. That is, if one twin gained a lot, so did the other. Bouchard et al. (1994) also studied identical twins who maintained their calorie intake but exercised 90 minutes a day for 100 days. Again, there was a large variation in weight lost (2 to 13 lb; 0.9 to 5.9 kg), but the loss by each set of twins was more similar. Therefore, personal trainers must realize that not all people respond the same way to diet and exercise and that genetic factors play a role.

There are some genetic disorders that affect appetite, metabolism, energy balance, and fat distribution (Karam & McFarlane, 2007). These relatively rare conditions require specific therapeutic strategies managed by a physician, along with healthful nutrition and exercise. Thus, genetic factors can be important for a few, but it is likely that lifestyle is more important for the majority of people.

HORMONES

Research has revealed that fat tissue (composed of **adipocyte** cells that specialize in fat storage) functions like other **endocrine** organs (i.e., glands that secrete **hormones**) in the body, sending signals to the brain that affect several intricate physiological mechanisms of EE regulation, **insulin sensitivity,** and **fat** and **carbohydrate** metabolism (Townsend & Tseng, 2012). Two key hormones related to energy metabolism regulation are **leptin** and **adiponectin,** while a host of other hormones are involved in immune reactions in the body.

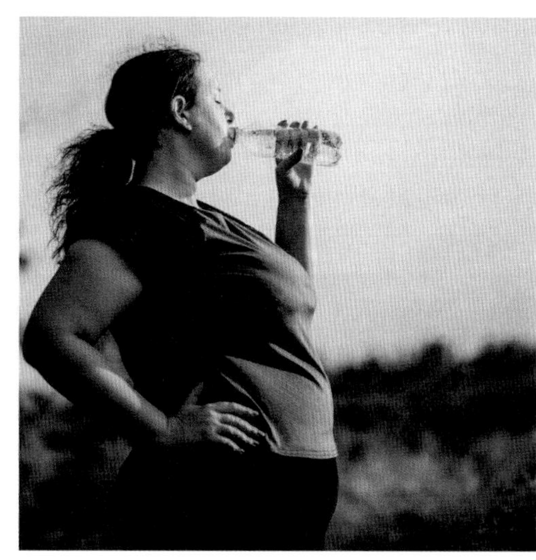

Leptin

Leptin resides in all fat cells and communicates directly with the hypothalamus in the brain, providing information about how much energy is currently stored in the body's fat cells. Leptin functions in what is referred to in biology as a **negative feedback loop.** For example, when fat cells decrease in size, leptin decreases, sending a message to the hypothalamus to direct the body to eat more. Similarly, when fat cells increase in size, leptin increases and the message sent to the hypothalamus is to instruct the body to eat less. However, it appears that the primary biological role of leptin is to facilitate EI when energy storage is low, as opposed to slowing down overconsumption when energy storage is high (Mantzoros et al., 2011).

Adiponectin

Another specialized hormone secreted by fat is adiponectin, which helps **insulin** by sending blood glucose into the body's cells for storage or use as fuel, thus increasing the cells' insulin sensitivity or glucose metabolism. It also helps decrease blood levels of **triglycerides** by working with insulin to stimulate fat breakdown. If a person has a lot of body fat, then he or she typically will have lower levels of adiponectin. This hormone is predictably low in individuals affected by overweight or obesity and especially low in individuals with **insulin resistance,** which occurs when the normal amount of insulin secreted by the pancreas is not able to transport glucose into cells. To maintain a normal blood glucose level, the pancreas secretes additional insulin. In some people, when the body cells resist or do not respond to even high levels of insulin, blood glucose increases, which may lead to type 2 diabetes.

Immune Hormones

It is known that fat tissue produces a number of immune-system hormones, such as tumor necrosis factor-alpha, interleukin-6, plasminogen activator inhibitor 1, angiotensin II, and other **cytokines** (Federico et al., 2010). Cytokines, which are hormone-like **proteins,** function largely as inflammatory proteins, reacting to areas of infection or injury in the body. However, persons with excess fat appear to have an overreaction in terms of the release of these inflammatory proteins. The concept of **inflammation** is one of the most critical in obesity biology. Both obesity and **diabetes** are associated with chronic low-grade inflammation (Wang et al., 2013). In addition, inflammation is understood to be a key risk factor in heart disease.

Appetite-regulating Hormones

Another component of the energy reserve regulation in the body involves some of the hormones that control feeding and appetite, which are located in the gastrointestinal tract. Specific hunger signals trigger eating, while **satiety** messages reduce appetite. These distinctive hormones are often referred to as the "gut hormones," one of which—**ghrelin**—has been proposed to be particularly associated with obesity (Koliaki et al., 2010). Ghrelin is secreted by the stomach and plays a chief role in appetite regulation. It is recognized as the "hunger hormone" and has garnered much attention due to its role in the prevalence of obesity.

In response to food intake, the hormone **peptide YY** (and other satiety hormones, such as cholecystokinin and glucagon-like peptide-1) is released from the intestines. It is particularly stimulated by **lipids** and carbohydrates. This gut hormone is thought to work with the **central nervous system** to regulate the cessation of appetite. Thus, when released, it provides a feeling of satiety. Research is ongoing related to the effectiveness of treating individuals with obesity with gut hormones, such as peptide YY, to help regulate food intake and energy **homeostasis** (Karra, Chandarana, & Batterham, 2009).

SLEEP

Obesity has been shown to interact with inadequate sleep quantity and poor sleep quality (Kahan, 2017). Over the past decades, there has been a rapid rise in obesity, in the number of people who get inadequate sleep (Liu et al., 2016), and in the number of people with poor sleep quality (Centers for Disease Control and Prevention, 2011). The reasons for this are varied and complex and have been associated with hunger, appetite, the immune system, stress, and inflammatory mediators (Kahan, 2017). In addition, Ogilvie and Patel (2017) suggest that there is fatigue and reduced physical activity with inadequate sleep.

It has been estimated that 58% of moderate-to-severe **obstructive sleep apnea (OSA)** is due to obesity (Newman et al., 2005). OSA is a common disorder that causes pauses in breathing during sleep associated with airway collapse or blockage. During this period of no breathing (**apnea**), blood oxygen levels decrease. Carbon dioxide levels increase to critical points and stimulate breathing, during which time the OSA sufferer may wake up. This cycle of breathing and non-breathing affects the quality of sleep and may cause snoring. It also can trigger the release of stress hormones, which then raise **heart rate** and the risk of hypertension, **myocardial infarction, stroke,** and **arrhythmias.** Although obesity is a major risk factor for OSA, there is also evidence that OSA can lead to rapid weight gain, resulting in a vicious cycle of increasing weight and worsening of OSA (Ong et al., 2013).

ENERGY BALANCE

Manore (2015) reviewed factors that influence weight loss and weight maintenance. She noted that many people have learned that there are about 3,500 kcal in 1 pound (0.45 kg) of fat. Therefore, if one can reduce EI by 250 kcal and increase EE by 250 kcal for a total deficit of 500 kcal daily, then one should lose 1 pound (0.45 kg) of fat after seven days. However, as Manore (2015) states, "We now know that the number of kilocalories required for 1 pound of weight loss changes depending on how long the dieting period lasts, what type of diet is fed, and whether participants engage in physical activity." She cites research by

Heymsfield et al. (2012) in which men and women with overweight dieted but did not increase their physical activity until they lost 15% of their body weight. During the first four weeks, the energy equivalent of 1 pound (0.45 kg) of weight loss was 2,208 kcal. This gradually increased until 20 weeks, when the energy equivalent of 1 pound (0.45 kg) of weight loss was near 3,500 kcal. How was this possible? If one loses water, lean tissue, or **glycogen,** the energy content is lower than if one loses all fat. More of these components are lost during the early phases of energy restriction, while mainly fat is lost during the latter phases. Adding exercise to dietary changes also can change the composition of the weight lost, the relative amounts of fat and carbohydrate used, and how fast the weight is lost.

With a change in body weight, there is also a change in EE. For example, if one eats more, the increased body weight causes a rise in **resting metabolic rate** and more energy is needed to move the bigger body. Eventually, the greater EE is similar to the greater EI and body weight stabilizes. Conversely, if one eats less or exercises more to lose weight, the resting metabolism goes down, less energy is needed to move the lighter body, and body weight will stabilize unless EI is less and/or EE is more. The actual amount of weight gained or lost also depends on the number of calories consumed, the composition of the diet, the type of exercise performed, and the level of daily physical activity (Manore, 2015). Figure 12-1 depicts many factors that affect both sides of the dynamic energy balance equation. Each person can respond to each factor in different ways (Galgani & Ravussin, 2008).

FIGURE 12-1
Key factors regulating and influencing energy balance

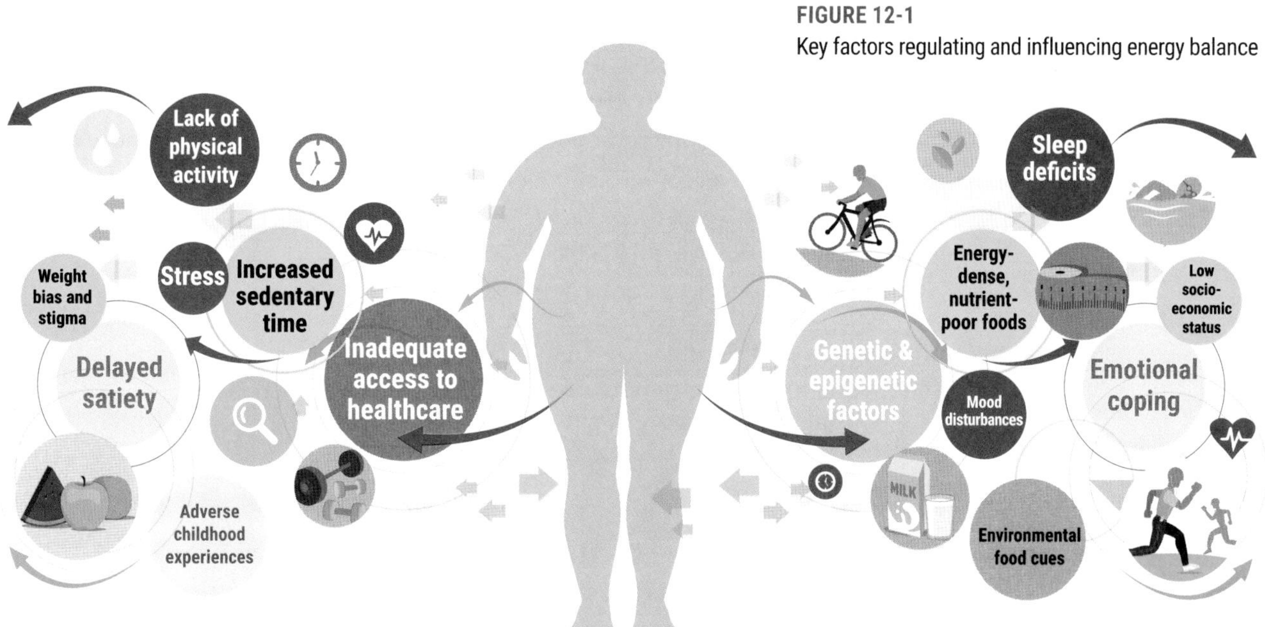

Nutritional Guidelines

Eating a low-calorie diet is the way many people try to lose weight. However, what happens during dietary restriction and why it occurs requires further clarification because the processes are complex and intertwined. Personal trainers who have a better understanding of these processes will be better able to assist their clients. Personal trainers should always be mindful of **scope of practice** when discussing nutrition with clients (see Chapter 6).

The American Dietetic Association (ADA, 2009) recommends reducing fat and/or carbohydrate intake to obtain a caloric deficit of 500 to 1,000 kcal per day to produce a weight loss of 1 to 2 pounds (0.45 to 0.9 kg) per week. However, this is based on the idea that ~3,500 kcal equals 1 pound (0.45 kg) of fat. The personal trainer should remember the information presented by Manore (2015) and not expect all of the weight loss to be fat, especially in the early stages of a program.

Other components of a recommended weight-loss program include:

- **Portion** control (providing information on serving sizes and the number of calories in various foods)
- Eating frequency (eating throughout the day, including breakfast, rather than mainly in the evening)
- Consuming foods high in nutrient density (nutrients per calorie of food) and low in energy density (calories per weight or volume of food)

The ADA (2009) also recommends assessing **resting energy expenditure (REE)** as a way to estimate the daily energy needs of clients. REE is measured at rest in the morning and is 60 to 75% of the body's **total energy expenditure (TEE)** (Wang et al., 2000). Because REE is such a major part of the TEE, it gives the personal trainer a general idea of how many calories are needed if the client remained at rest for 24 hours. Combined with a general idea of how active the client is, any proposed changes in EI can be estimated. Ideally, REE should be measured through **indirect calorimetry** in a clinical setting. If not, the Mifflin-St. Jeor equation (Mifflin et al., 1990), which uses actual body weight, is the most accurate equation for estimating REE for individuals with overweight and obesity (ADA, 2009; Frankenfield, Roth-Yousey, & Compher, 2005). The Mifflin-St. Jeor REE equations for men and women are as follows:

Males: REE (kcal/day) = (10 x Weight in kg) + (6.25 x Height in cm) – (5 x Age in yr) + 5
Females: REE (kcal/day) = (10 x Weight in kg) + (6.25 x Height in cm) – (5 x Age in yr) – 161

Conversions:
To convert from pounds to kilograms, divide by 2.2 (e.g., 140 lb/2.2 = 63.6 kg).
To covert from inches to centimeters, multiply by 2.54 (e.g., 66 inches x 2.54 = 167.6 cm)

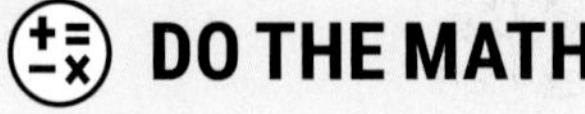

DO THE MATH

Barbara is a 35-year-old woman who is 5'3" tall and weighs 175 pounds. What is her estimated REE?

- **Convert pounds to kilograms: 175 lb/2.2 = 79.5 kg**
- **Convert inches to centimeters: 63 in x 2.54 = 160.0 cm**
- **REE = (10 x 79.5) + (6.25 x 160.0) – (5 x 35) – 161**
  - **REE = 795 + 1,000 – 175 –161**
  - **REE = 1,459 kcal/day**

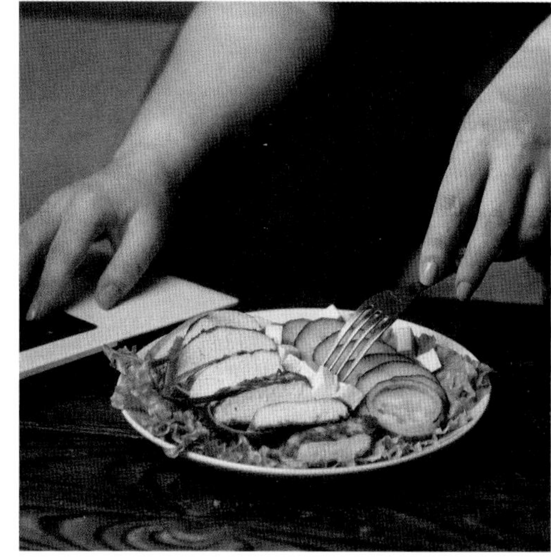

When a person eats an insufficient number of calories, some proteins may be used for energy. Thus, protein needs increase, while protein intake usually decreases. The current **Recommended Dietary Allowance (RDA)** for protein is 46 to 56 g/day, or 10 to 35% of total caloric intake, depending on age and sex (U.S. Department of Agriculture, 2015).

The goal should be to meet these recommended levels to help preserve lean tissue, especially if a person increases physical activity to lose more weight. Spreading food and protein intake throughout the day ensures that there will be adequate protein to build, repair, and maintain lean tissue. In addition, higher-protein diets tend to increase satiety (fullness) so that people will eat less (Weigle et al., 2005).

Low-energy-density food can help create feelings of satiety and curb hunger, increasing the chances of a successful weight-loss program (Rolls, 2012). Energy density is determined by measuring the amount of energy per gram of food (kilocalories per gram). A typical low-energy-density diet is high in fruits, vegetables, whole grains, legumes, and water, and low in fat, sweetened beverages, and alcohol. This type of whole-food, **plant-based diet** allows a person to consume a greater volume of food and feel satisfied while eating fewer calories.

The type and intensity of exercise can alter feelings of hunger and lower EI. Howe, Hand, and Manore (2014) report that acute exercise, especially when it is performed at greater than 60% of **maximal oxygen uptake ($\dot{V}O_2max$),** suppresses appetite by altering gut appetite-regulating hormones for two to 10 hours after exercise. However, such individual characteristics as body-fat percentage, level of fitness, age, and sex, as well as exercise duration, intensity, type, and mode, may also influence how exercise affects hunger. If there is appetite suppression after exercise, EI at the next meal and overall EI could be lower. For clients who exercise at a higher intensity while eating a low-energy-density diet, the appetite suppression due to exercise may help them manage hunger and reduce total EI, especially if both are done regularly.

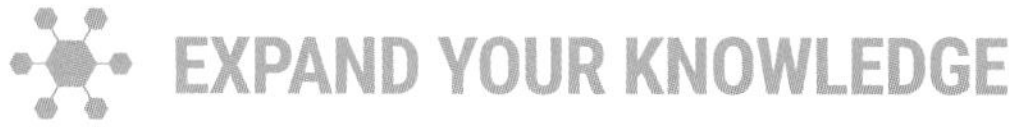

Evaluating Diets

Personal trainers can empower a client who is considering a new diet plan to critically evaluate whether a particular way of eating is a good choice. The client should be able to answer the following questions:

- **How does the diet cut calories?** For any diet to work, calories consumed (EI) need to be less than calories expended (EE). If clients want to lose weight, assist them in developing a plan that allows them to consume less energy and become more physically active in order to create a net caloric deficit.
- **What is the nutrient density of the diet?** The best diets will advocate up to nine servings daily of a variety of fruits and vegetables—low-calorie foods that provide most of the body's needed **vitamins, minerals,** and **phytochemicals** (a broad term for a variety of compounds produced by such plants

as fruits, vegetables, beans, and grains). Phytochemicals have been linked to decreasing the risk of infection and chronic diseases such as hypertension, stroke, and certain cancers (Boeing et al., 2012; Liu, 2003). **Fiber**-containing whole grains should also be encouraged. If the diet relies primarily on a supplement to assure sufficient vitamins and minerals, it probably is not the healthiest choice.

- **Does the diet recommend exercise?** Nutrition is only one component in making a long-term lifestyle change. Exercise not only supports weight loss by increasing caloric deficit, but is also essential in keeping the weight off.
- **Does it make sense?** Some diet plans make claims that often are based primarily on personal testimony. From promises to lose 10 or more pounds (4.5 kg) in the first two weeks of a diet to the promotion of supplements that supposedly speed weight and fat loss, diets are marketed as being so easy and effective that they are irresistible—at first. However, weight that is lost quickly is often regained quickly. Remember also that a good portion of initial, rapid weight loss is due to reduced body water (Manore, 2015).
- **Where is the evidence?** Research studies can be a rich source of information on the effectiveness and safety of different diets. When assessing research results, it is important to note the study limitations in addition to the results. For example, most of the diet research has been on middle-aged men and women who have obesity. Thus, the results may not apply to younger people or those who are simply trying to lose 5 or 10 pounds (2.3 to 4.5 kg) but who do not have obesity. Also, most diet studies are conducted over the course of one year or less. Therefore, the differences between different diets or the apparent benefits may not hold true for the long term.
- **Does it meet individual needs?** The client's health status and other individual factors must be considered when choosing an eating plan. Clients who have a history of unmanaged chronic disease such as diabetes or heart disease should talk with a physician or an appropriate healthcare professional before starting a diet or exercise regimen.
- **How much does it cost?** While clients may initially be able to afford an expensive weight-loss program, they may not be able to sustain the cost for an extended period of time. Help them plan ahead and understand their **readiness to change** and motivation to commit to a program before making huge lifestyle adjustments and financial sacrifices.
- **What kind of social support does the client have? Social support** is a key to successful weight loss. If a client's family is not supportive and committed to helping him or her make the healthy change, the client will likely struggle and will need to identify additional sources of social support.
- **How easy is it to adhere to the diet?** Long-term adherence to a program (i.e., lifestyle change) is the most important factor for sustainable weight-loss success. It is not necessary to select a specific diet to achieve long-term weight loss. Rather, individuals need to consume fewer calories while making healthy food choices they like and are likely able to maintain. Regardless of the weight-loss plan, most diets modestly reduce body weight and cardiovascular risk factors, but people who adhere to the diet over the long term have greater weight loss and risk-factor reductions (Dansinger et al., 2005). The problem is that most individuals struggle to adhere to restrictive eating plans. A landmark study conducted by the National Institutes of Health (1992) found that most dieters had regained one-third to two-thirds of the weight lost within one year, and dieters had regained almost all of the lost weight within five years. In addition, about one-third to two-thirds of dieters regained more weight than they initially lost (Mann et al., 2007). This reinforces the point that lasting lifestyle change is essential for successful weight loss and subsequent improved health.

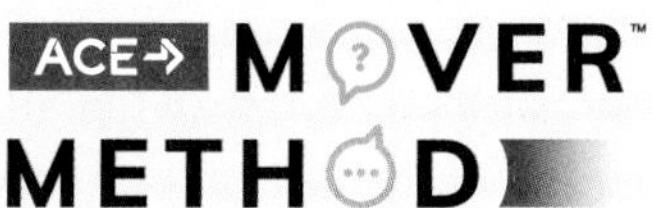

Handling Questions about Diets

During a recent session with your client James, he informs you that he is considering starting a new diet that he learned about online when researching new food preparation ideas. James has been your client for the past three months. He has been focused on becoming more active and had not previously mentioned making any dietary changes. James is curious to know if you have a specific diet you think he should be following and is interested in getting started soon.

ACE→ ABC APPROACH™

Following is an example of how the ACE Mover Method™ and the ACE ABC Approach™ can be used to address the topic of dieting with clients while staying within scope of practice and respecting the client's autonomy.

Ask: Use powerful open-ended questions to uncover what the client wants to achieve by starting a diet, and to keep the discussion moving in a positive direction while focusing on the client's expectations and preferences.

Personal Trainer: Thank you for sharing your nutrition aspirations with me. What do you hope to achieve by making changes to your diet?

Client: I would like to become more active and feel healthier. I know the combination of working out and proper nutrition will help me get the best results, so I want to eat healthier to support the physical activity I'm doing, and I want to get leaner. What diet do you think I should follow to do this?

Personal Trainer: That's a great question. If it's ok with you, I would like to learn a little more about your ideas about nutrition before I offer my thoughts. Is that ok?

Client: Yes, of course.

Personal Trainer: First off, I want to commend you for making this change and recognizing the relationship between diet and physical activity. You are correct: To achieve the best results, you want to eat a healthy balanced diet in combination with working out at an appropriate intensity and duration. Tell me, what does eating healthier mean to you?

Client: For me, eating healthier means I would be eating out less, eating more fruits and vegetables, and drinking more water.

Break down barriers: Continue asking open-ended questions and exploring what is hindering the client's progress toward his goal.

Personal Trainer: What, if anything, is preventing you from taking action on this right now?

Client: Eating out is convenient and takes less work. Right now, I don't eat many fruits or vegetables because I don't buy them, and meals I usually order when eating out don't include them. I know there are options where I eat out that do include fruits and vegetables, but I haven't tried them. I've made attempts in the past to drink more water, but I haven't been very successful, and I take in a lot of extra calories with the beverages I do drink. I suppose I could replace soda with water as an easy way to cut calories and increase my water intake.

Personal Trainer: That's an excellent starting point! What could you see yourself doing immediately to move closer to your healthy eating goal?

Client: I could start ordering fruits and vegetables when eating out, and I could buy some fruit to bring with me to work. I don't think I can replace all my soda and coffee with water, but I think I could replace some soda with water.

Collaborate: Work together with the client to develop next steps and solutions to potential barriers now that options have been identified. Ask more open-ended questions to ensure the client is playing a contributory role in the development of his program.

Personal Trainer: You asked if I had any specific recommendations for a diet you should follow, and together we uncovered some possible options to eating healthier. How do you see your goals for eating healthier unfolding over the next month?

Client: Over the next month, I will begin to incorporate more fruits and vegetables into my diet by buying apples and grapes at the beginning of each week and bringing them to work with me. I will also select food options with vegetables when I do eat out, and I'll buy a reusable water bottle and bring it to work and drink at least two full bottles per day.

Personal Trainer: Those are great ideas! If you decide you would like to try the diet plan you researched, here are some things to consider:

- How does the diet cut calories?
- What is the nutrient density of the diet?
- Does the diet recommend exercise?
- Does it make sense?
- Where is the evidence?
- Does it meet your individual needs?
- How much does it cost?
- What kind of social support does it provide?
- How easy is it to adhere to the diet?

If you decide it is right for you after answering all these questions, gradually work the changes into your daily routine rather than making all the changes at once.

In this scenario, the discussion began with a client asking for specific recommendations about what diet he should be following. By using the ACE ABC Approach, the personal trainer was able to find out what the client wants to achieve by following a diet. By creating the collaborative environment needed for the client to arrive at the appropriate next steps, the personal trainer was able to help this client improve his eating habits while staying within scope of practice (see Chapter 1).

Exercise Guidelines

Given that many people with overweight and obesity will walk to increase their EE because of the convenience, comfort, and accessibility of walking, it is important to know that there is a linear relationship between the usual walking speeds of 1.5 to 4.4 mph (2.4 to 7.1 km/h) and EE (Menier & Pugh, 1968). The importance of this relationship is that the total distance walked determines the EE. When one walks faster, more energy is used per minute but one exercises fewer minutes to walk the same distance.

There is also a linear relationship between running speeds ≥5 mph (≥8 km/h) and EE (Menier & Pugh, 1968). The EE of running is about 10% higher than that of walking because walking requires having one foot on the ground, while the body's **center of gravity** moves more with running when both feet are off the ground. Again, it is the total distance covered and not the speed of running that determines the total EE.

Given that the total EE is more important to the client wanting to lose or maintain weight, emphasis should be placed on the total distance or time walked or run. It is not necessary to do all of the walking in one session. Walking for 10 minutes three times requires roughly the same EE as one 30-minute walk, as long as the total distance covered is the same. This should make it easier for clients to find time during the day to walk, knowing that they do not have to exercise for a long period (i.e., it may be easier to make walking a part of their new lifestyle). For example, instead of having to find 30 minutes, clients can walk 15 minutes to lunch and 15 minutes back to work. One advantage of the shorter exercise intervals is that some people may decide to walk faster than they would if they had to walk 30+ minutes. Why is this important?

Duncan, Gordon, and Scott (1991) asked women with overweight to walk 3 miles (4.8 km) per session, five sessions per week for 24 weeks. One group (strollers) walked for 60 minutes at 3 mph (4.8 km/h), while the second group (brisk walkers) walked for 45 minutes at 4 mph (6.4 km/h), and the third group (aerobic walkers) walked for 36 minutes at 5 mph (8.1 km/h). Because there was no difference in the total distance walked, there was no difference in (1) the total EE, (2) body weight lost, or (3) the composition of the weight lost. However, those who walked faster (i.e., at a higher intensity) improved their fitness, as measured by $\dot{V}O_2$max, more so than those who walked more slowly.

Because the EE of walking or running is associated with transporting body weight, people with overweight and obesity will use more energy (kcal/min) when moving at the same speed as individuals of normal body weight. However, as they lose weight, there is less weight to transport and the EE will be reduced. For individuals with obesity, the EE may be even greater if they walk inefficiently due to their size (e.g., impaired gait). Once again, their EE will be less if they lose weight and/or walk more efficiently.

Personal trainers should also know that clients with obesity will likely experience challenges when they exercise in the heat. Because of their relative heat intolerance, these clients should train at lower intensities (especially in warm, humid environments) and will require a longer period to acclimatize to heat (Chung & Pin, 1996). They will also frequently have more problems with skin chafing, and the extra weight may exacerbate existing joint problems.

Swimming and water exercise place less stress on the joints, cause fewer problems with body-temperature regulation, and generate less friction and chafing. It is important, however, to also consider the potential psychological impact of water exercise, as clients with obesity may be self-conscious about their appearance and struggle with body-image issues. One disadvantage is that when exercising in the water, people with excess body fat are not transporting their body weight and will have a tendency to float, both of which will reduce EE. Nevertheless, water exercise is a good alternative, especially during the early stages of an exercise program to lose weight.

Some individuals with overweight and obesity have **mobility** and/or balance problems, such that some exercise equipment and physical-activity options may not be the best choices. For example, body-weight exercises performed on an unstable surface may not be a good option, while recumbent cycling may be more comfortable than exercising on a traditional upright bike due the larger seat and reduced balance requirements. Some machines may not accommodate larger sizes. Some individuals will have problems getting down to, and up from, the floor, or have problems while lying **supine** on the floor because the excess weight can make breathing more difficult. Like any client, individuals with obesity should always exercise within their physical capabilities, with good form, and through an appropriate **range of motion,** choosing forms of exercise they enjoy.

Another perspective that merits consideration for clients with obesity relates to lifestyle physical activity, which is any activity that is not a part of a structured period of exercise. For example, walking to work is lifestyle physical activity, but walking as part of an exercise program is not. A similar concept introduced by Levine et al. (2006) is that of **non-exercise activity thermogenesis (NEAT),** which is an important component of daily EE. It represents such common daily activities as fidgeting, walking, and standing. Implementing NEAT during leisure-time and occupational activities could be essential to maintaining a negative energy balance. NEAT can be promoted by being upright, ambulating, and redesigning workplace and leisure-time environments.

Adherence to formal exercise programs is typically poor among people with obesity (Dishman & Sallis, 1994). Lifestyle physical activity, which can be accumulated through daily activities at home and at work, may be an effective option for increasing EE and modifying body weight among people with obesity. Andersen et al. (1999) compared structured cardiorespiratory activity and moderate-intensity lifestyle physical activity and found that the weight loss from lifestyle physical activity was similar to that from cardiorespiratory exercise after 16 and 68 weeks of intervention.

Most adults spend a lot of time sitting at work, at home, or during their leisure time. This low level of EE results in a positive energy balance of about 100 kcal/day and is probably an important contributor to the obesity epidemic (Hill et al., 2003). Given that this low but constant positive energy balance may cause weight gain, finding ways to increase lifestyle physical activity or NEAT may produce a small but constant negative energy balance that can help clients lose, or at the very least maintain, weight. Personal trainers should empower clients to find more ways to move and be active each day (e.g., using stairs, standing instead of sitting, walking to a coworker's desk to talk rather than phoning or sending an email, or parking farther from the store or office).

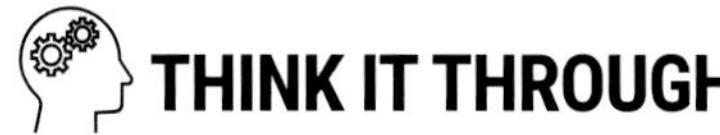

THINK IT THROUGH

Increasing Daily Physical Activity

Dave is a call-center manager who sits at his desk at least nine hours each day and enjoys watching TV during his time away from work. He makes it to the gym two days per week for exercise sessions with you but would like to be more physically active. How can you support Dave in exploring ways to increase his daily physical activity?

CARDIORESPIRATORY TRAINING

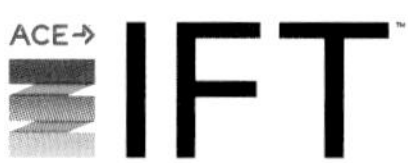

Personal trainers working with clients with obesity should be mindful of the key considerations outlined in this chapter as they utilize the ACE Integrated Fitness Training® (ACE IFT®) Model to design and implement safe, effective, and enjoyable exercise programming. It is important to note that the ACE IFT Model works in concert with the well-known FITT principle, where F = frequency, I = intensity, T = time, and T = type. The following is some general information about each component of a cardiorespiratory training program:

- *Frequency:* When starting out, be active on as many days of the week as possible and work up to at least five days per week. Any client who is not consistently performing moderate-intensity cardiorespiratory exercise on at least three days per week for bouts of at least 20 minutes will begin in the Base Training phase of Cardiorespiratory Training. Lifestyle activities should be done often throughout each day.
- *Intensity:* Exercise at a moderate level of intensity. To maximize EE, work at the highest intensity that can be sustained comfortably for an extended period of time. This intensity can be determined by using the **talk test.** When one begins to walk, run, or cycle at low intensities, heart rate and breathing increase, but it is possible to carry on a conversation. If clients can perform the exercise and talk comfortably, they are likely below the **first ventilatory threshold (VT1).** As the speed (intensity) increases, a point is reached where breathing is faster and deeper and it will be more difficult to talk. This is the intensity of exercise that is associated with VT1. When exercising below VT1, clients should be exercising at a moderate intensity. Clients should strive to increase duration and frequency of exercise bouts at this intensity to maximize EE. Personal trainers can also provide information to clients about use of the **rating of perceived exertion (RPE)** scale to monitor their intensity based on their subjective feelings. At the intensity where talking is comfortable, clients tend to give an RPE of "somewhat hard"; this would be 12 to 13 on the 6 to 20 scale and 3 to 4 on the 0 to 10 scale. This subjective feeling of "somewhat hard" could then be transferred to other activities to help clients maximize EE. Lifestyle activities are usually done at lower intensities to accumulate more time being active and less time sitting. See Chapter 8 for more information on the talk test, RPE, and other means of monitoring intensity.
- *Time:* Exercise 30 to 60 minutes per day. This can be done in one session or in multiple shorter bouts of exercise. Lifestyle activities are usually done in shorter segments throughout the day.
- *Type:* Perform low-impact, rhythmic exercises using large muscle groups. Exercise can be either weight-bearing (e.g., brisk walking) or non-weight-bearing (e.g., cycling and swimming).

Initial Programming Considerations

The most health benefits come when inactive people become moderately active. Making exercise a regular part of one's life can have a major impact on health. The key for personal trainers is to support their clients in choosing activities they enjoy and will continue to do until they meet their weight-loss goals, and beyond.

Moderate-intensity physical activity should be performed for 150 to 250 minutes each week to prevent significant weight gain, reduce associated chronic disease risk factors, and produce modest weight loss for individuals with overweight and obesity (ACSM, 2009). Greater amounts of physical activity (250 to 300 minutes/week or an EE of about 2,000 kcal/week) have been associated with clinically significant weight loss. To achieve this amount of physical activity, a person would have to walk about 20 miles/week (32 km/week) or about 3 miles/day (4.8 km/day) every day. Assuming a walking speed of 3 mph (4.8 km/h), this would require walking about one hour each day.

These recommendations present a problem in that many people with overweight or obesity have difficulty exercising enough to accumulate an EE of 2,000 kcal/week. Therefore, they should gradually increase the frequency, duration, and/or intensity of exercise over a long period (e.g., 20 weeks) to reach a point where they can achieve the recommended levels. Minimizing exercise-injury risk is an important consideration when designing physical-activity programs, and it is imperative to determine if an activity can be done independently or should initially be supervised by an exercise professional (Gordon et al., 2016). The risk of injury is usually greatest during the first few months of exercise or when there are abrupt increases in the total amount of exercise done (Skinner, 2005). Frequency and duration are probably the first components of an exercise program that should be gradually increased, because when intensity is increased too much or too soon, there is a greater risk of musculoskeletal injury (Skinner, 2005). Other recommendations to reduce the risk of injury include the inclusion of cross-training, gradual progression of exercise intensity and duration, use of low-impact or non-weight-bearing exercises, consideration of a person's injury history, selection of appropriate exercise environments and apparel to avoid heat-related complications, and incorporation of muscular and flexibility training into the exercise program.

Biomechanical Considerations for Cardiorespiratory Exercise

The preferred type of cardiorespiratory exercise for individuals with overweight or obesity is a combination of weight-bearing modes and non-weight-bearing modes. Exercise choices should be based on an individual's preferences and exercise history. Personal trainers can assist clients in finding modes of exercise with which they have a perceived comfort level with few barriers. The majority of the time exercising should be at a low-to-moderate intensity level to avoid joint stress and injury. Therefore, running, jumping, and high-impact types of movement are not recommended. These physical activities may lead to some musculoskeletal problems associated with body weight and impact forces from repeated (and forceful) foot strikes on the ground.

The emphasis of cardiorespiratory exercise should be on performing longer and/or more frequent bouts of exercise. It is important to monitor muscle soreness from exercise and ask clients if they are experiencing any orthopedic problems or discomfort. Stationary cycling is preferable to road cycling, because it eliminates any balance-related problems while also avoiding the hazards of traffic. Walking is considered a very good initial exercise because it requires no extra skill.

When clients embark on a walking or weight-bearing exercise regimen with or without the supervision of an exercise professional, it is important for them to keep a few things in mind.

Individuals with overweight or obesity need high-quality fitness shoes with good shock-absorbing qualities to minimize the chance of exacerbating orthopedic and joint problems.

Swimming and water exercise programs provide total-body exercise with little to no weight-bearing due to the buoyancy of water. Buoyancy is also a benefit for people with overweight or obesity who may have joint problems (e.g., arthritis of the hip, knee, or ankle or structural problems in these three joints).

Fitness facilities have a variety of exercise equipment for use. Personal trainers can assist clients in identifying exercise devices that are easy to use and that do not cause any back, knee, or ankle discomfort. For instance, recumbent bikes are good cycling options for individuals with obesity as compared with stationary or road cycling. Elliptical machines are also good choices for clients who can tolerate weight-bearing load because the low-impact nature of elliptical training may be easier on the knees compared with other forms of weight-bearing exercise, such as walking. For some clients, balance will be an additional challenge with some modes of exercise. If this is the case, clients should consider utilizing exercise devices that have handrails to minimize the risk of falling.

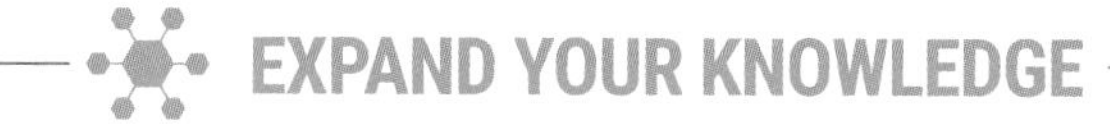

Realistic Anthropometric and Body Composition–related Outcomes with Weight Loss

Personal trainers can leverage numerous strategies to assist clients with exercise adherence, such as establishing attainable and personalized goals. However, implementation of this practical recommendation requires a clear understanding of the likely—and realistic—improvements in various outcomes that can be expected over a given period of training. Without this knowledge, attainable goals for the exercise program cannot be established and clients may become disenchanted with the program when they fall short of lofty goals.

A common goal for many clients initiating an exercise program is to lose weight or make other positive improvements to their physical appearance. Given both the widespread prevalence of obesity and the fact that excessive fat mass is associated with a myriad of unhealthy conditions, this is an admirable target. Regrettably, clients frequently establish weight-loss goals that are incongruent with what the scientific literature suggests are likely to occur with exercise training. In an ACE-sponsored study, participants with overweight/obesity (mean BMI = 30.3 kg/m^2) performed 13 weeks of personalized cardiorespiratory and muscular training based on the ACE IFT Model (Byrd et al., 2019). The anthropometric and body composition–related improvements in these individuals (N=20) are shown in Table 12-1. These research-substantiated outcomes provide personal trainers with an understanding of the expected changes in key anthropometric and body composition–related outcomes, as well as the expected timeframe to achieve these adaptations. Overall, this information can be integrated into a client-centered approach to working with clients with overweight/obesity.

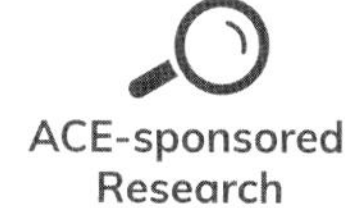

TABLE 12-1

Changes after 13 Weeks of Exercise in Clients with Overweight/Obesity

Outcome	Minimum Reduction	Maximum Reduction	Average Reduction
Weight	–0.5 lb (–0.2 kg)	–13.5 lb (–6.1 kg)	–4.0 (–1.8 kg)
Waist circumference	–0.25 inches (–0.6 cm)	–2.25 inches (–5.7 cm)	–1.0 (–2.5 cm)
Body fat (%)	–2.0	–8.0	–3.5

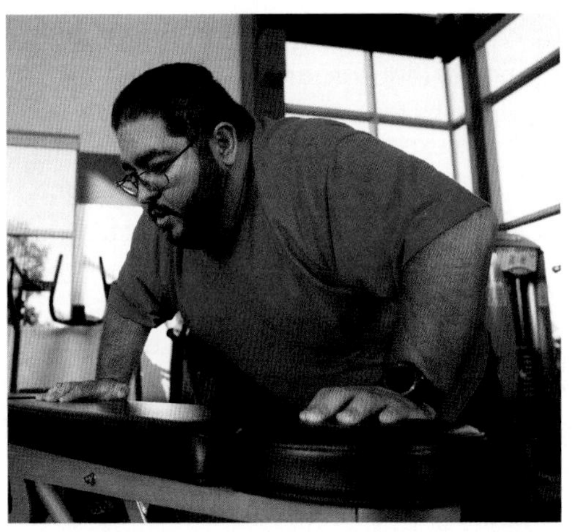

MUSCULAR TRAINING

Muscular training may not produce the greatest changes in terms of scale weight, but it offers many important benefits as part of a well-rounded weight-loss program, including improved body composition. Muscular training often creates a shift in the ratio of fat mass to lean mass that alters an individual's appearance. Because muscle tissue is denser and takes up less space than fat tissue, people often report looking better and feeling more comfortable in their clothing.

Muscular training's minimal direct impact on weight loss is probably due to the fact that the EE is not as large as that associated with cardiorespiratory exercise per unit of time. Nevertheless, muscular training may increase muscle mass, resulting in a greater 24-hour EE. Muscular training does improve **muscular strength** and **muscular endurance,** which may be especially beneficial in maintaining functional tasks for clients with obesity (e.g., getting out of a chair and lifting one's own body weight). This may facilitate adoption of a more active lifestyle in physically inactive individuals who struggle with obesity (Leermakers, Dunn, & Blair, 2000).

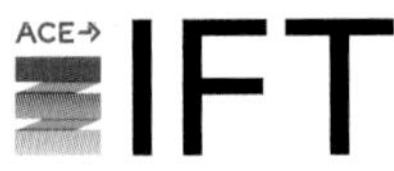

As with cardiorespiratory training, personal trainers can utilize the ACE IFT Model to develop muscular-training programs for clients with obesity, as long as they remain mindful of the modifications or considerations outlined in this chapter. The FITT recommendations for clients with obesity are as follows (ACSM, 2018):

- **Frequency:** Perform muscular training two to three days per week, with a day of rest between sessions.
- **Intensity:** Exercise at a moderate level [i.e., 60 to 70% of **one-repetition maximum (1-RM)**] for eight to 12 repetitions for two to four sets. Clients with obesity should focus on improving muscular strength and enhancing muscle mass so that daily activities will be less challenging.
- **Time:** This will depend on the number of exercises done and the number of sets completed. A full-body muscular-training program should require 20 to 30 minutes to complete.
- **Type:** Exercise all major muscle groups using free weights and/or machines. The decision regarding what form of resistance to use is largely a function of personal preference, training experience, and a client's goals.

Biomechanical Considerations for Muscular Training

There are some biomechanical concerns for people with overweight or obesity who perform muscular training. For some of these individuals, as well as older adults and those with mobility and/or balance challenges, seated exercise is a good option. This type of exercise can be useful in building basic muscular strength. While seated in a chair, individuals are able to do a variety of arm raises, leg lifts, and "bending" stretches. However, the seats on some exercise machines may not best accommodate individuals with obesity, which may limit the feasibility of using some equipment. In addition, weight benches are typically quite narrow, which could result in the loss of balance.

Another concern involves getting into and out from some resistance-training devices, which may be difficult based on an individual's specific body structure. It is sometimes preferable not to use exercise devices that are close to the floor (such as some abdominal-training devices) because a person with overweight or obesity may have great difficulty getting down to and up from the floor.

In addition, certain supine exercises may cause breathing difficulty for some clients with obesity (inhibiting the passage of air). Prudence should be taken in doing too much lunge and squat work because of possible knee and back discomfort and/or injury.

Exercise and Weight Management

Exercise plays an important role in the reduction of excess body weight and in achieving weight stability. Studies have shown a strong dose-response relationship between the volume (frequency, intensity, and duration) of cardiorespiratory and/or muscular exercise, and the amount of total and regional fat loss (Haskell et al., 2008). In the absence of concurrent caloric restriction, cardiorespiratory exercise in the range of 150 minutes per week has been associated with modest weight loss [4.4 to 6.6 lb (2.0 to 3.0 kg)], while 225 to 420 minutes per week results in a 11 to 16.5 lb loss (5.0 to 7.5 kg) in studies with durations ranging from 12 to 18 weeks (ACSM, 2009). Individuals seeking weight loss should include exercise as a key component of their programs, and adults with overweight and obesity should initially accumulate more than 150 minutes of moderate-intensity exercise each week and, when possible, more than 225 minutes per week (ACSM, 2018).

While it is generally accepted that people can lose weight, most cannot maintain significant weight loss over time. The exact amount of physical activity required to reduce or maintain weight remains unclear due to design flaws in many of the published studies. However, evidence suggests that "more is better" and that increased levels of physical activity are necessary to promote weight loss and weight stability. Stevens and colleagues (2006) defined weight stability as less than a 3% change in body weight; a change of 5% or more is considered clinically significant. For example, a 5% change for a 200-lb (90.1-kg) person would equate to a 10-lb (4.5-kg) change in weight. While the exact amount of physical activity required to maintain weight remains uncertain, research suggests that the gross EE required to achieve weight maintenance following substantial weight loss is approximately 2.0 kcal/lb (4.4 kcal/kg) per day [e.g., walking at 3 mph (4.8 km/h) for 80 minutes per day, walking at 4 mph (6.4 km/hr) for 54 minutes, or jogging at 6 mph (9.7 km/h) for 26 minutes] (Haskell et al., 2008). However, the research findings are not consistent and the amount may significantly vary among individuals. Because of these limitations, ACSM states that weight maintenance (weight fluctuation <3%) is likely to be associated with ~60 minutes of physical activity [~4 to 5 miles (6.4 to 8.0 km/h) of walking per day] at a moderate intensity (ACSM, 2009).

The combination of exercise and a sensible eating plan produces the best long-term weight-loss and weight-maintenance results. However, the key to successful, long-term weight stability is the adoption of lifelong physical activity and sensible eating habits.

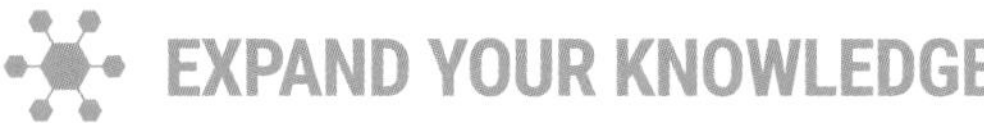

Not Gaining Is Winning

An important concept that personal trainers should consider while implementing programs for clients with overweight and obesity is that physical activity is a critical lifestyle behavior with the potential for impacting body composition and body weight, making it a key factor in both the prevention and treatment of overweight and obesity (Jakicic et al., 2017). While the focus of exercise programs often targets weight loss, the prevention of weight gain and weight-loss maintenance are also important goals influenced by physical activity (Jakicic et al., 2017). Physical activity supports the maintenance of a stable weight over time and can reduce the occurrence of obesity and the risk of excessive weight gain (U.S. Department of Health & Human Services, 2018). In other words, the prevention of further weight gain can be viewed as an achievement, especially during the first few weeks of a weight-loss program. The stoppage of additional weight gain means that the behavioral changes the client is attempting to make are working to the extent that the client has stopped the metabolic processes associated with adding more weight. Providing a client with this insight can be helpful if he or she becomes discouraged due to a lack of weight loss during the initial weeks of a behavior-change program.

Setting Body-weight Goals

Many people with overweight or obesity have unrealistic goals of how much weight they want to lose (e.g., 20 to 30%, when a more realistic goal would be 5 to 15%) (Fabricatore et al., 2007). Personal trainers should discuss with clients that a weight loss of 5 to 10% in people with overweight and obesity has been shown to significantly improve health-related outcomes for obesity-related **comorbidities,** including preventing and managing type 2 diabetes and improving abnormal lipids, high blood pressure, **osteoarthritis, stress incontinence,** and **gastroesophageal reflux disease (GERD)** (Cefalu et al., 2015).

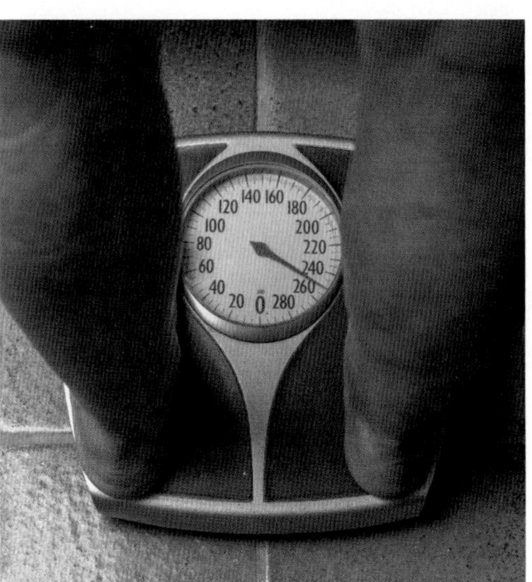

If a client starts out with a goal of going from 175 pounds (79.5 kg) to 135 pounds (61.4 kg), the amount of time and/or work that is needed may seem overwhelming. Instead, the personal trainer and client can collaboratively establish small, realistic, and attainable goals (e.g., reducing weight in one month by 2 to 3 lb or 0.9 to 1.4 kg).

Methods for predicting weight loss based on changes in dietary pattern and exercise are not precise (Manore, 2015). However, the NIH Body

Weight Planner is a simple web-based prediction model that the personal trainer can use to support clients in setting a goal weight or to determine what changes in physical activity or nutrition are needed to achieve the desired weight loss. See Chapter 6 for more information on the NIH Body Weight Planner.

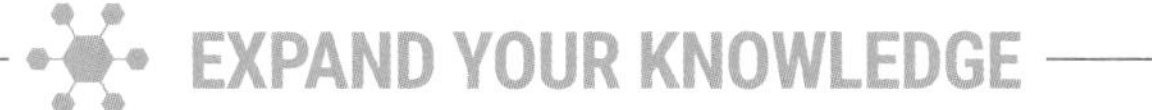

Fitness versus Fatness: Which Is More Important for Health?

Gaesser and Blair (2019) argue that many weight-control programs are ineffective, and that more emphasis should be put on adopting and maintaining a healthy lifestyle that includes more physical activity to increase fitness, rather than on weight loss alone. Jakicic, Rogers, and Donnelly (2019) counter by stating that the problems sustaining weight-control programs are not much different from those sustaining programs to increase physical activity, so the focus should remain on weight loss. Gaesser and Blair (2019) in turn counter by mentioning studies of the Diabetes Prevention Program, which found that about 50% more people were successful in meeting the physical-activity goal of ≥150 minutes per week than were successful in meeting the weight-loss goal of ≥7% body weight.

Relative to all-cause mortality, Gaesser and Blair (2019) report that fit people with overweight and obesity have about the same risk as fit people of normal weight but a lower risk than unfit people with overweight and obesity. In addition, unfit–normal weight people have a higher risk than fit people with overweight and obesity. Therefore, they state that fitness is more important than fatness. Jakicic, Rogers, and Donnelly (2019) mention that there are only a few studies on persons with severe obesity who have moderate-to-high levels of fitness and that persons with obesity may have problems being active enough to improve their fitness adequately. Therefore, they argue that weight loss may be more important. They also mention the results of a number of studies on the improvements in health when people with overweight and obesity lose adequate amounts of body weight.

Thus, while there is debate about whether maintaining an active lifestyle is more important than maintaining a healthy body weight, there are arguments for both and Gaesser and Blair (2019) and Jakicic, Rogers, and Donnelly (2019) agree that both are important.

What does this mean for the personal trainer? There is little question that obesity is associated with many health problems. Therefore, personal trainers should work with their clients to prevent weight gain, reduce excess weight, and improve their lifestyle through better nutrition and more physical activity. The personal trainer should also remember that genetic factors can influence how much weight their clients can lose (Bouchard et al., 1994; Bouchard et al., 1988) and how much they can improve their fitness (Bouchard, Rankinen, & Timmons, 2011). Therefore, rather than focusing on fitness or fatness, personal trainers should focus on improving those behaviors (physical activity and diet) that can positively affect fitness, fatness, and health.

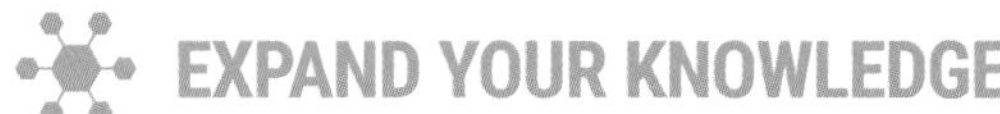

Metabolically Healthy Obese

Despite current estimates indicating that approximately 93 million U.S. adults have obesity (CDC, 2018), epidemiological data from the National Health and Nutrition Examination Survey (NHANES) suggest that a substantial portion of these individuals are essentially metabolically healthy (Wildman et al., 2008). This subset of individuals with obesity, often referred to as metabolically healthy but obese (MHO), appear to be more resistant to the adverse cardiometabolic consequences than their metabolically abnormal obese (MAO) peers often face (Karelis, 2008). For example, findings from a large prospective study demonstrated that the risks of all-cause and **cardiovascular disease (CVD)** mortality were 57% and 76% lower, respectively, in MHO compared with MAO adults (Ortega et al., 2013).

Although a universal definition of the MHO phenotype has not been established, it has been suggested that the remarkable protection against CVD and diabetes observed in this population is partly attributed to favorable metabolic profiles (Dalleck et al., 2014). It has been demonstrated that personalized, evidence-based exercise training can successfully transition MAO adults to metabolically healthy. Indeed, Dalleck and colleagues (2014) found that MAO adults who engaged in higher volumes of exercise and experienced the greatest increase in cardiorespiratory fitness were 22 and eight times more likely to transition from MAO to MHO, respectively. These findings are encouraging and underscore the importance of personal trainers implementing strategies that encourage active lifestyles and designing training programs with underpinning evidence for the improvement of cardiorespiratory fitness.

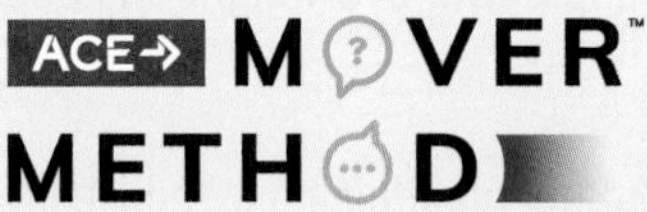

Reframing Long-term Goals

During a recent training session with your client Bill, he mentions feeling overwhelmed and frustrated when thinking about how much time, energy, and effort it will take to reach his goal of losing 45 pounds (20.5 kg). Bill has been successful at working toward a healthier lifestyle over the past five months and has already lost 15 pounds (6.8 kg). He shares with you that he has been working hard in many aspects of his life but feels like he still has a long way to go. Bill tells you that losing more weight is important to him and that reaching this goal is all he has been thinking about. He feels it will all be worth it once he gets to his goal weight, but for now, Bill feels like he has not accomplished much since he has so far to go. Bill would like to lose the weight as soon as possible and thinks it would be great if he could lose 10 to 15 pounds (4.5 to 6.8 kg) per month.

ACE→ ABC APPROACH

Following is an example of how the ACE Mover Method and the ACE ABC Approach can be used when working with a client who is focused only on his long-term goal [e.g., the **performance goal** of losing 45 pounds (20.5 kg)] and not feeling accomplished about what he has already achieved by adhering to **process goals.**

Ask: Use powerful open-ended questions to explore the client's specific goals and begin the process of working toward establishing smaller, more attainable goals.

Personal Trainer: You've started taking steps toward a healthier lifestyle and have lost 15 pounds (6.8 kg) over the past five months. How have you been so successful with your weight-loss journey up to this point?

Client: I have been meeting with you twice per week for our workout sessions, and I've made several other changes. I'm walking for 30 minutes during my lunch break five days per week, coming to the gym one additional time each week to work out on my own, and I've started making changes with what I'm eating. For example, I've been eating out less and tried a new recipe this week in addition to bringing lunch with me to work almost every day.

Personal Trainer: Increasing your physical-activity levels and planned exercise time while improving your nutrition have been key aspects of your success so far.

Client: Yes. I've tried losing weight in the past and never had as much success as I have been having this time. I think it's because of the walking and working out and being more aware of what I am eating. Things have been going pretty well so far, but lately I'm feeling burned out and not as consistent. Initially, the weight loss seemed to be happening quickly and I was motivated, but now the weight doesn't seem to be coming off and I'm losing motivation.

Break down barriers: Ask more open-ended questions to uncover what is impeding the client's consistency and motivation toward his current goals.

Personal Trainer: That's great that you've lost more weight now than you have during previous attempts! But, now the weight loss has slowed and you feel like you're losing some motivation. What do you think is contributing to this feeling?

Client: I think the main obstacle I am facing is that the overall time to reach this goal seems so long. Losing weight and having a healthier lifestyle is important to me, but when reaching the goal takes such a long time, it's hard to stay motivated, especially with how hard I am working. I thought I would be losing weight more quickly.

Collaborate: Work together to develop next steps and solutions to the barriers presented. The client has been implementing steps toward his goal, and now a plan will be established to shift the focus from the long-term goal of losing 45 pounds (20.5 kg) to setting clear and attainable short-term process and performance goals.

Personal Trainer: Focusing on losing 45 pounds (20.5 kg) is overwhelming because it will take a long time to reach the goal, but you've already made some significant changes that have resulted in weight loss. You would like to lose 15 pounds (6.8 kg) each month, and you are starting to feel discouraged because that is not happening. What do you know about healthy weight loss? Specifically, do you know how much weight you should lose each week in order to achieve safe and effective weight loss?

Client: I know that when I first started eating better and working out, I was losing more weight than I am now. I guess I'm not sure how much weight I should be trying to lose each week and I just figured the harder I worked the more weight I would lose and the quicker it would happen.

Personal Trainer: You're not alone; a lot of people believe that. However, safe and effective weight loss usually occurs at a rate of 1 or 2 pounds (0.45 to 0.9 kg) per week. If we look at a monthly level, a realistic goal would be to lose 4 to 8 pounds (1.8 to 3.6 kg). How does that sound to you?

Client: It seems like my goal of wanting to lose 45 pounds (20.5 kg) in three months may be out of reach. I've not been thinking of my goal in terms of monthly and weekly accomplishments and have only been thinking about losing weight as rapidly as possible.

Personal Trainer: Setting weekly goals may help with motivation and keep your focus on short-term success while still working toward your ultimate weight-loss goal. What specifically can you do this week to move forward with your weight-loss journey?

Client: I like the idea of taking things one week at a time and having something to accomplish each week. This week, I would like to continue to walk for 30 minutes five days per week, meet with you two times per week, and work out once on my own. I will also take my lunch to work with me each day and try to lose 1 to 2 pounds (0.45 to 0.9 kg) this week.

Focusing only on a long-term goal can be overwhelming, and it is important to work together with clients to break larger goals into smaller, more attainable steps. In this example, the personal trainer used open-ended questions and reflections to understand the client's position. The personal trainer also provided information about safe and effective weight loss and collaborated with the client on setting short-term goals that align with healthy weight-loss principles.

A Client-centered Approach to Working with Clients with Overweight/Obesity

Personal trainers should consider some of the methods used by health coaches, as these methods have been associated with significantly better weight-management success, increased physical activity, improved mental health status, and better management of chronic diseases (Kivela et al., 2014). Sherman, Peterson, and Guarino (2017) conducted a two-year weight-management study and found that primary care–integrated health coaching was cost-effective and resulted in significant weight loss in adults with overweight and obesity.

There are a number of strategies to help clients achieve and maintain weight loss. Lifestyle interventions designed to change eating behaviors and increase physical activity should be the first option used to manage weight, especially because of their low cost and low risk of complications [American College of Cardiology (ACC)/American Heart Association (AHA) Task Force, 2014].

APPLY WHAT YOU KNOW

Overcoming Weight Bias and Stigma

Given the prevalence of weight bias and stigma in society (Pachankis et al., 2018), personal trainers should realize that discussing body weight can be a sensitive issue for many clients. To ensure a safe and supportive environment, as well as to establish a positive and productive client–personal trainer relationship, personal trainers must take care to utilize inclusive language that makes clients feel comfortable and valued. Discussing weight should never be done in a way as to humiliate, blame, shame, degrade, or categorize people. This necessitates that personal trainers recognize and address their own implicit biases that may unintentionally impact the ability to see each client as being whole, resourceful, and capable of change. The personal trainer should ask permission to broach the subject of weight and to discuss the topic in a way that is comfortable for the client (e.g., "What words do you like to use when we talk about weight?"). Utilizing the skills of **motivational interviewing** can be helpful in discussing lifestyle changes in a way that enhances client **self-efficacy** and demonstrates the personal trainer's commitment to being a trusted partner in the journey of change (e.g., "What steps do you feel would be best to take to improve your health?") (see Chapter 4). Personal trainers should also exercise care when speaking about clients with other members of the care team, always utilizing people-first language (e.g., a client with obesity vs. an obese client).

In addition to increased EE and a modified diet with reduced EI, the American Dietetic Association (ADA, 2009) recommends that "a comprehensive weight management program should make maximum use of the multiple strategies for **cognitive behavioral therapy** (i.e., self-monitoring, stress management, stimulus control, problem solving, contingency management, cognitive restructuring, and social support)."

The three chief components of a behavioral weight-loss program are presented in Table 12-2.

The National Weight Control Registry (NWCR) has the largest database of individuals who successfully lost significant amounts of weight (30 lb; 13.6 kg) and maintained it for at least a year. Based on questionnaires, individuals in the registry who had effective maintenance after weight loss tended to engage in high levels of physical activity; eat a diet that was low in calories and fat; maintain a consistent eating pattern; and prevent small regains from turning into a larger regain (Wing & Phelan, 2005). A later analysis of data on lifestyle factors associated with achieving and maintaining weight loss showed the following: 98% modified their food intake; 94% increased physical activity (walking was the most common activity); 90% exercised on average for one hour each day; 78% ate breakfast every day; 75% weighed

TABLE 12-2

Chief Components of a Behavioral Weight-loss Program

Calorie Reduction	Personalized calorie goals to produce a 500- to 1,000-kcal daily deficit from baseline through reduced intake and increased physical activity: ▸ Assess caloric intake and support clients in devising a strategy to cut approximately 500 kcal per day (provided the client will maintain a healthy calorie level and is not at risk for nutrient deficiencies). ▸ Practice portion control. ▸ Reduce consumption of calorically dense foods, such as those with high fat and sugar content. ▸ Increase consumption of a variety of fruits and vegetables, which tend to be lower-calorie, nutrient-dense foods.
Physical Activity	Increases in moderate-intensity activities: ▸ Begin with 50 minutes/week (10-minute sessions on 5 days of the week) of cardiorespiratory activity, such as brisk walking.* ▸ Gradually increase to 150 minutes/week (30-minute sessions on 5 days in the week). ▸ For better maintenance of weight loss, increase further to 200 or 300 minutes/week. ▸ Perform muscular training at least twice/week. ▸ Increase non-exercise physical activity throughout the day (e.g., stand instead of sit, take the stairs, and walk or bike to do errands).
Behavioral Strategies	Behavioral strategies to increase adherence to the diet and activity goals: ▸ Practice self-monitoring (e.g., recording weight, nutritional intake, and activity through journaling or an app). ▸ Avoid tempting situations through stimulus control (e.g., removing high-calorie foods from the home and reducing time spent around friends and colleagues who have unhealthy eating habits and activity patterns). ▸ Spend more time around active, healthy individuals. ▸ Practice behavioral substitution (e.g., rather than eating an unhealthy snack, go for a short walk or practice yoga). ▸ Set SMART goals to transform vague intentions to specific plans for a healthier lifestyle (see Chapter 4).

*It should be noted that the starting amount of five 10-minute bouts of exercise per week is low and assumes that the individual with obesity is physically inactive. Please see the "Exercise Guidelines" section on page 567 for more information.

themselves weekly; 62% watched <10 hours of television weekly; and 55% lost weight with the help of a weight-loss program (NCWR, 2016). These data confirm that changes in eating patterns, physical activity, and other lifestyle behaviors are important elements to lose and maintain body weight.

Fruh (2017) states that structured lifestyle support is important for successful weight management. Of participants receiving structured lifestyle support from nurses who were trained in lifestyle behavior change, 34% achieved a weight loss of ≥5% over 12 weeks, compared to 19% who had usual care (Nanchahal et al., 2009).

Maintaining a food diary is one self-monitoring strategy that has been shown to be effective in long-term weight loss (Peterson et al., 2014). Similarly, recording physical activity and weight is also useful. This task can be facilitated by smart-phone applications, activity trackers, and wireless scales (ACC/AHA Task Force, 2014). Personal trainers can then collaboratively review a client's progress on a regular basis to provide encouragement and support in setting new goals and solving problems (ACC/AHA Task Force, 2014).

Another option is to refer clients to community programs (e.g., many YMCAs and fitness facilities offer a version of the Diabetes Prevention Program), established commercial weight-loss programs (e.g., Weight Watchers), and personalized dietary plans from **registered dietitians (RDs).** Lifestyle interventions using the telephone can result in about the same weight loss as in-person counseling (Appel et al., 2011). Web-based interventions that provide personalized feedback have been shown to result in a clinically meaningful amount of weight loss that is associated with a reduction in chronic disease risk (Harvey-Berino et al., 2010).

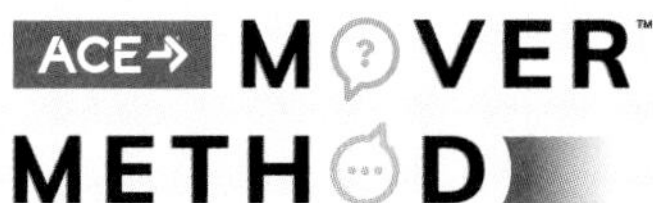

Journal Review

One of your clients, Sally, with whom you have been working for the past two months, tells you that she has been keeping a journal since beginning her health-improvement journey. In this journal, she records everything from her current physical-activity levels to food intake, weight, her feelings, and medical information. Last week, Sally mentioned that she wanted to review her activity and food entries at her next appointment. You both agreed to spend the last 30 minutes of the next session completing this review. Sally arrives prepared with her journal, including highlighted sections and marked pages. She has indicated food entries that she believes are areas that need improvement, has "starred" activity entries she is proud of, and highlighted days where she could have done more activity.

ACE ABC APPROACH

Following is an example of how to use the ACE Mover Method and the ACE ABC Approach to review a client's journal while remaining within your scope of practice.

Ask: Use powerful open-ended questions to discover what the client wants to achieve from the journal-review exercise.

Personal Trainer: You've been keeping track of your activity, food, weight, and feelings for the past two months. What specifically do you want to achieve by sharing this information with me?

Client: Mainly, I wanted to share with you some insights about my journey so far. My hope for today is to walk away with some action items and things to work on based on patterns I see in my journal. For example, if you look at this page, you can see that I highlighted all the times I consumed sugary beverages over one week. I drank two of these drinks per day, for a total of 14 in one week. I did some research and found that each one of these contains 140 calories, which means I am taking in almost 2,000 extra calories a week just from sugary beverages. I also learned that on days when I am feeling overwhelmed at work, I am less active. There are many days of the week where I do not move from my desk for almost the entire day. I wanted to highlight and share with you the main areas I want to focus on: decreasing sugary beverages and increasing my daily physical activity.

Break down barriers: Continue to use open-ended questions to assess what may get in the way of the client increasing physical-activity levels and decreasing sugary-beverage consumption.

Personal Trainer: Thank you for sharing that with me. Are there specific needs that are met by these current behavior patterns?

Client: I rely on sugary beverages to give me energy. In the past, if I forgot to bring them to work, I felt tired all day. When it comes to getting up and moving, I get so busy at work that I forget about my plans to walk, but I know I feel better when I do.

Personal Trainer: The drinks provide an energy boost, but they also contain a lot of excess calories from sugar. And when you do remember to walk during the day, you feel better, but often you get so busy that you forget to get away from your desk. What do you need to do more of, or less of, to be more in line with the changes you want to make?

Client: I think a good starting point would be to bring one canned drink to work with me instead of two and replace the second one with a bottle of water. For physical activity, I want to get away from my desk each day and go for a walk. I need some way of remembering to walk. Maybe an alarm or reminder on my phone will help.

Collaborate: Work together to develop next steps to help the client move toward her desired changes, while discussing strategies to overcome obstacles.

Personal Trainer: Drinking water in place of your energy drink and setting a reminder so that you get up and walk are great strategies! What specific action steps can you implement immediately to move forward with these changes?

Client: I've made up my mind that I can reduce sugary beverages from 14 per week to seven, and I will do this by replacing one sugary beverage with a bottle of water each day. Interestingly, in my journal, I have noted that on days when I am active, I have more energy, and perhaps the increased activity will make up for the loss of energy from the sugary drink. For physical activity, I will walk five days per week for 30 minutes each day by walking for 15 minutes during each of my breaks at work. Because I need a reminder, I can set this as an appointment on my calendar and an alert on my phone. I will also let my coworkers know about my plan to walk more and see if anyone would like to join me.

In this example, the personal trainer works with the client to review her food and activity journal. Since the client already has an idea of what she wants to achieve and is highly motivated, the personal trainer can address the client's expectations for the meeting. While keeping the conversation moving toward next steps and staying within scope of practice, the personal trainer can encourage the client to be the expert in setting goals that are specific to her ability and lifestyle.

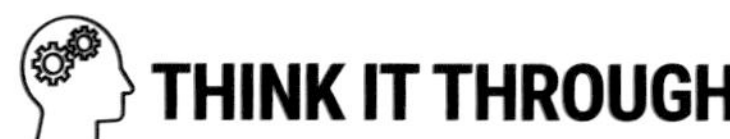

THINK IT THROUGH

Accurate Self-monitoring

One challenge with regard to health behavior change is that clients tend to underestimate how much they eat by approximately 30 to 50% (Fabricatore & Wadden, 2003) and overestimate their levels of physical activity (Dowd et al., 2018). As a result, they do not see a problem. Therefore, accurate self-monitoring is vital for the long-term success of a weight-management intervention. How can you support clients to accurately and honestly track their food consumption (EI) and their daily physical-activity levels (EE)?

Other Weight-loss Approaches

PHARMACOLOGICAL INTERVENTIONS

Lifestyle modification should be the main component of any weight-loss program and should be implemented before and during pharmacological therapy. If clients undergo intensive lifestyle intervention but cannot meet or maintain weight-loss goals and still have a BMI of ≥30 kg/m^2 (or a BMI ≥27 kg/m^2 with at least one obesity-related comorbidity), pharmacotherapy may be helpful and prescribed by their healthcare provider (ACC/AHA Task Force, 2014).

Currently approved drugs in the U.S. include phentermine for short-term use (<3 months) and five obesity pharmacotherapies that can be used longer (orlistat, lorcaserin, phentermine–topiramate, naltrexone–bupropion, and liraglutide 3.0 mg). For most of these long-term medications, the U.S. Food and Drug Administration (FDA) recommends discontinuation if there is <5% weight loss after 16 weeks, because it is unlikely that there will be further reductions. In addition, health status has to be monitored to minimize the risk of adverse effects (Golden, 2017).

Pharmacotherapy and lifestyle intervention should be used together. Wadden et al. (2005) studied the effects of lifestyle modification and/or pharmacotherapy on weight loss during a 52-week program. Those who did only pharmacotherapy had an average weight loss of about 11 pounds (5.0 kg), while those on lifestyle modification alone lost about 15 pounds (6.8 kg). Combining the two approaches resulted in a greater weight loss of about 26 pounds (11.8 kg).

Even after these interventions, regaining weight is common (Heymsfield & Wadden, 2017), which can be discouraging to patients and healthcare providers. Therefore, pharmacotherapy with lifestyle intervention also can be used to facilitate the maintenance of reduced weight. Weight loss achieved with pharmacotherapy is generally associated with improvements in risk factors and chronic diseases, as shown for **hemoglobin A1C** in patients with type 2 diabetes (Apovian et al., 2015). Clearly, a comprehensive behavioral weight-loss intervention needs to be fully implemented and sustained if a pharmacological intervention is to have any meaningful contribution to long-term weight-loss success.

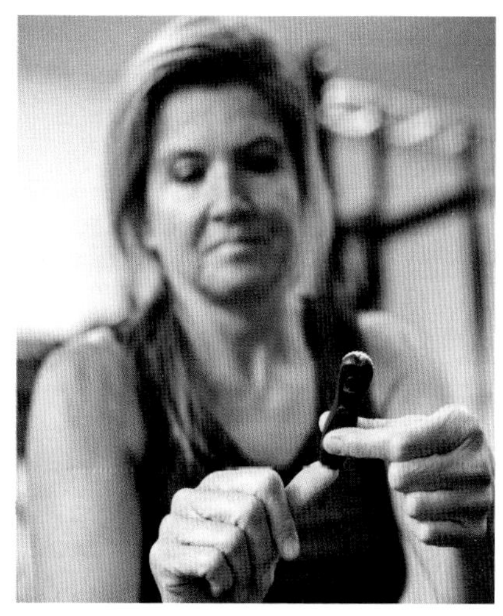

BARIATRIC SURGERY

Since high morbidity and mortality rates are associated with a BMI of 35 to 39 kg/m^2 in the presence of a coexisting condition, the use of surgical weight-loss procedures has increased. Although **bariatric surgery** is more effective than lifestyle and pharmacological interventions (Olson, Bond, & Wing, 2017), it is associated with greater risks (ACC/AHA Task Force, 2014). The ACC/AHA Task Force (2014) recommends this surgery for patients with a BMI ≥40 kg/m^2 or ≥35 kg/m^2 with at least one obesity-related comorbidity. Bariatric surgery is expensive, has short- and long-term complications [Longitudinal Assessment of Bariatric Surgery (LABS) Consortium, 2009], and about 5 to 20% of individuals regain weight (Schauer et al., 2014). Personal trainers may discuss with clients that bariatric surgery is not a cure for their obesity but a way to supplement or augment their behavior-change program, which they must continue to follow throughout their weight-management journey (Olson, Bond, & Wing, 2017).

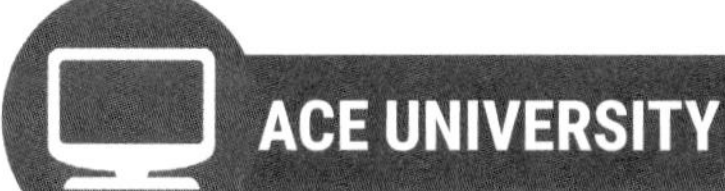

If your study program includes the ACE University, visit www.ACEfitness.org/MyACE and log in to your My ACE Account to take full advantage of the ACE Personal Trainer Study Program and online guided study experience.

A variety of media to support and expand on the material in this text is provided to facilitate learning and best prepare you for the ACE Personal Trainer Certification exam and a career as a personal trainer.

SUMMARY

Preventing overweight and obesity, as well as losing weight and keeping it off, is not easy, as there are a multitude of complex factors involved. Nevertheless, there is a great deal of evidence-based research showing that appropriate changes in lifestyle, dietary patterns, physical activity, and other health behaviors can prevent obesity at all ages and assist in efforts to lose weight and maintain a healthier body weight. However, weight loss should not be the only endpoint. There are important health-related benefits associated with adopting healthy lifestyle-behavior changes, including physical activity and healthful nutrition, even in the absence of large reductions in body weight. In fact, some of these important health-related benefits occur independent of changes in body weight.

REFERENCES

American College of Cardiology/American Heart Association Task Force on Practice Guidelines, Obesity Expert Panel, 2013 (2014). Expert Panel Report: Guidelines (2013) for the management of overweight and obesity in adults. *Obesity (Silver Spring)*, 22, Suppl. 2, S41–410.

American College of Sports Medicine (2018). *ACSM's Guidelines for Exercise Testing and Prescription* (10th ed.). Philadelphia: Wolters Kluwer.

American College of Sports Medicine (2009). Appropriate intervention strategies for weight loss and prevention of weight regain for adults. *Medicine & Science in Sports & Exercise*, 41, 2, 459–471.

American Dietetic Association (2009). Position of the American Dietetic Association: Weight management. *Journal of the American Dietetic Association*, 109, 2, 330–346.

Andersen, R.E. et al. (1999). Effects of lifestyle activity vs. structured aerobic exercise in obese women: A randomized trial. *Journal of the American Medical Association*, 281, 335–340.

Apovian, C.M. et al. (2015). Pharmacological management of obesity: An Endocrine Society clinical practice guideline. *Journal of Clinical Endocrinology and Metabolism*, 100, 342–362.

Appel, L.J. et al. (2011). Comparative effectiveness of weight-loss interventions in clinical practice. *New England Journal of Medicine*, 365, 1959–1968.

Boeing, H. et al. (2012). Critical review: Vegetables and fruit in the prevention of chronic diseases. *European Journal of Nutrition*, 51, 637–663.

Bouchard, C., Rankinen, T., & Timmons, J.A. (2011). Genomics and genetics in the biology of adaptation to exercise. *Comparative Physiology*, 1, 1603–1648.

Bouchard, C. et al. (1994). The response to exercise with constant energy intake in identical twins. *Obesity Research*, 2, 5, 400–410.

Bouchard, C. et al. (1988). Sensitivity to overfeeding: The Quebec experiment with identical twins. *Progress in Food & Nutrition Science*, 12, 1, 45–72.

Bray, M.S. et al. (2016). NIH working group report-using genomic information to guide weight management: From universal to precision treatment. *Obesity (Silver Spring)*, 24, 14–22.

ACE-sponsored Research

Byrd, B.R. et al. (2019). Personalized moderate-intensity exercise training combined with high-intensity interval training enhances training responsiveness. *International Journal of Environmental Research and Public Health*, 16, 12.

Cefalu, W.T. et al. (2015). Advances in the science, treatment, prevention of the disease of obesity: Reflections from a *Diabetes Care* editors' expert forum. *Diabetes Care*, 38, 8, 1567–1582.

Centers for Disease Control and Prevention (2018). *Adult Obesity Facts*. https://www.cdc.gov/obesity/data/adult.html

Centers for Disease Control and Prevention (2011). Unhealthy sleep-related behaviors: 12 states, 2009. *Morbidity and Mortality Weekly Reports*, 60, 8, 233–238.

Chung, N.K. & Pin, C.H. (1996). Obesity and the occurrence of heat disorders. *Military Medicine*, 161, 739–742.

Dalleck, L.C. et al. (2014). A community-based exercise intervention transitions metabolically abnormal obese adults to a metabolically healthy obese phenotype. *Diabetes, Metabolic Syndrome and Obesity: Target and Therapy*, 7, 369–380.

Dansinger, M.L. et al. (2005). Comparison of the Atkins, Ornish, Weight Watchers, and Zone diets for weight loss and heart disease risk reduction: A randomized trial. *Journal of the American Medical Association*, 293, 1, 43–53.

Dishman, R. & Sallis, J.F., Jr. (1994). Determinants and interventions for physical activity and exercise. In: Bouchard, C., Shephard, R.J., & Stephens, T. (Eds.) *Physical Activity, Fitness, and Health*. Champaign, Ill.: Human Kinetics, pp. 214–238.

Dowd, K.P. et al. (2018). A systematic literature review of reviews on techniques for physical activity measurement in adults: A DEDIPAC study. *International Journal of Behavioral Nutrition and Physical Activity*, 15, 15.

Duncan J.J., Gordon, N.F., & Scott, C.B. (1991). Women walking for health and fitness. How much is enough? *Journal of the American Medical Association*, 266, 23, 3295–3299.

Elkington, T.J. et al. (2017). Psychological responses to acute aerobic, resistance, or combined exercise in healthy and overweight individuals: A systematic review. *Clinical Medicine Insights: Cardiology*, DOI: 10.1177/1179546817701725

Fabricatore, A.N. & Wadden, T.A. (2003). Treatment of obesity. *Clinical Diabetes*, 21, 2, 67–72.

Fabricatore, A.N. et al. (2007). The role of patients' expectations and goals in the behavioral and pharmacological treatment of obesity. *International Journal of Obesity*, 31, 11, 1739–1745.

Federico, A. et al. (2010). Fat: A matter of disturbance for the immune system. *World Journal of Gastroenterology*, 16, 38, 4762–4772.

Frankenfield, D., Roth-Yousey, L., & Compher, C. (2005). Comparison of predictive equations for resting metabolic rate in healthy nonobese and obese adults: A systematic review. *Journal of the American Dietetic Association*, 105, 5, 775–789.

Fruh, S.M. (2017). Obesity: Risk factors, complications, and strategies for sustainable long-term weight management. *Journal of the American Association of Nurse Practitioners*, 29, Suppl. 1, S3–S14.

Gaesser, G.A. & Blair, S.N. (2019). The health risks of obesity have been exaggerated. *Medicine & Science in Sports & Exercise*, 51, 218–221.

Galgani, J. & Ravussin, E. (2008). Energy metabolism, fuel selection and bodyweight regulation. *International Journal of Obesity (London)*, 32, Suppl. 7, S109–S119.

Golden, A. (2017). Current pharmacotherapies for obesity: A practical perspective. *Journal of the American Association of Nurse Practitioners*, 29, S43–S52.

Gordon, B.T. et al. (2016). Basic physical activity and exercise recommendations for persons with chronic conditions. In: Moore, G.E., Durstine, J.L., & Painter, P.L. (Eds.) *ACSM's Exercise Management for Persons with Chronic Diseases and Disabilities* (4th ed.). Champaign, Ill.: Human Kinetics.

Harvey-Berino, J. et al. (2010). Internet delivered behavioral obesity treatment. *Preventive Medicine*, 51, 123–128.

Haskell, W.L. et al. (2008). *Physical Activity Guidelines Advisory Committee Report*. www.health.gov/paguidelines/Report/

Heymsfield, S.B. & Wadden, T.A. (2017). Mechanisms, pathophysiology and management of obesity. *New England Journal of Medicine*, 376, 254–266.

Heymsfield, S.B. et al. (2012). Energy content of weight loss: Kinetic features during voluntary caloric restriction. *Metabolism*, 61, 7, 937–943.

Hill, J.O. et al. (2003). Obesity and the environment: Where do we go from here? *Science*, 299, 853–855.

Howe, S.M., Hand, T.M., & Manore, M.M. (2014). Exercise-trained men and women: Role of exercise and diet on appetite and energy intake. *Nutrients*, 6, 11, 4935–4960.

Jakicic, J.M., Rogers, R.J., & Donnelly, J.E. (2019). The health risks of obesity have not been exaggerated. *Medicine & Science in Sports & Exercise*, 51, 222–225.

Jakicic, J.M. et al. (2018). Role of physical activity and exercise in treating patients with overweight and obesity. *Clinical Chemistry*, 64, 1, 1–9.

Kahan, S. (2017). Obesity and sleep: An evolving relationship. *Sleep Health*, 3, 5, 381–382.

Karam, J.G. & McFarlane, S.I. (2007). Secondary causes of obesity. *Therapy*, 4, 5, 641–656.

Karelis, A.D. (2008). Metabolically healthy but obese individuals. *Lancet*, 372, 1281–1283.

Karra, E., Chandarana, K., & Batterham, R.L. (2009). The role of peptide YY in appetite regulation and obesity. *Journal of Physiology*, 587, Pt. 1, 19–25.

Kivela, K. et al. (2014). The effects of health coaching on adult patients with chronic diseases: A systematic review. *Patient Education and Counseling*, 97, 147–157.

Koliaki, C. et al. (2010). The effect of ingested macronutrients on postprandial ghrelin response: A critical review of existing literature data. *International Journal of Peptides*, pii: 710852. DOI: 10.1155/2010/710852

Leermakers, E.A., Dunn, A.L., & Blair, S.N. (2000). Exercise management of obesity. *Medical Clinics of North America*, 84, 419–440.

Levine, J.A. et al. (2006). Nonexercise activity thermogenesis: The crouching tiger hidden dragon of societal weight gain. *Arteriosclerosis, Thrombosis, and Vascular Biology*, 26, 729–736.

Li, S. et al. (2010). Physical activity attenuates the genetic predisposition to obesity in 20,000 men and women from EPIC-Norfolk prospective population study. *PLoS Medicine*, 7, 8, e1000332.

Liu, R.H. (2003). Health benefits of fruit and vegetables are from additive and synergistic combinations of phytochemicals. *American Journal of Clinical Nutrition*, 78, Suppl., 517S–520S.

Liu, Y. et al. (2016). Prevalence of healthy sleep duration among adults – United States, 2014. *Morbidity and Mortality Weekly Reports*, 65, 6, 137–141.

Longitudinal Assessment of Bariatric Surgery (LABS) Consortium (2009). Perioperative safety in the longitudinal assessment of bariatric surgery. *New England Journal of Medicine*, 361, 445–454.

Mann, T. et al. (2007). Medicare's search for effective obesity treatments: Diets are not the answer. *American Psychologist*, 62, 3, 220–233.

Manore, M.M. (2015). Rethinking energy balance. Facts you need to know about weight loss and management. *ACSM's Health & Fitness Journal*, 19, 5, 9–15.

Mantzoros, C.S. et al. (2011). Leptin in human physiology and pathophysiology. *American Journal of Physiology–Endocrinology & Metabolism*, 301, 4, E567–E584.

Menier, D.R. & Pugh, L.G. (1968). The relation of oxygen intake and velocity of walking and running, in competition walkers. *Journal of Physiology*, 197, 3, 717–721.

Mifflin, M.D. et al. (1990). A new predictive equation for resting energy expenditure in healthy individuals. *American Journal of Clinical Nutrition*, 51, 241–247.

Nanchahal, K. et al. (2009). Weight-management interventions in primary care: A pilot randomized controlled trial. *British Journal of General Practice*, 59, 562, e157–e166.

National Institutes of Health (2012). *What Are Overweight and Obesity?* www.nhlbi.nih.gov/health/dci/Diseases/obe/obe_whatare.html

National Institutes of Health Technology Assessment Conference Panel (1992). Methods for voluntary weight loss and control. *Annals of Internal Medicine*, 116, 11, 942–949.

National Weight Control Registry (2016). *NCWR Facts*. https://www.ncwr.ws/

Newman, A.B. et al. (2005). Progression and regression of sleep-disordered breathing with changes in weight: The Sleep Heart Health Study. *Archives of Internal Medicine*, 165, 2408–2413.

Nguyen, D.M. & El-Serag, H.B. (2010). The epidemiology of obesity. *Gastroenterology Clinics of North America*, 39, 1, 1–7.

Ogilvie, R.P. & Patel, S.R. (2017). The epidemiology of sleep and obesity. *Sleep Health*, 3, 383–388.

Olson, K., Bond, D., & Wing, R.R. (2017). Behavioral approaches to the treatment of obesity. *Rhode Island Medical Journal*, 100, 2, 21–24

Ong, C.W. et al. (2013). The reciprocal interaction between obesity and obstructive sleep apnea. *Sleep Medicine Review*, 17, 123–131.

Ortega, F.B. et al. (2013). The intriguing metabolically healthy but obese phenotype: Cardiovascular prognosis and role of fitness. *European Heart Journal*, 34, 389–397.

Pachankis, J.E. et al. (2018). The burden of stigma on health and wellbeing: A taxonomy of concealment, course, disruptiveness, aesthetics, origin, and peril across 93 stigmas. *Personality and Social Psychology Bulletin*, 44, 4, 451–474.

Peterson, N.D. et al. (2014). Dietary self-monitoring and long-term success with weight management. *Obesity (Silver Spring)*, 22, 9, 1962–1967.

Pigeyre, M. et al. (2016). Recent progress in genetics, epigenetics and metagenomics unveils the pathophysiology of human obesity. *Clinical Science (London)*, 130, 943–986.

Rolls, B.J. (2012). Dietary strategies for weight management. *Nestle Nutrition Institute Workshop Series*, 73, 37–48.

Schauer, P.R. et al. (2014). Bariatric surgery versus intensive medical therapy for diabetes: 3-year outcomes. *New England Journal of Medicine*, 370, 2002–2013.

Sherman, R.P., Peterson, R., & Guarino, A.J. (2017). Primary care–based health coaching intervention for weight loss in overweight/obese adults: A 2-year experience. *American Journal of Lifestyle Medicine*, DOI: 10.1177/1559827617715218

Skinner, J.S. (2005). General principles of exercise prescription. In: Skinner, J.S. (Ed.) *Exercise Testing and Exercise Prescription for Special Cases* (3rd ed.). Philadelphia: Lippincott Williams & Wilkins, pp. 22–37.

Sominsky, L. & Spencer, S.J. (2014). Eating behavior and stress: A pathway to obesity. *Frontiers in Psychology*, 13, 5, 434–442.

Stevens, J. et al. (2006). The definition of weight maintenance. *International Journal of Obesity*, 30, 3, 391–399.

Townsend, K. & Tseng, Y-H. (2012). Brown adipose tissue: Recent insights into development, metabolic function and therapeutic potential. *Adipocyte*, 1, 1, 13–24.

U.S. Department of Agriculture (2015). *2015–2020 Dietary Guidelines for Americans* (8th ed.). www.health.gov/dietaryguidelines

U.S. Department of Health & Human Services (2018). *Physical Activity Guidelines for Americans* (2nd ed.). https://health.gov/paguidelines/second-edition/pdf/Physical_Activity_Guidelines_2nd_edition.pdf

Wadden, T.A. et al. (2005). Randomized trial of lifestyle modification and pharmacotherapy for obesity. *New England Journal of Medicine*, 353, 20, 2111–2120.

Wang, X. et al. (2013). Inflammatory markers and risk of type 2 diabetes: A systematic review and meta-analysis. *Diabetes Care*, 36, 1, 166–175.

Wang, Z. et al. (2000). Resting energy expenditure-fat free mass relationship: New insights provided by body composition modeling. *American Journal of Physiology, Endocrinology and Metabolism*, 279, E539–E545.

Weigle, D.S. et al. (2005). A high-protein diet induces sustained reductions in appetite, ad libitum caloric intake, and body weight despite compensatory changes in diurnal plasma leptin and ghrelin concentrations. *American Journal of Clinical Nutrition*, 82, 1, 41–48.

Wildman, R.P. et al. (2008). The obese without cardiometabolic risk factor clustering and the normal weight with cardiometabolic risk factor clustering: Prevalence and correlates of 2 phenotypes among the U.S. population (NHANES 1999–2004). *Archives of Internal Medicine*, 68, 1617–1624.

Wing, R.R. & Phelan, S. (2005). Long-term weight loss maintenance. *American Journal of Clinical Nutrition*, 82, Suppl., 222S–225S.

World Health Organization (2018). *Obesity and Overweight*. https://www.who.int/news-room/fact-sheets/detail/obesity-and-overweight

SUGGESTED READINGS

Heymsfield, S.B. & Wadden, T.A. (2017). Mechanisms, pathophysiology and management of obesity. *New England Journal of Medicine*, 376, 254–266.

Lavie, C.J. et al. (2018). Healthy weight and obesity prevention: JACC Health Promotion Series. *Journal of the American College of Cardiology*, 72, 13, 1506–1531.

Manore, M.M. (2015). Rethinking energy balance. Facts you need to know about weight loss and management. *ACSM's Health & Fitness Journal*, 19, 5, 9–15.

Olson, K., Bond, D., & Wing, R.R. (2017). Behavioral approaches to the treatment of obesity. *Rhode Island Medical Journal*, 100, 2, 21–24.

Trust for America's Health (2019). *The State of Obesity: Better Policies for a Healthier America 2019*. https://www.tfah.org/wp-content/uploads/2019/09/2019ObesityReportFINAL-1.pdf?fbclid=IwAR1dnsCKZQMrWu53STrlbJJsx6UisqrB0oF2hdAXUXj8N7_B6YoNBhw321g

Villablanca, P.A. et al. (2015). Nonexercise activity thermogenesis in obesity management. *Mayo Clinic Proceedings*, 90, 4, 509–519.

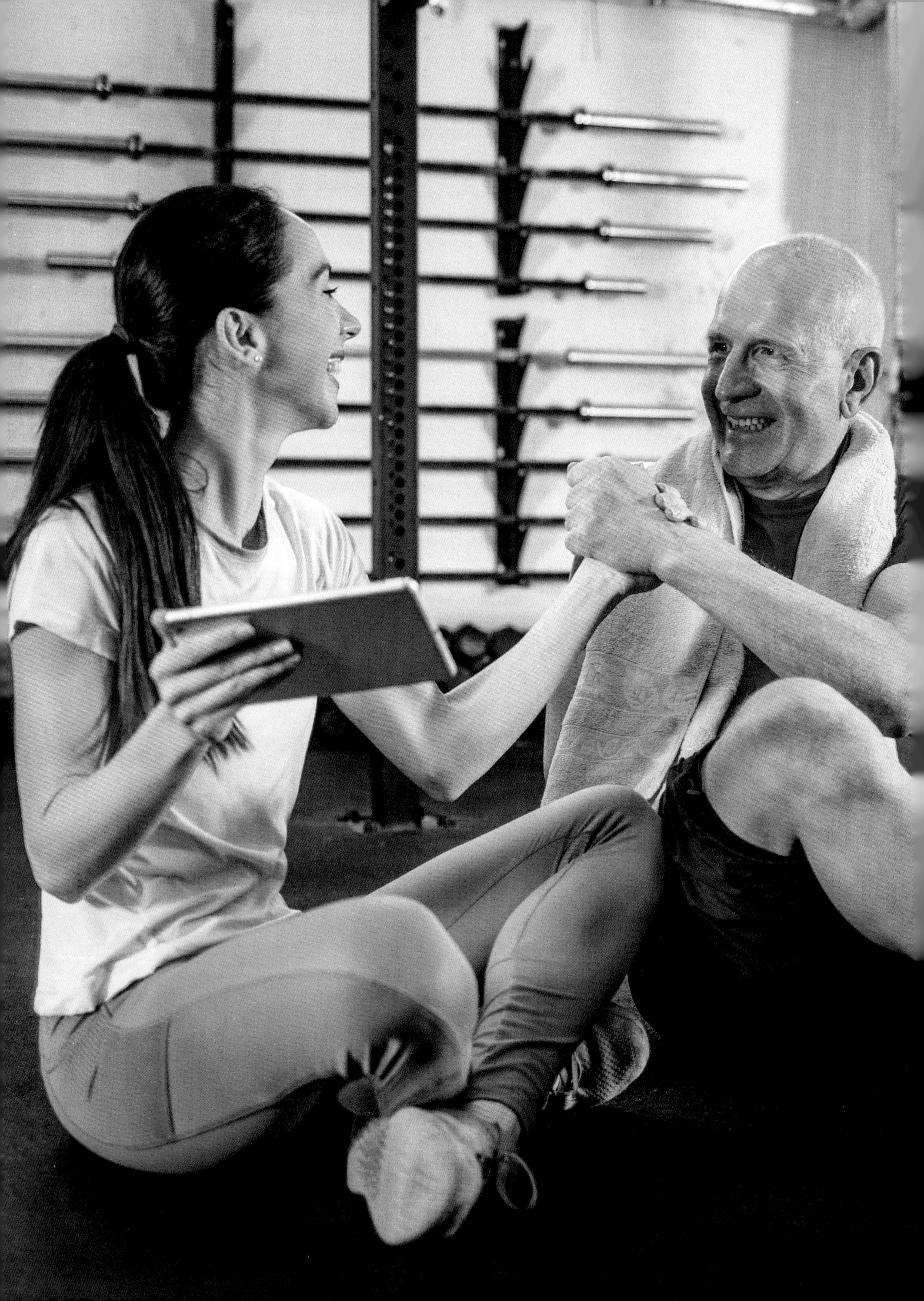

CHAPTER 13

Considerations for Clients with Chronic Disease

JAMES S. SKINNER, PhD
Senior Advisor for Exercise Science, American Council on Exercise; Professor Emeritus, Indiana University; Former President, American College of Sports Medicine

IN THIS CHAPTER

LEARNING OBJECTIVES:

Upon completion of this chapter, the reader will be able to:

- Explain that most chronic diseases in industrialized countries are associated with lifestyle choices
- Describe the role of personal trainers in improving the health and quality of life of clients through physical activity, healthy eating, and other lifestyle risk factors
- Explain how increased physical activity can influence other lifestyle risk factors
- Apply the general principles of training and exercise programming to specific chronic diseases and health conditions

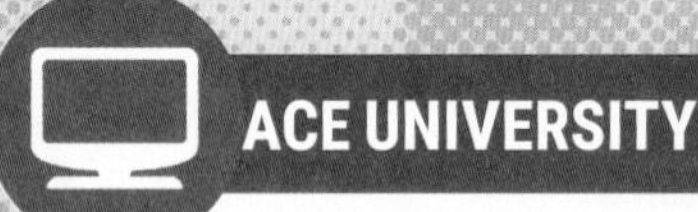

If your study program includes the ACE University, visit www.ACEfitness.org/MyACE and log in to your My ACE Account to take full advantage of the ACE Personal Trainer Study Program and online guided study experience.

A variety of media to support and expand on the material in this text is provided to facilitate learning and best prepare you for the ACE Personal Trainer Certification exam and a career as a personal trainer.

It is well known that regular exercise may help prevent a number of diseases or health conditions. Exercise is also useful to treat and manage these health problems once they are present [American College of Sports Medicine (ACSM), 2018]. Therefore, it is not unusual for personal trainers to work with clients who want to exercise to improve their physical and mental health.

Personal trainers should recognize that the same principles of exercise programming apply to persons who are apparently healthy and those with many **chronic diseases** or health conditions. Mainly, personal trainers should follow the general guidelines for apparently healthy persons as described in the ACE Integrated Fitness Training® Model, but modify them to specific clients using their best professional judgment. For example, the general guidelines apply to such conditions as uncomplicated **coronary artery disease (CAD), hypertension, dyslipidemia** (blood **lipid** disorder), **diabetes, metabolic syndrome (MetS), asthma,** cancer, and **osteoarthritis (OA).**

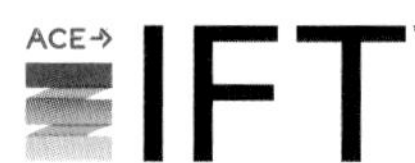

Any modifications that are needed should be based on such factors as:

- Characteristics of the disease
- Any restrictions that the disease places on clients and how they will respond to exercise
- Disease severity
- Safety concerns
- Activities to emphasize
- Activities to avoid

Cardiovascular disease (CVD), including **heart disease** and **stroke,** is the leading cause of death for men and women in the United States, as well as a leading cause of disability (Benjamin et al., 2019). Frequently thought of as conditions seen in older adults, metabolic diseases such as **obesity** and diabetes, and CVD **risk factors** such as hypertension, are becoming increasingly common in children and young adults. It is estimated that reducing three risk factors—poor diet, physical inactivity, and smoking—would dramatically reduce the incidence of chronic disease (Bauer et al., 2014).

Many healthcare professionals are not educated or trained to prescribe exercise for their patients who have, or may be at risk for, different health problems. Other than giving general recommendations to be more active, they may refer their patients to other professionals.

Personal trainers typically work with apparently healthy clients who do not need special instructions on what to do. Nevertheless, personal trainers should be aware of how exercise may help their clients who have, or are at risk for, health problems. They should know what types of exercise to emphasize or avoid, as well as the recommended frequencies, intensities, and durations of exercise.

It is important for ACE® Certified Personal Trainers to identify and discuss health conditions before working with a client. Such conditions may significantly influence exercise program development and should be part of the initial screening portion of the client–personal trainer interaction.

Once a client's medical and/or health conditions, including signs and symptoms, have been identified during the preparticipation health-screening process, the personal trainer will decide if a client needs approval from a healthcare professional before engaging in an exercise program. When needed, the personal trainer must obtain medical clearance before proceeding with assessments, exercise program design, and exercise participation (see Chapter 5). Along with physician approval, the personal trainer should request exercise guidelines and limitations. In many cases, a physician may choose to appoint another health professional to assist in providing exercise and educational guidelines. For example, this may be a nurse, physical therapist, clinical exercise physiologist, diabetes educator, and/or a **registered dietitian (RD).** Those personal trainers who have the advanced education and training that allows them to work with clients who have special needs must understand their role in relation to other healthcare professionals. It is important that the personal trainer adheres to the guidelines and restrictions provided and maintains close communication with the healthcare professional to have questions answered and to provide status reports at predetermined intervals. A personal trainer should regularly update client records to identify and effectively address changes in health status as they occur. Documentation of client encounters, health status, and progress is important for the personal trainer to appropriately adjust each client's program and prepare communication to other healthcare professionals.

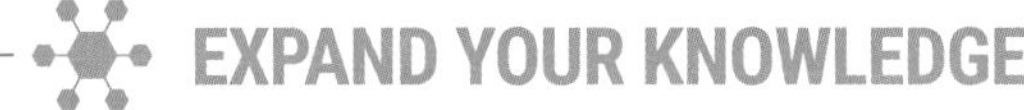

Using SOAP Notes to Document Client Progress

The **SOAP note** (an acronym for subjective, objective, assessment, and plan) is commonly used by healthcare providers to document patient progress. As used by exercise professionals, content for each section of the SOAP note is defined as follows:

- *Subjective:* Observations that include the client's own status report, a description of symptoms, challenges with the program, and progress made
- *Objective:* Measurements taken [e.g., **heart rate (HR), blood pressure (BP),** height, weight, age, **posture,** and results from assessments], as well as exercise and nutrition log information
- *Assessment:* A brief summary of the client's current status based on the subjective and objective observations and measurements
- *Plan:* A description of the next steps in the program based on the assessment

Wording in each section of the SOAP note should be concise and accurately reflect the activities documented. It is essential that every SOAP note is dated by the personal trainer. The SOAP note is an elegant and efficient way to communicate both what the client reports and what the personal trainer observes. Over time, SOAP notes document patterns of self-image versus actual performance and can be useful tools to provide feedback to the client. Personal trainers must be sure to protect sensitive client information when corresponding with a client's healthcare providers (see Chapter 16).

Typically, a client who has been released by his or her physician to take part in **independent activities of daily living** (including a limited exercise program) will also be cleared to work with a personal trainer who can provide additional guidance, motivation, and an appropriate rate of progression. An ACE Certified Personal Trainer must follow the guidelines provided by the healthcare provider. However, if there are only general recommendations to be more active, the personal trainer should know and follow established guidelines for each health condition and periodically inform the healthcare provider about what is being done, and what progress has been made.

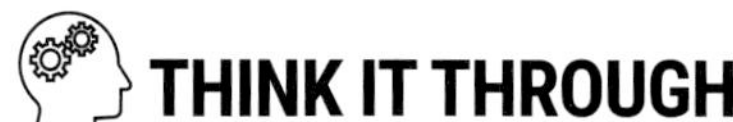

THINK IT THROUGH

Preparing to Work with Clients with Chronic Disease

Do you feel comfortable working with clients who have health issues? Given that the overall population is aging and becoming increasingly **overweight** and that with aging and/or obesity often comes an increased prevalence of health disorders, personal trainers must consider that their services will be offered to clients who are dealing with chronic diseases. Are you prepared to work with clients who have special considerations due to their health? How will you increase your knowledge, skills, and abilities in this important area? How will you promote your services to this clientele?

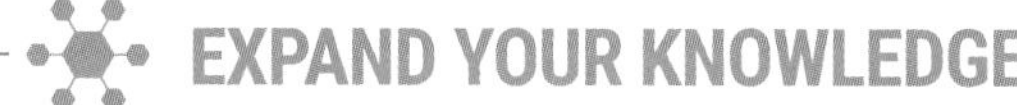

EXPAND YOUR KNOWLEDGE

Working with Clients with Multiple Chronic Diseases

While people are living longer, many are also dealing with multiple health challenges. The diagnosis of a disease can affect a person's sense of self and well-being. For some, the diagnosis comes after a catastrophic event, such as a heart attack or a stroke. For others, it is an insidious process that may be noticed only by loved ones. Reactions to a diagnosis can be as diverse as abject denial to a clear lifestyle alteration and is related to the person's coping mechanisms. Furthermore, physical and emotional health are related. Stress affects wellness physically and emotionally. It is appropriate to ask how a client is coping with the disease and how it impacts his or her life. This is a helpful step in establishing **rapport** and may alter the way a program is designed and modified. Some clients will experience a crisis and separate themselves from inappropriate life situations and/or experience a new appreciation for their friends and families. Others may feel helpless and unable to move toward better lifestyle decisions. Health challenges may require a change in habits, as the person's bodily functions and life circumstances change.

Although a disease is not necessarily a permanent state, clients may identify themselves by a diagnosis. For example, a client may say, "I am diabetic" rather than "I have diabetes." This disease identity is often one of the barriers that keeps clients from seeing themselves getting better. With more diagnoses, there may be **depression** and **chronic** pain. Depression may lead to decreased immunity and a greater predisposition to seasonal illnesses. The personal trainer should have frank discussions about a client's disease by identifying the client's knowledge of the disease, its signs and symptoms, the expectations of its progression or regression with an exercise program, and any concerns the client may have regarding how this disease impacts one's life. If a client has been traumatized by the sudden onset of the disease process, he or she may need a referral to a mental health professional to develop appropriate coping skills. Some clients will use humor as a way to minimize their reaction to their diagnosis. Others will have **anxiety** and need reassurance that their concerns are heard. It is important to separate the signs and symptoms of the disease from the client's sense of self. A focus on functional gains and separating the person from his or her diseases can dramatically impact a client's outlook in a positive way. By allowing clients to openly talk about their feelings, the personal trainer offers a way to discharge the negative impact of the health challenge prior to the workout, allowing for more productivity during the exercise session.

Many lifestyle-related diseases can be positively impacted by a combination of a healthy diet and a regular exercise program. While genetic predisposition can lead to increased risk of developing these diseases, lifestyle remains the single most influential factor in the incidence of these diseases. When working with clients with multiple health challenges, it is important to offer understanding regarding the effects of their disease processes, encourage transparency into their habits, and establish awareness of their choices (see Chapters 3 through 5).

There is a growing trend to employ multidisciplinary approaches to treating disease. Integral to this idea is teamwork that may involve the treating physician, patient/client, physical therapist, exercise professional, RD, and mental health professional. Once clearance has been obtained from the physician for an exercise program, the personal trainer has the option of recommending other team members. This multidisciplinary approach has been demonstrated to be more effective than medication alone or the use of any one aspect individually (Schultz et al., 2007; Li et al., 2006; Lillefjell, Krokstad, & Espnes, 2006).

Generally speaking, clients with one or more chronic diseases should follow a low- to moderate-intensity exercise program that gradually progresses. The exact nature of the program will depend on each person's current health status, physical condition, and other factors identified in the screening and referral process. The program must be personalized to the specific characteristics of the client, with appropriate modifications made to the activities that will enhance the safety and effectiveness of the exercise program. Many people with chronic health conditions have **comorbidities** (e.g., a person with heart disease and diabetes may also have overweight) that impact the exercise program. A personal trainer who chooses to train clients with chronic conditions has a responsibility to expand his or her knowledge and skills in this area through continuing education opportunities, advanced certifications, and close communication with healthcare professionals.

Cardiovascular and Cerebrovascular Disorders

CORONARY ARTERY DISEASE

Also called **atherosclerotic heart disease,** CAD is characterized by a narrowing of the coronary arteries that supply the heart muscle with blood and oxygen. The narrowing is an inflammatory response within the arterial walls resulting from an initial injury [due to high BP, elevated levels of **low-density lipoprotein (LDL)** cholesterol, elevated blood **glucose,** or other chemical agents such as those produced from cigarettes] and the deposition of lipid-rich plaque and calcified **cholesterol.** Heart attacks, or **myocardial infarctions (MI),** frequently result from the rupture of vulnerable plaques and the associated release of **thrombotic** (blood-clotting) substances that critically narrow or completely close the internal diameter of the artery.

Prevalence

The number-one cause of death in the U.S. is CVD (Benjamin et al., 2019). The American Heart Association (AHA) estimates that 121.5 million Americans have one or more types of cardiovascular disorders, including dyslipidemia, CAD, **congestive heart failure,** hypertension, stroke, and **peripheral arterial disease (PAD)** (Benjamin et al., 2019). CAD continues to be the leading cause of death in the developed world and for more than 100 years has caused more deaths in Americans than any other major cause.

Etiology

Atherosclerosis is also the underlying cause of cerebral and peripheral arterial diseases. Manifestations of atherosclerosis include **angina,** heart attack, stroke, and intermittent

claudication. Dyslipidemia significantly contributes to the development of atherosclerosis and associated disease conditions.

Well-established risk factors that contribute to CVD include family history, hypertension, diabetes, age, dyslipidemia, and lifestyle (i.e., poor diet, smoking, and physical inactivity) (Go et al., 2014a).

Nutrition

Diet has an important influence on the incidence and severity of CAD. One study estimated that 45% of U.S. deaths caused by heart disease, stroke, and **type 2 diabetes** in 2012 were attributable to dietary habits (Micha et al., 2017).

The AHA's 2020 Impact Goals to improve cardiovascular health suggest following a healthy diet pattern characterized by five primary and three secondary metrics (Benjamin et al., 2019). The primary dietary metrics are: fruits and vegetables (≥4.5 cups/day); fish and shellfish (≥2 3.5-oz servings/week); sodium (≤1500 mg/day); sugar-sweetened beverages (≤36 fl oz/ week); and whole grains (≥3 1-oz servings/day. The secondary dietary metrics are: 1 oz of nuts and seeds and ½ cup legumes (≥4 servings/week); processed meats (≤2 1.75-oz servings/ week); and **saturated fat** (≤7% of total daily energy intake).

Exercise

Physical inactivity is a major independent risk factor for CAD in both men and women. People participating in moderate amounts of physical activity have a 20% lower risk, while those undertaking higher amounts of exercise have a 30% or greater reduction in the risk of developing CAD (Haskell et al., 2008).

Exercise is also a critical part of the treatment regimen for people with CAD. For many years, heart attack patients were restricted to bed rest for six weeks or more. Unfortunately, this prolonged immobilization did not improve the healing process. Today, exercise training is an essential component of the therapeutic regimen for people with CAD. In almost all cases, an individual's recovery from an MI, cardiac surgery, or other cardiac procedure (e.g., **angioplasty** and stenting) will benefit from an appropriately designed and monitored exercise program.

Some clients with a history of CAD may be referred by their physicians to a supervised comprehensive cardiac rehabilitation program, before allowing them to start an exercise training program with a personal trainer. Most patients who have been released to take part in **activities of daily living (ADL)** will also have been given some basic activity guidelines. It is appropriate for the personal trainer to inform prospective clients that cardiac rehabilitation programs are available, and that clients should ask their physicians if participation is recommended. Unfortunately, many eligible patients are not referred to, or do not have access to, a cardiac rehabilitation program (Mayo Clinic Proceedings, 2016). In all cases, it is imperative that clients with known CAD or symptoms suggestive of CAD receive medical clearance prior to starting an exercise program with a personal trainer.

The physician or other designated health professional should provide the personal trainer with basic exercise program parameters such as heart-rate limits, exercise limitations, and other program recommendations. These guidelines will be based on the individual client's exercise test results, medical history, clinical status, and symptoms. Additionally, there are published guidelines available to assist the personal trainer in working with CAD clients and interacting with their healthcare team [ACSM, 2018; Wenger, 2008; Balady, 2007; American Association of Cardiovascular and Pulmonary Rehabilitation (AACVPR), 2013].

Exercise guidelines are based on the clinical status of the client, and it is most appropriate for personal trainers to work with low-risk CAD clients, who should have stable cardiovascular and physiological responses to exercise. The term low-risk is generally applied to clients who have the following characteristics:

- An uncomplicated clinical course in the hospital
- No evidence of resting or exercise-induced **ischemia**
- Functional capacity ≥7 **metabolic equivalents (METs)** three weeks following any medical event or treatment that required hospitalization (e.g., angina, heart attack, or cardiac surgery)
- Normal ventricular function with an **ejection fraction** greater than 50%
- No significant resting or exercise-induced **arrhythmias** (abnormal heart rhythms)

Most low-risk clients with CAD can also benefit from the improvement of **muscular strength** and **muscular endurance** that occurs with an appropriate muscular-training program. However, there are safety concerns that need to be considered by the personal trainer prior to implementing a muscular-training program with CAD clients, and physician clearance, recommendations, and limitations should be obtained before proceeding. Clients should be taught proper technique that includes breathing (avoiding a **Valsalva maneuver**) and moving through a full, pain-free **range of motion (ROM).** Begin with low-level exercises that use light weight (handheld weights or resistance tubing can be a good starting point) and gradually progress to weight machines. Many low-risk, stable CAD clients with whom a personal trainer will work have already undergone a course of cardiac rehabilitation that included muscular training, so the client may already be used to this type of exercise. Generally, clients should perform one to three sets of 10 to 15 repetitions using eight to 10 exercises that target all major muscle groups two to three times a week. HRs should not exceed the training target and/or a "somewhat hard" **rating of perceived exertion (RPE)** of 12 to 13 on the 6 to 20 scale, or the HR at the **first ventilatory threshold (VT1).** The client's physician or designated healthcare professional should provide initial guidelines for the client.

It is important for personal trainers to be knowledgeable about abnormal signs or symptoms that necessitate delaying or terminating the exercise session. Exercise should not continue if any abnormal signs or symptoms are observed, such as angina, **dyspnea,** lightheadedness or dizziness, pallor, or rapid HR above established targets. Personal trainers should communicate with clients and observe them for such signs and symptoms before, during, and immediately following each exercise session. If symptoms occur and persist, the emergency medical system should be activated and the client's physician notified. It is also important to teach clients to recognize signs and symptoms that indicate they should stop exercising and to report such experiences to their healthcare providers (see Chapter 5).

Table 13-1 provides an exercise guidelines summary for clients with cardiovascular disease.

TABLE 13-1

Exercise Guidelines Summary for Clients with Cardiovascular Disease

Cardiorespiratory Training	
Frequency	▸ At least 3, but preferably 5 or more days of the week ▸ Clients with limited exercise capacity can perform short, 1- to 10-minute sessions daily, as needed
Intensity	▸ Moderate to vigorous intensity* ▸ Intensity may be determined through the following methods: ▪ With an exercise test, use 40–80% HRR or $\dot{V}O_2R$ or $\dot{V}O_2$ peak ▪ Without an exercise test, use RPE of 12–16 (6–20 scale) or add 20–30 bpm to RHR ▪ HR should remain at least 10 bpm below the HR associated with the ischemic threshold (if exercise ischemic threshold has been determined) ▸ High-intensity interval training may be a safe and effective method for enhancing cardiorespiratory fitness for individuals with stable disease and a base level of conditioning.
Time	▸ Eventual goal of 20–60 minutes for cardiorespiratory training ▸ Warm-up and cool-down activities lasting 5–10 minutes should be included in each exercise session.
Type	▸ Rhythmic, large muscle group exercise that emphasizes whole-body conditioning and utilizes multiple activities and pieces of equipment, such as: ▪ Arm ergometer ▪ Upright and recumbent cycle ergometer ▪ Recumbent stepper ▪ Rower ▪ Elliptical ▪ Treadmill for walking
Progression	▸ Progress following the ACE Integrated Fitness Training Model based on client goals and availability. ▸ Sessions may include continuous or intermittent exercise.
Muscular Training	
Frequency	▸ 2–3 days per week with a minimum of 48 hours separating exercise for the same muscle group
Intensity	▸ 40–60% 1-RM, or a load that can be lifted 10–15 repetitions without straining ▸ RPE of 11–13 (6–20 scale)
Time	▸ No specific session duration has been found to be most effective
Type	▸ Various equipment can be used for resistance training, including: ▪ Elastic resistance ▪ Free weights ▪ Pulleys ▪ Selectorized machines ▸ Each major muscle group should be trained initially with one set ▸ Multiple-set routines may be introduced later, as tolerated

Continued on the next page

TABLE 13-1 *(continued)*

Muscular Training	
Progression	▸ Progress following the ACE Integrated Fitness Training Model based on client goals and availability. ▸ Progression can be introduced through increases in resistance, number of repetitions or sets, or decreasing rest periods between sets. ▸ Progression should be slow and dependent on tolerance. ▪ Volume can be increased 2–10% once clients comfortably complete 1–2 repetitions beyond the target range on two consecutive training sessions.

*Moderate intensity = Heart rates <VT1 where speech remains comfortable and is not affected by breathing; Vigorous intensity = Heart rates from ≥VT1 to <VT2 where clients feel unsure if speech is comfortable.

Note: HRR = Heart-rate reserve; $\dot{V}O_2R$ = Oxygen uptake reserve; RPE = Rating of perceived exertion; bpm = Beats per minute; HR = Heart rate; RHR = Resting heart rate; 1-RM = One-repetition maximum; VT1 = First ventilatory threshold; VT2 = Second ventilatory threshold

Source: American College of Sports Medicine (2018). *ACSM's Guidelines for Exercise Testing and Prescription* (10th ed.). Philadelphia: Wolters Kluwer.

HYPERTENSION

There are two types of hypertension. Most people with hypertension (90 to 95%) have what is designated **essential hypertension** or **primary hypertension** because there is no known or evident cause. In the other 5 to 10%, hypertension is the result of some identifiable cause (e.g., kidney disease) and is designated **secondary hypertension.**

Prevalence

In 2017, the American College of Cardiology (ACC) and the American Heart Association (AHA) released new guidelines for managing hypertension (Whelton et al., 2017). In these guidelines, they changed the definition of hypertension from a BP of ≥140/90 mmHg (32% of the population) to ≥130/80 mmHg (46% of the population) (Table 13-2). As a result, it is now estimated that approximately 103 million Americans require treatment. The majority of these

TABLE 13-2

Categories of Blood Pressure in Adults*

Category	Systolic Blood Pressure		Diastolic Blood Pressure
Normal	<120 mmHg	and	<80 mmHg
Elevated	120–129 mmHg	and	<80 mmHg
Hypertension			
Stage 1	130–139 mmHg	or	80–89 mmHg
Stage 2	≥140 mmHg	or	≥90 mmHg

*Individuals with systolic blood pressure and diastolic blood pressure in two different categories should be designated to the higher blood pressure category. Blood pressure is based on an average of two or more careful readings obtained on two or more occasions.

Reprinted with permission from Whelton, P.K. et al. (2017). 2017 ACC/AHA/AAPA/ABC/ACPM/AGS/APhA/ASH/ASPC/NMA/PCNA guideline for the prevention, detection, evaluation, and management of high blood pressure in adults: A report of the American College of Cardiology/American Heart Association Task Force on Clinical Practice Guidelines. *Journal of the American College of Cardiology*, Nov 7. pii: S0735-1097 (17) 41519-1.

patients can be treated with lifestyle changes instead of medication (Ioannidis, 2018), with the biggest impacts coming from changes in diet and exercise. This effectively shifts the emphasis of care for patients with hypertension from treatment to prevention. However, according to Ioannidis (2018), it is unclear whether patients and clinicians are ready for such a change and whether the many more people classified as having hypertension can find appropriate support and guidance for effective and sustainable lifestyle modifications. Thus, there is a great need for qualified healthcare professionals, including ACE Certified Personal Trainers, to help clients prevent and manage hypertension.

Hypertension is a key modifiable risk factor for CVD. It affects nearly one in three adults in the U.S. and contributes to one in seven deaths and nearly half of all CVD-related deaths in the U.S. (Chobanian et al., 2003).

Etiology

Essential hypertension is the result of genetic and environmental factors and their interactions. Risk factors include stress, body weight (especially excess **body fat**), and sleep, as well as age, excessive sodium intake, increased alcohol intake, and physical inactivity. A family history of hypertension increases the probability of developing hypertension, and men develop hypertension earlier than women (Whelton et al., 2017).

STRESS

There is a sufficient amount of evidence showing that psychological stress is a primary risk factor for hypertension (Cuffee et al., 2014). An increasing number of people have anxiety, depression, and chronic psychosocial stress because of global urbanization, cultural and socioeconomic changes, occupational stress, and a lack of physical activity and **social support** (Liu et al., 2017).

BODY WEIGHT

Body weight, especially excess body fat, is a risk factor for hypertension. One-third of Americans with obesity have been diagnosed with hypertension, compared to <20% of persons of normal weight (Saydah et al., 2014).

The association between obesity and hypertension is also apparent early in life, as the prevalence of both conditions has increased in children (Brady, 2017). Obesity-related hypertension is the most common form of hypertension among adolescents, as approximately 30% of adolescents with obesity also have hypertension (Falkner, 2017).

SLEEP

Inadequate sleep is becoming a problem for many adults (Covassin & Singh, 2016). Inadequate sleep (duration, complaints, and disorders) is associated with a higher risk of developing hypertension (Cuffee et al., 2014).

With the increased incidence of obesity, the most common sleep disorder is **obstructive sleep apnea (OSA)**. Numerous studies show a strong association between OSA and cardiovascular **morbidity** and **mortality,** as well as hypertension (Ahmad, Makati, & Akbar, 2017). Given that obesity is the most important risk factor for OSA, even modest reductions in weight will have a positive effect on the severity of OSA and OSA-induced hypertension.

GENETIC FACTORS

The contribution of genetic factors to the regulation of resting BP and the development of hypertension is long established (Williams et al., 1991). Research has identified a large number of genetic factors associated with BP. Even though genetic predisposition is a risk factor for hypertension, studies have shown that such behavioral factors as a **physically inactive** lifestyle are more important predictors (Douglas et al., 2003).

Although it is generally accepted that regular physical activity can lower BP, the magnitude of reduction varies greatly across controlled exercise training studies (Pescatello et al., 2004). Some of this variability is associated with genetic factors.

Treatment

Treatment for hypertension generally falls into two categories (Vamvakis et al., 2017): nonpharmacological (lifestyle) interventions and pharmacological interventions.

LIFESTYLE MODIFICATION

It is widely known that lifestyle behaviors contribute to hypertension and there is general agreement that lifestyle modification is important to prevent and manage hypertension (Mancia et al., 2013). Table 13-3 outlines the lifestyle changes recommended by the AHA (Chobanian et al., 2003).

TABLE 13-3

Lifestyle Modifications to Manage Hypertension*†

Modification	Recommendation	Approximate SBP Reduction (Range)
Weight reduction	Maintain normal body weight (body mass index 18.5–24.9 kg/m^2)	5–20 mmHg/10 kg weight loss
Adopt DASH eating plan	Consume a diet rich in fruits, vegetables, and low-fat dairy products with a reduced content of saturated and total fat	8–14 mmHg
Dietary sodium reduction	Reduce dietary sodium intake to no more than 100 mmol per day (2.4 g sodium or 6 g sodium chloride)	2–8 mmHg
Physical activity	Engage in regular aerobic physical activity such as brisk walking (at least 30 minutes per day, most days of the week)	4–9 mmHg
Moderation of alcohol	Limit consumption to no more than two drinks per day for most men and to no more than one drink per day for women and lighter-weight persons‡	2–4 mmHg

*For overall cardiovascular risk reduction, stop smoking.

†The effects of implementing these modifications are dose- and time-dependent, and could be greater for some individuals.

‡One drink is equivalent to 12 ounces of beer, 5 ounces of wine, or 1.5 ounces of hard liquor

Note: SBP = Systolic blood pressure; DASH = Dietary Approaches to Stop Hypertension

Source: Chobanian, A.V. et al. (2003). *JNC 7 Express: The Seventh Report of the Joint National Committee on Prevention, Detection, Evaluation, and Treatment of High Blood Pressure.* NIH Publication No. 03-5233. Washington, D.C.: National Institutes of Health & National Heart, Lung, and Blood Institute.

Included among the lifestyle modifications are losing weight (especially body fat), reducing intake of alcohol, exercising regularly, modifying diet (reducing salt intake and maintaining adequate levels of dietary potassium, magnesium, and calcium), and stopping the use of tobacco. Of these, nutrition, exercise, and reduced body weight are the major factors that can reduce BP (Appel, 2004). Caligiuri and Pierce (2017) reviewed the efficacy of diet, nutritional supplements, lifestyle modification, and medications for managing hypertension. They concluded that there is good evidence that the non-medication antihypertensive strategies can be just as effective as medications and, in some cases, even more effective.

Lifestyle modification can be beneficial for essentially everyone. People with normal BP levels can benefit from changing unhealthy habits that may increase the risk of developing hypertension. Those with elevated BP or **stage 1 hypertension** (see Table 13-2) are usually advised to modify their lifestyles to see if this will delay or prevent the need to take medication. The majority of individuals classified as having elevated BP or stage 1 hypertension can be treated with lifestyle changes instead of medications (Ioannidis, 2018). If lifestyle modifications fail to reduce BP after three to six months, then medications are usually prescribed. Even in persons with hypertension who are on medication, lifestyle changes that are maintained may reduce the amount of medication needed to control BP (Vamvakis et al., 2017). Thus, personal trainers should work with clients to effectively implement and sustain meaningful and lasting lifestyle changes.

Nutrition plays a significant role in preventing and managing hypertension. The AHA, ACC, and the Centers for Disease Control and Prevention (CDC) recommend the **Dietary Approaches to Stop Hypertension (DASH) eating plan** to all persons with hypertension, whether they are attempting to manage the disease with or without medication (Go et al., 2014a). The DASH eating plan advocates consuming **fiber** and potassium via fruits, vegetables, and whole grains, reducing sodium intake, reducing total and saturated fat, and getting adequate **protein** via lean meat and low-fat dairy products instead of high-fat or processed meat (Tyson et al., 2012) (see Chapter 6). Personal trainers can play an important role in partnering with clients to explore dietary changes to prevent and manage hypertension.

Exercise has both an acute and a chronic effect on BP, along with HR and various other physiological parameters. In individuals with hypertension and those with normal BP, a single exercise session lasting 10 to 50 minutes at intensities of 40 to 100% $\dot{V}O_2$**max** (moderate to very vigorous intensity) can acutely lower BP by 5 to 7 mmHg during the post-exercise period. However, the reduction is more pronounced in individuals with hypertension. This post-exercise decline in BP can persist for up to 24 hours (Pescatello et al., 2015). This effect has also been documented following resistance training, although the magnitude of BP change is not as great as it is following cardiorespiratory exercise. Combined cardiorespiratory and muscular training appears to produce a similar reduction in post-exercise BP as cardiorespiratory training alone (Keese et al., 2011). The take-home message is that participation in regular exercise is important for reducing BP and maintaining a normal BP.

The volume of regular cardiorespiratory exercise that has consistently been shown to reduce **systolic blood pressure (SBP)** and **diastolic blood pressure (DBP)** is 150 minutes per week or more, with the greatest reductions occurring in individuals with hypertension (Pescatello et al., 2015). This volume of activity is consistent with the *Physical Activity Guidelines for Americans* (U.S. Department of Health & Human Services, 2018) and recommendations from ACSM (2018). It is recommended that individuals with elevated BP and those with hypertension participate in regular exercise of moderate intensity for 30 minutes or more at least five days of the week. Cardiorespiratory activities such as walking, cycling, elliptical cross-training, stairclimbing, and swimming are excellent modes of exercise and should be supplemented with muscular training at least two times per week whenever possible.

Table 13-4 presents an exercise guidelines summary for clients with hypertension.

TABLE 13-4

Exercise Guidelines Summary for Clients with Hypertension

Cardiorespiratory Training	
Frequency	▸ Most, but preferably all, days of the week
Intensity	▸ Intensity may be determined through the following methods: ▪ 40–59% HRR or $\dot{V}O_2R$ ▪ RPE of 12–13 (6–20 scale) ▪ Below VT1 HR; can talk comfortably
Time	▸ Eventual goal of at least 30 minutes of continuous or accumulated exercise ▸ Clients with limited exercise capacity can accumulate bouts of intermittent exercise (10 minutes) throughout the day.
Type	▸ Emphasis should be placed on rhythmic, large-muscle-group activities: ▪ Walking ▪ Jogging ▪ Cycling ▪ Swimming
Progression	▸ Progress following the ACE Integrated Fitness Training Model based on client goals and availability. ▸ Progression should be personalized dependent on tolerance, client goals, and consideration of the following factors: ▪ Recent changes in antihypertensive drug therapy ▪ Medication-related adverse effects ▪ The presence of target-organ disease and/or other comorbidities
Muscular Training	
Frequency	▸ 2–3 days per week with a minimum of 48 hours separating exercise for the same muscle group
Intensity	▸ 60–80% 1-RM ▸ 40–50% 1-RM for older adults and novice exercisers
Time	▸ 2–4 sets of 8–12 repetitions ▸ Each major muscle group should be trained.

TABLE 13-4 *(continued)*

Muscular Training	
Type	▸ Either machine weights or free weights should be used to supplement cardiorespiratory training. ▸ Avoid the Valsalva maneuver during resistance training.
Progression	▸ Progress following the ACE Integrated Fitness Training Model based on client goals and availability.

Note: HRR = Heart-rate reserve; $\dot{V}O_2R$ = Oxygen uptake reserve; RPE = Rating of perceived exertion; VT1 = First ventilatory threshold; HR = Heart rate; 1-RM = One-repetition maximum

Source: American College of Sports Medicine (2018). *ACSM's Guidelines for Exercise Testing and Prescription* (10th ed.). Philadelphia: Wolters Kluwer.

Pharmacological Interventions

A number of medications prescribed to treat hypertension have a potential impact on the exercise and post-exercise responses. Some medications (e.g., **beta blockers** and **calcium channel blockers**) can blunt the heart-rate response and cause **orthostatic hypotension** and **post-exercise hypotension.** Individuals taking these medications should utilize RPE to monitor exercise intensity, change positions slowly, and conclude each exercise session with a gradual and prolonged cool-down period. Individuals should also be mindful to get up slowly from **supine** and/or seated positions to avoid a sudden drop in BP. **Diuretic** medications are commonly prescribed and may place certain individuals at increased risk for **dehydration** and post-exercise hypotension, especially in warm environments. It is important that people on diuretic medications maintain their hydration status and on very warm days appropriately adjust the intensity and/or duration of their activity. If orthostatic hypotension is a chronic problem, clients should be referred to their healthcare providers to have the dosage or class of antihypertensive medication reviewed and possibly changed.

STROKE

Strokes occur when the blood supply to the brain is compromised (**ischemic stroke**) or when a blood vessel in the brain bursts (**hemorrhagic stroke**). Like a heart attack, an ischemic stroke results from a blockage in a vessel—but instead of in the heart, it occurs in the brain. Ischemic strokes account for approximately 80% of all strokes and are usually caused by a fatty deposit in the lining of the vessel (atherosclerosis) (AHA, 2013; Go et al., 2014b). Hemorrhagic stroke is caused by the rupture of a blood vessel with bleeding out into the surrounding tissue (~20% of all cases). An **aneurysm** is a balloon-type bubble in the vessel at a weak spot that can rupture if left untreated. A malformation of blood vessels can also lead to a hemorrhagic stroke (AHA, 2013).

Etiology

The most important modifiable risk factor for stroke is hypertension. Other factors include smoking, heart disease, previous stroke, physical inactivity, and **transient ischemic attack (TIA).** A TIA can mimic the symptoms of a stroke but causes only temporary disability. Symptoms usually last less than one hour and may be relieved within 10 or 15 minutes. If a person has a TIA, he or she may be just as frightened as someone who has a stroke and should receive medical treatment to determine the cause. One-third of people who have a TIA will later have a stroke, many within the next month.

Prevalence

Strokes affect 795,000 Americans each year, resulting in more than 128,000 deaths. Stroke is the second leading cause of death globally and the number-one cause of disability (Feigin et al., 2014).

Nutrition

Many studies stress the benefits of a diet high in fruits and vegetables or in minerals such as potassium in the prevention and management of stroke (D'Elia et al., 2014; He, Nowson, & MacGregor, 2006). After a stroke, half of the survivors are considered malnourished, due to such risk factors as difficulty swallowing, old age, restricted upper limb movement, visuospatial impairment, and depression (Lieber et al., 2018).

Lifestyle

Important lifestyle factors to reduce the risk for stroke include reduced salt intake, not smoking, regular physical activity, and maintenance of normal body weight (Sarikaya, Ferro, & Arnold, 2015).

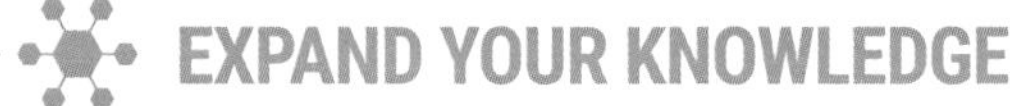

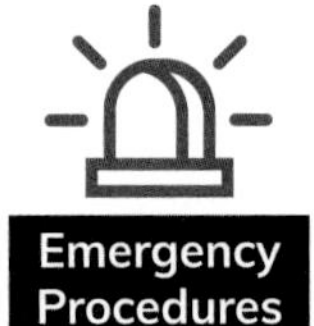

The Signs and Symptoms of Stroke

The brain controls various body functions, so symptoms of a stroke depend on what area of the brain is affected. Typical effects of a stroke include facial droop, weakness or paralysis of the body, vision problems, memory loss, and speech or language problems.

The personal trainer should be aware of the warning signs of a stroke:

- Sudden numbness or weakness of the face, arms, or legs
- Sudden confusion or trouble speaking or understanding others
- Sudden trouble seeing in one or both eyes
- Sudden walking problems, dizziness, or loss of **balance** and **coordination**
- Sudden severe headache with no known cause

The simple acronym FAST (facial drooping, arm weakness, speech difficulties, and time to call emergency services) serves as a mnemonic to help personal trainers to recognize and respond to the needs of a client having a stroke.

Exercise

Many people survive strokes, but not without damage, making it the leading cause of chronic disability (Feigin et al., 2014). Strokes can dramatically reduce a person's quality of life, robbing him or her of the ability to speak or utilize facial, arm, and leg muscles, and can cause other neurologic impairments. Additionally, people with stroke typically present in a severely deconditioned state, leading to a variety of metabolic disorders and significantly increased risk of recurrent stroke and MI. The deconditioning and associated metabolic changes, such as impaired glucose tolerance and type 2 diabetes, along with other risk factors, are typically worsened by physical inactivity.

Rehabilitation following stroke typically focuses on optimizing **basic activities of daily living** skills; regaining balance, coordination, and functional independence; and preventing complications and stroke reoccurrence. Unfortunately, this low-level rehabilitation does not provide adequate aerobic stimulus to reverse the physical deconditioning, muscular **atrophy,** increased cardiovascular risk resulting from stroke, and associated neurologic impairment. A number of studies have shown improved functional capacity resulting from a variety of exercise modalities, such as bicycle ergometer exercise, water exercise, and weight-supported treadmill exercise, as well as gait, balance, and coordination activities (Billinger et al., 2014). Exercise has also been shown to positively impact CVD risk factors in stroke patients (e.g., SBP, lipid profiles, **insulin sensitivity,** glucose metabolism, and **body composition**), reducing the overall risk of CAD and recurrent stroke. Additionally, exercise has been shown to improve fibrinolytic activity, the system responsible for dissolving blood clots.

For many years, clinicians considered the window for motor improvement following stroke to be within the first three to six months. However, there is evidence showing that exercise can improve selected motor performance even years after a stroke (Billinger et al., 2014). Therefore, people recovering from a stroke may gain additional benefit and improved quality of life by working with a personal trainer following release from a clinical rehabilitation program. Ideally, program guidelines for the personal trainer to utilize should come from the physical, occupational, and/or recreational therapist overseeing the clinical course of rehabilitation. Clients who are at risk for, or have experienced, a stroke, should follow the same guidelines and recommendations used for CAD and hypertension. Exercise activities may vary depending on the client's neurologic deficit profile, current functional capacity, and risk-factor status. Modalities such as using a cycle ergometer, walking/treadmill training, water exercise, and other exercise classes can be modified to accommodate clients who have survived a stroke. Activities that improve balance and coordination can also be helpful.

Table 13-5 presents an exercise guidelines summary for clients recovering from stroke.

TABLE 13-5

Exercise Guidelines Summary for Clients Recovering from Stroke

Cardiorespiratory Training	
Frequency	▸ 3 to 5 days per week
Intensity	▸ Light, moderate, or vigorous intensity* ▸ If HR data are available from recent GXT, use 40–70% HRR. ▸ In absence of GXT, or if atrial fibrillation is present, use RPE of 11–14 (6–20 scale).
Time	▸ Progressively increase from 20–60 minutes and consider multiple bouts of exercise throughout the day.
Type	▸ Considering functional and cognitive deficiencies, some use of equipment may need modifications. ▪ Cycle ergometry ▪ Recumbent seated steppers ▪ Treadmill walking
Progression	▸ Progress following the ACE Integrated Fitness Training Model based on client goals and availability.

Continued on the next page

TABLE 13-5 *(continued)*

Muscular Training	
Frequency	▸ 2 nonconsecutive days per week
Intensity	▸ 50–70% 1-RM
Time	▸ 1–3 sets of 8–15 repetitions
Type	▸ Use equipment and exercises that improve safety in those with deficits (e.g., machine versus free weights and seated versus standing)
Progression	▸ Progress following the ACE Integrated Fitness Training Model based on client goals and availability.

*Moderate intensity = Heart rates <VT1 where speech remains comfortable and is not affected by breathing; Vigorous intensity = Heart rates from ≥VT1 to <VT2 where clients feel unsure if speech is comfortable.

Note: HR = Heart rate; GXT = Graded exercise test; HRR = Heart-rate reserve; RPE = Rating of perceived exertion; 1-RM = One-repetition maximum; VT1 = First ventilatory threshold; VT2 = Second ventilatory threshold

Source: American College of Sports Medicine (2018). ACSM's *Guidelines for Exercise Testing and Prescription* (10th ed.). Philadelphia: Wolters Kluwer.

PERIPHERAL ARTERIAL DISEASE

PAD results from atherosclerosis of the arteries of the lower extremities. The most common sites for lower-extremity lesions include the abdominal aorta and the iliac, femoral, popliteal, and tibial arteries (see Figure 8-1, pages 252–253). Because there is narrowing of the arteries, blood flow **distal** to the lesion is reduced, significantly impacting the ability to walk. In general, the higher the lesion and the greater the narrowing, the greater the area that will be affected and the shorter the distance that a person can walk before having to stop due to ischemic pain.

Prevalence

PAD affects about 3 to 10% of adults. In persons older than 70 years, the prevalence rises to 15 to 20% (Dua & Lee, 2016). African Americans tend to have higher rates (6.7%) than Caucasians (3.5%) or Asians (3.7%). If diabetes is also present, these rates increase to 25%, 17%, and 10%, respectively (Vitalis et al., 2017).

Etiology

PAD is an important medical concern because of a high risk of concomitant CAD. Risk factors for PAD are similar to those of CAD and include dyslipidemia, smoking, hypertension, diabetes, family history, physical inactivity, obesity, and stress. The most prominent risk factors are smoking and diabetes (Creager & Libby, 2011).

PAD is characterized by muscular pain caused by ischemia, or lack of blood flow to the muscle. This ischemic pain is usually the result of spasms or arterial narrowing and is referred to as claudication. Most claudication pain is brought on by exercise, but more severe cases can also have pain at rest. Pain is frequently described as a dull, aching, and cramping pain and is usually reproducible at a given level of exercise. Many individuals with PAD can walk only a limited distance before needing to rest. Following a brief rest period, they usually are able to walk another short distance before stopping again.

Nutrition

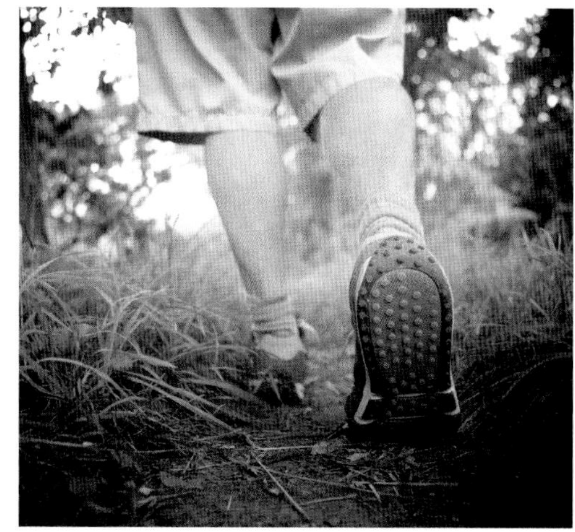

Given that PAD is common with persons with CAD, the general guidelines for both are similar (e.g., less meat and saturated fats, plus more fruits, vegetables and fiber). Older persons may have less access to nutritious foods, resulting in a greater risk of developing PAD (Redmond et al., 2016).

Exercise

Exercise consistently has been shown to be effective in improving walking distances in individuals with PAD (Olin et al., 2016). Improvement has been associated with better blood flow, as well as changes in blood viscosity and capillary and mitochondrial density, all of which improve oxygen utilization. Additionally, improved walking mechanics decreases oxygen demand at a given workload.

Before starting an exercise program, people with PAD should have a medical evaluation. The healthcare provider should give exercise clearance and provide basic exercise guidelines. Additional goals include modifying underlying risk factors and educating the client about PAD. Education is important because of the anxiety related to the pain associated with PAD.

Generally, walking is the exercise of choice because it uses the lower-leg muscles, effectively producing ischemia in the affected limb(s). This is important, as ischemia may be the primary stimulus for developing collateral circulation and other improvements in oxidative metabolism.

To improve exercise capacity, clients should walk to the point of pain, followed by rest until the pain subsides, and repeat. The process should initially be repeated for a total of 30 to 45 minutes with gradual progression to 60-minute sessions. The initial workload intensity should stimulate claudication pain within two to six minutes of walking. When eight to 12 minutes of continuous walking can be tolerated, consider increasing the walking pace or progressing the total activity time. However, caution should be taken to ensure that clients are free of cardiovascular symptoms and stay within moderate intensities.

It should be noted that "intensity" in this context refers more to the intensity of the pain (a 3 to 4 on the claudication pain/discomfort scale; Figure 13-1), and not to the energy expended relative to $\dot{V}O_2$max because these people cannot exercise enough to reach a maximum. In other words, there are peripheral limitations that do not allow them to tax the central cardiovascular system.

Some clients may develop CAD symptoms as walking distance and/or speed increase. In such cases, the exercise session should be discontinued until the client is evaluated by his or her physician and receives clearance to return to activity. Additionally, proper foot care is essential. The personal trainer should pay close attention to the client's feet, especially if the client has diabetes, and encourage proper footwear.

Table 13-6 presents an exercise guidelines summary for clients with PAD.

FIGURE 13-1
Claudication pain/discomfort scale

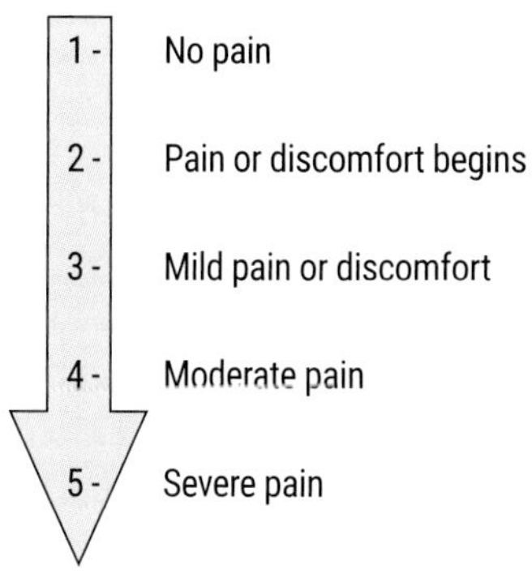

TABLE 13-6

Exercise Guidelines Summary for Clients with Peripheral Arterial Disease

Cardiorespiratory Training	
Frequency	▸ 3–5 days per week
Intensity	▸ Moderate intensity ▸ Below VT1 HR; can talk comfortably ▸ Walking speed and/or grade or workload that causes claudication pain within 2–6 minutes. Note that a percentage of HRR or $\dot{V}O_2R$ cannot be used because intensity is more closely associated with pain intensity. ▸ Do not exceed 3 to 4 on the claudication pain/discomfort scale.
Time	▸ 30–45 minutes (excluding rest periods) for up to 12 weeks ▸ May progress to 60 minutes
Type	▸ Weight-bearing ▪ Walking ▪ Intermittent exercise with seated rest when moderate pain (4 on the claudication pain/discomfort scale) is reached and resumption when pain dissipates
Progression	▸ Progress following the ACE Integrated Fitness Training Model based on client goals and availability.
Muscular Training	
Frequency	▸ At least 2 days per week performed on nonconsecutive days
Intensity	▸ 60–80% 1-RM
Time	▸ 2–3 sets of 8–12 repetitions ▸ 6–8 exercises targeting all major muscle groups
Type	▸ Whole body, focusing on large muscle groups ▸ Emphasize lower-limbs exercise if time is limited
Progression	▸ Progress following the ACE Integrated Fitness Training Model based on client goals and availability.

Note: VT1 = First ventilatory threshold; HR = Heart rate; $\dot{V}O_2R$ = Oxygen uptake reserve; HRR = Heart-rate reserve; 1-RM = One-repetition maximum

Source: American College of Sports Medicine (2018). *ACSM's Guidelines for Exercise Testing and Prescription* (10th ed.). Philadelphia: Wolters Kluwer.

Metabolic Disorders

DYSLIPIDEMIA

Lipids are a large group of organic compounds that are oily to the touch and insoluble in water and include **fatty acids,** oils, waxes, **sterols,** and **triglycerides (TG)**. Lipids are a source of stored energy and are a component of cell membranes. The most commonly measured lipids are TG and cholesterol.

The various lipids can be described as follows. **Chylomicrons** are large molecules of **fat** that mainly come from eating. TG form the major part of chylomicrons and can enter and accumulate in arterial walls. Cholesterol is a waxy, fat-like substance manufactured in the liver that is found in all cell membranes and is transported in the blood **plasma.** Cholesterol is an essential component of cell function and the production of **hormones,** vitamin D, and the bile acids that assist with fat digestion. However, while cholesterol is essential for life, undesirable levels are strongly associated with atherosclerosis and the development of CAD. Cholesterol travels through the body attached to a protein, referred to as a **lipoprotein.** The primary lipoproteins are characterized as follows:

- **Low-density lipoprotein (LDL)**: This is the major carrier of cholesterol in the blood, containing 60 to 70% of the body's total cholesterol. LDL is frequently referred to as the "bad" cholesterol because of its role in **atherogenesis,** the early stages of atherosclerosis.
- **Very low-density lipoprotein (VLDL)**: VLDL is the major carrier of TG and contains 10 to 15% of the body's total cholesterol.
- **Intermediate-density lipoprotein (IDL)**: Somewhat similar to LDL, IDL transports a variety of TG fats and cholesterol in the bloodstream and promotes atherogenesis. IDL are formed from the breakdown of VLDL.
- **High-density lipoprotein (HDL)**: Often referred to as the "good" cholesterol, HDL is produced in the small intestine and liver and normally contains 20 to 30% of the body's total cholesterol. HDL transports lipids to the liver for recycling and removal. HDL levels are inversely correlated to CAD (i.e., the higher the level of HDL, the lower the risk of developing CAD).
- **Non-HDL**: Non-HDL is defined as total cholesterol minus HDL, or put another way, the sum of the LDL, IDL, and VLDL. Non-HDL cholesterol is strongly associated with the development of CAD, and non-HDL levels appear to be equal or better than LDL levels at identifying atherogenic particles.

Dyslipidemia is defined as undesirable levels of these lipids. Elevated levels of total cholesterol and LDL cholesterol are the lipid parameters with the highest correlation to CAD, along with low levels of HDL and elevated levels of TG. Chronically elevated levels of TG have been associated with **endothelial dysfunction** and are considered an independent risk factor for CAD [Grundy et al., 2019; Grundy et al., 2004; National Cholesterol Education Program (NCEP), 2002].

Lipids may play a large role in the development of many chronic diseases, not just atherosclerosis and CAD. Examples include MetS, **abdominal obesity,** hypertension, **hyperglycemia, insulin resistance,** and type 2 diabetes (Pedersen & Saltin, 2006).

Table 13-7 presents the risk categories of LDL, total, and HDL cholesterol, while Table 13-8 shows the same for TG. Treatment for elevated total and LDL cholesterol and TG and/or low HDL is based on a person's overall CVD risk profile and blood lipid levels. Treatment generally involves diet, exercise, and medications. NCEP (2002) guidelines recommend at least six months of lifestyle-change therapy prior to initiating a medication regimen.

It should be noted that the levels in Table 13-8 are from blood samples taken after eight to 12 hours of fasting. When people eat meals and snacks, this produces higher levels of TG, which is known as **postprandial lipemia (PPL).**

Prevalence

The AHA reports that more than 28.5 million adults (11.9%) are estimated to have total blood cholesterol levels ≥240 mg/dL. The prevalence of high total cholesterol levels has decreased

TABLE 13-7

ATP III Classification of LDL, Total Cholesterol, and HDL Cholesterol (mg/dL)

LDL Cholesterol	
Optimal*	<100
Near optimal/above optimal	100–129
Borderline high	130–159
High	160–189
Very high	≥190

HDL Cholesterol	
Low	<40
High	≥60

Total Cholesterol	
Desirable	<200
Borderline high	200–239
High	≥240

*In high-risk individuals, use an LDL cholesterol threshold of 70 mg/dL.

Note: LDL = Low-density lipoprotein; HDL = High-density lipoprotein

Sources: Grundy, S.M. et al. (2019). 2018 AHA/ACC/AACVPR/AAPA/ABC/ACPM/ADA/AGS/APhA/ASPC/NLA/PCNA guideline on the management of blood cholesterol: Executive Summary. A Report of the American College of Cardiology/American Heart Association Task Force on Clinical Practice Guidelines. *Circulation*, 139, e1046–e1081; National Cholesterol Education Program (2002). Expert Panel on Detection, Evaluation and Treatment of High Blood Cholesterol in Adults: Summary of the second report of NCEP Expert Panel on Detection, Evaluation and Treatment of High Blood Cholesterol in Adults (Adult Treatment 31 Panel III). NIH Publication No. 02-5213. *Journal of the American Medical Association*, 285, 2486–2497.

TABLE 13-8

Classification of Triglycerides (mg/dL)

Normal	<150
Borderline high	150–199
High	200–499
Very high	≥500

Sources: Grundy, S.M. et al. (2019). 2018 AHA/ACC/AACVPR/AAPA/ABC/ACPM/ADA/AGS/APhA/ASPC/NLA/PCNA guideline on the management of blood cholesterol: Executive Summary. A Report of the American College of Cardiology/American Heart Association Task Force on Clinical Practice Guidelines. *Circulation*, 139, e1046–e1081; National Cholesterol Education Program (2002). Expert Panel on Detection, Evaluation and Treatment of High Blood Cholesterol in Adults: Summary of the second report of NCEP Expert Panel on Detection, Evaluation and Treatment of High Blood Cholesterol in Adults (Adult Treatment 31 Panel III). NIH Publication No. 02-5213. *Journal of the American Medical Association*, 285, 2486–2497.

over time (from 18.3% of adults in 1999 to 2000 to 11.0% of adults in 2013 to 2014), which appears to reflect a greater consumption of cholesterol-lowering medications (i.e., statin drugs), rather than changes in dietary patterns (Benjamin et al., 2019).

Etiology

Primary factors include genetics, sex, and age, along with secondary causes that contribute to dyslipidemia in varying degrees (e.g., body-fat distribution, cigarette smoking, some medications, dietary habits, and physical inactivity) (ACSM, 2018). In those who are genetically predisposed to dyslipidemia, problems with blood lipids may be exacerbated in the presence of significant secondary causes. For adults in developed countries, the most likely secondary cause is a physically inactive lifestyle with excessive dietary intake of saturated fat, cholesterol, and **trans fats.**

Nutrition

Dietary recommendations for managing dyslipidemia focus specifically on lowering the LDL cholesterol level. In a joint statement from the AHA and the American College of Cardiology (Eckel et al., 2013), the following guidelines are provided:

- Consume a dietary pattern that emphasizes vegetables, fruits, and whole grains; include low-fat dairy products, poultry, fish, legumes, non-tropical vegetable oils, and nuts; and limit intake of sweets, sugar-sweetened beverages, and red meats.
- Aim for a dietary pattern that achieves 5 to 6% of calories from saturated fat. Note: Reduce the percentage of calories from saturated fat in the diet, as any reduction may have a beneficial effect on the lipid profile.
- Reduce or eliminate the consumption of trans fat.

Exercise

While there are limited randomized, controlled studies investigating the lipid response to exercise, research generally suggests a benefit. Research from Gordon, Chen, & Durstine (2014) that looked at the effects of exercise training on the traditional lipid profile found that cardiorespiratory exercise combined with weight loss significantly reduces total blood cholesterol, LDL, VLDL, and TG, while improving HDL.

Relative to LDL, the results with cardiorespiratory training are inconsistent unless weight loss also occurs (Kelley, Kelley, & Tran, 2005). With muscular training, there is no change if there is no difference in weight, **lean body mass,** or body fat. Successful exercise programs for decreasing total and LDL cholesterol generally involve 250 to 300 minutes each week, expending approximately 2,000 calories. At this volume of exercise, most adults will lose weight and body fat.

For HDL, there are consistent improvements with cardiorespiratory training. If **cardiorespiratory fitness** improves, HDL generally increases. Although HDL can increase without a loss of weight or body fat, a greater rise in HDL is seen with fat loss. There is no convincing evidence that muscular training will have any effect on HDL. Programs with a high volume of exercise are generally successful for raising HDL. The frequency and duration of exercise appear to be more important than intensity, as long as the intensity is moderate to vigorous.

Unlike the various forms of cholesterol, TG can be used as fuel, especially during cardiorespiratory exercise. Cardiorespiratory training is most effective in persons with high TG and when the exercise intensity is moderate to vigorous. Muscular training has no effect, even with high levels of training. This is to be expected, however, since brief, high-intensity exercise is not aerobic and does not use fat as fuel.

Studies have shown that the TG levels of PPL are a better predictor of future CAD events than TG levels after fasting (Mora et al., 2008). The effects of exercise on PPL depend on the time elapsed since the last exercise session (i.e., 30 to 60 minutes of moderate-intensity exercise will lower TG levels for 12 to 36 hours, as well as improve the body's ability to respond to high-fat meals and reduce TG levels after meals) (Maraki & Sidossis, 2013). Therefore, clients should be encouraged to exercise at least every other day to keep their TG levels lower. The most effective programs include high volumes of moderate to vigorous exercise.

Table 13-9 presents an exercise guidelines summary for clients with dyslipidemia.

TABLE 13-9

Exercise Guidelines Summary for Clients with Dyslipidemia

Cardiorespiratory Training	
Frequency	▸ 5 or more days per week to maximize caloric expenditure
Intensity	▸ Below, at, and above VT1, but below VT2 ▸ 40–75% HRR or $\dot{V}O_2R$
Time	▸ 30–60 minutes per session ▸ However, a minimum of 50–60 minutes per day is recommended for weight loss or weight-loss maintenance
Type	▸ A variety of rhythmic large-muscle-group exercise
Progression	▸ Progress following the ACE Integrated Fitness Training Model based on client goals and availability.
Muscular Training	
Frequency	▸ 2–3 days per week
Intensity	▸ 50–85% 1-RM to improve muscular strength and <50% 1-RM to improve muscular endurance
Time	▸ 2–4 sets of 8–12 repetitions for muscular strength or 12–20 repetitions for muscular endurance
Type	▸ Resistance machines, free weights, and body weight
Progression	▸ Progress following the ACE Integrated Fitness Training Model based on client goals and availability.

Note: VT1 = First ventilatory threshold; VT2 = Second ventilatory threshold; $\dot{V}O_2R$ = Oxygen uptake reserve; HRR = Heart-rate reserve; 1-RM = One-repetition maximum

Source: American College of Sports Medicine (2018). *ACSM's Guidelines for Exercise Testing and Prescription* (10th ed.). Philadelphia: Wolters Kluwer.

DIABETES

Diabetes is a group of metabolic disorders involving an absolute or relative insufficiency of **insulin** secretion (Leon & Sanchez, 2005). Although there are several types of diabetes, the main ones are **type 1 diabetes** and type 2 diabetes. Table 13-10 compares the two types (Leon & Sanchez, 2005).

Worldwide, diabetes causes more than 3.2 million deaths per year. Many more deaths are likely related to health problems caused by diabetes but are attributed to a heart attack or stroke instead of being recognized as a diabetes-related death. Poorly managed diabetes has the potential to cause problems with almost every part of the body, including the heart, blood vessels, brain, kidneys, eyes, feet, nerves, muscles, and bones (Tang et al., 2013; Berry et al., 2012; Zoungas et al., 2012).

Type 1 Diabetes

ETIOLOGY AND PREVALENCE

About 5 to 10% of people, or around 1.25 million Americans, have type 1 diabetes [American Diabetes Association (ADA), 2017a; CDC, 2017]. This type of diabetes is caused by an

TABLE 13-10

Comparison of Type 1 and Type 2 Diabetes

Characteristics	Type 1	Type 2
Age of onset	Usually <35 years	Usually >40 years
Clinical onset	Abrupt	Gradual
Family history	Not always	Yes
Body composition	Normal or thin	Usually obese (central type)
Blood insulin levels	Reduced or absent	Normal or increased
Cell insulin resistance	Absent or minor	Present
Treatment for control of hyperglycemia	Insulin, diet, and/or exercise	Weight loss, diet, oral hypoglycemic drugs, or insulin

Source: Leon, A.S. & Sanchez, O.A. (2005). Diabetes mellitus. In: Skinner, J.S. (Ed.) *Exercise Testing and Exercise Prescription for Special Cases* (3rd ed.). Philadelphia: Lippincott Williams & Wilkins.

absolute insulin deficiency after the body's immune system attacks and destroys the **beta cells** of the pancreas, which make insulin (ADA, 2017a). Because of that destruction, insulin must be injected or infused to regulate blood sugar.

A person can develop type 1 diabetes at any age. Its rate of onset is quite variable, being rapid in infants and children, and slower in most adults. When pancreatic beta cells are down to about 10% of their usual function, symptoms of hyperglycemia first appear. Type 1 diabetes was once called "insulin-dependent" (as insulin is required) or "juvenile-onset" diabetes because three-quarters of all cases are diagnosed in individuals under 18 years of age (ADA, 2017b). However, most people currently living with type 1 diabetes are adults who either inject or pump insulin.

NUTRITION AND EXERCISE

Blood glucose levels are influenced by the interactions among diet, exercise, and insulin. Thus, if persons with type 1 diabetes eat or exercise, they would have to adjust the amount of insulin injected. Similarly, the timing of insulin injections influences when meals or snacks are eaten. As a result, it is complicated to control blood glucose and persons with type 1 diabetes have to be consistent as to when and how much (a) food is eaten, (b) exercise is performed, and (c) insulin is injected. If insulin levels are high, then blood glucose is low during and after exercise. If insulin levels are low, then there is a risk of high blood glucose and **ketosis** (a process that occurs when the body cannot use glucose and relies on incomplete **oxidation** of fats).

Now, with recent advances in insulin delivery systems and real-time continuous glucose monitoring, persons with type 1 diabetes can eat and exercise just as persons without the disease. In addition, the dietary and exercise guidelines to improve health are similar to those for the general population and the responses to training in persons with type 1 diabetes are also similar (Ostman et al., 2018). Unfortunately, about 60% of those with type 1 diabetes do not exercise sufficiently (Ostman et al., 2018). While this is not much different from the levels of participation of persons without type 1 diabetes, there is the additional barrier of fear of **hypoglycemia,** loss of glycemic control, and inadequate knowledge about exercise (Codella, Terruzzi, & Luzi, 2017; Riddell, 2017).

Persons with type 1 diabetes should reduce their insulin dose before exercise, take an easily absorbable **carbohydrate** before and during exercise, and adjust the infusion from the insulin pump during and after exercise (Codella, Terruzzi, & Luzi, 2017). Clients initiating an exercise program should consult their healthcare provider regarding which of the preceding actions they should take.

Type 2 Diabetes

More than 90% of people who have diabetes have type 2 diabetes. Type 2 diabetes is not due to inadequate levels of insulin, but more to the fact that the cells of the body are not sensitive (responsive) to insulin (i.e., relative insulin deficiency), such that more is needed for the same effect. Over time, the production of insulin cannot be increased enough and blood glucose levels rise.

PREVALENCE

The prevalence of type 2 diabetes in the U.S. in 2016 was 8.6%, or about 21 million people (Bullard et al., 2018).

ETIOLOGY

Type 2 diabetes is largely related to lifestyle habits (physically inactive and/or **sedentary** lifestyle, excess caloric intake, and nutritional deficiencies) that promote insulin resistance and **inflammation** resulting in hyperglycemia (ADA, 2017a). Type 2 diabetes is also associated with the following risk factors: family history, physical inactivity, overweight and obesity, high BP, abnormal lipids, high percentage of abdominal fat, and smoking (CDC, 2017).

Overweight and obesity are common among people with type 2 diabetes. A 5 to 7% decrease in body weight can reverse insulin resistance, even though individuals experiencing such losses seldom reach an ideal body weight (Hamdy et al., 2003). Improvements in insulin sensitivity appear to be more related to a reduction in systemic inflammation than to weight loss per se. However, obesity management can delay the progression from **prediabetes** to type 2 diabetes and may be beneficial to treat type 2 diabetes (ADA, 2017c), although not all forms of obesity are associated with insulin resistance (Hardy, Czech, & Corvera, 2012).

Highly characteristic of type 2 diabetes, insulin resistance is defined as the inability of insulin to effectively promote the uptake of glucose into cells to lower blood glucose levels. In people with this disease, this resistance is combined with a relative loss of beta cells (in the pancreas) that make insulin, which makes them unable to produce enough insulin to overcome their relative state of insulin resistance and leads to elevations in blood glucose. The majority of insulin resistance occurs in skeletal muscle. Some excess glucose may be lost in the urine, but the rest is usually converted into fat. Insulin resistance may be made worse by this excess fat being deposited in the **visceral fat** cells, liver, pancreas, and other intra-abdominal sites (Hardy, Czech, & Corvera, 2012). While many consider type 2 diabetes less severe than type 1 diabetes, its origin is more complex. Some people have an underlying genetic susceptibility that, when exposed to a variety of social, behavioral, and/or environmental factors, allows diabetes to develop. In other words, diabetes genes are triggered by a combination of factors, such as being inactive, eating poorly, gaining weight, being exposed to pollutants, stress, and more (ADA, 2017a).

Although lifestyle changes can assist in the management of type 2 diabetes (ADA, 2017d), many individuals also take diabetes medications and/or insulin to manage their blood

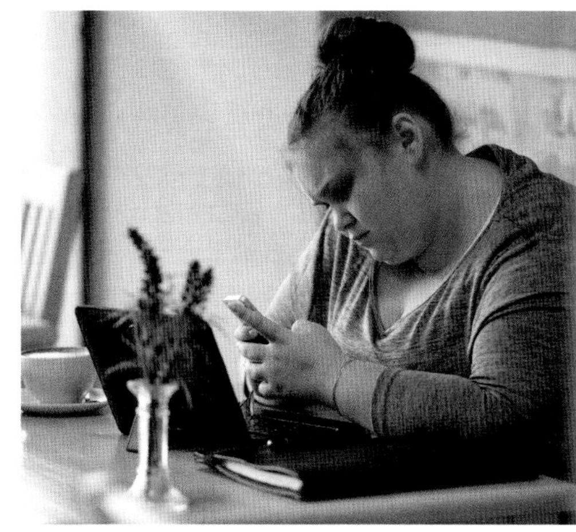

glucose. Most people with type 2 diabetes are adults, but the disease has become more common among teenagers and children with overweight or obesity (ADA, 2017b). Evidence suggests that type 2 diabetes in young people is more aggressive; this will lead to premature development of complications that will have adverse effects on quality of life and on long-term outcomes (Lascar et al., 2018).

For individuals born in the U.S. from the year 2000 forward, the probability of being diagnosed with type 2 diabetes at some point during their lives is substantial. Most people have at least a one-in-three chance and the prevalence is closer to 50% in ethnic and racial minorities (Narayan et al., 2003). Having a family history of type 2 diabetes increases the risk but a combination of lifestyle factors will also influence insulin resistance. Even in individuals with type 2 diabetes, pancreatic beta cells can lose some or all of their ability to release insulin when exposed to high levels of blood glucose over time (Abdul-Ghani et al., 2006), resulting in the need for insulin injections.

NUTRITION

Dietary improvements are a key component of managing body weight and blood glucose. Weight gain, loss, and maintenance are impacted by nutritional choices. Moreover, being active and eating more fiber are likely the two most important changes one can make to lower systemic inflammation and the risk of developing metabolic diseases (Herder et al., 2009). Eating well-balanced meals is essential for managing diabetes, and the *Dietary Guidelines for Americans* (www.health.gov/dietaryguidelines) and MyPlate guidelines (www.ChooseMyPlate.gov) include whole grains, vegetables and fruits, low-fat dairy, and lean proteins (U.S. Department of Agriculture, 2015). People with diabetes benefit from eating healthfully, just like everyone else.

While the **macronutrients** (i.e., carbohydrate, protein, and fat) each affect blood glucose differently, carbohydrates have the greatest impact because they are converted into blood glucose soon after being consumed. It is recommended that people check their blood glucose levels before and after meals to learn how foods, particularly those containing a lot of carbohydrate (e.g., potatoes, bread, rice, and pasta) affect them. The type of carbohydrate is also a factor to consider. **Simple carbohydrates** (i.e., sugars) are digested easily and are already available as glucose or can be converted quickly into glucose, resulting in spikes in blood glucose after eating. **Complex carbohydrates** (e.g., whole grains, potatoes, and starches) have to be broken down and most are released more slowly into the bloodstream. Blood glucose is generally at its highest one hour after eating, remains high for up to two hours, and then starts to fall. Checking blood glucose levels two hours after eating to see the effect of carbohydrates can be helpful. All macronutrients can cause weight gain when consumed in excess, but the greater release of, or need for, insulin due to excessive carbohydrate intake may contribute to weight gain due to the **anabolic** properties of insulin.

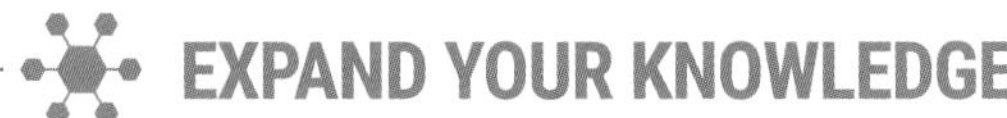

Fat Storage and Metabolic Dysfunction

The way that fat is distributed or stored across the body places a person at risk for cardiometabolic disease. **Subcutaneous** storage of fat is not as damaging to health as storing it in the liver or within the abdominal cavity (visceral fat); this may contribute to low-level inflammation, which can lead to insulin resistance, diabetes, heart disease, and other metabolic disorders. Visceral fat has long been associated with metabolic dysfunction, including insulin resistance, hypertension, elevated cholesterol and TG, and heart disease (Koska et al., 2008). In addition, whether the liver stores excess fat may prove to be a crucial link between weight gain and the development of prediabetes and type 2 diabetes (Koska et al., 2008). A fatty pancreas can also interfere with normal glucose metabolism (Ou et al., 2013). An insulin-resistant liver is often associated with elevated blood lipid levels that contribute to heart disease (Katsiki, Mikhailidis, & Mantzoros, 2016).

EXERCISE

All adults with diabetes or prediabetes should engage in at least 150 minutes of moderate-intensity or 75 minutes of vigorous-intensity cardiorespiratory exercise per week. Avoiding going more than two days in a row without exercising is important for blood glucose management. The main rationale for exercising at least every other day is that the effects of the last bout of cardiorespiratory activity on insulin sensitivity are lost after 24 to 48 hours in most cases, depending on the type, intensity, and duration of exercise (Colberg et al., 2016). Doing some type of muscular training at least twice per week helps make the body more sensitive to insulin and lowers blood glucose. Thus, if the person with diabetes or prediabetes engages in cardiorespiratory exercise three or four times a week and does muscular training exercise at least twice, the muscles could potentially maintain higher insulin sensitivity, resulting in better overall blood glucose management.

Table 13-11 presents an exercise guidelines summary for clients with diabetes.

TABLE 13-11
Exercise Guidelines Summary for Clients with Diabetes

Cardiorespiratory Training	
Frequency	▸ 3–7 days per week ▸ 3 days of vigorous or 5 days of moderate intensity (greater regularity may facilitate diabetes management)
Intensity	▸ Moderate intensity ▪ Below VT1 HR; can talk comfortably ▪ 40–59% HRR or $\dot{V}O_2R$ ▪ RPE 12–13 (6–20 scale) ▸ Vigorous intensity ▪ HR from VT1 to just below VT2 ▪ 60–89% HRR or $\dot{V}O_2R$ ▪ RPE 14–17 (6–20 scale)

TABLE 13-11 ***(continued)***

Cardiorespiratory Training	
Time	▸ Type 1 diabetes ▪ 150 minutes/week at moderate intensity; 75 minutes at vigorous intensity, or combination of both ▸ Type 2 diabetes ▪ 150 minutes/week at moderate intensity
Type	▸ A variety of rhythmic large-muscle-group exercises
Progression	▸ Progress following the ACE Integrated Fitness Training Model based on client goals and availability.
Muscular Training	
Frequency	▸ A minimum of 2 nonconsecutive days per week, preferably 3
Intensity	▸ 50–85% 1-RM (lower intensity to start)
Time	▸ 1–3 sets of 8–10 repetitions (10–15 repetitions to start)
Type	▸ All major muscle groups ▸ At least 8–10 exercises to near fatigue ▸ Resistance machines and free weights
Progression	▸ Progress following the ACE Integrated Fitness Training Model based on client goals and availability.

Note: VT1 = First ventilatory threshold; HR = Heart rate; HRR = Heart-rate reserve; $\dot{V}O_2R$ = Oxygen uptake reserve; RPE = Rating of perceived exertion; VT2 = Second ventilatory threshold; 1-RM = One-repetition maximum

Source: American College of Sports Medicine (2018). *ACSM's Guidelines for Exercise Testing and Prescription* (10th ed.). Philadelphia: Wolters Kluwer.

METABOLIC SYNDROME

MetS is not a disease but rather a cluster of conditions that increases a person's risk for developing heart disease, type 2 diabetes, and stroke. The AHA and the National Heart, Lung, and Blood Institute (NHLBI) recommend that MetS be identified by the presence of three or more of the following components (AHA/NHLBI, 2005):

- Elevated waist circumference
  - Men ≥40 inches (102 cm)
  - Women ≥35 inches (88 cm)
- Elevated TG
  - ≥150 mg/dL or on drug treatment
- Reduced HDL cholesterol
  - Men <40 mg/dL or on drug treatment
  - Women <50 mg/dL or on drug treatment
- Increased BP (systolic and/or diastolic)
  - ≥130/85 mmHg or on drug treatment
- Elevated fasting blood glucose
  - ≥100 mg/dL or on drug treatment

Prevalence

During the period of 2003 to 2012, the prevalence of MetS in the U.S. was 30.3% in men and 35.6% in women (Aguilar et al., 2015). Given that obesity and insulin resistance are present in most cases of MetS (Sherling, Perumareddi, & Hennekens, 2017; Samson & Garber, 2014) and that the rates of obesity and type 2 diabetes have increased over the past 15 years, it is likely that the prevalence of MetS is also higher. More African Americans, Hispanics, and Native Americans have MetS, as these ethnic groups also have more obesity, hypertension, and type 2 diabetes.

Etiology

MetS is identified by a number of other health states that are associated with obesity, type 2 diabetes, dyslipidemia, and high BP. MetS has been associated with physical inactivity, excessive caloric intake, obesity, genetics, and aging. Excess visceral fat is of particular concern and typically is the result of physical inactivity and poor nutritional habits.

Nutrition and Lifestyle

The primary treatment for MetS is to reduce the risk for developing CVD and type 2 diabetes. Lifestyle interventions, such as weight loss, increased physical activity, healthy eating (less saturated fat and cholesterol), and tobacco cessation are typically the initial strategies used. Research has shown that the negative energy balance induced by diet and exercise are necessary for achieving the metabolic benefits of weight loss (Tortosa et al., 2007; Klein et al., 2004).

Exercise

A variety of studies have shown that MetS is inversely associated with physical activity, with more active individuals having a lower incidence (Yang et al., 2008). The level of cardiorespiratory fitness has also been shown to independently influence the risk of premature mortality in people with increased body weight and/or the presence of MetS (Katzmarzyk, 2005). On the other hand, Stewart et al. (2005) examined whether the benefits of exercise on MetS risk factors were mediated by changes in fitness and body composition. After six months of training, they found no association among changes in fitness with risk factors for MetS, while reductions in total and abdominal fatness and increased leanness were more closely associated with risk factors for CVD, diabetes, and MetS.

Because many people with MetS also have obesity, the exercise program should be designed around guidelines for the treatment of clients with overweight or obesity [**body mass index (BMI)** 25 to 29.9 kg/m^2 and ≥30 kg/m^2, respectively] (ACSM, 2009; AHA/NHLBI, 2005) (see Chapter 12). However, additional factors such as underlying CAD, hypertension, dyslipidemia, and other risk factors should be evaluated and considered.

Exercise intensity will vary depending on the client's weight status, overall conditioning, and medical profile. Deconditioned individuals should begin at a lower intensity and gradually progress to moderate levels. Because a primary goal is weight loss, a frequency of five times per week or more is recommended and can consist of both continuous and intermittent activity.

Table 13-12 presents an exercise guidelines summary for clients with MetS.

TABLE 13-12

Exercise Guidelines Summary for Clients with Metabolic Syndrome

Cardiorespiratory Training	
Frequency	▸ 5 or more days per week to maximize caloric expenditure
Intensity	▸ 40–59% HRR or $\dot{V}O_2R$ ▸ Below VT1 HR; can talk comfortably ▸ RPE 12–13 (6–20 scale)
Time	▸ 30–60 minutes per session ▸ However, 50–60 minutes per session is recommended for weight loss or weight-loss maintenance. ▸ Intermittent exercise can be accumulated throughout the day as an alternative to continuous exercise.
Type	▸ A variety of rhythmic large-muscle-group exercises
Progression	▸ Progress following the ACE Integrated Fitness Training Model based on client goals and availability.
Muscular Training	
Frequency	▸ A minimum of 2 nonconsecutive days per week, preferably 3
Intensity	▸ 50–85% 1-RM (lower intensity to start)
Time	▸ 1–3 sets of 8–10 repetitions (10–15 repetitions to start)
Type	▸ All major muscle groups ▸ At least 8–10 exercises to near fatigue ▸ Resistance machines and free weights
Progression	▸ Progress following the ACE Integrated Fitness Training Model based on client goals and availability.

Note: $\dot{V}O_2R$ = Oxygen uptake reserve; HRR = Heart-rate reserve; RPE = Rating of perceived exertion; 1-RM = One-repetition maximum

Source: American College of Sports Medicine (2018). *ACSM's Guidelines for Exercise Testing and Prescription* (10th ed.). Philadelphia: Wolters Kluwer.

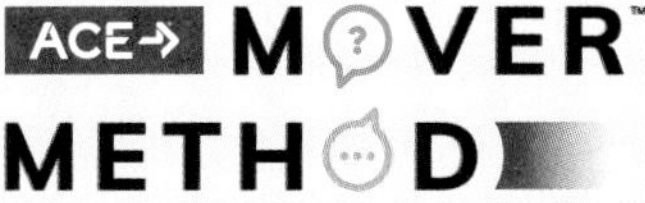

Initial Consultation with a Client with Multiple Chronic Diseases

Debbie is a 38-year-old banker who recently contacted you after viewing your personal-training website. Debbie has completed your online exercise preparticipation health screening and would like to meet with you to take advantage of your offer for a free initial consultation. The health-screening process revealed that Debbie is currently physically inactive. Furthermore, she recently had her first physical in three years. Her results indicated that she presents with type 2 diabetes, obesity, and high BP. Debbie also mentions that her doctor recommended beginning a moderate-intensity exercise program, as tolerated, and suggested adopting a healthy diet.

ACE→ ABC APPROACH™

Following is an example of how to use the principles of the ACE Mover Method™ and the ACE ABC Approach™ during an initial consultation. The objective of the meeting will be to build rapport, explore the client's needs, and to begin the collaborative, client-centered process of setting and working toward goals impacting the desired behavior change.

Ask: Start the initial consultation by asking powerful open-ended questions. This is a great way to explore the client's expectations and learn more about what she wants to achieve by working with a personal trainer.

Personal Trainer: Hi, Debbie, it's nice to meet you. I appreciate you taking the time to complete the online forms and scheduling this session to discuss your needs. What would you like to achieve by working together?

Client: I need to focus on the exercise aspect of managing my diabetes. Three weeks ago, my doctor told me that I have progressed from the overweight category to the obesity category. He also said that the insulin resistance he told me about three years ago has progressed to the point that I now have diabetes. My doctor mentioned that improving my lifestyle with exercise and eating better will help me manage the disease. So, I met with a registered dietitian last week and have already started following her suggestions. For a long time, I've known that my health status was moving in the wrong direction. Instead of facing reality, I ignored it to the point that things have become serious, and now I'm concerned.

Personal Trainer: It sounds like the diabetes diagnosis was a wake-up call for you and, as a result, you've started making changes to what you eat. In addition to diet changes, you would also like to start exercising to manage your diabetes. How will you define success? What needs to occur for you to be successful?

Client: For me, sticking to an exercise program would be a success! For that to happen, it would need to be fun and include things I enjoy, like being outdoors. More importantly, success would mean controlling my blood sugar.

Break down barriers: Spend time discussing potential barriers the client may encounter. Doing so prepares the client to overcome obstacles, which increases the likelihood of success.

Personal Trainer: Having fun, being outside, and managing your diabetes are some of the outcomes that will define success for you. What will be the most challenging part of this journey?

Client: I've not done any regular physical activity in over 10 years. I've thought about it a lot in the past five years and have tried to become more active, but I never stick with it.

Personal Trainer: What did you learn from those past attempts?

Client: The challenge I find is that I don't know what I'm doing when it comes to exercise and I don't feel confident with what I am doing. It's all so complicated: choosing the right exercises, knowing how hard I should work, how often to exercise, and things like that. Usually, after a few days, I decide it is easier to do nothing. Am I beyond help?

Personal Trainer: Absolutely not! The complexity of designing an exercise program can be intimidating. Because you are the expert in your own life, and I am here to provide you with the best exercise program that suits your unique needs, this will be a collaborative process. Together, we will create a program that is evidence-based, enjoyable, and focused on helping you manage your diabetes. Let's get some of your questions answered. Where would you like to start?

Client: To start, I'm not sure what my doctor means by doing moderate-intensity exercise as tolerated. I don't know what types of exercise to do, how long to do them, or how many times per week I should be doing them.

Personal Trainer: Excellent questions. Moderate-intensity means that you should be working at an intensity that allows you to speak comfortably and "as tolerated" means that you should do it for as long as you can. Generally, it is recommended to participate in moderate-intensity cardiorespiratory exercise for at least 150 minutes per week, but this is something we can work toward over time. A variety of cardiorespiratory, muscular, balance, and **flexibility** training can be beneficial, and we will incorporate all these aspects to create a well-rounded program. Lastly, when it comes to how many days per week, this is up to you, as any amount of physical activity will have a benefit. However, some of the benefits of exercise for people with diabetes are lost after 24 to 48 hours. So, exercising at a minimum of every other day can help to manage blood sugar levels. Does all of this make sense?

Client: Yes, it does. Thank you for the clarification. I've never thought of myself as an expert on me, but I get what you're saying. I have more skin in the game if I'm involved in creating the program with your guidance.

Collaborate: Work together with the client to identify next steps and **SMART goals** to find out how the client would like to get started.

Personal Trainer: Exactly! What is one small step you can see yourself taking to get started today?

Client: I'm motivated and ready! I think the right place to start would be to meet with you two times per week for private one-hour personal-training sessions. If your schedule allows for it, I would like to get started tomorrow!

Personal Trainer: That works great for me, and I do have some openings tomorrow.

In this scenario, notice how the personal trainer addresses the client's concerns, reminds the client that she is an expert on herself, and collaborates on realistic next steps. Taking the time to use the ACE ABC Approach allows for building rapport, creating a caring environment, and keeping the personal-training experience client-centered.

Pulmonary Disorders

Chronic obstructive pulmonary disease (COPD) is the result of chronic airway inflammation due to exposure to substances such as tobacco smoke and various other environmental and occupational pollutants. Symptoms include dyspnea, chronic cough and sputum, **sarcopenia**, and skeletal muscle dysfunction, which lead to ventilatory limitations, shortness of breath, and decreases in physical activity as a result of exercise intolerance (O'Donnell et al., 2017). The risk of falls is elevated in people with COPD, as lower-extremity muscle weakness and gait abnormalities are common (Voica et al., 2016).

There are several types of COPD, which suggests that all patients cannot be managed in a similar fashion. The three common obstructive diseases are asthma, **chronic bronchitis,** and **emphysema.**

ASTHMA

Asthma is a chronic inflammatory disorder of the airways in which many cells and cellular elements play a role. In susceptible individuals, this inflammation causes recurrent episodes of wheezing, breathlessness, chest tightness, and coughing, particularly at night or in the early morning. The inflammation also causes an associated increase in the existing bronchial hyper-responsiveness to a variety of stimuli, such as **allergens**, irritants (smoke, air pollution, strong odors and sprays, and pollens), viruses, stress, cold air, and exercise. These triggers can activate an inflammatory response that leads to airway hyper-responsiveness and airway obstruction due to constriction of smooth muscle around the airways, swelling of mucosal cells, and/or increased secretion of mucus.

When exercise provokes an asthma attack, there is a characteristic response. First, there is **bronchoconstriction,** which may last the duration of the activity or may persist for only a few minutes. This bronchoconstriction is followed by narrowing of the airways, an event that accelerates as soon as exercise is finished (Morton & Fitch, 2005).

Approximately 80% of people with asthma experience attacks during and/or after exercise; this is referred to as **exercise-induced bronchoconstriction (EIB)** (Morton & Fitch, 2005). EIB is characterized by a temporary narrowing of the airways following moderate to vigorous exercise. EIB typically occurs after breathing large quantities of air, especially dry, cold air that contains environmental allergens and/or pollutants. The severity of the response is related to the intensity of exercise (ventilatory requirement) and the environmental conditions. Symptoms usually peak five to 10 minutes after exercise and can last for 20 to 30 minutes. Some individuals also develop a hacking cough two to 12 hours after exercise that can last for one to two days. Between episodes of asthma, the cardiorespiratory system is normal in many people and does not interfere with physical performance.

Approximately 50% of those who have an EIB episode experience a relative refractory period, lasting for up to two hours, during which another exercise bout will not produce an EIB attack or will result in a less intense reaction (Morton & Fitch, 2005). Late asthmatic responses, six to eight hours after the initial bronchoconstriction, also occur in approximately half of individuals who experience EIB. These late responses are typically mild.

Prevalence

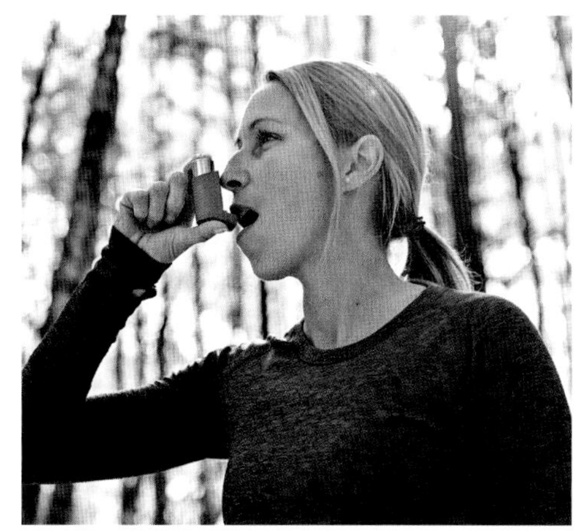

Asthma is one of the most common respiratory disorders. Its incidence is greatest in the first decade of life and it occurs among all races, with the first episode occurring at any age. Asthma affects more than 25 million children and adults in the United States [U.S. Environmental Protection Agency, 2018; Moorman et al., 2012; National Asthma Education and Prevention Program (NAEPP), 2007]. The disorder is responsible for nearly 500,000 hospitalizations, 2 million emergency room visits, and 3,400 deaths in the U.S. each year. Among children, boys have a higher prevalence than girls (11.1% vs. 7.8%) whereas among adults, men have lower prevalence than women (5.7% vs. 9.7%) (Moorman et al., 2012).

Etiology

Despite early recognition of the association between exercise and asthma and extensive research on EIB, no mechanism satisfactorily explains its occurrence. The best hypothesis is that EIB is caused by the release of a bronchoconstrictor substance that is thought to occur as a result of the loss of fluid from the airways during conditioning of inspired air.

Conditioning the air refers to the warming, humidifying, and filtering of inspired air and is important to prevent damage to delicate alveolar tissue that can occur when it is exposed to cold dry air. Most conditioning occurs in the nose, pharynx, and the first branches of the bronchi. Individuals with asthma should inhale through the nose during rest and light exercise to maximize this warming and humidification process. Even when dry air at 32° F (0° C) is inspired through the nose, it is modified so that it has been humidified and warmed to 98.6° F (37° C) by the time it reaches the alveolar membrane. This saturation of alveolar air occurs by absorbing water from the airways during its passage from the nose to alveolar regions.

Exercise

Regular exercise is an important component of disease management because of its beneficial effects on respiratory and circulatory function and on the psychological development of people with asthma, which is reflected in its effect on their social life. These training benefits are manifested in the improved working capacity due to an increased $\dot{V}O_2$max, as well as improved skill and efficiency during motor tasks. This means that the same tasks can be performed with less ventilation and thus less drying of the airways. In general, people with asthma should be able to participate in regular exercise and sports with minimal restriction, if correctly medicated.

Some people react to an EIB by avoiding exercise. As a result, their cardiorespiratory fitness gets worse and symptoms may occur with even lower levels of physical activity (Morton & Fitch, 2005). EIB can develop during exercise at 80% or more of maximum exertion (Parsons & Mastronarde, 2005). Although breathlessness is normal during high-intensity exercise, it is abnormal if it occurs during or after light exercise. Unfortunately, many people with asthma do not realize this fact and assume that dyspnea is just lack of cardiorespiratory fitness, fail to seek medical advice, and perform at a disadvantage because they lack appropriate medication.

Before starting an exercise program, a physician can provide guidance regarding potential triggers, medication use, and what to do in case of an asthmatic episode during and/or following exercise. Many people with asthma are placed on medications that lessen or prevent the EIB response, such as bronchodilators, anti-inflammatory agents, and a variety of other medications. It is important that clients review the use of these medications with their physician, especially prophylactic treatment prior to exercise.

Most people with controlled asthma will benefit from regular exercise and can follow exercise guidelines for the general population. Exercise conditioning can help to reduce the ventilatory requirement for various tasks, making it easier for people with asthma to participate in normal daily activities, recreational events, and competitive sports. Consistent participation in regular exercise can improve quality of life, reduce EIB severity, increase the level of exercise intensity triggering an attack, decrease EIB intensity, decrease medication usage, and lead to more symptom-free days (Rundell, 2016).

Because EIB is brought on by **hyperventilation,** individuals with asthma should be encouraged to perform a 10- to 15-minute warm-up consisting of vigorous or interval-type exercise to induce a refractory period and attenuate the EIB response (ACSM, 2018; Moore, Durstine, & Painter, 2016).

The following general activity guidelines will help the personal trainer develop, monitor, and progress an exercise program for clients with asthma.

- Clients should have **rescue medication** with them at all times and be instructed on how to use it should symptoms occur. Some physicians will also instruct their patients to prophylactically use a bronchodilating inhaler before exercise.
- Clients should drink plenty of fluids before, during, and after exercise to prevent dehydration.
- Clients should avoid asthma triggers during exercise and consider moving indoors on extremely hot or cold days or when pollen counts and/or air pollution are high. Some may benefit from wearing a face mask during exercise in the cold to keep inhaled air warm and moist.
- Clients should utilize prolonged warm-up and cool-down periods.
- It is important to keep the initial intensity low and gradually increase it over time. The peak exercise intensity should be determined by the client's state of conditioning and asthma severity. Clients should reduce the intensity if asthma symptoms begin to occur.
- Personal trainers should closely observe clients for early signs of EIB and respond immediately. They should reduce intensity and terminate the exercise session should symptoms worsen.
- If an asthma attack is not relieved by medication, the personal trainer should activate the emergency medical system.
- People with asthma often respond best to exercise in mid-to-late morning.
- Clients with well-controlled asthma can typically use the exercise guidelines for the general population for cardiorespiratory and muscular training.

Although exercise can induce an asthma attack, regular physical activity is an important component to manage the disease. Training can increase the maximal ventilation and reduce the ventilation needed for a given level of submaximal exercise. An aerobically trained person with asthma can cope better than an untrained person with asthma with the same degree of mild or moderate airway obstruction. In addition, it takes more provocation to produce symptoms in the aerobically trained person with asthma.

There are a number of effective medications to prevent and reverse EIB. The use of pre-exercise medication allows most people with asthma to perform exercise with little disadvantage.

Table 13-13 presents an exercise guidelines summary for clients with asthma.

Nutrition

Nutrition influences asthma in several ways. For example, dietary habits that result in overweight increase the risk of developing asthma. Obesity is associated with severity and

TABLE 13-13

Exercise Guidelines Summary for Clients with Asthma

Cardiorespiratory Training	
Frequency	▸ 3–5 days per week
Intensity	▸ Initially, below VT1 ▸ 40–59% HRR or $\dot{V}O_2R$. If well tolerated, progress to 60–70% HRR or $\dot{V}O_2R$ after 1 month. ▸ RPE 12–13 (6–20 scale)
Time	▸ Progressively increase to at least 30–40 minutes per session
Type	▸ Rhythmic large-muscle-group exercise such as: ▪ Walking ▪ Running ▪ Cycling ▪ Swimming in a nonchlorinated pool
Progression	▸ Progress following the ACE Integrated Fitness Training Model based on client goals and availability.
Muscular Training	
Frequency	▸ A minimum of 2 nonconsecutive days per week, preferably 3
Intensity	▸ 50–85% 1-RM (lower intensity to start)
Time	▸ 1–3 sets of 8–10 repetitions (10–15 repetitions to start)
Type	▸ All major muscle groups ▸ At least 8–10 exercises to near fatigue ▸ Resistance machines and free weights
Progression	▸ Progress following the ACE Integrated Fitness Training Model based on client goals and availability.

Note: VT1 = First ventilatory threshold; $\dot{V}O_2R$ = Oxygen uptake reserve; HRR = Heart-rate reserve; RPE = Rating of perceived exertion; 1-RM = One-repetition maximum

Source: American College of Sports Medicine (2018). *ACSM's Guidelines for Exercise Testing and Prescription* (10th ed.). Philadelphia: Wolters Kluwer.

frequency of asthma attacks (Wood, 2017). Food allergies are another possible trigger, as they increase inflammation and asthma attacks (Gupta & Verma, 2007).

Smoking

Smoking, including second-hand smoke, can influence the onset and severity of asthma. Vaping with electronic cigarettes (e-cigs) is gaining popularity. While there is little information on the potential long-term effect of e-cigs on the incidence or exacerbation of asthma, some ingredients are chemically similar to known airway irritants and have been reported to cause occupational asthma (Clapp & Jaspers, 2017).

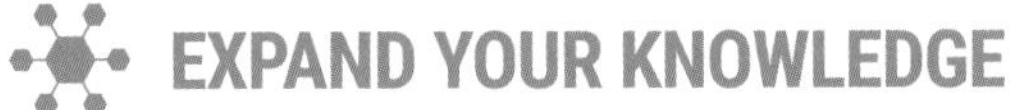

Chronic Bronchitis and Emphysema

Bronchitis is characterized by the chronic production of sputum, often resulting in airflow obstruction due mainly to thickened bronchial walls and secretions. Emphysema is characterized by distention and destruction of the alveoli. Because of a loss of pulmonary elastic recoil, there is obstruction due to dynamic airway narrowing.

It is unlikely that personal trainers will be involved with exercise programs for persons with chronic bronchitis and emphysema, except for those who are just beginning to have problems. For individuals who can walk fast and climb stairs, cardiorespiratory exercise programming is much the same as anyone with a low functional capacity (e.g., 20 to 60 minutes of moderate- to vigorous-intensity exercise at least three to five days per week, as tolerated). For those who can walk at a normal pace, exercise intensity and duration of exercise may be restricted, such that the person may have to exercise more than once a day every day for short periods before breathlessness restricts further activity (ACSM, 2018). Muscular training is an important part of an exercise plan for people with chronic bronchitis and emphysema, as it can be a potent intervention to address muscle weakness and balance problems. However, there are no evidence-based exercise guidelines specific to individuals with chronic bronchitis and emphysema (Maltais et al., 2014). Persons with severe, advanced chronic bronchitis and emphysema are so restricted that they are usually treated in hospitals and out-patient clinics and will not be seen by personal trainers.

There is general agreement that regular exercise training may effectively improve the ability to exercise and reduce dyspnea but will probably not affect the disease process or the person's pulmonary function (ACSM, 2018).

Table 13-14 presents an exercise guidelines summary for clients with chronic bronchitis and emphysema.

TABLE 13-14

Exercise Guidelines Summary for Clients with Chronic Bronchitis and Emphysema

Cardiorespiratory Training	
Frequency	▸ At least 3–5 days per week, ideally every day
Intensity	▸ Moderate to vigorous ▸ Below, at, and above VT1 but below VT2 HR ▸ 50–80% peak work rate ▸ RPE 4–6 (0–10 scale)
Time	▸ 20–60 minutes per session ▸ Intermittent exercise (i.e., interval training) may be used during initial sessions until longer durations are achieved.

TABLE 13-14 *(continued)*

Cardiorespiratory Training	
Type	▸ Walking or cycling, upper-body endurance activities to help improve activities of daily living
Progression	▸ Progress following the ACE Integrated Fitness Training Model based on client goals and availability.
Muscular Training	
Frequency	▸ 2–3 days per week
Intensity	▸ 60–70% of 1-RM for beginners' muscular strength ▸ >80% of 1-RM for experienced weight trainers' muscular strength ▸ <50% of 1-RM for muscular endurance
Time	▸ 2–4 sets of 8–12 repetitions for muscular strength ▸ ≤2 sets of 15–20 repetitions for muscular endurance
Type	▸ Weight machines, free weights, or body-weight exercise
Progression	▸ Progress following the ACE Integrated Fitness Training Model based on client goals and availability.

Note: VT1 = First ventilatory threshold; VT2 = Second ventilatory threshold; HR = Heart rate; RPE = Rating of perceived exertion; 1-RM = One-repetition maximum; Peak work rate measured in watts

Source: American College of Sports Medicine (2018). *ACSM's Guidelines for Exercise Testing and Prescription* (10th ed.). Philadelphia: Wolters Kluwer.

Other Chronic Conditions

CANCER

Cancer is a collection of approximately 200 related diseases characterized by the uncontrolled spread and growth of abnormal cells. Normally, cells grow and divide in an orderly, controlled fashion to produce new cells that replace old and/or damaged cells. Cancer cells develop when the **deoxyribonucleic acid (DNA)** of normal cells is damaged, producing mutations that affect the orderly, controlled process of growth and division. The damaged DNA and associated mutations result in uncontrolled cell growth. Some cancers form solid tumors, or masses of tissue. However, other types, such as cancers of the blood (e.g., leukemias), generally do not. When cancerous tumors are **malignant,** they can invade nearby tissues. A malignant tumor may also **metastasize,** which is the result of cancer cells breaking off from the original tumor and traveling to distant sites via the blood or the lymph system to form new tumors. Unlike malignant tumors, **benign** tumors do not spread to other tissues. Benign tumors typically do not grow back once surgically removed, whereas malignant tumors sometimes do. Metastatic tumors can severely disrupt bodily functions, and most cancer mortality is due to metastatic disease (National Cancer Institute, 2017).

The classification of different cancers is typically based on the cell type from which they originate. For example, cancer that develops in the endothelial cells that line many organs are called carcinomas and cancers of the blood cells are called leukemia. Cancers of the immune system or connective tissue and bones are termed lymphoma and sarcoma, respectively. Because cancer can develop from any type of cell and involve every organ system, it is not surprising that different cancers can produce a wide variety of challenges.

Prevalence

Cancer is the second-leading cause of morbidity and mortality worldwide. It was responsible for 8.8 million deaths in 2015, with a global death toll of nearly one in six (World Health Organization, 2017). Cancer disproportionally affects older people, with 87% of cases diagnosed in the U.S. 50 years of age or older (American Cancer Society, 2017). As such, adults diagnosed with cancer are also likely to have other chronic conditions (e.g., CVD, diabetes, **osteoporosis,** and arthritis). In the U.S., the lifetime risk of developing cancer for men is 41 out of 100, whereas the risk for women is 38 out of 100 (American Cancer Society, 2017).

Due to early detection and improved treatments, the U.S. has seen a 27% decline in cancer death over the past 10 years. As such, the number of cancer survivors has grown to over 15.5 million people in the U.S.—a figure that is expected to double by 2040 (Siegel, Miller, & Jemal, 2019). The three general phases of cancer survivorship are: (1) treatment and recovery; (2) living after recovery, including survivors who are disease-free or who have stable disease; and (3) advanced cancer and end of life (Rock et al., 2012). More and more cancer survivors are actively seeking out information about healthy behaviors (e.g., better diet and more physical activity) to improve their response to treatment, aid recovery, reduce their risk of recurrence, and improve their quality of life (Jones & Demark-Wahnefried, 2006).

Etiology

The cause of cancer is complex and linked to many factors, such as environmental exposures (e.g., pollutants, ultraviolet light, and chemicals), lifestyle practices (e.g., smoking, living a physically inactive lifestyle, and poor diet), medical interventions, viral infections, genetic traits, sex, and aging. It is estimated that around 30% of deaths from cancer are associated with the five leading behavioral and dietary risks: (1) high BMI (2) low consumption of fruits and vegetables, (3) physical inactivity, (4) tobacco use, and (5) alcohol intake (World Health Organization, 2017).

Nutrition

Traditionally, cancer was thought of as a disease associated with weight loss because patients undergoing treatment were often among those with late-stage cancer. The treatments tended to leave them with significant untreated nausea and vomiting, which led to decreased weight. Patients with cancer are now being diagnosed at earlier stages when treatments are more effective and more people have overweight or obesity when diagnosed (Pekmezi & Demark-Wahnefried, 2011). Significant weight loss and poor nutritional outcomes are still a concern in the early stages of some cancers, but malnutrition and weight loss vary widely across cancer types and stage at diagnosis (Fearon et al., 2011).

Nutrient requirements for macronutrients and **micronutrients** can be affected by metabolic and physiological changes caused by cancer. Common side effects of cancer and cancer treatment result in such symptoms as reduced appetite, early **satiety,** changes in taste and smell, and bowel disturbances, which can lead to low nutrient intake and subsequent malnutrition. Cancer treatments (e.g., surgery, radiation, and chemotherapy) can alter nutritional needs, disrupt eating habits, and adversely affect how the body digests, absorbs, and uses food (Schattner & Shike, 2006; McMahon & Brown, 2000). Consequently, nutritional assessment and dietary counseling from a qualified healthcare professional is recommended as soon after diagnosis as possible (McMahon & Brown, 2000). The overall goals of nutritional care are to prevent or resolve nutrient deficiencies, achieve or maintain a healthy weight, preserve lean body mass, minimize nutrition-related side effects, and maximize quality of life (Rock et al., 2012).

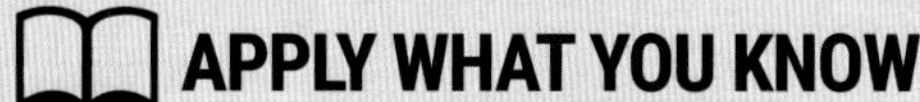

APPLY WHAT YOU KNOW

Suggestions for Locating Specialized Nutrition Counseling

Personal trainers who work with people with cancer must be aware of special nutrition considerations brought on by the disease and its treatment. The following strategies are recommended to help clients find appropriate professional nutrition support (Rock et al., 2012):

- Clients should ask their healthcare providers for a referral to see an RD, preferably one who is also a certified specialist in oncology.
- Survivors, caregivers, and providers may identify a local private-practice RD by consulting the Academy of Nutrition and Dietetics.

Exercise

Patients treated for cancer probably will have a decrease in lean body mass, muscular strength and muscular endurance, cardiorespiratory fitness, and flexibility, as well as an increase in body fat (Lane & McKenzie, 2005). As a result, they will be less able to or have less interest in performing ADL or becoming more active.

There exists a large body of epidemiologic evidence that concludes that those who participate in higher levels of physical activity have a reduced likelihood of developing a variety of cancers compared to those who engage in lower levels of physical activity (Brown et al., 2012). This protection for active people may be the result of balancing caloric intake with energy expenditure or by other means, including changes that positively affect the hormonal environments (Biswas et al., 2015; Schmid & Leitzmann, 2014). Regular activity also has a significant role in improving risk factors associated with cancer development. There is some evidence that physical activity improves immune function, and that this improvement may be an additional benefit of exercise in the prevention and treatment of some forms of cancer (Hojman, 2017).

Traditionally, during treatment for or recovery from cancer, patients were told to rest and limit their physical activity; this resulted in loss of strength, endurance, and **mobility,** which served only to intensify the deterioration of function and led to a worsening of signs and symptoms. Research has shown that exercise is not only safe and possible during cancer treatment, but also serves to improve common side effects of a cancer diagnosis and treatment—specifically anxiety, depressive symptoms, fatigue, health-related quality of life, and physical function (Campbell et al., 2019). Exercise benefits include preservation of muscle mass and an increase in muscular strength and muscular endurance; improved balance and overall physical function; reductions in fatigue, nausea, anxiety, and depression; and decreased risk for heart disease, osteoporosis, and diabetes.

The goal of exercise for individuals with cancer is to maintain and improve cardiovascular conditioning, achieve and/or maintain a healthy weight, prevent musculoskeletal deterioration, reduce symptoms such as nausea and fatigue, and improve mental health outlook and overall quality of life.

Table 13-15 presents an exercise guidelines summary for clients with cancer.

The specific exercise program undertaken should be tailored to the client's needs, type of cancer, treatments being done, and current medical and physical-fitness status (Rock et al., 2012). The training protocol should center on cardiorespiratory activities, light muscular

TABLE 13-15

Exercise Guidelines Summary for Clients with Cancer

Cardiorespiratory Training	
Frequency	▸ 3–5 days per week
Intensity	▸ Moderate ▪ 40–59% HRR or $\dot{V}O_2R$ ▪ Below VT1 HR; can talk comfortably ▪ RPE 12–13 (6 to 20 scale) ▸ May progress to vigorous ▪ 60–89% $\dot{V}O_2R$ or HRR ▪ Not sure if talking is comfortable; VT1 to just below VT2
Time	▸ 75 minutes per week of vigorous intensity or 150 minutes of moderate, or an equivalent combination of the two
Type	▸ Prolonged, rhythmic activities using large muscle groups ▪ Walking ▪ Cycling
Progression	▸ Progress following the ACE Integrated Fitness Training Model based on client goals and availability.
Muscular Training	
Frequency	▸ 2–3 days per week
Intensity	▸ Start with low resistance (<30% 1-RM) and progress with small increments (~5%)
Time	▸ At least 1 set of 8–12 repetitions
Type	▸ Free weights and resistance machines ▸ Weight-bearing functional tasks ▸ Target all major muscle groups
Progression	▸ Progress following the ACE Integrated Fitness Training Model based on client goals and availability.

Note: $\dot{V}O_2R$ = Oxygen uptake reserve; HRR = Heart-rate reserve; VT1 = First ventilatory threshold; HR = Heart rate; RPE = Rating of perceived exertion; VT2 = Second ventilatory threshold; 1-RM = One-repetition maximum

Source: American College of Sports Medicine (2018). *ACSM's Guidelines for Exercise Testing and Prescription* (10th ed.). Philadelphia: Wolters Kluwer.

training, and stretching, and be supplemented with recreational activities. People undergoing chemotherapy and/or radiation may be anemic and require reduced exercise intensity. Those with compromised skeletal integrity should minimize weight-bearing and heavy weight-lifting activities.

Following cancer treatment, weight management, regular physical activity, and a healthy diet are important to promote overall health, quality of life, and longevity (Coward, 2006). Individuals who have been diagnosed with cancer remain at a higher risk of developing second primary cancers and may also be at an increased risk for such chronic diseases as CVD, diabetes, and osteoporosis (Ng & Travis, 2008). As such, guidelines established to prevent these chronic diseases should be used.

Although healthy lifestyle practices are recommended to cancer survivors as supportive strategies for enhanced quality of life and longevity during and after treatment, obesity, inactivity, and poor-quality diets are common (Demark-Wahnefried et al., 2015). These unhealthy lifestyle behaviors tend to be present at cancer diagnosis and may become more pronounced with diagnosis and treatment. For many cancer survivors, CVD is a significant cause of death for which obesity, physical inactivity, and poor diet are established risk factors (Basen-Engquist et al., 2017).

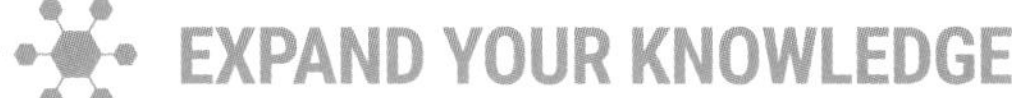

American Cancer Society Guidelines

Specialized diets for people who have been diagnosed with cancer should be prescribed and monitored by nutrition professionals, preferably RDs certified as oncology specialists. However, general guidelines from the American Cancer Society provide valuable information for personal trainers to keep in mind when collaborating with clients to develop behavior-change plans, particularly around areas of focus such as nutrition and physical activity. The following list describes evidence-informed actions that people with cancer can take to promote health (Rock et al., 2012):

- People diagnosed with cancer should aim for a healthy weight. The need to change body fat varies by the cancer site. For example, patients with head, neck, esophageal, and gastric cancer tend to be underweight, while many of those with breast and prostate cancer have overweight at diagnosis or after treatment.
- Participating in regular physical activity that includes at least 150 minutes per week of cardiorespiratory exercise, plus muscular-training exercises at least two days per week, is important. Those who have cancer should avoid inactivity and return to normal daily activities as soon as possible after diagnosis.
- Follow the American Cancer Society Guidelines on Nutrition and Physical Activity for Cancer Prevention (Rock et al., 2012):
    - Limit processed meat and red meat.
    - Consume 2.5 cups of vegetables and fruits daily.
    - Choose whole grains instead of refined grain products.
    - If alcoholic beverages are consumed, limit consumption to no more than one drink daily for women or two drinks daily for men.

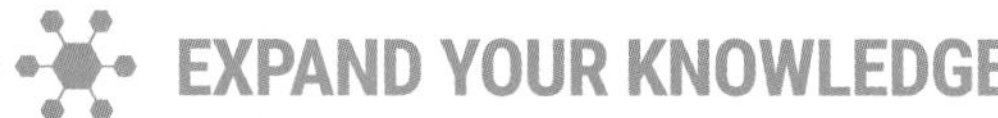

Physical Activity and Mental Health

While most people are aware of the link between physical activity and health, many overlook the connection between physical-activity levels and psychological well-being. Depression, anxiety, and other mental illnesses are ubiquitous in modern society, and individuals with chronic diseases are particularly prone to struggling with mental health (National Institute of Mental Health, 2019).

While a vicious cycle sometimes exists wherein declines in physical health, mental health, and levels of physical activity feed and negatively impact one another, the opposite is also true: increasing one's physical-activity level benefits both physical and mental health, thereby enabling the individual to be more physically active. In other words, the cycle can be both positive and negative.

Researchers have investigated the dose-response associations between physical activity and mental health (i.e., how much physical activity is needed to impact psychological well-being) in more than 8,000 individuals, as well as whether sedentary time affected these associations (Pacquito et al., 2018). They found that there was a significant correlation between time spent being physically active up to the point of approximately 50 minutes of moderate-to-vigorous physical activity or 16,000 steps per day. Beyond that point, the positive benefits started to decline. Importantly, they also found that sedentary time hampered the benefits of physical activity, meaning that 50 minutes of daily exercise may not be enough to improve mental health if an individual is otherwise largely sedentary (Pacquito et al., 2018). Personal trainers can empower their clients who are struggling with mental health to become more physically active while staying within **scope of practice,** as long as they are not diagnosing any illness or counseling their clients during sessions.

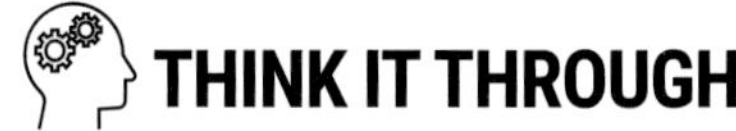

Collaborating with Clients to Enhance Emotional Well-being

For individuals undergoing cancer treatment, a decrease in quality of social support has been found to be a significant predictor of increased stress, depression, and negative affect (Fong et al., 2017). How can you as a personal trainer effectively collaborate with clients to identify and maintain high-quality social support to enhance emotional well-being?

OSTEOPOROSIS

Osteoporosis, characterized by low bone mass and disrupted microarchitecture, is one of the most prevalent public health issues in America. Defined as a **bone mineral density (BMD)** that is ≥2.5 standard deviations below the mean for young adults, osteoporosis affects more women than men. Low BMD and associated deterioration in bone microarchitecture result in structural weakness and increased risk for fracture. Women with a hip fracture have a fourfold risk of incurring another fracture [National Osteoporosis Foundation (NOF), 2017]. The most common fracture sites are the **proximal** femur (hip), vertebrae (spine), and distal forearm (wrist). The consequences of hip and spine fractures are significant, especially in older adults. Hip fractures are the most devastating because they are associated with severe disability and increased mortality. The incidence of hip fractures increases exponentially with age due to bone density declines, loss of muscular strength, and poor balance. Falls are responsible for more than 90% of all hip fractures (NOF, 2017).

A less severe condition, referred to as **osteopenia,** is defined as bone density between 1.0 and 2.5 standard deviations below the mean (NOF, 2017). Individuals with osteopenia are at a greater risk for fracture and further bone deterioration, advancing to osteoporosis. During the early growth years, the rate of **bone formation** is typically greater than the rate of **bone resorption,** resulting in an overall gain in bone mineral. This "remodeling" balance is disrupted as people age and the amount of bone formation no longer keeps pace with the amount of bone being resorbed.

Prevalence

An estimated 54 million Americans have, or are at risk for, osteoporosis. About one in two women and one in four men over the age of 50 will break a bone due to osteoporosis. By 2020, half of all Americans over age 50 are expected to have osteoporosis (NOF, 2017).

Etiology

Several health conditions (e.g., autoimmune, hematologic, endocrine, gastrointestinal, and neurological disorders; cancer; and mental illness) and/or their treatments can increase the likelihood of osteoporosis. If a client has any of these diseases or conditions, it would be prudent to learn more about his or her BMD and subsequent risk for osteoporosis.

Controllable factors that influence BMD include reproductive hormone levels, adequate levels of calcium and vitamin D, and physical activity. Uncontrollable factors include genetics, being female, being Caucasian or Asian, and being postmenopausal. Near or at the onset of menopause, there is a decline in **estrogen,** and bone loss accelerates from the typical rate of 0.5 to 1% to a rate of 2 to 6.5% per year (Winters-Stone & Snow, 2005).

Nutrition

An adequate intake of calcium and vitamin D are the two most important nutrients to consider in bone health. Lifelong adequate calcium intake is necessary for attaining peak BMD and maintaining bone health. The skeleton contains nearly all of the body's calcium stores. When a person's dietary intake of calcium is inadequate, bone tissue is resorbed from the skeleton to maintain blood calcium at a constant level. Vitamin D plays a major role in calcium absorption, bone health, muscle performance, and risk of falling.

Clinicians recommend a diet with adequate amounts of calcium (1,000 mg/day for men 50 to 70 years and 1,200 mg/day for women 51 and older and men 71 and older). For vitamin D, the recommended intake is 800 to 1,000 IU/day, including supplements if necessary for individuals age 50 and older (Cosman et al., 2014). Individuals with osteoporosis should be encouraged to meet with an RD or other qualified healthcare professional for recommendations on vitamin supplementation and appropriate diets.

Drinking alcohol in excessive amounts is detrimental to bone health. Moderate alcohol intake has no known negative effect on bone and may be associated with slightly higher bone density and lower risk of fracture in postmenopausal women. However, alcohol intake of more than two drinks per day for women or three drinks a day for men is associated with impaired bone health, increased risk of falling, and potential alcoholism (Maurel et al., 2012).

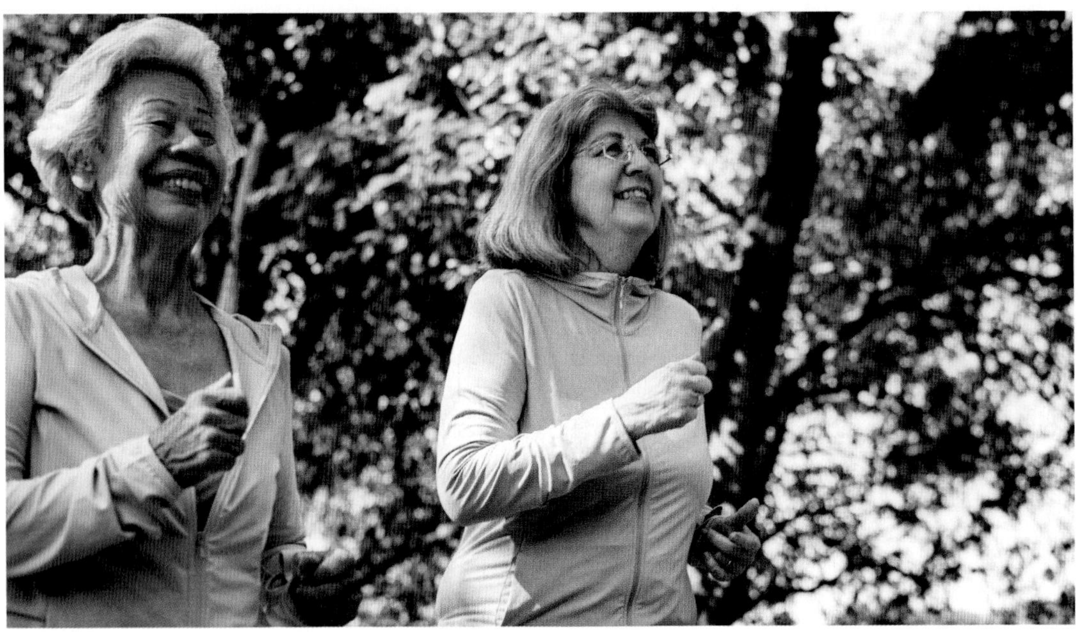

Exercise

Exercise is important to prevent and treat osteoporosis. The primary goal is to prevent the loss of bone mineral and to decrease the risk of falls and fractures. While the optimal strategy for preserving bone health remains unclear, it is known that physical stress influences the strength of bone. Mechanical stress applied to bone results in a small deformation of bone, which stimulates **bone deposition** and associated gains in bone mass and strength. There is compelling evidence that BMD will increase and the risk of falls and fractures will decrease with regular physical activity (Burr et al., 2012).

There are currently no established guidelines on contraindications for exercise for people with osteoporosis. However, the following exercise considerations are helpful for individuals who have, or are at risk for, osteoporosis (ACSM, 2018).

- Avoid excessive forward **flexion,** twisting, and compression movements of the spine. These types of activities may increase the risk of spine fracture. However, trunk **extension** and abdominal stabilization exercises may be beneficial.
- Engage in muscular training as well as weight-bearing (e.g., walking, jogging, and stair stepping) and impact (e.g., jumping) exercise, as they are most effective at stimulating bone mass and strength. Clients with osteoporosis can safely perform a variety of cardiorespiratory physical activities and muscular training. However, the intensity of the exercise sessions should initially be light to moderate and progressively increase based on the individual's capability.
- Incorporate activities that promote balance. Primary considerations should be exercises that improve strength in the muscles of the trunk, hips, and lower extremities, as these are important in balance.
- Avoid movements or environments that could lead to a fall. Quick, jarring movements or exercise on slick surfaces or around tripping hazards should be avoided to minimize the risk of a fall or fracture.

Table 13-16 presents an exercise guidelines summary for clients with osteoporosis.

TABLE 13-16

Exercise Guidelines Summary for Clients with Osteoporosis

Cardiorespiratory Training	
Frequency	▸ 4–5 days per week
Intensity	▸ Moderate (40–59% HRR or $\dot{V}O_2R$) intensity,* although some clients may be able to tolerate more intense exercise ▸ Below VT1 HR; can talk comfortably
Time	▸ Begin with 20 minutes and gradually progress to a minimum of 30 minutes and a maximum of 45–60 minutes
Type	▸ Emphasize weight-bearing, large-muscle-group activities, such as: ▪ Walking ▪ Stair climbing/descending
Progression	▸ Progress following the ACE Integrated Fitness Training Model based on client goals and availability.
Muscular Training	
Frequency	▸ Start with 1–2 nonconsecutive days and possibly progress to 2–3 days per week
Intensity	▸ Adjust resistance so that the last 2 repetitions are challenging to perform. ▸ High-intensity training is beneficial for those who can tolerate it.
Time	▸ Begin with 1 set of 8–12 repetitions and increase to 2 sets after approximately 2 weeks; no more than 8–10 exercises per session
Type	▸ Exercises involving each major muscle group with an emphasis on bone-loading forces ▸ Exercises while standing that emphasize balance, gait, and functional movements
Progression	▸ Progress following the ACE Integrated Fitness Training Model based on client goals and availability.

*Moderate intensity = Heart rates <VT1 where speech remains comfortable and is not affected by breathing; Vigorous intensity = Heart rates from ≥VT1 to <VT2 where clients feel unsure if speech is comfortable.

Note: HRR = Heart-rate reserve; $\dot{V}O_2R$ = Oxygen uptake reserve; VT1 = First ventilatory threshold; VT2 = Second ventilatory threshold

Source: American College of Sports Medicine (2018). *ACSM's Guidelines for Exercise Testing and Prescription* (10th ed.). Philadelphia: Wolters Kluwer.

Lifestyle

Lifestyle choices (e.g., being physically active, consuming adequate calcium and vitamin D, limiting alcohol intake, and avoiding smoking) influence 20 to 40% of adult peak bone mass (Weaver et al., 2016). An important issue with respect to smoking is its potential to negatively impact the acquisition of peak bone mass in adolescents and young adults. Therefore, optimizing lifestyle factors known to influence bone mass and strength is important to reduce risk of osteoporosis or low bone mass.

ARTHRITIS

Arthritis is a chronic degenerative condition of joints. The most common form is osteoarthritis (OA), followed by **rheumatoid arthritis (RA).** Other less-common forms include psoriatic arthritis (inflammation of the skin and joints), gout (build-up of uric acid crystals in a joint), and lupus (an **autoimmune disease** that can affect joints and many organs in the body). Note: Lupus is not a form of arthritis but does include arthritis as one of its most common symptoms.

Arthritis is not a simple disease, as it affects and is affected by other health states. For example:

- People with arthritis have higher rates of depression and anxiety.
- People with diabetes are almost twice as likely to have arthritis.
- Having arthritis increases the risk of developing CVD (Symmons & Gabriel, 2011). The higher risk of heart disease with OA is probably associated with excess body weight (Castrejon et al., 2017).
- The high levels of uric acid with gout is linked to a greater risk of hypertension (Grayson et al., 2011)
- Obesity increases the risk of developing OA because of the excess load on the joints. In addition, obesity makes OA worse.
- Obesity is also associated with RA and lupus (Castrejon et al., 2017).

OA is the leading cause of disability in the U.S. (U.S. Bone and Joint Initiative, 2014). RA is an autoimmune disease characterized by joint swelling, pain, and stiffness that can lead to severe motion impairment. It is also associated with an increased risk for CVD, high levels of fatigue, and depression (Metsios, Stavropoulos-Kalinoglou, & Kitas, 2015). Because it is a systemic disease, RA can affect many other areas of the body in addition to the joints (e.g., skin, eyes, lungs, heart, and blood vessels).

Prevalence

OA affects nearly 27 million Americans (Arthritis Foundation, 2017). In general, OA prevalence is significantly higher among women (26%) than among men (19.1%); persons with obesity (31%) compared with individuals who are normal/underweight (16%) and overweight (23%); and those who are older [people who are 65 years or older have a 49.6% prevalence compared to persons ages 45 to 64 years and 18 to 44 years (29.3% and 7.1%, respectively)] (Barbour et al., 2017). The treatment of OA can include medication, physical therapy, occupational therapy, and surgery, depending on the type and severity of arthritis.

RA affects 0.5 to 1% of the general population (Metsios, Stavropoulos-Kalinoglou, & Kitas, 2015) and about two-thirds of patients are women. RA can occur at any age, though it most commonly occurs between the ages of 20 and 50 years and the highest prevalence is found at the age of 70 years (Vuori, 2005). Although the prevalence of RA is relatively low, its burden is high because of its severely debilitating nature. The main symptom is chronic pain that often leads to depression, anxiety, feelings of helplessness, physical inactivity, and less social contact. Targeted treatment goals for RA are to maximize long-term health-related quality of life through control of symptoms, prevention of structural damage, and normalization of function (Smolen et al., 2010).

Etiology

OA results from overuse, trauma, obesity, or the degeneration of the joint **cartilage** that takes place with age. While some individuals will develop OA with no identifiable underlying cause, the majority of cases are secondary to trauma and/or obesity. OA is a degenerative joint condition that leads to deterioration of cartilage and the development of bony growths, or spurs, at the edges of joints. As the cartilage breaks down, pain, swelling, and lack of mobility at the affected joint may occur. Over time, bits of bone spurs or cartilage may chip off and float around in the joint. In response, there is an inflammatory process and **cytokines** and **enzymes** further damage the cartilage. Ultimately, as the cartilage wears away, the bones at the end of the joint rub against each other to cause joint damage and even more pain. The joints most often affected by OA are the cervical and lumbar spine, hip, knee, and the joints closest to the ends of the fingers. The risk of OA increases with age and is more common among women and individuals with overweight and obesity (Barbour et al., 2017). Usual symptoms are pain with motion, aggravation of pain with prolonged or intensive activity, and localized stiffness, especially in the morning or after periods of inactivity during the day (Vuori, 2005).

The risk of OA is higher in sports that have a high rate of injury, especially if combined with high impact and torsional movements (e.g., soccer and football). The highest risk is seen in elite players and in women. While running involves repetitive moderate-impact forces, there are not many injuries. In fact, several studies suggest that the risk of OA is not higher among runners (Vuori, 2005).

RA is the most crippling form of arthritis. While RA is classified as an autoimmune disease, the exact cause remains unknown. RA manifests in the **synovial tissue** that lines the outside of the joint and progresses to an erosion of articular cartilage and bone. In most instances, RA is more disabling than OA and causes greater joint deformity, typically in the hands (particularly the middle joints of the fingers and the knuckles), wrists, and feet. In severe cases, the **tendons**

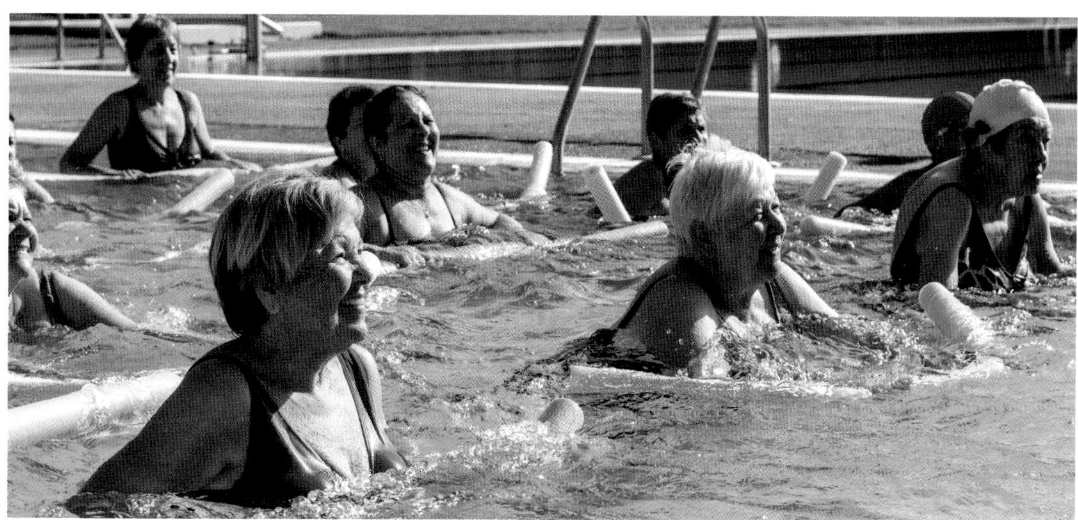

and occasionally the muscles that surround the joint also may become inflamed. Symptoms include joint pain, swelling, stiffness, and in some cases, **contractures.**

Nutrition

There are no established nutrition guidelines specifically for people with OA or RA. However, a diet rich in **omega-3 fatty acids, antioxidants,** and **phytochemicals** provides the body with powerful anti-inflammatory nutrients. A **Mediterranean-style eating plan** that includes ample fish, olive oil, fruits, vegetables, nuts/seeds, and beans may be helpful for individuals with arthritis (see Chapter 6). Small studies investigating the Mediterranean-style eating plan for its impact on RA symptoms have shown improvements in pain, morning stiffness, disease activity, and physical function. Researchers have found that cold-water fish high in omega-3 fatty acids along with oleocanthal, a key compound in extra virgin olive oil, have a positive and significant impact on inflammation, which may help reduce joint cartilage damage (Kinger, Kumar, & Kumar, 2017).

A combination of exercise and weight loss is the optimal approach in managing OA, particularly in those with overweight or obesity. Researchers have reported that weight loss can prevent the onset of OA, relieve symptoms, improve function, and increase quality of life in individuals who carry excess body weight (Bliddal, Leeds, & Christensen, 2014). On the other hand, persons with RA often have reduced appetite and greater **catabolism** and therefore lose weight (especially muscle).

Exercise

A comprehensive review of the literature strongly supports exercise as a cornerstone of therapy for persons with OA for improving pain and physical function (Golightly, Allen, & Caine, 2012). A consistent exercise program that promotes cardiorespiratory fitness, improved muscular strength and endurance, and joint mobility will decrease fatigue and significantly improve daily function and associated quality of life. Additional benefits include lower risk for CVD, improved psychosocial well-being, decreased pain and stiffness, and improved neuromuscular coordination. A comprehensive exercise program for OA should include education about the benefits of and need for regular exercise.

For RA, exercise is an integral part of treatment, as it has shown significant promise to improve arthritis-related and CVD outcomes, as well as fatigue and depression (Metsios, Stavropoulos-Kalinoglou, & Kitas, 2015). Goals of an exercise program are to reduce pain, maintain and increase joint function, prevent and correct joint deformities, maintain and increase muscle strength, and educate the client about managing the disease (Vuori, 2005). Because of the **catabolic** nature of RA, strengthening of the muscles around the affected joints is important. **Isometric** exercises are often recommended to avoid excess loading of the joints.

In general, recommendations for exercise for both types of arthritis are consistent with those for apparently healthy adults (see Chapters 8 through 11), with the additional consideration that the program must take into account the individual's current level of activity, pain, and functional limitations (ACSM, 2018). For individuals who have RA, low-impact exercises, using a limited ROM, performing exercise in warm water, and avoiding exercise during flare-ups may be beneficial. Exercise guidelines for those with RA should emphasize tailoring the program to the client's functional limits and baseline levels of cardiorespiratory fitness, as they tend to be less active (Tierney, Fraser, & Kennedy, 2012). The primary goals of the exercise program are to improve cardiorespiratory fitness and lower CAD risk, increase muscular endurance and strength, and maintain or, when indicated, improve ROM and flexibility around the affected joints.

Table 13-17 presents an exercise guidelines summary for clients with arthritis.

TABLE 13-17

Exercise Guidelines Summary for Clients with Arthritis

Cardiorespiratory Training	
Frequency	▸ 3–5 days per week
Intensity	▸ Below VT1 HR; can talk comfortably ▸ Moderate (40–59% HRR or $\dot{V}O_2R$) to vigorous (≥60% HRR or $\dot{V}O_2R$) intensity* ▸ Light intensity (e.g., 30–39% HRR or $\dot{V}O_2R$) may be necessary for deconditioned clients with arthritis.
Time	▸ Minutes per session will be dictated by the client's tolerance to exercise. ▸ At least 150 minutes per week of light or moderate intensity, 75 minutes of vigorous intensity, or a combination of the two
Type	▸ A variety of low-impact rhythmic large-muscle-group exercise: ▪ Walking ▪ Cycling ▪ Swimming ▸ High-impact activities such as running are not recommended for those with lower-extremity arthritis.
Progression	▸ Progress following the ACE Integrated Fitness Training Model based on client goals and availability.
Muscular Training	
Frequency	▸ 2–3 days per week
Intensity	▸ 50–80% 1-RM, with lower initial intensities
Time	▸ 2–4 sets of 8–12 repetitions
Type	▸ All major muscle groups ▸ Include machines, free weights, and body weight ▸ Perform all exercises within a pain-free range of motion.
Progression	▸ Progress following the ACE Integrated Fitness Training Model based on client goals and availability.

*Moderate intensity = Heart rates <VT1 where speech remains comfortable and is not affected by breathing; Vigorous intensity = Heart rates from ≥VT1 to <VT2 where clients feel unsure if speech is comfortable.

Note: HRR = Heart-rate reserve; $\dot{V}O_2R$ = Oxygen uptake reserve; 1-RM = One-repetition maximum; VT1 = First ventilatory threshold; VT2 = Second ventilatory threshold

Source: American College of Sports Medicine (2018). *ACSM's Guidelines for Exercise Testing and Prescription* (10th ed.). Philadelphia: Wolters Kluwer.

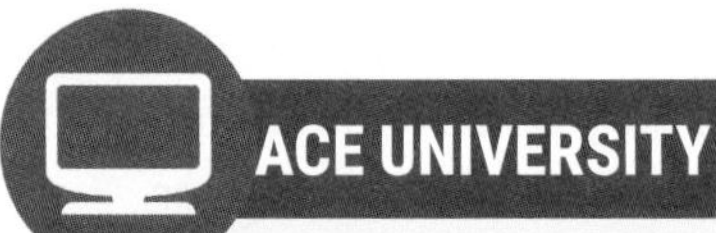

If your study program includes the ACE University, visit www.ACEfitness.org/MyACE and log in to your My ACE Account to take full advantage of the ACE Personal Trainer Study Program and online guided study experience.

A variety of media to support and expand on the material in this text is provided to facilitate learning and best prepare you for the ACE Personal Trainer Certification exam and a career as a personal trainer.

SUMMARY

Most chronic diseases are lifestyle-related diseases. What is the common characteristic of general recommendations to prevent and treat most lifestyle-related health problems? Moderation. In other words, if people had moderate intakes of certain nutrients and calories and did moderate amounts of exercise (frequency, intensity, and duration) most days of the week, the prevalence of many chronic diseases would be less and people would be healthier.

There is considerable evidence that regular physical activity reduces the risk of developing, and the mortality rates associated with, many chronic diseases. Therefore, personal trainers can have a major role in improving the health of their clients by helping them to be more active and to modify other lifestyle risk factors.

REFERENCES

Abdul-Ghani, M.A. et al. (2006). Insulin secretion and action in subjects with impaired fasting glucose and impaired glucose tolerance: Results from the Veterans Administration Genetic Epidemiology Study. *Diabetes*, 55, 1430–1435.

Aguilar, M. et al. (2015). Prevalence of the metabolic syndrome in the United States, 2003–2012. *Journal of the American Medical Association*, 313, 1973–1974.

Ahmad, M., Makati, D., & Akbar, S. (2017). Review and updates on hypertension in obstructive sleep apnea. *International Journal of Hypertension*, Article ID 1848375.

American Association of Cardiovascular and Pulmonary Rehabilitation (2013). *Guidelines for Cardiac Rehabilitation and Secondary Prevention Programs* (5th ed.). Champaign, Ill.: Human Kinetics.

American Cancer Society (2017). *Cancer Facts & Figures 2017*. Atlanta, Ga.: American Cancer Society.

American College of Sports Medicine (2018). *ACSM's Guidelines for Exercise Testing and Prescription* (10th ed.). Philadelphia: Wolters Kluwer.

American College of Sports Medicine (2009). Position stand: Appropriate physical activity intervention strategies for weight loss and prevention of weight regain for adults. *Medicine & Science in Sports & Exercise*, 41, 2, 459–471.

American Diabetes Association (2017a). Classification and diagnosis of diabetes. *Diabetes Care*, 40, S11–S24.

American Diabetes Association (2017b). Children and adolescents. *Diabetes Care*, 40, S105–S113.

American Diabetes Association (2017c). Lifestyle management. *Diabetes Care*, 40, S33–S43.

American Diabetes Association (2017d). Pharmacologic approaches to glycemic treatment. *Diabetes Care*, 40, S64–S74.

American Heart Association (2013). Heart disease and stroke statistics—2013 update: A report from the American Heart Association. *Circulation*, 127, e6–e245.

American Heart Association/National Heart, Lung, and Blood Institute (2005). Scientific statement: Diagnosis and management of the metabolic syndrome. *Circulation*, 112, e285–e290.

Appel, L.J. (2004). Lifestyle modification: Is it achievable and durable? The argument for. *Journal of Clinical Hypertension*, 6, 578–581.

Arthritis Foundation (2017). Osteoarthritis. www.arthritis.org/conditions-treatments/disease-center/osteoarthritis

Balady, G.J. (2007). Core components of cardiac rehabilitation. *Circulation*, 115, 2675–2682.

Barbour, K.E. et al. (2017). Vital signs: Prevalence of doctor-diagnosed arthritis and arthritis-attributable activity limitation, United States, 2013–2015. *Morbidity & Mortality Weekly Report*, March 7.

Basen-Engquist, K. et al. (2017). Agenda for translating physical activity, nutrition, and weight management interventions for cancer survivors into clinical and community practice. *Obesity (Silver Spring)*, 25, Suppl 2, S9–S22.

Bauer, U.E. et al. (2014). Prevention of chronic disease in the 21st century: Elimination of the leading preventable causes of premature death and disability in the USA. *Lancet*, 384, 9937, 45–52.

Benjamin, E.J. et al. (2019). Heart disease and stroke statistics – 2019 update: A report from the American Heart Association. *Circulation*, 139, e56–e528.

Berry, J.D. et al. (2012). Lifetime risks of cardiovascular disease. *New England Journal of Medicine*, 366, 321–329.

Billinger, S.A. et al. (2014). Physical activity and exercise recommendations for stroke survivors: A statement for healthcare professionals from the American Heart Association/American Stroke Association. *Stroke*, 45, 8, 2532–2553.

Biswas, A. et al. (2015). Sedentary time and its association with risk for disease incidence, mortality, and hospitalization in adults: A systematic review and meta-analysis. *Annals of Internal Medicine*, 162, 2, 123–132.

Bliddal, H., Leeds, A.R., & Christensen, R. (2014). Osteoarthritis, obesity and weight loss: Evidence, hypotheses and horizons—a scoping review. *Obesity Reviews*, 17, 7, 578–586.

Brady, T.M. (2017). Obesity-related hypertension in children. *Frontiers in Pediatrics*, 25, September.

Brown, J.C. et al. (2012). Cancer, physical activity, and exercise. *Comparative Physiology*, 2, 2775–2809.

Bullard, K.M. et al. (2018). Prevalence of diagnosed diabetes in adults by diabetes type – United States, 2016. *MMWR Morbidity and Mortality Weekly Reports*, 67, 359–361.

Burr, J. et al. (2012). Arthritis, osteoporosis, and low back pain: Evidence-based clinical risk assessment for physical activity and exercise clearance. *Canadian Family Physician*, 58, 59–62.

Caligiuri, S.P.B. & Pierce, G.N. (2017). A review of the relative efficacy of dietary, nutritional supplements, lifestyle, and drug therapies in the management of hypertension. *Critical Reviews in Nutrition and Food Science*, 57, 16, 3508–3527.

Campbell, K.L. et al. (2019). Exercise guidelines for cancer survivors: Consensus statement from International Multidisciplinary Roundtable. *Medicine & Science in Sports & Exercise*, 51, 11, 2375–2390.

Castrejon, I. et al. (2017). Higher rates of obesity and associations with poorer clinical status in patients with RA, OA, and SLE: A cross-sectional study from routine care. *Annals of the Rheumatic Diseases*, 76, Supplement 2, 1451.

Centers for Disease Control and Prevention (2017). *National Diabetes Statistics Report: Estimates of Diabetes and its Burden in the United States, 2017.* https://www.cdc.gov/diabetes/pdfs/data/statistics/national-diabetesstatistics-report.pdf

Chobanian, A.V. et al. (2003). Joint National Committee on Prevention, Detection, Evaluation, and Treatment of High Blood Pressure. National Heart, Lung, and Blood Institute, National High Blood Pressure Education Program Coordinating Committee. Seventh report of the Joint National Committee on Prevention, Detection, Evaluation, and Treatment of High Blood Pressure. *Hypertension*, 42, 6, 1206–1252.

Clapp, P.W. & Jaspers, I. (2017). Electronic cigarettes: Their constituents and potential links to asthma. *Current Allergy and Asthma Reports*, 17, 79–98.

Codella, R., Terruzzi, I., & Luzi, L. (2017). Why should people with type 1 diabetes exercise regularly? *Acta Diabetologica*, 54, 615–630.

Colberg, S.R. et al. (2016). Physical activity/exercise and diabetes: A position statement of the American Diabetes Association. *Diabetes Care*, 39, 2065–2079.

Cosman, F. et al. (2014). Clinician's guide to prevention and treatment of osteoporosis. *Osteoporosis International*, 25, 10, 2359–2381.

Covassin, N. & Singh, P. (2016). Sleep duration and cardiovascular disease risk: Epidemiologic and experimental evidence. *Sleep Medicine Clinics*, 11, 1, 81–89.

Coward, D.D. (2006). Supporting health promotion in adults with cancer. *Family & Community Health*, 29, Suppl. 1, 52S–60S.

Creager, M.A. & Libby, P. (2011). Peripheral arterial disease. In: Bonow, R.O. et al. (Eds.) *Braunwald's Heart Disease: A Textbook of Cardiovascular Medicine* (9th ed.). Philadelphia: Saunders.

Cuffee, Y. et al. (2014). Psychosocial risk factors for hypertension: An update of the literature. *Current Hypertension Reports*, 16, 10, 483.

D'Elia, L. et al. (2014). Potassium-rich diet and risk of stroke: Updated meta-analysis. *Nutrition, Metabolism, and Cardiovascular Disease*, 24, 585–587.

Demark-Wahnefried, W. et al. (2015). Practical clinical interventions for diet, physical activity, and weight control in cancer survivors. *CA: A Cancer Journal for Clinicians*, 65, 167–189.

Douglas, J.G. et al. (2003). Hypertension in African Americans. Working group of the International Society on Hypertension in Blacks. Management of high blood pressure in Americans. Consensus statement of the Hypertension in Africans and Americans Working Group of the International Society on Hypertension in Blacks. *Archives of Internal Medicine*, 163, 525–541.

Dua, A. & Lee, C.J. (2016). Epidemiology of peripheral arterial disease and chronic limb ischemia. *Techniques of Vascular Intervention and Radiology*, 19, 91–95.

Eckel, R.H. et al. (2013). American Heart Association/American College of Cardiology 2013 guidelines on lifestyle management to reduce cardiovascular risk. *Circulation*, 01.cir.0000437740.48606.d1.

Falkner, B. (2017). Monitoring and management of hypertension with obesity in adolescents. *Integrated Blood Pressure Control*, 10, 33–39.

Fearon, K. et al. (2011). Definition and classification of cancer cachexia: An international consensus. *The Lancet Oncology*, 12, 489–495.

Feigin, V.L. et al. (2014). Group global and regional burden of stroke during 1990–2010: Findings from the Global Burden of Disease Study 2010. *Lancet*, 383, 245–254.

Fong, A.J. et al. (2017). Changes in social support predict emotional well-being in breast cancer survivors. *Psychooncology*, 26, 5, 664–671.

Go, A.S. et al. (2014a). An effective approach to high blood pressure control: A science advisory from the American Heart Association, the American College of Cardiology, and the Centers for Disease Control and Prevention. *Hypertension*, 63, 878–885.

Go, A.S. et al. (2014b). Heart disease and stroke statistics – 2014 update: A report from the American Heart Association. *Circulation*, 29, e28–e292.

Golightly, Y.M., Allen, K.D., & Caine, D.J. (2012). A comprehensive review of the effectiveness of different exercise programs for patients with osteoarthritis. *The Physician & Sportsmedicine*, 40, 4, 52–65.

Gordon, B., Chen, S., & Durstine, J.L. (2014). The effects of exercise training on the traditional lipid profile and beyond. *Current Sports Medicine Reports*, 13, 253–259.

Grayson, P.C. et al. (2011). Hyperuricemia and incident hypertension: A systematic review and meta-analysis. *Arthritis Care and Research*, 63, 102–110.

Grundy, S.M. et al. (2019). 2018 AHA/ACC/AACVPR/AAPA/ABC/ACPM/ADA/AGS/APhA/ASPC/NLA/PCNA guideline on the management of blood cholesterol: Executive Summary. A Report of the American College of Cardiology/American Heart Association Task Force on Clinical Practice Guidelines. *Circulation*, 139, e1046–e1081.

Grundy, S.M. et al. (2004). Implication of recent clinical trials for the National Cholesterol Education Program Adult Treatment Panel III Guidelines. *Circulation*, 110, 227–239.

Gupta, K.B. & Verma, M. (2007). Nutrition and asthma. *Lung India*, 24, 105–114.

Hamdy, O. et al. (2003). Lifestyle modification improves endothelial function in obese subjects with the insulin resistance syndrome. *Diabetes Care*, 26, 2119–2125.

Hardy O.T., Czech, M.P., & Corvera, S. (2012). What causes the insulin resistance underlying obesity? *Current Opinion in Endocrinology, Diabetes and Obesity*, 19, 81–87.

Haskell, W.L. et al. (2008). *Physical Activity Guidelines Advisory Committee Report*. www.health.gov/paguidelines/Report/

He, F.J., Nowson, C.A., & MacGregor, G.A. (2006). Fruit and vegetable consumption and stroke: Meta-analysis of cohort studies. *Lancet*, 367, 320–326.

Herder, C. et al. (2009). Anti-inflammatory effect of lifestyle changes in the Finnish Diabetes Prevention Study. *Diabetologia*, 52, 433–442.

Hojman, P. (2017). Exercise protects from cancer through regulation of immune function and inflammation. *Biochemical Society Transactions*, 45, 905–911.

Ioannidis, J.P. (2018). Diagnosis and treatment of hypertension in the 2017 ACC/AHA guidelines and in the real world. *Journal of the American Medical Association*, 319, 115–116.

Jones, L.W. & Demark-Wahnefried, W. (2006). Diet, exercise, and complementary therapies after primary treatment for cancer. *The Lancet Oncology*, 7, 1017–1026.

Katsiki, N., Mikhailidis, D.P., & Mantzoros, C.S. (2016). Non-alcoholic fatty liver disease and dyslipidemia: A review. *Metabolism*, 65, 1109–1125.

Katzmarzyk, P.T. (2005). Metabolic syndrome, obesity, and mortality: Impact of cardiorespiratory fitness. *Diabetes Care*, 28, 2.

Keese, F. et al. (2011). A comparison of the immediate effects of resistance, aerobic, and concurrent exercise on post exercise hypotension. *Journal of Strength and Conditioning Research*, 25, 1429–1435.

Kelley, G.A., Kelley, K.S., & Tran, Z.V. (2005). Aerobic exercise, lipids and lipoproteins in overweight and obese adults: A meta-analysis of randomized controlled trials. *International Journal of Obesity (London)*, 29, 881–893.

Kinger, M., Kumar, S., & Kumar, V. (2017). Some important dietary polyphenolic compounds: An anti-inflammatory and immunoregulatory perspective. *Mini Reviews in Medicinal Chemistry*, DOI: 10.2174/1389557517666170208143410. [Epub ahead of print]

Klein, S. et al. (2004). Absence of an effect of liposuction on insulin action and risk factors for coronary heart disease. *New England Journal of Medicine*, 350, 25, 2549–2557.

Koska, J. et al. (2008). Increased fat accumulation in liver may link insulin resistance with subcutaneous abdominal adipocyte enlargement, visceral adiposity, and hypoadiponectinemia in obese individuals. *American Journal of Clinical Nutrition*, 87, 295–302.

Lane, K. & McKenzie, D.C. (2005). Cancer. In: Skinner, J.S. (Ed.) *Exercise Testing and Exercise Prescription for Special Cases* (3rd ed.). Philadelphia: Lippincott Williams & Wilkins.

Lascar, N. et al. (2018). Type 2 diabetes in adolescents and young adults. *Lancet Diabetes and Endocrinology*, 6, 69–80.

Leon, A.S. & Sanchez, O.A. (2005). Diabetes mellitus. In: Skinner, J.S. (Ed.) *Exercise Testing and Exercise Prescription for Special Cases* (3rd ed.). Philadelphia: Lippincott Williams & Wilkins.

Li, E.J.Q. et al. (2006) The effect of a "training on work readiness" program for workers with musculoskeletal injuries: A randomized control trial (RCT) study. *Journal of Occupational Rehabilitation*, 16, 4, 529–541.

Lieber, A.C. et al. (2018). Nutrition, energy expenditure, dysphagia, and self-efficacy in stroke rehabilitation: A review of the literature. *Brain Science*, 8, 218.

Lillefjell, M., Krokstad, S., & Espnes, G.A. (2006). Factors predicting work ability following multidisciplinary rehabilitation for chronic musculoskeletal pain. *Journal of Occupational Rehabilitation*, 16, 4, 543–555.

Liu, M.Y. et al. (2017). Association between psychosocial stress and hypertension: A systematic review and meta-analysis. *Neurological Research*, 39, 6, 573–580.

Maltais, F. et al. (2014). An Official American Thoracic Society/European Respiratory Society Statement: Update on limb muscle dysfunction in chronic obstructive pulmonary disease. *American Journal of Respiratory and Critical Care Medicine*, 189, 9, e15–e62.

Mancia, G. et al. (2013). ESH/ESC Guidelines for the management of arterial hypertension: The Task Force for the Management of Arterial Hypertension of the European Society of Hypertension (ESH) and of the European Society of Cardiology (ESC). *Journal of Hypertension*, 31, 1281–1357.

Maraki, M.I. & Sidossis, L.S. (2013). The latest on the effect of prior exercise on post-prandial lipaemia. *Sports Medicine*, 43, 463–481.

Maurel, D.B. et al. (2012). Alcohol and bone: Review of dose effects and mechanisms. Osteoporosis *International*, 23, 1, 1–16.

Mayo Clinic Proceedings (2016). Cardiac rehabilitation: The mandate grows. *Mayo Clinic Proceedings*, 91, 2, 125–128.

McMahon, K. & Brown, J.K. (2000). Nutritional screening and assessment. *Seminars in Oncology Nursing*, 16, 106–112.

Metsios, G.S., Stavropoulos-Kalinoglou, A., & Kitas, G.D. (2015). The role of exercise in the management of rheumatoid arthritis. *Expert Review of Clinical Immunology*, 11, 10, 1121–1130.

Micha, R. et al. (2017). Association between dietary factors and mortality from heart disease, stroke, and type 2 diabetes in the United States. *Journal of the American Medical Association*, 317, 912–924.

Moore, G.E., Durstine, J.L., & Painter, P.L. (Eds.) *ACSM's Exercise Management for Persons with Chronic Diseases and Disabilities* (4th ed.) Champaign, Ill.: Human Kinetics.

Moorman, J.E. et al. (2012). National surveillance for asthma—United States 2001–2010. National Center for Health Statistics. *Vital Health Statistics*, 3, 35.

Mora, S. et al. (2008). Fasting compared with nonfasting lipids and apolipoproteins for predicting incident cardiovascular events. *Circulation*, 118, 993–1001.

Morton, A.R. & Fitch, K.D. (2005). Asthma. In: Skinner, J.S. (Ed.) *Exercise Testing and Exercise Prescription for Special Cases* (3rd ed.). Philadelphia: Lippincott Williams & Wilkins.

Narayan, K.M. et al. (2003). Lifetime risk for diabetes mellitus in the United States. *Journal of the American Medical Association*, 290, 1884–1890.

National Asthma Education and Prevention Program (2007). *Expert Panel Report 3: Guidelines for the Diagnosis and Management of Asthma*. Bethesda, Md.: U.S. Department of Health & Human Services, Public Health Service, National Institutes of Health, National Heart, Lung, and Blood Institute; NIH publication number 08-4051.

National Cancer Institute (2017). *What Is Cancer?* https://www.cancer.gov/about-cancer/understanding/what-is-cancer

National Cholesterol Education Program (2002). Expert Panel on Detection, Evaluation and Treatment of High Blood Cholesterol in Adults: Summary of the second report of NCEP Expert Panel on Detection, Evaluation and Treatment of High Blood Cholesterol in Adults (Adult Treatment Panel III). NIH Publication No. 02-5213. *Journal of the American Medical Association*, 285, 2486–2497.

National Institute of Mental Health (2019). *Chronic Illness & Mental Health*. https://www.nimh.nih.gov/health/publications/chronic-illness-mental-health/index.shtml

National Osteoporosis Foundation (2017). *What is Osteoporosis and What Causes It?* https://www.nof.org/patients/what-is-osteoporosis/

Ng, A.K. & Travis, L.B. (2008). Second primary cancers: An overview. *Hematology/Oncology Clinics of North America*, 22, 271–289, vii.

O'Donnell, D.E. et al. (2017). Advances in the evaluation of respiratory pathophysiology during exercise in chronic lung diseases. *Frontiers in Physiology*, 8, 82.

Olin, J.S. et al. (2016). Peripheral artery disease. *Journal of the American College of Cardiology*, 67, 11, 1338–1357.

Ostman, C. et al. (2018). Clinical outcomes to exercise training in type 1 diabetes: A systematic review and meta-analysis. *Diabetes Research and Clinical Practice*, 139, 380–391.

Ou, H.Y. et al. (2013). The association between nonalcoholic fatty pancreas disease and diabetes. *PLoS One*, 8, e62561.

Pacquito, B. et al. (2018). Dose response association of objective physical activity with mental health in a representative national sample of adults: A cross-sectional study. *PloS One*, 13, 10, e0204682.

Parsons, J.P. & Mastronarde, J.G. (2005). Exercise-induced bronchoconstriction in athletes. *Chest*, 128, 3966–3974.

Pedersen, B.K. & Saltin, B. (2006). Evidence for prescribing exercise as therapy in chronic disease. *Scandinavian Journal of Medicine & Science in Sports*, 16, 3–63.

Pekmezi, D.W. & Demark-Wahnefried, W. (2011). Updated evidence in support of diet and exercise interventions in cancer survivors. *Acta Oncology*, 50, 167–178.

Pescatello, L.S. et al. (2015). Exercise for hypertension: A prescription update integrating existing recommendations with emerging research. *Current Hypertension Reports*, 17, 11, 87.

Pescatello, L.S. et al. (2004). American College of Sports Medicine position stand: Exercise and hypertension. *Medicine & Science in Sports & Exercise*, 36, 3, 533–553.

Redmond, M.L. et al. (2016). Food insecurity and peripheral arterial disease in older adult populations. *Journal of Nutrition, Health, and Aging*, 20, 989–995.

Riddell, M.C. (2017). Exercise management in type 1 diabetes: A consensus statement. *Lancet Diabetes and Endocrinology*, 5, 377–390.

Rock, C.L. et al. (2012). Nutrition and physical activity guidelines for cancer survivors. *CA: A Cancer Journal for Clinicians*, 62, 242–274.

Rundell, K.W. (2016). Asthma. In: Moore, G.E., Durstine, J.L., & Painter, P.L. (Eds.) *ACSM's Exercise Management for Persons with Chronic Diseases and Disabilities* (4th ed.) Champaign, Ill.: Human Kinetics. pp. 183–198.

Samson, S.L. & Garber, A.J. (2014). Metabolic syndrome. *Endocrinology and Metabolism Clinics of North America*, 43, 1–23.

Sarikaya, H., Ferro, J., & Arnold, M. (2015). Stroke prevention—medical and lifestyle measures. *European Neurology*, 73, 150–157.

Saydah, S. et al. (2014). Trends in cardiovascular disease risk factors by obesity level in adults in the United States, NHANES 1999–2010. *Obesity (Silver Spring)*, 22, 8, 1888–1895.

Schattner, M. & Shike, M. (2006). Nutrition support of the patient with cancer. In: Shils, M.E. et al. (Eds.) *Modern Nutrition in Health and Disease* (10th ed.). Philadelphia: Lippincott Williams & Wilkins.

Schmid, D. & Leitzmann, M.F. (2014). Television viewing and time spent sedentary in relation to cancer risk: A meta-analysis. *Journal of the National Cancer Institute*, 106, 7.

Schultz, I.Z. et al. (2007). Models of return to work for musculoskeletal disorders. *Journal of Occupational Rehabilitation*, 17, 4, 782.

Sherling, D.H., Perumareddi, P., & Hennekens, C.H. (2017). Metabolic syndrome. *Journal of Cardiovascular and Pharmacological Therapy*, 22, 365–367.

Siegel, R.L., Miller, K.D., & Jemal, A. (2019). Cancer statistics, 2019. *CA: A Cancer Journal for Clinicians*, 69, 1, 7–34.

Smolen, J.S. et al (2010). Treating rheumatoid arthritis to target: Recommendations of an international task force. *Annals of Rheumatic Diseases*, 69, 631–637.

Stewart, K.J. et al. (2005). Exercise and risk factors associated with metabolic syndrome in older adults. *American Journal of Preventive Medicine*, 28, 9–18.

Symmons, D.P.M. & Gabriel, S.E. (2011). Epidemiology of cardiovascular disease in rheumatic diseases with a focus on RA and SLE. *Nature Reviews, Rheumatology*, 7, 399–408.

Tang, M. et al. (2013). Autonomic neuropathy in young people with type 1 diabetes: A systematic review. *Pediatric Diabetes*, 14, 239–248.

Tierney, M., Fraser, A., & Kennedy, N. (2012). Physical activity in rheumatoid arthritis: A systematic review. *Journal of Physical Activity & Health*, 9, 1036–1048.

Tortosa, A. et al. (2007). Mediterranean diet inversely associated with the incidence of metabolic syndrome: The SUN prospective cohort. *Diabetes Care*, 30, 2957.

Tyson, C.C. et al. (2012). The Dietary Approaches to Stop Hypertension (DASH) eating pattern in special populations. *Current Hypertension Reports*, 14, 388–396.

U.S. Bone and Joint Initiative (2014). *The Burden of Musculoskeletal Diseases in the United States (BMUS)* (3rd ed.). Rosemont, Ill: United States Bone and Joint Initiative.

U.S. Department of Agriculture (2015). *2015-2020 Dietary Guidelines for Americans* (8th ed.). www.health.gov/dietaryguidelines

U.S. Department of Health & Human Services (2018). *Physical Activity Guidelines for Americans* (2nd ed.). www.health.gov/paguidelines

U.S. Environmental Protection Agency (2018). *Asthma Facts*. www.epa.gov/asthma

Vamvakis, A. et al. (2017). Beneficial effects of nonpharmacological interventions in the management of essential hypertension. *Journal of the Royal Society of Medicine Cardiovascular Disease*, 6, 1–6.

Vitalis, A. et al. (2017). Ethnic differences in the prevalence of peripheral arterial disease: A systematic review and meta-analysis. *Expert Reviews of Cardiovascular Therapy*, 15, 327–338.

Voica, A.S. et al. (2016). Chronic obstructive pulmonary disease phenotypes and balance impairment. *International Journal of Chronic Obstructive Pulmonary Disease*, 11, 919–925.

Vuori, I. (2005). Arthritis. In: Skinner, J.S. (Ed.) *Exercise Testing and Exercise Prescription for Special Cases* (3rd ed.). Philadelphia: Lippincott Williams & Wilkins.

Weaver, C.M. et al. (2016). The National Osteoporosis Foundation's position statement on peak bone mass development and lifestyle factors: A systematic review and implementation recommendations. *Osteoporosis International*, 27, 1281–1386.

Wenger, N.K. (2008). Current status of cardiac rehabilitation. *Journal of the American College of Cardiology*, 51, 1619–1631.

Whelton, P.K. et al. (2017). 2017 ACC/AHA/AAPA/ABC/ACPM/AGS/APhA/ASH/ASPC/NMA/PCNA guideline for the prevention, detection, evaluation, and management of high blood pressure in adults: A report of the American College of Cardiology/American Heart Association Task Force on Clinical Practice Guidelines. *Journal of the American College of Cardiology*, Nov 7. pii: S0735-1097 (17) 41519-1.

Williams, R.R. et al. (1991). Are there interactions and relations between genetic and environmental factors predisposing to high blood pressure? *Hypertension*, 18 (Suppl. I), I29–I37.

Winters-Stone, K.M. & Snow, C.M. (2005). Osteoporosis. In: Skinner, J.S. (Ed.) *Exercise Testing and Exercise Prescription for Special Cases* (3rd ed.). Philadelphia: Lippincott Williams & Wilkins.

Wood, L.G. (2017). Diet, obesity, and asthma. *Annals of the American Thoracic Society*, 14 (Suppl. 5), S332–S338.

World Health Organization (2017). *Cancer Fact Sheet, February 2017*. http://www.who.int/mediacentre/factsheets/fs297/en/

Yang, X. et al. (2008). The longitudinal effects of physical activity history on metabolic syndrome. *Medicine & Science in Sports & Exercise*, 40, 8, 1424–1431.

Zoungas, S. et al. (2012). Association of HbA1c levels with vascular complications and death in patients with type 2 diabetes: Evidence of glycaemic thresholds. *Diabetologia*, 55, 636–643.

SUGGESTED READINGS

Campbell, K.L. et al. (2019). Exercise guidelines for cancer survivors: Consensus statement from International Multidisciplinary Roundtable. *Medicine & Science in Sports & Exercise*, 51, 11, 2375–2390.

Colberg, S.R. (2018). *Diabetes and Keeping Fit for Dummies*. New York: Wiley Publishing.

Colberg, S.R. (2013). *Exercise and Diabetes: A Clinician's Guide to Prescribing Physical Activity*. Alexandria, Va.: American Diabetes Association.

Lennon, S.L. et al. (2017). 2015 Evidence analysis library: Evidence-based nutrition practice guidelines for the management of hypertension in adults. *Journal of the Academy of Nutrition and Dietetics*, 117, 1445–1458.

Pescatello, L.S. et al. (2004). American College of Sports Medicine position stand: Exercise and hypertension. *Medicine & Science in Sports & Exercise*, 36, 3, 533–553.

Skinner, J.S. (2005). Hypertension. In: Skinner, J.S. (Ed.) *Exercise Testing and Exercise Prescription for Special Cases* (3rd ed.). Philadelphia: Lippincott, Williams & Wilkins.

Whelton, P.K. et al. (2017). 2017 ACC/AHA/AAPA/ABC/ACPM/AGS/APhA/ASH/ASPC/NMA/PCNA guideline for the prevention, detection, evaluation, and management of high blood pressure in adults: A report of the American College of Cardiology/American Heart Association Task Force on Clinical Practice Guidelines. *Journal of the American College of Cardiology*, Nov 7. pii:S0735-1097 (17) 41519-1.

Whelton, S.P. et al. (2002). Effect of aerobic exercise on blood pressure: A meta-analysis of randomized, controlled trials. *Annals of Internal Medicine*, 136, 493–503.

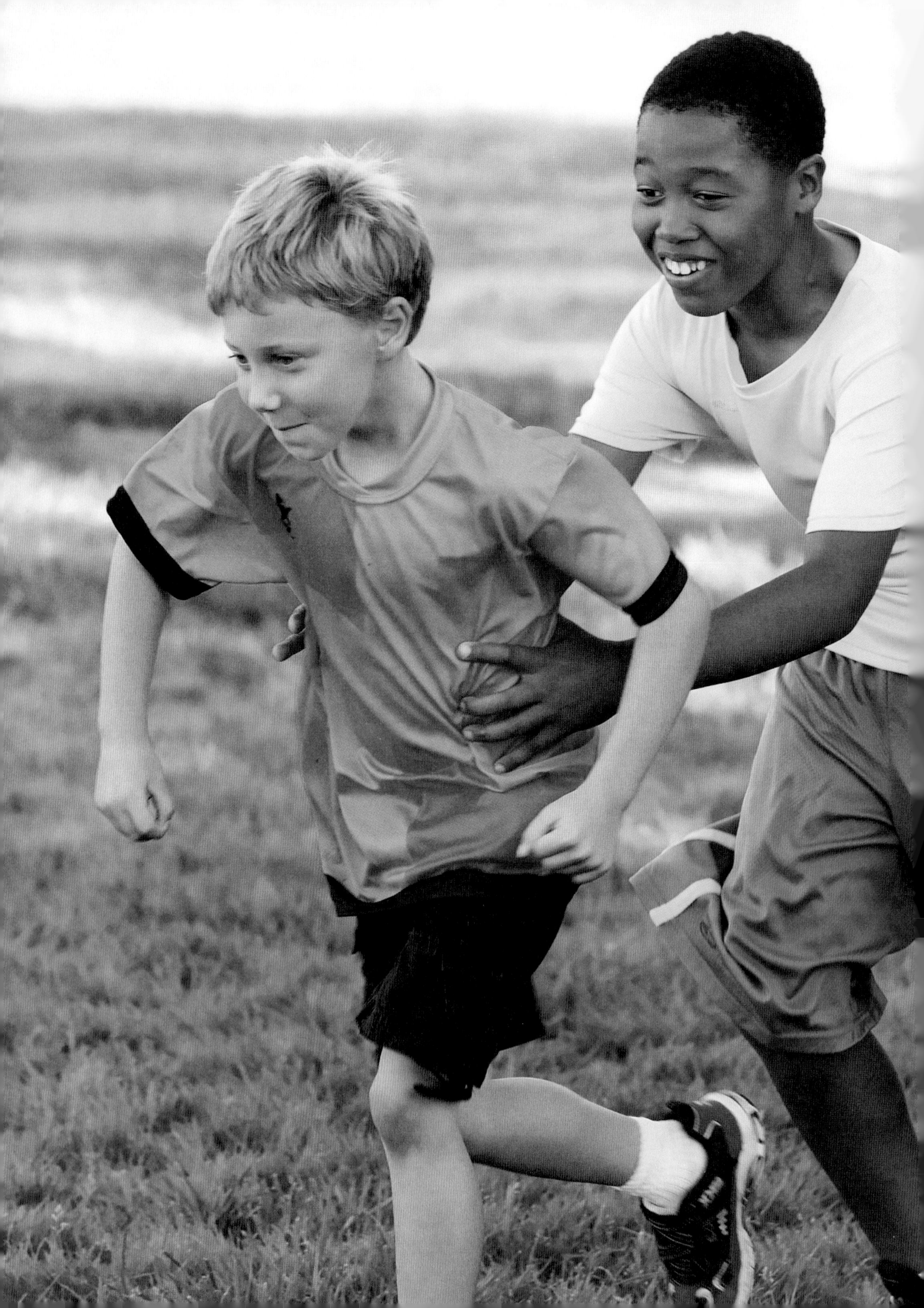

CHAPTER 14

Exercise Considerations across the Lifespan

LAUREN SHROYER, MS, ATC
Senior Director for Product Development for the American Council on Exercise; NATA-BOC Certified Athletic Trainer

IN THIS CHAPTER

LEARNING OBJECTIVES:

Upon completion of this chapter, the reader will be able to:

- Describe the recommended exercise guidelines for youth, women during pregnancy and the postpartum period, and older adults
- List the risk factors for exercises for women during pregnancy and the postpartum period
- Apply the ACE Integrated Fitness Training Model to youth, women during pregnancy and the postpartum period, and older adults
- Explain the unique benefits of muscular and cardiorespiratory training for youth, women during pregnancy and the postpartum period, and older adults
- Describe some typical physiological and structural changes that occur due to aging

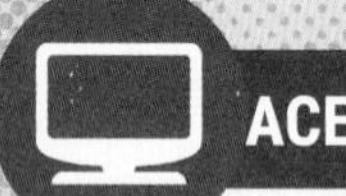

ACE UNIVERSITY

If your study program includes the ACE University, visit www.ACEfitness.org/MyACE and log in to your My ACE Account to take full advantage of the ACE Personal Trainer Study Program and online guided study experience.

A variety of media to support and expand on the material in this text is provided to facilitate learning and best prepare you for the ACE Personal Trainer Certification exam and a career as a personal trainer.

Research establishing the health benefits of regular exercise has prompted healthcare professionals to broadly recommend physical activity as a component of a healthy lifestyle across the lifespan. The needs, goals, and capabilities of people change as they move through life and it is essential that ACE® Certified Personal Trainers be mindful of the guidelines and key considerations presented in this chapter when they design and implement exercise programs for youth, women during pregnancy and the postpartum period, and older adults. This chapter also presents the current knowledge on exercise programming for these populations.

Exercise and Youth

Regular physical activity is important for overall health and wellness, and activity is as important for children and adolescents as it is for adults. Unfortunately, millions of American youth do not get the recommended amount of physical activity, which puts them at greater risk for developing inactivity-related diseases in their adult years. The *2018 United States Report Card on Physical Activity for Children and Youth* gives overall physical activity in the United States a grade of D–, with only 20 to 26% of youth meeting recommended levels of physical activity (National Physical Activity Plan, 2018). Average grades for both overall physical activity and **sedentary** behavior for youth around the world are a D (Aubert, S. et al., 2018).

Many causes for this decline in physical activity exist. In most of the U.S., youth have been negatively impacted by the decline in physical-activity requirements in schools. Around the globe, this is coupled with an increase in sedentary recreational activities like viewing social media and streaming video, computer gaming, and watching television (National Physical Activity Plan, 2018). While younger children report fewer hours of daily screen time and children ages 6 to 11 are more likely to meet screen-time recommendations, almost 45% of high school–aged children report using a computer or electronic device for more than three hours per day (National Physical Activity Plan, 2018). Some children living in high crime areas lack access to safe neighborhood streets and parks, effectively confining them to their homes and schools. The National Physical Activity Plan (2018) also noted that physical-activity levels drop significantly with age, with only 5% of 16- to 19-year-olds meeting physical-activity recommendations, with girls participating in activity at significantly lower rates than boys.

The negative health consequences of physical inactivity, poor dietary habits, and associated weight gain include childhood **obesity, hypertension, type 2 diabetes, osteoporosis,** and the development of **atherosclerosis.** Furthermore, behaviors established at a young age have a high probability of persisting into adulthood, making it likely that **physically inactive** youth will remain inactive as adults, placing them at risk for premature death. The inactivity patterns of adults are mirrored by their children, thus perpetuating a cycle of physical inactivity passed from parent to child (Jago et al., 2010).

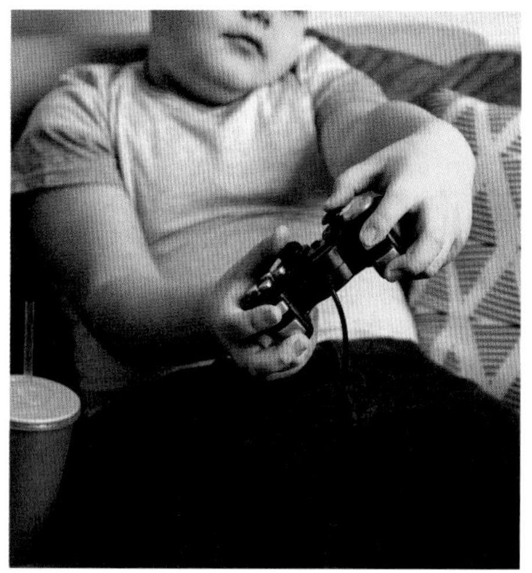

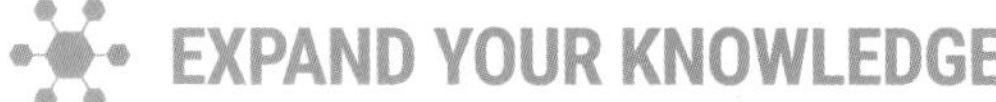

Physical Literacy—A Call to Action

Physical literacy is defined as the ability, confidence, and desire to by physically active for life (The Aspen Institute, 2015). In recent years, there have been a variety of initiatives launched to establish physical literacy among youth in response to declining rates of physical activity. This lack of physical activity impairs quality of life, drains economies, and sets in motion a cycle in which parents who are inactive are nearly six times more likely to have inactive children (The Aspen Institute, 2015). The goal of these initiatives is to help children develop the motor skills to run, jump, balance, and perform other basic skills needed to live an active life, as well as the mindset to use those skills, thereby setting them up to enjoy a variety of physical activities throughout their lives.

The Aspen Institute (2015) makes a call to action to a number of sectors that are well-positioned to play key roles in advancing physical literacy, including education, healthcare and medical providers, and parents/guardians. Specific to the fitness world, strategies include making physical literacy the basis of programming for families, taking gym classes for kids to schools and community centers, and prioritizing effort, not performance. Personal trainers should be mindful of the need for physical literacy when developing exercise programs for youth.

EXERCISE GUIDELINES FOR YOUTH

With the increased need for organized youth activity, the number of youth-focused fitness facilities and exercise programs is increasing. Youth can achieve substantial health benefits by performing bouts of moderate- and vigorous-intensity physical activity that add up to 60 minutes or more each day (U.S. Department of Health & Human Services, 2018). This should include cardiorespiratory activities as well as age-appropriate muscle- and bone-strengthening exercises. As with adults, it appears that the total amount of physical activity accumulated each week is more important for achieving health benefits than is any one component (frequency, intensity, or duration). However, bone-strengthening activities are especially critical for children and young adolescents, because the greatest gains in bone mass occur during the period just before and during puberty (U.S. Department of Health & Human Services, 2018).

Inspiring children to be more active requires understanding the child and his or her interests and motivations. While recreational and competitive sports are a great way to provide opportunities to be active, for some children, especially those whose motor skills are less developed or who have **overweight** or obesity, the competitive atmosphere can be defeating. A personal trainer can have a positive impact on a child's perception of exercise by ensuring that activities are fun for the child and appeal to his or her unique interests. A child interested in science may enjoy a hike to collect flower or rock specimens, while a child with a high sense of adventure may enjoy bouldering or rock climbing. Activities like dancing, bouncing on a trampoline, and riding a bike or skateboard are all fun ways to increase cardiorespiratory activity. Personal trainers can encourage children to try new modalities and experiment as they look for activities they find pleasurable. It is important that children understand that exercise involves simply moving the body and that everyone can enjoy movement.

Muscle-strengthening activities are an important part of an activity program for youth. They do not have to be structured (e.g., resistance training), but can instead be incorporated into play and games (e.g., climbing trees, tug of war, or jumping). Research demonstrating increases in strength following structured muscular training in children is mounting [American College of Sports Medicine (ACSM), 2018; Faigenbaum & Westcott, 2013]. These studies indicate that strength increases in children are similar to those observed in older age groups. Furthermore, the safety and efficacy of muscular-training programs for prepubescent children has been well-documented.

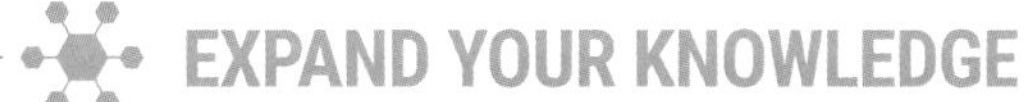

Can Youth Safely Perform Muscular Training?

Some people believe that preadolescents are too young to perform muscular training and that doing so will damage their bones. Evidence has dispelled that myth, showing that children can significantly increase their muscular strength and physical abilities through properly designed programs of progressive muscular exercise (Faigenbaum et al., 2009).

In fact, muscular training is the most effective means for young people to build bone density. In one study, nine-year old girls who performed 10 months of simple muscular-training exercise increased their **bone mineral density** four times as much as nine-year old girls who did not strength train (6.2% increase vs. 1.4% increase) (Morris et al., 1997).

With respect to safety, there has never been research published indicating that growth retardation, skeletal damage, or even substantial injury in youth muscular-training programs occurs when qualified adult supervision is provided, evidence-based recommendations are followed, equipment is used properly, and appropriate loads are used. In a study of sports-related injuries, muscular training had a much better safety record than other athletic activities (Hamill, 1994). Youth who perform regular muscular exercise may experience numerous health and fitness benefits, including an improved cardiovascular-risk profile, better **body composition** and weight control, stronger bones, more proficient motor-skill performance, reduced injury risk, and enhanced positive psychosocial outcomes (Faigenbaum et al., 2009).

Injuries can occur in any sport or strenuous physical activity. Importantly, children have different risk factors than adults. The epiphyseal plate, or growth plate, is a cartilaginous area of the bone that is not fully formed in youth. Improper form, repetitive impact, and torque may increase the risk of injury to this area. To minimize the risk of injury during muscular training, personal trainers should adhere to the following guidelines:

- Children should be properly supervised and use proper exercise technique at all times. Note that traditional exercise machines may not provide the appropriate **lever** arm for children and, therefore, may increase the incidence of injury. Free weights or body-weight exercises may be preferred.
- Never encourage children to perform single maximal lifts, sudden explosive movements, or compete with other children while performing muscular training.
- Teach children how to breathe properly during exercise movements.
- Encourage children to drink plenty of fluids before, during, and after exercise.

- Tell children that they need to communicate with a personal trainer, coach, parent, or teacher when they feel tired or fatigued, or when they feel discomfort or pain.
- Create a dynamic, fun, and age-appropriate muscular-training program.

As stated in **Wolff's Law,** bone strengthening occurs when bones are acted upon by forces to which they are unaccustomed. Table 14-1 shows examples of moderate- and vigorous-intensity cardiorespiratory activities, as well as examples of activities that promote the strengthening of bone and muscle.

TABLE 14-1

Examples of Physical Activities for Youth

Type of Physical Activity	Preschool-aged Children	School-aged Children	Adolescents
Moderate-intensity aerobic	▸ Games such as tag or follow the leader ▸ Playing on a playground ▸ Tricycle or bicycle riding ▸ Walking, running, skipping, jumping, dancing ▸ Swimming ▸ Playing games that require catching, throwing, and kicking ▸ Gymnastics or tumbling	▸ Brisk walking ▸ Bicycle riding ▸ Active recreation, such as hiking, riding a scooter without a motor, swimming ▸ Playing games that require catching and throwing, such as baseball and softball	▸ Brisk walking ▸ Bicycle riding ▸ Active recreation, such as kayaking, hiking, swimming ▸ Playing games that require catching and throwing, such as baseball and softball ▸ House and yard work, such as sweeping or pushing a lawn mower ▸ Some video games that include continuous movement
Vigorous-intensity aerobic	▸ Games such as tag or follow the leader ▸ Playing on a playground ▸ Tricycle or bicycle riding ▸ Walking, running, skipping, jumping, dancing ▸ Swimming ▸ Playing games that require catching, throwing, and kicking ▸ Gymnastics or tumbling	▸ Running ▸ Bicycle riding ▸ Active games involving running and chasing, such as tag or flag football ▸ Jumping rope ▸ Cross-country skiing ▸ Sports such as soccer, basketball, swimming, tennis ▸ Martial arts ▸ Vigorous dancing	▸ Running ▸ Bicycle riding ▸ Active games involving running and chasing, such as flag football ▸ Jumping rope ▸ Cross-country skiing ▸ Sports such as soccer, basketball, swimming, tennis ▸ Martial arts ▸ Vigorous dancing
Muscle strengthening	▸ Games such as tug of war ▸ Climbing on playground equipment ▸ Gymnastics	▸ Games such as tug of war ▸ Resistance exercises using body weight or resistance bands ▸ Rope or tree climbing ▸ Climbing on playground equipment ▸ Some forms of yoga	▸ Games such as tug of war ▸ Resistance exercises using body weight, resistance bands, weight machines, hand-held weights ▸ Some forms of yoga

TABLE 14-1 *(continued)*

Type of Physical Activity	Preschool-aged Children	School-aged Children	Adolescents
Bone strengthening	▸ Hopping, skipping, jumping ▸ Jumping rope ▸ Running ▸ Gymnastics	▸ Hopping, skipping, jumping ▸ Jumping rope ▸ Running ▸ Sports that involve jumping or rapid change in direction	▸ Jumping rope ▸ Running ▸ Sports that involve jumping or rapid change in direction

Note: Some activities, such as bicycling or swimming, can be moderate or vigorous intensity, depending upon level of effort. For preschool-aged children, aerobic activities listed can be either moderate or vigorous intensity.

Source: U.S. Department of Health & Human Services (2018). *Physical Activity Guidelines for Americans* (2nd ed.). www.health.gov/paguidelines/

Personal trainers working with youth with health challenges (e.g., **asthma** and **diabetes**) should communicate with their healthcare providers to understand the types and amounts of physical activity that are appropriate for the child. The personal trainer should apply a thoughtful approach to program design to create gradual increases in activity that have a positive impact on the child's overall health and wellness.

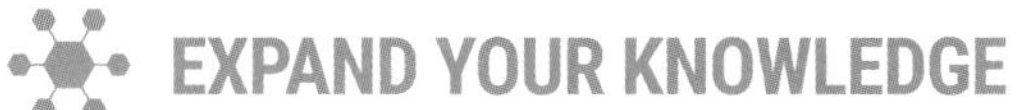

Precautions for Youth when Exercising in the Heat or Cold

Research suggests that children and adults are relatively similar in terms of risk for heat-related illness and that no maturational differences exist in thermal balance or endurance performance during exercise in the heat (Falke & Dotan, 2008; Naughton & Carlson, 2008; Rowland, 2008; Rowland et al., 2008). However, concern exists that children may be at greater risk of heat-related illnesses than adults due to their:

- Higher ratio of body surface area to mass
- Lower exercise economy
- Diminished sweating capacity
- Lower **cardiac output** at a similar workload

These greater risk factors should be considered, especially when children are playing sports that require padding.

Children exercising in extremely cold temperatures are at increased risk of **dehydration, hypothermia,** and **frostbite.** Careful attention should be given to ensure proper hydration and layering of clothing when exercising in cold conditions. In extremely cold conditions, personal trainers should consider moving activities indoors. Note that cold air lacks moisture and an individual with asthma or **exercise-induced bronchoconstriction** may be at a greater risk for exacerbation in these conditions. Precautions regarding exercise in the heat and cold should also be recognized (see Chapter 8).

In recent years, local weather services have begun issuing heat and cold warnings when conditions are not optimal for prolonged outdoor activity. These are well-informed warnings and should be considered by personal trainers before deciding on an outdoor exercise session.

Though physical inactivity is a threat to youth, **overuse injuries** and sports-related traumatic injuries can occur due to the increase in "sport specialization" and year-round single-sport play. This singular focus increases repetitive forces on the growing body, sometimes resulting in overuse injury. This is often accompanied by a loss of fun and ultimately a decline in participation or burnout. Vigorous exercise is good for youth. However, it must be age-appropriate and not so strenuous that it increases injury risk. Additionally, the variability of multiple sports and activities provides the most well-rounded opportunity for a child to improve overall athleticism by increasing proprioceptive capability, along with multidimensional strength, agility, endurance, speed, and confidence.

Consider these sport-specific differences—baseball and softball rely on mental focus and quick reactions; while gymnastics requires strength, coordination, and balance; and biking and climbing incorporate independence and cardiorespiratory and muscular fitness. A schedule that alternates fun, independent activity with a variety of organized sports will improve the skills in even the most talented athlete. A personal trainer must also remember the principles of **periodization** (see Chapter 11), which should be applied to children involved with organized sport; professional and Olympic athletes do not compete year-round, but instead vary their routine to increase performance and minimize risk of injury. Youth should do the same.

A personal trainer can have a meaningful impact on the health of children by leading appropriate exercise programs; incorporating cardiorespiratory training, muscle- and bone-strengthening activities, and stretching; and by progressively increasing activity levels while taking into consideration the health and fitness levels of the child.

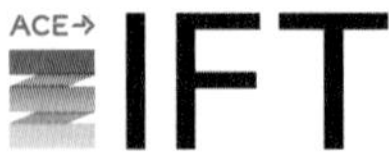

APPLYING THE ACE INTEGRATED FITNESS TRAINING MODEL TO YOUTH

Especially when working with youth who are inactive or have overweight or obesity, it is important to structure movement assessments as fun activities and remain noncritical of movement. However, the assessments themselves need not vary from those used for adults. Setting up children for success and celebrating each of their achievements are important in improving confidence and enjoyment of exercise.

A program that includes fun, playful movements is often engaging, even for older teens. Vary the equipment to keep the workout fun, while maintaining attention to detailed and varied program design. A training program for youth should include movement in all three **planes of motion** and use different pieces of equipment throughout the workout. Exercises should be selected for their benefits to balance, coordination, muscle and bone strengthening, as well as their fun and engaging nature. Due to increased hours sitting at a keyboard, playing video games, or using a mobile phone, youth are prone to forward-head and rounded-shoulder postures. The cool-down is a great time to teach stretches that can be done daily to benefit postural alignment.

If personal trainers remain mindful of the guidelines and key considerations presented in this chapter, their apparently healthy youth clients can participate in exercise plans aligned with the ACE IFT Model Exercise Programming Template presented in Chapter 11 (see pages 518–519). The FITT recommendations for children and adolescents are presented in Table 14-2.

TABLE 14-2

FITT Recommendations for Children and Adolescents

	Aerobic	Resistance	Bone Strengthening
Frequency	Daily	≥3 days/week	≥3 days/week
Intensity	Most should be moderate (noticeable increase in HR and breathing) to vigorous intensity (substantial increase in HR and breathing). Include vigorous intensity at least 3 days/week.*	Use of body weight as resistance or 8–15 submaximal repetitions of an exercise to the point of moderate fatigue with good mechanical form	N/A
Time	As part of ≥60 minutes/day of exercise	As part of ≥60 minutes/day of exercise	As part of ≥60 minutes/day of exercise
Type	Enjoyable and developmentally appropriate activities, including running, brisk walking, swimming, dancing, bicycling, and sports such as soccer, basketball, or tennis	Muscle-strengthening physical activities can be unstructured (e.g., playing on playground equipment, climbing trees, tug of war) or structured (e.g., lifting weights, working with resistance bands)	Bone-strengthening activities include running, jump rope, basketball, tennis, resistance training, and hopscotch

Note: FITT = Frequency, intensity, time, and type; HR = Heart rate

*Moderate intensity = Heart rates <VT1 where speech remains comfortable and is not affected by breathing; Vigorous intensity = Heart rates from ≥VT1 to <VT2 where clients feel unsure if speech is comfortable; VT1 = First ventilatory threshold; VT2 = Second ventilatory threshold

Reprinted with permission from American College of Sports Medicine (2018). *ACSM's Guidelines for Exercise Testing and Prescription* (10th ed.). Philadelphia: Wolters Kluwer.

Exercise for Women during Pregnancy and the Postpartum Period

It used to be that the medical community encouraged pregnant women to reduce their physical-activity levels and refrain from starting vigorous exercise programs due to concerns that exercise might harm the fetus. Since the mid-1990s, an increasing amount of research on exercise during pregnancy has shown that pregnant women can exercise safely without harming the fetus. In their most recent guidelines, the American College of Obstetricians and Gynecologists (ACOG, 2015) announced in reference to women exercising during pregnancy, "The World Health Organization and the American College of Sports Medicine have issued evidence-based recommendations indicating that the beneficial effects of exercise in most adults are indisputable and that the benefits far outweigh the risks." Furthermore, studies indicate regular exercise is associated with reduced rates of **preeclampsia, gestational diabetes mellitus,** Caesarean section (C-section), low-back pain, **anxiety,** nausea, heartburn, **insomnia,** leg cramps, and possibly control of excessive weight gain (Lamina & Agbanusi, 2013).

It is important that personal trainers request medical clearance from the client's physician if the woman also has severe obesity, gestational diabetes, or hypertension. Some chronic conditions may worsen during pregnancy or can be difficult to control. Doctors may determine that poorly controlled **anemia,** hypertension, seizure disorder, or **hyperthyroidism** are contraindications to activity during pregnancy.

PHYSICAL AND PHYSIOLOGICAL CHANGES DURING PREGNANCY

Women undergo a variety of physical changes during pregnancy that must be considered. During a healthy pregnancy, it is recommended a woman gain 25 to 35 pounds (11.4 to 15.9 kg), though that recommendation may change if a woman has underweight, overweight, or obesity prior to the pregnancy (ACOG, 2013). Because the majority of additional weight gain during pregnancy contributes to an increase in abdominal circumference, additional stress is placed on the back, pelvis, hips, and legs. As the fetus grows and weight gain occurs, a woman's **center of gravity (COG)** moves upward and forward. The changes in weight and COG may result in low-back discomfort and affect balance and coordination. A focus early in the pregnancy on increased **posterior** leg and trunk strength through properly performed squat, lunge, and deadlift exercise programming, can help ready the body for the increased weight and change in the COG.

Throughout the pregnancy, women will experience a change in **hormone** levels, which may cause nausea and fatigue. This is most common in the first trimester but may occur at any stage during the pregnancy. A personal trainer must be sensitive to the needs of the client and adjust programming intensity and rest periods to meet such needs during each session.

An increase in the hormone **relaxin** will increase joint **laxity.** This is an important development of pregnancy, as relaxin allows the increased widening of the pelvis and, therefore, the birth canal to facilitate delivery. However, it is important to remember that the increase in this hormone affects the laxity of all joints and women may see a flare-up of an old injury or simply feel more discomfort due to joint instability. Training for strength and stability is effective in providing additional stabilization as the body changes throughout the course of the pregnancy.

Cardiac reserve, or the difference between resting and maximal cardiac function, is reduced in pregnant women. During the early months of pregnancy, hormonal signals stimulate increases in **heart rate,** blood volume, **stroke volume,** and cardiac output. As pregnancy progresses, these cardiovascular changes can make increased physical demands more difficult than normal. Women may feel out of breath after short bouts of moderate-intensity exercise or tire more easily in general. Personal trainers should allow for increased rest periods at these times. Motionless postures such as those common in yoga and the **supine** lying position should be avoided as much as possible because they may result in decreased **venous return** and **hypotension.**

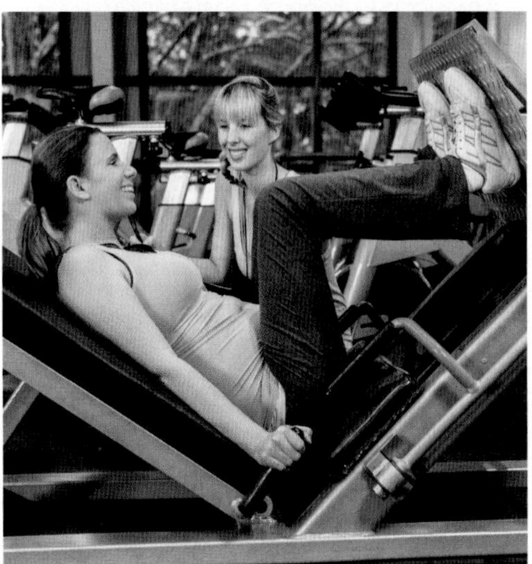

The thermoregulatory system is also affected by pregnancy, resulting in a slight improvement in women's ability to dissipate heat. This may be due to increased blood flow to the skin and increases in tidal volume. However, it is critical that the pregnant exerciser is aware of the **ambient temperature** prior to each workout. Exercise increases body temperature, so increased ambient temperature and/or humidity may significantly affect the woman's ability to dissipate heat and could result in **hyperthermia.** However, there have been no reports that hyperthermia associated with exercise causes malformations of the embryo or fetus.

EXERCISE GUIDELINES FOR WOMEN DURING PREGNANCY

Guidelines for exercise are updated as new research is conducted and reviewed. It is important that personal trainers review updated ACOG guidelines whenever training a client during pregnancy and include the PARmed-X for Pregnancy physical activity readiness evaluation form as part of the preparticipation health screening process (www.csep.ca). Current recommendations support moderate-intensity exercise for at least 150 minutes over a minimum of three days per week during a normal pregnancy, as this amount and intensity of exercise poses minimal risk for the fetus and offers beneficial metabolic and cardiorespiratory effects for the exercising woman. ACSM, ACOG, and others have concluded that physician-guided exercise is beneficial during and following pregnancy for all women, regardless of prenatal exercise history, and women should include a combination of cardiorespiratory and muscular training in their programs (ACSM, 2018; ACOG, 2015). Note: ACOG's 2015 guidelines were reaffirmed by the organization in 2017.

According to ACOG, in the absence of complications or contraindications, exercise during pregnancy is safe and desirable. Obstetric care providers are responsible for ensuring that there are no conditions present that would limit activity, such as risk factors for preterm labor, vaginal bleeding, premature labor, rupture of membranes, or severe anemia. It is important that personal trainers are aware of warning signs to discontinue exercise while pregnant. Should any of the following occur, the exercise session should be postponed and the client should discuss the condition with her physician prior to resuming exercise training (ACOG, 2015):

- Vaginal bleeding
- Regular painful contractions
- Amniotic fluid leakage
- **Dyspnea** before exertion
- Dizziness or feeling faint
- Headache
- Chest pain
- Muscle weakness affecting balance
- Calf pain or swelling

Personal trainers should be empathetic to the changes of the body during pregnancy, which can be tiring and the decrease in exercise capacity may be frustrating for some women. Creating programs should take into account a client's goals and the day-to-day energy fluctuations of the individual, and should adhere to the following guidelines:

- Women who have been previously active may continue their exercise program. The upper level of safe exercise intensity has not been established. ACOG (2015) guidelines state that women with healthy uncomplicated pregnancies should be able to maintain their previous level of exercise intensity, as tolerated.

- Women who have not previously been physically active should begin slowly and progress to a moderate level of exercise. Some women may need to begin with low intensity and shorter durations (<10 minutes) and/or perform intermittent activity.
- Using the **talk test** will ensure a more effective means than heart rate to monitor exercise intensity (see Chapter 8). Staying below the **first ventilatory threshold (VT1)** indicates a moderate level of cardiorespiratory intensity.
- Avoid activities with high risk of abdominal trauma from contact or fall (e.g., contact sports, skiing, and surfing). In addition, exercise performed in extreme heat (e.g., "hot" yoga) should be avoided. Certain exercises (e.g., jogging, running, racquet sports, and muscular training) may be safe to initiate or continue with during pregnancy, while other activities may need to be modified or discussed with an obstetric care provider before participation.
- Focus on hydration and balancing caloric intake with the metabolic demands of exercise and pregnancy.
- Some pregnant women may benefit from a small snack prior to exercise to help avoid **hypoglycemia,** especially when exercising at a moderate intensity for longer than 45 minutes.

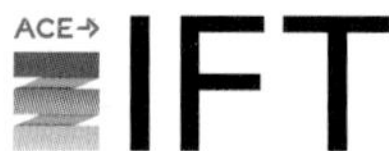

APPLYING THE ACE INTEGRATED FITNESS TRAINING MODEL DURING PREGNANCY

It is not unusual for a personal trainer to have a client who becomes pregnant during their time working together. This is an appropriate time for the personal trainer to review updated ACOG guidelines and share these resources with the client. It is also a good opportunity for the personal trainer to connect with the client's physician (once permission has been granted by the client) to discuss any health considerations. By taking these steps, a personal trainer will increase the client's confidence that she can continue personal-training sessions throughout her pregnancy.

Women may seek out a personal trainer early in pregnancy for a variety of reasons. She may have received such a recommendation from her doctor or she may wish to remain active and want an expert supervising her program to ensure that it is safe. Alternately, she may have led a physically inactive lifestyle prior to pregnancy and has decided that improving her health is important at this time in her life.

The intensity of the exercise program for a pregnant woman will depend on the previous exercise habits of the client. Whenever creating a program for a woman during pregnancy, a few considerations should be kept in mind:

- Consider recommending shorter sessions (e.g., 30 minutes versus 60 minutes) for new clients who have not exercised before pregnancy and then slowly increase duration and intensity over the course of the program.
- Choose exercises to support the changing COG, such as squats, stiff-legged deadlifts, side lunges, lat pull-downs, seated rows, and bird dog exercises.
- Encourage clients to discuss their energy level, aches and pains, and exercise warning signs in real time so the program can be modified accordingly.
- Individualize intensity level and rest time as needed. These requirements may change daily.

Cardiorespiratory exercise programming should avoid risk to the abdomen. Exercises like walking, running, riding a stationary bike, and using elliptical machines are excellent forms of exercise. As body weight increases, women may find they enjoy spending time in the pool. Swimming, water exercise, and walking or running in the pool can take strain off the low back and legs while providing cardiorespiratory benefits.

If personal trainers conduct a thorough preparticipation health screening including the completion of the PARmed-X for Pregnancy and remain mindful of the guidelines and key considerations presented in this chapter, they can create a safe and effective exercise plan aligned with the ACE IFT Model Exercise Programming Template presented in Chapter 11 (see pages 518–519). The FITT recommendations for women who are pregnant are presented in Table 14-3.

TABLE 14-3

FITT Recommendations for Women Who Are Pregnant

	Aerobic	Resistance	Flexibility
Frequency	≥3–5 days/week	2–3 nonconsecutive days/week	≥2–3 days/week, with daily being most effective
Intensity	Moderate intensity (3–5.9 METs; RPE of 12–13 on the 6–20 scale); vigorous-intensity exercise (≥6 METs; RPE 14–17 on the 6–20 scale) for women who were highly active prior to pregnancy or for women who progress to higher fitness levels during pregnancy*	Intensity that permits multiple submaximal repetitions (i.e., 8–10 or 12–15 repetitions) to be performed to a point of moderate fatigue	Stretch to the point of feeling tightness or slight discomfort
Time	~30 minutes/day of accumulated moderate-intensity exercise to total at least 150 minutes/week or 75 minutes/week of vigorous-intensity aerobic exercise	One set for beginners; two to three sets for intermediate and advanced; target major muscle groups	Hold static stretch for 10–30 seconds
Type	A variety of weight- and non-weight-bearing activities are well tolerated during pregnancy (e.g., hiking, group exercise, swimming).	A variety of machines, free weights, and body-weight exercises are well tolerated during pregnancy (e.g., upright chest press, dumbbells, lunges).	A series of static (i.e., active or passive) and dynamic flexibility exercises for each muscle-tendon unit.

Note: FITT = Frequency, intensity, time, and type; METs = Metabolic equivalents; RPE = Rating of perceived exertion

*Moderate intensity = Heart rates <VT1 where speech remains comfortable and is not affected by breathing; Vigorous intensity = Heart rates from ≥VT1 to <VT2 where clients feel unsure if speech is comfortable; VT1 = First ventilatory threshold; VT2 = Second ventilatory threshold

Reprinted with permission from American College of Sports Medicine (2018). *ACSM's Guidelines for Exercise Testing and Prescription* (10th ed.). Philadelphia: Wolters Kluwer.

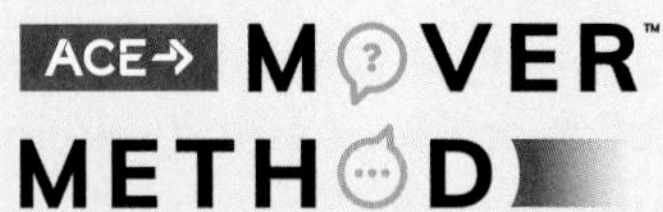

Exercise Consistency Throughout Pregnancy

Michelle, a client with whom you have been working for the past six months, informs you that she is seven weeks pregnant. She is very excited about the pregnancy and has already discussed continuing her exercise program with her doctor. The doctor advised Michelle that continuing with her current exercise program is a great idea, as long as the pregnancy remains uncomplicated. Michelle is aware of the benefits derived from physical activity during pregnancy, so she was pleased to receive her doctor's clearance. Michelle wants to discuss her goals with you, as she has newfound motivation to continue her journey toward a healthy lifestyle.

ACE ABC APPROACH

Following is an example of how the ACE Mover Method™ philosophy can be used along with the ACE ABC Approach™ to establish goals with a client to promote an environment that is conducive to maintaining **adherence** and enjoyment as the body physiologically changes with pregnancy.

Ask: Use powerful **open-ended questions** during the conversation to find out what Michelle hopes to accomplish by continuing her work with you as her pregnancy progresses.

Personal Trainer: Congratulations on your exciting news! For the past six months, you have been working toward leading a healthier life, and exercise has been the foundation of this change. With the news of your pregnancy, leading a healthy lifestyle has become even more relevant to you.

Client: Leading a healthier life was important to me before I got pregnant, and now I realize the choices I make are not just impacting my life, but the life of my baby as well. I spoke with my doctor and learned that working out can enhance my overall feelings of well-being, maintain my cardiorespiratory health, decrease my chances of developing diabetes and **depression,** help prepare me for the challenges of becoming a mom, and help me manage my weight after the baby is born. Plus, I've worked hard over the past six months, and I do not want to lose my progress.

Personal Trainer: Becoming healthier is still important to you, and your doctor has also communicated to you the benefits of remaining physically active. What do you want to achieve by working with me during your pregnancy?

Client: I know I have not always been consistent with my training, but I would like to work with you to meet the physical-activity guidelines my doctor gave me, which means my priorities will shift to placing greater focus on my health and my baby's health. My doctor also said it is okay to continue working at the same intensity I have been, and she suggested incorporating muscle-strengthening activity.

Break down barriers: At this point, you may ask more open-ended questions to learn what may be interfering with Michelle's consistency. You can also uncover what potential obstacles may impede her progress.

Personal Trainer: Not being consistent with your program has been an obstacle to reaching your goals. What has prevented you from reaching the level of consistency you would like?

Client: I don't exercise as much as I plan to because I can always think of reasons not to do it. Sometimes I feel like if I take time for myself to exercise, I am not making time for my husband, my work, my friends, or my family. I sometimes skip my workouts to be with my friends or husband.

Personal Trainer: Exercise is important to you, and spending time with your family and friends is also important. In an ideal world, what would it look like to have a perfect balance of friends, family, and exercise?

Client: My ideal situation would be that my friends and family would come alongside me and support my goals. It's not that they don't support my goals, but I guess I haven't expressed to them how important being healthier is to me. One thing my ideal world would include is doing exercise with my friends and family. It would be great to take a walk or go to the gym with my husband.

Personal Trainer: What could you start doing now to move closer to your goals and your ideal vision?

Client: I need to start letting those people who are closest to me know how important becoming healthier is. There are lots of opportunities for me to be active throughout my day, and having support and encouragement from friends, family, and coworkers would help. I want to start inviting my coworkers to walk with me on breaks, and I want to encourage my husband to be active with me. I want to do cardio throughout the week for a total of 150 minutes and meet with you twice per week to focus on muscle-strengthening activities.

Collaborate: After you've worked together to identify barriers and goals, the focus of this collaborative process can switch to eliciting action items from the client, so that she feels ownership over the program.

Personal Trainer: You would like to do cardio for 150 minutes per week and meet with me twice per week to do muscle-strengthening activities. Support from friends and family is vital to your success. What can you do within the next week to get started?

Client: First, I would like to schedule our sessions together on Tuesday and Thursday mornings at 7:00 if you still have this spot available. Next, I will walk for 30 minutes a day for five days per week while on my lunch break at work. To be successful with this, I will let my friends and coworkers know about my plan and invite them to join me. This week, I will also set up a date night with my husband that involves being active, and I will talk to him about my desire to be active together.

Personal Trainer: That sounds like a solid plan! I do still have Tuesday and Thursday mornings available, and it would be my pleasure to schedule you for that time. **Social support** is an important element of your success, and I look forward to hearing about the response you get from your friends and family when we meet next week. Thank you again for sharing your exciting news with me. I will see you on Tuesday!

In this example, Michelle is motivated to continue her behavior-change journey and become more consistent after learning she is seven weeks pregnant. Using the ACE Mover Method philosophy and the ACE ABC Approach, the personal trainer and client can co-create specific action steps. By using open-ended questions, affirmations, reflections, and summary statements, the personal trainer helped Michelle identify and overcome barriers while collaborating with her to develop a program that is specific to her individual needs.

POSTPARTUM EXERCISE GUIDELINES

Each woman's delivery experience is unique and many factors contribute to her readiness to exercise following delivery. As with during pregnancy, hormone levels continue to shift. Fatigue remains a factor from the changing hormones and demands on the body, as well as the interrupted sleep that is common when caring for a newborn. Likewise, postpartum anemia is common and is associated with an impaired quality of life, reduced **cognitive** abilities, emotional instability, and depression (Milman, 2011). In the days and weeks following delivery, a woman should gradually increase exercise as she feels ready and as her doctor recommends. She should be aware that, though fatigue is normal, it may indicate another condition and she should not be shy about asking her doctor for advice. Women who have had a C-section will require additional recovery time, as this is a highly invasive surgery that requires incision through the skin, **fascia,** uterine tissue, and occasionally muscle tissue. Healing time will vary, and the physician should be consulted for a return-to-activity protocol.

Miscarriage and stillbirth are sad realities of pregnancy; an estimated 25% of pregnancies end in miscarriage and 1% end in stillbirth (Dugas & Slane, 2019; Hoyert & Gregory, 2016). It is important for personal trainers to recognize that after the loss of a pregnancy, a woman may be dealing with intense grief. Though most miscarriages are caused by chromosomal defect and 50% of stillbirths are caused by disorders of the placenta (Hoyert & Gregory, 2016), there are many misconceptions in the general population, including the belief that exercise or **activities of daily living (ADL)** may have caused the loss of a wanted pregnancy. In many cases, a woman may be dealing with feelings of guilt, thinking that her actions were at fault. A personal trainer can support a woman in

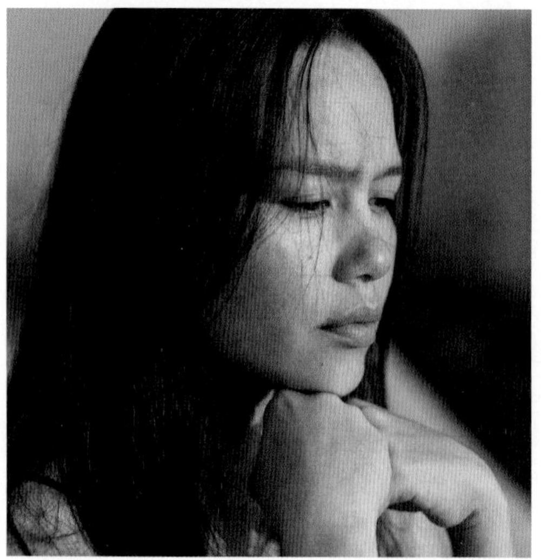

this situation by maintaining professional distance yet checking in on how she is feeling during sessions and showing care and **empathy** for her loss.

Nutrition is another important consideration, as breastfeeding women have increased caloric and nutrient requirements, which is vital to support activity levels and adequate milk production. Personal trainers can help support women by emphasizing their overall health and reminding them that healthy habits are essential to maintaining the energy and confidence for parenting a newborn.

Occasionally, a woman may wish to resume exercise shortly after delivery. Personal trainers should create programs that adhere to the following general guidelines:

- Obtain physician clearance and/or guidelines prior to resuming or starting an exercise program if medical or surgical complications are present.
- Begin slowly and gradually increase duration, frequency, and then intensity. Depending on their personal goals and energy levels, women may increase their activity levels until moderate-intensity activity or pre-pregnancy activity levels have been met.
- ACOG (2015) recommends at least 20 to 30 minutes of activity daily, including walking and simple exercises to strengthen major muscle groups. A woman may progress in activity as she feels ready and as her physician recommends.
- A woman should stop the exercise session if unusual pain is experienced and consult her physician, especially following an **episiotomy** or C-section.
- Stop the exercise session and seek medical evaluation if bright red vaginal bleeding occurs that is heavier than a normal menstrual period.
- Drink plenty of water and eat healthfully, taking into account energy needs for physical activity and lactation.

Lack of childcare and changing schedules may make it difficult for women to get to the gym or attend regular personal-training appointments in the months following the birth of a baby. A personal trainer can support a client's goals by creating simple exercise programs that can be performed in 10-minute time blocks. Encouraging walking is appealing, as the mother can take the child with her on walks.

When a woman is breastfeeding, sitting with a child frequently and for long periods during the day can contribute to forward-rounded shoulders. Back and posterior shoulder exercises (e.g., seated row) as well as **anterior** shoulder and pectoralis stretches (e.g., anterior shoulder and chest wall stretch) should be included in the exercise program design.

Exercises that promote trunk strength and stability can be included in the program design. It is essential to take into consideration a healing C-section incision or the presence of **diastasis recti.**

Personal trainers can further support women by reminding them that their pre-pregnancy exercise intensity levels have been changing for nine months or longer. To remain realistic, an expectation should be set for women to return to pre-pregnancy exercise-intensity levels over the subsequent nine to 12 months.

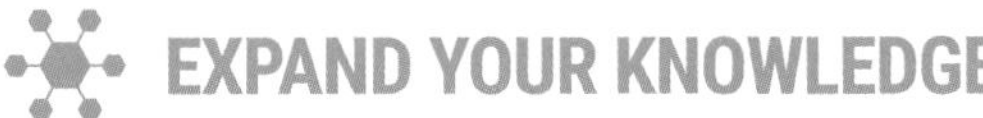

Diastasis Recti and Appropriate Exercise Considerations

Diastasis recti is the separation of the two muscle bellies of the rectus abdominis (see Figure 9-34, page 362) that may be up to 1 to 2 inches (2.5 to 5.1 cm) in width. Though there is little research on the incidence, one study found that the incidence was as high as 45% during pregnancy and 33% 12 months postpartum (Sperstad et al., 2016).

The change in appearance may be apparent in some women and, though surgical repair is not essential for health reasons, it may be pursued for cosmetic reasons. Occasionally, the incidence of diastasis recti may correlate to low-back or sacroiliac joint pain. In these cases, research has mixed results on whether diastasis recti is the cause of such pain (Sperstad et al., 2016). Additionally, more research needs to be done to evaluate the effectiveness of abdominal, pelvic floor, and postural exercises in correcting diastasis recti. However, a systematic review of the literature concluded that exercise performed prior to and during pregnancy reduced the presence of diastasis recti by 35% and suggested that diastasis recti width may be reduced by exercising during pregnancy and the postpartum period (Benjamin, Van de Water, & Peiris, 2014). Some research supports that exercises such as **isometric** contractions of the transverse abdominis and pelvic floor, as well as strength exercises for postural muscles and the abdomen result in a reduction of diastasis recti (Benjamin, Van de Water, & Peiris, 2014; Sharma, Lobo, & Keller, 2014). The exercises presented in Figures 14-1 through 14-5 can be incorporated into a pregnancy and postpartum exercise routine to reduce the risk of diastasis recti and support the low back and pelvic floor.

FIGURE 14-1
Quadruped transverse abdominis isometric contraction

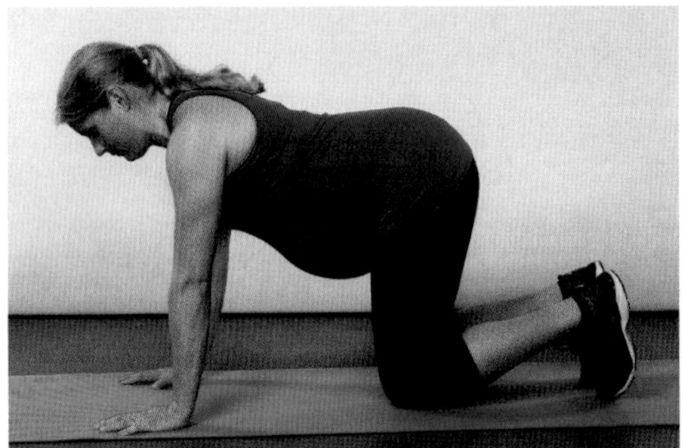
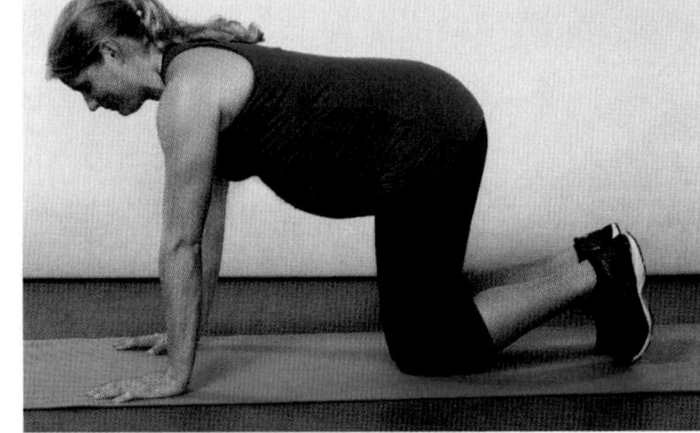

FIGURE 14-2
Wide-stance squats with dumbbell

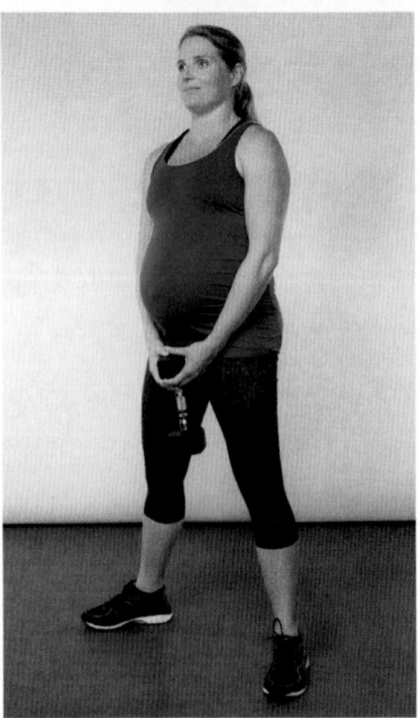
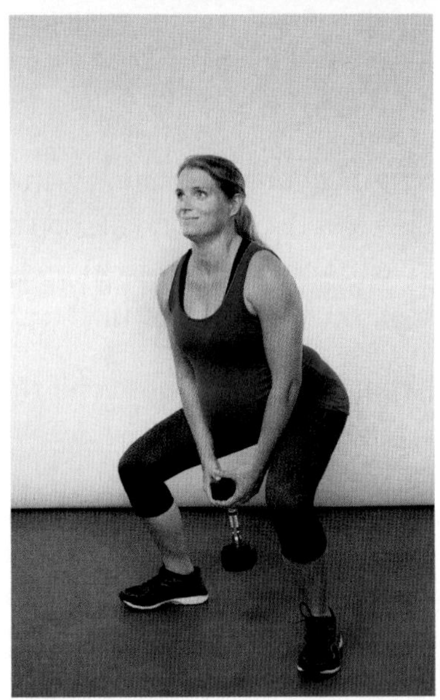

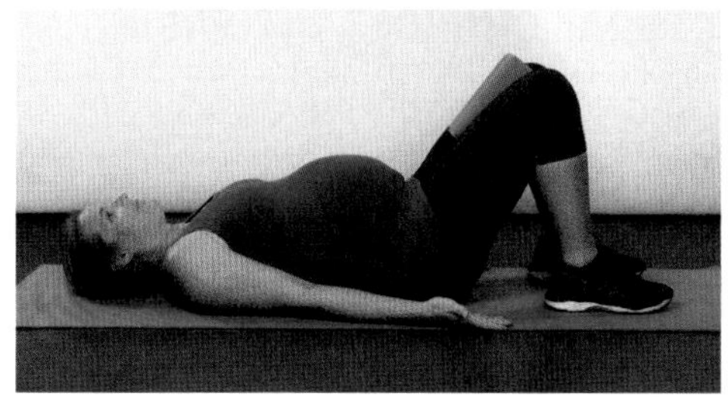
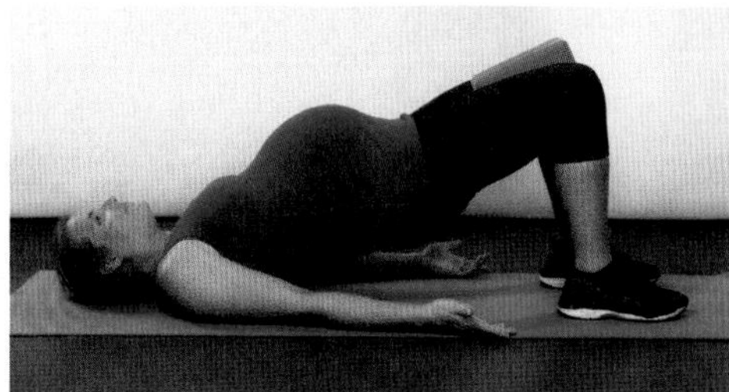

FIGURE 14-3
Bridges (with yoga block between thighs)

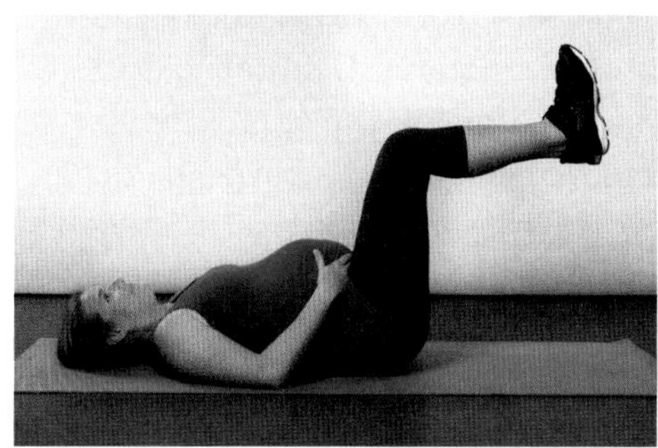
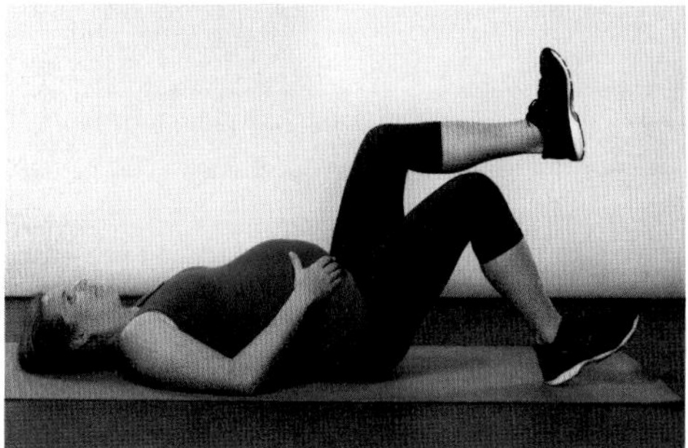

FIGURE 14-4
Bent-knee, alternate-leg heel taps (dead bugs)

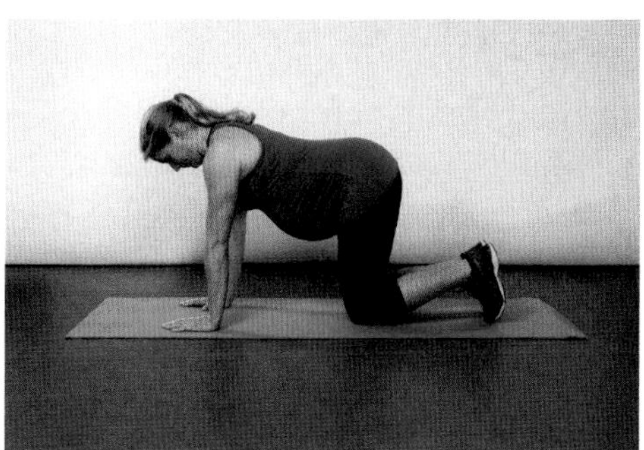
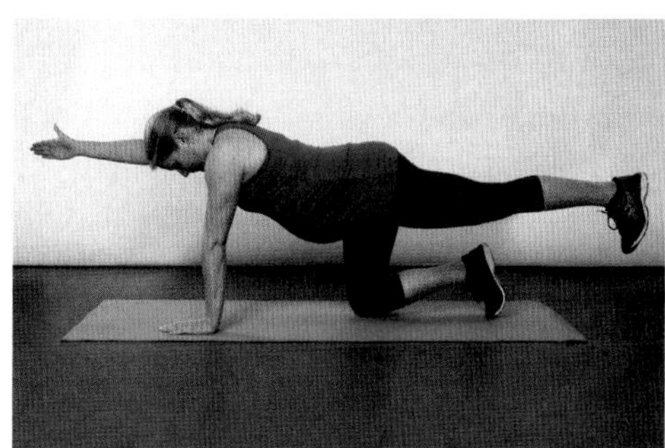

FIGURE 14-5
Bird dog

Exercise and Older Adults

Regular physical activity is essential for everyone, including older adults (i.e., individuals ≥65 years of age). According to the U.S. Census Bureau (2017), the Baby Boomer generation (in 2016, ages 52 to 70) numbered 74 million people in the U.S. This population has an increasing awareness of health and a desire to maintain independence and quality of life as they age. The expectations of this generation are that they will remain active well into their later years. For some, ADL become strenuous due to the development of chronic conditions and the associated loss of physical function, resulting in a loss of independence. To achieve the aim of remaining independent and active, regular exercise, healthful eating, and not smoking become even more important as people age.

Physiological results of aging typically include a decline in fitness levels, loss of height, reduced **lean body mass,** loss of skin and connective tissue **elasticity,** slower healing, changes in eyesight, and reduced coordination. Additionally, there are noticeable changes in the cardiovascular, endocrine, respiratory, and musculoskeletal systems. These natural effects of aging may be compounded by the presence of chronic disease, as discussed in Chapter 13.

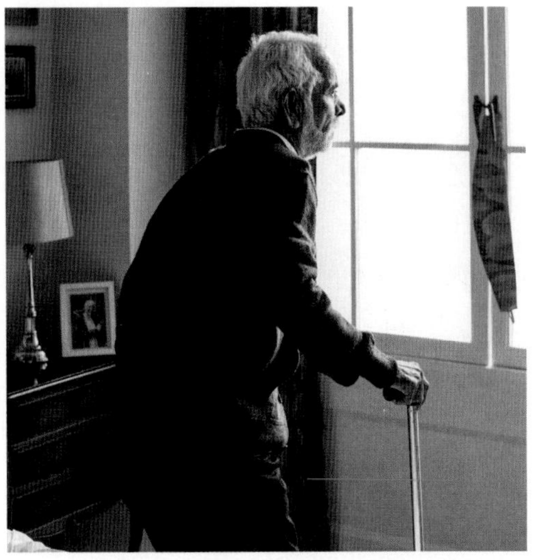

STRUCTURAL CHANGES WITH AGING

Muscle mass declines with age, resulting in reduced muscular strength and endurance. This is primarily attributed to changes in lifestyle (e.g., reduced physical activity) and decreased effectiveness of the neuromuscular system. The aging process also affects bones, as they become more fragile and porous with advancing years, placing older adults at a greater risk of **fractures.** Debilitating fractures become more common and approximately 20% of older individuals who sustain a hip fracture will die of related complications (National Osteoporosis Foundation, 2019). With age, loss of calcium results in decreased bone mass, but weight-bearing and muscular-training exercises can help maintain bone mass. Increased muscle and sustained bone mass result from exercise later in life, further supporting the need for muscular training throughout the lifespan.

As lean body mass declines with age, **body fat** typically increases. These changes in body composition are primarily due to decreased muscle mass and **basal metabolic rate,** and insufficient physical activity. Regular physical activity helps to stimulate **protein** synthesis, preserve lean body mass, and decrease **fat** stores.

STABILITY AND BALANCE FOR OLDER ADULTS

As people age, balance and coordination tend to decline, increasing the risk of falls and fall-associated injury. This is due to the loss of muscle mass and associated strength and a decline in **proprioception.** The **visual system, vestibular system,** and **somatosensory system** provide essential information to the **central nervous system** to maintain balance. Each of these systems is negatively affected by aging. Vision is a primary proprioceptive input and typically declines as people age, impacting balance. Declines in the function of the vestibular system, which provides information regarding the position of the head in space, and the somatosensory system (e.g., muscle and joint proprioceptors, and cutaneous and pressure receptors) also significantly impact balance and coordination. Physical activity can positively impact balance and coordination in older adults.

EXERCISE GUIDELINES FOR OLDER ADULTS

When working with older adults, personal trainers should recognize that energy levels will fluctuate and, especially if a person is experiencing cognitive decline, so may balance, attention, and focus. This can be frustrating for the client, and the personal trainer should recognize this, highlighting areas of success and improvement whenever possible. The U.S. Department of Health & Human Services (2018) recommends that older adults participate in exercise at the same level as other adults, performing moderate-intensity cardiorespiratory physical activity for a minimum of 150 to 300 minutes each week or vigorous-intensity cardiorespiratory activity for a minimum of 75 to 150 minutes each week, or an equivalent combination of both, preferably spread throughout the week. These guidelines also note that additional benefits are gained by engaging in more physical activity and that some exercise is better than none. In the absence of a regular exercise program, older adults should move more and sit less throughout the day. Likewise, muscular training is recommended at least twice each week to maintain or increase muscular strength and endurance using the major muscles of the body. Balance training should be incorporated into exercise programs to improve proprioception and decrease the risk of falls. Personal trainers should program exercises for older adults with medical conditions as is appropriate to the condition (see Chapter 13).

APPLYING THE ACE INTEGRATED FITNESS TRAINING MODEL FOR OLDER ADULTS

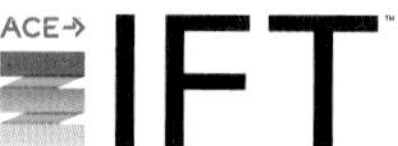

As individuals age, their motivations to begin, continue, or modify an exercise program may change. A competitive athlete may increase his or her interest in injury prevention, an occasional exerciser may choose to introduce more consistency to improve bone density, and a **previously physically inactive** individual may elect to begin a program to improve declining health markers. Often, older adults have more time and sufficient financial stability to work with a personal trainer in creating a safe and effective exercise program, which makes serving this population a great business opportunity for personal trainers.

Though exercise guidelines for older adults are similar to those for the general population, the initial fitness levels and abilities of an older client may be adversely affected by chronic disease. Accordingly, a thorough exercise preparticipation health screening must be conducted by the personal trainer (see Chapter 5) and may require that movement assessments be modified (if they are deemed necessary to include through a collaboration between the client and personal trainer).

Arthritis, among other joint injuries or conditions, is prevalent in this population [i.e., 49.6% of those over 65 years of age have the disease (Barbour et al., 2017)], so it is wise to begin with posture and **flexibility** assessments before progressing to the movement assessment. Coupling the results of these assessments with the information provided on an exercise preparticipation health-screening questionnaire, a personal trainer can modify movement assessments to mitigate pain and increase the confidence of the client by allowing him or her to complete a successful first workout. For instance, a client who has arthritis in the knee may not be asked to perform a body-weight squat, but instead be asked to sit and stand up from a chair to evaluate form and strength.

Balance training is recommended for the older adult population (U.S. Department of Health & Human Services, 2018). When assessing balance, it is important to provide a safe environment. Instead of starting with the Y balance test, it may be more prudent to begin with a unipedal stance test (see Chapter 10). For some individuals, it is ideal to begin by holding onto, or being near, an external stabilizer like a wall or doorframe on which to place a hand. It is also advised that the personal trainer stay close by, with hands outstretched, so the client may grasp them as needed. The client may progress to holding a cane, walking stick, or dowel rod while balancing on one leg. These external supports are less stable than a wall but provide some assistance. Balancing without any external support is the next step in exercise progression. If the individual remains capable, the Y balance test may be modified by using an external support or can be skipped altogether if the risk-benefit ratio is unacceptable.

Through an appropriate movement assessment, a personal trainer can establish the baseline capability of the client, which, along with taking the client's goals into consideration, ensures that the program focus is appropriate. As with any population, when a client who was previously physically inactive begins an exercise program, a slow increase in activity duration and overall volume is essential to preventing injury and improving the likelihood of adherence. It is essential that the personal trainer, while carefully considering previous exercise history, not impose limits on the client, and instead challenge the client's sense of adventure and achievement by selecting exercises that aim for continued gradual improvement toward whichever goals the client has outlined for him- or herself. Though chronic disease considerations are more likely to be present with this population, fitness levels will vary, and the goal-setting process remains a collaborative effort between client and personal trainer.

A warm-up to enhance **range of motion** becomes increasingly important as individuals age, due to overall decreased **collagen** content and concomitant reductions in elasticity of **connective tissue.** A thorough warm-up may further reduce the risk of injury. Likewise, the cool-down period can be used for static stretching when muscle tightness hampers **mobility** or the performance of ADL. Focusing the workout on elements of Functional Training is essential in this population. Balance exercises should be introduced early in the session, so that the client has the highest amount of strength and mental focus, reducing the risk of injury.

Another important consideration for this population is to determine whether the client is able to get down onto and up from the floor. In many clubs and studios, there is a massage table or bench available to provide an alternative option for those clients who have a harder time with ground-to-standing movement. For some older adults, playing with grandchildren on the floor may be a goal and a personal trainer may work with them to improve balance, strength, and mobility to achieve this meaningful personal goal.

Cardiorespiratory training will remain a high priority for older adults, as the risk and incidence of **cardiovascular disease** and other chronic diseases will be prevalent and are positively impacted by this type of exercise. As balance and vision decline with age, personal trainers should consider realistic recommendations for their clients' capabilities. Weight-bearing exercise is preferred, if tolerated, for bone strength. Stationary or recumbent bikes are also excellent options. For those who struggle with hip and knee mobility and/or balance, find a bike situated in an easy-to-access area of the gym. Additionally, many recumbent bikes are built with a low center bar, which allows for easier entry. Accommodations like these are important for a personal trainer to consider.

Building thoughtful and comprehensive programs using the ACE Integrated Fitness Training Model will allow older clients to achieve heightened fitness, health, and improved quality of life.

If personal trainers remain mindful of client goals and the guidelines and key considerations presented in this chapter, they can create and implement a meaningful, safe, and effective exercise program aligned with the ACE IFT Model Exercise Programming Template presented in Chapter 11 (see pages 518–519). The FITT recommendations for older adults are presented in Table 14-4.

TABLE 14-4
FITT Recommendations for Older Adults

	Aerobic	Resistance	Flexibility
Frequency	≥5 days/week for moderate intensity; ≥3 days/week for vigorous intensity; 3–5 days/week for a combination of moderate and vigorous intensity	≥2 days/week	≥2 days/week
Intensity	On a scale of 0–10 for level of physical exertion, 5–6 for moderate intensity and 7–8 for vigorous intensity*	Light intensity (i.e., 40–50% 1-RM) for beginners; progress to moderate-to-vigorous intensity (60–80% 1-RM); alternatively, moderate (5–6) to vigorous (7–8) intensity on a 0–10 scale	Stretch to the point of feeling tightness or slight discomfort.
Time	30–60 minutes/day of moderate-intensity exercise; 20–30 minutes/day of vigorous-intensity exercise; or an equivalent combination of moderate- and vigorous-intensity exercise; may be accumulated in bouts of at least 10 minutes each	8–10 exercise involving the major muscle groups; 1–3 sets of 8–12 repetitions each	Hold stretch for 30–60 seconds.
Type	Any modality that does not impose excessive orthopedic stress such as walking. Aquatic exercise and stationary cycle exercise may be advantageous for those with limited tolerance for weight-bearing activity.	Progressive weight-training programs or weight-bearing calisthenics, stair climbing, and other strengthening activities that use the major muscle groups	Any physical activities that maintain or increase flexibility using slow movements that terminate in static stretches for each muscle group rather than rapid ballistic movements

Note: FITT = Frequency, intensity, time, and type; 1-RM = One-repetition maximum

*Moderate intensity = Heart rates <VT1 where speech remains comfortable and is not affected by breathing; Vigorous intensity = Heart rates from ≥VT1 to <VT2 where clients feel unsure if speech is comfortable; VT1 = First ventilatory threshold; VT2 = Second ventilatory threshold

Reprinted with permission from American College of Sports Medicine (2018). *ACSM's Guidelines for Exercise Testing and Prescription* (10th ed.). Philadelphia: Wolters Kluwer.

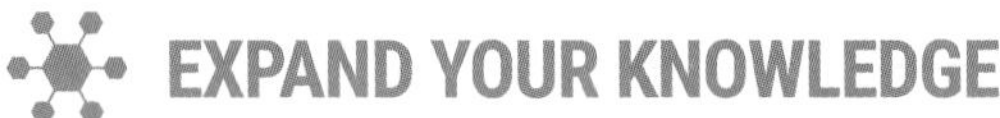

How Exercise Affects Cognitive Decline and Mental Health Risks in Older Adults

While cognitive decline is associated with aging, there is some evidence that physical activity prevents or delays cognitive impairment and disability. In a systematic review of 43 research articles, Northey and colleagues (2018) concluded that physical activity improves cognitive function in people over the age of 50 regardless of the cognitive status at onset. These findings were consistent with cardiorespiratory and muscular training (Northey et al., 2018).

As people age, depression and anxiety disorders increase. Furthermore, there is a natural loss of family, friends, and acquaintances as people age, which leads to a decline in socialization and can lead to depression. In addition to the physiological benefits of exercise on mental health, physical activity provides an avenue for older adults to have regular social interaction through their gyms, community centers, exercises classes, or interactions with a personal trainer.

The value of exercise extends well beyond physical benefits in all populations. In particular, for older adults, exercise provides mental and cognitive benefits as well as challenges and goals that may be missing in other parts of life. A fitness facility can provide a place for a social network that supports and cares for the well-being of the individual, providing important human connection and socialization.

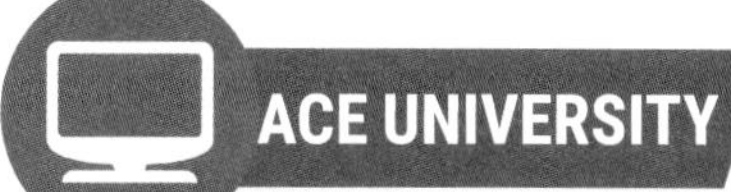

If your study program includes the ACE University, visit www.ACEfitness.org/MyACE and log in to your My ACE Account to take full advantage of the ACE Personal Trainer Study Program and online guided study experience.

A variety of media to support and expand on the material in this text is provided to facilitate learning and best prepare you for the ACE Personal Trainer Certification exam and a career as a personal trainer.

SUMMARY

Exercise has physical and mental health benefits across the lifespan and exercise guidelines vary nominally across the lifespan. It should be the focus of the personal trainer to understand both the capabilities and limitations of the individual in achieving overall fitness and enhanced quality of life and health through exercise. By observing movement and collaborating with clients to determine goals, the personal trainer can customize programs to focus on their needs and wants, and create an engaging, safe, and effective exercise program for clients across the lifespan.

REFERENCES

The Aspen Institute (2015). *Physical Literacy in the United States: A Model, Strategic Plan, and Call to Action.* https://www.aspeninstitute.org/publications/physical-literacy-model-strategic-plan-call-action/

Aubert, S. et al. (2018). Global matrix 3.0 physical activity report card grades for children and youth: Results and analysis from 49 countries. *Journal of Physical Activity and Health*, 15 (Suppl. 2), S251–S273.

American College of Obstetricians and Gynecologists (2015). Physical activity and exercise during pregnancy and the postpartum period. Committee Opinion No. 650. *Obstetrics & Gynecology*, 126, e135–142.

American College of Obstetricians and Gynecologists (2013). Weight gain during pregnancy. Committee Opinion No. 548. *Obstetrics & Gynecology*, 121, 1, 210–212.

American College of Sports Medicine (2018). *ACSM's Guidelines for Exercise Testing and Prescription* (10th ed.). Philadelphia: Wolters Kluwer.

Barbour, K.E. et al. (2017). Vital signs: Prevalence of doctor-diagnosed arthritis and arthritis-attributable activity limitation, United States, 2013–2015. *Morbidity & Mortality Weekly Report*, March 7.

Benjamin, D.R., Van de Water, A.T.M., & Peiris, C.L. (2014). Effects of exercise on diastasis of the rectus abdominis muscle in the antenatal and postnatal periods: A systematic review. *Physiotherapy*, 100, 1, 1–8.

Dugas, C. & Slane, V.H. (2019). *Miscarriage*. Treasure Island, Fla.: StatPearls Publishing.

Faigenbaum, A.D. & Westcott, W.L. (2013). *ACE Youth Fitness Manual*. San Diego, Calif.: American Council on Exercise.

Faigenbaum, A.D. et al. (2009). Youth resistance training: Updated position paper from the National Strength and Conditioning Association. *Journal of Strength and Conditioning Research*, 23, 4, 1–20.

Falke, B. & Dotan, R. (2008). Children's thermoregulation. *Applied Physiology, Nutrition, and Metabolism*, 33, 2, 420–427.

Hamill, B. (1994). Relative safety of weight lifting and weight training. *Journal of Strength and Conditioning Research*, 8, 53–57.

Hoyert, D.L. & Gregory, E.C.W. (2016). Cause of fetal death: Data from the Fetal Death Report, 2014. *National Vital Statistics Reports*, 65, 7, 1–25.

Jago, R. et al. (2010). Parent and child physical activity and sedentary time: Do active parents foster active children? *BMC Public Health*, 10, 194.

Lamina, S. & Agbanusi, E.C. (2013). Effect of aerobic exercise training on maternal weight gain in pregnancy: A meta-analysis of randomized controlled trials. *Ethiopian Journal of Health Sciences*, 23, 1, 59–64.

Milman, N. (2011). Postpartum anemia I: Definition, prevalence, causes, and consequences. *Annals of Hematology*, 90, 11, 1247.

Morris, F. et al. (1997). Prospective ten-month exercise intervention in premenarcheal girls: Positive effects on bone and lean mass. *Journal of Bone and Mineral Research*, 12, 9, 1453–1462.

National Osteoporosis Foundation (2019). *What Is Osteoporosis and What Causes It?* https://www.nof.org/patients/what-is-osteoporosis/

National Physical Activity Plan (2018). *The 2018 United States Report Card on Physical Activity for Children and Youth.* Washington, D.C.: National Physical Activity Plan Alliance.

Naughton, G.A. & Carlson, J.S. (2008). Reducing the risk of heat-related decrements to physical activity in young people. *Journal of Science and Medicine in Sport*, 11, 1, 58–65.

Northey, J.M. et al. (2018) Exercise interventions for cognitive function in adults older than 50: A systematic review with meta-analysis. *British Journal of Sports Medicine*, 52, 154–160.

Rowland, T. (2008). Thermoregulation during exercise in the heat in children: Old concepts revisited. *Journal of Applied Physiology*, 105, 2, 718–724.

Rowland, T. et al. (2008). Exercise tolerance and thermoregulatory responses during cycling in boys and men. *Medicine & Science in Sports & Exercise*, 40, 2, 282–287.

Sharma, G., Lobo, T., & Keller, L. (2014). Postnatal exercise can reverse diastasis recti. *Obstetrics & Gynecology*, 123, Suppl. 1, 171S.

Sperstad, J.B. et al. (2016). Diastasis recti abdominis during pregnancy and 12 months after childbirth: Prevalence, risk factors and report of lumbopelvic pain. *British Journal of Sports Medicine*, 50, 1092–1096.

U.S. Census Bureau (2017). *2014 National Population Projections Datasets.* https://www.census.gov/programs-surveys/popproj/data/datasets.html

U.S. Department of Health & Human Services (2018). *Physical Activity Guidelines for Americans* (2nd ed.). www.health.gov/paguidelines/

SUGGESTED READINGS

American College of Obstetricians and Gynecologists (2015). Physical activity and exercise during pregnancy and the postpartum period. Committee Opinion No. 650. *Obstetrics & Gynecology*, 126, e135–142.

American Council on Exercise (2014). *Senior Fitness Manual*. San Diego: American Council on Exercise.

Cadore, E. L. et al. (2014). Strength and endurance training prescription in healthy and frail elderly. *Aging and Disease*, 5, 3, 183–195.

Faigenbaum, A.D. & Westcott, W.L. (2013). *ACE Youth Fitness Manual*. San Diego, Calif.: American Council on Exercise.

Jago, R. et al. (2010). Parent and child physical activity and sedentary time: Do active parents foster active children? *BMC Public Health*, 10, 194.

Jo, S. (2015). Prenatal and postpartum exercise. In: American Council on Exercise. *Medical Exercise Specialist Manual*. San Diego: American Council on Exercise.

National Physical Activity Plan (2018). *The 2018 United States Report Card on Physical Activity for Children and Youth*. Washington, D.C.: National Physical Activity Plan Alliance.

Northey, J.M. et al. (2018) Exercise interventions for cognitive function in adults older than 50: A systematic review with meta-analysis. *British Journal of Sports Medicine*, 52, 154–160.

Sharma, G., Lobo, T., & Keller, L. (2014). Postnatal exercise can reverse diastasis recti. *Obstetrics & Gynecology*, 123, Suppl. 1, 171S.

U.S. Department of Health & Human Services (2018). *Physical Activity Guidelines for Americans* (2nd ed.). www.health.gov/paguidelines/

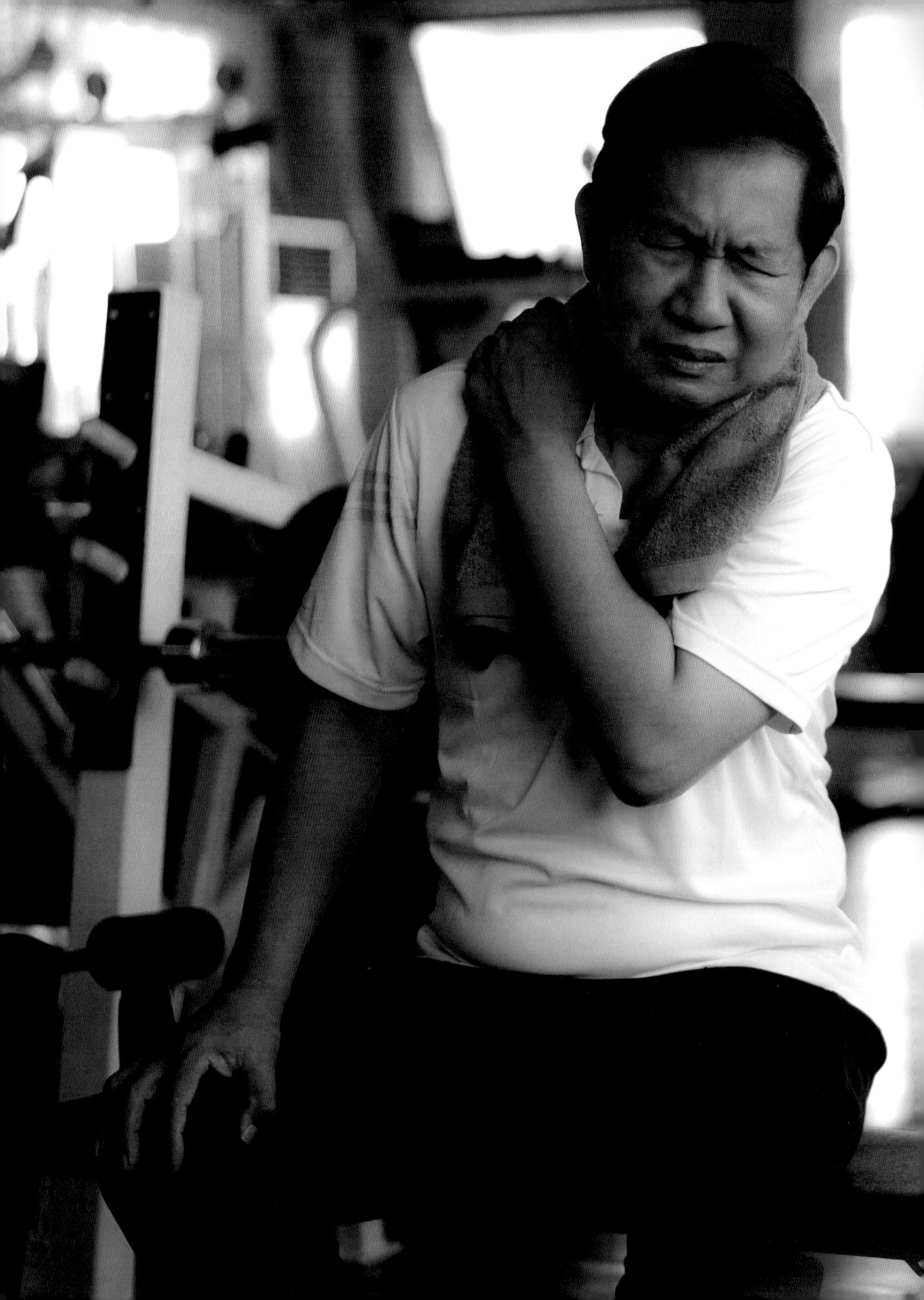

CHAPTER 15

Considerations for Clients with Musculoskeletal Issues

LAUREN SHROYER, MS, ATC
Senior Director for Product Development for the American Council on Exercise;
NATA-BOC Certified Athletic Trainer

IN THIS CHAPTER

LEARNING OBJECTIVES:

Upon completion of this chapter, the reader will be able to:

- Describe the role and scope of a personal trainer in working with clients who have or have had musculoskeletal injuries
- Explain the role of pain and how to communicate with clients in pain
- Recognize acute injuries and respond through the application of emergency response protocols
- Identify signs of chronic injuries or conditions
- Recognize when referral to a healthcare professional is indicated
- Design safe and effective exercise programs for clients with a history of common musculoskeletal injuries
- Apply appropriate exercise programming to avoid injury during workouts

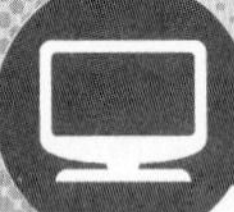

ACE UNIVERSITY

If your study program includes the ACE University, visit www.ACEfitness.org/MyACE and log in to your My ACE Account to take full advantage of the ACE Personal Trainer Study Program and online guided study experience.

A variety of media to support and expand on the material in this text is provided to facilitate learning and best prepare you for the ACE Personal Trainer Certification exam and a career as a personal trainer.

Throughout any personal-training career, professionals may see clients who report pain during exercise or arrive to workouts with a new injury. Through careful exercise program design and implementation, personal trainers can have a considerable effect on the overall health of the **connective tissue** as well as **muscular endurance,** thereby positively impacting clients with musculoskeletal conditions. The role of a personal trainer in these situations does not change with experience, but the ability to skillfully create, implement, and modify exercise programs to address such situations can be enhanced with continued education.

A personal trainer may observe inefficiencies in movement during an assessment, or clients may report pain during movement. It is important that a personal trainer recognize the difference between pain associated with injury versus physical discomfort during exercise, while keeping in mind that the **scope of practice** of a personal trainer does not include evaluation, assessment, or diagnosis of muscle or joint pain. In cases of pain or injury, it is essential that clients are referred to an appropriate healthcare provider.

Physicians have at their disposal diagnostic tools such as **magnetic resonance imaging (MRI),** x-ray, and **computed tomography** to identify injury or illness. No amount of posture or movement assessment can replace these tools, and it is important that personal trainers help clients understand how their skills are best used within their scope of practice. Likewise, it is important for a personal trainer to be proficient at communicating with healthcare professionals when a client is under medical supervision.

Additionally, medical referrals afford the opportunity for personal trainers to reach out to medical professionals to learn the current exercise restrictions and return-to-activity protocols for a previously injured client. This opportunity to work in conjunction with medical professionals is the best way to support a client in safely achieving his or her goals. As an added bonus, introducing oneself as an ACE® Certified Personal Trainer to physicians, physical therapists, chiropractors, and other health professionals as a conscientious and collaborative professional broadens one's professional network, which can lead to client referrals.

Common Injuries and Reactions to Healing

Exercise is important to overall health and **wellness** and individuals often seek out a personal trainer with the expectation of learning safe and effective exercise techniques. These same people may be new to exercise and **physically inactive.** The risks of injury increase with deconditioning, whether it stems from a **sedentary** day at a desk or a lifetime of exercise avoidance. Thus, having a basic understanding of common musculoskeletal injuries will help the personal trainer provide safe and effective exercise programming and make appropriate referrals to the healthcare team when warranted.

ACUTE AND CHRONIC INJURIES: THE PHYSIOLOGY OF HEALING

Injuries may occur in an instant or manifest progressively over time. An **acute** injury has an onset that may be identified by a single instance. For example, the popping sensation of a torn **ligament** or the breaking of a bone indicate the occurrence of an acute injury. On the other hand, a **chronic** injury or condition is one with an onset that is harder to pinpoint. For example, low-back pain that is consistent for more than six months is a chronic injury and **osteoarthritis** of the knee is a chronic condition that often takes several years to develop.

When a soft-tissue injury occurs, the body goes through a systematic process with three distinct phases. When an injury fails to progress through the stages and acute **inflammation** is present for months, the condition is termed chronic. Often, chronic injury can be avoided by proper care of an acute injury, as continued microtrauma to an area may result in a chronic condition.

Phase I: Inflammation

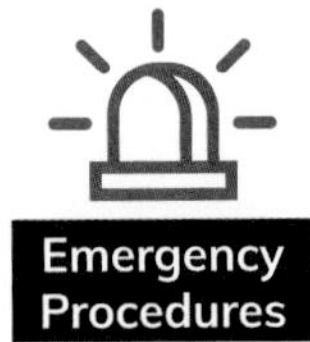

The first phase is the acute inflammatory phase, which lasts approximately three to four days after injury, depending on the severity. This phase is marked by the cardinal signs of inflammation—redness, swelling, pain, and localized increased temperature (Figure 15-1). The swelling causes stiffness, which helps to stabilize the injured area to prevent further injury while initiating the healing process. While other methods of acute injury treatment are being researched, it is still standard practice during this phase to implement **RICE,** which stands for rest or restricted activity, ice, compression, and elevation (van den Bekerom et al., 2012).

FIGURE 15-1
Inflammation of the ankle joint

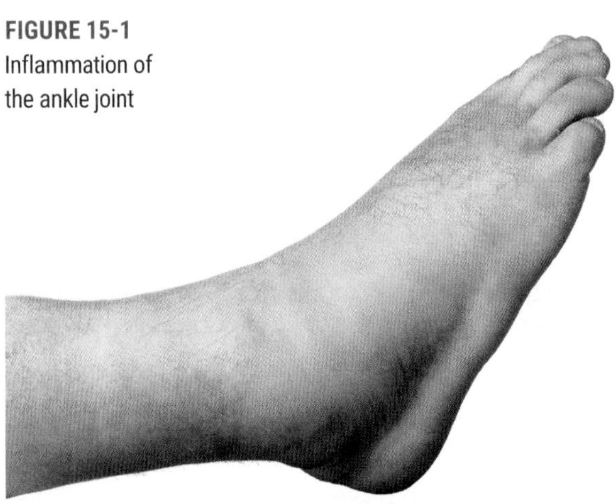

Rest or restricted activity is essential to prevent re-injury to the tissue. For lower-extremity injuries, it can be helpful to use crutches through this phase until walking without a limp is possible. The standard recommendation is that ice be applied indirectly to the skin (e.g., with a cloth between the ice and the skin) for no longer than 20 minutes at a time to relieve swelling and pain (Pek, 2017). Although different theories exist, ice (not heat) is usually used in the first 24 to 48 hours. Compression comes in many forms, but for acute injury refers to the application of an elastic bandage to an injured area. The purpose of the bandage is to control the amount of swelling during the inflammation stage. The bandage should be wrapped firmly, but not tightly, as a tight bandage may block **venous return,** resulting in trapped inflammation **inferior** to the injury site. Elevation of the injury above the level of the heart assists venous return. This can be done while applying ice or any time one is sitting or lying down.

Phase II: Repair

The inflammation phase gives way to the repair phase, which consists of both repair and regeneration of tissue. This phase may overlap with the inflammation phase and lasts approximately six weeks. The body heals through the formation of scar tissue. Though a normal result of healing, excessive scar tissue can become adhesive and cause movement restriction. Within two to three weeks, the injured area can resist normal stresses, but the strength of the injured area continues to build for several months (Buganza-Tepole & Kuhl, 2013). Challenging the tissue with pain-free, non-weight-bearing movement can lead to less adhesive scarring and stronger tissue while preventing re-injury. It is important, however, that personal trainers work together with the healthcare team to determine specific exercise recommendations and restrictions during this phase.

Phase III: Remodeling

The **remodeling** phase overlaps with the repair phase at about three to six weeks post-injury. Healing, especially of ligament and bone, can last one to two years. In this phase, scar tissue continues to strengthen. As during the repair phase, an adhesive scar can be avoided through movement during this phase.

Table 15-1 offers a summary of the three stages of healing.

TABLE 15-1

Three Stages of Healing

	Time	Characteristics	Movement	Contraindications
Phase I: Inflammation	First 3–4 days	Redness, swelling, pain, and local heat	Non–weight bearing, active range of motion	Exercise and movement is contraindicated when pain and/or swelling is present at the site of injury.
Phase II: Repair	3 days to 6 weeks	Initial formation of scar	Weight bearing as tolerated Gentle, pain-free movement	
Phase III: Remodeling	4 weeks to 2 years	Increased strength of scar tissue	Progressive, pain-free exercise	

Exercise Progression after Injury

Exercise progression must always be conservative when working with individuals recovering from a musculoskeletal injury. It is common for personal trainers to conduct sessions with clients whose injuries are in the repair and remodeling phases. It is essential that trainers stay in contact with the client's physician or physical therapist to obtain recommendations for contraindicated movements and recommended return-to-activity protocols. If a client asks about an injury, the personal trainer should refer him or her to an appropriate healthcare provider.

With conscientious application of pain-free exercise programming, tissue remodeling post-injury can result in complete and **asymptomatic** function. Given that tissue remodels to the strength of the forces imposed upon it, appropriate progression protocols can lead to improved strength of tissue after healing. With most common injuries, personal trainers can continue to move clients toward their physical-activity goals. At the same time, it is essential to understand that pain at the injury site marks a stopping point for exercise.

THE ESSENTIAL ROLE OF PAIN

The body uses pain as a quick and clear signal, indicating the need to stop whatever one is doing to determine the cause of the pain and proceed by decreasing stress on the painful area.

Pushing through the pain of an injury can prolong healing, promote further damage, or cause an acute injury to become chronic. While healing from an injury, the injury site is weaker and will become overloaded before the surrounding structures, causing pain. It is important to honor the body's need to stop.

It is also important to acknowledge that a client may experience some trepidation in returning to exercise, so the personal trainer should keep the lines of communication open by explaining the importance of stopping exercises that cause pain and use a perceived pain scale to gauge the stopping point. Application of these concepts is discussed in depth later in this chapter.

COMMON ACUTE INJURIES: RECOGNITION AND ACTION

Exercise and sport have an inherent risk of injury. A personal trainer must be able to recognize when a client sustains an injury and discontinue the session when it is necessary. In the event of an injury that occurs during a personal-training session, the personal trainer must assess the situation, administer appropriate first aid, and document the injury. Some acute injuries may require that emergency medical services (EMS) be called to the scene. If EMS is not needed or is refused by the client, it is essential that the personal trainer recommend that the client see his or her physician for evaluation and treatment.

Muscle Strains

Muscle **strains** are among the more common injuries and can occur during any type of exertion. Muscle strains are injuries in which the muscle works beyond its capacity, resulting in tears of the muscle fibers. A grading system exists to categorize the severity of strains:

- Grade I strains are mild. A client will likely report an acute episode of mild pain or intense local soreness or cramping of the muscle. Some swelling may be present, though it may be mild or hard to see depending on the thickness of the surrounding muscle and **adipose** tissue. Though tender or painful, strength of the muscle remains normal.
- Grade II strains are moderate and are characterized by more severe pain and swelling that will likely cause weakness and decreased **range of motion (ROM).** When the hip or lower-extremity musculature is involved, a limp is likely to be present.
- Grade III strains are severe injuries and indicate a complete tear of the muscle. In these severe cases, the client may report feeling a sudden "tear" or "pop" accompanied by immediate pain and loss of function. Pain, swelling, and discoloration may also be present. There may be a noticeable deformation of the area as the muscle separates and each end pulls closer to its bony attachment site. Though rare overall, a grade III strain is more common in the older adult population as the collagenous tissue loses **elasticity** with aging, making it more susceptible to tear.

Ligament Sprains

While muscle strains are likely a result of unprepared exertion, ligament **sprains** more frequently occur as a result of an external force that applies sufficient pressure to stretch the ligament to the point of injury. This force is referred to as the **mechanism of injury.** While external forces, especially in sport, are outside the control of the athlete, ligament sprains can also be caused by **ground reaction force** when an individual has insufficient strength,

coordination, or **stability** to maintain control of the joint during movement. These injuries are referred to as **non-contact injuries.** For example, tears of the **anterior cruciate ligament (ACL)** (Figure 15-2) may occur as either a contact or non-contact injury. The mechanism of injury for an ACL tear is a hyperextension and/or twisting of the knee joint. In contact sports, like rugby or American football, a blow to the front and outside of the knee joint can cause enough **shearing** force to tear the ACL. In activities such as basketball or volleyball, planting the foot against the unyielding surface of the floor, accompanied by a sudden cutting and twisting motion, can cause a non-contact ACL tear. A muscular training program that includes multidirectional strength and stability can reduce the risk of non-contact injury (Sugimoto et al., 2015).

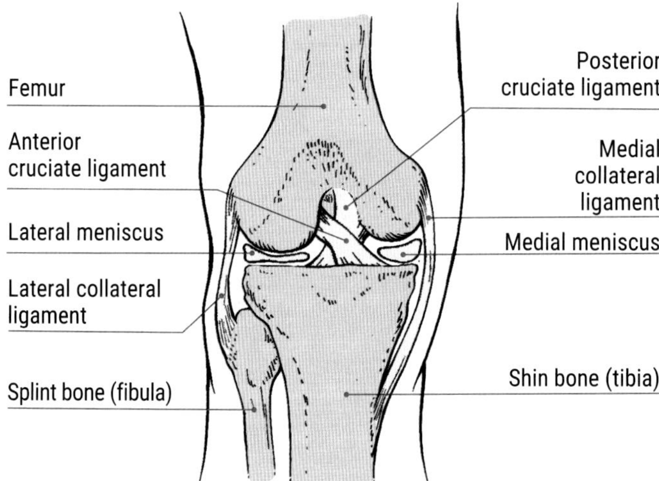

FIGURE 15-2
Knee joint anatomy depicting the anterior cruciate ligament (ACL), the medial collateral ligament (MCL), the posterior cruciate ligament (PCL), the lateral collateral ligament (LCL), and the medial and lateral menisci

Degrees of sprain also follow a grading system. Similar to the grading system for muscle strain, the grades of ligament sprain range from Grade I (minimal) to Grade III (severe). Signs and symptoms of each grade are presented in Table 15-2.

TABLE 15-2
Grading System for Ligament Sprains

Severity	Physical Examination Findings	Impairment	Pathophysiology	Acute Care
Grade I	Minimal tenderness Minimal swelling	Minimal	Microscopic tearing of collagen fibers	RICE
Grade II	Moderate tenderness Moderate swelling Decreased ROM Possible instability	Moderate	Complete tears of some, but not all, collagen fibers in the ligament	RICE Physician evaluation
Grade III	Significant swelling Significant tenderness Instability	Severe	Complete tear/rupture of ligament	Immobilization with air splint RICE Prompt physician evaluation

Note: ROM = Range of motion; RICE = Rest or restricted activity, ice, compression, and elevation

Source: American College of Sports Medicine (2013). *ACSM's Resource Manual for Guidelines for Exercise Testing and Prescription* (7th ed.). Baltimore: Wolters Kluwer/Lippincott Williams & Wilkins.

When a ligament sprain occurs, the client may report having heard a "popping" sound followed by immediate pain and swelling. In the case of a Grade III sprain, one will experience instability, decreased ROM, and a loss of function.

Healing

The healing time of muscle strains and ligament sprains are dependent upon severity. In the case of a grade I injury, the phases of healing may persist for several days to a few weeks. As the injury increases in severity, so does the length of time to heal. A grade III strain or sprain may require surgical intervention for one to regain full strength and function. It is important to note that as people age, even mild muscle strains and ligament sprains may take longer to heal.

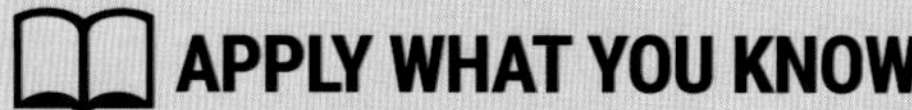

Responding to a Strain or Sprain

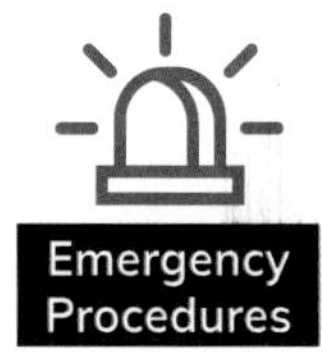

If an acute strain or sprain occurs in the gym or during a personal-training session, the client should not be physically moved unless he or she is in danger from the surrounding environment. If the client is able to move him- or herself, it is wise to have the client move to a comfortable location where the injured area may be evaluated. In any case, ice may be applied and, when necessary, EMS may be called to transport the individual to a hospital. Refer to your employer's established first-aid protocols and reporting procedures.

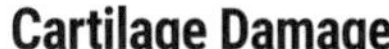

Cartilage Damage

Cartilage, which is found between bony surfaces, is a collagenous structure that provides shock absorption, stability, joint congruency, lubrication, and **proprioception.** The mechanism of injury for cartilage damage is compression of the joint coupled with a shearing motion. Though cartilage can be found in all joint spaces, and injuries can occur to any of these, the knee is predisposed to this type of injury because it is a weight-bearing joint with relatively large degrees of freedom for movement. Therefore, it is not uncommon to come across a client with such an injury. Further, compared to their younger counterparts, older individuals with degeneration of the joint cartilage are more predisposed to tears with less force (Eleftherios et al., 2011).

When a client has a cartilage tear, he or she may complain of symptoms such as joint stiffness, clicking or popping with weight-bearing activities, giving way, catching, and/or locking. Other signs and symptoms may include joint pain, swelling, and muscle weakness.

Cartilage is largely **avascular** (without blood flow). Without nutrient delivery from the blood, cartilage cannot heal; therefore, surgical intervention is often required to remove the sheared bits of cartilage from the joint space. Occasionally, cartilage can be surgically repaired in areas of sufficient vascularity, like the outer one-third of the **menisci.** This procedure requires prolonged post-surgical non–weight bearing to allow time for sufficient healing.

Bone Fractures

While acute bone **fractures** may be less common in a personal-training setting, it is important to recognize that **osteoporosis,** infection, cancer, radiation treatment, and less-conditioned bones are more susceptible to both acute and stress fracture.

A bone fracture is caused by impact or stress to the bone. This stress may be applied by a compressive force like a straight-leg landing on a hard surface, a torsional force like a rotation and compression, or a direct impact to the bone.

When a fracture occurs, an individual may experience an audible snap. The area may appear deformed and/or swollen and discolored and will be painful or tender to the touch.

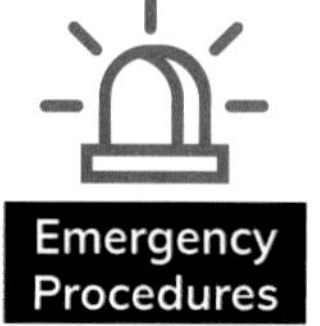

Immediate care for a client with a suspected fracture involves preventing further injury to the bone and soft tissue and providing first aid for shock, if necessary. If a personal trainer suspects a fracture, he or she should activate EMS immediately and control the surrounding environment so the client may rest quietly until emergency crews arrive. Note that in the event of a fracture, applying ice may increase pain at the injury site.

Splinting or immobilizing a fractured limb is only necessary if the incident occurs in a remote area and EMS is not readily available. In such cases, a personal trainer should rely on his or her first-aid skills.

Head, Neck, and Back Injuries

Acute head, neck, and back injuries can be catastrophic. Recognition of these injuries and referral to a physician is essential.

CONCUSSION

A **concussion** is a brain injury that causes a change in mental status. Concussions can occur during contact sports, car accidents, or as the result of falls or blows to the head. There may or may not be an accompanying temporary loss of consciousness.

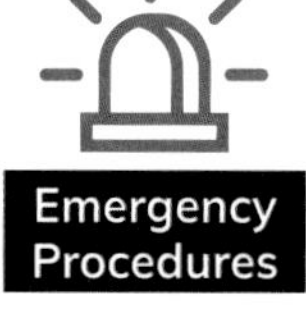

The first signs of a concussion are often confusion and disorientation. The person may not be able to explain what happened and may experience memory loss that causes him or her to ask the same question repeatedly or be unable to recognize people or places. Speech may be slow or slurred and the person may be uncoordinated and have a headache or nausea/vomiting. In addition, the person may look less alert, display impaired balance or be dizzy, or even experience a seizure, experience numbness in the limbs, or lose consciousness. Following a concussion, the brain is in a particularly vulnerable state and a second injury could be debilitating. In some instances, a second injury can lead to **second-impact syndrome,** which can be life-threatening. For this reason, it is imperative that individuals who have experienced a concussion are removed immediately from activity.

Individuals who experience any concussion symptoms should be kept from activity until given permission to return by a qualified healthcare professional with experience treating head injury. This permission should be accompanied by a written return-to-activity protocol. Gradual return to activity is essential and a personal trainer should be watchful for the reemergence of any concussion signs and symptoms during this period.

ACUTE NECK AND BACK INJURIES

Neck and back injuries are often muscle strains that may be sustained during exercise. In these cases, the injury is treated as any other strain. Occasionally, a client may suffer a disc injury. The vertebral disc (Figure 15-3) sits between two vertebrae and provides shock absorption, support, and stability for the spine. Discs are made of **collagen,** which may deteriorate for a variety of reasons, putting the disc at increased risk of injury. Disc injuries, like cartilage injuries, are most often a consequence of combined compression and shearing forces. The disc is also at increased risk when an individual is performing the **Valsalva maneuver.** Though this may be avoidable during exercise, sneezing and coughing produce this same internal force. Sufficient force may cause a tear in the annulus fibrosus layer, resulting in the gelatinous fluid of the nucleus pulposus to leak, creating a bulge of the outer layers of the disc tissue. This bulging layer may compress nerves or be caught between the vertebrae. Both can cause considerable pain and may cause nerve spasm, resulting in referred or shooting pain along the nerve.

FIGURE 15-3
Anatomy of a vertebral disc
© Fotosearch
www.fotosearch.com

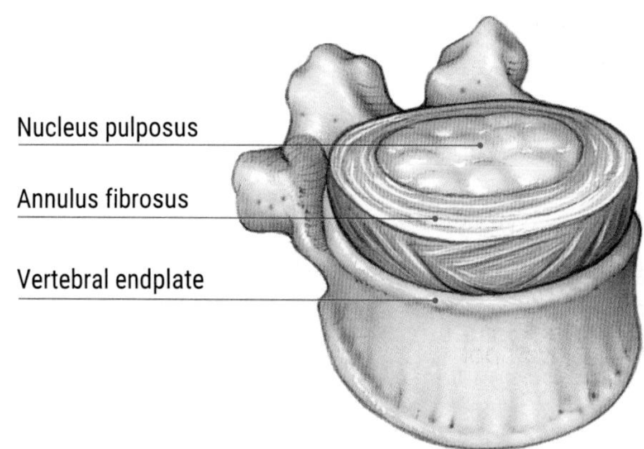

In any of these cases, ice may help alleviate pain, but immediate referral to a doctor is needed. Pain may be such that the client is unable to walk, and EMS will need to be contacted for transport to the emergency room.

COMMON OVERUSE CONDITIONS

Overuse conditions occur when tissues cannot withstand the forces put upon them over time. Overuse injuries may be caused by repetitive movements or faulty body mechanics.

Tendinitis, Bursitis, and Fasciitis

Excessive demands during physical activity may result in overuse conditions such as **tendinitis, bursitis,** and **fasciitis.** The suffix "itis" means "inflammation of." Tendinitis, or inflammation of the tendon, is a common diagnosis. Even injuries caused by overuse go through the inflammatory process. For example, acute tendinitis refers to tendinitis in the inflammation phase of healing. These conditions can each become chronic if the condition is not treated properly.

Bursitis is an inflammation of the **bursa** sac. Though sometimes due to acute trauma, bursitis is more frequently the result of repetitive stress, muscle imbalance, or muscle tightness surrounding the bursa.

Lastly, fasciitis is inflammation of the connective tissue called **fascia.** Two common conditions are **plantar fasciitis** and **iliotibial band (IT band) friction syndrome,** both of which are covered later in this chapter.

Stress Fracture

Stress fractures occur where there is an imbalance in **bone formation** and **bone resorption.** These fractures are a result of compression forces that put repetitive stress on a bone that is not strong enough to withstand these forces. Stress fractures can occur in any bone, are sometimes found in the femoral neck, but occur most frequently in the tibia. Tibial stress fractures are often mistaken as **shin splints** and may go misdiagnosed or ignored. Due to the mechanism of injury, distance runners are at increased risk, especially those who increase mileage when the bone has not had sufficient time for osteoblastic activity to adapt and increase bone density.

Unlike shin splints, stress fractures will have point tenderness in a single spot on the bone. Pain will be focal and progressive and will worsen with weight-bearing activity. In some cases, individuals will experience aching pain at rest or during sleep and may even show local swelling.

Continued activity when a stress fracture is present will lead to worsening symptoms and can lead to complete fracture of the bone. It is essential that any client showing symptoms of an acute or stress fracture be referred to a physician for diagnosis and treatment. It is important to note that symptoms of bone cancer can be similar to those of stress fractures and early diagnosis of the disease is important.

Preventing Musculoskeletal Injury

Conscientious program design and **periodization** are essential to prevent injury. A personal trainer should be cognizant that certain clients may be at a greater risk of injury due to age, previous injury history, deconditioned musculature, and/or disease.

FLEXIBILITY AND ELASTICITY

Tissue becomes inelastic for many reasons. For example, post-injury scar tissue is not pliable and will cause a decrease in the elasticity of a muscle's surrounding connective tissue, as well as its capacity to lengthen. Other causes of inelasticity include tissue **adhesion** from scar formation, disuse, radiation treatment, decreased collagen production due to age, and acute or chronic injury.

Decreases in elasticity and **flexibility** may be the cause or consequence of injury. This type of physiological dysfunction in the muscle not only compromises ROM, but also compromises the ability to generate force. Additionally, it may be the cause of postural muscle imbalances (see Chapter 10) and may result in misuse or overuse injury elsewhere.

To address inflexibility and help prevent further injury, personal trainers commonly develop flexibility programs for their clients. When a client is returning from injury, the doctor and/or physical therapist should be consulted for any movement restrictions. See Chapter 11 for various types of stretching, along with recommendations for including them in exercise programming.

WARM-UP

Readying the body for a workout is an essential first step of any personal-training session and proper execution may help reduce the risk of injury. A warm-up specifically focuses on preparing the body for movement and should take into account all **planes of motion,** as well as the various exercises that will be performed in the upcoming training session.

With any client, but especially with those who are deconditioned, even the **nervous system** needs to be prepared for movement. By focusing on function and movement at the start of each workout, the **proprioceptors,** which are frequently affected during injury, are activated, thereby improving **balance** and coordination. Moreover, the muscles begin to receive increased blood flow, and connective tissues benefit from enhanced elasticity. The warm-up presented in the Figure 11-32, pages 521–530 (i.e., the ACE IFT Model Exercise Programming Template for a busy mom who wants to run a 5K race) includes an appropriate exercise sequence that could help reduce musculoskeletal injury risk. This combination of movements, which can be performed unweighted or with minimal resistance depending on client capacity, ensures that the musculature surrounding the hip, knee, and ankle have been moved through a functional ROM and in all three planes of motion. Increasing tendon and muscle elasticity in all directions, while stimulating the **proprioceptive nervous system,** prepares the body to take on the demands of progressively weighted squats. In considering this multidimensional approach to the warm-up, the preparatory sequence of addressing movement patterns to improve elasticity and neuromuscular readiness is preferred to a warm-up including single-plane activities, such as walking or biking.

RECOVERY

Allowing time for adequate restoration between exercise sessions is essential for tissue recovery. In addition, stretching and **self–myofascial release** techniques may provide relief for stiff muscles that have worked hard in previous workouts. The average exerciser should ensure that recovery includes adequate rest between training sessions and variability in the exercise program. See Chapter 11 for more on recovery.

Programming Considerations for Clients with Musculoskeletal Issues

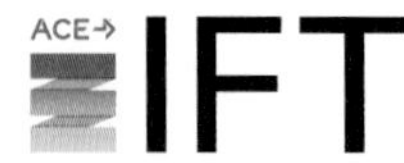

Within the scope of practice of a personal trainer is the opportunity to assess movement and create an exercise program. Personal trainers working with clients with musculoskeletal injuries should be mindful of the key considerations outlined in this chapter as they utilize the ACE Integrated Fitness Training® (ACE IFT®) Model to design and implement safe, effective, and enjoyable exercise programming. By programming using the ACE IFT Model, a personal trainer can have a positive impact on the overall health and wellness of clients with acute and/or chronic musculoskeletal issues.

WHEN PAIN IS PRESENT

Clinically, pain is a physical event marked by neural firing, but pain itself is a subjective sensation. The perceived pain scale is a method of quantifying the level of pain by rating the pain on a 0 to 10 scale, where an indication of 0 is no pain and 10 is equivalent to the worst pain ever experienced (Figure 15-4). When clients indicate that pain is above a 3, the exercise should stop and a modification to that exercise or a different exercise should be chosen. A pain level of 3 is used as a threshold because at that point the perception of pain is not yet discomforting or distressing. This allows the client to feel comfortable with the movement and for the personal trainer to maintain a level of confidence that further damage is not occurring at the injury site. A client may indicate that he or she can continue even as pain increases, at which time the personal trainer should explain that overexerting the injury site may cause a setback to healing or result in an overuse or chronic injury.

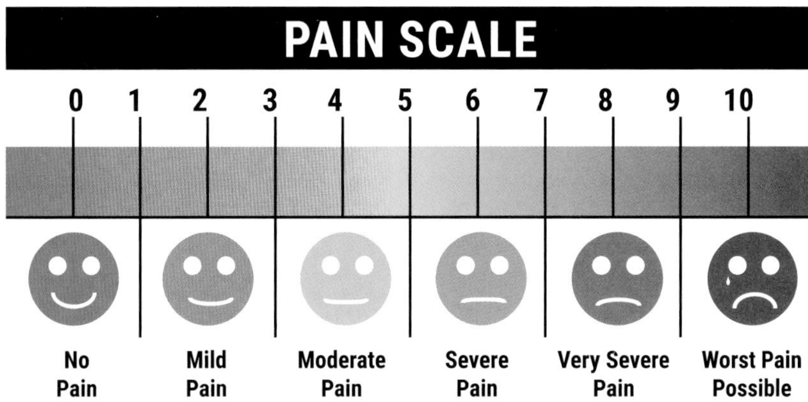

FIGURE 15-4
Perceived pain scale

Personal trainers can follow a few quick steps to prepare a client for a conversation about pain management during a workout:

- Explain to the client before starting an exercise that the affected area may be challenged.
- Explain the perceived pain scale (see Figure 15-4).
- Explain that the exercise will discontinue if pain exceeds a 3 on the scale, or if the client feels uncomfortable continuing.
- Encourage the client to communicate any amount of pain.
- Ask the client to assess pain prior to exercise and throughout the session to ensure that pain has not surpassed a 3.

Relationship and trust building cannot be overemphasized, especially when a client is experiencing chronic pain. Though a physical sensation, chronic pain has biological, psychological, and emotional impacts that may cause feelings of anger, hopelessness, and sadness, or clinically manifest as **depression** and **anxiety** (Hooten, 2016). In some cases, the health professional referring to a personal trainer may be a mental health professional. The American Psychological Association (2019) recommends exercise and staying active as strategies for coping with chronic pain.

Acknowledging a client's feelings about exercise is an important validating step. A personal trainer is working in partnership with clients, which requires sincere and consistent communication about how they are feeling during the exercise program. Listening ensures clients feel respected and supported in their goals and remain engaged in the exercise program. This leads to improved **adherence** and results, as well as a long-lasting and trusting professional relationship.

Addressing a Client's Concerns about Pain

Olivia is a new client. While discussing her goals and health history, she mentions that she is interested in working with a personal trainer because of a recommendation made by her psychologist. Olivia tells you that she has been struggling with chronic pain for the past eight years due to a **herniated disc** she sustained when she lifted a box of printer paper off the floor at work. She informs you that she has followed her doctor's recommendations, including physical therapy, but the pain has remained constant. Currently, Olivia has no physical-activity restrictions and was surprised that her doctor recommended exercise and physical activity for coping with her long-term pain. When asked to use the perceived pain scale to average her pain level over the past few months, she rates herself at a 2 and notes being in a constant state of mild pain with occasional flare-ups that bring her to a 5 or 6, during which she says that her pain is severe. Olivia is open to learning more and participating in exercise but associates movement with pain, is anxious about exercise, and does not see how lifting weights will make things better.

ACE ABC APPROACH™

Following is an example of how using the ACE Mover Method™ and the ACE ABC Approach™ can benefit a client who has been experiencing chronic pain.

Ask: Asking powerful open-ended questions helps you gain a better understanding of what the client would like to accomplish by working with a personal trainer.

Personal Trainer: I understand that managing pain has been a significant part of your life for the past eight years and, even though you have followed all your doctor's recommendations, the pain has persisted at a constant mild state with occasional flare-ups that feel severe. What do you want to achieve by working with a personal trainer?

Client: Before I got hurt, I enjoyed being active. After completing physical therapy for my back, I haven't been active because I am afraid I might get hurt again. So, I would like to be able to start exercising again—slowly—and see if it helps my pain.

Personal Trainer: You hurt your back while doing something active at work, and you now associate physical activity with an increased risk of making your pain worse. What are the three best reasons to become more active?

Client: First, I've forgotten what being pain-free feels like. Second, my pain has limited my ability to advance at work. And third, my pain has interfered with personal relationships. I want to be more active, so I can better cope with the pain and get back to living my life again.

Personal Trainer: You mentioned enjoying physical activity before your injury. What types of activities did you enjoy and what can you see yourself doing now?

Client: When I was younger, I participated in formal sports like soccer and softball and as I got into high school I enjoyed running cross country and being active with friends at the beach and parks on the weekends. After my injury, I've not been spending much time outdoors, so I could see myself doing outdoor activities of some type.

Break down barriers: Ask more open-ended questions to discover any potential barriers that may get in the way of becoming more physically active.

Personal Trainer: Getting back to a life without pain, advancing at work, and developing personal relationships are reasons you have for becoming more active. What are possible obstacles to reaching your goal of becoming more physically active?

Client: The main obstacle I can think of is the pain. When my pain level is bad, I don't want to be active. Also, I am still a little nervous about exercising because I am afraid lifting weights will cause me to hurt my back again.

Personal Trainer: Pain is a reality for you, and if you are in pain you will not be active. On the other hand, being more active can help you cope with the pain you have.

Client: Yes. My concern is that I won't know which activities will help me manage my pain compared to those that will cause more pain.

Personal Trainer: My role as an exercise professional will be to work with you to figure out which activities are safe, appropriate, and enjoyable. Initially, this may involve observing how you move and asking questions to find out what movements you can do without making the pain worse. In the beginning, we will start slow and continue to adjust your plan as necessary, to ensure you are becoming more active while still being respectful of any pain you may be experiencing. How does that sound?

Collaborate: Working together with the client on goals and solutions is the next step now that you have set the stage. The client has told you why being active is important to her, explained what her potential barriers are, and you have defined what your role will be.

Client: I'm glad to hear about the safe and enjoyable approach. I'm open to getting started with a program, but as I mentioned earlier, I've not been active for a long time and I'm not sure where to begin.

Personal Trainer: What might you imagine as a first step?

Client: I know I want to sign up for some sessions with you, and I need to get some appropriate clothes and shoes for exercise, so my first step will be to get some exercise clothing and shoes and to schedule our appointment for next week.

Using the ACE ABC Approach allowed the client and personal trainer to engage in a client-centered conversation. This approach encourages respect for the client's feelings and beliefs while providing reflections to demonstrate that you understand her point of view.

ACUTE INJURIES

In all stages post-injury, a personal trainer must defer to the return-to-activity protocol provided by the physician or physical therapist. When a physician has cleared the client to proceed with exercise as tolerated, the personal trainer is then at liberty to select exercise programming within any limits set by the physician.

A client may wish not to regress on the gains in his or her overall fitness or performance and will require guidance to safely continue to exercise while dealing with a recent injury. Table 15-3 lists acceptable types of muscular training and cardiorespiratory training, as well as movements to avoid while keeping a client active during healing. Even when working within these guidelines, if the client indicates pain in the affected area, the exercise should stop immediately.

TABLE 15-3
Muscular and Cardiorespiratory Training Considerations for Post-rehabilitation

Type of Acute Injury	Muscular Training	Cardiorespiratory Training	Avoid:
Lower-extremity Injury: A lower-extremity injury will affect the kinetic chain in all weight-bearing movements but leaves opportunity for upper-body strength training. Buoyancy in water exercise offers a cardiorespiratory challenge while unloading the joints.	▸ Upper body: Seated or lying exercises ▸ Lower body: Exercises as prescribed by a physical therapist or physician ▸ Spine and core: Exercises that do not involve the affected limb	▸ Water exercise ▸ Upper-body ergometer ▸ Recumbent or stationary bike	▸ Any movements that cause pain ▸ Weight-bearing exercise until cleared by a physician and/or physical therapist
Upper-extremity Injury: An upper-extremity injury has a lesser effect on maintaining good cardiorespiratory health, but the kinetic chain effect must be considered. For example, if a cast or sling is worn, axial rotation during bipedal movement will be compromised.	▸ Lower body: Exercises that do not involve the affected limb ▸ Upper body: Exercises as prescribed by a physical therapist or physician ▸ Spine and core: Exercises that do not involve the affected limb	▸ Walking ▸ Recumbent or stationary bike ▸ Elliptical machine	▸ Any movements that cause pain ▸ Running, as the impact on the kinetic chain can cause pain in the affected limb ▸ Exercise that requires both hands for stability
Back/Spinal Injury: Back/spinal injury can be quite debilitating, but movement can provide relief as well.	▸ Exercises and stretches as prescribed by a physical therapist or physician ▸ Body-weight exercises as tolerated	▸ Water exercise ▸ Walking ▸ Recumbent or stationary bike	▸ Any movements that cause pain ▸ High-repetition sets (keep repetitions between 8 and 10 to avoid fatigue) ▸ Weighted spinal rotation ▸ Exercises that require the client to get onto the floor. Use a raised surface or massage table when available.

Note: The client's physician or physical therapist should be consulted in all cases, but especially when the affected area is challenged in any way.

CHRONIC INJURIES AND CONDITIONS

Overuse injury, chronic injury, chronic muscle pain, and recurring injury—these terms and phrases are all used to describe a physical condition that involves pain and/or inflammation of soft tissue, bone, and/or the nerve structures and affects strength, balance, and/or function and efficiency of movement. There are a variety of reasons these conditions may occur. Osteoarthritis and **rheumatoid arthritis** are disease states, while a herniated disc is a chronic condition caused by an acute episode. While it is outside the scope of practice for a personal trainer to assess or diagnose these conditions, a personal trainer can recognize the effect of these conditions on movement and exercise and train clients accordingly. When a client has not been exercising regularly, a careful exercise program design can result in improved strength, flexibility, balance, and efficiency in movement, which also may result in decreased pain—a rewarding outcome for both client and personal trainer.

For discovering the presence of chronic injuries and conditions, the role of the **lifestyle and health-history questionnaire** becomes an important focus of communication (see Figure 5-4, pages 150–153). The client should indicate any injuries or surgeries as well as any known limitations of movement. When reviewing the lifestyle and health-history questionnaire, a personal trainer should see these notes as a cue to have a deeper conversation, collecting a verbal history of the injury and treatment. The following is a list of important questions that can be asked and discussed during an initial goal-setting session.

- History:
  - How did you sustain the original injury? Was it a slow progression or did something happen to cause it?
  - What was the original treatment?
  - What other treatments or exercises have you tried?
  - What is your current diagnosis?
  - Are you currently seeing any medical professionals for this condition?
  - Do you mind if I speak to them?
- Pain:
  - How often do you experience pain?
  - How severe is the pain when you experience it?
  - Does the pain stop you from doing things that you would like to do? If so, what kinds of things does it stop you from doing?
  - Are there certain movements or activities that cause pain? If so, tell me more about those movements or activities.
- Activity and treatment:
  - Is your ROM limited in any way?
  - Do you ever use a brace/sling/immobilizer to manage the injury? If so, was it recommended by your doctor?
  - Are you taking any medications for pain?

- Have you tried, or do you use, ice or heat to manage pain or discomfort?
- Are you doing any stretches or exercises currently that were recommended by a medical professional? If so, tell me more about those.
- Were you ever given stretches or exercises that seemed to help? If so, tell me more about those.
- What hesitations, if any, do you have about starting an exercise program, as it relates to this injury/condition?
- Is there anything else you think I should know about this injury, the treatments you have tried, or how you are feeling?

APPLY WHAT YOU KNOW

Assessing Clients with Chronic Musculoskeletal Conditions

Assessment (whether administered formally via established protocols and shared with the client, or informally conducted through observations of basic movements during an initial workout) is a critical piece of creating an appropriate program design for any client, especially when the client is struggling with a chronic or overuse injury or condition. When working with these clients, the personal trainer is looking for additional cues during the assessment, including wincing, hesitancy to begin, slowed or erratic pace, balance, and/or jerkiness during movement. Each of these indicates either pain or **neurological inhibition.** If any of these is observed during the assessment, the personal trainer should ask if the client is experiencing pain. If so, at what point in the movement does the pain begin, and exactly where does the pain originate?

Remembering that chronic pain takes an emotional toll as well as a physical one, it is essential that the personal trainer remain empathetic and avoid judgement. The experience of pain is different for everyone.

When a client has experienced chronic pain or an overuse injury, ROM may be affected due to inflammation, scar tissue or adhesions, or by the sensation of pain at the end range of a joint. Taking a few minutes to assess posture and flexibility prior to activity will alert both the client and personal trainer to limitations in movement. Use of the static posture and flexibility assessments described in Chapter 10 will allow you to understand these limitations before beginning the exercise program. Observations made during the assessment of primary movements may help determine which ROM assessments should be administered.

Before beginning an assessment with a client following injury, it is important to put the client at ease. Explaining each movement and how it may challenge the area of injury and reiterating that the client may stop at any time will go a long way in easing the mind of the client. Before the first assessment, the personal trainer should:

- Explain that the assessment is going to help determine a starting point for safe exercise programming.
- Tell the client that he or she may request a modification for any movement.
- Explain the perceived pain scale (see Figure 15-4) and ask the client to share whenever he or she is in pain.
- Inform the client that he or she should move only within a pain-free ROM.
- Ask the client if he or she has any questions or concerns.
- Remind the client that he or she can ask questions at any time.

Using the ACE IFT Model, a personal trainer can build an effective program design progression that slowly and effectively addresses deficiencies in ROM or movement quality while remaining mindful of the injury and avoiding exacerbation.

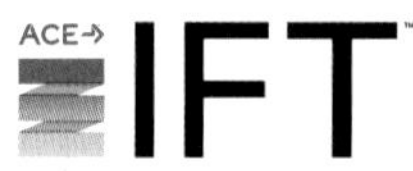

Warm-up

The warm-up is an essential part of the workout for any client. When working with a client who has had a chronic injury or condition, this step must be even more mindful and, in some cases, additional sets and/or multiple exercises addressing a specific movement pattern may be needed before the warm-up is complete.

In general, focused attention to activating the nervous system is an important part of the warm-up. Increased blood flow and elasticity should be achieved with the warm-up sequence, which should include multidirectional movements that prepare the client for exercises planned for the rest of the workout. The goal is to increase connective tissue elasticity in all planes of motion, while stimulating the proprioceptors.

Remembering the **kinetic chain,** the personal trainer must ensure that the joints **superior** and inferior to the previously injured site have sufficient ROM and stability following the movement prep sequence. Movement at these adjacent joints can be affected. During each exercise, the perceived pain scale should be referenced to ensure that there is no pain at the injury site.

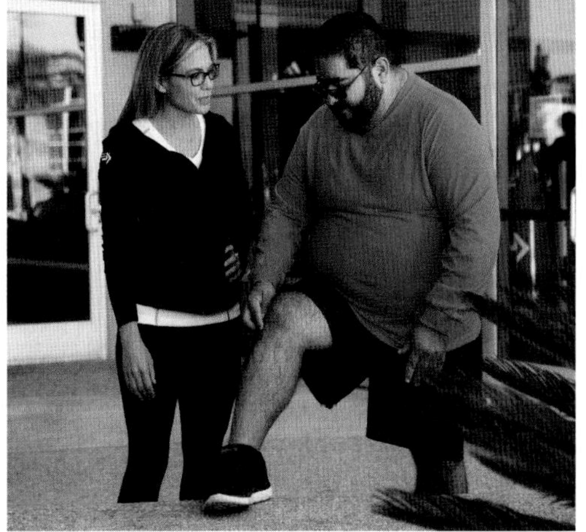

Establishing Goals

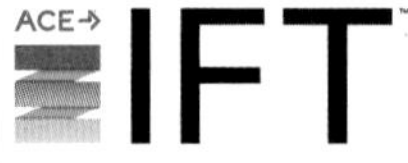

During the investigation stage, the client and personal trainer will together determine whether Functional, Movement, or Load/Speed is the appropriate starting phase for Muscular Training. At times, a client's goals may seem in conflict with his or her assessment or injury history. In these cases, it is important for the personal trainer to honor the client's goals while finding a safe, balanced exercise and recovery program to address both what he or she wants *and* needs. To accomplish this, it is essential that the personal trainer identify which exercises the client can do without causing pain.

A client who has a chronic injury or condition may not have a goal of improved function as it relates to the condition. In this case, including exercises to support the needs as related to the injury could be included as a secondary goal. These exercises can be added to the latter part of the training session or included during periods of active rest between exercises. For instance, when working with a client struggling with issues related to exaggerated **kyphosis,** upper-back strengthening exercises could be inserted between sets of lunges, giving the legs a break while improving muscular endurance to better support the thoracic spine.

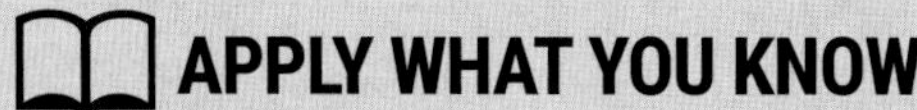

Collaborating on Goals with a Client with Low-back Pain

A client with occasional low-back pain may indicate that weight loss is his or her primary goal. In this case, the low-back pain is a condition that the personal trainer should keep in mind. However, the client may not spend a significant amount of time during the training session performing **static stretching** to improve **mobility,** as that will not address the client's primary goal. Instead, perhaps the client is pain-free on an elliptical machine, in which case intermittent intervals on the machine may more directly address the weight-loss goal and avoid overloading the low back with jarring exercise. The low-back condition would be addressed through exercises during the warm-up and, potentially, during the active rest periods of the program design. Additionally, it is appropriate to recommend a targeted stretching routine for the client to perform on recovery days.

In some instances, the client's primary goal will be to reduce pain, increase ROM, or remain physically independent in the face of a chronic condition. The program design will be whole-body in nature, with the specific focus on improving function in terms of postural stability and kinetic chain mobility by using exercises to improve joint function through flexibility, muscular endurance, core function, and balance. Once postural stability and kinetic chain mobility are achieved, the focus may shift toward developing good movement patterns.

Finally, in some cases, exercise may cause injury or the condition to flare up. It is important for the personal trainer to acknowledge this challenge with **empathy** while clearly outlining plans to shift the focus of the workout program. These can be the most challenging conversations for a personal trainer to have with a client. The client may feel defeated by the injury or condition and frustrated that he or she cannot exercise at the desired intensity. In these cases, an empathetic personal trainer can provide a great deal of reassurance to the client that the program being created is unique to his or her personal goals based on current ability levels and desired outcomes.

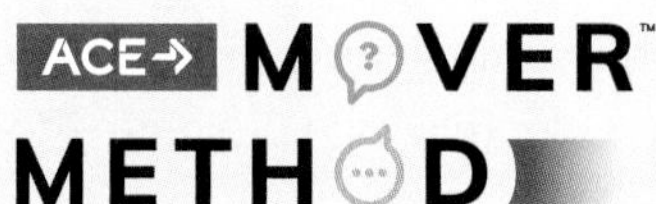

Helping a Client with Pain Reframe Exercise Intensity

Julio, a client who you have been working with for the past three months, shares with you that he is feeling frustrated and defeated. He tells you that he wants to get in better shape, but the level of his consistent pain is preventing him from working out as hard and as often as he would like. Julio enjoys working with you and has not missed or been late for a single session for the entire time you have been his personal trainer. He mentioned being a dedicated, hard-working athlete when he was younger. Now, when he sees other people in the gym working hard, he is frustrated that he cannot work as hard due to his pain.

ACE ABC APPROACH™

Following is an example of how the ACE Mover Method and the ACE ABC Approach can be used when working with clients experiencing pain and feeling discouraged about the inability to perform at an expected level.

Ask: Asking powerful open-ended questions and reflecting on what the client is saying will help you gain a better understanding of what the client wants to achieve.

Personal Trainer: You're feeling frustrated and defeated because your pain is preventing you from being as active as you would like to be. Beyond what we have been working on for the past three months, how do you envision me helping to support you?

Client: Over the past three months, I know I've made progress and have even been feeling better, both physically and emotionally. But, I'm still frustrated! When I worked out before and played sports, I trained at such a high intensity; it felt good to push myself like that. Now, it seems like I am taking baby steps and sometimes I want to give up. I guess the support I need is for you to help me get back to that level of training.

Personal Trainer: So, in the past, you felt like you had good workouts, but now you feel like giving up because you can't train as hard. But, you also reported that our current workouts have led to you feeling better emotionally and physically.

Client: That's correct. I know what we are doing is working for me, and I want to continue, but I sure wish I could get to a higher intensity of training.

Break down barriers: Continue this conversation and ask more open-ended questions to find out what obstacles are getting in the way of this client's goals.

Personal Trainer: What were your workouts like in the past, before your pain limited you?

Client: I was able to train as hard and as often as my schedule and body would let me! After each workout, I felt like I had achieved something meaningful. I had a great program, I pushed heavy weights, I was lean and cut, and my blood pressure was low. I just felt healthy and strong. But now, this pain prevents that kind of training.

Personal Trainer: The pain has caused you to change the way you think about working out, and if you were not in pain, you would be working out at a much higher intensity. Coping with pain is challenging you to think differently about health and exercise. Considering your pain, what could you do now to get that same meaningful experience out of your current exercise program?

Client: I think I need to consider my current reality and acknowledge that now is not the right time to compare myself to where I used to be or to others at the gym. I know I'm feeling healthier, both physically and emotionally, but I want to feel like I am getting more out of my exercise program.

Personal Trainer: What does that look like for you?

Client: I'm a competitive person, so I like to see improvement. I understand there may not be visible changes within each exercise session, but if I had something to compare myself to and could see changes in scores or values in addition to my personal feelings about improving emotionally, that might make things seem more meaningful to me.

Personal Trainer: Thank you for sharing that with me. It will help me ensure that our time together is focused on achieving what is most important to you, and it enables me to support you in a way that will be meaningful to you. Since we began working together three months ago, I have recorded assessment information, observations, and progress you've made. If it would be helpful to you, I can put together a summary of this information and share it with you at our next session.

Client: That would be great!

Collaborate: Working together with the client on goals and solutions is the next step once the client's feelings have been expressed. During this step, the personal trainer and client will work together to set action items to follow up on at an agreed upon time.

Personal Trainer: So far, we have decided that we will go over a summary report of your progress at our next session. Being as specific as possible, how will you know if this exercise program is successful?

Client: If my pain levels decrease and I can see improvement on specific assessments and tests, I think that will reduce my feelings of defeat. Maybe it's my competitive nature or the fact that I can't do the things I want to because of pain, but I think having more assessment and test results to track my progress will motivate me.

Personal Trainer: Having less pain and seeing improvement on paper will make your exercise sessions feel more meaningful to you, and the added challenge might work with your competitive nature. Based on our work together and what I know about movements that elicit your pain, I can compile a list of assessments we can review together next week to see if any of them seem like a good starting point. Once we agree on the right assessments for you, how do you see things unfolding over the next few months?

Client: I would like to continue working with you three times per week to increase my physical and emotional well-being. Also, I would like to schedule some regularly occurring assessments so I can track the numbers. I think monitoring my progress in this way will motivate me and help take the focus off the pain.

In this scenario, the client and personal trainer work together to establish what would make the exercise program more useful to the client. Even if a personal trainer has created an effective exercise program, if the client does not find it valuable and is feeling discouraged about his current situation, this may lead to poor adherence. Working together, the client and personal trainer can uncover new ways to create a more meaningful experience. In this scenario, the personal trainer respects the client's feelings and does not try to tell him his feelings are right or wrong, but instead asks questions, breaks down barriers, and collaborates on next steps, while affirming that the client is the expert in his own life. This method allows the personal trainer to focus on program design and assessment selection and administration.

Cool-down

Static stretching takes on a specific and meaningful purpose when a client exhibits ROM restriction. The use of this kind of stretching can have an impact on overall flexibility of the muscle. Static stretching is used primarily at the end of a workout because studies have demonstrated neural inhibition and a decrease in strength after a prolonged stretch (Page, 2012). Alternatively, when the goal is to inhibit an overactive muscle or address posture at the beginning of the workout, static stretching may be employed first (after a brief warm-up).

While the warm-up readies a client for activity, the cool-down is the opportunity to focus on stress reduction, returning the **heart rate** to resting levels and initiating relaxation and the recovery process. Including static stretching during the cool-down period can inhibit overactive muscles and improve flexibility, using static stretching to gently inhibit a potentially highly active nervous system and improve ROM.

Recovery

Because recovery is essential to preventing injury, creating an **active recovery** program for an individual with a history of chronic injuries or conditions is an important part of designing a successful program. As such, the client's injury history must be taken into consideration. While gentle walking daily may be an appropriate activity for an individual with low-back pain, this may be aggravating to a client with knee arthritis, who may be better served by walking in the pool or riding a recumbent bike.

Recovery days should be spent addressing the health of the tissue, along with ROM of the joints. A program of self–myofascial release and stretching after light activity on non-exercise days may promote healthy tissue recovery.

Common Conditions of the Upper Extremity

Whether an injury is acute or chronic in nature, post-rehabilitative exercise of the upper extremity should take into account the **activities of daily living (ADL)** of the client. An individual who spends considerable time sitting at a desk may struggle with forward-head position and/or forward-rounded shoulders. In this case, strengthening the postural muscles becomes an essential part of the exercise program. Proper posture provides a strong base of support for extremity movement.

A client who participates in regular activity that requires unilateral repetitive motion, like playing tennis or the violin, may have an upper-body imbalance between the right and left sides, which should be addressed to create more equal strength and ROM among limbs.

It is common for personal trainers to notice these imbalances in a movement assessment and it is within the scope of practice to address them. However, the personal trainer must remember that regardless of what is observed in the movement assessment, the goals of the client must be prioritized while accounting for the injury and/or muscle imbalance strategically throughout the workout.

Creating an appropriate program for clients with common musculoskeletal conditions, once cleared by their physician, is a common role of the personal trainer. It is essential that the personal trainer remain within his or her scope of practice and avoid assessing the injury or postulating on the cause.

SHOULDER

The anatomical configuration of the shoulder allows for a large ROM and thus leaves it vulnerable to injury. The shoulder joint has the largest ROM of any joint in the body. It is the shallow articular surface of the glenoid fossa that allows such motion. As such, it also offers a lack of bony stability. The cartilage of the glenoid fossa deepens the joint, creating a flexible cup in which the humeral head sits, called the glenoid labrum. The joint is further stabilized by ligamentous tissue, the articular capsule, and the rotator cuff muscles (Figure 15-5). If strength and stability of the surrounding musculature are not present, the humerus may become unstable in the socket joint such that the supraspinatus tendon and subacromial bursa may

FIGURE 15-5
Rotator cuff muscles

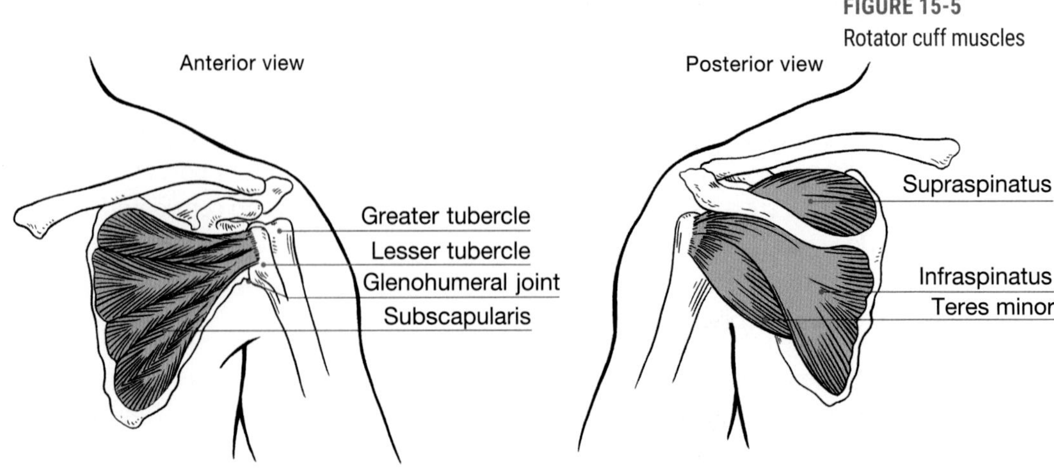

be compressed between the humeral head and the acromion process. If complicated by faulty posture, including forward-rounded shoulders and/or exaggerated kyphosis of the thoracic vertebrae, the scapulae will sit superior and **anterior** to its ideal position and the space between the humerus and acromion process is made even smaller.

The compression and subsequent inflammation of the supraspinatus tendon and subacromial bursa is called **impingement syndrome.** This condition sometimes includes the inflammation of the long head of the biceps tendon (Figure 15-6). In cases where this condition is prolonged, damage to the rotator cuff muscles can cause decreased elasticity and may lead to rotator cuff muscle tendon tear. The incidence of rotator cuff muscle tear increases with age (Park et al., 2016).

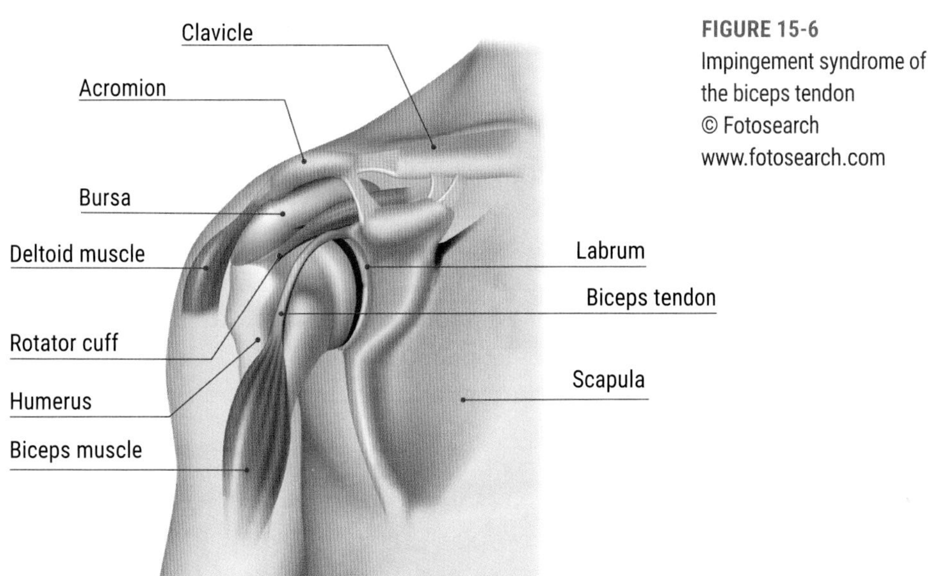

FIGURE 15-6
Impingement syndrome of the biceps tendon
© Fotosearch www.fotosearch.com

The function of the rotator cuff muscles is to decelerate forward movement of the humerus during overhead activity (e.g., the serving motion in tennis or throwing a baseball or football) and to stabilize the humerus in the glenoid fossa. For most individuals, these functions can be compensated for by other soft tissue. For this reason, individuals may elect conservative treatment and physical therapy over surgical repair, even with a full-thickness rotator cuff tear. In this case, general upper-body strength, stability, and ROM exercise should become part of a regular routine to prevent pain and loss of function.

When working with a client who has shoulder dysfunction, the personal trainer should avoid exercises that require overhead movement, as these movements require stability and strength that is beyond the capability of a client with a compromised shoulder. Further, overhead movement places the humeral head in closer contact with the acromion process, increasing risk of impingement.

Program Design for the Shoulder

The exercise program should emphasize strength and posture that opens the subacromial space while regaining stability of the joint. To open the subacromial space, the anterior shoulder and chest can be stretched to allow for proper scapular positioning. In this case, the

FIGURE 15-7
Superficial and deep muscles that act at the scapulothoracic articulation

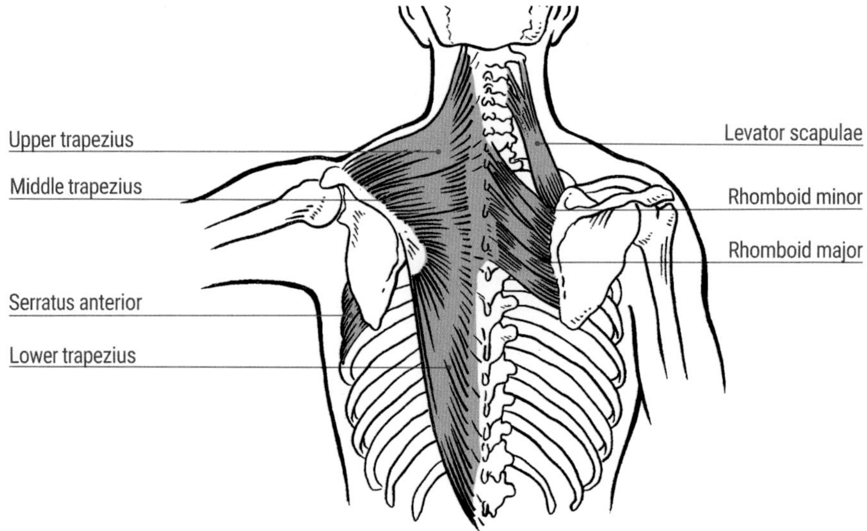

program design aim is to inhibit these muscles, so this stretch may be done during the warm-up. A muscular-training program should focus on the muscles that stabilize the scapulae, specifically exercises that target the lower trapezius, rhomboids, and serratus anterior (Figure 15-7) [e.g., seated row (see Figure 9-41, page 372) and serratus punch (Figure 15-8)]. To stimulate the stabilization capacity of the rotator cuff muscles, closed-chain weight-bearing exercises like the bird dog (see Figure 15-19, page 711) and open-chain exercises like the farmer carry (Figure 15-9) will activate the rotator cuff muscles without aggravating the tissue.

Consider the following steps when selecting exercises for improving shoulder function:

- First, address postural imbalances that may cause a decrease in space between the acromion process and humeral head (e.g., forward rounded shoulders or exaggerated kyphosis).
- Next, strengthen the scapular stabilizing muscles, including the rotator cuff.
- Then, improve strength of the anterior shoulder muscles and pectoralis major through controlled pushing motion.
- Finally, begin to introduce overhead activities as is functionally appropriate and, if using overhead press movements, instruct clients to perform the exercise in the scapular plane (i.e., shoulder positioned 30 degrees anterior to the frontal plane) to prevent impingement (i.e., pinching) of shoulder structures (Figure 15-10).

FIGURE 15-8
Serratus punch

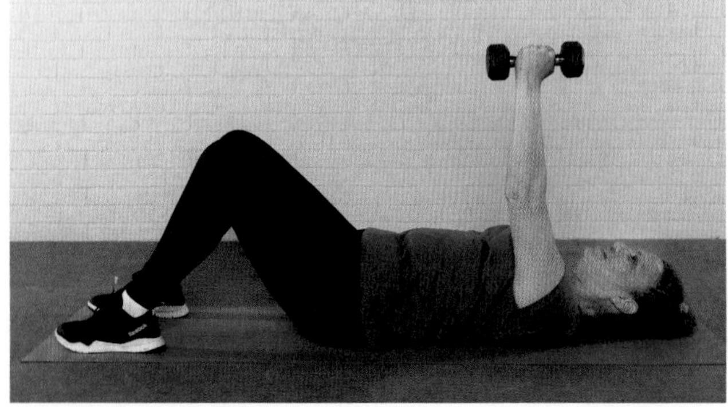

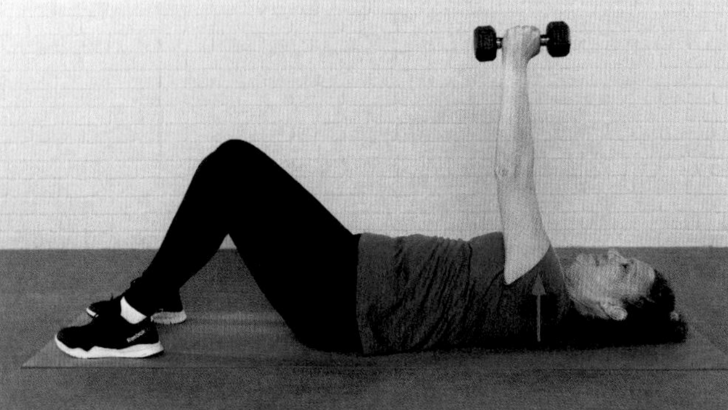

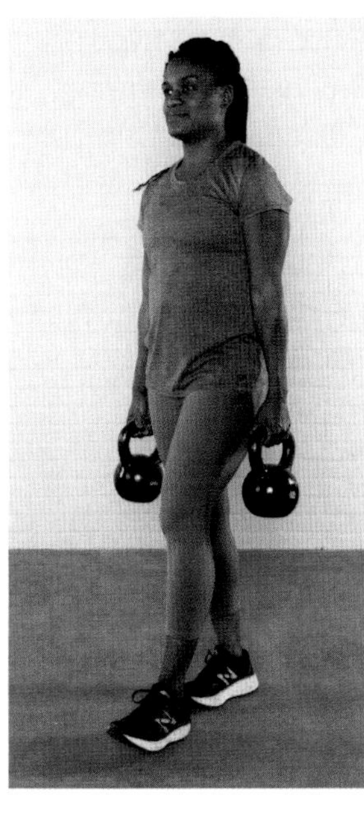
FIGURE 15-9
Farmer carry

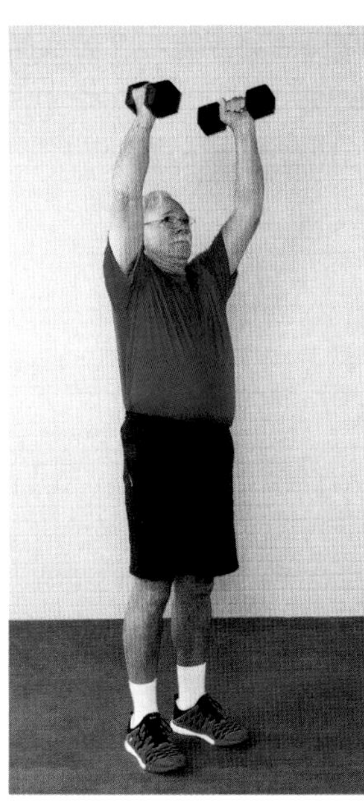
FIGURE 15-10
Overhead press in the scapular plane

ELBOW, WRIST, AND HAND

Overuse injuries associated with prolonged use of a computer mouse and keyboard both at work and in recreation are on the rise. Prolonged static load and improper workstation set-up contribute to these conditions (Baba & Daruis, 2016). The elbow, wrist, and hand are commonly affected.

Tendinitis of both the extensor and flexor muscle tendons of the elbow and wrist can occur with overuse of the upper extremity. Two of the most common injuries are **lateral epicondylitis** and **medial epicondylitis.**

Lateral epicondylitis, which is commonly called tennis elbow, is defined as an overuse or repetitive-trauma injury of the wrist extensor muscle tendons near their origin on the lateral epicondyle of the humerus (Figure 15-11) (Bisset, Coombes, & Vicenzino, 2011).

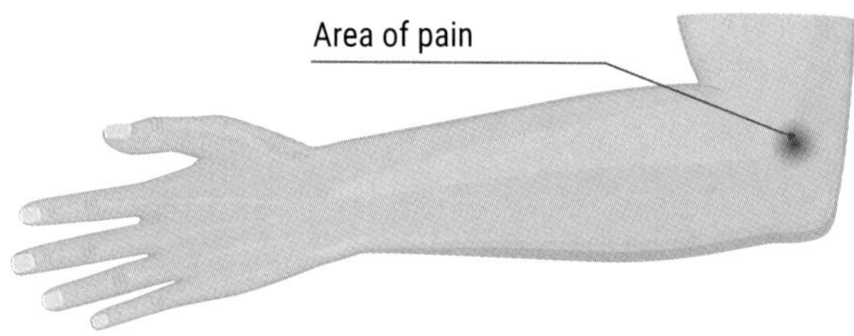

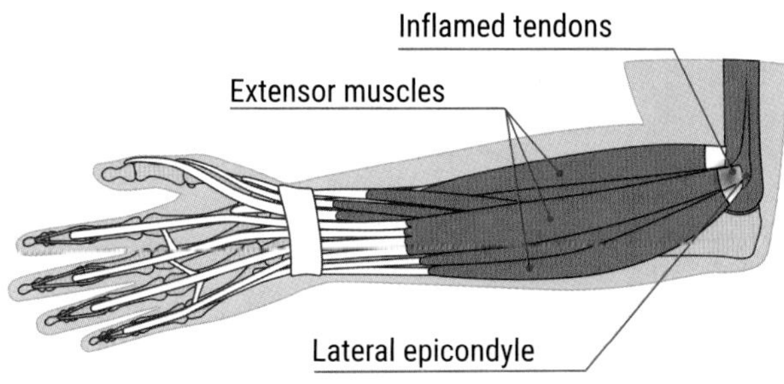

FIGURE 15-11
Lateral epicondylitis, or "tennis elbow"

Medial epicondylitis, which is sometimes called golfer's elbow, is an overuse or repetitive-trauma injury of the wrist flexor muscle tendons near their origin on the medial epicondyle of the humerus (Figure 15-12). These conditions are common in adults 30 to 55 years old (Taylor & Hannafin, 2012).

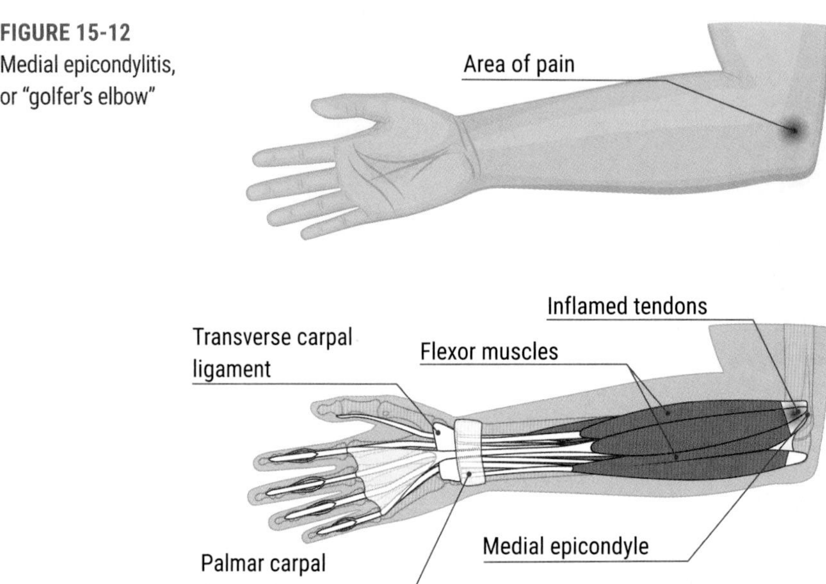

FIGURE 15-12
Medial epicondylitis, or "golfer's elbow"

When the tendons are inflamed, a personal trainer should avoid adding stress, eliminating anything that causes pain or discomfort. Exercises that require wrist **flexion, extension,** or gripping may need to be modified.

Carpal tunnel syndrome is caused by an inflammation of the flexor tendons that pass under the flexor retinaculum at the wrist. This inflammation in the small space between the bones of the wrist and the flexor retinaculum, dubbed the carpal tunnel, eventually compresses the median nerve (Figure 15-13), causing pain and numbness. In such cases, it would be appropriate for the personal trainer to recommend that the client request a workstation **ergonomic** assessment from his or her human resources department.

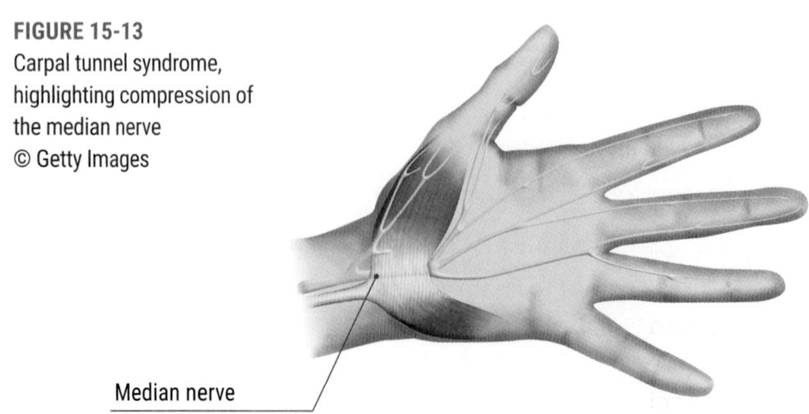

FIGURE 15-13
Carpal tunnel syndrome, highlighting compression of the median nerve
© Getty Images

The same cautions appropriate for elbow tendinitis are applicable when training a client with diagnosed carpal tunnel syndrome, or carpal tunnel syndrome–like symptoms. Avoiding exercises that require gripping or wrist extension is important. Due to the prolonged nature of this condition, it may be wise to find modifications for these exercises that keep the wrist in a neutral position. For example, push-ups can be done using neutral-grip handles and the need for grip strength can be minimized by using wrist straps to assist in holding the handle during pulling exercises.

Program Design for the Elbow, Wrist, and Hand

Conditions of the elbow, wrist, and hand may benefit from splinting or using an orthosis during exercise, especially when a client is struggling with persistent pain. Such bracing is at the discretion of a doctor, so a personal trainer should consider discussing a referral to a physician for evaluation. The client should wear the prescribed wrist splint during activity as recommended by the physician and follow any guidelines provided for the client by the physician. A program for clients struggling with elbow, wrist, or hand dysfunction should focus on commonly compromised mobility and stability related to all upper-extremity function.

Consider the following steps when selecting exercises for improving elbow, wrist, and hand function:

- First, limit overuse by introducing various grips for comfort and/or wearing gloves to increase friction between the hand and handle or device when doing pulling exercises, which will lessen the workload on injured tissue.
- Next, increase ROM through gentle stretches in all planes of motion.
- Then, improve strength of the wrist and hand through exercises such as a wall push-up and wrist flexion and extension.
- Finally, remove grips or gloves and slowly introduce volume to pulling exercises, as tolerated.

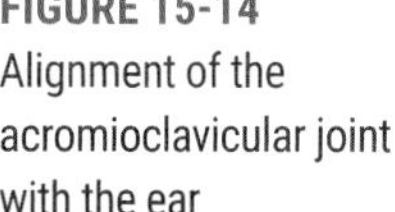

FIGURE 15-14 Alignment of the acromioclavicular joint with the ear

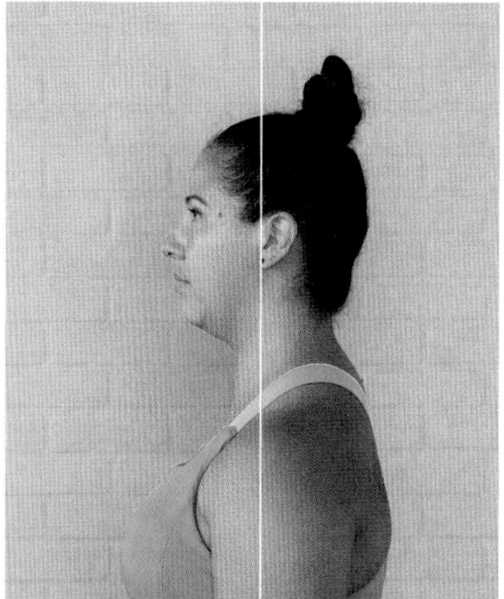

Postural alignment

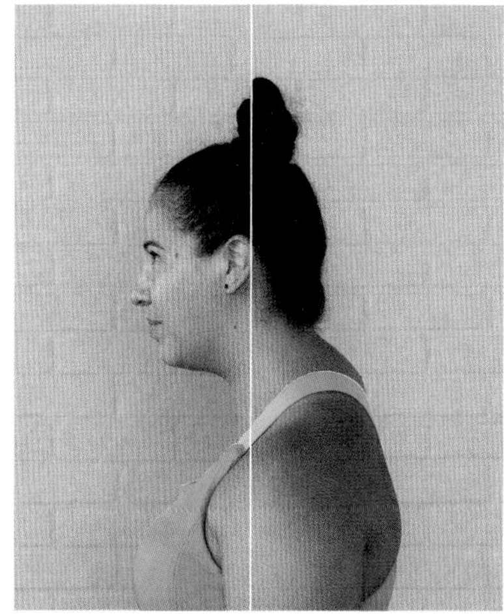

Forward-head position

Common Conditions of the Spine

Personal trainers will frequently encounter clients who struggle with neck, mid-back, or low-back problems. As much as overuse activity can cause these issues, a physically inactive lifestyle, coupled with desk sitting and computer work, also makes a person particularly vulnerable to muscle stiffness or injury along the spine. Thoughtful program design can have a marked impact on tissue health and improve mobility, postural alignment, and strength of the muscles along the spine.

NECK

Like the shoulder, the neck is vulnerable when postural alignment is altered. An exaggerated posterior curve of the thoracic spine will result in forward-head posture, putting an abnormal stress on the muscles of the neck (Figure 15-14). In this case, it is essential to address the postural alignment to improve head and cervical spine position.

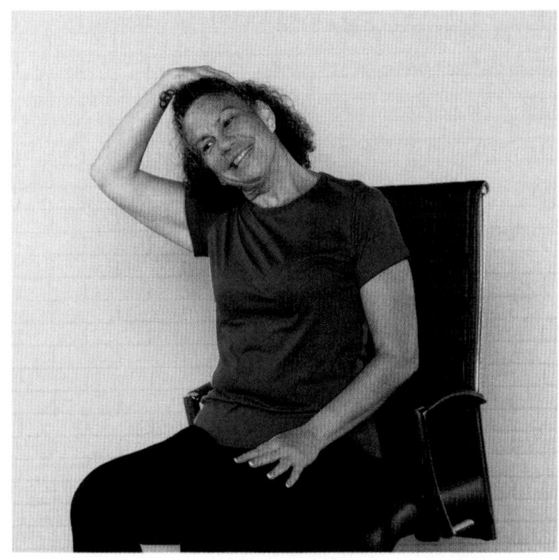

FIGURE 15-15
Lateral neck stretch

It is also important to remember that the spine is connected through bony protuberances and soft tissue. When there is a misalignment anywhere along the spine, there is a chain reaction that may cause pain farther away. An example of this involves muscle tightness in the right erector spinae, causing right-side lateral flexion and resulting in an elevation of the left shoulder and subsequent left-side neck pain. It is important to address the shortened tissue along the length of the kinetic chain, not just the affected area, to achieve the greatest result. In this example, stretching only the shortened muscles along the left side of the neck while neglecting the muscles along the thoracic spine would not address the primary problem. As such, strengthening the neck muscles in isolation should not be the goal of a personal-training session. Instead, focus should be on exercises that support postural alignment (see Chapter 10 to review static posture assessment and proper spine alignment).

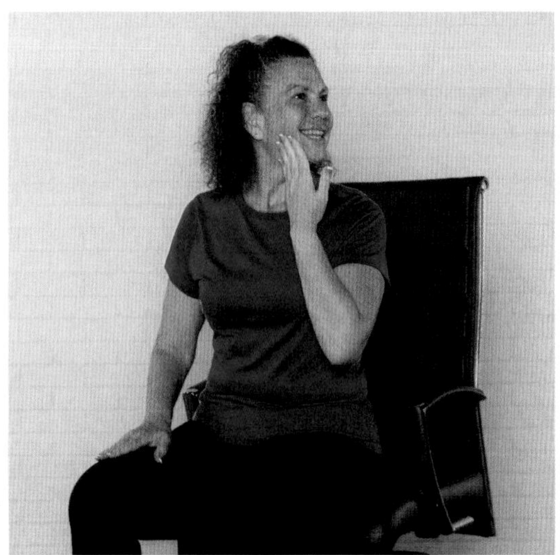

FIGURE 15-16
Rotational neck stretch

Consider the following steps when selecting exercises for improving neck function:

- First, observe the relationship of neck position to that of the thoracic spine and shoulder. Forward-rounded shoulders and exaggerated kyphosis will be especially common. If faulty posture is observed, address the spine and shoulder position first (see recommendations for those specific joints in this chapter).
- Next, introduce gentle movement and stretching that can be executed by the client at any time of day when discomfort occurs (e.g., lateral and rotational neck stretches; Figures 15-15 and 15-16).
- Finally, refer to a physician if pain is severe or persistent.

LOW BACK

Low-back pain most often occurs in individuals between 30 and 50 years of age. Some researchers report that up to 80% of adults will experience low-back pain at some point (Peng, 2013), and in 30% of cases, acute low-back pain becomes chronic (Strong et al., 2013). This is a major cause of disability and an important driver of healthcare costs in the U.S. and other countries.

Low-back pain has a variety of causes, including muscle strain, soft-tissue stress from prolonged faulty static posture, poor physical fitness, disc disease, as well as other conditions like osteoarthritis, rheumatoid arthritis, **ankylosing spondylitis,** and cancer (American College of Sports Medicine, 2013; Whiting & Zernicke, 2008).

A common postural dysfunction associated with low-back pain is exaggerated **lordosis.** Depending on the cause of pain, correcting this postural dysfunction may play a part in decreasing the stress on the structures of the low back. Exaggerated lordosis is characterized by tight erector spinae in the lumbar region, tight hip flexors, and potential weakness in the muscles of the **posterior chain** (e.g., calves, hamstrings, gluteal muscles, and erector spinae). This combination may cause stiffness or pain in the low-back region.

When disc injury is present, it commonly occurs in the lumbar spine. In this case, the client may develop signs of sciatica or other nerve **radiculopathy.** A client will often report a shooting sensation of pain, numbness, and/or tingling along the affected nerve and into the foot.

Though causes of low-back pain differ, the physical needs of each individual struggling with this condition are similar. Lack of hip mobility often leads to increased ROM between the vertebrae of the lumbar spine, which should ideally be more stable than mobile.

Similarly, the muscles of the lumbar spine are frequently overused. The erector spinae work as spinal stabilizers, not powerful muscles of extension. On the other hand, the muscles of the posterior hip and thigh are powerful extensors of the hip and should perform as such during movement.

Program design should include static stretching to inhibit overactive muscles that might be contributing to postural dysfunction, as well as exercises to improve ROM of the hips and strengthening of the gluteal muscles, hamstrings, rectus abdominis, and internal and external obliques (see Figures 9-15 and 9-34, pages 340 and 362) (Table 15-4).

TABLE 15-4

Select Muscles and Muscle Groups and Their Contributions to Trunk and Pelvic Stability

Muscle Group	Function to Support Low-back Pain
Gluteus maximus	Hip extensor; provides support for pelvic and trunk stability; contributes to proper pelvic position
Hamstrings	Hip extensors; provide support for pelvic and trunk stability; contribute to proper pelvic position Tight muscles inhibit hip hinge and may cause posterior tilt.
Rectus abdominis	Trunk stabilizer; contributes to proper pelvic position
Internal and external obliques	Trunk stabilizers; contribute to proper pelvic position
Latissimus dorsi	Provides stabilization of lumbar spine through its attachment at the thoracolumbar fascia
Internal rotators of the hip	Tight muscles inhibit hip hinge and may contribute to anterior pelvic tilt
External rotators of the hip	Tight muscles inhibit hip hinge and may contribute to posterior pelvic tilt
Hip flexors	Tight muscles inhibit hip hinge and may contribute to anterior pelvic tilt

Program Design for the Spine

When working with a client who struggles with neck, shoulder, or low-back dysfunction, beginning a training program by addressing faulty posture and ROM restriction can provide meaningful results.

APPLY WHAT YOU KNOW

Daily Routine for Enhancing Low-back Health

While there is a common belief that exercise sessions should be performed at least three times per week, it appears that low-back exercises have the most beneficial effect when performed daily. When selecting exercises for low-back strength and stability, more repetitions of less-demanding exercises will assist in the enhancement of postural endurance and strength (McGill, 2016). Given that endurance has protective value to these slow-twitch postural muscles, strength gains should not be overemphasized at the expense of endurance.

The following exercises are a simple daily routine that can be recommended to a client to strengthen the stabilizing musculature of the spine and enhance motor control to ensure that spine stability is maintained in all activities. These exercises may be included when training within the Functional Training phase of the Muscular Training component of the ACE IFT Model. Keep in mind that these are only examples of well-designed exercises and may not be for everyone; the initial challenge may or may not be appropriate for every individual, nor will the graded progression be the same for all clients. These are simply examples of exercises that challenge the muscles of the torso, improving fluidity of movement and postural stabilization.

Cat-cow

The routine begins with the cat-cow exercise (spine flexion-extension cycles) to improve flexibility and warm the tissue with rhythmic motion (Figure 15-17). Note that the cat-cow is intended as a motion exercise—not a stretch—so the emphasis is on motion rather than "pushing" at the end

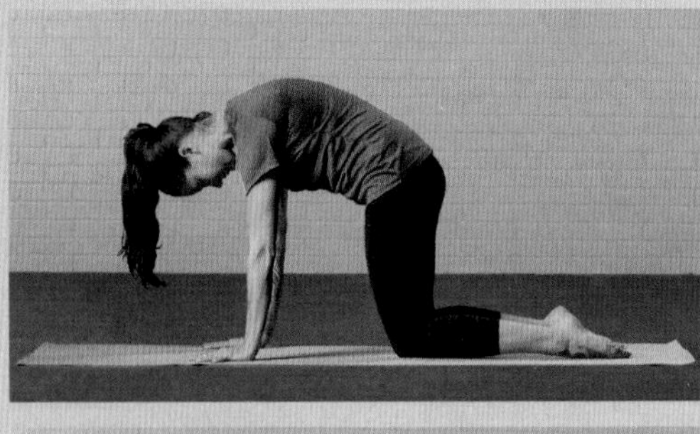

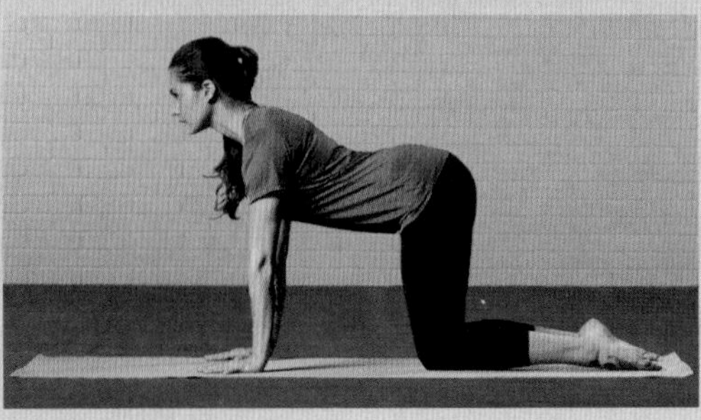

FIGURE 15-17
Cat-cow

ranges of flexion and extension. As the client moves into the cat position, he or she should slowly exhale; as the client moves into the cow position he or she should inhale. The neutral spine, or center point of the movement, is the time to transition the breathing.

Modified Curl-up

The cat-camel motion exercise is followed by anterior abdominal exercises, in this case the modified curl-up (Figure 15-18). The hands or a rolled towel are placed under the lumbar spine to preserve a neutral spine posture. Do not allow the client to flatten the back to the floor, as doing so flexes the lumbar spine, violates the neutral spine principle, and increases the loads on the discs and ligaments. One knee is flexed but the other leg is straight to lock the pelvis–lumbar spine and minimize the loss of a neutral lumbar posture. Have clients alternate the bent leg (right to left) midway through the repetitions.

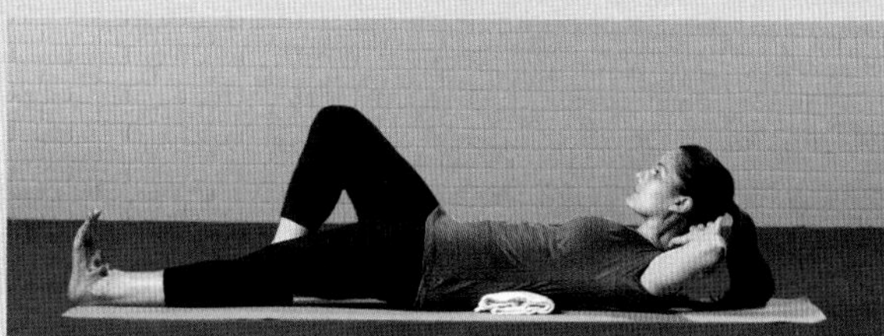

FIGURE 15-18
Modified curl-up

Bird Dog

The extensor component of the program consists of the bird dog exercise (Figure 15-19). Starting with the hands placed directly under the shoulders and the knees directly under the hips, the personal trainer should instruct the client in finding a neutral spine position. Stabilization through the abdominal musculature is needed to ensure consistent neutral spine position while the opposite arm and leg are lifted in unison. If a client is not ready to stabilize this load, he or she can start with one arm or one leg and progress to the full exercise. Holding the position for 5 to 8 seconds for each repetition is recommended to improve muscular endurance before alternating sides (McGill, 2016).

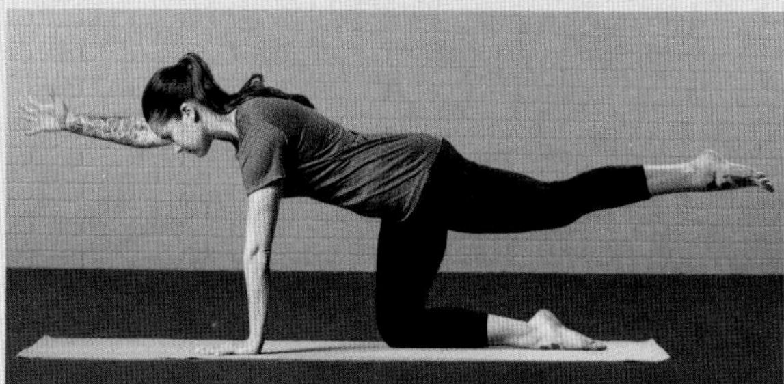

FIGURE 15-19
Bird dog

Side Bridge

The lateral muscles of the torso (i.e., quadratus lumborum and abdominal obliques) are important for optimal stability and are targeted with the side bridge exercise. The beginner level of this exercise involves bridging the torso between the elbow and the knees (Figure 15-20a). Once this is mastered and well-tolerated, the challenge is increased by bridging using the elbow and the feet (Figure 15-20b). It is important when performing the side bridge exercise to maintain a neutral neck and spine position. Holding the position for 5 to 8 seconds for each repetition before alternating sides is recommended to improve muscular endurance (McGill, 2016).

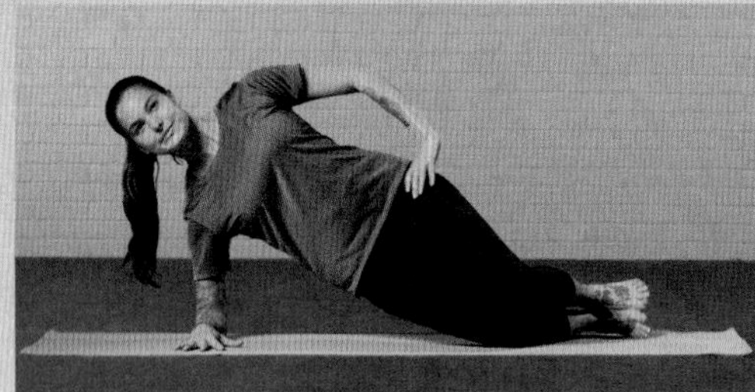

a. Basic

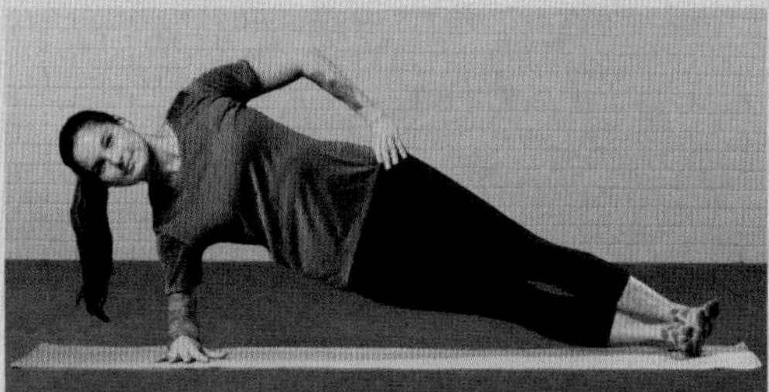

b. Progression

FIGURE 15-20
Side bridge

Consider the following steps when selecting exercises for improving low-back function:

- First, address any imbalance between the right and left sides.
- Next, address any anterior/posterior postural imbalance (e.g., anterior or posterior pelvic tilt).
- Then, increase functional internal and external rotation of the hip [e.g., wood chop exercises (see Figure 11-70, page 538) promote internal rotation of the hip in the downward movement and external rotation of the same hip in the upward movement].
- Finally, strengthen the posterior chain, especially the hamstrings and gluteal muscles, to provide powerful support.

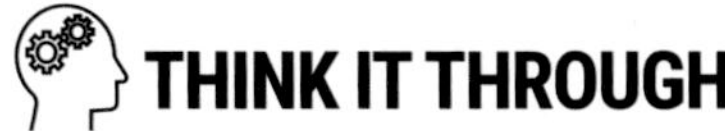

Programming for a Client with Low-back Dysfunction

Considering the exercise recommendations for an individual with a history of low-back dysfunction, create cardiorespiratory- and muscular-training programs for the following client:

- 45-year-old man who works as a computer engineer
- Has experienced low-back pain intermittently for the past two years
- Enjoys gardening and coaching soccer for his 8- and 10-year-old children
- Goal: To be strong enough to do weekly gardening and yard work without back pain and be an active coach for his soccer teams
- Has committed to muscular training for 60 minutes twice per week and cardiorespiratory training for 30 minutes twice per week

Common Conditions of the Lower Extremity

The lower extremities control the transmission of all ground reaction forces through the body. From the ground up, the muscles and joints work in concert to stabilize the body, control movement, and distribute ground reaction forces through the kinetic chain. Injury to the lower extremity can lead to compensations that result in other overuse syndromes.

HIP

Like the shoulder, the hip is a ball-and-socket joint that allows multidirectional movement. However, the acetabulum of the hip is a deep bony socket that limits ROM and, along with the joint capsule and muscle structure, provides significant joint stability. When there is an acute or chronic injury affecting the joint, the dysfunction can cause kinetic chain implications upward, into the low back, or downward, into the knee. Likewise, it is not uncommon for clients to struggle with hip pain when they lead an inactive lifestyle. Prolonged sitting leaves the muscles of the anterior hip shortened and the posterior hip lengthened. This imbalance could negatively impact the ability to execute a proper hip hinge. This chapter covers the more common conditions of the hip, including **piriformis syndrome,** hip arthritis, and hip replacement.

Piriformis Syndrome

Piriformis syndrome is a condition where the piriformis muscle becomes tight, taut, or inflamed, causing compression of the sciatic nerve that runs between it and the **gemelli** (Figure 15-21). In as much as 22% of the population, the sciatic nerve splits (i.e., runs through) the piriformis, making people with this anatomical variation more prone to the condition (Boyajian-O'Neill et al., 2008). Nerve compression may cause radiculopathy similar to the symptoms of lumbar disc injury. It is estimated that at least 6% of patients diagnosed with low-back pain actually have piriformis syndrome (Boyajian-O'Neill et al., 2008). The function of the piriformis muscle is as an external rotator of the hip and stabilizer of the femoral head during **gait** (Figure 15-22).

The pelvis is formed by the sacrum and right and left ilium (see Figure 9-1, page 323). The sacroiliac joints and the pubic symphysis are mobile, but tightly held into position by strong ligamentous and cartilaginous structures. When performing an assessment on someone with hip dysfunction, it is important to assess the position of the pelvis and associated relative position of the femur. As the joint with the most ROM and muscular support in the lower extremity, the hip absorbs a great deal of ground reaction force. Dysfunction at the hip may be caused by lack of strength, stability, or mobility.

In a static posture assessment, evaluate the pelvic position by paying special attention to the height of the iliac crests. For example, while performing an assessment on a client who complains of pain in the left hip, the left iliac crest may be higher than the right, in which case the left femur is in adduction relative to the pelvis. If the foot is still pointing forward, it is also in relative internal rotation. This relative positioning causes the muscles of the left hip to be pulled taut (i.e., put on chronic stretch), especially the IT band, the external rotator group, and the gluteus maximus. Remembering that the sciatic nerve travels between two external rotators or through the piriformis, this position may cause compression on the sciatic nerve and/or localized aching or pain. This *taut* position can

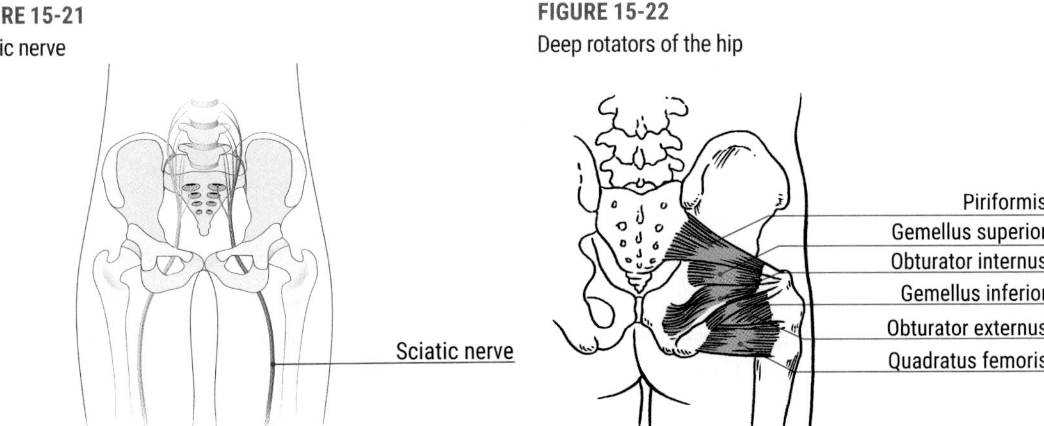

FIGURE 15-21
Sciatic nerve

FIGURE 15-22
Deep rotators of the hip

be likened to a rubber band pulled to the limit of its stretch. It cannot absorb further stretch and the position puts great strain on its structural integrity. Alternatively, a chronically *tight* muscle resists lengthening and cannot stretch to its fullest capacity due to decreased elasticity.

Because the pelvis is a closed loop, the relative position of the femur on the right side will likely be the opposite of the femur on the left side, where the external rotators of the right hip will be tight. The proper progression of exercises consists of static stretching for the right side, while working on active ROM on both sides with a concerted effort toward improved strength and stability on the left hip abductors and external rotators.

Program design for clients with piriformis syndrome should focus on balancing the position of the right and left pelvis via static stretching of the tight muscles and conditioning of the taut muscles. The program also includes closed-chain internal and external hip rotation exercises to improve both mobility and stability of the hip.

Hip Arthritis and Hip Replacement

Arthritis is a chronic condition characterized by joint pain and inflammation, which, especially in advanced stages, may lead to decreases in ROM, stability, and strength (see Chapter 13). A physically inactive lifestyle will only worsen the condition. An exercise program can improve mobility and function when executed appropriately. However, these symptoms can be exacerbated by exercise when the program puts undue stress on the joint structure. It is essential to progress slowly, mindfully, and in consideration of the client's readiness.

Hip replacement surgery, or total hip arthroplasty, is recommended by orthopedic surgeons when physical therapy and medication cease to have a positive effect and the performance of ADL is impacted. In a review done by Kremers et al. (2015), it was estimated that 2.5 million people in the U.S. were living with a hip replacement (1.4 million women and 1.1 million men) in 2010, some up to 25 years after initial hip replacement. The data collected in this study show an increase in incidence of hip arthritis as individuals age, as well as an increase in elective surgery at a younger age.

In the first several months post-surgery, a client should engage in regular physical therapy sessions, and the physical therapist will share progression of exercise programming and

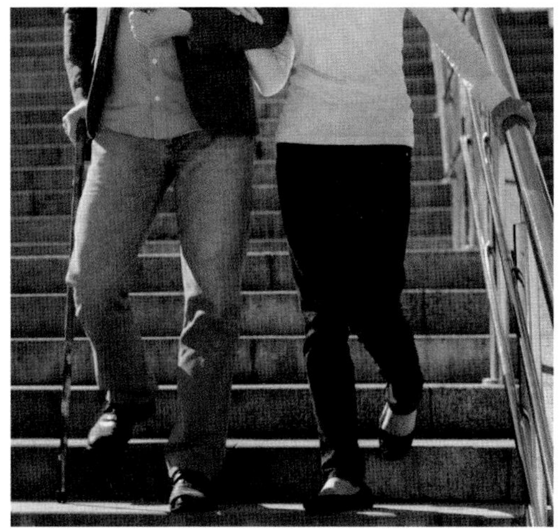

limitations in each stage of recovery. Once a client has been released from physical therapy, ROM of the hip may not be equal to the nonsurgical side. Though equal ROM is ideal, it is not necessary and may not be possible after surgery. Gentle stretching and dynamic ROM exercises are encouraged, but the expectations of the personal trainer and the client must remain realistic.

The recumbent bike is an excellent modality to improve cardiorespiratory fitness, ROM, and quadriceps strength. Cycling on a stationary bike is effective for improving cardiorespiratory fitness and quadriceps strength, but requires less flexion at the hip and knee, and so will not challenge ROM to the same degree. Therefore, the stationary bike may be more appropriate for those who are struggling to regain full ROM.

Program Design for the Hip

Regardless of the dysfunction of the hip, the approach to program design remains the same. Conduct ROM and movement assessments to identify areas that require improved ROM, stability, and/or strength. During a standing postural assessment, a personal trainer should identify imbalances between the left and right sides, paying particular attention to the position of the pelvis. Before designing the exercise program, the personal trainer should review the client's goals to ensure that they are appropriately addressed through the exercise program.

Consider the following steps when selecting exercises for improving hip function:

- First, address any imbalance between the right and left sides.
- Next, improve ROM in hip internal and external rotation, as well as single-leg stance stability.
- Then, improve hip-hinge mobility and stability.
- Lastly, improve the strength of the muscles of the posterior chain.

When addressing muscle imbalances, the personal trainer must remember that the exercises and stretches will be different for each side because of the closed loop created at the pelvis. Tight muscles on one side should be stretched while the weak muscles of the opposite side should be strengthened. When creating a program, include static stretching early in the workout (after a brief warm-up) to inhibit tight muscles to allow for increased ROM, thereby maximizing the effects of the exercises.

KNEE

The bony structure of the knee is a classic hinge joint; however, rotation has been measured at this joint from 2 to 23 degrees (Shamaei & Dollar, 2011). Though the joint is supported by strong ligamentous and fascial structures, it is highly mobile, allowing up to 130 degrees of flexion. The only muscle belly that crosses the knee is the popliteus (see Figure 9-31, page 362).

Otherwise, the muscles that move and stabilize the knee cross the joint as tendinous tissue. As mentioned earlier, cartilage damage and ligament sprains are common in the knee. Other common conditions include iliotibial band (IT band) friction syndrome, tendinitis, **patellofemoral pain syndrome (PFPS),** and **chondromalacia.**

Iliotibial Band Friction Syndrome

IT band friction syndrome is a repetitive overuse condition that occurs when the **distal** portion of the IT band rubs against the lateral femoral epicondyle, causing burning or pain at the lateral aspect of the knee, which may be described as sharp or stabbing (Figure 15-23). IT band friction syndrome is common among active individuals 15 to 50 years of age and is primarily caused by poor training form, lack of recovery, or poor technique in runners, cyclists, volleyball players, and weight lifters (Martinez & Honsik, 2006). Risk factors may include the following: overuse, improper footwear or equipment use, changes in running surface, muscle imbalance (e.g., weakness or tightness), or structural abnormalities like **pes planus** (flat feet), knee **valgus,** and leg-length discrepancy (Houglum, 2016; Martinez & Honsik, 2006).

FIGURE 15-23
Iliotibial band friction syndrome

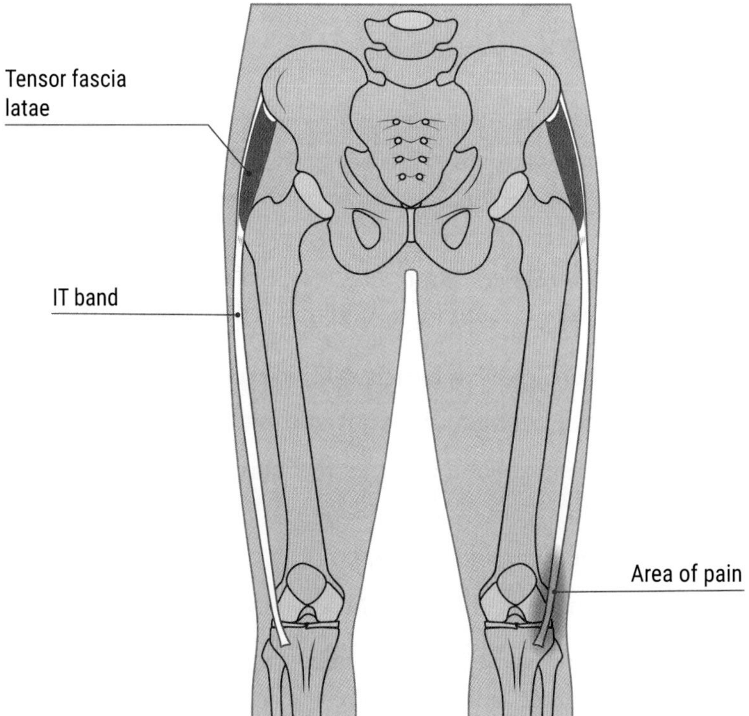

Conducting a static posture assessment is useful for observing positional imbalances of the pelvis. As discussed with piriformis syndrome, the IT band may be held taut due to an imbalance in the pelvis. If the left side of the pelvis is higher than the right, the IT band on the left is held taut, which could lead to increased contact between the IT band and lateral femoral epicondyle. Alternatively, if the right tensor fascia latae is tight, it could contribute to symptoms because such tightness can also cause increased contact between the IT band and lateral femoral epicondyle. In either case, it would be correct to use self–myofascial release and static stretching (Figures 15-24 and 15-25) on the right side (the tight side), to increase ROM and correct the right/left imbalance.

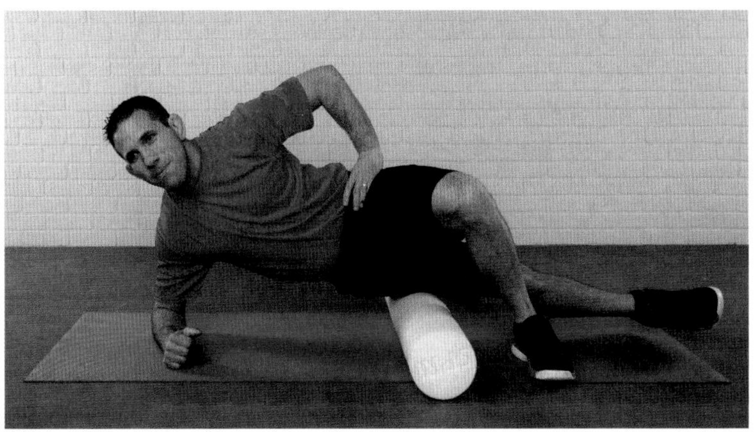

FIGURE 15-24
Self-myofascial release of the iliotibial band

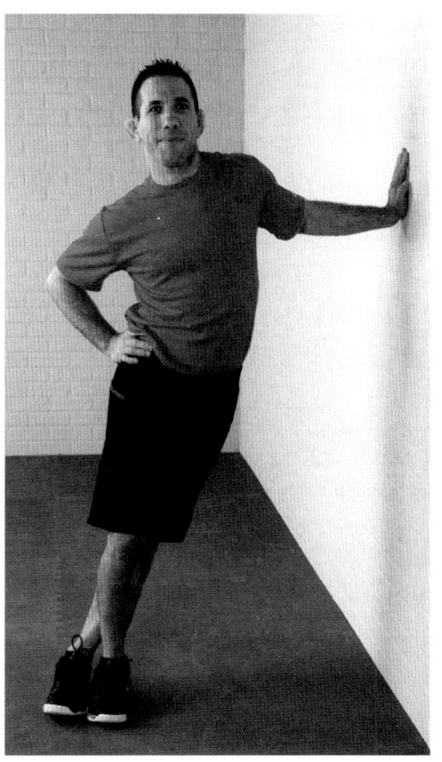

FIGURE 15-25
Static stretch for the iliotibial band

Tendinitis

Tendinitis is an inflammation of the tendon that may be progressing through the stages of healing or can be categorized as chronic. In addition to the patellar tendon, the pes anserine tendons and quadriceps tendon are common areas for tendinitis to occur (Figure 15-26). Each is characterized by pain at the tendon site. Because tendinitis pain is common during activities

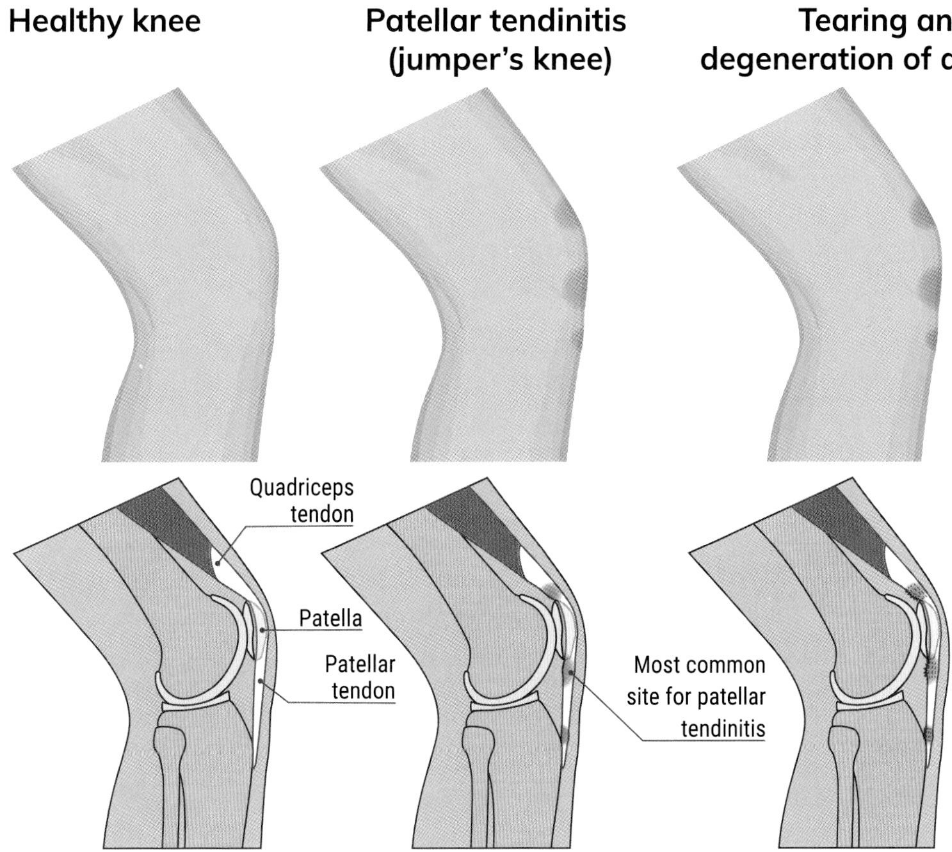

FIGURE 15-26
Common sites of knee tendinitis

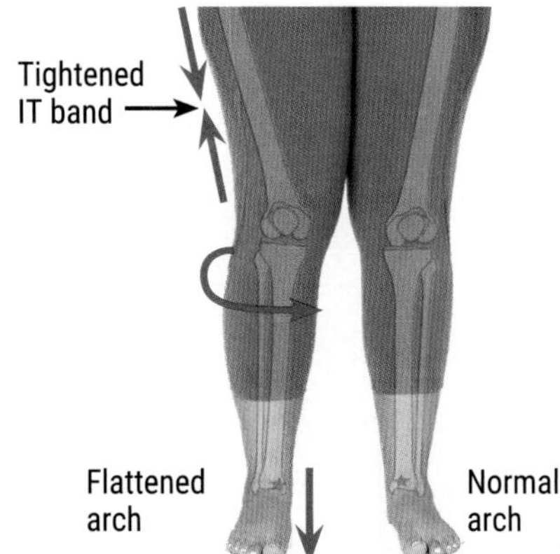

FIGURE 15-27
Example of foot-position effects on the kinetic chain of the lower extremity

like running, walking up or down stairs, or squatting, it is essential that a personal trainer stay in communication with his or her client regarding their pain levels and recommend avoiding exercise when pain is present to limit exacerbation of the condition (Tiemessen et al., 2009).

When observing movement in the presence of knee dysfunction, pay close attention to the hip, ankle, and foot. Because the knee has limited bony or soft-tissue support, it relies on the structures of the adjacent joints for stability and to absorb ground reaction forces. Observe the feet and ankles during a static posture assessment for **pronation** or **supination** in the foot (Figure 15-27). Once any foot, ankle, or hip imbalances have been identified, select the appropriate exercises to enhance ROM or strengthening.

With patellar tendinitis, there is likely tightness in the quadriceps. If the quadriceps muscles are tight, there will be additional strain on the patellar tendon and increased pressure between the patella and the femoral condyles. This can be addressed through self–myofascial release and stretching (Figures 15-28 and 15-29). Muscular-training exercise should focus on restoring strength in the posterior chain, which includes the calf, hamstrings, and gluteal muscle groups.

Patellofemoral Pain Syndrome

PFPS, which is sometimes referred to as patella femoral tracking syndrome, can be caused by various factors including overuse, altered biomechanics, and muscle dysfunction. As with all overuse conditions, lack of proper programming can cause diffuse inflammation of the soft tissue surrounding the patella, resulting in generalized patellofemoral pain. PFPS can occur when repetitive loading activities cause abnormal stress to the knee joint, leading to pain and dysfunction. The excessive loading exceeds the body's physiological balance, which leads to tissue trauma, injury, and pain (Dixit et al., 2007). Recent changes in intensity, frequency, duration, and training environment (e.g., surface) may contribute to this condition.

The patella acts to lengthen the **lever** arm of the quadriceps, allowing the development of more force in concentric and eccentric knee extension. The anatomy of the patellofemoral

FIGURE 15-28
Self–myofascial release of the quadriceps

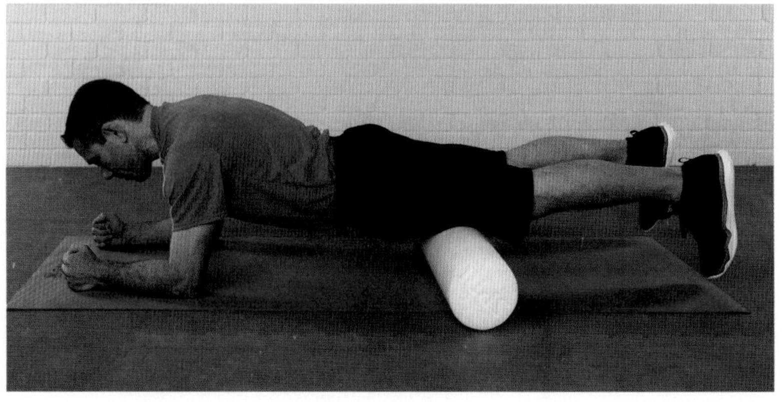

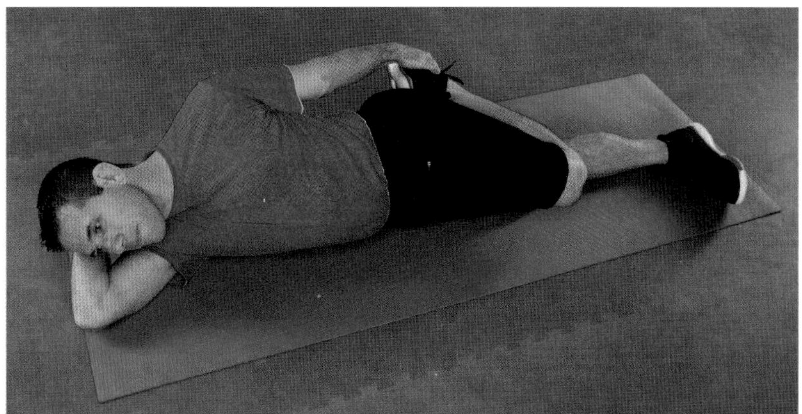

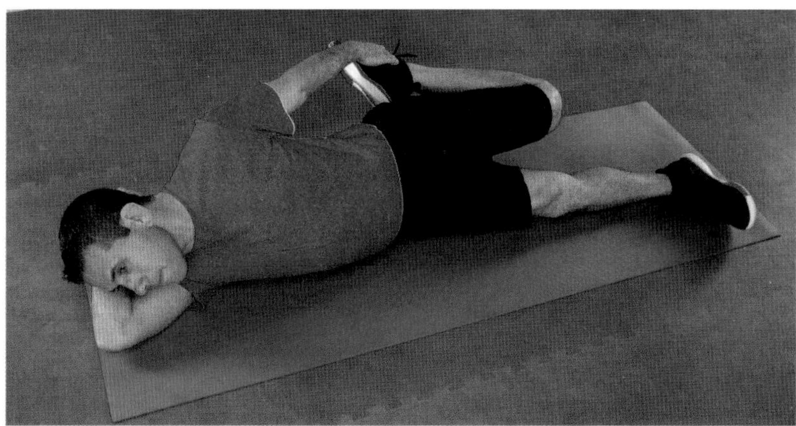

FIGURE 15-29
Quadriceps stretch

joint makes this joint particularly vulnerable (Figure 15-30). When properly positioned, the patella travels superiorly and inferiorly through the trochlear groove. When misaligned, the patella will rub against the lateral epicondyle of the femur, causing pain. PFPS occurs with a lack of control of internal rotation of the femur during knee flexion, when postural malalignment keeps the femur in chronic internal rotation (**genu valgum,** or

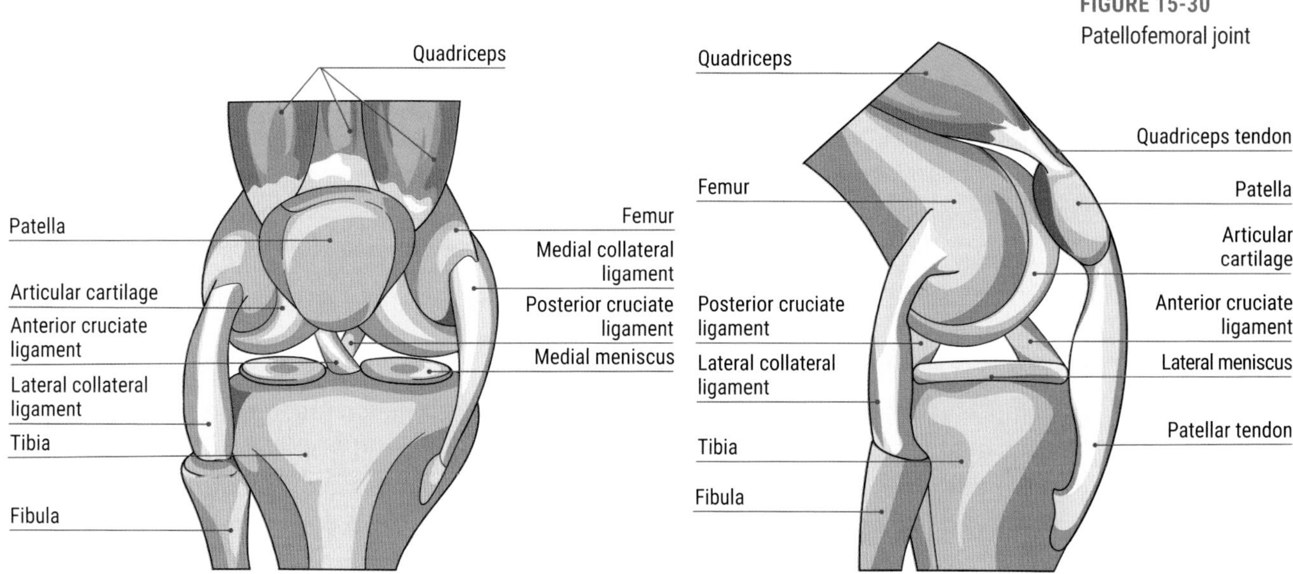

FIGURE 15-30
Patellofemoral joint

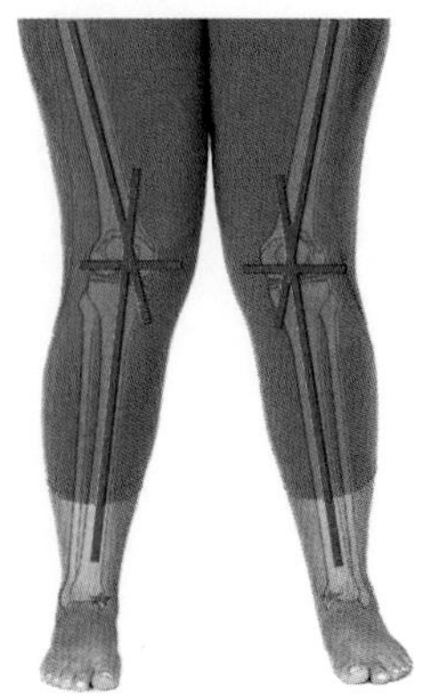

FIGURE 15-31
Bilateral genu valgum, or "knock knees"

"knock knees") (Figure 15-31), or when muscle tightness pulls the patella out of the trochlear groove during knee flexion. If this condition continues uncorrected, over time the cartilage on the posterior aspect of the patella and the femoral condyle can be damaged, causing **chondromalacia patella.** This condition, which may cause swelling and pain, often occurs during activity and is often described as a stabbing pain that occurs intermittently during activity. Commonly, this pain occurs when walking down stairs or down a steep hill.

Biomechanical abnormalities can alter tracking of the patella and/or increase patellofemoral joint stress. Pes planus has been associated with PFPS because it alters the alignment of the knee, causing a compensatory internal rotation of the tibia or femur that alters the dynamics of the patellofemoral joint.

Muscle tightness and length deficits have been associated with PFPS. Tightness in the IT band causes an excessive lateral force to the patella via its fascial connection. Also, tightness in the gastrocnemius/soleus complex (see Figure 9-31, page 362) can lead to compensatory pronation during walking and excessive posterior force that results in increased patellofemoral contact pressure. Muscle weakness in the quadriceps and hip musculature has been associated with PFPS. In fact, research has shown that hip abductor and external rotator weakness can be present in individuals with PFPS (Bolgla & Boling, 2010; Boling, Padua, & Creighton, 2009; Souza & Powers, 2009). This weakness can cause femoral internal rotation and abnormal knee valgus during activity, which can cause abnormal patellofemoral tracking (Boling, Padua, & Creighton, 2009).

During activities that require the quadriceps to decelerate knee flexion, like walking down stairs and walking or running downhill, the natural space between the patella and femur decreases. Often, these activities are painful for clients with PFPS and aggravate inflammation. Personal trainers should be cautious of recommending such exercises.

After identifying areas of tightness, instability, or postural malalignment, the personal trainer can plan exercises accordingly, paying special attention to improving strength in the corresponding hip, thereby improving overall stability.

Knee Arthritis and Knee Replacement

Knee arthritis is a common condition of the knee. Similar to clients who suffer from hip arthritis, stability and strengthening exercises can improve movement and ease efficiency in the performance of ADL. Knee replacement or total knee arthroplasty is recommended for individuals when conservative treatment has failed.

Program Design for the Knee

Approaching program design for clients with knee dysfunction first requires ROM and movement assessments to identify areas that need improved mobility, stability, and/or strength. During a static postural assessment, a personal trainer should identify imbalances between the left and right sides, paying particular attention to the hip, ankle, and foot to determine if any faulty alignment at these important supporting joints are

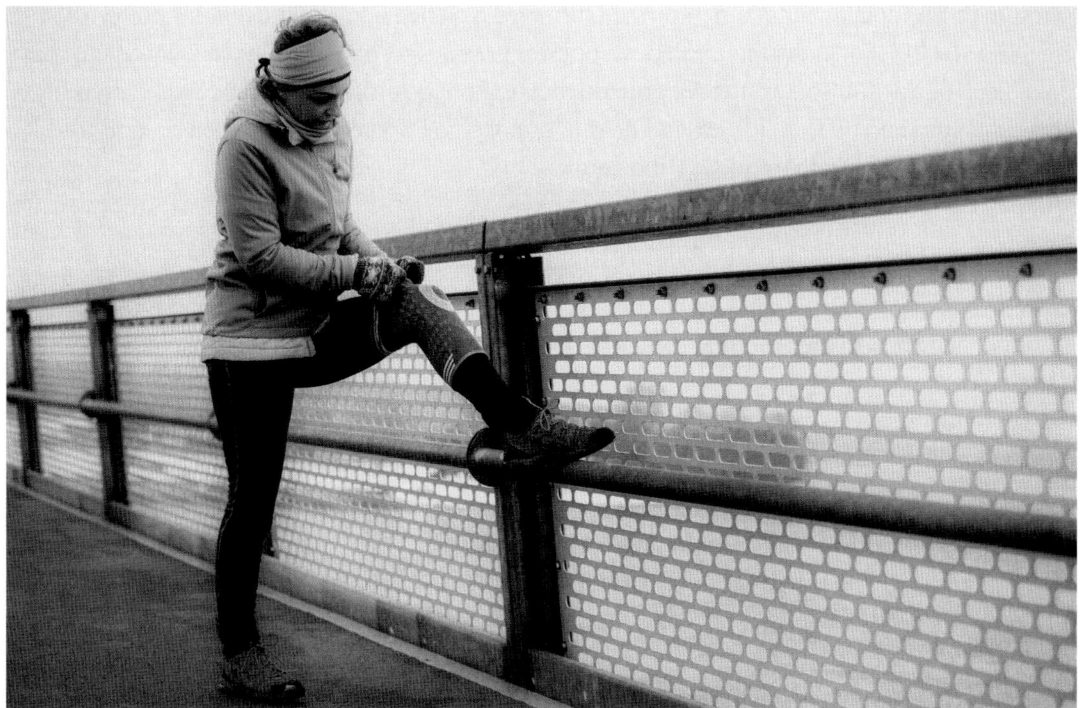

contributing to knee dysfunction. In general, knee pain is exacerbated by open-chain extension exercises (e.g., seated knee extensions). Therefore, these exercises should be avoided in favor of weight-bearing, closed-chain exercises.

As with hip conditions, the stationary bike and recumbent bike are often used to increase ROM and strength for clients with these knee conditions. After a knee replacement, strengthening the quadriceps muscles is an important focus and frequent exercise sessions on a bike can be beneficial. It is also important to ensure mobility in hip hinging and strengthening of the muscles of the posterior chain. Importantly, full-knee ROM may not return. Squatting is an important movement pattern, but ROM at the knee may limit how deep an individual can squat while maintaining proper technique. Once appropriate rhythm in hip hinging is mastered, the stiff-legged deadlift is an excellent exercise for increasing strength in the muscles of the posterior chain.

Consider the following steps when selecting exercises for improving knee function:

- First, address any imbalance between the right and left sides.
- Next, address any tightness and instability in the hip, ankle, and foot that may be contributing to femoral internal rotation.
- Then, improve hip-hinge mobility and stability.
- Lastly, improve the strength of the muscles of the posterior chain.

When designing a program to improve balance among the muscles on opposite sides of the body, personal trainers must remember that the exercises and stretches will be different for each side. Tight muscles on one side should be stretched while the weak muscles of the opposite side should be strengthened. When creating a program, include static stretching early in the workout (after a brief warm-up) to allow for increased ROM, thereby maximizing the effects of the exercises.

A return to full function means a return to efficiency in all five primary movement patterns (see Chapter 10). For individuals with low-back or lower-extremity dysfunction, squatting may be difficult or painful. Squatting is a required movement pattern in most ADL. Sitting onto a chair and standing up from it, getting into and out of a car, and even getting on and off the toilet require the strength and ROM of a squat.

In some cases, a client may be hesitant to squat because of concerns about placing a weighted barbell on his or her back. Instead, a personal trainer might explain that these exercises will start with body weight and be progressed to improve strength and ROM in common activities. In fact, a barbell squat may not ever be included in the program, especially if the client prefers not to do it. Lack of coordination during hip hinging and lack of strength in the posterior chain are common deficiencies involved in squatting. Both are evident in clients who initiate the lowering phase of a squat by driving the knees forward over the toes, often resulting in knee pain. Additionally, when the knees shift past the toes it does not maximize the lever arm for the strong muscles of the posterior chain. Without the strength of the hamstrings and gluteus maximus adequately contributing during the squat, the low back is put under unnecessary stress.

Choosing the right modification depends on the capability of the client. For example, a client who struggles with stability will benefit from holding onto a fixed object or a wall for balance, while a client who struggles with strength will benefit from holding onto the same fixed object for the assistance of using his or her arm strength during the squat. A client who struggles with ROM will benefit from a partial ROM–exercise progression.

Chair Sit:

- This exercise is good for clients who struggle with stability, strength, and/or ROM. The chair sit is an excellent starting point for any client. It can even replace the body-weight squat assessment when the client is not ready for the unsupported movement. This exercise teaches the client to hinge at the hip and maintain a neutral spine while functionally challenging the posterior chain.

FIGURE 15-32
Chair sit with support

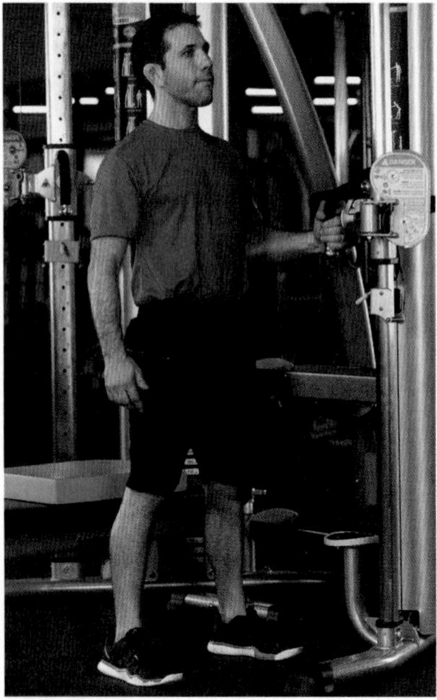

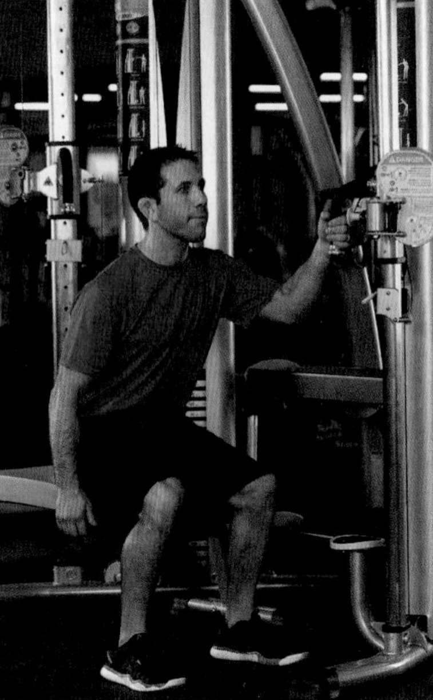

- While holding onto something fixed and stable and standing in front of a box or bench, the client uses his or her hands to assist in sitting back and down onto the bench (Figure 15-32). Holding onto a fixed bar or handle allows the client to use upper-body strength to slow him- or herself down during sitting and to pull during standing.
- The personal trainer should cue the client to flex at the hips first, pushing the hips back as he or she bends the knees. This cue prompts movement to initiate at the hips and encourages proper alignment of the knees and ankles.

- If the client is not strong enough or does not have enough ROM to maintain control throughout the movement, the personal trainer can choose a higher bench or add a pad to the bench to make the seat higher.
- To return to standing, the client should shift the torso forward moving from the hips, with the spine long, and assist with his or her arms to return to a standing position.
- The personal trainer should cue the client to push the feet firmly into the ground. This cue teaches the proper neurological firing of the kinetic chain as a whole.
- To advance this exercise, decrease the reliance on the fixed support by coaching the client to pull less with the arm. The ROM can be increased by lowering the box height.

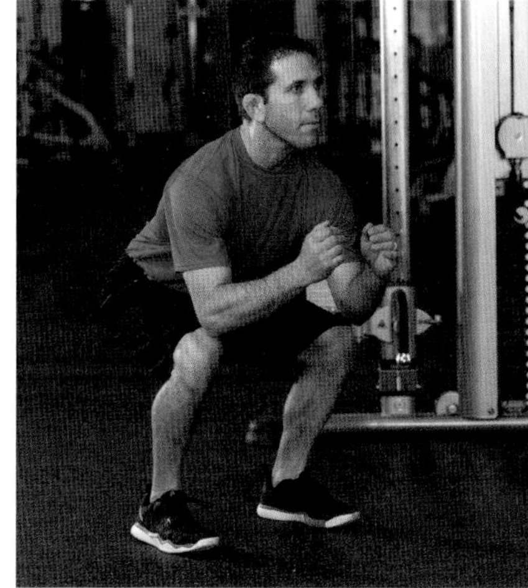

FIGURE 15-33
Body-weight squat

Body-weight Squat:

- This exercise is good for clients who struggle less with stability, strength, and/or ROM. Once a client performs well on the chair sit, he or she is ready for the more unsupported body-weight squat.
- The movement is executed as any other squat would be, with a focus on encouraging a proper hip hinge and maintaining knee alignment (Figure 15-33).
- Consider the assistance of a fixed object, which will act as a counterbalance to those who are having trouble keeping their knees in line with their ankles. As with the chair sit, the client will hold onto the fixed object, which provides more stability when pushing the hips back to squat.
- Cue the client to keep the spine long and press the feet firmly into the ground to return to standing.
- If the knees drift into genu valgum during a squat, cueing the client to push harder into the floor will often correct this position, as it activates more stabilizing musculature.

Cable Squat:

- This exercise is good for clients who are ready to improve posterior chain strength, but not ready for weighted barbell or dumbbell squats.
- Similar to the fixed-object assistance in the chair sit, the client can use a weighted cable to slightly offset his or her weight, giving more support in pushing the hips backward (Figure 15-34).
- Additionally, the weight pulling forward throughout the movement requires the body to counterbalance through the posterior chain and spinal stabilizing muscles, thereby increasing activation of these muscles.

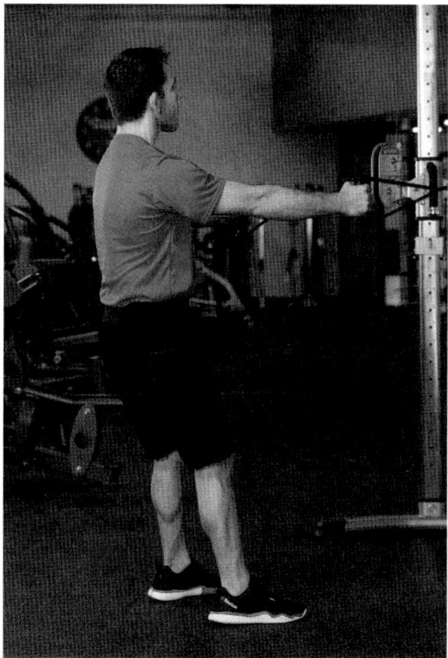

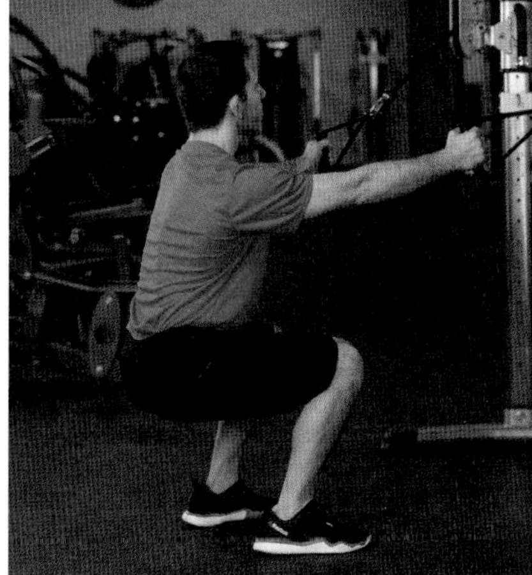

FIGURE 15-34
Cable squat

ANKLE AND LOWER LEG

Shin Splints

"Shin splints" is a general term used to describe exertional, lower-leg pain (Houglum, 2016). Shin splints are typically classified as one of two specific conditions: **medial tibial stress syndrome (MTSS),** which is also called **posterior shin splints,** and **anterior shin splints** (Figure 15-35).

FIGURE 15-35
Site of pain for anterior and posterior shin splints

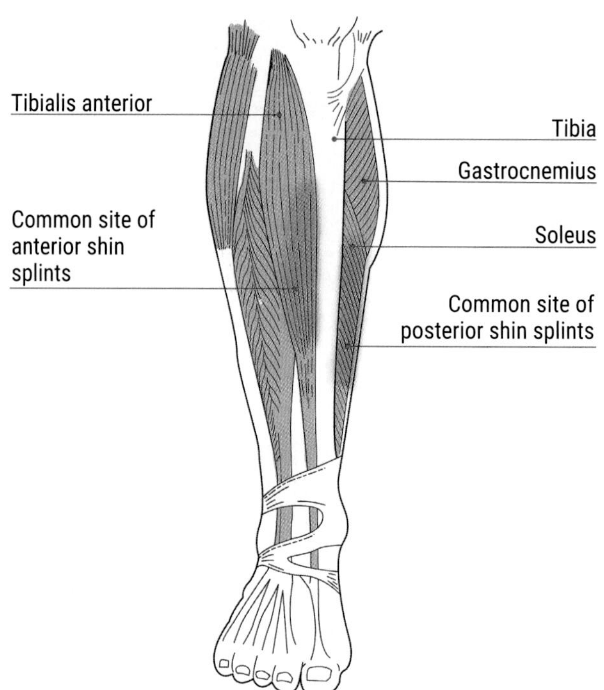

MTSS, an overuse injury that occurs in the active population, is an exercise-induced condition that is often triggered by a sudden change in activity. MTSS is actually **periostitis,** or inflammation of the **periosteum** (connective tissue covering the bone). MTSS is a frequently diagnosed injury in runners, dancers, and military personnel (Brewer & Gregory, 2012). MTSS affects the posterior compartment muscles of the leg (i.e., posterior tibialis, flexor digitorum longus, flexor hallucis longus, and popliteus) (Figure 15-36).

Anterior shin splints are also common in the active population, and pain often occurs in the anterior compartment of the leg. The cause of anterior shin splints is not completely known, but it is often associated with exertional activity. The anterior compartment muscles of the leg (i.e., anterior tibialis, extensor digitorum longus, and extensor hallucis longus), along with the fascia and periosteal lining, are often affected (see Figure 15-36).

Unlike stress fractures, shin splints usually do not require complete rest and clinicians most often recommend a modification to the exercise program. Active individuals may seek out a personal trainer to help them create a safe and effective exercise routine so they can continue working out without exacerbating the condition.

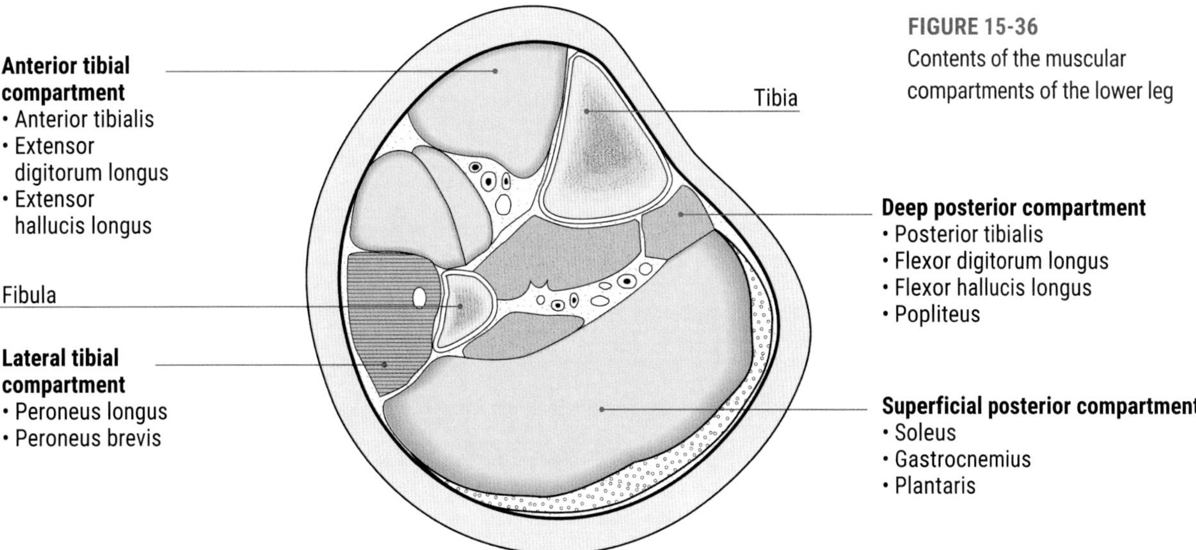

FIGURE 15-36
Contents of the muscular compartments of the lower leg

The personal trainer will need to modify training by offering lower-impact/lower-mileage options and cross-training alternatives to allow the areas to rest and heal. This may require a period of restricted activity, like eliminating running in favor of biking or swimming, where the personal trainer will need to slowly introduce full activity without inciting a return of symptoms. Pain-free stretching of the calf muscles, especially the soleus, has been shown to be effective in relieving symptoms related to MTSS (Brewer & Gregory, 2012) (Figures 15-37 and 15-38).

Static posture and movement assessments may uncover misalignment or instability in the foot or ankle, which may translate up the kinetic chain and contribute to this overuse syndrome. If this is the case, proper return to activity will include improving flexibility and stability in the foot and ankle.

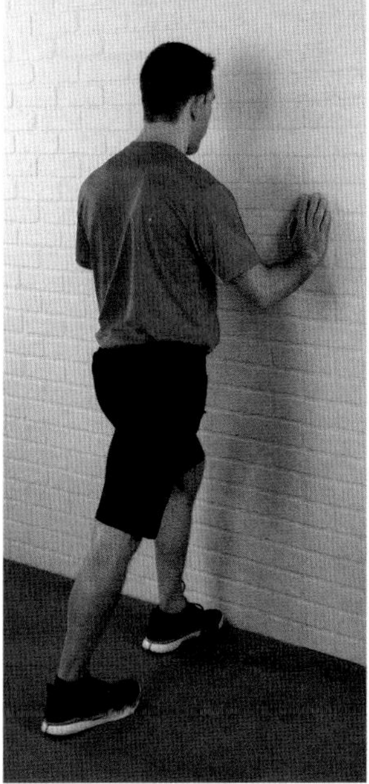

a. Gastrocnemius stretch

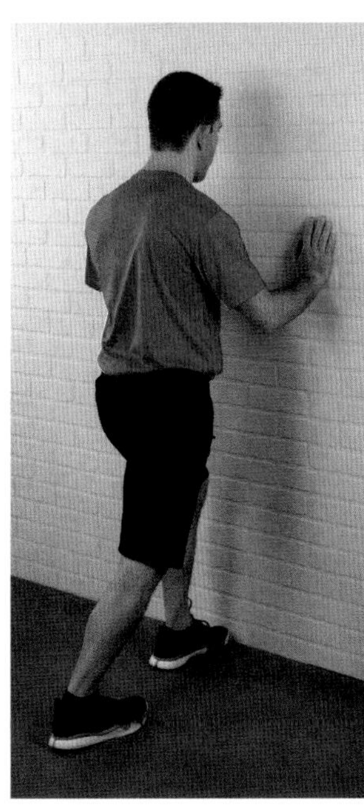

b. Soleus stretch

FIGURE 15-37
Standing calf stretches

Note that slight flexion of the knee joint of the rear leg shifts the emphasis of the stretch from the gastrocnemius to the soleus.

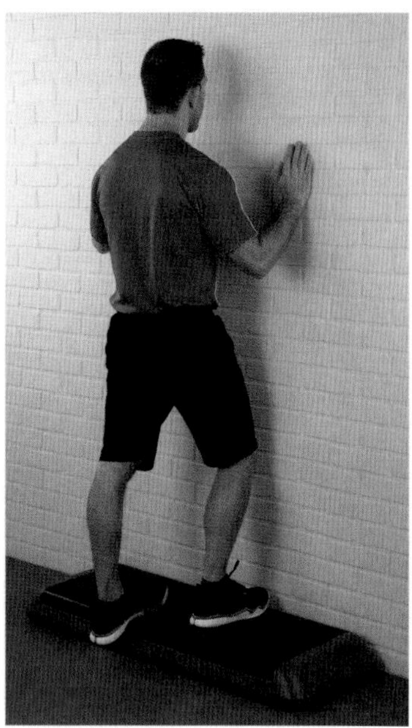

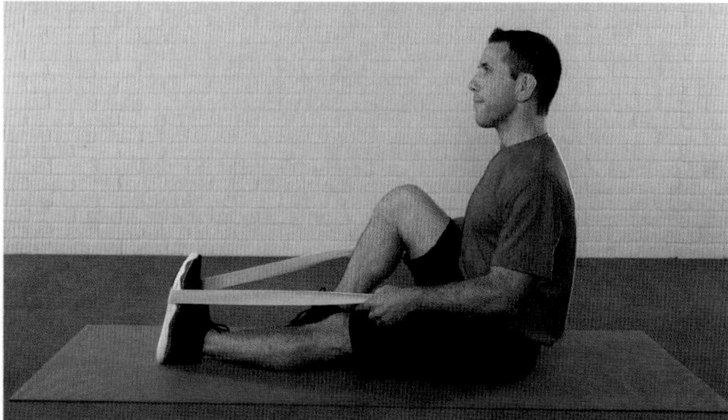

FIGURE 15-38
Calf stretch modifications

Ankle Sprains

Ankle sprains are common injuries affecting about 2 million people in the U.S. each year and only half of these injuries occur in atletic and highly active populations (Herzog et al., 2019). Lateral, or **inversion** ankle sprains are most common while medial, or **eversion** ankle sprains are relatively rare. Of this high incidence, 70% of lateral ankle sprains lead to repetitive sprains and chronic symptoms (Herzog et al., 2019).

Lateral ankle sprains are so named because they effect the ligaments on the lateral side of the ankle, which include the anterior talofibular ligament, calcaneofibular ligament, and posterior talofibular ligament (Figure 15-39). In fact, most ankle sprains (approximately 75%) are to the lateral structures of the ankle (Herzog et al., 2019). These are commonly referred to as inversion ankle sprains, which describes the mechanism of injury—excessive **plantar flexion** and inversion.

Medial, or eversion, ankle sprains are relatively rare because the fibular head on the lateral side reinforces the ankle in eversion. The medial deltoid ligament is the most common structure involved in an eversion sprain, and injury often requires further medical examination to rule out a fracture (Fong et al., 2009).

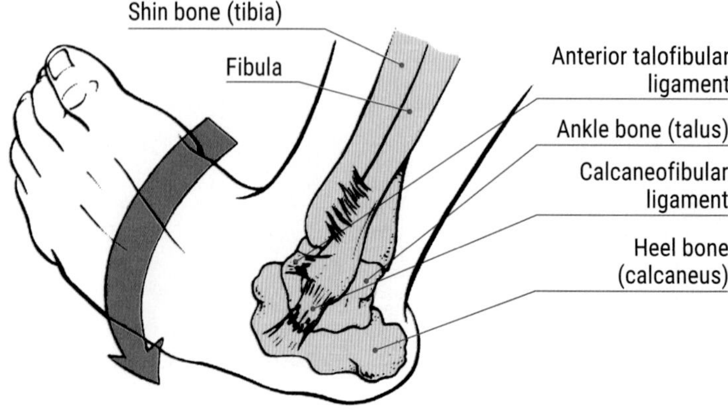

FIGURE 15-39
Lateral ankle sprain

A personal trainer should follow the same return-to-activity guidelines as with any other sprain. As a weight-bearing joint, an ankle sprain may require a slower return to activity, depending on the severity of the injury. Crutches may be indicated in the early phases of healing and a physician may require a brace once the client returns to activity. Remember, the client can return to exercise for non-injured regions, such as the upper body. The injured area should always be protected during activity to avoid re-injury.

Once the client is released from physical therapy to return to exercise, restoring proper proprioception, flexibility, and strength is an important first step. The ligaments contain essential sources of proprioceptive feedback for balance and joint position (Houglum, 2016). Progressing single-leg exercises is an excellent way to promote proprioceptive training. Personal trainers should limit exercises on unstable surfaces like half-foam rollers or mini-trampolines, which can overload the proprioceptive system, especially in a symptomatic or initial post-injury state. Lateral movements create opening of the lateral ankle joint and may create undue strain, so a personal trainer should use caution to ensure that the client is ready to challenge the injury site before recommending exercises in the **frontal plane** (Figure 15-40).

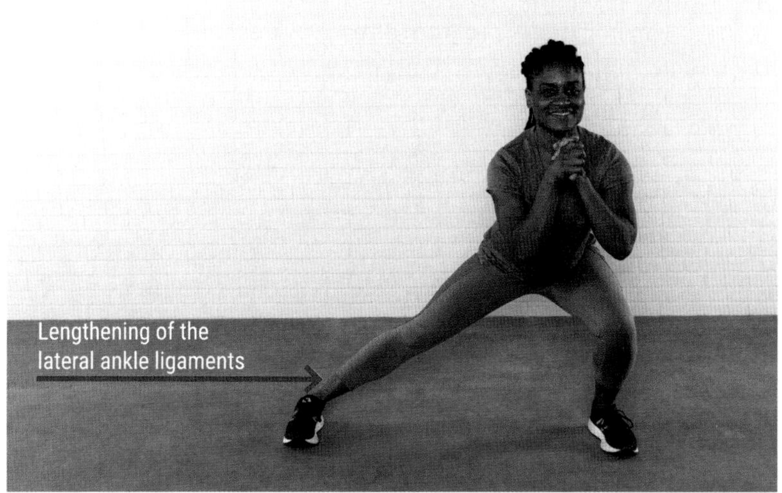

FIGURE 15-40
Lateral movements create opening of the lateral ankle

Achilles Tendinitis

Achilles tendinitis (inflammation of the Achilles tendon) is a common condition that can be a risk factor for a grade II or grade III muscle strain, especially for clients over the age of 45 years (Kettunen et al., 2006). A grade III strain to the Achilles tendon is called an Achilles tendon rupture. Grade II and III strains most commonly occur as a result of chronic Achilles tendinitis. The mechanism of injury is most frequently a sudden start from a standing position, like leaving first base in a softball game. To reduce the risk of injury, a personal trainer can include specific exercises in program design that foster progressively improved elasticity. Any exercise that requires multiplanar quickness and toe-off propulsion will accomplish this goal. Consider the client's capacity when starting out. A simple heel raise may be the appropriate starting point before progressing to drills with an agility ladder.

Some common structural factors that may lead to Achilles tendinitis include **pes cavus** (high arches), pes planus (flat feet), leg-length discrepancies, and lateral ankle instability (Gallo, Plakke, & Silvis, 2012). Fitness-related factors may include poor training mechanics, poor footwear, muscle weakness, and poor flexibility (Gallo, Plakke, & Silvis, 2012).

Regaining calf flexibility is a key strategy in managing this problem, though overstretching of the Achilles tendon can cause irritation to the musculotendinous unit and should be avoided. Instead, gentle dynamic stretching should be a part of the warm-up routine. In particular, when stretching the calf in a standing position, the client should keep the foot in a neutral position to avoid excessive pronation or supination. The client should be taught to properly position the foot to point straight ahead, which will ensure that the target tissues will be stretched (see Figures 15-37 and 15-38).

Both mobility and stability exercises will benefit the client who struggles with Achilles tendinitis. Progressively regaining ROM and strength in **dorsiflexion** and power during the push-off phase of gait is important for these clients.

Plantar Fasciitis

Plantar fasciitis is an inflammation of the connective tissue (plantar fascia) on the bottom, or plantar surface, of the foot (Figure 15-41). A client with plantar fasciitis may be cleared to exercise, possibly with restrictions from his or her medical professional. The goal is to design a program that challenges the client but does not excessively load the foot. Integrating specific foot exercises into the client's general fitness program often provides the best results. This allows the client to work toward his or her fitness goals as well as address the foot problems.

FIGURE 15-41
Plantar fascia

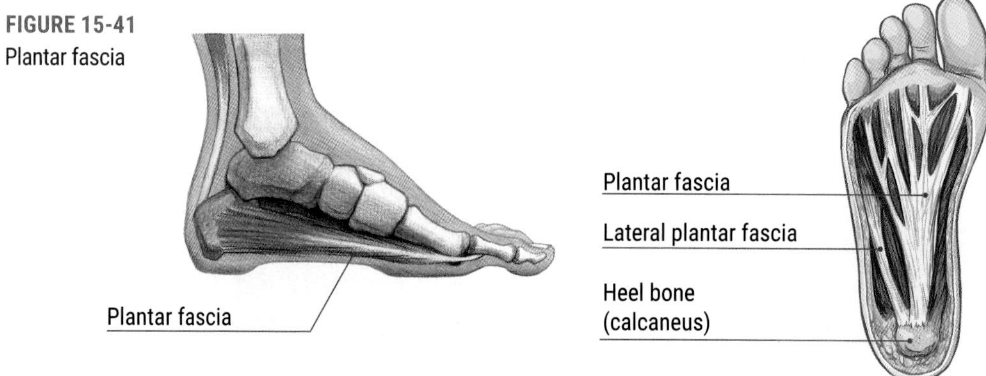

Stretching of the gastrocnemius, soleus (see Figures 15-37 and 15-38), and plantar fascia (Figure 15-42) is beneficial and has been shown to help relieve symptoms. Self-myofascial release techniques, which include rolling the foot over a tennis ball, self-myofascial release ball, or golf ball has been shown to increase ROM in dorsiflexion (Stanek, Sullivan, & Davis, 2018) and relieve pain in the plantar fascia. Other studies have shown that applying self-myofascial release techniques to the entire posterior chain may increase ROM in dorsiflexion (Do, Kim, & Yim, 2018). Strengthening the foot's intrinsic muscles may help to improve arch stability and help decrease the stresses imposed across the plantar fascia.

Program Design for the Foot, Ankle, and Lower Leg

Program-design considerations that provide the most support for the foot, ankle, and lower leg depend on the client's barefoot position while standing. Clients with pes planus (flat feet) or pes cavus (high arches) are not necessarily symptomatic. This is most noticeable when observed from behind, as the Achilles tendon will appear bowed.

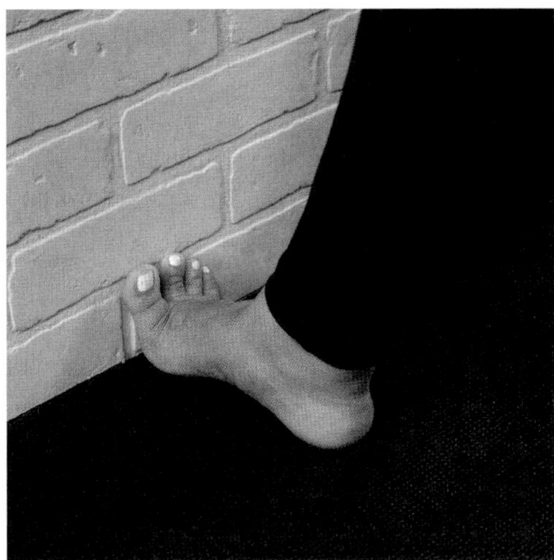
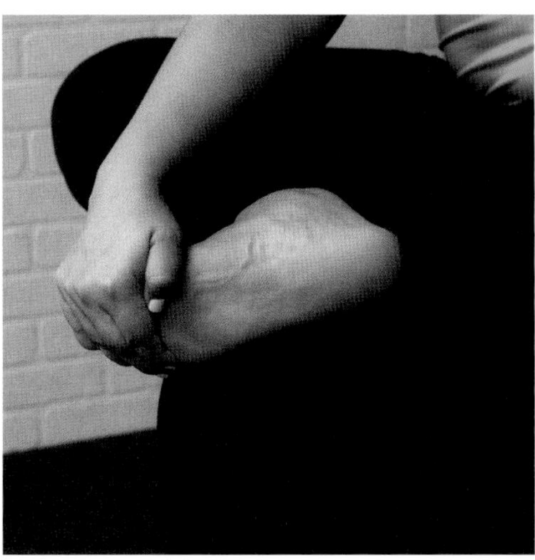

FIGURE 15-42
Plantar fascia stretches

The first step to addressing these conditions is improving function through increased mobility and stability. Stretching of these muscles is most effective when done daily or even twice daily. A stretching program can be recommended for a client to do on his or her own. Simply using a tennis ball for self–myofascial release of the plantar fascia is of benefit regardless of the lower leg and/or foot dysfunction.

Balance work can also be executed daily without risk of overuse. A simple recommendation is that clients work on balance by standing on the affected leg while brushing their teeth. This habit will ensure that clients are getting one to two minutes of proprioceptive training twice daily.

Consider the following steps when selecting exercises for improving foot and ankle function:

- First, address mobility and stability in the foot and ankle.
- Next, improve strength in the muscles that control movement in the **sagittal plane.**
- Then, improve strength in the muscles that control movement in the **transverse plane** and frontal plane.
- Lastly, improve strength in the muscles of the posterior chain.

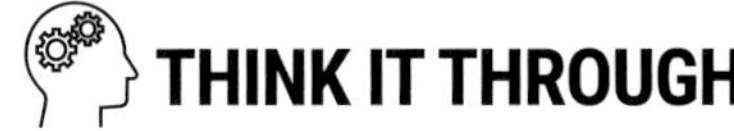

THINK IT THROUGH

Programming for a Client with Pain

Designing a safe and effective exercise program to support the goals of clients with pain and/or injury is a challenging yet essential function of a personal trainer. Using the ACE Mover Method and ACE IFT Model Exercise Programming Template found in Chapter 11, create an exercise program and potential next steps for a client presenting with an injury or condition from this chapter.

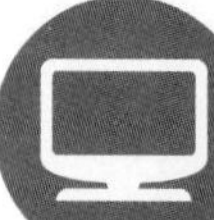

ACE UNIVERSITY

If your study program includes the ACE University, visit www.ACEfitness.org/MyACE and log in to your My ACE Account to take full advantage of the ACE Personal Trainer Study Program and online guided study experience.

A variety of media to support and expand on the material in this text is provided to facilitate learning and best prepare you for the ACE Personal Trainer Certification exam and a career as a personal trainer.

SUMMARY

A personal trainer may work with clients who have had various musculoskeletal injuries. It is important for a personal trainer to understand that his or her scope of practice includes movement assessment, but not injury assessment, and instructions from a medical professional must always be followed. In developing exercise programs for clients in the inflammation phase of injury healing, program design should avoid challenging the injured tissue. As healing progresses into later stages, exercise may challenge the tissue enough for strengthening adaptation, but not so much that the injury is aggravated. A personal trainer should remember too that an injury or chronic condition may present an emotional challenge for the client. A client-centered approach, rooted in non-judgement, empathy, and understanding, should always be employed, progressing only as the client is ready to do so. Working with clients who have suffered from injuries presents an opportunity for the personal trainer to enter into discussion and collaboration with other health professionals who may be involved in post-injury rehabilitation.

REFERENCES

American College of Sports Medicine (2013). *ACSM's Resource Manual for Guidelines for Exercise Testing and Prescription* (7th ed.). Philadelphia: Wolters Kluwer/Lippincott Williams & Wilkins.

American Psychological Association (2019). *Managing Chronic Pain: How Psychologists Can Help with Pain Management.* https://www.apa.org/helpcenter/pain-management

Baba, N.H. & Daruis, D. (2016). Repetitive Strain Injury (RSI) among computer users: A case study in telecommunication company. *Malaysian Journal of Public Health Medicine,* 48–52.

Bisset L., Coombes B., & Vicenzino, B. (2011). Tennis elbow. *Clinical Evidence (Online),* pii: 1117.

Bolgla, L.A. & Boling, M.C. (2011). An update for the conservative management of patellofemoral pain syndrome: A systematic review of the literature from 2000 to 2010. *International Journal of Sports Physical Therapy,* 6, 2, 112–125.

Boling, M.C., Padua, D.A., & Creighton, R. (2009). Concentric and eccentric torque of the hip musculature in individuals with and without patellofemoral pain. *Journal of Athletic Training,* 44, 1, 7–13.

Boyajian-O'Neill, L.A. et al. (2008). Diagnosis and management of piriformis syndrome: An osteopathic approach. *Journal of the American Osteopathic Association,* 108, 11, 657–664.

Brewer, R.B. & Gregory, A.J.M. (2012). Chronic lower leg pain in athletes: A guide for the differential diagnosis, evaluation, and treatment. *Sports Health,* 4, 2, 121–127.

Buganza-Tepole, A. & Kuhl, E. (2013). Systems-based approaches toward wound healing. *Pediatric Research,* 73, 553–563.

Dixit, S. et al. (2007). Management of patellofemoral pain syndrome. *American Family Physician,* 75, 194–204.

Do, K., Kim, J. & Yim, J. (2018). Acute effect of self-myofascial release using a foam roller on the plantar fascia on hamstring and lumbar spine superficial back line flexibility. *Physical Therapy Rehabilitation Science,* 7, 35–40.

Eleftherios A. et al. (2011). The knee meniscus: Structure-function, pathophysiology, current repair techniques, and prospects for regeneration. *Biomaterials,* 32, 30, 7411–7431.

Fong, D.T.P. et al. (2009). Understanding acute ankle ligamentous sprain injury in sports. *Sports Medicine, Arthroscopy, Rehabilitation, Therapy & Technology,* 1, 14.

Gallo, R.A., Plakke, M., & Silvis, M.L. (2012). Common leg injuries of long-distance runners: Anatomical and biomechanical approach. *Sports Health,* 4, 6, 485–495.

Herzog, M.M. et al. (2019). Epidemiology of ankle sprains and chronic ankle instability. *Journal of Athletic Training,* 54, 6, 603–610.

Hooten, W.M. (2016). Chronic pain and mental health disorders. *Mayo Clinic Proceedings,* 91, 7, 955–970.

Houglum, P.A. (2016). *Therapeutic Exercise for Musculoskeletal Injuries* (4th ed.). Champaign, Ill.: Human Kinetics.

Kettunen, J.A. et al. (2006). Health of master track and field athletes: A 16-year follow-up study. *Clinical Journal of Sports Medicine,* 16, 2, 142–148.

Kremers, M. H. et al. (2015). Prevalence of total hip and knee replacement in the United States. *The Journal of Bone and Joint Surgery, American Volume,* 97, 17, 1386–1397.

Martinez, J.M. & Honsik, K. (2006). Iliotibial band syndrome. *E-Medicine Online Journal* (Web MD), Dec 6, 1–14.

McGill, S.M. (2016). *Low Back Disorders: Evidence Based Prevention and Rehabilitation* (3rd ed.). Champaign, Ill.: Human Kinetics.

Page P. (2012). Current concepts in muscle stretching for exercise and rehabilitation. *International Journal of Sports Physical Therapy,* 7, 1, 109–119.

Park, G.W. et al. (2016). Rotator cuff repair in patients over 75 years of age: Clinical outcome and repair integrity. *Clinics in Orthopedic Surgery,* 8, 4, 420–427.

Pek, J.H. (2017). Guidelines for bystander first aid 2016. *Singapore Medical Journal,* 58, 7, 411–417.

Peng, B-G. (2013). Pathophysiology, diagnosis, and treatment of discogenic low back pain. *World Journal of Orthopaedics,* 4, 2, 42–52.

Shamaei, K. & Dollar, A.M. (2011). On the mechanics of the knee during the stance phase of the gait. *IEEE International Conference on Rehabilitation Robotics.* DOI: 10.1109/ICORR.2011.5975478

Souza, R.B. & Powers, C.M. (2009). Differences in hip kinematics, muscle strength, and muscle activation between subjects with and without patellofemoral pain. *Journal of Orthopaedic and Sports Physical Therapy*, 39, 1, 12–19.

Stanek, J., Sullivan, T., & Davis, S. (2018). Comparison of compressive myofascial release and the Graston technique for improving ankle-dorsiflexion range of motion. *Journal of Athletic Training*, 53, 2, 160–167.

Strong, J.A. et al. (2013). Preclinical studies of low back pain. *Molecular Pain*, 9, 17.

Sugimoto, D. et al. (2015). Specific exercise effects of preventive neuromuscular training intervention on anterior cruciate ligament injury risk reduction in young females: Meta-analysis and subgroup analysis. *British Journal of Sports Medicine*, 49, 282–289.

Taylor, S.A. & Hannafin, J.A. (2012). Evaluation and management of elbow tendinopathy. *Sports Health*, 4, 5, 384–393.

Tiemessen, I.J.H. et al. (2009). Risk factors for developing jumper's knee in sport and occupation: A review. *BMC Research Notes*, 2, 127.

van den Bekerom, M.P. et al. (2012). What is the evidence for rest, ice, compression, and elevation therapy in the treatment of ankle sprains in adults? *Journal of Athletic Training*, 47, 4, 435–443.

Whiting, W.C. & Zernicke, R.F. (2008). *Biomechanics of Musculoskeletal Injury* (2nd ed.). Champaign, Ill.: Human Kinetics.

SUGGESTED READINGS

American Council on Exercise (2015). *Medical Exercise Specialist Manual*. San Diego: American Council on Exercise

American Heart Association (2016). *Heartsaver First Aid CPR AED*. Jackson, Tenn.: Ingram.

American Red Cross (2014). *First Aid/CPR/AED Participant's Manual* (2nd ed.). Washington, D.C.: American Red Cross.

Kendall, F.P. et al. (2005). *Muscles: Testing and Function with Posture and Pain* (5th ed.). Philadelphia: Lippincott Williams & Wilkins.

SECTION V

Professional Responsibilities

CHAPTER 16
Legal Guidelines and Business Considerations

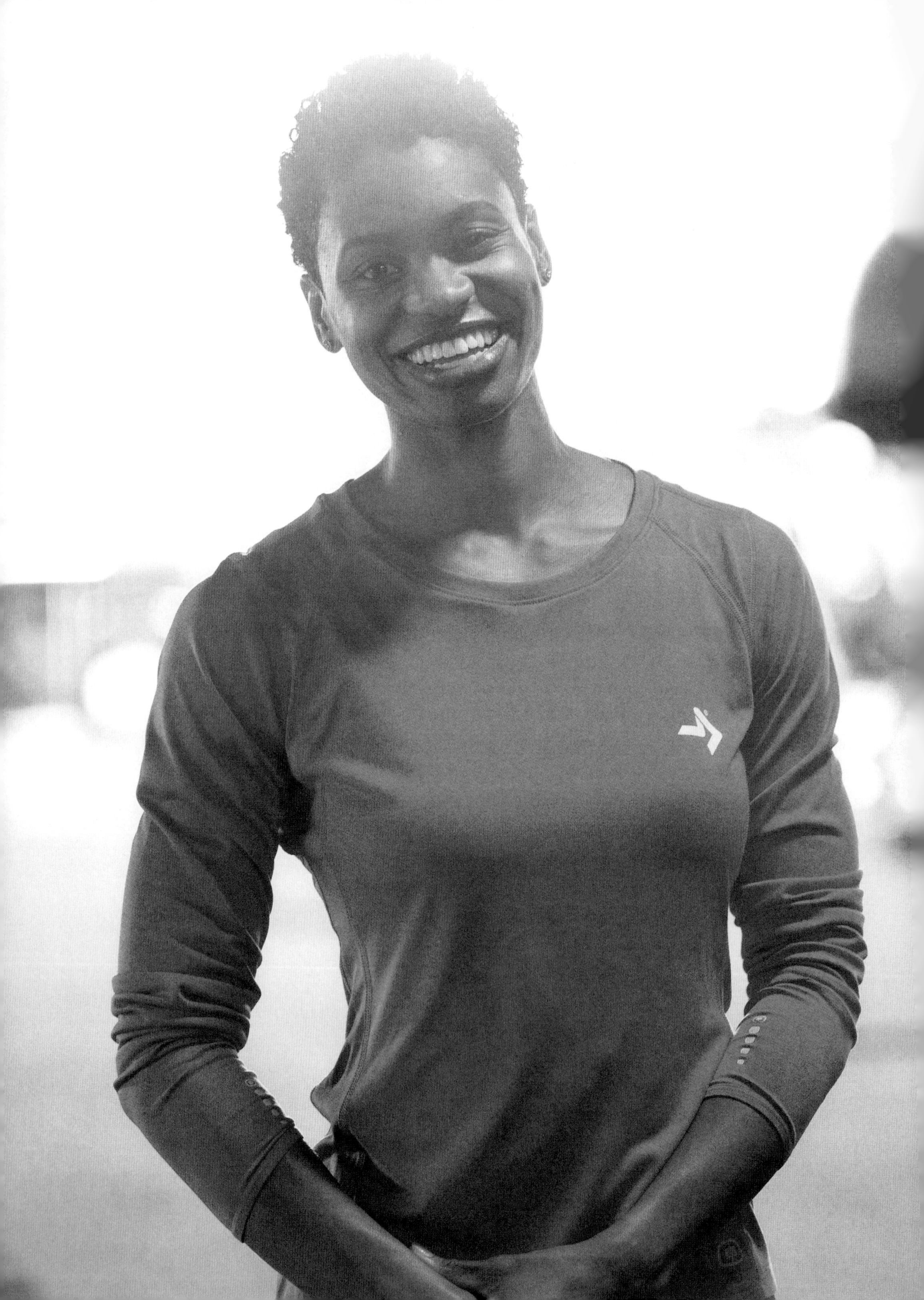

CHAPTER 16

Legal Guidelines and Business Considerations

MARK S. NAGEL, EDD
Professor, Sport and Entertainment Management Department, University of South Carolina

IN THIS CHAPTER

LEARNING OBJECTIVES:

Upon completion of this chapter, the reader will be able to:

- Identify the advantages and disadvantages of various business structures as well as employee versus independent contractor status
- Explain the proper use of contracts, agreements to participate, informed consent, and waivers
- Describe the legal responsibilities of a personal trainer, including those related to facilities, equipment, supervision, and instruction
- Identify the legal implications of various business practices, including marketing activities and social media use
- Implement an appropriate risk-management protocol to not only mitigate potential legal liability, but also to ensure a safe environment for clients

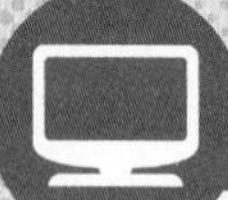

ACE UNIVERSITY

If your study program includes the ACE University, visit www.ACEfitness.org/MyACE and log in to your My ACE Account to take full advantage of the ACE Personal Trainer Study Program and online guided study experience.

A variety of media to support and expand on the material in this text is provided to facilitate learning and best prepare you for the ACE Personal Trainer Certification exam and a career as a personal trainer.

ACE® Certified Personal Trainers typically do not need to be reminded of the importance of studying the latest research related to physical activity and nutrition. Most personal trainers know that it is essential to spend considerable time and energy developing exercise programs to help clients achieve their goals. However, the majority of personal trainers often neglect the legal issues pertinent to operating a fitness business. Far too often, filed lawsuits are the first indication that a personal trainer has not adhered to established legal guidelines. In the vast majority of these cases, a simple understanding of the law and a personal trainer's responsibilities could have prevented the lawsuit or mitigated the potential damages.

This chapter addresses many of the standard legal and business concerns that personal trainers may have regarding business structure, employment status, **contracts,** insurance, and **risk management.** It also addresses the **scope of practice** in personal training and summarizes legal responsibilities.

The guidelines offered, while based on sport law and the experience of exercise professionals, are not intended as legal advice, but rather as guidance. Every personal trainer should utilize these principles when conferring with attorneys who specialize in the appropriate areas. As a personal trainer's knowledge of the law increases, the ability to anticipate potential legal concerns is heightened, which not only helps to decrease potential litigation, but also provides a better environment for clients, vendors, and **employees.**

Ideally, personal trainers will regularly consult with an attorney who is aware of the unique laws governing the personal trainer's city, state, and county to remain abreast of recent legal developments. In addition, personal trainers should diligently read publications and attend conference presentations that address legal issues, as the **standard of care** and accepted business practices can be altered through legislation or case law.

Do not open a personal-training business without first consulting with an attorney who understands the fitness industry and its unique legal standing within your state.

Business Structure

Much of the personal-training industry is comprised of entrepreneurs—individuals who undertake new financial ventures. Many personal trainers start their careers as an offshoot of their own physical training. New personal trainers often begin by working with close friends and family members before expanding their businesses to a greater assortment of clients. Most personal trainers, like many entrepreneurs in other industries, do not realize that the moment they begin providing advice in exchange for financial considerations they have created a business. Every business "owner," even one who is working part-time in a "hobby," should understand the ramifications of business structure.

Each personal trainer must decide the type of business structure under which he or she will operate. Each type retains certain legal and financial advantages and disadvantages. The size and scope of the business—in both the short- and long-term—will be important factors in the initial selection of the business entity. The business can be altered if conditions warrant, but personal trainers must understand that legal issues arising at a time when one structure

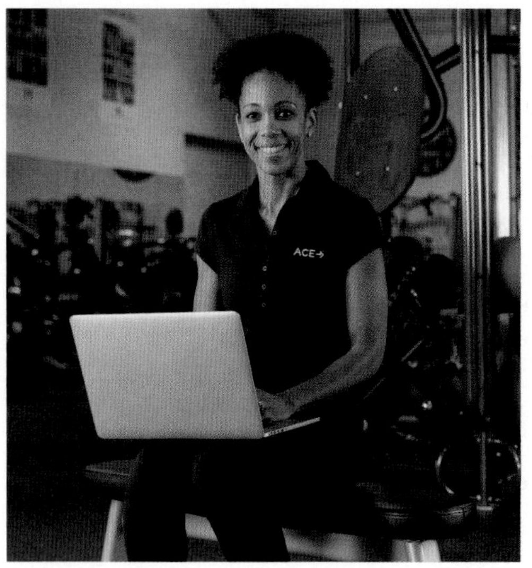

was utilized cannot simply be mitigated by then switching to a different structure. The business entity employed at the time of the incident will usually be utilized by the courts in the event of a lawsuit. Typically, for-profit businesses* operate under one of the following structures: **sole proprietorship, partnership,** or **corporation.**

SOLE PROPRIETORSHIP

The vast majority of for-profit businesses in the United States operate as sole proprietorships. As the name implies, a sole proprietorship is a business owned and operated by one person. Since the individual owner operates the business, extensive meetings to determine strategy and company direction are not necessary, as the owner can simply make decisions. Creating a sole proprietorship does not require any formal paperwork and there is minimal ongoing paperwork necessary (compared to other business types) to sustain the business. It exists as long as the owner operates the business, and profits from the business belong to the owner. However, financial losses and liabilities are also the sole responsibility of the owner. In a sole proprietorship, there is no **corporate veil** that shields the actions of the business from the personal responsibility of the owner, even if the owner conducts business under a different company name. Personal training involves extensive physical movement, which often results in injuries even when proper techniques are utilized. The likelihood of injuries results in a greater opportunity for clients to potentially seek financial remuneration. One successful lawsuit against a sole proprietor could destroy not only the business's finances, but also the owner's personal finances, as courts have often required sole proprietors to sell assets, including their homes, to pay for incurred debts or court judgments.

There are other potential drawbacks to operating a personal-training business as a sole proprietorship. Since the business is owned by one individual, it can be more difficult to raise capital. In addition, though sole proprietorships may certainly hire employees, often the business cannot effectively function without the presence of the owner. Most personal trainers directly work with all of their clients, so if the owner takes a vacation, incoming revenue is potentially decreased. In addition, newly established personal trainers often maintain consistent contact with their clients to ensure that they do not have any reason to seek other potential trainers. This can create difficulties if the personal trainer is sick or has to attend to an emergency.

---

* Though this chapter primarily focuses on for-profit businesses, there are government-operated businesses as well as nonprofit organizations that operate with different legal and financial constraints. Even though a personal trainer may be training a client at a government-operated business (e.g., a community recreation center) or a nonprofit organization (e.g., a YMCA fitness center), the personal trainer may retain a different business structure for liability purposes. Personal trainers should consult legal counsel prior to training any client.

PARTNERSHIP

Two or more people who agree to operate a business and share profits and losses may form a partnership. Two personal trainers, for example, could form a company, or a personal trainer could become part owner of a fitness facility. Although partnerships may be created without filing paperwork, any partnership should have legal documents that establish the rules of operation. This agreement should clearly define and explain the structure for authority, the partners' rights, expected performance and contributions from each partner, buy-out clauses, income distribution, and responsibility for debts. Operating a partnership without a partnership agreement—even when it involves family members or close personal friends—is asking for potential disaster. Even partnerships that begin based on strong relationships can become strained as the business develops. Furthermore, even if the partners maintain a solid personal or professional relationship, other non-business-related occurrences can cause tremendous stress on the company. If one partner becomes divorced or deceased, other family members may become involved in the ownership and operation of the partnership. In extreme cases, the lack of a partnership agreement can result in the courts requiring the business to be dissolved to settle financial disputes. Partnership paperwork should be designed to address any eventuality, including the death or incapacity of one of the partners.

Do not assume a partnership will exist forever and that the partners will remain compatible and cordial throughout their business relationship.

As potential partners plan and design their business, the type of partnership utilized should be identified. **General partnerships** are merely the joining of two or more individuals to own and operate a business. A general-partnership agreement could divide ownership equally or unequally. Most attorneys will advise against operating a business as a 50-50 partnership, even if it involves owners from the same family. A 50-50 partnership can result in a stalemate, because neither partner can institute policy without the permission of the other, since business decisions must be approved by a majority (50.1%) of the owners. However, disproportionate ownership positions in partnerships can also present problems for the **minority partner** or partners. If a two-person partnership is owned with a 60-40 split, the minority partner is only entitled to 40% of the profits and retains only 40% input regarding company decisions. That particular partner could be out-voted on any organizational issue. Some investors in partnerships who will take a minority position are not as likely to invest as much money as they would if they received operating control.

General partnerships can be established either formally or informally. An **express partnership** can be created by a contract between the parties. However, an **implied partnership** can be created and recognized by the judicial system if individuals act as partners (such as by sharing a company checking account or jointly signing for a business loan). It is critical that owners understand the consequences of their actions when operating a business, as the courts will likely examine the activities of the owners when determining potential liabilities if there is no clearly defined partnership agreement.

A partnership retains the same potential detriments as a sole proprietorship. Personal **liability** for company losses or judgments is retained by the partners. In some cases, minority partners may be personally liable for a greater share of the companies' liabilities than their percentage

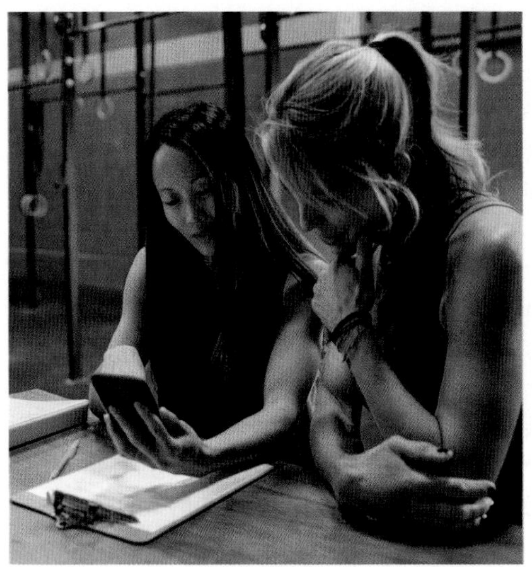

of ownership. If a partner who owns 55% of a business files for bankruptcy, a judgment against the business may result in the minority partner being required to cover the financial obligation of the insolvent general partner, even though the minority partner owns only 45% of the company. For this reason, some partnerships involve **limited partners.** While a general partner typically retains personal liability, limited partners are only liable for their direct financial contribution.

However, in exchange for this limited liability, limited partners do not retain any formal managerial input regarding the operation of the business. Limited partners must also remember that the general partner or partners still retain personal liability and they should ensure that a judgment or other financial loss will not bankrupt the general partners, and hence the overall company. It is important to note that limited partners may retain more than 50% of the ownership in the company. For example, a limited partner who owns 70% of the organization still does not have any formal input into the company's operation but is entitled to 70% of the company's profits.

At some point in a personal trainer's career, decisions regarding partnerships are likely to be contemplated. As personal trainers expand their client base, it may become difficult to organize a time for individual face-to-face interaction with each client. The personal trainer could elect to hire an employee or find a partner who could alleviate some concerns if multiple clients desire to work out at the same time. Personal training also involves marketing and advertising, as well as scheduling clients. Some personal trainers have entered into partnership agreements where one partner does the "hands-on" training while the other coordinates the "office" activities. These particular types of partnerships are especially prone to problems, as one partner may not understand or fully value the importance of the other partner's duties and activities. Ultimately, any potential partnership can become contentious and should not be entered into without considerable contemplation, and only after seeking personalized legal advice.

A partnership ends when a partner dies or becomes bankrupt, or its partners engage in any illegal activity. A partnership could also be discontinued by the courts if one of the partners is deemed to be mentally incapacitated. One difficulty that sometimes arises when terminating partnerships is if the business is not making any money. Ultimately, if the business cannot make money, the partnership will be dissolved. However, in some cases, one or more partners may have differing opinions about the future financial viability of the company. If one or more partners wish to continue the business, but one or more other partners do not, a resolution must occur. In many cases, these split decisions regarding continuing the business will require court intervention to dissolve the partnership or to determine how, and at what compensation, one or more partners may exit.

Though sole proprietorships and partnerships offer potential problems due to personal liability for the business's actions, they usually provide potential benefits from **flow-through taxation.**

Typically, profits are taxed at lower personal rates rather than higher corporate rates. In addition, yearly losses can flow through to be used by the owner to offset profits from other income. Potential investors, who will be providing money rather than day-to-day labor, will often desire to take positions as limited partners in a business. The limited partnership protects them from personal liability (beyond their initial investment) and allows them to have a low tax rate on profits if the business is successful or to use the losses during poorly performing periods to offset income from other investments.

CORPORATIONS

Corporations are designed to create a "separate" entity from the investors and operators of a business. Regulated by state and federal (and in some cases international) laws, corporations exist as distinct legal entities. Investors own shares of the corporation, which limits the investors' personal liability. As long as the corporation and the investors maintain "separate" existences, the corporate veil protects investors from personal liability. It is critical that investors in a corporation do not "act" as the corporation or the corporate veil may be pierced. For example, if an investor mixes his personal checking account with that of the corporation, he or she may be deemed by the courts to be acting as the corporation and therefore be personally liable for potential corporate debts and judgments.

Forming and maintaining a corporation is much more burdensome than a sole proprietorship or partnership. Corporations are formed and registered in the office of the secretary of state (typically in the state where the business operates). Different states have various requirements, so a corporation that will operate in multiple states must determine the "best" state for short- and long-term operation. A person forming a corporation must select a name that has not previously been registered in that state. The appropriate notice of incorporation forms must be completed, fees must be paid, and a registered agent must be identified. The registered agent is the contact person in the event a lawsuit is filed against the corporation. Typically, it is one of the corporation's founders or it may be an attorney who represents the corporation. It is important that the person "registered" as the agent for the corporation be readily accessible. After being notified of a lawsuit, the registered agent must notify personnel to take appropriate action. In some cases, the registered agent must be a resident of the state in which the corporation operates. The secretary of state's office can help individuals complete the appropriate paperwork, but some entrepreneurs seek legal guidance to diminish the time and potential aggravation of incorporating.

Once the incorporation is complete, the corporation is recognized as a distinct legal entity. The shareholders will elect a board of directors who in turn will hire the executive management team. In cases where there are few shareholders in the corporation, such as when the corporation is first created, investors may fill all of the corporate positions. Once established, the company must annually complete and file operational paperwork with the state, and it also must file tax returns with appropriate local, state, and federal governments.

There are a variety of corporate structures and potential types of shareholders (e.g., preferred and common), and any personal trainer who is considering forming a corporation should seek legal advice to ensure that the proper corporate entity is created for both short- and long-term plans. Corporations can change their form, but this can require considerable time and may involve extensive (and costly) paperwork. In general, some of the main corporate structures include **subchapter S-corporations, limited liability companies (LLCs), limited liability partnerships (LLPs),** and **C-corporations,** as well as **franchise** operation business models.

Subchapter S-Corporations

The main financial advantage of subchapter S-corporations (often called sub-S corps or simply S-corps) is that profits flow through the business to the shareholders and are taxed as ordinary income. S-corps are the most "typical" type of corporation used by personal-training businesses that do not operate as a sole proprietorship or partnership.

Shareholders in S-corps are shielded from personal liability—beyond their investment—by the corporate veil. S-corps can own subsidiaries that operate independently (from a legal standpoint), which enables the S-corp to be shielded from liability. S-corps do have some significant drawbacks, particularly if the business is going to grow and seek a wide variety of investors. S-corps must be based in the United States, can only have up to 100 total investors, and all of the investors must be from the United States. An S-corp can only issue one form of stock, meaning that every share must have the same voting rights and dividend allotments. Many businesses that do not anticipate having a large diversified ownership structure or operating in other countries choose to be incorporated as S-corps.

Limited Liability Companies and Limited Liability Partnerships

Forming and operating a subchapter S-corporation requires extensive paperwork and attention to detail. For this reason, many small business owners have chosen to operate as LLCs or LLPs. An LLC or LLP operates in many ways like a subchapter S-corporation. Profits flow through to the investors and are taxed as ordinary income. The LLC and LLP also provide a corporate veil against personal liability. However, LLCs and LLPs typically can be established by filing simple paperwork in the state where the LLC/LLP will initially operate. Forms for taxes are also much easier to fill out and file than those for an S-corp. However, unlike S-corps, which have been in existence for many decades, there are not any national standards regarding the operation of LLCs or LLPs, which are relatively new business entities. Individual states govern LLCs/LLPs in a variety of ways. In some states, the rules regarding LLCs/LLPs have been determined through legislative or judicial action. However, rules and operating procedures have not been firmly established in all states. In addition, some states have different laws regarding taxes owed by the owners of LLCs/LLPs. It is critical that investors seek financial and legal advice regarding the formation and operation of LLCs/LLPs. As consistent guidelines regarding LLCs and LLPs are established, they will likely become the preferred operating structures for personal trainers, as they combine the limited liability and flow-through taxation of the S-corp with easier creation and operation requirements.

C-Corporations

It is highly unlikely that most personal trainers will ever create a subchapter C-corporation (often called C-corporations or C-corps). Many, though not all, of the 500 largest companies in the United States operate as C-corps. The primary reason is that C-corps are structured in a manner that allows the company to seek investors and conduct business activities around the world. In addition, companies organized as C-corps do not have limits on the number of potential shareholders, different classifications of stock may be issued, and stock can be sold to foreign nationals and institutional investors. A company wishing to operate as a C-corp must annually file extensive paperwork in its home state and in countries where it conducts business. Companies classified as C-corps retain the corporate veil that protects investors from company liability. However, unlike an S-corp, C-corps are taxed as a company first and then any profits that are remaining may be provided to shareholders. Since the shareholders must then pay taxes on their dividends, C-corps are said to provide **double taxation.**

Personal trainers must contemplate the advantages and disadvantages of their business structure (Table 16-1). Ideally, personal trainers should seek the advice of an attorney and an accountant who have experience with helping a number of clients establish and expand businesses. In most cases, consultation with an attorney who specializes in business formation and risk management can assist in reducing potential liability, while conferring with an accountant can mitigate potential tax payments. Working with an experienced attorney and an accountant to determine the most appropriate business structure will help alleviate potential issues when establishing a business and properly prepare the personal trainer for expanding the business if necessary.

TABLE 16-1

Advantages and Disadvantages of Various Business Structures

Type	Advantages	Disadvantages
Sole proprietorship	▸ Easily created and managed ▸ Flow-through taxation	▸ Personal liability ▸ Raising capital
Partnership	▸ Easily created ▸ Flow-through taxation	▸ Potential management disputes ▸ Personal liability (except limited partners)
S-corps	▸ Flow-through taxation ▸ Limited liability	▸ Limited number of potential investors ▸ Costs of formation and operation
LLC/LLP	▸ Flow-through taxation ▸ Limited liability	▸ Operating standards not defined in all states
C-corps	▸ Limited liability ▸ Unlimited number of investors	▸ Cost of formation and operation ▸ Double taxation

Note: S-corps = Subchapter S-corporation; LLC = Limited liability company; LLP = Limited liability partnership; C-corps = Subchapter C-corporation

Franchise Operation Business Models

Personal-training studio franchise opportunities are another option for personal trainers looking to open their own fitness businesses. Owning and operating a franchise provides some of the advantages of both an independent operation and a multiple-facility operation. The franchising model is based on the principle that local business owners will have greater success connecting their facilities to the local communities and more commitment to making them successful if they have an ownership stake in the business. A franchisee (the owner of a franchise) has the right to use an established brand name, trademark, logo, and business model. These individuals benefit from being associated with a recognized brand and a central franchising organization that provides operational and marketing assistance. A franchisee can purchase a specific location or the rights to open a number of locations for a specific market. The expectation is that the franchisee will meet certain financial requirements to make an investment in an individual franchise. Most franchise operations charge an individual franchisee an upfront fee that can range up to $25,000 and annual fees of a percentage of revenue earned from the business. There are other costs associated with owning a franchise, including the cost of purchasing operational and retail products through the franchiser's business structure. Table 16-2 presents the advantages and disadvantages of being a franchisee.

TABLE 16-2
Advantages and Disadvantages of Owning and Operating a Franchise

Advantages	Disadvantages
▸ Obtaining the rights to a recognized brand name that will assist the personal trainer in creating a strong presence in a specific market ▸ Access to the business and operating systems created by the franchiser, such as floor plans, equipment layouts, discounts on equipment purchases, operating plans, and marketing information ▸ Access to national advertising programs and the ability to share costs associated with marketing and brand identity with other franchise owners ▸ The ability to control the business, as long as the needs and requirements of the parent franchise company are met ▸ Franchisers will provide training and advice on all aspects of marketing and operating the business, since it is in their best interest for each individual franchisee to be successful	▸ The upfront costs for the franchise fee and the ongoing costs to maintain the association with the parent brand of the franchise ▸ The annual costs of maintaining the franchise, which include making necessary purchases through the franchise system ▸ An association with a particular brand, which could be a drawback if other franchisees within the network perform badly or engage in unethical business practices ▸ The franchisee agrees to follow the franchise's operating model, which could limit the franchisee's ability to adapt to changing market forces

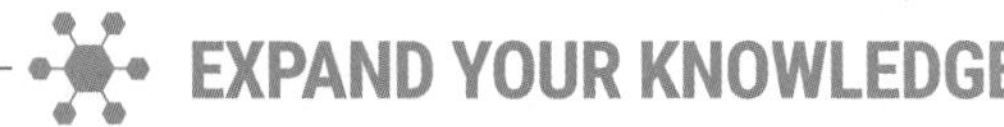

Be Aware of Licensee, Affiliate, and Franchisee Status

Over the past 10 years, the number of "easy to open" fitness facilities has expanded greatly. A few very popular companies have advertised that just about anyone can take a training course and be "certified" to operate their own fitness facility. These venues may not be franchises, but rather operate as a **licensee** or as an **affiliate,** where little support beyond the use of the parent company's name is provided. In some cases, the offered training courses are rudimentary and may not focus on a complete understanding of what is needed to maximize client health while also maintaining a safe environment.

For some companies, this has created a wide discrepancy in the overall quality of instruction at various gym locations that have the same corporate name. In some cases, these companies have encountered significant criticism when patrons undertake exercises for which they have not been adequately trained, especially if there is a lack of proper supervision by an employee who has limited exercise experience. There is certainly nothing inherently wrong with fitness companies that operate as licensees, affiliates, or franchises, but personal trainers need to investigate not only the corporate name of the parent company, but also the individual location to determine if the business is providing adequate and proper training to its clients.

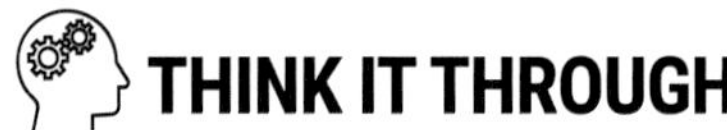

Business Structures

Consider which business structure is best suited for your current situation. Why do you think that is the best option? Do you foresee your business structure changing in the future as you expand your offerings or discover your niche in your local market?

Independent Contractors versus Employees

Once the business structure has been selected and established, personal trainers need to address other legal concerns. Of particular note for personal trainers is the definition of an employee versus an **independent contractor.** Employees "regularly" work for their employer, while independent contractors typically are hired on a short-term basis to perform a specific task or series of tasks. Once the specific identified tasks are complete, the independent contractor is compensated and then is no longer needed. A classic example of an independent contractor occurs when a homeowner has a leaking sink. The homeowner identifies the problem, hires a plumber, and pays the plumber once the leak is fixed. The plumber does not have an *expectation* of consistent work. Alternatively, an employer–employee relationship is created when a business hires a plumber full-time to address ongoing problems. In this case, the plumber would report to work daily, take direction from the employer regarding tasks, and be compensated on a regular basis (e.g., weekly, biweekly, or monthly) rather than at the completion of each job.

The classification of a worker as an independent contractor versus an employee has numerous ramifications. In most cases, employers are responsible to train and supervise their employees and to maintain records regarding their employees' work. Employers usually must also withhold and match the employees' FICA (Federal Insurance Contributions Act) taxes for Social Security and Medicare. The employer usually offers and pays for unemployment coverage, workers' compensation coverage, and medical benefits. These requirements typically consume a tremendous amount of time and financial resources. In addition, employers often must provide justification for firing an employee. Conversely, someone hiring an independent contractor simply negotiates the job and the final compensation, and the independent contractor completes the work. If the independent contractor does not complete the work to the payer's satisfaction, the independent contractor will likely not be rehired in the future.

The main criteria the judicial system will utilize when addressing a potential complaint regarding independent contractor status is "control." In most cases, if the hiring authority maintains control over the worker, an employer–employee relationship has likely been established. A comparison of independent contractor and employee status is presented in Table 16-3.

Certainly, most businesses would like to operate by limiting the number of employees and maximizing the number of independent contractors they retain. The time and expense necessary to adhere to laws regarding employer–employee relationships have caused some businesses to attempt to utilize *only* independent contractors. However, simply *designating* someone an independent contractor does not necessarily mean that an individual is *acting* as an independent contractor. Some companies have been penalized by the government for improperly classifying an employee as an independent contractor to avoid their financial and administrative duties. Companies should ensure that they are properly classifying and utilizing independent contractors at all times.

TABLE 16-3
Independent Contractors versus Employees*

	Independent Contractor Status	Employee Status
Work Details	Independent contractors have more control over work details.	Employers will create schedules, require specific materials to be utilized, and oversee procedures.
Payment	Payment by the "job"	Regularly scheduled payments
Length of Relationship	Hired for short periods of time (typically a few weeks or less)	Ongoing relationship
Training and Retraining	Require no initial or ongoing training	Initial and ongoing training is expected
Equipment	Provide their own equipment	Equipment is provided by the employer
Number of Clients	Serve multiple clients	Typically work for only one employer
Nature of the Work	The specific type of work is typically performed by independent contractors.	The work is integral to the core function of the business, meaning in most cases immediate attention is required.

*It is important to note that each of these areas in and of itself will typically not be the sole criteria utilized by the courts when adjudicating a potential status dispute. The courts will examine the entire relationship and the extent to which the potential employer "control" is present. While the intent of the parties is a factor, it will certainly not be the only or deciding factor in the eventual classification.

There are multiple issues that personal trainers and business owners must consider regarding the classification or status of employees. In most cases, personal trainers act as independent contractors. Personal trainers typically do not have long-term commitments to their clients to perform services beyond the immediate future. In addition, personal trainers provide the expertise during the workout, with the client utilizing the personal trainer's guidance. However, since the majority of personal trainers will work with clients at an established fitness center, the relationship between the center and the personal trainer needs to be clearly defined. Unlike a plumber who brings tools to complete a job, personal trainers who work with clients at fitness centers typically do not provide their own equipment (unless they own the center). Another potential concern is the solicitation of clients. A personal trainer who brings clients to a fitness center is operating in a different environment than one who arrives at the center and trains whoever has signed up that day.

Even though a personal trainer who is an independent contractor will adhere to the fitness center's general rules, he or she should be able to:

- Choose when and where to work
- Charge variable fees for different situations
- Begin working without extensive guidance
- Maintain autonomy in training decisions

Do not assume that because a worker is called an independent contractor that he or she is actually acting as one or would be automatically recognized as one by the legal system.

By comparison, a fitness center employee will adhere to the general and specific guidelines of the employer when providing services. In many cases, a personal trainer who operates as an independent contractor retains greater personal and financial risk, while an employee exchanges the potential risks and rewards for the security of being an employee.

Both independent contractors and employees must be certain that every detail of their agreement is clear from the beginning of their professional relationship with a fitness facility. Often, the legal nature of the relationship is ambiguous, and personal trainers have filed lawsuits attempting to collect worker's compensation or unemployment insurance from clubs that consider them independent contractors. Other personal trainers who assumed that they were employees have been forced to pay back taxes and penalties for neglected FICA responsibilities once they were identified by the government as independent contractors. Ultimately, it is the responsibility of all parties to clearly define the relationship and ensure that the actions of the fitness center and the personal trainer adhere to guidelines that govern the actions of independent contractors or employees.

Contracts

Some personal trainers who are starting a business may feel that written contracts are unnecessary and that a brief chat and a handshake are sufficient when negotiating agreements. In the case of scheduling clients, that is often the standard practice. However, a potential miscommunication or misunderstanding may result in some difficulties, as any oral contract is subject to misinterpretation by the involved parties, and therefore is potentially dangerous. In the event of an oral contract dispute necessitating legal intervention, conflicting stories may be settled in a courtroom without sufficient evidence to support the personal trainer's account of what transpired.

Contracts are the best method to ensure that all aspects of a relationship are properly established. Whether a personal trainer works as an independent contractor or an employee, the basic tenets of contract law should be understood. The following elements are necessary to create a binding contract:

- An offer and acceptance with a mutual agreement of terms
- Consideration (an exchange of valuable items, such as money for services)
- Legality (acceptable under the law)
- Ability of the parties to enter into a contract with respect to legal age and mental capacity

For example, a personal trainer may talk to a prospective client and mention potential services, such as designing personalized exercise sessions. The personal trainer and client may agree on dates and times for specific workouts. This negotiation constitutes an offer and an acceptance. Stating a fee of $50 per hour for services establishes an exchange of consideration (i.e., training services for money). Once these negotiations are

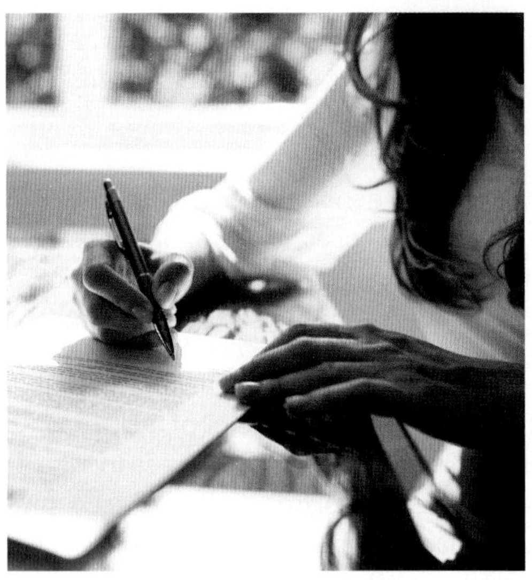

settled, the personal trainer should prepare a written contract by filling out a basic contract form or by having one specifically written for each agreement. Regardless of the type of form, legal counsel should be consulted to ensure that the written form is valid under contract law before it is utilized. This document becomes a valid contract when signed by both the personal trainer and the client, assuming both parties are of legal age to enter into contracts. Certainly, difficulty can arise if a minor seeks to retain a personal trainer's services. Since minors may not legally sign a contract, the personal trainer is retaining some risk in this situation. Having the parents sign the contract to perform services may mitigate, but not completely solve, this potential problem.

In addition to scheduling, written contracts should be utilized to establish payment terms before any session occurs. There should also be considerations for issues such as rescheduling, bounced checks, agreements to follow instructions and adhere to proper techniques, confidentiality, termination of the agreement, and other aspects critical to the session. These terms not only establish what the client must do for the personal trainer, but also what the personal trainer must do for the client. For example, both parties should have full knowledge of the rules regarding a cancelled session. Will the client be required to pay for a session even if he or she cancels with at least 24 hours' notice? Will the personal trainer be required to provide additional concessions beside a make-up session if he or she is forced to cancel a session? The client–personal trainer relationship can become strained if both parties are not aware of the contract stipulations and one party feels that the "proposed solution" to an unusual circumstance is unfair. Providing contract details enables both parties to maintain a professional relationship, as they can refer to the contract when such a situation arises.

Personal trainers should insist upon a written contract not only with clients, but also with fitness centers, vendors, and any other entities with which they conduct business. In any case in which the agreement involves real estate or goods or services worth $500 or more, or requires more than one year to complete, the **statute of frauds** requires that there be a written contract if the agreement is to be valid. The courts will not intervene in a potential oral contract dispute if the contract violates the statute of frauds—it will simply invalidate the agreement.

Using valid contracts can save businesses money and mitigate a tremendous amount of time and stress. Far too often, personal trainers neglect to understand the importance of operating with valid contracts. In addition, they often fail to thoroughly read and understand the contracts presented to them by fitness centers and other vendors. A visit to an attorney's office is advisable before signing any contract, but it is particularly important in cases where an employer–employee relationship is established or an ongoing time or financial commitment is created. Long-term contracts should be examined with particular scrutiny, since much can change over time.

Negligence

One of the most important aspects of personal training is the adherence to established professional guidelines. Failing to perform as a reasonable and prudent person would under similar circumstances is considered **negligence.** In the case of personal trainers, a reasonable and prudent person is someone who adheres to the established standard of care, or the expected behavior for a professional faced with a similar set of circumstances. Attainment of ACE **certification** indicates that the personal trainer has demonstrated an acceptable level of competence and understanding of the established standards. Since standards of care can and do change, it is critical that personal trainers stay abreast of new guidelines. A negligent act can occur if a personal trainer fails to act (act of omission) or acts inappropriately (act of commission). For example, a personal trainer could be successfully sued for neglecting to spot a client during a free-weight bench press (omission), or for programming straight-leg sit-ups for a client with known lower-back problems (commission). These actions would likely be found inappropriate as compared to what a reasonable and prudent professional would do in a similar situation.

In 2016, a $10.875 million verdict was awarded to plaintiffs Chetan Vaid and his wife Sreemoee Mukherjee after a Connecticut court determined Vaid's personal trainer, Joseph Dominguez, and his employer, Equinox Fitness, were responsible for a stroke that occurred due to negligence (*Vaid v. Equinox*, 2016). Industry observers have noted that the judgement is believed to be one of the largest ever awarded in a fitness industry case (Stromgren, 2016). Vaid had been required by Dominguez to continue strenuous exercise even after complaining of significant physical issues, including dizziness and blurred vision. In addition, it was determined that Dominguez had not developed a gradual exercise program that would have better suited Vaid's physical capabilities. The significance of the financial award reinforced to many in the fitness industry that adhering to the standard of care and providing personalized programming that incorporates client feedback is of the utmost importance.

To substantiate a charge of negligence in court, the plaintiff must establish four elements:

- The defendant had a duty to protect the plaintiff from injury.
- The defendant failed to uphold the standard of care necessary to perform that duty.
- Damage or injury to the plaintiff occurred.
- The damage or injury was caused by the defendant's breach of duty (proximate causation).

Negligence in personal training could occur, for example, if a personal trainer agreed to provide instruction and supervision for a cardiorespiratory training regimen. The agreement between the personal trainer and the client establishes a legal duty that would not be present if both parties were simply working out at a fitness center at the same time. Certainly, there may be a moral duty to help a fellow patron in need, but there is not a legal duty to do so absent a special relationship such as parent–child.

If the personal trainer does not provide proper instruction while a client is using a treadmill for the first time, the personal trainer has breached his or her duty to the client. If the client is injured as a direct result of the breach, which can happen if a person who has never walked, let alone run, on a treadmill, is asked to start at a rapid pace. In this case, the client will likely have a successful lawsuit for negligence against the personal trainer. The courts would examine the situation, the expected standard of care, the extent of the injury, and the result of the injury (e.g., medical bills or lost time at work) when assessing potential damages.

Important Legal Forms

There are a variety of potential contracts that personal trainers may utilize in their day-to-day operations. Of particular importance are contracts detailing the relationship between the personal trainer and the client as they pertain to the potential rigors and injuries associated with physical activity.

Personal trainers should understand the concept and use of **agreements to participate, informed consent,** and **waivers,** as they can be important defenses to litigation for negligence. Ideally, each of these forms should be printed (avoid handwritten agreements) and signed by all clients before beginning the first exercise session. It is important to note that these forms can be combined in some instances. For example, an informed consent and waiver are often very similar, with the primary difference being the inclusion of an **exculpatory clause** in a waiver. However, personal trainers should not make such changes themselves and should always work with an attorney in their state to ensure that the forms they are using are valid.

Before a personal trainer begins using any of the documents presented in this chapter, it is critical that legal counsel specializing in health and exercise in the personal trainer's state be consulted.

AGREEMENTS TO PARTICIPATE

An agreement to participate is designed to protect the personal trainer from a client claiming to be unaware of the potential risks of physical activity (Figure 16-1). An agreement to participate is not typically considered a formal contract, but rather serves to demonstrate that the client was made aware of the "normal" outcomes of certain types of physical activity and willingly assumed the risks of participation. Typically, the agreement to participate is utilized for "class" settings (e.g., bootcamp and group cycling) rather than for individualized personal-training situations. The agreement to participate should detail the nature of the activity, the potential risks to be encountered, and the expected behaviors of the participant (Cotten & Cotten, 2016). This last consideration is important, as the participant recognizes that he or she may need to follow instructions while participating.

Personal trainers should have a process to formally warn their clients about the potential dangers of exercise.

FIGURE 16-1
Sample agreement to participate

"I, ______________________, have enrolled in a program of strenuous physical activity including, but not limited to, high-intensity interval training, weight training, stationary bicycling, and the use of various aerobic-conditioning machinery offered by [name of personal trainer and/or business]. I am aware that participating in these types of activities, even when completed properly, can be dangerous. I agree to follow the verbal instructions issued by the personal trainer. I am aware that potential risks associated with these types of activities include, but are not limited to, death, serious neck and spinal injuries that may result in complete or partial paralysis or brain damage, serious injury to virtually all bones, joints, ligaments, muscles, tendons, and other aspects of the musculoskeletal system, and serious injury or impairment to other aspects of my body, general health, and well-being.

Because of the dangers of participating, I recognize the importance of following the personal trainer's instructions regarding proper techniques and training, as well as other organization rules.

I am in good health and have provided verification from a licensed physician that I am able to undertake a general fitness-training program. I hereby consent to first aid, emergency medical care, and admission to an accredited hospital or an emergency care center when necessary for executing such care and for treatment of injuries that I may sustain while participating in an exercise-training program.

I understand that I am responsible for my own medical insurance and will maintain that insurance throughout my entire period of participation with [name of personal trainer and/or business].
I will assume any additional expenses incurred that go beyond my health coverage. I will notify [name of personal trainer and/or business] of any significant injury or change in health status that requires medical attention (such as emergency care, hospitalization, etc.).

Signed ______________________

Printed Name ______________________

Phone Number ______________________

Address ______________________

Emergency Contact ______________________

Contact Phone Number ______________________

Insurance Company ______________________

Policy # ______________________

Effective Date ______________________

Name of Policy Holder ______________________

Note: This document has been prepared to serve as a guide to improve understanding. Personal trainers should not assume that this sample form will provide adequate protection in the event of a lawsuit. Please see an attorney before creating, distributing, and collecting any agreements to participate, informed consent forms, or waivers.

Typically, agreements to participate are incorporated into other documents, such as informed consent forms and waivers. One potential consideration for each of these documents is a general request, or in some cases a requirement, that participants consult with a doctor prior to beginning any exercise routine. This practice is particularly important if vigorous-intensity exercise is to be performed. Though most personal trainers know to "start slowly" with new clients, personal trainers cannot evaluate the overall health of a client in the same manner as a medical doctor. Some agreements to participate also ask that health insurance information be provided. This not only lets the personal trainer know that the client has coverage, but also enables the personal trainer to provide that information if a client were in need of medical attention.

INFORMED CONSENT

An informed consent form can be utilized by a personal trainer to demonstrate that a client acknowledges that he or she has been specifically informed about the risks associated with the activity in which he or she is about to engage (Figure 16-2). It is primarily intended to communicate the potential benefits and dangers of the program or exercise-testing procedures to the client. Informed consent forms should detail the possible discomforts involved and potential alternatives. Personal trainers should remember that many potential clients will be unaccustomed to straining their bodies through physical exertion. The informed consent form, combined with oral communication, prepares the client for the positive and negative effects of certain types of exercise.

FIGURE 16-2
Sample informed consent form

CARDIORESPIRATORY FITNESS TEST

Informed Consent for Exercise Testing of Apparently Healthy Adults
(without known heart disease)

Name ______________________________

1. Purpose and Explanation of Test

I hereby consent to voluntarily engage in an exercise test to determine my cardiorespiratory fitness. It is my understanding that the information obtained will help me evaluate future physical activities and sports activities in which I may engage.

Before I undergo the test, I certify that I am in good health and have had a physical examination conducted by a licensed medical physician within the past ________ months. Further, I hereby represent and inform the facility that I have accurately completed the pre-test health-history questionnaire or interview presented to me by the facility staff and have provided correct responses to the questions as indicated on the health-history form or as supplied to the interviewer. It is my understanding that I will be interviewed by a physician or other person prior to my undergoing the test who will in the course of interviewing me determine if there are any reasons that would make it undesirable or unsafe for me to take the test. Consequently,

Initial: _____

FIGURE 16-2
(continued)

I understand that it is important that I provide complete and accurate responses to the interviewer and recognize that my failure to do so could lead to possible unnecessary injury to myself during the test.

The test that I will undergo will be performed on a motor-driven treadmill or bicycle ergometer with the amount of effort gradually increasing. As I understand it, this increase in effort will continue until I feel and verbally report to the operator any symptoms such as fatigue, shortness of breath, or chest discomfort that I may experience. It is my understanding and I have been clearly advised that it is my right to request that a test be stopped at any point if I feel unusual discomfort or fatigue. I have been advised that I should, immediately upon experiencing any such symptoms or if I so choose, inform the operator that I wish to stop the test at that or any other point. My wishes in this regard shall be absolutely carried out.

During the test itself, it is my understanding that a trained observer will monitor my responses continuously and take frequent readings of blood pressure, the electrocardiogram, and my expressed feelings of effort. I realize that a true determination of my exercise capacity depends on progressing the test to the point of fatigue.

Once the test has been completed, but before I am released from the test area, I will be given special instructions about showering and recognition of certain symptoms that may appear within the first 24 hours after the test. I agree to follow these instructions and promptly contact the facility personnel or medical providers if such symptoms develop.

2. Risks

It is my understanding and I have been informed that there exists the possibility of adverse changes during the actual test. I have been informed that these changes could include abnormal blood pressure, fainting, disorders of heart rhythm, stroke, and very rare instances of heart attack or even death. Every effort, I have been told, will be made to minimize these occurrences by preliminary examination and by precautions and observations taken during the test. I have also been informed that emergency equipment and personnel are readily available to deal with these unusual situations should they occur. I understand that there is a risk of injury, heart attack, stroke, or even death as a result of my performance of this test, but knowing those risks, it is my desire to proceed to take the test as herein indicated.

3. Benefits to Be Expected and Alternatives Available to the Exercise Testing Procedure

The results of this test may or may not benefit me. Potential benefits relate mainly to my personal motives for taking the test (e.g., knowing my exercise capacity in relation to the general population, understanding my fitness for certain sports and recreational activities, planning my physical conditioning program, or evaluating the effects of my recent physical habits). Although

Initial: _____

Continued on the next page

FIGURE 16-2
(continued)

my fitness might also be evaluated by alternative means (e.g., a bench step test or an outdoor running test), such tests do not provide as accurate a fitness assessment as the treadmill or bike test, nor do those options allow equally effective monitoring of my responses.

4. Confidentiality and Use of Information

I have been informed that the information that is obtained from this exercise test will be treated as privileged and confidential and will consequently not be released or revealed to any person without my express written consent or as required by law. I do, however, agree to the use of any information for research or statistical purposes so long as same does not provide facts that could lead to the identification of my person. Any other information obtained, however, will be used only by the facility staff to evaluate my exercise status or needs.

5. Inquiries and Freedom of Consent

I have been given an opportunity to ask questions about the procedure. Generally, these requests, which have been noted by the testing staff, and their responses are as follows:

____

____

I further understand that there are also other remote risks that may be associated with this procedure. Despite the fact that a complete accounting of all remote risks is not entirely possible, I am satisfied with the review of these risks, which was provided to me, and it is still my desire to proceed with the test.

I acknowledge that I have read this document in its entirety or that it has been read to me if I have been unable to read same.

I consent to the rendition of all services and procedures as explained herein by all facility personnel.

Date ________________________________

Client's Signature __________________________

Witness' Signature __________________________

Test Supervisor's Signature ______________________

Modified with permission from Herbert, D.L. & Herbert, W.G. (2002). *Legal Aspects of Preventive, Rehabilitative, and Recreational Exercise Programs* (4th ed.). Canton, Oh.: PRC Publishing. Pages 467–470.

Note: This document has been prepared to serve as a guide to improve understanding. Personal trainers should not assume that this sample form will provide adequate protection in the event of a lawsuit. Please see an attorney before creating, distributing, and collecting any agreements to participate, informed consent forms, or waivers.

WAIVERS

Personal trainers who hire employees need to understand the concept of **vicarious liability** (also known as **respondeat superior**). Employers are responsible for the employment actions of their employees. If an employee is negligent while working within the normal scope of employment, it is likely that the injured party will sue not only the employee who breached the duty to cause injury, but also the employer or employers. Since employees often do not have the financial resources of employers, courts have typically upheld the right of the injured party to seek damages from the employer's "deep pockets." In most cases, litigants name every possible entity linked to the employee when negligence occurs.

The use of waivers is critical in personal training, as a properly worded exculpatory clause bars the injured party from potential recovery (Figure 16-3). There are some potential issues that every personal trainer must investigate with an attorney prior to crafting a waiver. Each state has slightly different rules regarding the validity of waivers, meaning that a waiver that is valid in one state may not be valid in another. In addition,

FIGURE 16-3
Sample waiver

I, ________________________________, through the purchase of training sessions, have agreed to voluntarily participate in an exercise program, including, but not limited to, cardiorespiratory, muscular, and flexibility training under the guidance of [name of personal trainer and/or business]. I hereby stipulate and agree that I am physically and mentally sound and currently have no physical conditions that would be aggravated by my involvement in an exercise program. I have provided verification from a licensed physician that I am able to undertake a general fitness-training program.

I understand and am aware that physical-fitness activities, including the use of equipment, are potentially hazardous activities. I am aware that participating in these types of activities, even when performed properly, can be dangerous. I agree to follow the verbal instructions issued by the personal trainer. I am aware that potential risks associated with these types of activities include, but are not limited to: death, fainting, disorders in heartbeat, serious neck and spinal injuries that may result in complete or partial paralysis or brain damage, serious injury to virtually all bones, joints, ligaments, muscles, tendons, and other aspects of the musculoskeletal system, and serious injury or impairment to other aspects of my body, general health, and well-being.

I understand that I am responsible for my own medical insurance and will maintain that insurance throughout my entire period of participation with [name of personal trainer and/or business]. I will assume any additional expenses incurred that go beyond my health coverage. I will notify the [name of personal trainer and/or business] of any significant injury or change in health status that requires medical attention (such as emergency care, hospitalization, etc.).

[name of personal trainer or business] or I will provide the equipment to be used in connection with workouts, including, but not limited to, benches, dumbbells, barbells, and similar items. I represent and warrant any and all equipment I provide for training sessions is for personal

Continued on the next page

FIGURE 16-3
(*continued*)

use only. [name of personal trainer or business] has not inspected my equipment and has no knowledge of its condition. I understand that I take sole responsibility for my equipment. I acknowledge that although [name of personal trainer and/or business] takes precautions to maintain the equipment, any equipment may malfunction and/or cause potential injuries. I take sole responsibility to inspect any and all of my or [name of personal trainer and/or business]'s equipment prior to use.

Although [name of personal trainer and/or business] will take precautions to ensure my safety, I expressly assume and accept sole responsibility for my safety and for any and all injuries that may occur. In consideration of the acceptance of this entry, **I, for myself and for my executors, administrators, and assigns, waive and release any and all claims against [name of personal trainer and/or business] and any of their staffs, officers, officials, volunteers, sponsors, agents, representatives, successors, or assigns and agree to hold them harmless from any claims or losses, including but not limited to claims for negligence for any injuries or expenses that I may incur while exercising or while traveling to and from training sessions.** These exculpatory clauses are intended to apply to any and all activities occurring during the time for which I have contracted with [name of personal trainer and/or company].

I represent and warrant I am signing this agreement freely and willfully and not under fraud or duress.

HAVING READ THE ABOVE TERMS AND INTENDING TO BE LEGALLY BOUND HEREBY AND UNDERSTANDING THIS DOCUMENT TO BE A COMPLETE WAIVER AND DISCLAIMER IN FAVOR OF [name of personal trainer and/or business], I HEREBY AFFIX MY SIGNATURE HERETO.

____

Client's name (please print clearly)

____________________________ Date: ____________

Client's signature

____

Client's address

____________________________ Date: ____________

Parent/guardian signature (if applicable)

____________________________ Date: ____________

Personal trainer's signature

Note: This document has been prepared to serve as a guide to improve understanding. Personal trainers should not assume that this sample form will provide adequate protection in the event of a lawsuit. Please see an attorney before creating, distributing, and collecting any agreements to participate, informed consent forms, or waivers.

confusion and litigation can arise when a fitness club utilizes personal trainers who are not employees. Consider the following court case, which addressed the situation in which a member of a health club signed a supplemental contract for personal-training services in the club setting. When the client was injured in a session with the personal trainer, she contended that the waiver signed with her membership contract did not extend and cover the services of the personal trainer. The court disagreed and ruled that the services of the personal trainer were part of the activities and benefits offered at the club and were therefore covered by the original waiver (Cotten, 2000a). Despite the outcome of this case, personal trainers should utilize their own waivers in addition to the ones potentially already signed when the client joined the fitness center or club.

Waivers also must detail the types of activities and potential risks of injury that would be barred from recovering remuneration in a court of law. A client must knowingly understand the nature of the activities and the potential risks before he or she can waive the right to potentially sue for injuries occurring during participation. Waivers also typically do not protect the personal trainer from injuries directly caused by **gross negligence**—an action that demonstrates recklessness or a willful disregard for the safety of others. As a general rule, gross negligence occurs when someone deliberately acts in a manner that extends beyond the scope of employment or fails to meet the accepted standard of care. For example, a correctly worded waiver would likely protect a personal trainer who did not properly spot a client completing an overhead press, as spotting would likely be considered part of the normal activities conducted during the course of personal training. However, if the personal trainer knowingly and intentionally used a piece of equipment after a safety screw was removed for use on another machine from the seat prior to the client's arrival, the waiver would likely not apply, because using a machine without the proper safety equipment in place is something that should *never* occur during the normal course of a personal trainer's activities. Ultimately, the use of proper waivers protects the personal trainer from lawsuits that arise not only from injuries that typically occur during exercises, but also from injuries that might occur due to mistakes the personal trainer may make while interacting with clients. Hopefully, mistakes are mitigated, injuries are limited, and potential lawsuits are completely avoided.

Even if a waiver is not utilized properly, a personal trainer may successfully defend against a negligence lawsuit in certain situations, even if he or she is partially at fault. Courts will typically examine every aspect of the scenario to determine who was at fault. In some cases, the client may have contributed to the potential injury. In certain states, **contributory negligence** laws prevent a plaintiff in a lawsuit who has played some role in the injury from receiving *any* remuneration. For example, if a client failed to notify a personal trainer that the soles of one of his shoes had been slipping, he would be partially to blame if his foot slipped while conducting a squat exercise, even if the personal trainer did not properly spot the client. The clients' improper actions bar him from recovering any money, even though the personal trainer was partially at fault.

The majority of states do not use the contributory negligence standard, instead utilizing **comparative negligence** when deciding negligence cases. When multiple parties may have caused injuries, the court will apportion guilt and any subsequent award for damages. For instance, in the earlier example the client may be deemed to be 40% at fault for the injury (for failing to inform the personal trainer of the issue with his shoes) and the personal trainer 60% at fault (for failing to spot the client during the lift). If the court were to normally award $100,000 in damages, the award would be lowered to $60,000 (i.e., 60% of the damages). There are a variety of state standards regarding comparative negligence and its potential impact upon monetary awards.

INHERENT RISKS

Agreements to participate and informed consent forms, though potentially important in the defense against a lawsuit, primarily cover the **inherent risks** of participation in an activity. For instance, even if proper stretching and lifting techniques are utilized, injuries can occur to ligaments, tendons, muscles, and other parts of the body. An agreement to participate and an informed consent form would help to protect the personal trainer in the event that a lawsuit is filed by an injured client. However, it is often difficult to determine an inherent risk of participation and what might have been caused, in whole or in part, by the actions of the personal trainer. A client may claim that a personal trainer did not provide proper spotting during an exercise and that this action specifically caused an injury. The personal trainer might counter that an injury was unfortunate, but part of the normal, safe lifting process, and that the spotting provided was well within the normal standard of care. This dispute would likely be settled in court. To potentially avoid this type of a scenario, personal trainers should have all clients sign a waiver prior to beginning any exercise routine. The waiver (sometimes called a release) will not only typically incorporate similar language included in an agreement to participate and an informed consent form but will also include an exculpatory clause that bars the clients from seeking damages for injuries caused by the inherent risk of activities and by the ordinary negligence of the personal trainer and his or her employees and agents (see boldface text in Figure 16-3).

PROCEDURES

Valid agreements to participate, informed consent forms, and waivers must be administered properly to clients. There should not be any underhanded attempt to hide the true nature of these agreements prior to a client signing the document. Though some states permit **group waivers** that have a list of spaces for multiple patrons to sign below the waiver, it is advisable to have a stand-alone document for each client. Often, personal trainers properly insist that a new client sign a waiver prior to the first session, but then fail to allow sufficient time for the new client to read, understand, and ask questions about the document. Requiring a client to rush when reviewing a waiver can result in a court invalidating an otherwise properly crafted waiver. In addition, though courts have typically found that individuals who cannot read English retain the responsibility to have someone translate the waiver prior to signing, it is a good practice to have someone available to assist with the translation if needed (Cotten & Cotten, 2016). If the document is multiple pages, a space for the client to initial the bottom of each page should be provided (see Figure 16-2 as an example).

Minors cannot legally sign a contract, so in most cases a waiver signed by a child will be invalidated by the courts. However, some states do allow parents to sign paperwork

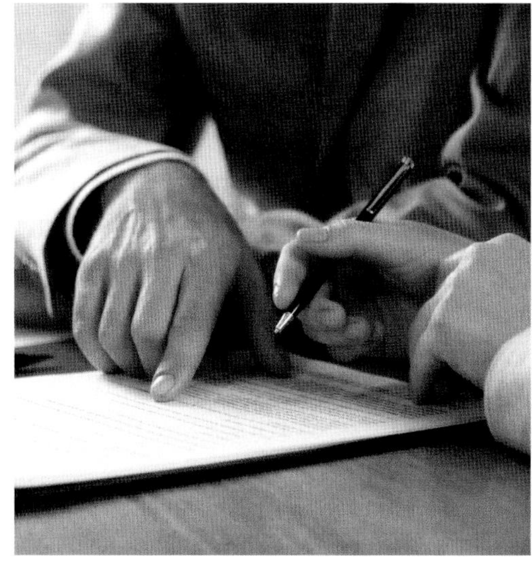

that may provide limited protection for the personal trainer. An attorney specializing in this area should be consulted if children will be utilizing a personal trainer's services. A waiver signed by one spouse may not cover the other spouse (Cotten, 2000b). Once agreements to participate, informed consent forms, and waivers have been signed, the personal trainer should retain the paperwork on file at least until the **statute of limitations**—the time allotted to sue for damages—has elapsed. Some attorneys even recommend retaining records past the statute of limitations to ensure that a sudden change in the law does not negatively impact the ability of a service provider to defend against potential litigation.

Ultimately, the goal of any personal trainer should be to eliminate all client injuries. However, even in the safest conditions, physical activity will likely result in some physical injuries, even when proper care is provided. Personal trainers should utilize paperwork to notify new clients of *all* risks and potential dangers. This creates a situation in which the client knows and assumes the risks of participation. Personal trainers should then also utilize waivers to protect against costly lawsuits that arise both from the normal physical injuries associated with physical activity and from mistakes that may occur during personal-training sessions.

Record Keeping

Keeping current and accurate records for every client is essential for a personal trainer. The important legal principle to remember is that if information is not written down, then from the perspective of the court system, it did not occur and does not exist.

MEDICAL HISTORY

A personal trainer must maintain current records of each client's medical conditions. A personal trainer should document a client's condition prior to beginning any exercise. This will provide the personal trainer with a baseline to compare to in the future. It is advisable for the personal trainer to update each client's records every time new information is provided or observed. Positive changes from the baseline can be used for motivation and goal development.

EXERCISE RECORD

A client's exercise record needs to stay current with specific notations for any changes, such as a new onset of pain. This will provide the personal trainer with an accurate record of any program changes and when the incident occurred. A good practice is to write down some important details of every single session.

INCIDENT REPORT

If an injury does occur during a workout session, it needs to be recognized and addressed appropriately. The client's injury will need immediate medical attention. This may include minor first aid or, potentially, something drastic like the activation of emergency medical services. Client safety is the number-one priority throughout the entire process. After the client is safe and stable, a formal written account of the incident needs to be documented. Most organizations will have a specific "incident" report that is completed after an injury has occurred. Copies of these reports are typically distributed to all pertinent parties. However, to protect their interests and to support their memory of the incident and the response, the personal trainer needs to keep his or her own account of what occurred and maintain any pertinent documentation. This will help ensure that an accurate account of the incident is maintained.

CORRESPONDENCE

Since the passage of the 1996 **Health Insurance Portability and Accountability Act (HIPAA),** maintaining the privacy of medical records has not only been a good ethical practice, but it has also been mandated by law. **Protected health information** includes any identifiable health information that is kept or communicated in any form. Like any other healthcare professional, personal trainers cannot print, email, or discuss a client's health information unless the client has granted written permission to do so. Though most personal trainers inherently know to protect the confidentiality of written health information, some have become lax in their approach to conversations with other personal trainers, facility employees, or even other clients. If there is any chance for someone to be able to determine which client's health information is being discussed, the personal trainer should refrain from engaging in such conversations. If outside consultation is deemed by the personal trainer to be necessary, he or she should obtain written permission from the client. In cases where permission has been granted, the personal trainer should document all conversations and sharing of information. This will help ensure protection of the client's personal information. See Figure 16-4 for a sample HIPAA permission form and refer to the Appendix for the ACE Code of Ethics.

Legal Responsibilities

The use of proper paperwork prior to working with clients can mitigate some of the potential for litigation against the personal trainer. But even if clients waive their right to potentially sue, the personal trainer should still prepare for each training session with safety as the first priority. Not only is this a professional requirement, but it also provides a better experience for the client and increases the likelihood that the client will continue to utilize the personal trainer's services. One of the most important things a personal trainer can do is establish plans to regularly inspect facilities and equipment and review protocols regarding supervision and instruction.

FACILITIES

Personal trainers have an obligation to ensure that the facilities used are free from unreasonable hazards. At the very least, the physical environment should be inspected

I, ______________________________, direct my healthcare and medical service provider
[client]

______________________________ to disclose and release my protected health
[healthcare provider]

information that is *pertinent* and *necessary* for ______________________________, acting
[personal trainer]

as my personal trainer, to design, implement, and supervise an exercise program. Further, I permit my personal trainer and my healthcare provider to discuss my medical condition as it pertains to my general health and my ongoing participation in said designed fitness program.

Health Information to be disclosed upon the request of the person named above (Check either A or B):

☐ A. Disclose my complete health record (including but not limited to diagnoses, lab tests, prognosis, treatment, and billing, for all conditions) **OR**

☐ B. Disclose my health record, as above, BUT do not disclose the following (check as appropriate):

- ☐ Mental health records
- ☐ Communicable diseases (including HIV and AIDS)
- ☐ Alcohol/drug abuse treatment
- ☐ Other (please specify): ______________________________

This authorization shall be effective until (Check one):

☐ All past, present, and future periods, **OR**

☐ Date or event: ____________________ unless I revoke it. (NOTE: You may revoke this authorization in writing at any time by notifying your healthcare provider and personal trainer, preferably in writing.)

Printed Name of the Individual Granting this Authorization ______________________________

Date of birth ____________________

Signature of the Individual Granting this Authorization ______________________________

Medical Personnel Name and Contact Information

____

____

Personal Trainer Name and Contact Information

____

____

FIGURE 16-4
Sample HIPAA permission form for a medical doctor and personal trainer to disclose information

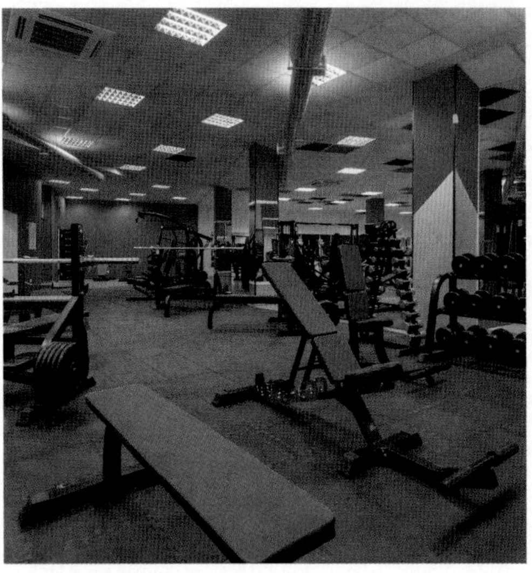

each day prior to beginning any training session, especially when the training area has been used by other patrons after the personal trainer last was present. Inspecting the facilities can be a problem if training sessions are conducted outdoors or in a client's home. Personal trainers should allocate sufficient time to inspect the environment prior to the workout. In some cases, clients will recognize these inspections of the facility as a genuine concern for their well-being, which can have a positive impact on client retention and may generate new clients through referrals. The inspection should consider the following issues:

- Falls, often due to uneven floor surfaces or slick surfaces, are one of the most common safety concerns while exercising. The personal trainer should inspect the training area for potential trip hazards.
- Different floor surfaces are designed for different activities. Personal trainers should ensure that floor surfaces will cushion the feet, knees, and legs from excessive stress.
- There should be sufficient free space available to protect the client from other patrons and from hurting him- or herself on equipment.
- Functional lighting must be sufficient for chosen exercises.
- There must be functional heating and air conditioning systems.
- Proximity to drinking fountains and bathrooms is important for some clients.

Because a personal trainer's primary responsibility is the client's safety, regular inspection using a safety checklist is recommended. If an unsafe condition is noticed, the personal trainer should notify the facility's management and avoid that area until it has been addressed. If a fitness club owner does not repair the problem and the client is injured, the personal trainer can still be held partially liable. Though juries have often looked favorably on independent contractors or employees who have tried unsuccessfully to persuade management to correct dangerous conditions, there is always a potential risk when training in an unsafe environment. For this reason, personal trainers should develop relationships with reputable fitness centers that focus on safety. In addition, personal trainers should develop contingency plans (outside of canceling the session and losing potential revenue) for unsafe facilities.

Working with clients in their homes can pose potential safety problems as well. Often, the client may be reluctant to alter the environment or change the overall décor. Though this type of situation may shift some or all of the responsibility for safety from the personal trainer to the client, an attorney should always be consulted in these instances.

Another consideration for training is the use of public spaces, especially the outdoors. For many personal trainers and clients, it is much more enjoyable to walk or run on a trail than on a treadmill in a fitness center. However, in some jurisdictions it is illegal to train clients on public beaches, parks, or trails. It is the personal trainer's responsibility to know the local laws prior to using these areas. Once a "legal" outdoor area has been identified and selected for a training session, the personal trainer should be sure to understand the potential dangers of the area before meeting the client. Outdoor areas pose specific risks. Running on a public street may involve evading oncoming vehicular traffic, while running on a mountain trail could involve dodging loose rocks or tree roots. Training outdoors certainly can be an enjoyable experience, but it is the personal trainer's responsibility to ensure that the activities will not pose a significant risk for clients.

While most courts recognize that outdoor activities pose certain risks that a typical person would assume (such as loose dirt or rocks on a hiking trail), the personal trainer should inspect the area to identify any particularly unusual dangers. In addition, certain aspects of the environment may impact the choice to utilize it for a training session. If a client has never run on a specific outdoor trail, it is advisable to walk the trail with the client the first time rather than expecting an all-out initial effort. The safety of outdoor activities is also impacted by the weather. The courts often will remove a person's potential liability for acts of God (e.g., earthquakes and mudslides), but if the weather forecast indicates heightened dangers, the personal trainer should not engage in the activity. For example, though earthquakes and lightning storms are both acts of God, in many cases a lightning storm can be predicted. Courts might be willing to absolve personal trainers of potential liability from injuries caused by an earthquake, but they are less likely to rule in favor of a personal trainer if he or she knew, or should have known, that a lightning storm was in the area. In all outdoor training situations, extreme weather conditions such as excessive heat and humidity or freezing cold should be avoided. Acceptable exercise routines in 75° F (24° C) weather may not be acceptable in 95° F (35° C) or 35° F (2° C) weather conditions (see Chapter 8).

Some personal trainers use fitness centers without informing the management that there will be a training session. This is certainly not an ethical business practice, and in many areas is a violation of the law. In addition to adhering to the law and using good ethical behavior, personal trainers should work toward developing a formal relationship with the fitness facility that may eventually result in an expanded client base from fitness center referrals. An attorney should be consulted prior to establishing any formal relationship with a fitness center.

EQUIPMENT

Fitness programs may utilize a variety of equipment, and injuries from the use of exercise equipment are often a source of litigation in the fitness industry. All equipment should meet the highest safety and design standards and should be purchased from a reputable manufacturer. In most cases, the use of homemade equipment should be avoided, since designing and manufacturing are not considered part of the "normal" duties of a personal trainer. Equipment must be regularly inspected and properly maintained. Of particular concern is the protocol utilized when broken equipment is discovered. Once something is deemed unsafe, the personal trainer should immediately remove the equipment from the training area. If quick removal is not feasible, the equipment should be disabled to prevent further use until repaired. Unfortunately, broken equipment is often only marked with a sign that says "do not use." Far too often, these signs easily fall off and unsuspecting patrons may be injured when trying to use the broken equipment. Manufacturers typically

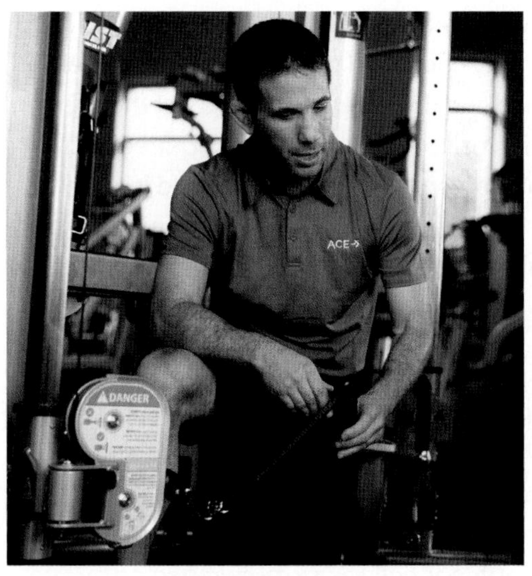

provide maintenance schedules for equipment that personal trainers and club operators should follow. Regular maintenance should be logged and records retained for future referral in the event of a lawsuit.

The use of equipment owned by a client may create a conflict between professional practice and legal protection. A conservative legal stance would be to avoid any contact with the client's equipment, but most personal trainers accept some liability by using their expertise to adjust a client's equipment or recommend maintenance. For example, a personal trainer may arrive at a client's home for an initial fitness session and find a leg extension machine with a frayed cable. The personal trainer should inform the client that the equipment needs repairs, suggest that he or she call the company to order a replacement part, and then conduct sessions without using this equipment until it has been repaired.

Personal trainers should also understand the importance of non-exercise equipment when working with clients. Personal trainers should require that proper clothing and shoes be worn by their clients during sessions. Failure to stop a client from exercising with improper shoes may be deemed an endorsement of a bad practice. If the training sessions will be conducted outdoors, the personal trainer should provide water in containers that will be sufficient for the time, intensity, and temperature during the workout.

The use of safety equipment, such as **automated external defibrillators (AEDs),** has gained considerable attention in recent years. These devices can be found in many places of public assembly (e.g., airports, shopping malls, and amusement parks) and are rapidly becoming standard emergency equipment in health and fitness facilities, not only because they can save lives, but also because they are legally *required* for fitness centers in many states (Agoglia, 2005). Even in states where AEDs are not required in fitness centers, courts can rule in favor of plaintiffs and change the standard of care (*Fowler v. Bally Total Fitness,* 2008). It is important for personal trainers (as well as every other staff member at a fitness facility) to know where the AED is located. In an emergency, there is limited time to save a client's life. A case involving a former professional football player who was exercising at a fitness facility demonstrates the importance of preparation. After he went into cardiac arrest while exercising, the staff was delayed in finding the facility's AED. Once located, the AED was not sufficiently charged, which his family claimed contributed to his death (Dominic, 2016).

Personal trainers will familiarize themselves with AEDs through adult **cardiopulmonary resuscitation (CPR)** and AED courses, which are required prior to registering for an ACE certification exam and need to be kept current to maintain active certification status. Personal trainers may want to consider purchasing an AED for use in their own studios or when working with clients in their homes, particularly if state or local laws require having such equipment available. Though a national standard has not yet been established, it is likely that future legislation will continue to expand the requirements to have AEDs, and eventually they will become a standard piece of equipment for personal trainers working with clients in all settings. Every personal trainer should consult with his or her attorney to understand the local laws that may apply to a specific situation.

Do not assume that any piece of equipment, particularly an AED or other life-saving device, is ready for use. Always regularly inspect and maintain equipment so it is ready for use.

SUPERVISION

General supervision involves overseeing a group of people, such as when a group fitness instructor leads a large class. **Specific supervision** occurs when an individual is supervised while performing a specific activity, such as what typically occurs during a personal-training session. When working with clients, personal trainers need to remember that most personal-training activities require specific supervision for safety purposes. A personal trainer should never leave a client when there is a potential for injury (such as when a spotter is needed on a bench press). Personal trainers who work with two or more clients during the same session may choose to design the workouts to alternate between activities requiring general and specific supervision. For example, while the personal trainer provides specific supervision to one client (e.g., spotting), the other client can briefly rest or work on an activity that requires only general supervision (e.g., stretching or cardiorespiratory exercises). Personal trainers should eliminate any time that a client is not in their direct view, as this is when injuries can quickly occur. A personal trainer should never leave a client during a session.

With the proliferation of online content, a number of personal trainers have begun to train clients remotely. This can certainly provide a service for clients who might not be able to meet in person with the personal trainer. Though online training may provide convenience for both the personal trainer and clients, there are some concerns. A view of a client exercising online may not provide the complete perspective of the physical movements undertaken, as the camera will only show movement from one perspective. Personal trainers may also not be able to notice the entire environment through a narrow camera view.

Personal trainers should consult with their attorneys prior to implementing any online sessions, particularly if those sessions will be undertaken with the client in a different state or country. Negligence laws and personal trainer responsibility may be different in various jurisdictions and there may be special stipulations regarding online training. Further, if a signed waiver is valid in one state and the client travels to another state and participates in an online training session, the language of the waiver may be invalid in the second state. In addition, professional liability insurance purchased by the personal trainer may not cover online training sessions.

Before beginning any session, the personal trainer must adequately plan for any emergencies that may arise. A client's emergency medical information should be immediately available in the event of an accident. This will eliminate the need to search for critical information about the client (such as emergency contact numbers) in the event of an emergency. If training is to occur in a remote area, cell phone coverage should be checked prior to the exercise session to ensure that 9-1-1 may be reached if necessary.

Proper supervision involves not only clients, but also employees. Personal trainers need to be aware of the actions of their employees. This awareness includes properly screening potential employees prior to hiring them. It is the responsibility of an employer to determine if the potential employee would pose a specific danger to clients due to his or her past history. Each employee should be trained regarding the unique aspects of the employer's operation and then supervised and retrained at regular intervals. Employers should conduct written performance evaluations with each of their employees and should retain those files even after an employee has stopped working for the employer.

INSTRUCTION

Personal trainers should utilize instructional techniques that are consistent with current professional practices. If one fails to demonstrate a movement or give proper instructions regarding how to use a piece of equipment and the client is injured, the personal trainer may be found negligent. Legal standards require that clients be given "adequate and proper" instruction before and during an activity. In a courtroom, an expert witness could be asked to assess "proper" or factually correct instruction. Adequate and proper instruction also means avoiding high-risk exercises, or those not recommended by professional peers. Advocating dangerous or controversial exercises puts the personal trainer at risk for a successful lawsuit if a client is injured. In one case, a personal trainer put his client on a treadmill, but failed to appropriately adjust the speed for this first-time user or explain how to adjust the speed or stop the belt (*Corrigan v. Musclemakers, Inc.*, 1999). The client could not keep pace, and she was catapulted backward and fractured her ankle in the ensuing fall.

Proper instruction also means individualizing workout routines for each client. An exercise may be appropriate for one client but completely inappropriate for another due to a variety of circumstances. In a reported case in the media, a personal trainer was sued for causing injuries to his client. The personal trainer admitted to using the same workout routine with all of his clients. The injured woman was 42 years old and was not in proper physical condition to perform the same exercises as the personal trainer's other clients, who were much younger, healthier, and more advanced in their exercise training. After only her second workout, she was admitted to a hospital for nearly two weeks.

Personal trainers should insist on proper use of equipment and correct completion of activities at all times. Many personal trainers remember to properly demonstrate how to operate equipment the first time a client uses it, but if the client uses poor form in the future, personal trainers often become lax in terms of maintaining proper standards of performance. Personal trainers should demonstrate proper instruction by always using good technique during their own workouts. If a client is not corrected when using bad form or sees a personal trainer "bending the rules," the client may be more likely to exercise improperly, which can increase the likelihood of injury.

A relatively new aspect of instructional liability concerns the physical touching of clients. Personal trainers should avoid touching clients unless it is essential for proper instruction and explicit permission is obtained from the client. Clients should be informed about the purpose of potential touching before it occurs. If a client objects or does not give explicit permission for the personal trainer to touch him or her, an alternative exercise should be utilized. Charges of sexual assault, even if groundless, can have disastrous consequences for a personal trainer's career.

APPLY WHAT YOU KNOW

Safety Guidelines

In reference to the aforementioned areas of responsibility, personal trainers should adhere to the following safety guidelines in the conduct of their activities:

- Be sure that all sessions are well-planned, appropriate, and documented.
- Communicate and enforce all safety rules for equipment use.
- Ensure that equipment meets or exceeds all industry standards.
- Inspect all equipment prior to use and document adherence to maintenance schedules.
- Never allow unsupervised activity by the client.
- Limit participation to those under contract (i.e., no friends or family members).
- Clearly warn clients about the specific risks of planned activities.
- Only select activities within the defined scope of practice and appropriate areas of expertise.
- Ensure that clients wear any necessary protective equipment.
- Review the emergency plan [access to a phone and 9-1-1 for emergency medical services (EMS)].
- Stay up to date with certifications and education in the field.

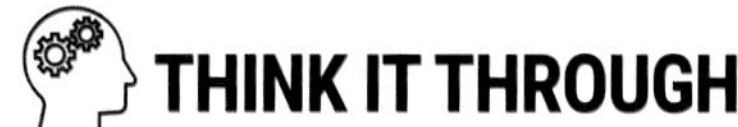

Safety Guidelines

Review the list of safety guidelines above. Do you take all of those steps to ensure the safety of your clients? If not, why not? What can you do to improve these practices in your business?

Scope of Practice

One of the biggest difficulties for a personal trainer—particularly one who constantly spends time seeking to learn new information—is to remember the extent of one's professional qualifications (see Table 1-2, page 12). An ACE certification signifies the attainment of a specific level of knowledge, but it is narrowly focused in certain areas. Certainly, the more one learns, the greater the ability to help clients, but there is a danger that personal trainers may extend their service offerings beyond their area of established expertise or scope of practice. Many states allow exercise "prescriptions" to be developed only by a licensed doctor. Therefore, it is important that personal trainers who are not also credentialled in the medical community provide exercise programs, not exercise prescriptions. Although the difference between these terms may sound like a technicality, it could become an important issue in a courtroom. Personal trainers should attempt to develop a network of doctors and other allied health professionals, such as dietitians and physical therapists, who can provide meaningful information and services to their clients. Clients who need

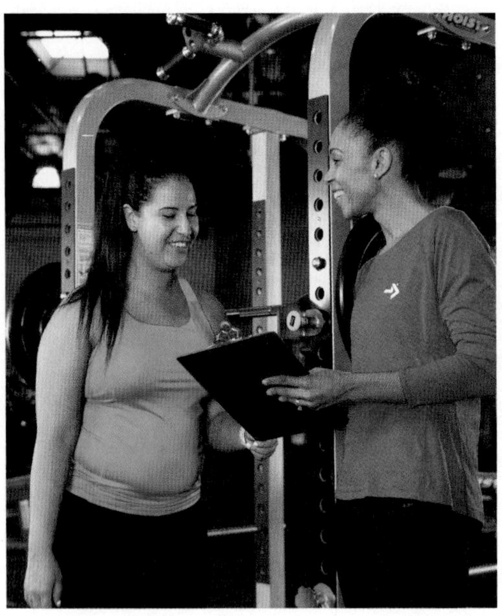

the specialized services of these allied health professionals should be referred for treatment and counseling. In turn, these professionals may refer clients to the personal trainer.

In addition to referring new clients for medical clearance when appropriate prior to beginning an exercise regimen with a personal trainer, it is also important for the personal trainer to have a completed **lifestyle and health-history questionnaire** (see Figure 5–4, pages 150–153). However, these documents should be utilized for the determination of an individual's level of fitness, rather than for the purpose of providing or recommending treatment for specific medical conditions.

Personal trainers should use the lifestyle and health-history questionnaire to screen the client for appropriate placement in a fitness program. In cases where significant risk is indicated, the client should be referred to a physician for clearance before the program begins. If personal trainers were to use the lifestyle and health-history questionnaire to recommend treatment, they could be accused of practicing medicine without a license. Ideally, clients will have a physician sign a physician's clearance form and produce a letter on the doctor's letterhead prior to beginning exercise. However, if a client fakes a physician's signature to obtain acceptance to a fitness program, the personal trainer probably would not be held liable, unless, possibly, the personal trainer had knowledge of the forgery prior to the client's participation.

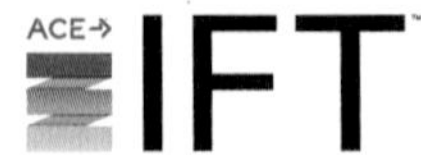

Personal trainers must understand how to use the information collected on the lifestyle and health-history questionnaire, asking only those questions that they can interpret and apply. Personal trainers must read and fully understand the answers the client provides. The forms are designed to alert the personal trainer to any potential problems that could occur; therefore, the personal trainer should not just see the completed form as an item to "cross off the checklist." Personal trainers should incorporate the information on the forms into the fitness programs they design for their clients. Creating and implementing safe and effective exercise programs for clients can be accomplished effectively through the guidelines set forth in the ACE Integrated Fitness Training® Model, which include asking important questions during the initial interview, selecting appropriate assessments, developing programs that are informed by the results of those assessments, and progressing clients as appropriate.

Personal trainers may administer fitness assessments if they are recognized by a professional organization as appropriate for the intended use and are within the scope of the personal trainers' qualifications and training. For example, the American College of Sports Medicine (ACSM, 2018) has established protocols for assessing a client's health-related physical fitness to collect baseline data that may be helpful for initial exercise program design and creating reasonable and attainable fitness goals. Personal trainers should carefully follow preparticipation health-screening and fitness-assessment procedures and should never attempt to administer an assessment without proper training. In some cases, a qualified physician or other trained medical personnel must be present. It is important for personal trainers to operate only within their areas of expertise, particularly when exercise testing is conducted.

Most personal trainers can easily recognize certain situations in which they do not have the needed expertise. For example, most personal trainers would know immediately that a client who asked to have a sample of his or her blood drawn and analyzed would likely need to see a physician. However, in other situations, personal trainers may not recognize that they are providing advice beyond their qualifications. The unique close and personal relationship that often develops between personal trainers and their clients can cause potential areas of concern. Many clients view their personal trainer not only as their fitness advisor, but also as their physical therapist, dietitian, marriage counselor, or psychologist. When these types of perceived relationships develop, the personal trainer must pay particular attention to comments that may be construed as qualified professional advice. It is important for personal trainers to always stay within their scope of practice when providing professional advice or providing a personal opinion that could be taken as professional advice. Though personal trainers may never wish to purposely hurt their clients, careless or misunderstood comments and actions can cause considerable pain, both physical and psychological.

When clients seek recommendations about exercise equipment, clothing, or shoes, it is important for personal trainers to remain cautious when responding, particularly when they may have a pre-existing endorsement arrangement with a service provider. Before giving advice, personal trainers should become knowledgeable about the products and equipment available, as well as their advantages and disadvantages. Another option would be to limit potential liability by referring clients to their choice of retail sporting goods stores. Advice based solely on personal experience should be given with that express qualification.

Though the choice of shoes and other equipment is important, of far greater concern and consequence is the solicitation of advice regarding nutrition and supplements (refer to Chapter 6 for the ACE Position Statement on Nutrition Scope of Practice for Personal Trainers). One of the most noteworthy cases in this area concerned a personal trainer who suggested dietary supplements for a client (*Capati v. Crunch Fitness*, 2002). The client died from a brain hemorrhage due to complications from an adverse interaction between the supplements and other medication she was taking. Unless personal trainers have received specific medical or nutritional training and have earned appropriate professional licenses, credentials, or certifications (e.g., medical doctor or **registered dietitian**), they should not provide advice in these areas. Most personal trainers know and understand this potential area of concern, but they often unwittingly provide advice to their clients. For example, there is a distinct difference between telling a client that a certain food, beverage, or supplement contains a high amount of **vitamins** and **minerals** and specifically telling a client to eat more of a particular food, beverage, or supplement. When a client is told to do something, it creates a potential liability for the personal trainer.

Personal trainers should also learn to recognize physical problems that their clients may be having. Unfortunately, impulsive behaviors regarding diet and exercise can lead some clients to engage in potentially destructive behaviors. It is important to learn to recognize signs indicative

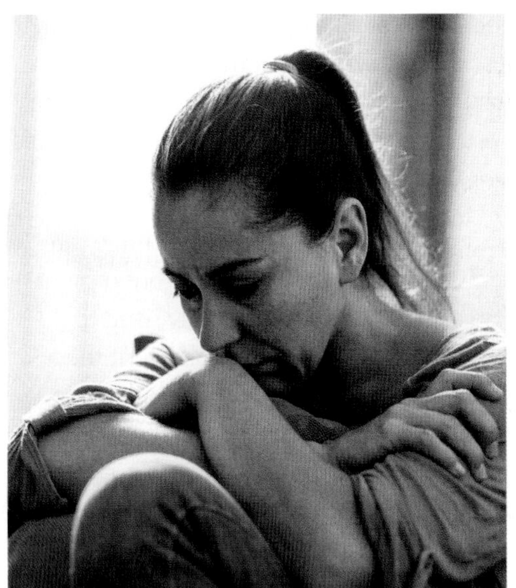

of eating disorders such as **anorexia**, **bulimia,** and **binge eating disorder.** In addition, despite various potential side effects, the use and overuse of supplements, steroids, and **growth hormone** has become more common. Personal trainers should never state, or even insinuate, that they support their client's use of these products. When personal trainers recognize potential problems in their clients, they should have a plan to address the situation. Personal trainers should seek the advice of experts in the field when developing these protocols and should seek legal counsel when necessary.

Though a client–personal trainer relationship does not legally require the same standards for confidentiality as a physician–patient or attorney–client relationship, personal trainers should maintain that same level of expectation. It is inappropriate for personal trainers to discuss their client's workout regimens, strength and flexibility achievements, and weight loss with others. Violating a client's privacy is not only unethical but can also lead to significant negative repercussions (refer to the Appendix for the ACE Code of Ethics).

Liability Insurance

Even after taking precautions, it is important for personal trainers to be aware of the importance of insurance. The recent rise in litigation throughout the healthcare industry has caused nearly every personal trainer to seek some sort of insurance. The need for insurance is always present, but as personal trainers and their businesses become more financially successful, the importance of insurance also increases. Unfortunately, potential plaintiffs and their lawyers often "target" successful businesses, since there is a greater likelihood of "winning" a substantial financial reward. Though most trial attorneys will agree to work on a contingency fee basis, some unscrupulous attorneys will take meritless cases simply with the hope that they will be "successful" in convincing a judge or jury that their client deserves compensation. Judgments for millions of dollars are not uncommon, and few individuals or businesses could survive such a substantial financial loss. Insurance protection provides some peace of mind, as personal trainers can be secure in the knowledge that if someone were to be injured as a result of their actions or if a meritless lawsuit were to occur, insurance coverage would be adequate to recompense that individual for his or her losses. There are a variety of important insurance aspects to understand.

Generally, an insurance policy is a contract designed to protect personal trainers and their assets from litigation. There is, however, some truth to the saying that insurance companies are in the business of collecting premiums and denying claims. It is important to understand the basic components of insurance coverage before soliciting guidance from an insurance agent. Agents are in the business of selling policies, which means some agents will focus more on the potential sale than on providing accurate advice. Though it is important to never be "underinsured," personal trainers can purchase too much insurance given their unique situation. Talking with established personal trainers or seeking information from trusted industry organizations such as ACE can be a great way to be referred to a successful insurance agent who understands the unique aspects of the fitness industry. Not all insurance carriers are equal in their experience, acumen, and financial resources. The most reputable insurance carriers have a national affiliation, are licensed, have strong financial backing, have a reinsurer (corporate policy to ensure that policy holders' claims will be met even if their business collapses), and have not had any claims filed against them by the Better Business Bureau. It is the personal trainer's responsibility to investigate insurance carriers and coverage prior to beginning training sessions. This investigation should not be conducted only upon initial purchase, as the performance and financial resources of insurance carriers can change each year. It is important that the personal trainer is aware of potential alterations in the ability of the insurance company to meet its obligations.

In general, personal trainers should not assume that any of their typically established personal insurance (e.g., auto and home) extends to their professional activities. For example, most homeowner's insurance has general liability to cover slips, trips, and falls that may occur while guests are visiting a person's home. This type of coverage would likely not cover a client who fell while being trained, since the training would be considered a business activity.

Personal trainers need to secure **professional liability insurance** that is specifically designed to cover activities related to their health and fitness business. The selected liability insurance policy should cover personal injuries that can occur as a result of a training session. Injured clients may sue not only for medical expenses, but also for a variety of other compensation, such as lost wages from being unable to work, pain and suffering, and loss of consortium. ACE recommends retaining at least $1 million in coverage, as medical expenses can easily cost hundreds of thousands of dollars. In some instances, a higher liability coverage amount may be advisable.

The American Council on Exercise has an established relationship with a reputable insurance carrier who specializes in the fitness industry. Visit www.ACEfitness.org/insurancecenter/ for more information.

Personal trainers must understand the specific insurance needs that may arise given the location of the training activities. Home-based training has become popular, as many clients prefer to work with personal trainers in their own residence. In addition, some personal trainers would rather use their homes for training activities than maintain a formal relationship with a fitness center. General liability policies may not cover a personal trainer who works with clients in a private residence or for those who provide instruction and supervision online. Owners who will use their own home or a client's home should ensure that a specific insurance **rider**—a special addition to typical policy provisions—will cover those activities. In addition, specific language should provide liability protection for personal trainers who utilize outdoor settings for their training activities. In cases where personal trainers will work outside of a fitness center, it is imperative that the insurance carrier is aware of the professional activities that will occur. In most cases,

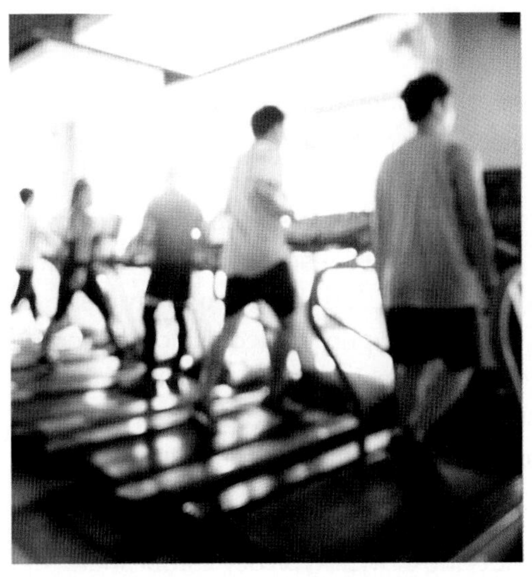

home-based or outdoor training will require insurance (typically at higher rates) that specifically covers the personal trainer for these locations. For personal trainers who own their own fitness clubs, insurance should be retained that covers potential problems with the facility as well as the instruction and supervision of the personal trainer.

Most insurance agents now recommend that all professionals purchase an **umbrella liability policy.** The umbrella policy provides added coverage for all of the other insurance (e.g., auto, home, and professional liability) that a person may have in place. For example, if a personal trainer was sued and the judgment exceeded his or her professional liability coverage, the umbrella policy would cover the insurance shortfall. When purchasing an umbrella policy, personal trainers should be sure that it covers professional activities associated with personal training. In addition, every liability policy should be examined to ensure that it covers the personal trainer while working in various locations (e.g., fitness center, personal home, client's home, online, and outdoors).

Personal trainers who sell products may need to secure **product liability insurance** in the event a product fails to perform properly. This is particularly important for personal trainers who own and operate fitness centers. Though the manufacturer of a product retains most of the liability for design flaws, manufacturing defects, and product malfunctions, there have been cases where the "middleman" was also successfully sued.

Personal trainers who form partnerships or corporations may wish to investigate the purchase of **keyman insurance.** A keyman insurance policy is designed to compensate the business for the loss of a person who performs a unique and valuable function. If a business will experience significant financial trouble if one person has an extended illness or dies, keyman insurance should be purchased. Keyman insurance pays a specified amount to assist the business in its recovery from losing a critical human resource.

EMPLOYEES AND INDEPENDENT CONTRACTORS

Many health and fitness industry employers now require their employees to demonstrate proof of liability insurance when they are hired, even though they will be potentially covered under the fitness center's insurance. Employers should ensure that employees renew and verify their policies annually. Potential employees may wish to verify that the fitness center has adequate coverage and that the employer's insurance will assist them in defending a potential lawsuit. It is *critical* that independent contractors working for fitness clubs or other facilities maintain adequate insurance, as the facility's legal representatives would likely seek to separate the facility itself from the actions of the personal trainer if a lawsuit occurs. The employment or independent contractor contract between the fitness center and the personal trainer should contain language detailing insurance requirements and responsibilities.

One important aspect of insurance is to obligate the insurance carrier to pay in the event of a loss. The following statement, or some version of it, should be included in any basic agreement:

> *We agree to pay those sums that the insured becomes legally obligated to pay as damages because of bodily injury or property damage to which this insurance applies, and these will include damages arising out of any negligent act, error, or omission in rendering or failing to render professional services described in this policy.*

One of the key provisions is that the insurance company will pay even if the personal trainer fails to provide a service. For example, if an injured person needed first-aid attention and the personal trainer did not provide it, the policy should still provide protection. If "failure to render" or "omission" is not specified, the policy covers the personal trainer only if the services provided were inadequate or improper.

A critical component of an insurance policy is related to coverage of legal fees, settlements, and defense charges. Personal trainers should look for the following type of clause in their policy:

> *We will have the right and duty to defend any suit seeking damages under this policy, even if the allegations are groundless, false, or fraudulent and may, at our discretion, make such investigation and settlement of any claim or suit deemed expedient.*

The best policies cover the cost of a legal defense *and* any claims awarded. Policies that only cover an amount equal to awarded damages are not recommended, as the personal trainer will be covered for the final judgment, but all of the trial expenses incurred will be the personal trainer's responsibility. One of the realities of insurance litigation is that the insurance company may make a strategic decision to settle rather than fight the case in court. It is important to have a policy that covers the cost of litigation, but the personal trainer should not necessarily be disappointed if the insurance company elects to settle a lawsuit out of court.

While it is important to identify and understand what is covered in the insurance policy, it is also critical to know what is not covered. Most policies delineate specific exclusions. The following liabilities are often excluded in exercise professional policies: abuse, molestation, cancer (resulting from tanning), libel, and slander. Personal trainers should also inquire whether bodily insurance coverage will cover lawsuits alleging mental stress. Most policies differentiate between the two, and a standard bodily injury clause does not necessarily include mental injuries. A client filing a suit might claim that the personal trainer was overly critical and, as a result, mental injuries were suffered. Mental injuries are difficult to define and determine. The courts are split on the issue of inclusion.

Most policies exclude coverage for acts committed before the policy was purchased. Coverage also might be excluded for claims that occurred during the policy period but are filed after the coverage has been terminated. These issues are related to the "claims-made basis" of a policy. Though it can be expensive, "prior acts coverage" can be purchased from most insurance carriers for an additional cost if a personal trainer has made the ill-advised decision to have begun training without insurance coverage. An "extended reporting endorsement" will ensure that claims made in the future for injuries during the policy period will be covered even if the policy is cancelled.

Ideally, insurance coverage should be maintained until after the statute of limitations has expired for anyone who has been a client of a personal trainer.

Understanding insurance policies initially can be difficult. Proper research of potential insurance agents is critical. Once an insurance carrier has been identified, the personal trainer should maintain an open line of communication with his or her agent. Ultimately, the agent and the insurance company work for the personal trainer, but it is the personal trainer's responsibility to maintain open communication. Any changes in business activity should be immediately relayed to the insurance company so that appropriate changes in the policy can be made. Adequate levels of insurance can change as a personal trainer's client list, employees, and income increase.

Other Business Concerns with Legal Implications

In addition to the legal responsibilities in the areas of business structure, scope of practice, facilities, equipment, testing, instruction, and supervision, personal trainers must be aware of the implications of certain other potential legal issues.

MARKETING ACTIVITIES

Identifying and procuring clients is the lifeblood of any business. Though many personal trainers maintain high ethical standards, some health clubs and fitness centers have relatively little concern for ethical behavior. Unfortunately, it has become common for some fitness centers to utilize improper marketing tactics and long-term contracts that contain devious language to attract and retain clients. In some extreme cases, fitness centers have even misused direct deposit agreements to commit fraud. Personal trainers should understand the marketing and operating activities that their fitness centers may utilize. If a fitness center is behaving unethically or illegally, the personal trainer may be "associated" with those practices, even if he or she had no direct involvement in the improper behavior. The widespread use of the Internet has enabled customer complaints to be relayed to current and potential clients, as well as to the Better Business Bureau. Since a significant portion of a personal trainer's business is related to reputation, it is important to only associate with fitness facilities that maintain high legal and ethical standards.

SOCIAL MEDIA

Social media has become a powerful tool to reach and influence current and potential customers. When utilizing various social media platforms, personal trainers must remember that laws do apply, particularly in the area of clients' right to privacy. Though a personal trainer may take photos of a client exercising, using those photos in a social media marketing campaign may violate the person's right to protect his or her name, image, and likeness. In most cases, it is necessary to have a client (or anyone whose face may be recognizable in a photo) to sign a release granting permission to utilize the image to further the marketing activities of the personal trainer. In addition, the use of social media does not enable the personal trainer to share information regarding the health or performance of an individual. Posting comments regarding the progress a client is making, even if done with good intentions, may violate the person's privacy and leave the personal trainer susceptible to a lawsuit.

INTELLECTUAL PROPERTY

Music recordings sold commercially are intended strictly for the private, noncommercial use of the purchaser. In addition, there are rules regarding the use of television programming as a key component of any non-food or beverage service business. This means that in many cases copyright violations occur when a fitness center utilizes music or television broadcasts as a key component of its business. Although two groups in America, the **American Society of Composers, Authors, and Publishers (ASCAP)** and **Broadcast Music, Inc. (BMI),** as well as the **Society of European Stage Authors and Composers (SESAC),** will issue licenses for the commercial use of broadcasts and recordings, their fees may be prohibitive in many situations. When training clients in their homes, personal trainers can have clients provide the music for each session. In effect, the clients are then using these recording for their own private, non-commercial enjoyment during exercise.

Some personal trainers may seek copyright or trademark protection for their own creative works. Personal trainers who develop specific routines or who write books or other materials may wish to profit from their creativity. For example, a book or instruction manual can be copyrighted so that any future sales provide a **royalty** to the author. Personal trainers who develop a company name or slogan may seek trademark protection so that other individuals or businesses cannot utilize that name or slogan without permission.

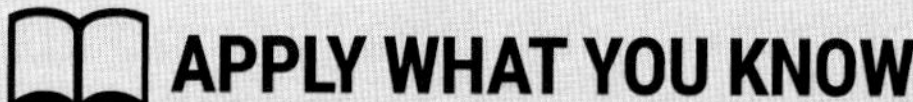

Proper Use of the ACE Name and Logo

ACE is an internationally recognized brand that has garnered a high level of respect from leaders in the health and fitness industry, healthcare, business, and government over the past several decades. If you identify yourself as an ACE® Certified Professional in your marketing materials, you will benefit from the reputation the organization has built. To preserve the integrity of the ACE name and enhance the status of both the organization and the professionals it serves, certifies, and represents, ACE has developed a trademark usage program. As an ACE Certified Professional, we ask that you follow the guidelines set by ACE when it comes to utilizing the organization's trademarks. The trademarks you are authorized to use, as well as guidelines that ACE provides so you utilize them properly, are available in your My ACE Account (once you earn your ACE Certification) on ACEfitness.org. In general, a trademark should not be used as a noun but rather an adjective to describe a product or service. In addition, you need to disclose that ACE is the owner of their trademarks. You can do so by stating in your marketing materials that feature the ACE logo or name, "ACE is a registered trademark of the American Council on Exercise."

TRANSPORTATION

In most cases, personal trainers will meet their clients at a fitness center or some other location. However, there may be a situation where the personal trainer provides transportation for the client to or from a training session. Personal trainers should be aware that many "standard" automobile insurance policies may not cover injuries sustained by clients riding in the personal trainer's vehicle. If the personal trainer is going to provide a ride to a client, the personal trainer should check with his or her auto insurance company to ensure that potential injuries from accidents are covered.

FINANCING

As personal trainers create and expand their businesses, they may need to seek financing for certain activities. Even if the personal trainer is operating as an LLC/LLP or S-corp, banks and other lenders usually will only loan money if it is personally guaranteed by an individual. Unfortunately, many companies have advertised "business loans" that are in fact personal loans.

Personal trainers who thought that only their businesses were liable for the financial obligation later learned that the lender was able to pursue the personal trainer for unpaid debts. Personal trainers should read and understand the "fine print" of any loan (or, better yet, hire an attorney to review the documents) prior to signing.

Risk Management

One of the most important aspects of any business is risk management. There are risks associated with any activity, but exercise programs carry specific risks due to the physical movement and exertion often required. Personal trainers should constantly search for methods to make the environment safer for their clients. Periodically reviewing programs, facilities, and equipment to evaluate potential dangers allows the personal trainer to decide the best way to reduce potentially costly injuries in each situation.

Most authorities recommend a risk-management protocol that consists of the following five steps:

- **Risk identification:** This step involves the specification of all risks that may be encountered in the areas of instruction, supervision, facilities, equipment, contracts, and business structure.
- **Risk evaluation:** The personal trainer must review each risk, with consideration given to the probability that the risk could occur and, if so, what would be the conceivable severity. Table 16-4 can be used to assess the identified risks.
- **Selection of an approach for managing each risk:** Several approaches are available to the personal trainer for managing and reducing the identified risks:
  - **Avoidance:** Remove the possibility of danger and injury by eliminating the activity.
  - **Transfer:** Move the risk to others through waivers, insurance policies, etc.
  - **Reduction:** Modify the risks by removing or altering part of the activity.
  - **Retention:** Often, there are risks that will be retained, especially if the removal of the risk would eliminate a potential benefit (e.g., no risks will occur if exercise

is eliminated, but then no health benefits can be accrued). The recommended approach for extreme risks is to avoid the activity completely. Risks that fall into one of the high categories can be managed either through insurance or viable actions to reduce the likelihood of occurrence or severity of outcome. Reduction is also the preferred method for addressing risks in the medium category, while risks with low impact can be retained (see Table 16-4).

- **Implementation:** Institute the plan.
- **Evaluation:** Continually assess the outcome of risk-management endeavors. The standard of care regarding some risks may change over time. Therefore, risk-management approaches may need to be altered.

TABLE 16-4
Evaluating Risk Based on Frequency and Severity

Severity of Injury or Financial Impact	Frequency of Occurrence		
	High or Often	**Medium or Infrequent**	**Low or Seldom**
High or Vital	Avoid	Avoid or transfer	Transfer
Medium or Significant	Avoid or transfer	Transfer, reduce, or retain	Transfer, reduce, or retain
Low or Insignificant	Retain	Retain	Retain

Personal trainers can also manage risk by examining procedures and policies and developing conduct and safety guidelines for clients' use of equipment. Strict safety guidelines for each activity, accompanied by procedures for emergencies, are particularly important. Personal trainers must not only develop these policies, but also become thoroughly familiar with them by mentally practicing emergency plans. Several lawsuits have resulted in substantial judgments against exercise professionals who failed to respond to the emergency medical needs of clients. In some cases, the initial injury was not a major concern, but the failure to adequately address the initial problem was the focus of the litigation. When an incident occurs, the personal trainer should first ensure the safety of all individuals involved. Once the immediate concern for safety has passed, the personal trainer should complete an incident report. The personal trainer should note any facts related to the incident and solicit information from any witnesses. When collecting information from witnesses, it is critical to get phone numbers, physical addresses, email addresses, and signatures for future verification and follow-up. This information should be retained in a secure location for future reference in the event of a lawsuit or when reviewing past performance and emergency-management procedures.

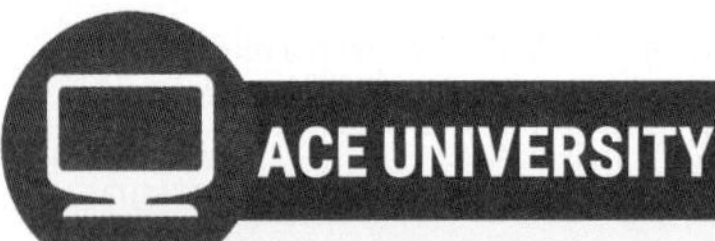

If your study program includes the ACE University, visit www.ACEfitness.org/MyACE and log in to your My ACE Account to take full advantage of the ACE Personal Trainer Study Program and online guided study experience.

A variety of media to support and expand on the material in this text is provided to facilitate learning and best prepare you for the ACE Personal Trainer Certification exam and a career as a personal trainer.

SUMMARY

Although often overlooked when considering the technical aspects of providing quality personalized fitness instruction, legal and business concerns are of paramount importance. This chapter provided a summary overview of the legal and professional responsibilities of personal trainers. In every instance, personal trainers should seek the guidance of qualified attorneys who specialize in the fitness industry. Personal trainers should establish their businesses in the proper structure, understand and utilize contracts, know the changing nature of their legal responsibilities, secure proper insurance, and implement a comprehensive risk-management plan. Ultimately, it is the personal trainer's responsibility to not only continually educate him- or herself regarding the "science" of personal training, but also to thoroughly understand the legal guidelines that must be followed to create a safe and enjoyable environment for clients.

REFERENCES

Agoglia, J. (2005). *The AED Agenda.* www.clubindustry.com/mag/aed-agenda

American College of Sports Medicine (2018). *ACSM's Guidelines for Exercise Testing and Prescription* (10th ed.). Philadelphia: Wolters Kluwer.

Capati v. Crunch Fitness International, Inc. et al. (N.Y. App. 2002). 295 A.D.2d 181.

Corrigan v. Musclemakers, Inc. (1999). 686 N.Y.S. 2d 143.

Cotten, D.J. (2000a). Carefully worded liability waiver protects Bally's from liability for personal trainer negligence. *Exercise Standards and Malpractice Reporter,* 14, 5, 65.

Cotten, D.J. (2000b). Non-signing spouses: Are they bound by a waiver signed by the other spouse? *Exercise Standards and Malpractice Reporter,* 14, 2, 18.

Cotten, D.J. & Cotten, M.B. (2016). *Waivers & Releases of Liability* (9th ed.). Scotts Valley, Calif.: CreateSpace Independent Publishing.

Dominic, A. (2016). *24 Hour Fitness Sued in Death of Former San Diego Charger.* https://www.clubindustry.com/commercial-clubs/24-hour-fitness-sued-death-former-san-diego-charger

Fowler v. Bally Total Fitness (2008). Maryland Case No. 07 L 12258.

Herbert, D.L. & Herbert, W.G. (2002). *Legal Aspects of Preventive and Rehabilitative Exercise Programs* (4th ed.). Canton, Ohio: PRC Publishing.

Stromgren, E. (2016). *Connecticut Jury Finds Equinox, Personal Trainer Negligent in $10.875 Million Injury Case.* https://www.clubindustry.com/equinox/connecticut-jury-finds-equinox-personal-trainer-negligent-10875-million-injury-case

Vaid v. Equinox Greenwich Old Track Road, Inc., et al., Superior Court, J.D. of Stamford/Norwalk, D.N. FST CV 13 6019426 S (February 16, 2016).

SUGGESTED READINGS

Broadcast Music, Inc. (2014). *Music Licensing for Fitness & Health Clubs.* www.bmi.com/licensing/entry/fitness_clubs

DeMers, J. (2014). *Don't Post Pictures of Your Customers Online without Reading This.* https://www.forbes.com/sites/jaysondemers/2014/09/04/dont-post-pictures-of-your-customers-online-without-reading-this/#352bab633cc3

National Conference of State Legislatures (2017). *State Laws on Cardiac Arrest & Defibrillators.* www.ncsl.org/research/health/laws-on-cardiac-arrest-and-defibrillators-aeds.aspx

Rabe, A. (2017). *Legal Risks and Issues to Consider for Fitness Trainers Working Online.* https://fitlegally.com/legal-risks-issues-consider-fitness-trainers-working-online/

APPENDIX

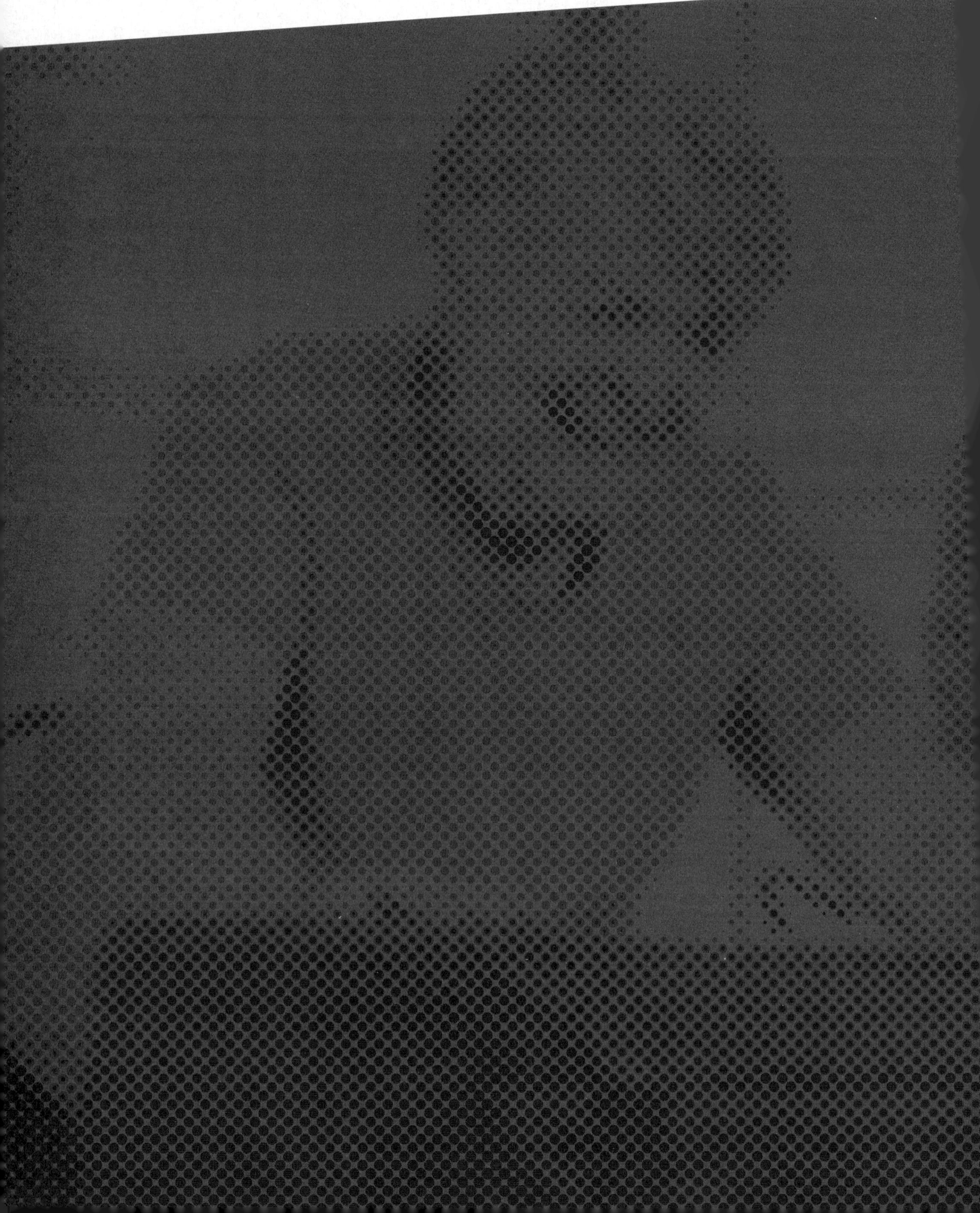

APPENDIX
ACE Code of Ethics

GLOSSARY

INDEX

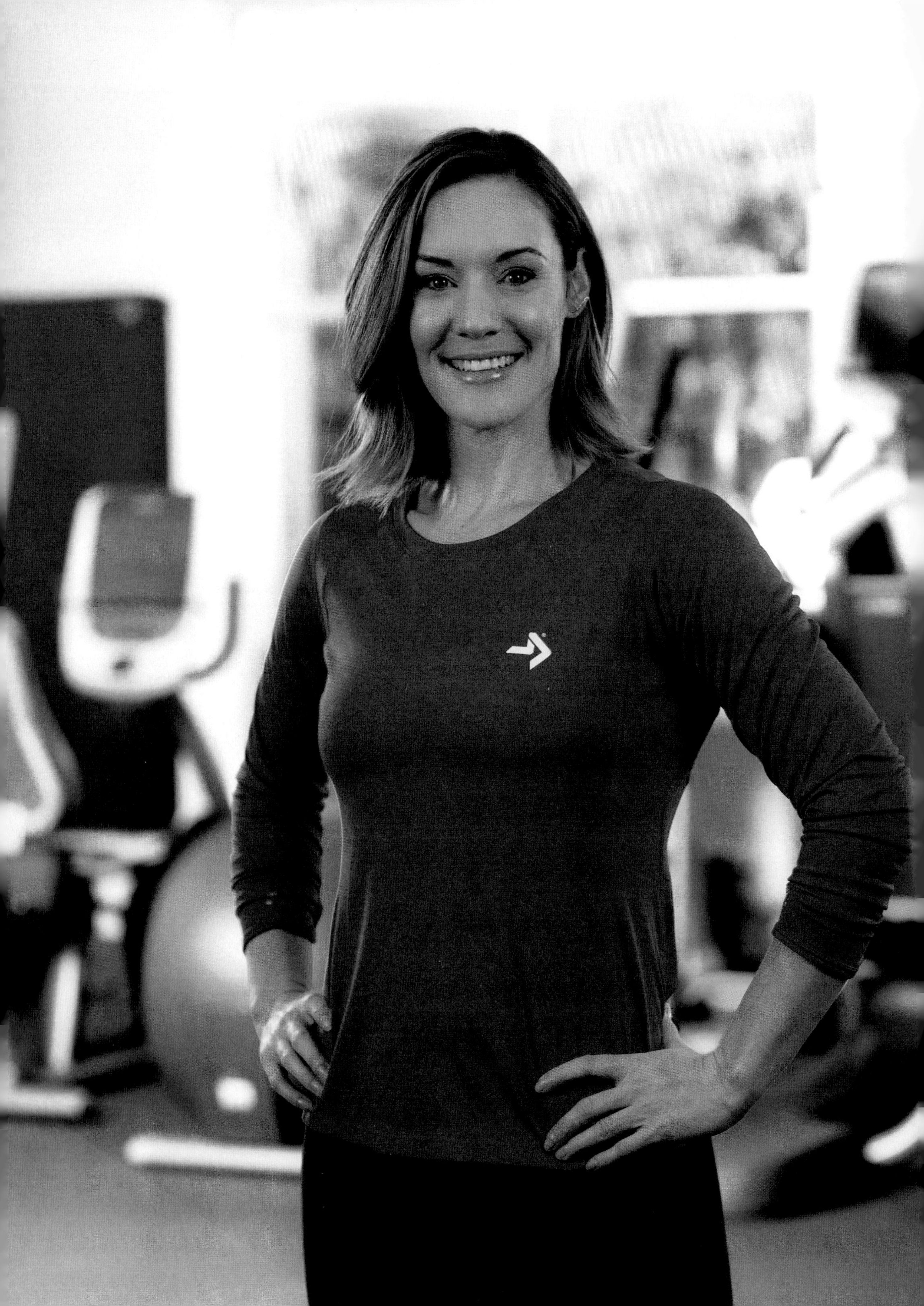

APPENDIX

ACE Code of Ethics

PROVIDE SAFE AND EFFECTIVE INSTRUCTION

Providing safe and effective instruction involves a variety of responsibilities for ACE Certified Professionals. Safe means that the instruction will not result in physical, mental, emotional, or financial harm to the client/participant. Effective means that the instruction or coaching has a purposeful, intended, and desired effect toward the client's/participant's goal. Great effort and care must be taken in carrying out the responsibilities that are essential in creating a positive and enjoyable exercise experience for all clients/participants.

Preparticipation Health Screening

ACE Certified Professionals should have all potential clients/participants complete an industry-recognized health-screening tool to ensure safe and enjoyable exercise participation. If significant risk factors or signs and symptoms suggestive of chronic disease are identified, refer the client/participant to a physician or primary healthcare practitioner for medical clearance and guidance regarding which types of assessments, activities, or exercises are indicated, contraindicated, or deemed high risk. If an individual does not want to obtain medical clearance, it may be prudent to have that individual sign a legally prepared document that releases you and the facility in which you work from any liability related to any injury that may result from exercise participation or assessment. Once the client/participant has been cleared for exercise and you have a full understanding of the client's/participant's health status and medical history, including his or her current use of medications, a formal risk-management plan for potential emergencies must be prepared and reviewed periodically.

Assessments

The main objective of a health and fitness assessment is to establish the client's/participant's current health and fitness levels in order to design an appropriate exercise program. Explain the risks and benefits of each assessment and provide the client/participant with any pertinent instructions. Prior to conducting any type of assessment, the client/participant must be given an opportunity to ask questions and read and sign an informed consent. The types and order of assessments are dictated by the client's/participant's health status, fitness level, symptoms, and/or use of medications. Remember that each assessment has specific protocols and only those within your scope of practice should be administered. Once the assessments are completed, evaluate and discuss the results objectively as they relate to the client's/participant's health condition and goals. Educate the client/participant and emphasize how an exercise program will benefit the client/participant.

Program Design

You must not prescribe exercise, diet, or treatment, as doing so is outside your scope of practice and implies ordering or advising a medicine or treatment. Instead, it is appropriate for you to design exercise programs that improve components of physical fitness and wellness while adhering to the limitations of a previous injury or condition as determined by a certified, registered, or licensed allied health professional. Because nutritional laws and the practice of dietetics vary in each state, province, and country, understand what type of basic nutritional information is appropriate and legal for you to disseminate to your client/participant. The client's/participant's preferences, and short- and long-term goals, as well as current industry standards and guidelines, must be taken into consideration as you develop an engaging and realistic program to facilitate desired physical activity, behavior change, and other health and fitness outcomes. Provide as much detail for all exercise parameters such as frequency, intensity, type of exercise, duration, volume, progression, and termination points.

Program Implementation

Do not underestimate your ability to influence the client/participant to become active for a lifetime. Be sure that each class or session is well-planned, sequential, and documented. Instruct the client/participant how to safely and properly perform the appropriate exercises and communicate this in a manner that the client/participant will understand and retain. Each client/participant has a different learning curve that will require different levels of attention, learning aids, and repetition. Supervise the client/participant closely, especially when spotting or cueing is needed. If supervising a group of two or more, ensure that you can supervise and provide the appropriate amount of attention to each individual at all times. Ideally, the group will have similar goals and will be performing similar exercises or activities. Position yourself so that you do not have to turn your back to any client/participant performing an exercise.

Facilities and Non-Facility Spaces

Although the condition of a facility, or non-facility, space may not always be within your control, you are still obligated to ensure a hazard-free environment to maximize safety. If you notice potential hazards in the exercise space, communicate these hazards to the client/participant and/or the facility management. For example, if you notice that the clamps that keep the weights on the barbells are getting rusty and loose, it would be prudent of you to remove them from the training area and alert management that immediate repair is required.

Equipment

Obtain equipment that meets or exceeds industry standards and utilize the equipment only for its intended use. Arrange exercise equipment and stations so that adequate space exists between equipment, participants, and foot traffic. Schedule regular maintenance and inspect equipment prior to use to ensure it is in proper working condition. Avoid the use of homemade equipment, as your liability is greater if it causes injury to a person exercising under your supervision.

PROVIDE EQUAL AND FAIR TREATMENT TO ALL CLIENTS/PARTICIPANTS

ACE Certified Professionals are obligated to provide fair and equal treatment for each client/participant without bias, preference, or discrimination against gender, ethnic background, age, national origin, basis of religion, or physical disability.

The Americans with Disabilities Act protects individuals with disabilities against any type of unlawful discrimination. A disability can be either physical or mental, such as epilepsy, paralysis, HIV infection, AIDS, a significant hearing or visual impairment, mental retardation, or a specific learning disability. ACE Certified Professionals should, at a minimum, provide reasonable accommodations to each individual with a disability. Reasonable simply means that you are able to provide accommodations that do not cause you any undue hardship that requires additional or significant expense or difficulty. Making an existing facility accessible by modifying equipment or devices, assessments, or training materials are a few examples of providing reasonable accommodations. However, providing the use of personal items or providing items at your own expense may not be considered reasonable.

This ethical consideration of providing fair and equal treatment is not limited to behavioral interactions with clients/

participants, but also extends to exercise programming and other business-related services such as communication, scheduling, billing, cancellation policies, and dispute resolution.

STAY UP-TO-DATE ON THE LATEST HEALTH AND FITNESS RESEARCH AND UNDERSTAND ITS PRACTICAL APPLICATION

Obtaining an ACE certification required you to have broad-based knowledge of many disciplines; however, this credential should not be viewed as the end of your professional development and education. Instead, it should be viewed as the beginning or foundation. The dynamic nature of the health and fitness industry requires you to maintain an understanding of the latest research and professional standards and guidelines and their impact on the design and implementation of exercise programming. To stay informed, make time to review a variety of industry resources such as professional journals, position statements, trade and lay periodicals, and correspondence courses, as well as to attend professional meetings, conferences, and educational workshops.

An additional benefit of staying up-to-date is that it also fulfills your certification renewal requirements for continuing education credit (CEC). To maintain your ACE Certified status, you must obtain an established amount of CECs every two years. CECs are granted for structured learning that takes place within the educational portion of a course related to the profession and presented by a qualified health or exercise professional.

MAINTAIN CURRENT CPR AND AED CERTIFICATION AND KNOWLEDGE OF FIRST-AID SERVICES

ACE Certified Professionals must be prepared to recognize and respond to heart attacks and other life-threatening emergencies. Emergency response is enhanced by training and maintaining skills in cardiopulmonary resuscitation (CPR) and using automated external defibrillators (AEDs), which have become more widely available. An AED is a portable electronic device used to restore normal heart rhythm in a person experiencing a cardiac arrest and can reduce the time to defibrillation before emergency medical services (EMS) personnel arrive. For each minute that defibrillation is delayed, the victim's chance of survival is reduced by 7 to 10%. Thus, survival from cardiac arrest is improved dramatically when CPR and defibrillation are started early.

COMPLY WITH ALL APPLICABLE BUSINESS, EMPLOYMENT, AND INTELLECTUAL PROPERTY LAWS

As an ACE Certified Professional, you are expected to maintain a high level of integrity by complying with all applicable business, employment, copyright, and intellectual property laws. Be truthful and forthcoming with communication to clients/participants, coworkers, and other health and exercise professionals in advertising, marketing, and business practices. Do not create false or misleading impressions of credentials, claims, or sponsorships, or perform services outside of your scope of practice that are illegal, deceptive, or fraudulent.

All information regarding your business must be clear, accurate, and easy to understand for all potential clients/participants. Provide disclosure about the name of your business, physical address, and contact information, and maintain a working phone number and email address. So that clients/participants can make an informed choice about paying for your services, provide detailed information regarding schedules, prices, payment terms, time limits, and conditions. Cancellation, refund, and rescheduling information must also be clearly stated and easy to understand. Allow the client/participant an opportunity to ask questions and review this information before formally agreeing to your services and terms.

Because employment laws vary in each city, state, province, and country, familiarize yourself with the applicable employment regulations and standards to which your business must conform. Examples of this may include conforming to specific building codes and zoning ordinances or making sure that your place of business is accessible to individuals with a disability.

The understanding of intellectual property law and the proper use of copyrighted materials is an important legal issue for all ACE Certified Professionals. Intellectual property laws protect the creations of authors, artists, software programmers, and others with copyrighted materials. The most common infringement of intellectual property law in the fitness industry is the use of music in an exercise class. When commercial music is played in a for-profit exercise class, without a performance or blanket license, it is considered a public performance and a violation of intellectual property law. Therefore, make sure that any music, handouts, or educational materials are either exempt from intellectual property law or permissible under laws by reason of fair use, or obtain express written consent from the copyright holder for distribution, adaptation, or use. When in doubt, obtain permission first or consult with a qualified legal professional who has intellectual property law expertise.

MAINTAIN THE CONFIDENTIALITY OF ALL CLIENT/PARTICIPANT INFORMATION

Every client/participant has the right to expect that all personal data and discussions with an ACE Certified Professional will be safeguarded and not disclosed without the client's/participant's express written consent or acknowledgment. Therefore, protect the confidentiality of all client/participant information such as contact data, medical records, health history, progress notes, and meeting details. Even when confidentiality is not required by law, continue to preserve the confidentiality of such information.

Any breach of confidentiality, intentional or unintentional, potentially harms the productivity and trust of your client/participant and undermines your effectiveness as an exercise professional or health coach. This also puts you at risk for potential litigation and puts your client/participant at risk for public embarrassment and fraudulent activity such as identity theft.

Most breaches of confidentiality are unintentional and occur because of carelessness and lack of awareness. The most common breach of confidentiality is exposing or storing a client's personal data in a location that is not secure. This occurs when a client's/participant's file or information is left on a desk, or filed in a cabinet that has no lock or is accessible to others. Breaches of confidentiality may also occur when you have conversations regarding a client's/participant's performance or medical/health history with staff or others and the client's/participant's first name or other identifying details are used.

Post and adhere to a privacy policy that communicates how client/participant information will be used and secured and how a client's/participant's preference regarding unsolicited mail and email will be respected. When a client/participant provides you with any personal data, new or updated, make it a habit to immediately secure this information and ensure that only you and/or the appropriate individuals have access to it. Also, the client's/participant's files must only be accessed and used for purposes related to health and fitness services. If client/participant information is stored on a personal computer, restrict access by using a protected password. Should you receive any inquiries from family members or other individuals regarding the progress of a client/participant or other personal information, state that you cannot provide any information without the client's/participant's permission. If and when a client/participant permits you to release confidential information to an authorized individual or party, utilize secure methods of communication such as certified mail, sending and receiving information on a dedicated private fax line, or email with encryption.

REFER CLIENTS/PARTICIPANTS TO MORE QUALIFIED HEALTH OR MEDICAL PROFESSIONALS WHEN APPROPRIATE

It is vitally important that ACE Certified Professionals refer their clients/participants to a more qualified professional (e.g., physician, physical therapist, registered dietitian, psychologist, or attorney) when warranted. Doing so not only benefits your clients/participants by making sure that they receive the appropriate attention and care, but also enhances your credibility and reduces liability by defining your scope of practice and clarifying what services you can and cannot reasonably provide.

Knowing when to refer a client/participant is, however, as important as choosing to which professional to refer. For instance, when a client/participant complains of symptoms of muscle soreness or discomfort or exhibits signs of fatigue or lack of energy, it is not an absolute indication to refer your client/participant to a physician. Because continual referrals such as this are not practical, familiarize and educate yourself on expected signs and symptoms, taking into consideration the client's/participant's fitness level, health status, chronic disease, disability, and/or background as he or she is screened and as he or she begins and progresses with an exercise program. This helps you better discern between emergent and non-emergent situations and know when to refuse to offer your services, continue to monitor, and/or make an immediate referral.

It is important that you know the scope of practice for various health professionals and which types of referrals are appropriate. For example, some states require that a referring physician first approve visits to a physical therapist, while other states allow individuals to see a physical therapist directly. Only registered or licensed dietitians or physicians may provide specific dietary recommendations or diet plans; however, a client/participant who is suspected of an eating disorder should be referred to an eating disorders specialist. Refer clients/participants to a clinical psychologist if they wish to discuss family or marital problems or exhibit addictive behaviors such as substance abuse.

Network and develop rapport with potential allied health professionals in your area before you refer clients/participants to them. This demonstrates good will and respect for their expertise and will most likely result in reciprocal referrals for your services and fitness expertise.

UPHOLD AND ENHANCE PUBLIC APPRECIATION AND TRUST FOR THE HEALTH AND FITNESS INDUSTRY

The best way for ACE Certified Professionals to uphold and enhance public appreciation and trust for the health and fitness industry is to represent themselves in a dignified and professional manner. As the public is inundated with misinformation and false claims about fitness products and services, your expertise must be utilized to dispel myths and half-truths about current trends and fads that are potentially harmful to the public.

When appropriate, mentor and dispense knowledge and training to less-experienced exercise professionals and health coaches. Novice exercise professionals and health coaches can benefit from your experience and skill as you assist them in establishing a foundation based on exercise science, from both theoretical and practical standpoints. Therefore, it is a disservice if you fail to provide helpful or corrective information—especially when an individual, the public, or other exercise professionals or health coaches are at risk for injury or increased liability. For example, if you observe an individual using momentum to perform a strength-training exercise, the prudent course of action would be to suggest a modification. Likewise, if you observe an exercise professional in your workplace consistently failing to obtain informed consents before clients/participants undergo fitness testing or begin an exercise program, recommend that he or she consider implementing these forms to minimize liability.

Finally, do not represent yourself in an overly commercial or misleading manner. Consider the exercise professional who places an advertisement in a local newspaper stating: "Lose 10 pounds in 10 days or your money back!" It is inappropriate to lend credibility to or endorse a product, service, or program founded upon unsubstantiated or misleading claims; thus a solicitation such as this must be avoided, as it undermines the public's trust of exercise professionals and health coaches.

ESTABLISH AND MAINTAIN CLEAR PROFESSIONAL BOUNDARIES

Working in the fitness profession requires you to come in contact with many different people. It is imperative that a professional distance be maintained in relationships with all clients/participants. Exercise professionals and health coaches are responsible for setting and monitoring the boundaries between a working relationship and friendship with their clients/participants. To that end, ACE Certified Professionals should:

- Never initiate or encourage discussion of a sexual nature
- Avoid touching clients/participants unless it is essential to instruction
- Inform clients/participants about the purpose of touching and find an alternative if the client/participant objects
- Discontinue all touching if it appears to make the client/participant uncomfortable
- Take all reasonable steps to ensure that any personal and social contacts between themselves and their clients/participants do not have an adverse impact on the personal trainer–client, coach–client, or instructor–participant relationship

If you are unable to maintain appropriate professional boundaries with a client/participant (whether due to your attitudes and actions or those of the client/participant), the prudent course of action is to terminate the relationship and, perhaps, refer the client/participant to another professional. Keep in mind that charges of sexual harassment or assault, even if groundless, can have disastrous effects on your career.

Glossary

Abdominal fat See Visceral fat.

Abdominal obesity Excessive storage of abdominal fat. Usually indicated by a waist circumference of ≥40 inches (102 cm) in men and ≥35 inches (88 cm) in women.

Abduction Movement away from the midline of the body.

Absolute strength The maximal amount of weight an individual can lift one time.

Absorption The uptake of nutrients across a tissue or membrane by the gastrointestinal tract.

Acceptable Macronutrient Distribution Range (AMDR) The range of intake for a particular energy source that is associated with reduced risk of chronic disease while providing intakes of essential nutrients.

Acclimatization Physiological adaptation to an unfamiliar environment and achievement of a new steady state. For example, the body can adjust to a high altitude or a hot climate and gain an increased capacity to work in those conditions.

Acetylcholine A white crystalline neurotransmitter and derivative of choline that is released at the ends of nerve fibers in the somatic and parasympathetic nervous systems and is involved in the transmission of nerve impulses in the body.

Actin Thin contractile protein in a myofibril.

Action The stage of the transtheoretical model of behavior change during which the individual is actively engaging in a behavior that was started less than six months ago.

Active listening Mode of listening in which the listener is concerned about the content, intent, and feelings of the message.

Active recovery Continuing to move immediately after an exercise segment is completed but at a lower intensity.

Activities of daily living (ADL) Activities normally performed for hygiene, bathing, household chores, walking, shopping, and similar activities.

Acute Descriptive of a condition that usually has a rapid onset and a relatively short and severe course; opposite of chronic.

Acute myocardial infarction (AMI) A myocardial infarction resulting from acute obstruction of a coronary artery. *See also* Myocardial infarction.

Adduction Movement toward the midline of the body.

Adenosine triphosphate (ATP) A high-energy phosphate molecule required to provide energy for cellular function. Produced both aerobically and anaerobically and stored in the body.

Adequate Intake (AI) A recommended nutrient intake level that, based on research, appears to be sufficient for good health.

Adherence The extent to which people follow their plans or treatment recommendations. Exercise adherence is the extent to which people follow an exercise program.

Adhesion A fibrous band of scar tissue forming between two surfaces.

Adipocyte A fat cell.

Adiponectin A hormone related to energy metabolism regulation that facilitates the action of insulin by sending blood glucose into the body's cells for storage or use as fuel, thus increasing the cells' insulin sensitivity or glucose metabolism.

Adipose Fat cells stored in fatty tissues in the body.

Adulterated A supplement is considered adulterated if it, or one of its ingredients, presents a "significant or unreasonable risk of illness or injury" when used as directed, or under normal circumstances.

Aerobic In the presence of oxygen.

Affiliate A facility or business that is connected or attached to a larger organization or company.

Affirmation A positive statement to accentuate a client's strengths or effort.

Agility The ability to move quickly and easily; a skill-related component of physical fitness.

Agonist The muscle directly responsible for observed movement; also called the prime mover.

Agreement to participate Signed document that indicates that the client is aware of inherent risks and potential injuries that can occur from participation.

Air displacement plethysmography (ADP) A body-composition assessment technique based on the same body volume measurement principle as hydrostatic weighing; uses air instead of water.

Allergen A substance that can cause an allergic reaction by stimulating type-1 hypersensitivity in genetically susceptible individuals.

Altitude sickness An altitude-induced illness caused by exercising at a moderate to high altitude without acclimatizing to the decreased partial pressure of oxygen in the air, resulting in less oxygen being carried in the blood. Symptoms include shortness of breath, headache, lightheadedness, and nausea.

Alveoli Spherical extensions of the respiratory bronchioles and the primary sites of gas exchange between the lungs and the blood.

Ambient temperature The temperature of the surrounding air; room temperature.

Ambivalence A state of having mixed feelings about a change; arguing both for and against change simultaneously.

American Society of Composers, Authors, and Publishers (ASCAP) One of two performing rights societies in the United States that represent music publishers in negotiating and collecting fees for the nondramatic performance of music.

Amino acid Nitrogen-containing compound that is one of the building blocks of protein.

Amortization phase The transition period between the eccentric and concentric actions during plyometrics; a crucial part of the stretch-shortening cycle that contributes to power development.

Anabolic Muscle-building effects.

Anaerobic Without the presence of oxygen.

Anaerobic efficiency The ability to use the energy systems that do not require the presence of oxygen to contribute to the total energy needs during physical activity.

Anaerobic glycolysis The metabolic pathway that uses glucose for energy production without requiring oxygen. Sometimes referred to as the lactic acid system or anaerobic glucose system, it produces lactic acid as a by-product.

Anatomical position Standing erect with the arms hanging by the side and the head, eyes, feet, and palms facing forward.

Android Adipose tissue or body fat distributed in the abdominal area (apple-shaped individuals).

Anemia A reduction in the number of red blood cells and/or quantity of hemoglobin per volume of blood below normal values.

Anemic See Anemia.

Aneurysm A localized abnormal dilation of a blood vessel; associated with a stroke when the aneurysm bursts.

Angina A common symptom of coronary artery disease characterized by chest pain, tightness, or radiating pain resulting from a lack of blood flow to the heart muscle.

Angioplasty A surgical procedure that involves inserting a catheter into a blocked coronary artery. A narrow balloon is then inflated inside the artery, to widen the artery. Also called percutaneous transluminal coronary angioplasty (PTCA).

Angiotensin II receptor antagonist A class of drugs used to treat high blood pressure and other conditions by preventing angiotensin II from binding to angiotensin II receptors, thereby allowing blood vessels to dilate; also referred to as angiotensin-receptor blockers.

Angiotensin-converting enzyme (ACE) inhibitor A class of drugs used to treat high blood pressure and other conditions by reducing the activity of angiotensin converting enzyme, which converts angiotensin I to angiotensin II.

Ankylosing spondylitis Inflammatory arthritis of the spine, resembling rheumatoid arthritis, that may progress to bony ankylosis with slipping of vertebral margins; the disease is more common in males.

Anorexia An eating disorder characterized by a restriction of energy intake leading to a significant low body weight relative to normative values for sex, age, physical health, and developmental trajectory; intense fear of gaining weight or persistent behavior that interferes with weight gain.

Antagonist The muscle that acts in opposition to the contraction produced by an agonist (prime mover) muscle.

Antecedent Variable or factor that precedes and influences a client's behavior.

Anterior Anatomical term meaning toward the front. Same as ventral; opposite of posterior.

Anterior cruciate ligament (ACL) A primary stabilizing ligament of the knee that travels from the medial border of the lateral femoral condyle to its point of insertion anterolaterally to the medial tibial spine.

Anterior shin splints Pain in the anterior compartment muscles of the lower leg, fascia, and periosteal lining. Often induced by exertional or sudden changes in activity.

Anthropometry The measurement of the size and proportions of the human body.

Antihistamine A class of drugs that blocks histamine receptors involved in the allergic response.

Antioxidant A substance that prevents or repairs oxidative damage; includes vitamins C and E, some carotenoids, selenium, ubiquinones, and bioflavonoids.

Anxiety A state of uneasiness and apprehension; occurs in some mental disorders.

Aorta The major artery of the cardiovascular system; arises from the left ventricle of the heart.

Apnea A temporary absence or cessation of breathing; when this condition occurs during sleep it is called sleep apnea.

Appendicular skeleton The bones of the upper and lower limbs and the pectoral (shoulder) and pelvic (hip) girdles.

Applied force An external force acting on a system (body or body segment).

Arrhythmia A disturbance in the rate or rhythm of the heartbeat. Some can be symptoms of serious heart disease; may not be of medical significance until symptoms appear.

Arteriole Small-diameter blood vessel that extends and branches out from an artery and leads to capillaries; the primary site of vascular resistance.

Arteriosclerosis A chronic disease in which thickening, hardening, and loss of elasticity of the arterial walls result in impaired blood circulation; develops with aging, and in hypertension, diabetes, hyperlipidemia, and other conditions.

Artery A blood vessel that carries oxygenated blood away from the heart to vital organs and the extremities.

Arthritis Inflammation of a joint; a state characterized by the inflammation of joints.

Articulation A joint.

Associative stage of learning The second stage of learning a motor skill, when performers begin to master the fundamentals and can concentrate on skill refinement.

Asthma A chronic inflammatory disorder of the airways that affects genetically susceptible individuals in response to various environmental triggers such as allergens, viral infection, exercise, cold, and stress.

Asymptomatic Without the presence of symptoms.

Ataxia Failure of muscular coordination; irregularity of muscular action.

Atherogenesis Formation of atheromatous deposits, especially on the innermost layer of arterial walls.

Atherosclerosis A specific form of arteriosclerosis characterized by the accumulation of fatty material on the inner walls of the arteries, causing them to harden, thicken, and lose elasticity.

Atherosclerotic heart disease The end result of the accumulation of atherosclerotic plaques within the coronary arteries that supply the muscle of the heart with oxygen and nutrients.

Athletic trainer A healthcare professional who collaborates with physicians and specializes in providing immediate intervention when injuries occur and helping athletes and clients in the prevention, assessment, treatment, and rehabilitation of emergency, acute, and chronic medical conditions involving injury, impairment, functional limitations, and disabilities.

Atria One of the two upper chambers of the heart (right and left atrium).

Atrium See Atria.

Atrophy A reduction in muscle size (muscle wasting) due to inactivity or immobilization.

Auscultation Listening to the internal sounds of the body (such as the heartbeat), usually using a stethoscope.

Autogenic inhibition An automatic reflex relaxation caused by stimulation of the Golgi tendon organ.

Autoimmune disease Any of a group of disorders in which tissue injury is associated with the body's responses to its own constituents; they may be systemic (e.g., systemic lupus erythematosus) or organ-specific (e.g., autoimmune thyroiditis).

Automated external defibrillator (AED) A portable electronic device used to restore normal heart rhythms in victims of sudden cardiac arrest.

Autonomic nervous system The part of the nervous system that regulates involuntary body functions, including the activity of the cardiac muscle, smooth muscles, and glands. It has two divisions: the sympathetic nervous system and the parasympathetic nervous system.

Autonomous motivation Engaging in an activity out of free will and the desire to do so.

Autonomous stage of learning The third stage of learning a motor skill, when the skill has become habitual or automatic for the performer.

Autonomy The capacity of a rational individual to make an informed, un-coerced decision.

Avascular Characterized by a lack of blood vessels.

Axial skeleton The bones of the head, neck, and trunk.

Axis of rotation The imaginary line or point about which an object, such as a joint, rotates.

Axon A nerve fiber that conducts a nerve impulse away from the neuron cell body; efferent nerve fiber.

Balance The ability to maintain the body's position over its base of support within stability limits, both statically and dynamically; a health-related component of physical fitness.

Ballistic stretching Dynamic stretching characterized by rhythmic bobbing or bouncing motions representing relatively high-force, short-duration movements.

Bariatric surgery A variety of surgical procedures (e.g., gastric bypass, sleeve gastrectomy, and adjustable gastric band) to induce weight loss.

Basal metabolic rate (BMR) The energy required to complete the sum total of life-sustaining processes, including ion transport (40% BMR), protein synthesis (20% BMR), and daily functioning such as breathing, circulation, and nutrient processing (40% BMR).

Base of support (BOS) The areas of contact between the feet and their supporting surface and the area between the feet.

Basic activities of daily living Any daily activity performed for self-care, including personal hygiene, dressing and undressing, eating, transferring from bed to chair and back, voluntarily controlling urinary and fecal discharge, elimination, and moving around (as opposed to being bedridden).

Behavior chain A sequence of events in which variables both preceding and following a target behavior help to explain and reinforce the target behavior, such as participation in an exercise session.

Benign Pertaining to a non-cancerous growth or tumor; mild disease or condition that is not life threatening.

Beta blocker Medication that "blocks" or limits sympathetic nervous system stimulation. Acts to slow the heart rate and decrease maximal heart rate and is used for cardiovascular and other medical conditions.

Beta cell Endocrine cell in the islets of Langerhans of the pancreas responsible for synthesizing and secreting the hormone insulin, which lowers the glucose levels in the blood.

Binge eating disorder An eating disorder characterized by frequent binge eating (without purging) and feelings of being out of control when eating.

Bioavailability The degree to which a substance can be absorbed and efficiently utilized by the body.

Bioelectrical impedance analysis (BIA) A noninvasive, low cost, and a commonly used approach for body-composition measurement and assessment. This measurement is based on the obstruction of flow of an alternating current as it moves through parts of the body.

Blood pressure (BP) The pressure exerted by the blood on the walls of the arteries; measured in millimeters of mercury (mmHg) with a sphygmomanometer.

Body composition The makeup of the body in terms of the relative percentage of fat-free mass and body fat; a health-related component of physical fitness.

Body fat A component of the body, the primary role of which is to store energy for later use.

Body-fat percentage The proportion of body composition representing the relative percentage of body fat. Calculated by dividing the fat mass by the total body mass, then multiplying by 100.

Body mass index (BMI) A relative measure of body height to body weight used to determine levels of weight, from underweight to extreme obesity.

Bolus A food and saliva digestive mix that is swallowed and then moved through the digestive tract.

Bone density See Bone mineral density.

Bone deposition A process in which calcium, phosphate, and other ions are taken from blood plasma and deposited in bone tissue.

Bone formation The processes resulting in the formation of normal, healthy bone tissue, including remodeling and resorption.

Bone mineral density (BMD) A measure of the amount of minerals (mainly calcium) contained in a certain volume of bone.

Bone resorption The dissolving of bone.

Branched-chain amino acid (BCAA) An essential amino acid that inhibits muscle protein breakdown and aids in muscle glycogen storage. The BCAAs are valine, leucine, and isoleucine.

Broadcast Music, Inc. (BMI) One of two performing rights societies in the U.S. that represent music publishers in negotiating and collecting fees for the nondramatic performance of music.

Bronchi The two large branches of the trachea leading into the lungs.

Bronchiole The smallest tubes that supply air to the alveoli (air sacs) of the lungs.

Bronchitis Acute or chronic inflammation of the bronchial tubes.

Bronchoconstriction The constriction of the airways in the lungs caused by the tightening of surrounding smooth muscle, with consequent coughing, wheezing, and shortness of breath.

Bronchodilator Medication inhaled to dilate (enlarge) and relax the constricted bronchial smooth muscle.

Buffering capacity The ability of muscles to neutralize the acid that accumulates in them during high-intensity exercise, thus delaying the onset of fatigue.

Bulimia An eating disorder characterized by recurrent episodes of uncontrolled binge eating; recurrent inappropriate compensatory behavior such as self-induced vomiting, laxative misuse, diuretics, or enemas (purging type), or fasting and/or excessive exercise (nonpurging type); episodes of binge eating and compensatory behaviors occur at least twice per week for three months; self-evaluation that is heavily influenced by body shape and weight; and episodes that do not occur exclusively with episodes of anorexia.

Bursa A sac of fluid that is present in areas of the body that are potential sites of friction.

Bursitis Swelling and inflammation in the bursa that results from overuse.

Calcaneal eversion Movement of the plantar surface of the calcaneus laterally away from the midline of the body.

Calcium channel blocker A class of blood pressure medication that relaxes and widens the blood vessels.

Calorie A measurement of the amount of energy in a food available after digestion.

The amount of energy needed to increase 1 kilogram of water by 1 degree Celsius. Also called a kilocalorie.

Capillary The smallest type of blood vessel that supplies blood to the tissues, and the site of all gas and nutrient exchange in the cardiovascular system. Capillaries connect the arterial and venous systems.

Carbohydrate The body's preferred energy source. Dietary sources include sugars (simple) and grains, rice, potatoes, and beans (complex). Carbohydrate is stored as glycogen in the muscles and liver and is transported in the blood as glucose.

Carbohydrate loading Up to a week-long regimen of manipulating intensity of training and carbohydrate intake to achieve maximum glycogen storage for an endurance event.

Cardiac cycle The period from the beginning of one heartbeat to the beginning of the next heartbeat; the systolic and diastolic phases and the interval in between.

Cardiac muscle A type of involuntary, striated muscle tissue that makes up the walls of the heart and provides the continuous rhythmic action known as heart contractions.

Cardiac output The amount of blood pumped by the heart per minute; usually expressed in liters of blood per minute.

Cardiac reserve The work that the heart is able to perform beyond that required of it under ordinary circumstances.

Cardiopulmonary resuscitation (CPR) A procedure to support and maintain breathing and circulation for a person who has stopped breathing (respiratory arrest) and/or whose heart has stopped (cardiac arrest).

Cardiorespiratory fitness The ability to perform large muscle movement over a sustained period; related to the capacity of the heart-lung system to deliver oxygen for sustained energy production. Also called cardiorespiratory endurance or aerobic fitness.

Cardiovascular disease (CVD) A general term for any disease of the heart, blood vessels, or circulation.

Cardiovascular drift Changes in observed cardiovascular variables that occur during prolonged, submaximal exercise without a change in workload.

Carpal tunnel syndrome A pathology of the wrist and hand that occurs when the median nerve, which extends from the forearm into the hand, becomes compressed at the wrist.

Cartilage A smooth, semi-opaque material that absorbs shock and reduces friction between the bones of a joint.

Casein The main protein found in milk and other dairy products.

Catabolic Pertaining to the breaking down of tissue, or catabolism. Catabolism generally refers to a decrease in lean tissue, particularly muscle.

Catabolism Metabolic pathways that break down molecules into smaller units and release energy.

Catecholamine Hormone (e.g., epinephrine and norepinephrine) released as part of the sympathetic response to exercise.

C-corporation A corporation that is designed to operate in multiple countries and with various types of investors.

Cellular acidosis A decrease in muscle pH (below 7) caused by the accumulation of protons in a muscle cell. These protons come from the splitting of adenosine triphosphate (ATP) into adenosine diphosphate (ADP) and inorganic phosphate. Each time this splitting takes place, one hydrogen ion (proton) is released.

Center of gravity (COG) See Center of mass (COM).

Center of mass (COM) The point around which all weight is evenly distributed; also called center of gravity.

Central nervous system (CNS) The brain and spinal cord.

Cerebral vascular disease One of a group of brain dysfunctions related to disease of the blood vessels supplying the brain.

Certification A credential attesting that an individual or organization has met a specific set of standards.

Change talk Statements reflecting a desire to change.

Cholesterol A fatlike substance found in the blood and body tissues and in certain foods. Can accumulate in the arteries and lead to a narrowing of the vessels (atherosclerosis).

Chondromalacia A gradual softening and degeneration of the articular cartilage, usually involving the back surface of the patella (kneecap). This condition may produce pain and swelling or a grinding sound or sensation when the knee is flexed and extended.

Chondromalacia patella Inflammation of the underside of the patella (kneecap) and softening of the cartilage that is associated with knee pain.

Chronic Descriptive of a condition that persists over a long period of time; opposite of acute.

Chronic bronchitis Characterized by inflamed bronchiole tubes, increased mucus secretion, and a productive cough lasting several months to several years.

Chronic disease Any disease state that persists over an extended period of time.

Chronic obstructive pulmonary disease (COPD) A condition, such as asthma, bronchitis, or emphysema, in which there is chronic obstruction of air flow. See Asthma, Bronchitis, *and* Emphysema.

Chylomicron A large lipoprotein particle that transfers fat from food from the small intestine to the liver and adipose tissue.

Circuit training A form of training that takes the participant through a series of exercise stations, sometimes with brief rest intervals in between; can emphasize muscular endurance, aerobic conditioning, muscular strength, or a combination of all three.

Claudication Cramplike pains in the calves caused by poor circulation of blood to the leg muscles; frequently associated with peripheral vascular disease.

Closed-kinetic-chain exercise Movements where the distal segment of the target body part is more fixed; generally considered more functional, as they mimic daily activities closely.

co-contraction The mutual coordination of antagonist muscles (such as flexors and extensors) to maintain a position.

Cognition Current thought or feeling that can function as an antecedent or consequence for overt behaviors.

Cognitive Pertaining to, or characterized by, that operation of the mind by which we become aware of objects of thought or perception; includes all aspects of perceiving, thinking, and remembering.

Cognitive behavior therapy A form of psychotherapy that focuses on how thoughts and feelings influence behavior.

Cognitive distortion Unproductive thought process that can paralyze a client when making a positive and lasting behavioral change.

Cognitive domain One of the three domains of learning; describes intellectual activities and involves the learning of knowledge.

Cognitive stage of learning The first stage of learning a motor skill when performers make many gross errors and have extremely variable performances.

Collagen The main constituent of connective tissue, such as ligaments, tendons, and muscles.

Comorbidity Disorder (or disease) in addition to a primary disease or disorder.

Comparative negligence A system used in legal defenses to distribute fault between an injured party and any defendant.

Competence Having the necessary ability, knowledge, or skill to do something successfully; one of the three basic psychological needs that influence motivation, according to self-determination theory.

Complex carbohydrate A long chain of sugar that takes more time to digest than a simple carbohydrate.

Compound set A resistance-training approach involving the performance of two or more exercises for the same muscle or muscle group in rapid succession.

Computed tomography (CT) A development of x-ray technology to examine the soft tissues of the body. Involves recording "slices" of the body with a CT scanner. A cross-sectional image is then formed by computer integration.

Concentric A type of isotonic muscle contraction in which the muscle develops tension and shortens when stimulated.

Concussion A type of traumatic brain injury caused by a bump, blow, or jolt to the head or by a hit to the body that causes the head and brain to move rapidly back and forth.

Conduction The direct flow of heat through a material resulting from physical contact.

Congestive heart failure Inability of the heart to pump blood at a sufficient rate to meet the metabolic demand or the ability to do so only when the cardiac filling pressures are abnormally high, frequently resulting in lung congestion.

Connective tissue The tissue that binds together and supports various structures of the body. Ligaments and tendons are connective tissues.

Consequence Variable that occurs following a target behavior, such as exercise, that influences a person's future behavior-change decisions and efforts.

Contemplation The stage of the transtheoretical model of behavior change during which the individual is weighing the pros and cons of behavioral change.

Contract A binding agreement between two or more persons that is enforceable by law. Composed of an offer, acceptance, and consideration (or what each party puts forth to make the agreement worthwhile).

Contractile protein The protein myofilaments that are essential for muscle contraction.

Contracture An abnormal and usually permanent contraction of a muscle characterized by a high resistance to passive stretching.

Contraindication Any condition that renders some particular movement, activity, or treatment improper or undesirable.

Contributory negligence A legal defense used in claims or suits when the plaintiff's negligence contributed to the act in dispute.

Controlled motivation Doing a task with a sense of pressure, demand, or coercion.

Convection The transfer of heat through surrounding air or water molecules.

Coordination The ability to use different parts of the body together efficiently; a skill-related component of physical fitness.

Coronary artery disease (CAD) The major form of cardiovascular disease; results when the coronary arteries are narrowed or occluded, most commonly by atherosclerotic deposits of fibrous and fatty tissue; also called coronary heart disease.

Corporate veil A legal doctrine that shields individual investors in a corporation from financial or legal liability beyond their initial investment.

Corporation A legal entity, independent of its owners and regulated by state laws; any number of people may own a corporation through shares issued by the business.

Cortical bone Compact, dense bone that is found in the shafts of long bones and the vertebral endplates.

Cortisol A hormone that is often referred to as the "stress hormone," as it is involved in the response to stress. It increases blood pressure and blood glucose levels and has an immunosuppressive action.

Creatine phosphate A storage form of high-energy phosphate in muscle cells that can be used to immediately resynthesize adenosine triphosphate (ATP).

Creep The tendency of connective tissue to slowly deform permanently (or lengthen) under the influence of applied stress such as a stretching force.

Crimp The zigzag structure of collagen, which gradually straightens out when the tissue is subjected to high tensile forces.

Cultural competence The ability to communicate and work effectively with people from different cultures.

Cyanosis A bluish discoloration, especially of the skin and mucous membranes, due to reduced hemoglobin in the blood.

Cytokine Hormone-like low molecular weight proteins, secreted by many different cell types, which regulate the intensity and duration of immune responses and are involved in cell-to-cell communication.

Decisional balance One of the four components of the transtheoretical model of behavioral change; refers to the numbers of pros and cons an individual perceives regarding adopting and/or maintaining an activity program.

Deep Anatomical term meaning internal; that is, located further beneath the body surface than the superficial structures.

Dehydration The process of losing body water; when severe can cause serious, life-threatening consequences.

Delayed-onset muscle soreness (DOMS) Soreness that occurs 24 to 48 hours after strenuous exercise, the exact cause of which is unknown.

Dendrite The portion of a nerve fiber that transmits impulses toward a nerve cell body; receptive portion of a nerve cell.

Deoxyribonucleic acid (DNA) A large, double-stranded, helical molecule that is the carrier of genetic information.

Depression 1. The action of lowering a muscle or bone or movement in an inferior or downward direction. 2. A condition of general emotional dejection and withdrawal; sadness greater and more prolonged than that warranted by any objective reason.

Detraining Reversal of adaptation to exercise.

Diabetes A disease of carbohydrate metabolism in which an absolute or relative deficiency of insulin results in an inability to metabolize carbohydrates normally.

Diaphragm The most important muscle of inspiration; the only skeletal muscle considered essential for life.

Diaphysis The shaft of a long bone.

Diastasis recti A separation of the recti abdominal muscles along the midline of the body.

Diastole The period of filling of the heart between contractions; resting phase of the heart.

Diastolic blood pressure (DBP) The pressure in the arteries during the relaxation phase (diastole) of the cardiac cycle; indicative of total peripheral resistance.

Dietary Approaches to Stop Hypertension (DASH) eating plan An eating plan designed to reduce blood pressure; also serves as an overall healthy way of eating that can be adopted by nearly anyone; may also lower risk of coronary heart disease.

Dietary Reference Intake (DRI) A generic term used to refer to three types of nutrient reference values: Recommended Dietary Allowance (RDA), Estimated Average Requirement (EAR), and Tolerable Upper Intake Level (UL).

Dietary supplement A product (other than tobacco) that functions to supplement the diet and contains one or more of the following ingredients: a vitamin, mineral, herb or other botanical, amino acid, dietary substance that increases total daily intake, metabolite, constituent, extract, or some combination of these ingredients.

Dietary Supplement Health and Education Act (DSHEA) A bill passed by Congress in 1994 that sets forth regulations and guidelines for dietary supplements.

Digestion The process of breaking down food into small enough units for absorption.

Diminishing returns Principle stating that after a certain level of performance has been achieved, there will be a decline in the effectiveness of training at furthering a person's performance level.

Directing style A communication style in which the personal trainer leads, tells, and decides; the personal trainer is the main player and the client is a passive player. Triggers the "righting reflex."

Distal Farthest from the midline of the body, or from the point of origin of a muscle.

Diuretic Medication that produces an increase in urine volume and sodium excretion.

Dorsiflexion Movement of the foot up toward the shin.

Dose-response relationship Direct association between the amount of a stimulus and the magnitude of the desired outcome (e.g., amount of physical activity and good health).

Double-progression training protocol Progressing the intensity of a muscular-training program using first an increase in the number of repetitions performed with a given load and second an increase in the amount of weight lifted using increments of 5%.

Double taxation The imposition of taxation on corporate earnings at both the corporate level and again as a stockholder dividend.

Dual-energy X-ray absorptiometry (DXA) An imaging technique that uses a very low dose of radiation to measure bone density. Also can be used to measure overall body fat and regional differences in body fat.

Dynamic balance The act of maintaining postural control while moving.

Dynamic stretching Type of stretching that involves taking the joints through their ranges of motion while continuously moving. Often beneficial in warming up for a particular sport or activity that involves the same joint movements.

Dyslipidemia A condition characterized by abnormal blood lipid profiles; may include elevated cholesterol, triglyceride, or low-density lipoprotein (LDL) levels and/or low high-density lipoprotein (HDL) levels.

Dyspnea Shortness of breath; a subjective difficulty or distress in breathing.

Eating disorder Disturbed eating behavior that jeopardizes a person's physical or psychological health.

Eccentric A type of isotonic muscle contraction in which the muscle lengthens against a resistance when it is stimulated; sometimes called "negative work" or "negative reps."

Edema Swelling resulting from an excessive accumulation of fluid in the tissues of the body.

Ejection fraction The percentage of the total volume of blood that is pumped out of the left ventricle during the systolic contraction of the heart.

Elasticity Temporary or recoverable elongation of connective tissue.

Elastin A protein, similar to collagen, found in connective tissue that has elastic properties.

Electrolyte A mineral that exists as a charged ion in the body and that is extremely important for normal cellular function.

Emotional arousal A state of heightened physiological activity, emotions, and emotional behavior.

Empathy Understanding what another person is experiencing from his or her perspective.

Emphysema An obstructive pulmonary disease characterized by the gradual destruction of lung alveoli and the surrounding connective tissue, in addition to airway inflammation, leading to reduced ability to effectively inhale and exhale.

Employee A person who works for another person in exchange for financial compensation. An employee complies with the instructions and directions of his or her employer and reports to them on a regular basis.

End-diastolic volume The volume of blood in a ventricle at the end of the cardiac filling cycle (diastole).

Endocrine Refers to either the gland that secretes directly into the systemic circulation or the substance secreted.

Endomysium A layer of connective tissue that surrounds individual muscle fibers and contains capillaries, nerves, and lymphatics.

Endosteum A soft tissue lining the internal surface of the diaphysis on a long bone.

Endothelial dysfunction An imbalance between vasodilating and vasoconstricting substances produced by (or acting on) the endothelium (the inner lining of blood vessels), which can lead to atherosclerosis.

Enzyme A protein that speeds up a specific chemical reaction.

Epimysium A layer of connective tissue that encloses the entire muscle and is continuous with fascia and other connective-tissue wrappings of muscle, including the endomysium and perimysium.

Epinephrine A hormone released as part of the sympathetic response to exercise; also called adrenaline.

Epiphyseal cartilage Cartilaginous layer between the head and shaft of a long bone where bone growth occurs. Also called a growth plate.

Epiphysis The end of a long bone, usually wider than the shaft (plural: epiphyses).

Episiotomy An incision made in the perineum—the tissue between the vaginal opening and the anus—during childbirth.

Ergogenic Intended to enhance physical performance, stamina, or recovery.

Ergonomic Designed for efficiency and comfort in the working environment.

Essential amino acid One of the eight to 10 of the 23 different amino acids needed to make proteins. Called essential because the body cannot manufacture them; they must be obtained from the diet.

Essential body fat Fat thought to be necessary for maintenance of life and reproductive function.

Essential hypertension Hypertension without an identifiable cause; also called primary hypertension.

Estimated Average Requirement (EAR) An adequate intake in 50% of an age- and sex-specific group.

Estrogen Generic term for estrus-producing steroid compounds produced primarily in the ovaries; the female sex hormones.

Euhydration A state of "normal" body water content.

Evaporation The process by which molecules in a liquid state (e.g., water) spontaneously become gaseous (e.g., water vapor).

Eversion Rotation of the foot to direct the plantar surface outward; occurs in the frontal plane.

Evidence-based practice Making informed decisions and taking action based on the best available evidence.

Exculpatory clause A clause within a waiver that bars the potential plaintiff from recovery.

Exercise-induced bronchoconstriction (EIB) The narrowing of the airways causing difficulty moving air out of the lungs during exercise. Caused by the loss of heat, water, or both from the airways during exercise when quickly breathing in air that is drier than what is already in the body. Symptoms typically appear within a few minutes after exercise begins and may continue for 10 to 15 minutes after a workout is complete.

Expiration The act of expelling air from the lungs; exhalation.

Express partnership A partnership created through formal paperwork.

Extension The act of straightening or extending a joint, usually applied to the muscular movement of a limb.

External rotation Outward turning about the vertical axis of bone.

Extinction The removal of a positive stimulus that has in the past followed a behavior.

Extrinsic feedback Information received from an external source (such as another person) about a completed task (such as an exercise).

Extrinsic motivation Motivation that comes from external (outside of the self) rewards, such as material or social rewards.

Fartlek training A form of training during which the exerciser randomly changes the aerobic intensity based on how he or she is feeling. Also called speed play.

Fascia Strong connective tissue that performs a number of functions, including developing and isolating the muscles of the body and providing structural support and protection (plural: fasciae).

Fasciae See Fascia.

Fascicle A bundle of skeletal muscle fibers surrounded by perimysium.

Fasciitis An inflammation of the fascia.

Fast-twitch muscle fiber One of several types of muscle fibers found in skeletal muscle tissue; also called type II fibers and characterized as having a low oxidative capacity but a high gylcolytic capacity; recruited for rapid, powerful movements such as jumping, throwing, and sprinting.

Fat An essential nutrient that provides energy, energy storage, insulation, and contour to the body. 1 gram of fat equals 9 kcal.

Fat oxidation The metabolic pathway that, in the presence of oxygen, breaks down fatty acids to produce energy in the form of adenosine triphosphate (ATP).

Fat-free mass (FFM) That part of the body composition that represents everything but fat—blood, bones, connective tissue, organs, and muscle; also called lean body mass.

Fatty acid A long hydrocarbon chain with an even number of carbons and varying degrees of saturation with hydrogen.

Feedback An internal response within a learner; during information processing, it is the correctness or incorrectness of a response that is stored in memory to be used for future reference. Also, verbal or nonverbal information about current behavior that can be used to improve future performance.

Femoral anteversion A congenital condition in which the femur is rotated inward (medially).

Fiber Carbohydrate chains the body cannot break down for use and which pass through the body undigested.

First ventilatory threshold (VT1) Intensity of aerobic exercise at which ventilation starts to increase in a nonlinear fashion in response to an accumulation of metabolic by-products in the blood.

Flexibility The ability to move joints through their normal full ranges of motion; a health-related component of physical fitness.

Flexion The act of moving a joint so that the two bones forming it are brought closer together.

Flow-through taxation Financial profits and losses flow from the business directly to the investors. The business does not pay any taxes; rather, business profits are taxed on the investors' individual tax return and losses can be utilized by the investors to offset other personal income.

Foramina Holes or openings in a bone or between body cavities.

Force-couple relationship A situation in which muscles work as a group to provide opposing, directional, or contralateral pulls to achieve balanced movement.

Fracture Any break in the continuity of a bone, ranging from a simple crack to a severe shatter of the bone with multiple fracture fragments.

Franchise A type of license that a party (franchisee) acquires to allow them to have access to a business's (franchisor) proprietary knowledge, processes, and trademarks in order to allow the party to sell a product or provide a service under the business's name.

Free radical A chemical group that has unshared electrons available for a reaction. Free radicals can damage the integrity of deoxyribonucleic acid (DNA) and have been implicated as a cause of cancers.

Frontal plane A longitudinal section that runs at a right angle to the sagittal plane, dividing the body into anterior and posterior portions.

Frostbite An injury caused by freezing of the skin and underlying tissues. First the skin becomes very cold and red, then numb, hard and pale.

Fructose Fruit sugar; the sweetest of the monosaccharides; found in varying levels in different types of fruits.

Gait The manner or style of walking.

Ganglia A group of nerve cell bodies usually located in the peripheral nervous system.

Gastroesophageal reflux disease (GERD) A chronic condition in which the lower esophageal sphincter allows gastric acids to reflux into the esophagus, causing heartburn, acid indigestion, and possible injury to the esophageal lining.

Gastrointestinal tract A long hollow tube from mouth to anus where digestion and absorption occur.

Gemelli Plural term for the gemellus inferior and superior, which are both posterior hip muscles that when activated contribute to external rotation of the femur in the acetabulum.

General partnership A type of business arrangement in which each partner assumes management responsibility and unlimited liability and must have at least a 1% interest in profit and loss.

General supervision A method of supervision where the worker (or trainee) does not require the constant attendance of the supervisor (or trainer).

Genu valgum A knock-knee deformity in which the angulation distal to the knee is away from the midline of the body.

Gestational diabetes mellitus An inability to maintain normal glucose, or any degree of glucose intolerance, during pregnancy, despite being treated with either diet or insulin.

Ghrelin A hormone produced in the stomach that is responsible for stimulating appetite.

Glucose A simple sugar; the form in which all carbohydrates are used as the body's principal energy source.

Glycogen The chief carbohydrate storage material; formed by the liver and stored in the liver and muscle.

Glycogen sparing The use of non-carbohydrates as a source of energy during exercise so that the depletion of muscle glycogen stores is delayed. If fat, for example, makes a greater contribution to an athlete's efforts during the initial stages of a race, more glycogen will be available for the later stages and muscle fatigue will be delayed.

Glycolysis The breakdown of glucose or of its storage form glycogen.

Goal-setting theory A theory of motivation developed by psychologists Edwin Locke and Gary Latham that identified a connection between the establishment of goals and task performance.

Golgi-Mazzoni corpuscle A specialized mechanoreceptor located in the joint capsule responsible for detecting joint compression. Any weight-bearing activity stimulates these receptors.

Golgi tendon organ (GTO) A sensory organ within a tendon that, when stimulated, causes an inhibition of the entire muscle group to protect against too much force.

Green exercise Exercise performed in natural environments.

Gross negligence A form of negligence that is worse than normal negligence. Generally, a waiver clause cannot prevent a suit for gross negligence or for wanton or recklessness or intentional misconduct in any state or jurisdiction.

Ground reaction force The force exerted by the ground on a body in contact with it.

Group waiver Waiver that includes lines for multiple signatures.

Growth hormone A hormone secreted by the pituitary gland that facilitates protein synthesis in the body.

Guiding style A communication style in which the personal trainer helps to motivate, encourage, support, and assist a client in making a change; the personal trainer is engaged but the client is the main player.

Gynoid Adipose tissue or body fat distributed on the hips and in the lower body (pear-shaped individuals).

Health belief model A model to explain health-related behaviors that suggests that an individual's decision to adopt healthy behaviors is based largely upon his or her perception of susceptibility to an illness and the probable severity of the illness. The person's view of the benefits and costs of the change also are considered.

Health claim A statement that describes a relationship between a food or food component and the prevention or treatment of a disease or health-related condition.

Health equity A fair and equal opportunity for every individual to attain their highest level of health.

Health Insurance Portability and Accountability Act (HIPAA) Enacted by the U.S. Congress in 1996, HIPAA requires the U.S. Department of Health and Human Services (HHS) to establish national standards for electronic health care information to facilitate efficient and secure exchange of private health data. The Standards for Privacy of Individually Identifiable Health Information ("Privacy Rule"), issued by the HHS, addresses the use and disclosure of individuals' health information—called "protected health information"—by providing federal protections and giving patients an array of rights with respect to personal health information while permitting the disclosure of information needed for patient care and other important purposes.

Healthy Mediterranean-Style Eating Pattern One of three USDA Food Patterns featured in the *Dietary Guidelines for Americans;* modified from the Healthy U.S.-Style Eating Pattern to more closely reflect eating patterns that have been associated with positive health outcomes in studies of Mediterranean-style diets.

Healthy U.S.-Style Eating Pattern One of three USDA Food Patterns featured in the *Dietary Guidelines for Americans;* based on the types and proportions of foods Americans typically consume, but in nutrient-dense forms and appropriate amounts.

Healthy Vegetarian Eating Pattern One of three USDA Food Patterns featured in the *Dietary Guidelines for Americans;* modified from the Healthy U.S.-Style Eating Pattern to more closely reflect eating patterns reported by self-identified vegetarians.

Heart disease A structural or functional abnormality of the heart or of the blood vessels supplying the heart that impairs its normal functioning.

Heart rate (HR) The number of heartbeats per minute.

Heart-rate reserve (HRR) The reserve capacity of the heart; the difference between maximal heart rate and resting heart rate. It reflects the heart's ability to increase the rate of beating and cardiac output above resting level to maximal intensity.

Heat exhaustion The most common heat-related illness; usually the result of intense exercise in a hot, humid environment and characterized by profuse sweating, which results in fluid and electrolyte loss, a drop in blood pressure, lightheadedness, nausea, vomiting, decreased coordination, and often syncope (fainting).

Heat stroke A medical emergency that is the most serious form of heat illness due to heat overload and/or impairment of the body's ability to dissipate heat; characterized by high body temperature (>104° F or 40° C), dry, red skin, altered level of consciousness, seizures, coma, and possibly death.

Hemoglobin (Hb) The protein molecule in red blood cells specifically adapted to carry oxygen molecules (by bonding with them).

Hemoglobin A1C The amount of hemoglobin with attached glucose over the preceding three months; a measure of long-term blood sugar control.

Hemopoiesis The formation of blood cells.

Hemorrhagic stroke Disruption of blood flow to the brain caused by the presence of a blood clot or hematoma.

Herniated disc Rupture of the outer layers of fibers that surround the gelatinous portion of the disc.

High-density lipoprotein (HDL) A lipoprotein that carries excess cholesterol from the arteries to the liver.

High-intensity interval training (HIIT) An exercise strategy alternating periods of short, intense anaerobic exercise with less-intense recovery periods.

Homeostasis An internal state of physiological balance.

Hormone A chemical substance produced and released by an endocrine gland and transported through the blood to a target organ.

HR turnpoint The point during incremental aerobic exercise at which the heart rate no longer increases linearly, but rather shows a curvilinear response; also called the heart rate deflection point and is related to the onset of blood lactate accumulation.

Hydrogen ion Also known as a proton, a hydrogen ion is the nucleus of a hydrogen atom separated from it accompanying electron. In the context of exercise, hydrogen ions accumulate in the blood during times of vigorous exercise through hydrolysis when adenosine triphosphate (ATP) is broken down into adenosine diphosphate (ADP) and inorganic phosphate. One hydrogen ion is released each time an ATP molecule is split for energy.

Hydrolysate A product of hydrolysis, in which water reacts with a compound to produce other compounds.

Hydrostatic weighing Weighing a person fully submerged in water. The difference between the person's mass in air and in water is used to calculate body density, which can be used to estimate the proportion of fat in the body.

Hypercholesterolemia An excess of cholesterol in the blood.

Hyperglycemia An abnormally high content of glucose (sugar) in the blood.

Hyperlipidemia An excess of lipids in the blood that could be primary, as in disorders of lipid metabolism, or secondary, as in uncontrolled diabetes.

Hypertension High blood pressure, or the elevation of resting blood pressure above 130/80 mmHg.

Hyperthermia Abnormally high body temperature.

Hyperthyroidism A condition characterized by hyperactivity of the thyroid gland; the metabolic processes of the body are accelerated.

Hypertonic (1) Having extreme muscular tension; (2) Having a solute concentration that is greater than the concentration of human blood.

Hypertrophy An increase in the cross-sectional size of a muscle in response to progressive muscular training.

Hyperventilation A greater-than-normal rate of breathing that results in an abnormal loss of carbon dioxide from the blood; dizziness may occur.

Hypoglycemia A deficiency of glucose in the blood commonly caused by too much insulin, too little glucose, or too much exercise. Most commonly found in the insulin-dependent diabetic and characterized by symptoms such as fatigue, dizziness, confusion, headache, nausea, or anxiety.

Hyponatremia Abnormally low levels of sodium ions circulating in the blood; severe hyponatremia can lead to brain swelling and death.

Hypotension Low blood pressure.

Hypothalamus An organ in the brain situated below the thalamus that coordinates both autonomic nervous system function and pituitary activity.

Hypothermia Abnormally low body temperature.

Iliotibial band (IT band) friction syndrome A repetitive overuse condition that occurs when the distal portion of the iliotibial band rubs against the lateral femoral epicondyle.

Impingement syndrome Reduction of space for the supraspinatus muscle and/or the long head of the biceps tendon to pass under the anterior edge of the acromion and coracoacromial ligament; attributed to muscle hypertrophy and inflammation caused by microtraumas.

Implied partnership A partnership lacking a written agreement, but in which the parties involved conduct business like a partnership.

Independent activities of daily living Activities often performed by a person who is living independently in a community setting during the course of a normal day, such as managing money, shopping, telephone use, traveling within the community, housekeeping, preparing meals, and taking medications correctly.

Independent contractor A person who conducts business on his or her own on a contract basis and is not an employee of an organization.

Indirect calorimetry A method used to predict resting metabolic rate. Since oxygen is used in the metabolic process to create energy, a person's metabolic rate can be determined by measuring how much oxygen he or she consumes when breathing.

Inextensibility The property of a tissue that makes it unable to be extended; tissues (e.g., ligaments) contribute to limiting the range of motion of a joint when they are inextensible.

Inferior Located below.

Inflammation A protective tissue response to injury or destruction of tissues, which serves to destroy, dilute, or wall off both the injurious agent and the injured tissues; classic signs include pain, heat, redness, swelling, and loss of function.

Informed consent A written statement signed by a client prior to testing that informs him or her of testing purposes, processes, and all potential risks and discomforts.

Inherent risk Risks that can occur through normal participation in the stated activity. Inherent risks can only be avoided by declining to participate.

Insomnia Inability to sleep; abnormal wakefulness.

Inspiration The drawing of air into the lungs; inhalation.

Insulin A hormone released from the pancreas that allows cells to take up glucose.

Insulin resistance An inability of muscle tissue to effectively use insulin, where the action of insulin is "resisted" by insulin-sensitive tissues.

Insulin sensitivity The degree of sensitivity of a receptor site on a tissue cell for insulin, which functions to allow glucose to enter the cell.

Intermediate-density lipoprotein (IDL) Formed from the degradation of very low-density lipoproteins; enables fats and cholesterol to move within the bloodstream.

Intermittent claudication Muscle pain (e.g., ache, cramp, numbness, or sense of fatigue), classically in the calf muscle, which occurs during exercise, such as walking, and is relieved by a short period of rest.

Interstitial fluid Fluid between the cells or body parts.

Intrinsic feedback Feedback provided by the clients themselves; the most important type of feedback for long-term program adherence.

Intrinsic motivation Motivation that comes from internal states, such as enjoyment or personal satisfaction.

Inversion Rotation of the foot to direct the plantar surface inward; occurs in the frontal plane.

Ion A single atom or small molecule containing a net positive or negative charge due to an excess of either protons (positive) or electrons (negative).

Ischemia A decrease in the blood supply to a bodily organ, tissue, or part caused by constriction or obstruction of the blood vessels.

Ischemic stroke A sudden disruption of cerebral circulation in which blood supply to the brain is either interrupted or diminished.

Isometric A type of muscular action in which the muscle is stimulated to generate tension but little or no joint movement occurs.

Ketosis An abnormal increase of ketone bodies in the body; usually the result of a low-carbohydrate diet, fasting, or starvation.

Keyman insurance Insurance that compensates a company for the loss of a representative of the company who was performing unique and valuable functions.

Kinetic chain The concept that joints and segments have an effect on one another during movement.

Knowledge of results The motivational impact of feedback provided to a person learning a new task or behavior indicating the outcomes of performance.

Korotkoff sounds Five different sounds created by the pulsing of the blood through the brachial artery; proper distinction of the sounds is necessary to determine blood pressure.

Kyphosis Excessive posterior curvature of the spine, typically seen in the thoracic region.

Lactate A chemical derivative of lactic acid, which is formed when sugars are broken down for energy without the presence of oxygen.

Lactate threshold The point during exercise of increasing intensity at which blood lactate begins to accumulate above resting levels, where lactate clearance is no longer able to keep up with lactate production.

Lactose A disaccharide; the principal sugar found in milk.

Lapse An expected slip or mistake that is usually a discreet event and is a normal part of the behavior-change process.

Larynx The organ of the voice; located between the trachea and the base of the tongue.

Lateral Away from the midline of the body, or the outside.

Lateral epicondylitis An injury resulting from the repetitive overloading of the wrist and finger extensors that originate at the lateral epicondyle; often referred to as "tennis elbow."

Laxity Lacking in strength, firmness, or resilience; joints that have been injured or overstretched may exhibit laxity.

Lean body mass The components of the body (apart from fat), including muscles, bones, nervous tissue, skin, blood, and organs.

Length-tension relationship Refers to the relationship between the length of the sarcomere or muscle fiber and the ability to produce force/tension. An optimal length of the muscle fiber for producing force exists. Lengths that are above or below this optimal length result in reduced force production when stimulated.

Leptin A hormone released from fat cells that acts on the hypothalamus to regulate energy intake. Low leptin levels stimulate hunger and subsequent fat consumption.

Lever A rigid bar that rotates around a fixed support (fulcrum) in response to an applied force.

Liability Legal responsibility.

Licensee Any business, organization, or individual that has been granted legal permission by another entity to engage in an activity.

Lifestyle and health-history questionnaire A type of form utilized by personal trainers and healthcare professionals that gathers an individual's personal medical information, family health history, and individual health behaviors.

Ligament A strong, fibrous tissue that connects one bone to another.

Limited liability company (LLC) A company that limits investors' personal financial and legal liabilities but provides flow-through taxation for investors. It is not limited to a certain number of shareholders and owners do not have to be U.S. citizens.

Limited liability partnership (LLP) A partnership in which some or all partners (depending on the jurisdiction) have limited liability; exhibits elements of both partnerships and corporations.

Limited partner An individual who retains no legal liability beyond his or her initial investment and does not have any formal input regarding partnership operations.

Line of gravity A theoretical vertical line passing through the center of gravity, dissecting the body into two hemispheres.

Linear periodization A form of periodization used in resistance training that provides a consistent training protocol within each microcycle and changes the training variables after each microcycle.

Lipid The name for fats used in the body and bloodstream.

Lipoprotein An assembly of a lipid and protein that serves as a transport vehicle for fatty acids and cholesterol in the blood and lymph.

Locus of control The degree to which people attribute outcomes to internal factors, such as effort and ability, as opposed to external factors, such as luck or the actions of others. People who tend to attribute events and outcomes to internal factors are said to have an internal locus of control, while those who generally attribute outcomes to external factors are said to have an external locus of control.

Lordosis Excessive anterior curvature of the spine that typically occurs at the low back (may also occur at the neck).

Low-density lipoprotein (LDL) A lipoprotein that transports cholesterol and triglycerides from the liver and small intestine to cells and tissues; high levels may cause atherosclerosis.

Macrocycle The longest timeframe in a periodized training program, usually a period of six months to one year. The goals of a macrocycle are long-term and require multiple steps to be achieved.

Macronutrient A nutrient that is needed in large quantities for normal growth and development.

Magnetic resonance imaging (MRI) A diagnostic modality in which the patient is placed within a strong magnetic field and the effect of high-frequency radio waves on water molecules within the tissues is recorded. High-speed computers are used to analyze the absorption of radio waves and create a cross-sectional image based upon the variation in tissue signal.

Maintenance The stage of the transtheoretical model of behavior change during which the individual is incorporating the new behavior into his or her lifestyle and has been doing so for more than six months.

Malignant Pertaining to a cancerous tumor characterized by progressive and uncontrolled growth.

Maximal heart rate (MHR) The highest heart rate a person can attain. Sometimes abbreviated as HRmax.

Maximal oxygen uptake ($\dot{V}O_2$max) The maximum capacity for the body to take in, transport, and use oxygen during exercise; a common indicator of physical fitness.

Mechanism of injury The manner in which a physical injury occurred. Describes how energy is transferred to an individual and results in an injury.

Medial epicondylitis An injury that results from an overload of the wrist flexors and forearm pronators. Sometimes called golfer's elbow.

Medial tibial stress syndrome (MTSS) Inflammation of the periosteum (connective tissue covering of the bone). Often induced by a sudden change in activity and has been associated with pes planus.

Mediastinum The portion of the thoracic cavity between the lungs.

Medical nutrition therapy Disease management through nutritional diagnostic, therapy, and counseling services provided by a registered dietitian or nutrition professional.

Mediterranean-style eating plan An eating plan generally characterized by increased consumption of olive oil, complex carbohydrates, vegetables, and fish, and decreased red meat and pork consumption.

Meissner's corpuscle A specialized mechanoreceptor located in the superficial aspect of the skin responsible for detecting light touch; occur abundantly in the skin of the fingertips, palms, soles, lips, tongue, and face.

Menisci The plural form of meniscus; cartilage disks that act as a cushion between the ends of bones that meet in the knee joint.

Mesocycle The mid-length timeframe of a periodized training program, usually two weeks to a few months long. The goals of a mesocycle are designed to be steps on the way to the overall goal of the macrocycle.

Metabolic equivalents (METs) A simplified system for classifying physical activities where one MET is equal to the resting oxygen consumption, which is approximately 3.5 milliliters of oxygen per kilogram of body weight per minute (3.5 mL/kg/min).

Metabolic syndrome (MetS) A cluster of factors associated with increased risk for coronary heart disease and diabetes—abdominal obesity indicated by a waist circumference ≥40 inches (102 cm) in men and ≥35 inches (88 cm) in women; levels of triglyceride ≥150 mg/dL (1.7 mmol/L); high-density lipoprotein levels <40 and 50 mg/dL (1.0 and 1.3 mmol/L) in men and women, respectively; blood-pressure levels ≥130/85 mmHg; and fasting blood glucose levels ≥110 mg/dL (6.1 mmol/L).

Metabolite Any substance produced during metabolism.

Metastasize To spread to other sites in the body.

Micelle An aggregate of lipid- and water-soluble compounds in which the hydrophobic portions are oriented toward the center and the hydrophilic portions are oriented outwardly.

Microcycle The shortest timeframe in a periodized training program, usually one to four weeks long. The goals of a microcycle are short-term and are designed to be steps on the way to the overall goal of the mesocycle.

Micronutrient A nutrient that is needed in small quantities for normal growth and development.

Mineral An inorganic substance needed in the diet in small amounts to help regulate bodily functions.

Minority partner A partner holding less than 50% of the company's ownership shares.

Minute ventilation ($\dot{V}_E$) A measure of the amount of air that passes through the lungs in one minute; calculated as the tidal volume multiplied by the ventilatory rate.

Mitochondria The "power plant" of the cells where aerobic metabolism occurs.

Mobility The degree to which an articulation is allowed to move before being restricted by surrounding tissues.

Moderate-intensity continuous training (MICT) Exercise performed continuously at a moderate intensity (50–75% of $\dot{V}O_2$max, 50–75% of heart-rate reserve, or 50–80% of maximal heart rate).

Monocarboxylate transport (MCT) proteins Proteins acting as carriers for lactate, pyruvate, and ketone bodies.

Monounsaturated fat A type of unsaturated fat (liquid at room temperature) that has one open spot on the fatty acid for the addition of a hydrogen atom (e.g., oleic acid in olive oil).

Morbidity The disease rate; the ratio of sick to well persons in a community.

Mortality The death rate; the ratio of deaths that take place to expected deaths.

Motivational interviewing (MI) A person-centered conversation style that encourages clients to honestly examine beliefs and behaviors, and that motivates clients to make a decision to change a particular behavior.

Motor learning The process of acquiring and improving motor skills.

Motor unit A motor nerve and all of the muscle fibers it stimulates.

Muscle spindle The sensory organ within a muscle that is sensitive to stretch and thus protects the muscle against too much stretch.

Muscular endurance The ability of a muscle or muscle group to exert force against a resistance over a sustained period of time; a health-related component of physical fitness.

Muscular fitness Having appropriate levels of both muscular strength and muscular endurance.

Muscular strength The maximal force a muscle or muscle group can exert during contraction; a health-related component of physical fitness.

Myelin The fatty insulation of nerve fibers that is important for the conduction of nerve impulses. These fibers are damaged in individuals with multiple sclerosis.

Myocardial infarction (MI) An episode in which some of the heart's blood supply is severely cut off or restricted, causing the heart muscle to suffer and die from lack of oxygen. Commonly known as a heart attack.

Myocardial ischemia The result of an imbalance between myocardial oxygen supply and demand, most often caused by atherosclerotic plaques that narrow and sometimes completely block the blood supply to the heart.

Myofibril The portion of the muscle containing the thick (myosin) and thin (actin) contractile filaments; a series of sarcomeres where the repeating pattern of the contractile proteins gives the striated appearance to skeletal muscle.

Myofibrillar hypertrophy The increase in the size of muscle cells (myofibrils).

Myoglobin A compound similar to hemoglobin, which aids in the storage and transport of oxygen in the muscle cells.

Myosin Thick contractile protein in a myofibril.

Near-infrared interactance Body-composition assessment method that involves the use of light absorption and reflection to estimate percent fat and percent fat-free mass. It is based on the principle that body fat absorbs light while lean body mass reflects light.

Negative affect A broad concept that can be summarized as feelings of emotional distress. More specifically, it is a construct that is defined by the common variance between anxiety, sadness, fear, anger, guilt, shame, irritability, and other unpleasant emotions.

Negative feedback loop A bodily reaction that causes a decrease in function because of some kind of stimulus.

Negative reinforcement The removal or absence of aversive stimuli following a desired behavior. This increases the likelihood that the behavior will occur again.

Negligence Failure of a person to perform as a reasonable and prudent professional would perform under similar circumstances.

Nervous system A complex collection of nerves and specialized cells known as neurons that collect information about conditions in relation to the body's external state and transmit signals between different parts of the body.

Neurological inhibition The suppression of normal nervous system function, often leading to jerkiness and erratic movement patterns and sequences.

Neuromotor Involving motor skills such as agility, gait, coordination, and balance. Neuromotor training is sometimes referred to as balance training.

Neuromuscular efficiency The ability of the neuromuscular system to allow muscles that produce movement and muscles that provide stability to work together synergistically as an integrated functional unit.

Neuromuscular junction The site at which a motor neuron transmits information to a muscle fiber.

Neuromuscular system The nervous and muscular systems, which work together to control, direct, and allow movement of the body.

Neuron The basic anatomical unit of the nervous system; the nerve cell.

Neurotransmitter A chemical substance such as acetylcholine or dopamine that transmits nerve impulses across synapses.

Niacin A B vitamin found in meat, wheat germ, dairy products, and yeast; used to treat and prevent pellagra.

Noncommunicable disease (NCD) A medical condition or disease that is noninfectious and non-transmissible among people.

Non-contact injury Refers to an injury that occurs through a non-contact mechanism and is not the result of contact from another person or piece of equipment. These injuries may be the result of compressive forces, ground reaction forces, muscular imbalances, impingement, overuse, and alignment of the body.

Non-exercise activity thermogenesis (NEAT) Physiological processes that produce heat; a relative newly discovered component of energy expenditure.

Non-HDL Cholesterol other than high-density lipoprotein (HDL) circulating in the blood.

Nonshivering thermogenesis Generation or production of heat, especially by physiological processes.

Nonsteroidal anti-inflammatory drug (NSAID) A drug with analgesic, antipyretic, and anti-inflammatory effects. The term "nonsteroidal" is used to distinguish these drugs from steroids, which have similar actions.

Norepinephrine A hormone released as part of the sympathetic response to exercise.

Nutrient A component of food needed by the body. There are six classes of nutrients: water, minerals, vitamins, fats, carbohydrates, and protein.

Nutrient content claim Statement of the implied health benefits of a product that describes the level of a nutrient in a product using terms like "free," "high," or "low," or compared to another product using terms like "more," "reduced," and "lite."

OARS A tool used to explore a client's values; stands for Open-ended questions, Affirmations, Reflections, and Summarizing.

Obesity An excessive accumulation of body fat. Usually defined as more than 20% above ideal weight, or over 25% body fat for men and over 32% body fat for women; also can be defined as a body mass index of >30 kg/m^2 or a waist girth of >40 inches (102 cm) in men and >35 inches (89 cm) in women.

Obesogenic An environment that tends to generate or create a state of obesity.

Obstructive sleep apnea (OSA) A condition in which breathing stops for more than 10 seconds during sleep due to part of the airway being closed off while a person is trying to inhale during sleep.

Occupational therapist A healthcare provider specializing in treatments that help people who suffer from mentally, physically, developmentally, or emotionally disabling conditions to develop, recover, or maintain daily living and work skills that include improving basic motor functions and reasoning abilities.

Omega-3 fatty acid An essential fatty acid that promotes a healthy immune system and helps protect against heart disease and other diseases; found in egg yolk and cold water fish and shellfish like tuna, salmon, mackerel, cod, crab, shrimp, and oyster. Also known as linolenic acid.

One-repetition maximum (1-RM) The amount of resistance that can be moved through the range of motion one time before the muscle is temporarily fatigued.

Onset of blood lactate accumulation (OBLA) The point in time during high-intensity exercise at which the production of lactic acid exceeds the body's capacity to eliminate it; after this point, oxygen is insufficient at meeting the body's demands for energy. Also referred to as the second ventilatory threshold (VT2).

Open-ended question A question that does not allow for a simple one-word answer (yes/no); designed to encourage a full, meaningful answer using the subject's own knowledge and/or feelings.

Open-kinetic-chain exercise Exercises in which the distal end of a limb (kinetic chain) is free to move. Examples of open-kinetic-chain exercises include the seated leg extension and biceps curl with dumbbells. Typically, these movements involve isolated, single-joint movements.

Operant conditioning A learning approach that considers the manner in which behaviors are influenced by their consequences.

Orthopnea Form of dyspnea in which the person can breathe comfortably only when standing or sitting erect; associated with asthma, emphysema, and angina.

Orthostatic hypotension A drop in blood pressure associated with rising to an upright position.

Osteoarthritis (OA) A degenerative disease involving a wearing away of joint cartilage. This degenerative joint disease occurs chiefly in older persons.

Osteoblast A bone-forming cell.

Osteoclast A cell that reabsorbs or erodes bone mineral.

Osteopenia A disorder in which bone density is below average, classified as 1.5 to 2.5 standard deviations below peak bone density.

Osteoporosis A disorder, primarily affecting postmenopausal women, in which bone mineral density decreases and susceptibility to fractures increases.

Outcome goal A goal that can be assessed via a measured outcome [e.g., weight loss of 5 pounds (2.3 kg)].

Overfat The presence of excess body fat that can impair health, even for normal weight non-obese individuals.

Overload The principle that a physiological system subjected to above-normal stress will respond by increasing in strength or function accordingly.

Overtraining syndrome The result of constant intense training that does not provide adequate time for recovery; symptoms include increased resting heart rate, impaired physical performance, reduced enthusiasm and desire for training, increased incidence of injuries and illness, altered appetite, disturbed sleep patterns, and irritability.

Overuse condition Refers to a state of repetitive movements and faulty body mechanics leading to excessive forces being applied beyond what tissues can normally withstand and, over time, may lead to overuse injuries.

Overuse injury An injury caused by activity that places too much stress on one area of the body over an extended period.

Overweight A term to describe an excessive amount of weight for a given height, using height-to-weight ratios.

Oxidation Process of oxidizing, or the addition of oxygen to a compound with a resulting loss of electrons.

Oxygen uptake ($\dot{V}O_2$) The process by which oxygen is used to produce energy for cellular work.

Pacinian corpuscle A specialized bulblike mechanoreceptor located in the subcutaneous tissue of the skin responsible for detecting pressure; occur abundantly in the skin of palms, soles, and joints.

Palpation The use of hands and/or fingers to detect anatomical structures or an arterial pulse (e.g., carotid pulse).

Palpitation A rapid and irregular heartbeat.

Parasympathetic nervous system A subdivision of the autonomic nervous system that is involved in regulating the routine functions of the body, such as heartbeat, digestion, and sleeping. Opposes the physiological effects of the sympathetic nervous system (e.g., stimulates digestive secretions, slows the heart, constricts the pupils, and dilates blood vessels).

Paroxysmal nocturnal dyspnea Attacks of severe shortness of breath and coughing that generally occur at night.

Partial pressure The pressure of each gas in a multiple gas system, such as air, which is composed of nitrogen, oxygen, and CO_2.

Partnership A business entity in which two or more people agree to operate a business and share profits and losses.

Passive recovery Complete rest; no activity at all.

Patellofemoral pain syndrome (PFPS) A degenerative condition of the posterior surface of the patella, which may result from acute injury to the patella or from chronic friction between the patella and the groove in the femur through which it passes during motion of the knee.

Peptide YY A satiety hormone that is released from the intestines.

Perceived seriousness An individual's feelings regarding the severity associated with developing an illness or disease. This is one of the four constructs of the health belief model.

Perceived susceptibility An individual's perception of the risk of personal vulnerability to illness or disease. This is one of the four constructs of the health belief model.

Percent daily value (PDV) A replacement for the percent Recommended Dietary Allowance (RDA) on the newer food labels. Gives information on whether a food item has a significant amount of a particular nutrient based on a 2,000-calorie diet.

Performance goal A goal that represents change in a measurable variable, such as increases in strength scores, reductions in resting heart rate, or weight loss.

Perfusion The passage of fluid through a tissue, such as the transport of blood through vessels from the heart to internal organs and other tissues.

Perimysium A sheath of connective tissue that covers a bundle of muscle fibers.

Periodization The systematic application of overload through the pre-planned variation of program components to optimize gains in strength (or any specific component of fitness), while preventing overuse, staleness, overtraining, and plateaus.

Periosteum A double-layered connective tissue sheath surrounding the outer surface of the diaphysis of a long bone; serves to cover and nourish the bone.

Periostitis Inflammation of the membrane of connective tissue that closely surrounds a bone.

Peripheral arterial disease (PAD) Any disease caused by the obstruction of large peripheral arteries, which can result from atherosclerosis, inflammatory processes leading to stenosis, an embolism, or thrombus formation.

Peripheral nervous system (PNS) The parts of the nervous system that are outside the brain and spinal cord (central nervous system).

Peripheral resistance The resistance of the arteries to blood flow. As the arteries constrict, the resistance increases; as they dilate, resistance decreases.

Peripheral vascular disease A painful and often debilitating condition, characterized by muscular pain caused by ischemia to the working muscles. The ischemic pain is usually due to atherosclerotic blockages or arterial spasms, referred to as claudication. Also called peripheral vascular occlusive disease (PVOD).

Peripheral vasoconstriction The narrowing of blood vessels resulting from contraction of the muscular wall of the vessels, particularly in the periphery of the body (limbs).

Peripheral vasodilation The widening of the blood vessels (vasodilation) of the peripheral vasculature in the systemic circulation.

Person-centered care Healthcare services that are tailored to individuals' needs and provided in partnership with them.

Pes cavus High arches of the feet.

Pes planus Flat feet.

Pharynx The muscular, membranous tube extending from the base of the skull to the esophagus.

Phosphagen High-energy phosphate compounds found in muscle tissue, including adenosine triphosphate (ATP) and creatine phosphate, that can be broken down for immediate use by the cells.

Phosphagen energy system A system of transfer of chemical energy from the breakdown of creatine phosphate to regenerate adenosine triphosphate (ATP).

Physical Activity Readiness Questionnaire for Everyone (PAR-Q+) A brief, self-administered medical questionnaire recognized as a safe pre-exercise screening measure for low-to-moderate (but not vigorous) exercise training.

Physical inactivity Not meeting the recommended levels of regular physical activity.

Physical literacy The development of fundamental movement skills and fundamental sport skills that permit a child to move confidently and with control in a wide range of physical activity, rhythmic (dance), and sport situations.

Physical therapist A healthcare provider specializing in treatments that help restore function, improve mobility, relieve pain, and prevent or limit permanent physical disabilities in patients of all ages suffering from medical problems, injuries, diseases, disabilities, or other health-related conditions.

Physically active Meeting the recommended levels of regular physical activity.

Physically inactive Not getting any moderate- or vigorous-intensity physical activity beyond basic movement from daily life activities.

Phytochemical A biologically active, non-nutrient component found in plants; includes antioxidants.

Piriformis syndrome A neuromuscular condition characterized by hip and buttock pain (and potentially leg pain) caused by the piriformis muscles compressing the sciatic nerve.

Planes of motion The conceptual planes in which the body moves; called the sagittal, frontal, and transverse planes; often used as a way to describe anatomical movement.

Plantar fasciitis Inflammation of the plantar fascia, a broad band of connective tissue running along the sole of the foot; caused by stretching or tearing the tissue, usually near the attachment at the heel.

Plantar flexion Distal movement of the plantar surface of the foot; opposite of dorsiflexion.

Plant-based diet An eating pattern that emphasizes the consumption of whole, minimally processed foods derived primarily from plants, including vegetables, fruits, whole grains, nuts, seeds, and legumes; also referred to as a whole food, plant-based diet.

Plasma The liquid portion of the blood.

Plasticity Capable of undergoing continuous deformation without rupture or relaxation.

Platelet One of the disc-shaped components of the blood; involved in clotting.

Plyometrics High-intensity movements, such as jumping, involving high-force loading of body weight during the landing phase of the movement that take advantage of the stretch-shortening cycle.

Polyunsaturated fat A type of unsaturated fat (liquid at room temperature) that has two or more spots on the fatty acid available for hydrogen (e.g., corn, safflower, and soybean oils).

Portion The amount of a food or beverage consumed by an individual in one sitting.

Positive reinforcement The presentation of a positive stimulus following a desired behavior. This increases the likelihood that the behavior will occur again.

Posterior Toward the back or dorsal side.

Posterior chain A group of muscles, tendons, and ligaments on the posterior kinetic chain of the body (e.g., biceps femoris, gluteus maximus, erector spinae, trapezius, and posterior deltoids).

Posterior shin splints An overuse injury that occurs in the active population. This is an exercise-induced condition that is often triggered by a sudden change in activity and has been associated with pes planus.

Post-exercise hypotension Acute post-exercise reduction in both systolic and diastolic blood pressure.

Postprandial lipemia (PPL) The transient excess of lipids in the blood occurring after the ingestion of foods with a large content of fat; hyperlipemia.

Posture The arrangement of the body and its limbs.

Power The capacity to move with a combination of speed and force; a skill-related component of physical fitness.

Precontemplation The stage of the transtheoretical model of behavior change during which the individual is not intending to change within the next six months.

Prediabetes The state in which some but not all of the diagnostic criteria for diabetes are met (e.g., blood glucose levels are higher than normal but are not high enough for a diagnosis of diabetes).

Preeclampsia A pregnancy complication characterized by high blood pressure and signs of damage to another organ system, most often the liver and kidneys. Usually begins after 20 weeks of pregnancy in women whose blood pressure had been normal.

Preparation The stage of the transtheoretical model of behavior change during which the individual is getting ready to make a change.

Previously physically inactive Describes an individual who previously was not meeting the recommendations for regular physical activity.

Primary hypertension See Essential hypertension.

Prime mover A muscle responsible for a specific movement. Also called an agonist.

Process goal A goal a person achieves by doing something, such as completing an exercise session or attending a talk on stress management.

Product liability insurance Insurance that covers damages occurring due to product failure.

Professional liability insurance Insurance to protect a personal trainer against professional negligence or failure to perform as a competent and prudent professional would under similar circumstances.

Pronation Internal rotation of the forearm causing the radius to cross diagonally over the ulna and the palm to face posteriorly.

Prone Lying flat, with the anterior aspect of the body facing downward.

Proprioception Sensation and awareness of body position and movements.

Proprioceptive nervous system A combination of the vestibular (eyes and inner ears), subcutaneous (beneath and within the skin), and kinesthetic (muscles and joints) sensors that enables an individual to determine body position and its movement in space.

Proprioceptive neuromuscular facilitation (PNF) A method of promoting the response of neuromuscular mechanisms through the stimulation of proprioceptors in an attempt to gain more stretch in a muscle; often referred to as a contract/relax method of stretching.

Proprioceptor Somatic sensory receptor in muscles, tendons, ligaments, joint capsules, and skin that gathers information about body position and the direction and velocity of movement.

Protected health information Health data created, received, stored, or transmitted by the Health Insurance Portability and Accountability Act (HIPAA)–covered entities and their business associates in relation to the provision of healthcare, healthcare operations, and payment for healthcare services. Protected health information includes individually identifiable health information, including demographic data, medical histories, test results, insurance information, and other information used to identify clients or provide healthcare services or healthcare coverage. 'Protected' means the information is protected under the HIPAA Privacy Rule.

Protein A compound composed of a combination 20 amino acids that is the major structural component of all body tissue.

Proton In bioenergetics, refers to a hydrogen ion.

Proximal Nearest to the midline of the body or point of origin of a muscle.

Pulmonary circuit The circulatory vessels of the lungs; involved in the circulation of blood from the right ventricle of the heart to the lungs and back to the left atrium of the heart.

Pulmonary ventilation The total volume of gas inspired or expired per minute.

Punishment The presentation of aversive stimuli following any behavior, good or bad. Decreases the likelihood that the behavior will occur again.

Quickness The quality of moving fast.

Radiation Heat transferred from one body to another which are not in contact, such as heat transferring from the sun to a roof.

Radiculopathy Dysfunction of a nerve root that can cause numbness or tingling, muscle weakness, or loss of reflex associated with that nerve.

Range of motion (ROM) The number of degrees that an articulation will allow one of its segments to move.

Rapport A relationship marked by mutual understanding and trust.

Rating of perceived exertion (RPE) A scale, originally developed by noted Swedish psychologist Gunnar Borg, that provides a standard means for evaluating a participant's perception of exercise effort. The original scale ranged from 6 to 20; a revised category ratio scale ranges from 0 to 10.

Reaction time The amount of time required to respond to a stimulus; a skill-related component of physical fitness.

Reactivity The ability to rapidly respond to stimuli; generally, includes the time needed to process sensory information, plus the time needed to generate and execute the appropriate motor response.

Readiness to change A reference to how likely someone is to make a behavioral change based on their current stage of change (precontemplation, contemplation, preparation, action, or maintenance) according to the transtheoretical model of behavior change.

Reciprocal inhibition The reflex inhibition of the motor neurons of antagonists when the agonists are contracted.

Recommended Dietary Allowance (RDA) The levels of intake of essential nutrients that, on the basis of scientific knowledge, are judged by the Food and Nutrition Board to be adequate to meet the known needs of practically all healthy persons.

Reduced-exertion high-intensity interval training (REHIT) A modified form of high-intensity interval training (HIIT) that shortens the traditional HIIT workout by using fewer and shorter sprints, though those sprints are at a supra-maximal intensity.

Reflective listening A communication strategy that involves paying respectful attention to the content and feeling expressed by a speaker.

Registered dietitian (RD) A food and nutrition expert who has met the following criteria: completed a minimum of a bachelor's degree at a U.S. accredited university, or other college coursework approved by the Commission on Accreditation for Dietetics Education (CADE); completed a CADE-accredited supervised practice program; passed a national examination; and completed continuing education requirements to maintain registration.

Relapse In behavioral change, the return of an original problem after many lapses (i.e., slips or mistakes) have occurred.

Relatedness A sense of belonging and connectedness with others; one of the three basic psychological needs that influence motivation, according to self-determination theory.

Relative strength The ratio of the amount of weight lifted to the total body weight of the person. It can be used to compare the strength of different individuals.

Relaxin A hormone of pregnancy that relaxes the pelvic ligaments and other connective tissue in the body.

Remodeling A phase of healing that begins three to six weeks after the onset of an injury and can last for one year or more, during which the tissue attempts to restore structure and increase the strength of scar tissue.

Rescue medication Quick-relief or fast-acting inhaled medications taken by individuals with asthma to quickly stop symptoms.

Residual volume (RV) The volume of air remaining in the lungs following a maximal expiration.

Respiratory compensation threshold See Second ventilatory threshold (VT2).

Respondeat superior A legal doctrine wherein the actions of an employee can subject the employer to liability; Latin for "Let the master answer."

Resting energy expenditure (REE) The amount of energy expended at rest; represents 60 to 75% of the body's total energy expenditure.

Resting heart rate (RHR) The number of heartbeats per minute when the body is at complete rest; usually counted first thing in the morning before any physical activity.

Resting metabolic rate (RMR) The number of calories expended per unit time at rest; measured early in the morning after an overnight fast and at least eight hours of sleep; approximated with various formulas.

Reversibility The principle of exercise training that suggests that any improvement in physical fitness due to physical activity is entirely reversible with the discontinuation of the training program.

Rheumatoid arthritis (RA) An autoimmune disease that causes inflammation of connective tissues and joints.

Riboflavin A yellow, water-soluble, B vitamin that occurs in green vegetables, germinating seeds, and in milk, fish, egg yolk, liver, and kidney; essential for the carbohydrate metabolism of cells.

RICE An immediate treatment for injury: Stands for Rest or Restricted activity, Ice, Compression, and Elevation.

Rider Specific additions to a standard insurance policy.

Righting reflex The tendency to give advice, push recommendations, and offer solutions; makes sustainable behavior change less likely for a client who is ambivalent about change.

Risk factor A characteristic, inherited trait, or behavior related to the presence or development of a condition or disease.

Risk management Minimizing the risks of potential legal liability.

Royalty A payment made to the owner of a copyright, patent, or trademark in exchange for use of the protected intellectual property; typically a percentage of each sale.

Sagittal plane The longitudinal plane that divides the body into right and left portions.

SAID principle A training principle that states that the body will adapt to the specific challenges imposed upon it, as long as the program progressively overloads the system being trained; SAID stands for "specific adaptation to imposed demands."

Sarcomere The basic functional unit of the myofibril containing the contractile proteins that generate skeletal muscle movements.

Sarcopenia Decreased muscle mass; often used to refer specifically to an age-related decline in muscle mass or lean-body tissue.

Sarcoplasm A gelatin-like tissue surrounding the sarcomere.

Sarcoplasmic hypertrophy An increase in muscle size due to an increase in the volume of sarcoplasmic fluid as a result of high-repetition weight-lifting sets. See Transient hypertrophy.

Sarcoplasmic reticulum The form of endoplasmic reticulum where calcium is stored to be used for muscle activation; located in striated muscle fibers.

Satiety A feeling of fullness.

Saturated fat A fatty acid that contains no double bonds between carbon atoms; typically solid at room temperature and very stable.

Scapulohumeral rhythm Combined action of scapular and humeral movement. For every 2 degrees of humeral motion, 1 degree of scapular motion takes places throughout the available range of motion for flexion/extension and abduction/adduction.

Scoliosis Excessive lateral curvature of the spine.

Scope of practice The range and limit of responsibilities normally associated with a specific job or profession.

Secondary hypertension Hypertension resulting from an identifiable cause.

Second ventilatory threshold (VT2) A metabolic marker that represents the point at which high-intensity exercise can no longer be sustained due to an accumulation of lactate.

Second-impact syndrome A condition in which an individual experiences a second head injury before complete recovery from an initial head injury

Sedentary Doing or requiring much sitting; minimal activity.

Self-determination theory A psychological theory suggesting that people need to feel competent, autonomous, and connected to others in the many domains of life.

Self-efficacy One's perception of his or her ability to change or to perform specific behaviors (e.g., exercise).

Self–myofascial release The act of rolling one's own body on a round foam roll or other training tool, massaging away restrictions to normal soft-tissue extensibility.

Serving The amount of food used as a reference on the nutrition label of that food; the recommended portion of food to be eaten.

Shearing force Any force that causes slippage between a pair of contiguous joints or tissues in a direction that parallels the plane in which they contact.

Shin splint A general term for any pain or discomfort on the front or side of the lower leg in the region of the shin bone (tibia).

Shivering A rapid, involuntary cycle of contraction and relaxation of skeletal muscles, which can increase the body's rate of heat production by four to five times.

Simple carbohydrate A short chain of sugar that is rapidly digested.

Skeletal muscle A type of voluntary, striated muscle tissue attached to the skeleton that provides movement at the joints when it contracts.

Skeletal muscle milieu The biochemical substances that make up the setting in which skeletal muscles are located.

Slow-twitch muscle fiber A muscle fiber type designed for use of aerobic glycolysis and fatty acid oxidation, recruited for low-intensity, longer-duration activities such as walking and swimming.

Small intestine The part of the gastrointestinal system that is the site of the majority of food digestion and absorption.

SMART goal A properly designed goal; SMART stands for Specific, Measurable, Attainable, Relevant, and Time-bound.

Smooth muscle A type of involuntary, nonstriated muscle tissue responsible for the contractility of hollow organs, such as the blood vessels, gastrointestinal tract, bladder, or uterus.

SOAP note A communication tool used among healthcare professionals; SOAP stands for Subjective, Objective, Assessment, and Plan.

Social cognitive theory A behavior-change theory that posits that all health behaviors are goal-driven through anticipation of outcomes.

Social support The perceived comfort, caring, esteem, or help an individual receives from other people.

Society of European Stage Authors and Composers (SESAC) A performing rights organization designed to represent songwriters and publishers and their right to be compensated for having their music performed in public.

Socio-ecological model A framework that examines interrelationships between individuals and the environments in which they live and work, as well as the many levels at which individuals are influenced, both in terms of support for health behaviors and barriers to improving health behavior.

Sole proprietorship A business owned and operated by one person.

Somatic nervous system Division of the peripheral nervous system that conducts signals from sensory receptors to the central nervous system (afferent signals) and signals from the central nervous system to skeletal muscles (efferent signals).

Somatosensory system The physiological system relating to the perception of sensory stimuli from the skin and internal organs.

Specific supervision A method of supervision where the worker (or trainee) requires direct involvement of the supervisor (or trainer).

Specificity Exercise training principle explaining that specific exercise demands made on the body produce specific responses by the body; also called exercise specificity.

Speed Rate of movement; a skill-related component of physical fitness.

Speed-endurance The ability of an individual to maintain maximal velocity over an extended time period.

Speed-strength The ability to develop force at high velocities.

Sprain A traumatic joint twist that results in stretching or tearing of the stabilizing connective tissues; mainly involves ligaments or joint capsules, and causes discoloration, swelling, and pain.

Sprint interval training (SIT) A type of interval training characterized by repeated bouts of 20 -to 30-second all-out supramaximal sprints.

Stability Characteristic of the body's joints or posture that represents resistance to change of position.

Stabilizer A muscle that acts to maintain a position of or fixate a joint.

Stadiometer A device for measuring height that typically consists of a vertical ruler with a sliding horizontal rod or paddle that is adjusted to rest on the top of the head.

Stage 1 hypertension A systolic blood pressure of 130–139 mmHg or a diastolic blood pressure of 80–89 mmHg.

Stages-of-change model A lifestyle-modification model that suggests that people go through distinct, predictable stages when making lifestyle changes: precontemplation, contemplation, preparation, action, and maintenance. The process is not always linear.

Standard of care Appropriateness of an exercise professional's actions in light of current professional standards and based on the age, condition, and knowledge of the client or participant.

Static balance The ability to maintain the body's center of mass (COM) within its base of support (BOS).

Static stretching Holding a nonmoving (static) position to immobilize a joint in a position that places the desired muscles and connective tissues passively at their greatest possible length.

Statute of frauds A contract that must be in writing in order to be enforceable.

Statute of limitations A formal regulation limiting the period within which a specific legal action may be taken.

Steady state Constant submaximal exercise below the lactate threshold where the oxygen consumption is meeting the energy requirements of the activity.

Sterol Naturally occurring unsaturated steroid alcohols, typically waxy solids.

Stimulus control A means to break the connection between events or other stimuli and a behavior; in behavioral science, sometimes called "cue extinction."

Strain A stretch, tear, or rip in the muscle or adjacent tissue such as the fascia or tendon.

Stress incontinence Pressure (or stress) on the bladder resulting from physical movement or activity, such as coughing, sneezing, running, or heavy lifting. Not related to psychological stress.

Stretch reflex An involuntary motor response that, when stimulated, causes a suddenly stretched muscle to respond with a corresponding contraction.

Stretch-shortening cycle An active stretch (eccentric action) of a muscle followed by an immediate shortening (concentric action) of that same muscle. A component of plyometrics.

Stroke A sudden and often severe attack due to blockage of an artery into the brain.

Stroke volume (SV) The amount of blood pumped from the left ventricle of the heart with each beat.

Structure/function claim A statement that relates a nutrient or dietary ingredient to normal human structure or function such as "calcium builds strong bones," or describes a benefit related to a nutrient deficiency. It must state a disclaimer that the

U.S. Food and Drug Administration has not evaluated the claim and that the supplement is not intended to treat, cure, or prevent any disease.

Subchapter S-corporation A corporation that does not pay any income taxes. Instead, the corporation's income or losses are divided among and passed through to its shareholders.

Subcutaneous fat Fatty deposit or pad of storage fat found under the skin.

Sudden cardiac death (SCD) Immediate death resulting from a sudden change in the rhythm of the heart usually caused by heart rhythms that are too fast. This condition is also called cardiac arrest.

Summarizing A feature of active listening in which the personal trainer states back to a client what the personal trainer perceives to be the main points of what the client has said.

Superficial External; located close to or on the body surface.

Superior Located above.

Superset Alternating exercises for opposing muscle groups with little rest between sets.

Supination External rotation of the forearm (radioulnar joint) that causes the palm to face anteriorly.

Supine Lying face up (on the back).

Sustain talk Statements reflecting a desire not to change.

Sympathetic nervous system A branch of the autonomic nervous system responsible for mobilizing the body's energy and resources during times of stress and arousal (i.e., the fight or flight response). Opposes the physiological effects of the parasympathetic nervous system (e.g., reduces digestive secretions, speeds the heart, contracts blood vessels).

Sympathomimetic A characteristic of medications that mimic the effects of the sympathetic nervous system.

Synapse The region of communication between neurons.

Syncope A transient state of unconsciousness during which a person collapses to the floor as a result of lack of oxygen to the brain; commonly known as fainting.

Synergist A muscle that assists another muscle in function.

Synovial tissue Connective tissue that makes up the membranes surrounding joints and the sheaths protecting tendons.

Systemic circuit The circulatory vessels of the body.

Systole The contraction phase of the cardiac cycle.

Systolic blood pressure (SBP) The pressure exerted by the blood on the vessel walls during ventricular contraction.

Tachycardia Elevated heart rate over 100 beats per minute.

Talk test A method for measuring exercise intensity using observation of respiration effort and the ability to talk while exercising.

Target heart rate Number of heartbeats per minute that indicates appropriate exercise intensity levels for each individual; also called training heart rate.

Tendinitis Inflammation of a tendon.

Tendon A band of fibrous tissue forming the termination of a muscle and attaching the muscle to a bone.

Tensile strength The amount of longitudinal pulling stress that a material (e.g., soft tissue) can withstand before being pulled apart.

Testosterone In males, the steroid hormone produced in the testes; involved in growth and development of reproductive tissues, sperm, and secondary male sex characteristics.

Thermoregulation Regulation of the body's temperature.

Thiamin A water-soluble B vitamin found in meat, yeast, and the bran coat of grains; necessary for carbohydrate metabolism and normal neural activity.

Thorax The portion of the trunk above the diaphragm and below the neck.

Thrombotic Pertaining to thrombosis, which is blood clotting within blood vessels.

Tidal volume The volume of air inspired per breath.

Tolerable Upper Intake Level (UL) The maximum intake of a nutrient that is unlikely to pose risk of adverse health effects to almost all individuals in an age- and sex-specific group.

Torsion The rotation or twisting of a joint by the exertion of a lateral force tending to turn it about a longitudinal axis.

Total body electrical conductivity (TOBEC) A noninvasive measurement technique used to estimate body composition in human subjects, in which the whole body is placed in a chamber surrounded by a conductive coil. Based on the principle that electrical conductivity travels at different rates through lean and fat tissue.

Total energy expenditure (TEE) Amount of energy expended in a 24-hour period, which includes basal metabolism, physical activity, and dietary-induced thermogenesis.

Trabecular bone Spongy or cancellous bone composed of thin plates that form a honeycomb pattern; predominantly found in the ends of long bones and the vertebral bodies.

Trans fat An unsaturated fatty acid that is converted into a saturated fat to increase the shelf life of some products.

Transient hypertrophy The "pumping" up of muscle that happens during a single exercise bout, resulting mainly from fluid accumulation in the interstitial and intracellular spaces of the muscle. *See* Sarcoplasmic hypertrophy.

Transient ischemic attack (TIA) Momentary dizziness, loss of consciousness, or forgetfulness caused by a short-lived lack of oxygen (blood) to the brain; usually due to a partial blockage of an artery, it is a warning sign for a stroke.

Transtheoretical model of behavior change (TTM) A theory of behavior that examines one's readiness to change and identifies five stages: precontemplation, contemplation, preparation, action, and maintenance. Also called the stages-of-change model.

Transverse plane Anatomical term for the imaginary line that divides the body, or any of its parts, into upper (superior) and lower (inferior) parts. Also called the horizontal plane.

Triglyceride (TG) Three fatty acids joined to a glycerol (carbon and hydrogen structure) backbone; how fat is stored in the body.

Type 1 diabetes Form of diabetes caused by the destruction of the insulin-producing beta cells in the pancreas, which leads to little or no insulin secretion; generally develops in childhood and requires regular insulin injections; formerly known as insulin-dependent diabetes mellitus (IDDM) and childhood-onset diabetes.

Type 2 diabetes Most common form of diabetes; typically develops in adulthood and is characterized by a reduced sensitivity of the insulin target cells to available insulin; usually associated with obesity; formerly known as non-insulin-dependent diabetes mellitus (NIDDM) and adult-onset diabetes.

Type I muscle fiber See Slow-twitch muscle fiber.

Type II muscle fiber See Fast-twitch muscle fiber.

Umbrella liability policy Insurance that provides additional coverage beyond other insurance such as professional liability, home, automobile, etc.

Undulating periodization A form of periodization used in resistance training that provides different training protocols adjusting the volume and intensity during the microcycles in addition to changing the training variables after each microcycle.

Valgus Characterized by an abnormal outward turning of a bone, especially of the hip, knee, or foot.

Valsalva maneuver A strong exhaling effort against a closed glottis, which builds pressure in the chest cavity that interferes with the return of the blood to the heart; may deprive the brain of blood and cause lightheadedness or fainting.

Vascular disease Any disease of the blood vessels.

Vasoconstriction Narrowing of the opening of blood vessels (notably the smaller arterioles) caused by contraction of the smooth muscle lining the vessels.

Vasodilation Increase in diameter of the blood vessels, especially dilation of arterioles leading to increased blood flow to a part of the body.

Vasodilator Any drug that causes dilation of blood vessels; typically prescribed for the treatment of hypertension.

Vasovagal response A response that occurs from pressure placed on the vagus nerve, which slows the heart rate and can cause fainting.

Vegan A vegetarian who does not consume any animal products, including dairy products such as milk and cheese.

Vegetarian A person who does not eat meat, fish, poultry, or products containing these foods.

Vein Blood vessels that carry deoxygenated blood toward the heart from vital organs and the extremities.

Venous return Return to the heart of the circulatory fluids by way of the veins.

Ventilatory threshold (VT) Point of transition between predominantly aerobic energy production to anaerobic energy production; involves recruitment of fast-twitch muscle fibers and is identified via gas exchange during exercise testing.

Ventral Relating to or situated on or close to the anterior aspect of the human body.

Ventricle The two lower chambers of the heart (right and left ventricles).

Venule Smaller divisions of veins.

Very low-density lipoprotein (VLDL) Synthesized in the liver, this is the major carrier of triglyceride and cholesterol to the peripheral tissues.

Vestibular system Part of the central nervous system that coordinates reflexes of the eyes, neck, and body to maintain equilibrium in accordance with posture and movement of the head.

Vicarious liability Legal term meaning that employers are responsible for the workplace conduct of their employees.

Viscera The collective internal organs of the abdominal cavity.

Visceral fat Excess fat located deep in the abdomen that surrounds the vital organs; closely related to abdominal girth. Its accumulation is associated with insulin resistance, glucose intolerance, dyslipidemia, hypertension, and coronary artery disease. Abdominal girth measured at the level of the umbilicus with values >40 inches (102 cm) in men and >35 inches (89 cm) in women are strong indicators of visceral obesity.

Viscoelasticity The property that allows tissues to exhibit both plastic and elastic behaviors.

Visual system The series of structures by which visual sensations are received from the environment and conveyed as signals to the central nervous system.

Vitamin An organic micronutrient that is essential for normal physiologic function.

$\dot{V}O_2$max Considered the best indicator of cardiovascular endurance, it is the maximum amount of oxygen (mL) that a person can use in one minute per kilogram of body weight. Also called maximal oxygen uptake and maximal aerobic capacity.

$\dot{V}O_2$reserve ($\dot{V}O_2$R) The difference between $\dot{V}O_2$max and $\dot{V}O_2$ at rest; used for programming aerobic exercise intensity.

Waist-to-hip ratio (WHR) A useful measure for determining health risk due to the site of fat storage. Calculated by dividing the ratio of abdominal girth (waist measurement) by the hip measurement.

Waiver Voluntary abandonment of a right to file suit; not always legally binding.

Wellness Dynamic process of realizing one's full potential in various aspects of life, including physically, mentally, emotionally, socially, and spiritually.

Whey The liquid remaining after milk has been curdled and strained; high in protein and carbohydrates.

Wolff's law A principle stating that bone is capable of increasing its strength in response to stress (e.g., exercise) by laying down more bone.

Index

Figures, tables, and boxes are indicated by f, t, and b, respectively, following the page number.

D

E

G

I

M

N

O

Q

R

S

U